Second Edition

NEUROLOGICAL SURGERY *Volume 1*

A Comprehensive Reference Guide to the Diagnosis and Management of Neurosurgical Problems

Edited by

JULIAN R. YOUMANS, M.D., Ph.D.

Professor, Department of Neurological Surgery,
School of Medicine, University of California
Davis, California

W. B. SAUNDERS COMPANY

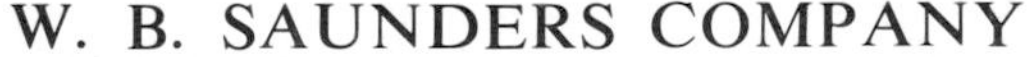

Philadelphia • London • Toronto • Mexico City • Rio de Janeiro • Syd

W. B. Saunders Company: West Washington Square
Philadelphia, PA 19105

1 St. Anne's Road
Eastbourne, East Sussex BN21 3UN, England

1 Goldthorne Avenue
Toronto, Ontario M8Z 5T9, Canada

Apartado 26370—Cedro 512
Mexico 4, D.F., Mexico

Rua Coronel Cabrita, 8
Sao Cristovao Caixa Postal 21176
Rio de Janeiro, Brazil

9 Waltham Street
Artarmon, N.S.W. 2064, Australia

Ichibancho, Central Bldg., 22-1 Ichibancho
Chiyoda-Ku, Tokyo 102, Japan

Library of Congress Cataloging in Publication Data

Youmans, Julian Ray, 1928–
Neurological surgery.

1. Nervous system—Surgery. I. Title.
[DNLM: 1. Neurosurgery. WL368 N4945]
RD593.Y68 1980 617'.48
ISBN 0-7216-9662-7 (v. 1) 80-21368

	Volume 1	ISBN	0-7216-9662-7
	Volume 2	ISBN	0-7216-9663-5
	Volume 3	ISBN	0-7216-9664-3
	Volume 4	ISBN	0-7216-9665-1
	Volume 5	ISBN	0-7216-9666-X
	Volume 6	ISBN	0-7216-9667-8
Neurological Surgery—Volume One	Six Volume Set	ISBN	0-7216-9658-9

Last digit is the print number: 9 8 7 6 5 4 3 2

The Editor dedicates this book
to his parents,

John

and

Jennie Lou,

and his sons,

Reed Nesbit,

John Edward,

and

Julian Milton

Contributors

MAURICE S. ALBIN, M.D.

Ultrasound in Neurosurgery

Professor of Anesthesiology and Neurological Surgery, Department of Anesthesiology, University of Texas Health Science Center at San Antonio. Attending Anesthesiologist, Bexar County Hospital and Audie Murphy Veterans Administration Hospital, San Antonio, Texas.

JOHN F. ALKSNE, M.D.

Cerebral Death

Professor of Neurological Surgery, Chairman of the Division of Neurological Surgery, University of California at San Diego, School of Medicine. Attending Neurological Surgeon, University of California at San Diego Medical Center; Chairman of the Department of Neurological Surgery, Kaiser Medical Center, San Diego, California. Chairman of the Department of Neurological Surgery, Veterans Administration Medical Center, La Jolla, California.

MARSHALL B. ALLEN, JR., M.D., F.A.C.S.

Intracerebral and Intracerebellar Hemorrhage, Sympathectomy

Chairman of Department of Neurological Surgery, Medical College of Georgia. Chief of Neurological Surgery, Eugene Talmadge Memorial Hospital; Consultant, University Hospital and Veterans Administration Hospital, Augusta, Georgia; Dwight D. Eisenhower Army Medical Center, Fort Gordon, Georgia; and Central State Hospital, Milledgeville, Georgia.

EHUD ARBIT, M.D.

Extradural Dorsal Spinal Lesions

Instructor in Neurological Surgery, Cornell University Medical College. Neurological Surgeon, The New York Hospital Cornell Medical Center, New York.

NANCY JANE AUER, M.D.

Extracranial Arterial Occlusive Disease

Associate Resident in Neurological Surgery, Baptist Memorial Hospital, Memphis, Tennessee.

DONALD P. BECKER, M.D., F.A.C.S.

Pathophysiology, Diagnosis, Treatment, and Outcome of Head Injury in Adults

Professor of Neurological Surgery, Chairman of Division of Neurological Surgery, Virginia Commonwealth University, Medical College of Virginia. Chief of Neurological Surgery, Medical College of Virginia Hospitals; Consultant, McGuire Veterans Administration Hospital and St. Mary's Hospital, Richmond, Virginia.

JOHN R. BENTSON, M.D.

Acoustic Neuromas

Associate Professor of Radiology, University of California at Los Angeles. Chief of Section of Neuroradiology, University of California Los Angeles Medical Center, Los Angeles, California.

LESLIE BERNSTEIN, M.D., D.D.S., M.B. B.Ch., D.L.O., F.A.C.S.

Neurotology

Professor of Otorhinolaryngology, Chairman of Department of Otorhinolaryngology, University of California, School of Medicine at Davis, Davis, California. Chief of Otorhinolaryngology, University of California Davis Medical Center at Sacramento, Sacramento, California.

HENRY BERRY, M.D., M.R.C.P.(U.K.), F.R.C.P.(C.)

Peripheral Nerve Entrapment

Associate Professor of Medicine (Neurology), University of Toronto School of Medicine. Director, Clinical Neurophysiology Laboratory, St. Michael's Hospital, Toronto, Ontario.

GILLES G. P. BERTRAND, M.D., F.R.C.S.(C.)

Anomalies of Craniovertebral Junction

Professor of Neurological Surgery, McGill University Faculty of Medicine. Neurological Surgeon-in-Chief, Montreal Neurological Institute and Hospital, Montreal, Quebec.

PETER McL. BLACK, M.D., Ph.D.

Hydrocephalus in Adults

Assistant Professor of Surgery, Harvard Medical School. Assistant in Neurosurgery, Massachusetts General Hospital, Boston, Massachusetts.

ROGER BOLES, M.D., F.A.C.S.

Cranial Nerve Injury in Basilar Skull Fractures

Professor of Otolaryngology, Chairman of Department of Otolaryngology, School of Medicine, University of California at San Francisco. Chief of Otolaryngology Services, University of California at San Francisco General Hospital; Attending Staff, San Francisco General Hospital and Veterans Administration Hospital; Consultant, Letterman Army Hospital, San Francisco, California; Consultant in Otolaryngology to Surgeon General of the United States Air Force, San Francisco, California; Consultant, United States Naval Hospital, Oakland, California.

ROGER CONLEY BONE, M.D.

Pulmonary Care and Complications

Associate Professor of Medicine, University of Arkansas School of Medicine. Chief of Pulmonary Medicine, University of Arkansas Medical Center; Consultant, Veterans Administration Hospital, Little Rock, Arkansas.

CHARLES E. BRACKETT, M.D., F.A.C.S.

Pulmonary Care and Complications, Arachnoid Cysts, Subarachnoid Hemorrhage, Post-Traumatic Arachnoid Cysts, Cordotomy

Professor of Neurological Surgery, Chairman of Department of Neurological Surgery, University of Kansas Medical Center, College of Health Sciences and Hospital. Chief of Neurological Surgery Service, University of Kansas Medical Center; Attending Staff, Kansas City Veterans Administration Hospital, Kansas City, Missouri.

VERNE L. BRECHNER, M.D., F.A.C.A.

Conduction Anesthesia Techniques

Clinical Professor of Anesthesiology, School of Medicine, University of California at Los Angeles. Attending Staff in Anesthesiology, Center for Health Sciences, University of California at Los Angeles, Los Angeles, California; Medical Director, Centinela Pain Management Center, Inglewood, California.

ROBERT W. BRENNAN, M.D.

Differential Diagnosis of Altered States of Consciousness

Professor of Medicine, Pennsylvania State University College of Medicine. Chief of Division of Neurology, The Milton S. Hershey Medical Center, Hershey, Pennsylvania.

WILLIAM H. BROOKS, M.D.

Classification and Biology of Brain Tumors

Assistant Professor of Neurological Surgery, University of Kentucky College of Medicine. Chief of Neurological Surgery, Veterans Administration Hospital, Lexington, Kentucky.

DONALD DEANE BURROW, M.B., B.S., F.R.A.C.P.

Pathophysiology and Evaluation of Ischemic Vascular Disease

Lecturer in Medicine, School of Medicine, University of Adelaide. Senior Visiting Neurologist, Royal Adelaide Hospital and Repatriation General Hospital, Adelaide, South Australia.

ALBERT B. BUTLER, M.D.

Classification and Biology of Brain Tumors

Professor of Neurological Surgery, School of Medicine, University of Virginia. Attending Surgeon, University of Virginia Hospital, Charlottesville, Virginia.

FERNANDO CABIESES, M.D., Ph.D., F.A.C.S.

Parasitic and Fungal Infections

Professor of Neurological Surgery (Ret.), School of Medicine, Universidad de San Marcos. Chief, Neurological Surgery Unit, Peruvian Armed Forces, Anglo-American Hospital, and Hospital 2 de Mayo, Lima, Peru.

SHELLEY N. CHOU, M.D., Ph.D., F.A.C.S.

Urological Problems; Scoliosis, Kyphosis, and Lordosis; Tumors of Skull

Professor of Neurological Surgery, Head of Department of Neurological Surgery, University of Minnesota Medical School. Chief of Neurological Surgery Service, University of Minnesota Hospitals; Consultant, Minneapolis Veterans Administration Hospital, Minneapolis, Minnesota.

KEMP CLARK, M.D., F.A.C.S.

Cervical, Thoracic, and Lumbar Spinal Injury; Anterior Operative Approach to Cervical Spine

Professor of Neurological Surgery, Chairman of Division of Neurological Surgery, University of Texas Health Science Center at Dallas. Director of Neurological Surgery Service, Parkland Memorial Hospital; Chief of Neurological Surgery Service, Children's Medical Center, Dallas, Texas.

CULLY A. COBB, III, M.D., F.A.C.S.

Glial and Neuronal Tumors, Lymphomas, Sarcomas and Vascular Tumors, Tumors of Disordered Embryogenesis

Assistant Clinical Professor of Neurological Surgery, University of California, School of Medicine at Davis, Davis, California. Attending Neurological Surgeon, Sutter Community Hospitals and University of California Davis Medical Center at Sacramento, Sacramento, California.

WILLIAM M. COCKE, JR., M.D., F.A.C.S.

Scalp Injuries, Tumors of Scalp

Professor of Surgery, Chief of Plastic and Reconstructive Surgery, School of Medicine, Texas Technical University. Chief of Plastic Surgery, Health Sciences Center; Attending Staff, St. Mary's of the Plains, Lubbock, Texas; Consultant, Veterans Administration Hospital, Big Springs, Texas.

WILLIAM F. COLLINS, M.D., F.A.C.S.

Physiology of Pain

Harvey and Kate Cushing Professor of Surgery, Chief of Section of Neurological Surgery, Yale University School of Medicine. Neurological Surgeon-in-Chief, Yale–New Haven Medical Center, New Haven, Connecticut.

EDWARD S. CONNOLLY, M.D., F.A.C.S.

Spinal Cord Tumors in Adults

Clinical Professor of Neurological Surgery, Tulane University School of Medicine; Associate Professor of Neurological Surgery, Louisiana State University School of

Medicine. Chairman of Department of Neurological Surgery, Ochsner Clinic, New Orleans, Louisiana.

GUY CORKILL, M.B., B.Ch., F.R.C.S., F.R.C.S.(E.), F.R.A.C.S.

Craniofacial Neoplasia

Professor of Neurological Surgery, University of California, School of Medicine at Davis, Davis, California. Attending Neurological Surgeon, University of California Davis Medical Center at Sacramento, Sacramento, California; Consultant in Neurological Surgery, Martinez Veterans Administration Hospital, Martinez, California; David Grant Medical Center, Travis Air Force Base, Travis, California.

WILLIAM S. COXE, M.D., F.A.C.S.

Viral Encephalitis

Professor of Neurological Surgery, Washington University School of Medicine. Assistant Neurological Surgeon, Barnes and Allied Hospitals; Attending Neurological Surgeon, St. Louis City Hospital; Consultant, Veterans Administration Hospital, St. Louis, Missouri.

BENJAMIN L. CRUE, JR., M.D.

Stereotaxic Mesencephalotomy, Trigeminal Tractotomy

Clinical Professor of Surgery (Neurological Surgery), University of California, School of Medicine at Los Angeles, Los Angeles, California. Director, New Hope Pain Center, Alhambra Community Hospital, Alhambra, California.

COURTLAND H. DAVIS, JR., M.D., F.A.C.S.

Extradural Lumbar Spinal Lesions

Professor of Surgery (Neurological Surgery), Bowman Gray School of Medicine, Wake Forest University. Staff Neurological Surgeon, North Carolina Baptist Hospital, Winston-Salem, North Carolina.

DAVID O. DAVIS, M.D.

Computed Tomography

Professor of Radiology, Chairman of Department of Radiology, The George Washington University School of Medicine. Chairman of Radiology, The George Washington University Hospital, Washington, District of Columbia.

ARTHUR L. DAY, M.D., F.A.C.S.

Intracavernous Carotid Aneurysms and Fistulae

Assistant Professor of Neurological Surgery, University of Florida College of Medicine. Attending Neurological Surgeon, Shands Teaching Hospital; Assistant Chief, Section of Neurological Surgery, Veterans Administration Medical Center, Gainesville, Florida.

IRA C. DENTON, JR., M.D.

Ventriculography

Chief of Neurological Surgery, St. Paul Hospital, Dallas, Texas; Attending Neurological Surgeon at St. Paul Hospital; Consulting Neurological Surgeon, Irving Community Hospital and Medical Arts Hospital, Dallas, Texas, and Lewisville Hospital, Lewisville, Texas.

RICHARD A. DE VAUL, M.D.

Pain Refractory to Therapy

Associate Professor of Psychiatry, The University of Texas Medical School at Houston. Attending Staff, Hermann Hospital and Memorial Southwest Hospital, Houston, Texas.

DONALD D. DIRKS, Ph.D.

Acoustic Neuromas

Professor of Head and Neck Surgery, University of California at Los Angeles, School of Medicine. Staff, Head and Neck Surgery, University of California at Los Angeles Hospital, Los Angeles, California.

MICHEL DJINDJIAN

Spinal Angiography

Neurochirurgien Assistant, Service de Neurochirurgie, Hôpital Henri Mondor, Creteil, France.

RÉNÉ DJINDJIAN

Spinal Angiography

Professeur Feu de Neuroradiologie à la Faculté de Médécine de Paris. Chef Feu du Service de Neurochirurgie, Hôpital Lariboisière, Paris, France.

PAUL J. DONALD, M.D., F.R.C.S.(C.), F.A.C.S.

Craniofacial Neoplasia

Associate Professor of Otorhinolaryngology, Vice Chairman of Department of Otorhinolaryngology, University of California, School of Medicine at Davis, Davis, California. Attending Staff, Department of Otorhinolaryngology, University of California Davis Medical Center at Sacramento, Sacramento, California.

CHARLES G. DRAKE, M.D., F.R.C.S.(C.), F.A.C.S.

Aneurysms of Posterior Circulation

Professor of Surgery, Chairman of Department of Surgery, Faculty of Medicine, The University of Western Ontario. Chief of Surgery, Victoria and St. Joseph's Hospitals, London, Ontario.

PIERRE M. DREYFUS, M.D.

Diagnostic Biopsy

Professor of Neurology, Chairman of Department of Neurology, University of California, School of Medicine at Davis, Davis, California. Chief of Neurology Service, University of California Medical Center at Sacramento, Sacramento, California.

ARTHUR B. DUBLIN, M.D.

Spinal Angiography

Associate Professor of Diagnostic Radiology, Department of Diagnostic Radiology, University of California, School of Medicine at Davis, Davis, California. Chief of Neuroradiology Section and Staff Neuroradiologist, University of California Davis Medical Center at Sacramento, Sacramento, California.

STEWART B. DUNSKER, M.D.

Hyperextension-Hyperflexion Injuries

Adjunct Associate Professor of Anatomy, University of Cincinnati College of Medicine. Assistant Attending Neurological Surgeon, University of Cincinnati Hospital; Attending Neurological Surgeon, Good Samaritan Hospital and Christ Hospital, Cincinnati, Ohio.

PETER DYCK, M.D., F.A.C.S.

Echoencephalography

Clinical Professor of Neurological Surgery, University of Southern California. Consultant, St. Vincent's Medical Center, Good Samaritan, Queen of Angels, and Los Angeles Orthopedic Hospitals, and Ross-Loos Medical Center, Los Angeles, California.

MICHAEL J. EBERSOLD, M.D.

Meningeal Tumors of Brain

Instructor in Neurological Surgery, Mayo Medical School. Consultant, Department of Neurological Surgery, Mayo Clinic; Attending Neurological Surgeon, St. Marys Hospital and Rochester Methodist Hospital, Rochester, Minnesota.

GEORGE EHNI, M.D., M.S., F.A.C.S.

Extradural Cervical Spinal Injuries

Professor of Neurological Surgery, Baylor College of Medicine. Senior Attending Staff, Methodist, St. Luke's, Ben Taub, and Veterans Administration Hospitals, Houston, Texas.

WILLIAM G. ELLIS, M.D.

Diagnostic Biopsy

Associate Professor of Pathology and Neurology, University of California, School of Medicine at Davis, Davis, California. Attending Neuropathologist, University of California Davis Medical Center at Sacramento, Sacramento, California.

ALAN S. FLEISHER, M.D.

Carotid Artery Occlusion for Aneurysms

Associate Professor of Neurological Surgery, Emory University School of Medicine. Chief of Neurological Surgery, Grady Memorial Hospital, Atlanta, Georgia.

ELDON L. FOLTZ, M.D., F.A.C.S.

Affective Disorders Involving Pain

Professor of Neurological Surgery, School of Medicine, University of California at Irvine. Chief of Section of Neurological Surgery, University of California Medical Center, Irvine, California.

BARRY N. FRENCH, M.D., F.R.C.S.(C.), F.A.C.S.

Midline Fusion Defects

Associate Professor of Neurological Surgery, University of California, School of Medicine at Davis, Davis, California. Attending Staff, University of California Davis Medical Center at Sacramento and Sutter Community Hospitals of Sacramento, Sacramento, California; Consultant in Neurological Surgery, Veterans Administration Hospital, Martinez, California.

ANDREW J. GABOR, M.D., Ph.D.

Post-Traumatic Epilepsy

Associate Professor of Neurology, University of California, School of Medicine at Davis, Davis, California. Director, Laboratory of Electroencephalography and Clinical Neurophysiology, University of California Davis Medical Center at Sacramento, Sacramento, California.

FRANCIS W. GAMACHE, JR., M.D.

Metastatic Brain Tumors

Assistant Professor of Neurological Surgery, Cornell University Medical College. Attending Neurological Surgeon, New York Hospital–Cornell Medical Center, New York, New York.

TAHER EL GAMMAL, M.B., Ch.B., F.F.R.

Intracerebral and Intracerebellar Hemorrhage

Professor of Radiology, Medical College of Georgia. Chief of Neuroradiology, Eugene Talmadge Memorial Hospital; Attending Staff, Veterans Administration Hospital, Augusta, Georgia.

PHILIP L. GILDENBERG, M.D., Ph.D., F.A.C.S.

Pain Refractory to Therapy

Professor of Neurological Surgery and Chief of Division of Neurological Surgery, University of Texas Medical School at Houston. Chief of Neurological Surgery, Hermann Hospital, Houston, Texas.

SIDNEY GOLDRING, M.D., F.A.C.S.

Epilepsy in Adults

Professor of Neurological Surgery and Co-Head of Department of Neurology and Neurological Surgery, Washington University School of Medicine. Neurosurgeon-in-Chief, Barnes Hospital and St. Louis Children's Hospital, St. Louis, Missouri.

STANLEY J. GOODMAN, M.D., F.A.C.S.

Bacterial Infections

Associate Clinical Professor of Neurological Surgery, University of California, School of Medicine at Los Angeles, Los Angeles, California. Attending Staff, South Bay Hospital; San Pedro Peninsula Community Hospital, San Pedro, California; Community Hospital of Gardena, Gardena, California; Kaiser Hospital, Harbor City, California; Wadsworth Veterans Administration Hospital, Los Angeles, California; Little Company of Mary Hospital and Harbor General Hospital, Torrance, California.

JACK KNIGHT GOODRICH, M.D., F.A.C.R., F.A.C.N.P.

Radionuclide Imaging Studies

Formerly Professor of Radiology, School of Medicine, Duke University. Director of Nuclear Medicine Service, Hamot Medical Center; Radiologist, Radiology Associates of Erie, Erie, Pennsylvania.

JOHN R. GREEN, M.D., F.A.C.S.

Epilepsy in Children

Adjunct Professor of Surgery (Neurological Surgery), University of Arizona College of Medicine, Tucson, Arizona. Director, Barrow Neurological Institute of St. Joseph's Hospital and Medical Center, Phoenix, Arizona.

RICHARD PAUL GREENBERG, M.D., Ph.D.

Diagnosis, Treatment, and Outcome of Head Injury in Adults

Assistant Professor of Neurological Surgery, Medical College of Virginia, Virginia Commonwealth University. Attending in Neurological Surgery, Medical College of Virginia Hospitals, Richmond, Virginia.

MELVIN GREER, M.D.

Pseudotumor Cerebri

Professor of Neurology, Chairman of Department of Neurology, University of Florida College of Medicine. Chief of Neurology, University of Florida Teaching Hospitals and Clinics, Gainesville, Florida.

GERALD A. GRONERT, M.D.

Neuroanesthesia

Professor of Anesthesiology, Mayo Medical School. Consultant, Anesthesiology, Mayo Clinic; Attending Staff, St. Marys Hospital, Rochester, Minnesota.

MUTAZ B. HABAL, M.D., F.R.C.S.(C.), F.A.C.S.

Craniofacial Malformations

Adjunct Professor, University of Florida, Gainesville, Florida; Courtesy Professor, University of South Florida, Tampa, Florida. Director, Tampa Bay Center for Craniofacial Surgery; Attending Surgeon, Tampa General Hospital and University Community Hospital, Tampa, Florida; All Children's Hospital, St. Petersburg, Florida.

JULES HARDY, M.D., F.R.C.S.(C.), F.A.C.S.

Indications for and Results of Hypophysectomy, Transsphenoidal Hypophysectomy

Professor of Neurological Surgery, Chairman of Division of Neurological Surgery, University of Montreal Faculty of Medicine. Neurosurgeon, Notre Dame Hospital and University of Montreal Hospital, Montreal, Quebec.

LAWRENCE C. HARTLAGE, Ph.D., F.A.P.A., F.A.A.M.D., F.A.O.A.

Psychological Testing

Professor of Neurology and Pediatrics, Medical College of Georgia, Neuropsychologist, Talmadge Memorial Hospital; Consultant, University Hospital and Veterans Administration Hospitals, Augusta, Georgia, and Eisenhower Army Medical Center, Fort Gordon, Georgia.

PATRICIA L. HARTLAGE, M.D.

Psychological Testing

Associate Professor of Neurology and Pediatrics, Medical College of Georgia. Attending Staff, Talmadge Memorial Hospital; Consulting Staff, University Hospital and Gracewood State School and Hospital, Augusta, Georgia.

NELSON HENDLER, M.D.

Psychiatric Aspects of Pain

Assistant Professor of Psychiatry, The Johns Hopkins University School of Medicine. Psychiatric Consultant, Chronic Pain Treatment Center, Johns Hopkins Hospital, Baltimore, Maryland; Clinical Director, Mensana Clinic, Stevenson, Maryland.

E. B. HENDRICK, M.D., F.R.C.S.(C.)

Spinal Cord Tumors in Children

Professor of Surgery, University of Toronto. Neurosurgeon in Chief, The Hospital for Sick Children; Consultant in Neurological Surgery, Queensway General Hospital and Ontario Society for Crippled Children; Active Staff in Neurological Surgery, Toronto Western Hospital; Consultant Neurosurgeon, North York General Hospital, Toronto, Ontario.

SADEK K. HILAL, M.D., Ph.D

Interventional Neuroradiology, Tumors of Orbit

Professor of Radiology, Columbia University College of Physicians and Surgeons. Attending Radiologist, Presbyterian Hospital; Director of Neuroradiology, Neuroradiological Institute of New York, New York, New York.

ROBERT EDGAR HODGES, M.D.

Nutrition and Parenteral Therapy

Professor of Internal Medicine, University of Nebraska College of Medicine. Chief of Clinical Nutrition Section, University of Nebraska Medical Center, Omaha, Nebraska.

STEPHEN F. HODGSON, M.D.

Empty Sella Syndrome

Assistant Professor of Medicine, Mayo Medical School. Consultant in Internal Medicine and Endocrinology, Mayo Clinic; Attending Physician, St. Marys Hospital and Rochester Methodist Hospital, Rochester, Minnesota.

HAROLD J. HOFFMAN, M.D., F.R.C.S.(C.), F.A.C.S.

Supratentorial Tumors in Children

Associate Professor of Surgery, University of Toronto Faculty of Medicine. Neurological Surgeon, The Hospital for Sick Children, Toronto, Ontario.

GWENDOLYN R. HOGAN, M.D.

Clinical Examination of Children

Professor of Pediatrics, Professor of Neurology, University of Mississippi School of Medicine. Chief of Pediatric Neurology Service, University of Mississippi Medical Center, Jackson, Mississippi.

TAKAO HOSHINO, M.D., D.M.Sc.

Chemotherapy of Brain Tumors

Associate Professor of Neurological Surgery, School of Medicine, University of California at San Francisco. Research Associate, Laboratory of Radiobiology, School of Medicine, University of California at San Francisco, San Francisco, California.

EDGAR M. HOUSEPIAN, M.D., F.A.C.S

Tumors of Orbit

Professor of Clinical Neurological Surgery, Columbia University College of Physicians and Surgeons. Attending Neurological Surgeon, Columbia–Presbyterian Medical Center, New York, New York.

ALAN R. HUDSON, M.D., Ch.B., F.R.C.S.(Ed.), F.R.C.S.(C.)

Peripheral Nerve Entrapment

Professor of Neurological Surgery, Chairman of Division of Neurological Surgery, University of Toronto. Neurological Surgeon-in-Chief, St. Michael's Hospital, Toronto, Ontario.

ROBIN P. HUMPHREYS, M.D., F.R.C.S.(C.)

Posterior Fossa Tumors in Children

Assistant Professor of Neurological Surgery, University of Toronto Faculty of Medicine. Neurological Surgeon, The Hospital for Sick Children; Consultant, North York General Hospital and Ontario Crippled Children's Center, Toronto, Ontario.

WARREN Y. ISHIDA, M.D.

Peripheral and Sympathetic Nerve Tumors

Attending Neurological Surgeon, Kapiolani Children's Hospital, Queen's Medical Center, St. Francis Hospital, and Kuakini Medical Center, Honolulu, Hawaii.

FREDERICK A. JAKOBIEC, M.D., D.Sc.

Tumors of Orbit

Professor of Ophthalmology and Pathology, Cornell University Medical College. Director of Laboratories, Manhattan Eye, Ear and Throat Hospital, New York, New York.

PETER J. JANNETTA, M.D.

Micro-Operative Decompression for Trigeminal Neuralgia, Cranial Rhizopathies

Professor of Neurological Surgery, Chairman of Department of Neurological Surgery, University of Pittsburgh. Active Staff, Presbyterian–University Hospital and Children's Hospital of Pittsburgh; Senior Attending Neurological Surgeon, Montefiore Hospital; Senior Consultant, Veterans Administration Hospital, Pittsburgh, Pennsylvania.

THOMAS McNEESE KELLER, M.D.

Cerebral Death

Attending Neurological Surgeon, Santa Rosa Memorial Hospital, Community Hospital, and Warrack Hospital, Santa Rosa, California.

LUDWIG G. KEMPE, M.D., F.A.C.S.

Glomus Jugulare Tumors

Professor of Neurological Surgery and Anatomy, Medical University of South Carolina. Staff, Veterans Administration Medical Center, Charleston, South Carolina.

STEPHEN A. KIEFFER, M.D.

Tumors of Skull

Professor of Radiology, Chairman of Department of Radiology, State University of New York at Syracuse. Chief of Radiology, University Hospital, Syracuse, New York.

DAVID J. KIENER, M.D.

Neurotology

Assistant Professor of Otolaryngology, University of California, School of Medicine at Davis, Davis, California. Attending Staff, University of California Davis Medical Center at Sacramento, Sacramento, California.

ROBERT B. KING, M.D., F.A.C.S.

Cephalic Pain

Professor of Neurological Surgery, Chairman of Department of Neurological Surgery, State University of New York, Upstate Medical Center College of Medicine, Syracuse, New York. Chief of Neurological Surgery, State University Hospital of Upstate Medical Center; Attending Neurological Surgeon, Crouse-Irving Memorial Hospital; Consultant, Neurological Surgery, Veterans Administration Hospital. Syracuse, New York.

PULLA R. S. KISHORE, M.D.

Head Injury in Adults

Professor of Radiology, Medical College of Virginia, Virginia Commonwealth University, Richmond, Virginia. Director of Neuroradiology, Medical College of Virginia Hospitals; Consultant in Radiology, McGuire Veterans Administration Hospital, Richmond, Virginia.

DAVID G. KLINE, M.D., F.A.C.S.

Peripheral Nerve Injuries

Professor of Neurological Surgery, Head of Department of Neurological Surgery, Louisiana State University School of Medicine; Chief of Louisiana State University Neurological Surgery Service. Attending Staff, Touro and Hotel Dieu Hospitals; Academic Staff, Ochsner Clinic; Consultant, United States Public Health, Veterans Administration Hospital, New Orleans, Louisiana, and Biloxi Air Force Base Hospital, Biloxi, Mississippi.

ARTHUR I. KOBRINE, M.D., Ph.D., F.A.C.S.

Computed Tomography

Professor of Neurological Surgery, George Washington University School of Medicine. Attending Neurological Surgeon, George Washington University Hospital, Washington Hospital Center, Children's Hospital and National Medical Center, Washington, District of Columbia.

CAROLE C. LA MOTTE, Ph.D.

Physiology of Pain

Assistant Professor of Neuroanatomy and Neurological Surgery, Sections of Neuroanatomy and Neurological Surgery, Yale University School of Medicine, New Haven, Connecticut.

ALEX M. LANDOLT, M.D.

Sellar and Parasellar Tumors

Privatdozent, Neurosurgical Clinic, Kantonsspital, University of Zurich, Zurich, Switzerland.

THOMAS WILLIAM LANGFITT, M.D., F.A.C.S.

Increased Intracranial Pressure

Charles Harrison Frazier Professor of Neurosurgery, Director of Division of Neurological Surgery, University of Pennsylvania School of Medicine. Vice President for Health Affairs, University of Pennsylvania, Philadelphia, Pennsylvania.

EDWARD R. LAWS, M.D., F.A.C.S.

Empty Sella Syndrome

Professor of Neurological Surgery, Mayo Medical School. Neurological Surgeon, Mayo Clinic; Attending Neurological Surgeon, St. Marys Hospital and Rochester Methodist Hospital, Rochester, Minnesota.

HUN JAE LEE, M.D.

Parasitic and Fungal Infections

Late Professor of Neurological Surgery, Chairman of Department of Neurological Surgery, Yonsei University College of Medicine. Late Chief of Neurological Surgery, Yonsei Medical Center, Seoul, Korea.

VICTOR A. LEVIN, M.D.

Chemotherapy of Brain Tumors

Associate Professor of Neurological Surgery, Pharmacology and Pharmaceutical Chemistry, Schools of Medicine and Pharmacy, University of California at San Francisco. Associate Director, Brain Tumor Research Center; Chief, Neuro-Oncology Service, Department of Neurological Surgery, San Francisco, California.

JAMES S. LIEBERMAN, M.D.

Neuromuscular Electrodiagnosis

Professor of Physical Medicine and Rehabilitation and Neurology. University of California, School of Medicine at Davis, Davis, California. Attending Physiatrist and Neurologist, University of California Davis Medical Center at Sacramento, Sacramento, California.

JOHN D. LOESER, M.D.

Dorsal Rhizotomy

Professor of Neurological Surgery, University of Washington School of Medicine. Attending Physician, University Hospital, Veterans Administration Hospital, Harborview Medical Center, and Children's Orthopedic Hospital, Seattle, Washington.

DONLIN M. LONG, M.D., Ph.D., F.A.C.S.

Tumors of Skull, Chronic Pain, Pain of Spinal Origin, Pain of Visceral Origin, Peripheral Nerve Pain

Professor of Neurological Surgery, Chairman of Department of Neurological Surgery, The Johns Hopkins School of Medicine. Neurological Surgeon-in-Chief, Johns Hopkins Hospital, Baltimore, Maryland.

JOHN E. LONSTEIN, M.D., F.A.C.S.

Scoliosis, Kyphosis, and Lordosis

Assistant Professor of Orthopedic Surgery, University of Minnesota Medical School.

Attending Surgeon, Minneapolis Fairview Hospital, Minneapolis, Minnesota; Gillette Children's Hospital, St. Paul, Minnesota.

COLLIN S. MacCARTY, M.D., F.A.C.S.

Meningeal Tumors of Brain

Emeritus Professor of Neurological Surgery, Mayo Medical School. Consultant, Department of Neurological Surgery, Mayo Clinic, Rochester, Minnesota.

LEONARD I. MALIS, M.D., F.A.C.S.

Arteriovenous Malformations of Brain and Spinal Cord

Professor of Neurological Surgery, Chairman of Department of Neurological Surgery, City University of New York, Mount Sinai School of Medicine. Neurosurgeon-in-Chief, Department of Neurological Surgery, Mount Sinai Hospital, New York, New York.

JACK E. MANISCALCO, M.D., F.A.C.S.

Craniofacial Malformations

Clinical Assistant Professor of Surgery, University of South Florida College of Medicine. Attending Neurological Surgeon, St. Joseph's Hospital and Tampa General Hospital, Tampa, Florida.

JOSEPH C. MAROON, M.D., F.A.C.S.

Ultrasound in Neurosurgery

Professor of Neurological Surgery, University of Pittsburgh School of Medicine. Attending Neurological Surgeon, Presbyterian–University Hospital, Pittsburgh, Pennsylvania.

JOSE GERARDO MARTIN-RODRIGUES, M.D.

Tuberculoma and Syphilitic Gumma

Head of Neurosurgical Service, Department "Sixto Obrador," Centro Especial "RAMON Y CAJAL," Ministry of Health and Social Security, Madrid, Spain.

FRANK H. MAYFIELD, M.D., F.A.C.S.

Peripheral Nerve Entrapment

Clinical Professor of Neurological Surgery, Emeritus, University of Cincinnati School of Medicine. Director, Department of Neurological Surgery, Christ Hospital; Senior Attending Staff, Good Samaritan Hospital, Cincinnati, Ohio.

J. A. McCRARY, III, M.D.

Neurophthalmology

Associate Professor of Ophthalmology and Neurological Surgery, Baylor College of Medicine. Attending Staff, Methodist Hospital and St. Luke's Episcopal Hospital; Consultant, Houston Veterans Administration Hospital and Ben Taub Hospital, Houston, Texas.

ROBERT L. McLAURIN, M.D., F.A.C.S.

Head Injury in Children, Post-Traumatic Syndrome

Professor of Surgery and Neurological Surgery, University of Cincinnati College of Medicine. Chief of Neurological Surgery, University of Cincinnati Medical Center, University Hospital, and Children's Hospital Medical Center; Consultant, Veterans Administration Hospital, Jewish Hospital, and Christ Hospital; Attending Neurological Surgeon, Good Samaritan Hospital, and Bethesda Hospital, Cincinnati, Ohio.

JAMES E. McLENNAN, M.D., F.A.C.S.

Head Injury in Children

Assistant Professor of Surgery and Neurological Surgery, University of Cincinnati School of Medicine. Attending Neurological Surgeon, University of Cincinnati Hospital and Children's Hospital, Cincinnati, Ohio.

CAROL A. McMURTRY, M.A.

Neurotology

Clinical Instructor of Audiology, Department of Otorhinolaryngology, University of California, School of Medicine at Davis, Davis, California. Senior Audiologist, University of California Davis Medical Center at Sacramento, Sacramento, California.

W. JOST MICHELSEN, M.D., F.A.C.S.

Interventional Neuroradiology

Associate Professor of Neurological Surgery, Columbia University College of Physicians and Surgeons. Associate Attending Neurological Surgeon, Columbia–Presbyterian Hospital, New York, New York.

JOHN D. MICHENFELDER, M.D.

Neuroanesthesia

Professor of Anesthesiology, Mayo Medical School. Consultant Neuroanesthesiologist, Mayo Clinic; Attending Neuroanesthesiologist, St. Marys Hospital and Rochester Methodist Hospital, Rochester, Minnesota.

JAMES DOUGLAS MILLER, M.D., M.B., Ch.B., Ph.D., F.R.C.S.(Ed.), F.A.C.S.

Diagnosis, Treatment, and Outcome of Head Injury in Adults

Forbes Professor of Surgical Neurology and Chairman of Department of Surgical Neurology, University of Edinburgh School of Medicine. Chairman of Department of Surgical Neurology, Royal Infirmary and Western General Hospital, Edinburgh, Scotland.

THOMAS J. MIMS, JR., M.D.

Trauma to Carotid Arteries

Resident in Neurological Surgery, Baylor College of Medicine Affiliated Hospitals, Houston, Texas.

ROBERT A. MORANTZ, M.D., F.A.C.S.

Special Problems with Subarachnoid Hemorrhage

Associate Professor of Neurological Surgery, University of Kansas School of Medicine. Attending Staff, University of Kansas Medical Center; Consulting Staff Neurological Surgeon, Kansas City Veterans Administration Hospital, Kansas City, Missouri.

WILLIAM H. MORETZ, M.D., F.A.C.S.

Sympathectomy

President, Medical College of Georgia; Professor of Surgery, Medical College of Georgia. Attending Surgeon, Eugene Talmadge Memorial Hospital and University Hospital, Augusta, Georgia.

DONALD E. MORGAN, Ph.D.

Acoustic Neuromas

Associate Professor of Head and Neck Surgery, University of California at Los Angeles, School of Medicine. Director of Audiology Clinic, University of California at Los Angeles Hospital, Los Angeles, California.

BLAINE SANDERS NASHOLD, JR., M.D., F.A.C.S.

Stereotaxic Mesencephalotomy, Trigeminal Tractotomy

Professor of Neurological Surgery, Duke University School of Medicine. Attending Neurological Surgeon, Duke University Hospital, Durham, North Carolina.

MARTIN G. NETSKY, M.D.

Classification and Biology of Brain Tumors

Professor of Pathology, Vanderbilt University School of Medicine. Attending Pathologist, Vanderbilt University Hospital, Nashville, Tennessee.

CARL-HENRIK NORDSTRÖM, M.D., Ph.D.

Cerebral Metabolism

Teaching Staff, Department of Neurological Surgery, University Hospital, Lund, Sweden.

FRANK E. NULSEN, M.D., F.A.C.S.

Peripheral Nerve Injuries

Professor of Neurological Surgery, Chairman of Neurological Surgery, Case Western Reserve University. Director of Neurological Surgery Division, University Hospitals of Cleveland; Consulting Neurological Surgeon, Veterans Administration Hospital and Cleveland Metropolitan General Hospital, Cleveland, Ohio.

SIXTO OBRADOR, M.D.

Tuberculoma and Syphilitic Gumma

Late Professor of Neurological Surgery, Facultad de Medicina, Universidad Autonoma. Late Director and Chief of Department of Neurological Surgery, Centro Especial "RAMON Y CAJAL" of the Spanish Social Security, Madrid, Spain.

MARK STEPHEN O'BRIEN, M.D., F.A.C.S., F.A.A.P.

Hydrocephalus in Children

Professor of Surgery, Emory University School of Medicine. Chief of Neurological Surgery, Henrietta Egleston Hospital for Children, Atlanta, Georgia.

GUY L. ODOM, M.D., F.A.C.S.

General Operative Technique

James B. Duke Professor of Neurological Surgery, Duke University School of Medicine. Attending Neurological Surgeon, Duke University Hospital, Durham, North Carolina.

GEORGE A. OJEMANN, M.D.

Abnormal Movement Disorders

Professor of Neurological Surgery, University of Washington School of Medicine. Attending Physician, University Hospital and Harborview Medical Center; Consultant, Veterans Administration Hospital, Seattle, Washington.

ROBERT G. OJEMANN, M.D., F.A.C.S.

Hydrocephalus in Adults

Professor of Surgery, Harvard Medical School. Visiting Neurological Surgeon, Massachusetts General Hospital, Boston, Massachusetts.

AYUB K. OMMAYA, M.D., F.R.C.S., F.A.C.S.

Mechanisms of Cerebral Trauma

Clinical Professor of Neurological Surgery, George Washington University School of Medicine. Attending Neurological Surgeon, George Washington University Medical Center, Washington, District of Columbia. Chief Medical Adviser, National Highway Traffic Safety Administration, Department of Transportation; Former Chief of Applied Research in Neurological Surgery, Clinical Center, National Institutes of Health, Bethesda, Maryland.

DWIGHT PARKINSON, M.D., F.R.C.S.(C.), F.A.C.S.

Cavernous Plexus Lesions

Professor of Neurological Surgery, University of Manitoba. Chief of Section of Neurological Surgery, Health Sciences Centre, Winnipeg, Manitoba.

RUSSELL H. PATTERSON, JR., M.D., F.A.C.S.

Extradural Dorsal Spinal Lesions, Metastatic Brain Tumors, Hypophysectomy by Craniotomy

Professor of Neurological Surgery, Cornell University Medical College. Attending Surgeon-in-Charge, Department of Neurological Surgery, The New York Hospital, New York, New York.

S. J. PEERLESS, M.D., F.R.C.S.(C.)

Aneurysms of Posterior Circulation

Professor of Neurological Surgery, The University of Western Ontario. Chairman of Division of Neurological Surgery in the Department of Clinical Neurological Sciences, University Hospital and Victoria Hospital; Chief of Division of Neurological Surgery, University Hospital, London, Ontario.

DAVID GEORGE PIEPGRAS, M.D.

Operative Management of Intracranial Occlusive Disease, Meningeal Tumors of Brain

Assistant Professor of Neurological Surgery, Mayo Medical School. Consultant, Department of Neurological Surgery, Mayo Clinic; Attending Neurological Surgeon, St. Marys Hospital and Rochester Methodist Hospital, Rochester, Minnesota.

FRED PLUM, M.D.

Differential Diagnosis of Altered States of Consciousness

Professor of Neurology, Chairman of Department of Neurology, Cornell University Medical College. Neurologist-in-Chief, The New York Hospital, New York, New York.

JEROME B. POSNER, M.D.

Metastatic Brain Tumors

Professor of Neurology, Cornell University Medical College. Chairman of Department of Neurology, Memorial Sloan–Kettering Cancer Center, New York, New York.

MORRIS W. PULLIAM, M.D., F.A.C.S.

Problems with Multiple Trauma

Assistant Clinical Professor of Neurological Surgery, University of North Dakota School of Medicine. Staff Neurological Surgeon, Department of Neurosciences, Quain and Ramstad Clinic; Attending Neurological Surgeon, Bismarck Hospital and St. Alexius Hospital, Bismarck, North Dakota.

ROBERT W. RAND, M.D., Ph.D., J.D., F.A.C.S.

Acoustic Neuromas

Professor of Neurological Surgery, University of California, Los Angeles, School of Medicine; Attending Neurological Surgeon, University of California Hospital, Los Angeles, California.

RAYMOND V. RANDALL, M.D., F.A.C.P.

Neuroendocrinology, Empty Sella Syndrome

Professor of Medicine, Mayo Medical School. Senior Consultant, Mayo Clinic; Consultant Physician, St. Marys Hospital and Rochester Methodist Hospital, Rochester, Minnesota.

ROBERT A. RATCHESON, M.D., F.A.C.S.

Stereotaxic Surgery

Harvey Huntington Brown, Jr., Professor of Neurological Surgery; Director of Division of Neurological Surgery, Case Western Reserve University School of Medicine. Director of Division of Neurological Surgery, University Hospitals of Cleveland, Cleveland, Ohio.

KAI REHDER, M.D.

Neuroanesthesia

Professor of Anesthesiology and Physiology, Department of Anesthesiology and Department of Physiology and Biophysics, Mayo Medical School. Anesthesiologist, Department of Anesthesiology, Mayo Clinic; Attending Anesthesiologist, St. Marys Hospital and Rochester Methodist Hospital, Rochester, Minnesota.

O. HOWARD REICHMAN, M.D., F.A.C.S.

Extracranial to Intracranial Arterial Anastomosis

Professor of Neurological Surgery. Chief of Division of Neurological Surgery, Loyola University of Chicago. Chief of Neurological Surgery, Foster G. McGaw Hospital of Loyola University, Maywood, Illinois; Consulting Physician, Hines Veterans Administration Hospital, Hines, Illinois.

MICHAEL H. REID, Ph.D., M.D.

Ultrasound in Neurosurgery

Associate Professor of Radiology, University of California, School of Medicine at Davis, Davis, California. Chief, Section of Computerized Tomography; Chief, Section of Mammography; Staff Radiologist, University of California Davis Medical Center at Sacramento, Sacramento, California.

RALPH M. REITAN, Ph.D.

Psychological Testing After Craniocerebral Injury

Professor of Psychology, University of Arizona, Tucson, Arizona.

SETTI S. RENGACHARY, M.D.

Arachnoid Cysts, Post-Traumatic Arachnoid Cysts

Associate Professor of Neurological Surgery, The University of Kansas Medical Center, College of Health Sciences. Chief, Neurological Surgery Service at Kansas City Veterans Administration Hospital, Kansas City, Kansas.

ALBERT L. RHOTON, JR., M.D., R.D., F.A.C.S.

Micro-Operative Technique, Intracavernous Carotid Aneurysms and Fistulae

Keene Family Professor of Neurological Surgery, University of Florida College of Medicine. Chairman of Department of Neurological Surgery, University of Florida Teaching Hospitals and Clinics; Consultant, Veterans Administration Hospital, Gainesville, Florida.

JAMES THOMAS ROBERTSON, M.D.

Ventriculography, Extracranial Arterial Occlusive Disease

Professor of Neurological Surgery, Chairman of Department of Neurological Surgery, University of Tennessee Center for the Health Sciences. Chief of Neurological Surgery Service, Baptist Memorial Hospital and City of Memphis Hospitals, Memphis, Tennessee.

GAYLAN L. ROCKSWOLD, M.D., Ph.D.

Urological Problems

Associate Professor of Neurological Surgery, University of Minnesota Medical School. Chief of Neurological Surgery, Hennepin County Medical Center, Minneapolis, Minnesota.

MICHAEL JOHN ROSNER, M.D.

Head Injury in Adults

Assistant Professor of Neurological Surgery, Medical College of Virginia, Virginia Commonwealth University. Attending Neurological Surgeon, Medical College of Virginia Hospitals; Assistant Chief of Neurological Surgery, McGuire Veterans Administration Hospital, Richmond, Virginia.

HUBERT L. ROSOMOFF, M.D., D. Med. Sc., F.A.C.S.

Stereotaxic Cordotomy

Professor of Neurological Surgery, Chairman of Department of Neurological Surgery, University of Miami School of Medicine. Chief of Neurosurgical Service, Jackson Memorial Hospital; Attending Neurological Surgeon, Veterans Administration Hospital; Medical Director, Pain and Back Rehabilitation Program, University of Miami Hospital and Diagnostic Clinic, Miami, Florida.

FRANK A. ROWE, M.D.

Parasitic and Fungal Infections

Resident, Neurological Surgery, University of California at Davis Medical Center at Sacramento, Sacramento, California.

HOWARD A. RUSK, M.D., F.A.C.P.

Rehabilitation

Distinguished University Professor, New York University. Founder, Institute of Rehabilitation Medicine, New York, New York.

NELL J. RYAN, M.D.

Clinical Examination of Children

Associate Professor of Pediatrics, Assistant Professor of Neurology, University of Mississippi, School of Medicine. Director, Birth Defects Clinic, University of Mississippi Medical Center, Jackson, Mississippi.

ENRIQUE E. SAJOR, M.D.

Radiology of Spine

Chief, Neuroradiology Section, Sinai Hospital of Baltimore, Baltimore, Maryland.

MANNIE M. SCHECHTER, M.D.

Radiology of Skull, Cerebral Angiography, Encephalography, Radiology of Spine

Professor of Radiology, Albert Einstein College of Medicine. Radiologist, Beth Israel Medical Center, New York, New York.

RICHARD CARLTON SCHULTZ, M.D., F.A.C.S.

Maxillofacial Injuries

Professor of Surgery, Head of Division of Plastic Surgery, University of Illinois Abraham Lincoln College of Medicine. Chief of Division of Plastic Surgery and President of Medical Staff, Lutheran General Hospital; Attending Staff, University of Illinois Hospital, Chicago, Illinois.

JOHN BERNARD SELHORST, M.D.

Head Injury in Adults

Associate Professor of Neurology, Medical College of Virginia, Virginia Commonwealth University. Attending Neurologist, Richmond Eye Hospital and Medical College of Virginia Hospital; Consultant Neurologist, McGuire Veterans Administration Hospital, Richmond, Virginia, and Central State Hospital, Petersburg, Virginia; Eastern State Hospital, Williamsburg, Virginia.

GEORGE HEINRICH SELL, M.D.

Rehabilitation

Late Associate Professor of Clinical Rehabilitation Medicine, New York University School of Medicine. Late Acting Clinical Director, Institute of Rehabilitation Medicine, New York University Medical Center; Late Associate Attending Physician, Bellevue Medical Center, New York, New York.

FRANK W. SHARBROUGH, M.D.

Electroencephalography

Associate Professor of Neurology, Mayo Medical School. Consultant, Department of Neurology, Mayo Clinic; Attending Neurologist, St. Marys Hospital and Rochester Methodist Hospital, Rochester, Minnesota.

GLENN E. SHELINE, Ph.D., M.D., F.A.C.R.

Radiation Therapy of Brain, Pituitary, and Spinal Cord Tumors

Professor of Radiation Oncology, Vice-Chairman of Radiation Oncology, University of California, School of Medicine at San Francisco. Attending Radiologist, Mount Zion Hospital, Franklin Hospital, and Ft. Miley Veterans Administration Hospital, San Francisco, California.

JOHN SHILLITO, JR., M.D., F.A.C.S.

Craniosynostosis

Professor of Surgery, Harvard Medical School. Associate Chief of Neurosurgery, Children's Hospital Medical Center; Neurological Surgeon, Peter Bent Brigham Hospital, Boston, Massachusetts.

ROBERT J. SHORR, M.D.

Cerebrospinal Fluid

Resident in Neurology, Veterans Administration Wadsworth Medical Center. Post-Doctoral Trainee, University of California, School of Medicine at Los Angeles, Los Angeles, California.

ALVIN D. SIDELL, M.D.

Epilepsy in Children

Senior Pediatric Neurologist, Director of Electroencephalography Laboratory, Barrow Neurological Institute, St. Joseph's Hospital and Medical Center, Phoenix, Arizona.

BO U. SIESJÖ, M.D., Ph.D.

Cerebral Metabolism

Professor, Medical Research Council Cerebral Metabolism Group, Research Department of University Hospital, University of Lund, Lund, Sweden.

JOHN S. SILVERTON, M.D., F.R.C.S., F.R.C.S.(Ed.)

Tumors of Scalp

Assistant Clinical Professor of Plastic Surgery, University of California, School of Medicine at Davis, Davis, California. Consultant, Department of Plastic Surgery, University of California Davis Medical Center at Sacramento, Sacramento, California; Plastic Surgery Consultant, Veterans Administration Hospital, Martinez, California; Attending Staff, St. Joseph's Hospital and Dameron Hospital, Stockton, California; Lodi Memorial Hospital and Lodi Community Hospital, Lodi, California.

ROBERT R. SMITH, M.D., F.A.C.S.

Pathophysiology and Nonoperative Treatment of Subarachnoid Hemorrhage

Professor of Neurological Surgery, Chairman of Department of Neurological Surgery, University of Mississippi School of Medicine. Chief of Neurological Surgery Services, University Hospital and Veterans Administration Hospital; Consultant, Methodist Rehabilitation Center, Jackson, Mississippi.

ROGER D. SMITH, M.D.

Aneurysms of Anterior Circulation

Assistant Professor of Neurological Surgery, Department of Neurosurgery, Louisiana State University School of Medicine, New Orleans. Visiting Neurological Surgeon, Charity Hospital, Hotel Dieu Hospital, Southern Baptist Hospital, and West Jefferson Hospital, New Orleans, Louisiana.

ROBERT F. SPETZLER, M.D., F.A.C.S.

Dural Fistulae

Associate Professor of Neurological Surgery, Case Western Reserve University. Attending Neurological Surgeon, University Hospitals, Case Western Reserve University, Cleveland, Ohio; Veterans Administration; Consultant, Lakewood Hospital, Lakewood, Ohio.

BENNETT M. STEIN, M.D., F.A.C.S.

Pineal Tumors

Byron Stookey Professor of Neurological Surgery, Chairman of Department of Neurological Surgery, Columbia University College of Physicians and Surgeons. Director of Neurological Surgery, The Neurological Institute, New York, New York.

W. EUGENE STERN, M.D., F.A.C.S.

Preoperative Evaluation, Prevention and Treatment of Complications; Bacterial Infections

Professor of Surgery/Neurological Surgery, University of California, School of Medicine at Los Angeles, Los Angeles, California. Chief of Neurological Surgery, University of California Los Angeles Center for Health Sciences; Neurological Surgeon Consultant, Wadsworth Veterans Administration Hospital, Harbor General Hospital, St. John's Hospital, Los Angeles, California, and Santa Monica Hospital, Santa Monica, California.

THORALF M. SUNDT, JR., M.D., F.A.C.S.

Electroencephalography, Operative Management of Intracranial Occlusive Disease

Professor of Neurological Surgery, Mayo Medical School. Consultant, Department of Neurological Surgery, Mayo Clinic; Attending Neurological Surgeon, St. Marys Hospital and Rochester Methodist Hospital, Rochester, Minnesota.

WILLIAM H. SWEET, M.D., D.Sc., D.H.C., F.A.C.S.

Intracerebral Stimulation for Pain, Primary Affective Disorders

Emeritus Professor of Surgery, Harvard Medical School. Senior Neurosurgeon, Massachusetts General Hospital; Consulting Neurosurgeon, New England Deaconess Hospital, Massachusetts Eye and Ear Infirmary, Waltham Hospital, and Milton Hospital, Boston, Massachusetts.

O. RHETT TALBERT, M.D., F.A.C.P.

Clinical Examination

Clinical Professor of Neurology, School of Medicine, Medical University of South Carolina; Attending Neurologist, Roper Hospital and Medical College Hospital, Charleston, South Carolina.

JOHN M. TEW, JR., M.D., F.A.C.S.

Percutaneous Rhizotomy for Trigeminal, Glossopharyngeal and Vagal Pain

Adjunct Professor of Anatomy, University of Cincinnati College of Medicine. Chairman of Department of Neurological Surgery, Good Samaritan Hospital; Attending Neurological Surgeon, Christ Hospital, Cincinnati, Ohio.

ROBERT L. TIMMONS, M.D., F.A.C.S.

Cranial Defects

Clinical Professor of Surgery, East Carolina University School of Medicine, Attending Neurological Surgeon, Pitt County Memorial Hospital, Greenville, North Carolina.

GEORGE T. TINDALL, M.D.

Carotid Artery Occlusion for Aneurysms

Professor of Neurological Surgery, Emory University School of Medicine. Chief of Department of Neurological Surgery, Emory University Hospital, Atlanta, Georgia.

JAMES L. TITCHENER, M.D.

Post-Traumatic Syndrome

Professor of Psychiatry, University of Cincinnati Medical Center. Attending Staff, Cincinnati General Hospital; Consultant, Veterans Administration Hospital, Cincinnati, Ohio.

ALEXANDER B. TODOROV, M.D.

Genetic Aspects of Anomalies

Associate Professor of Neurology, College of Community Health Sciences, The University of Alabama. University, Alabama.

JAMES FRANCIS TOOLE, M.D., L.L.B., F.A.C.P.

Pathophysiology and Evaluation of Ischemic Vascular Disease

Professor of Neurology, Chairman of Department of Neurology, Bowman Gray School of Medicine, Wake Forest University. Chief of Neurology, North Carolina Baptist Hospital, Winston-Salem, North Carolina.

WALLACE W. TOURTELLOTTE, M.D., Ph.D.

Cerebrospinal Fluid

Professor of Neurology, Vice-Chairman of Department of Neurology, University of California, School of Medicine at Los Angeles. Chief of Neurology, Veterans Administration Wadsworth Medical Center, Los Angeles, California.

STEPHEN L. TROKEL, M.D.

Tumors of Orbit

Associate Professor of Clinical Ophthalmology, Columbia University College of Physicians and Surgeons. Attending Ophthalmologist, Edward S. Harkness Eye Institute, Columbia–Presbyterian Medical Center, New York, New York.

JOHN S. TYTUS, M.D., F.A.C.S.

Medical Therapy, Minor Procedures, and Craniotomy for Trigeminal Neuralgia; Glossopharyngeal and Geniculate Neuralgias

Clinical Associate Professor of Neurological Surgery, University of Washington School of Medicine. Attending Neurological Surgeon, Virginia Mason Hospital, King County Hospital, and Children's Orthopedic Hospital, Seattle, Washington.

JOHN M. VAN BUREN, M.D., Ph.D.

Stereotaxic Surgery

Professor of Neurological Surgery, University of Miami School of Medicine. Chief of Neurological Surgery, Veterans Administration Hospital; Attending Neurological Surgeon, Jackson Memorial Hospital, Miami, Florida.

WILLIAM M. WARA, M.D.

Radiation Therapy of Brain, Pituitary, and Spinal Cord Tumors

Associate Professor of Radiation Oncology, University of San Francisco, School of Medicine at San Francisco; Attending Radiologist, University of California Hospital, San Francisco, California.

ARTHUR A. WARD, JR., M.D.

Abnormal Movement Disorders

Professor of Neurological Surgery, Chairman of Department of Neurological Surgery, University of Washington School of Medicine. Attending Neurological Surgeon, University Hospital, Harborview Medical Center; Consultant, Veterans Administration Hospital, Children's Orthopedic Hospital, Seattle, Washington.

JOHN D. WARD, M.D.

Head Injury in Adults

Assistant Professor of Neurological Surgery, Medical College of Virginia Hospital, Virginia Commonwealth University. Chief, Pediatric Neurological Surgery, Medical College of Virginia Hospital, Richmond, Virginia.

CLARK C. WATTS, M.D., F.A.C.S.

Problems with Multiple Trauma

Professor of Neurological Surgery, University of Missouri School of Medicine. Chief of Neurological Surgery, University Hospital, University of Missouri/Columbia Health Sciences Center; Consultant, Harry S Truman Memorial Veterans Administration Hospital, Columbia, Missouri.

PHILIP RALPH WEINSTEIN, M.D., F.A.C.S.

Indications for and Results of Hypophysectomy, Stereotaxic Hypophysectomy

Professor of Neurological Surgery, University of Arizona School of Medicine. Chief of Neurological Surgery, University of Arizona Hospital; Attending Neurological Surgeon, Tucson Medical Center; Consultant, Barrow Neurological Institute, St. Joseph's Hospital, Tucson, Arizona.

KEASLEY WELCH, M.D., M.S., F.A.C.S.

Sensory Root Section for Trigeminal Neuralgia

Franc D. Ingraham Professor of Neurosurgery, Harvard Medical School, Neurosurgeon-in-Chief, Children's Hospital Medical Center; Division Chief (Neurosurgery), Department of Surgery, Peter Bent Brigham Hospital and Women's Hospital, Boston, Massachusetts.

MICHAEL WEST, M.D., Ph.D., F.R.C.S.(C.)

Cavernous Plexus Lesions

Lecturer in Physiology, Department of Physiology, University of Manitoba. Staff Neurosurgeon, St. Boniface General Hospital, Winnipeg, Manitoba.

LOWELL E. WHITE, JR., M.D.

Affective Disorders Involving Pain

Professor of Neuroscience, University of South Alabama. Attending Neurological Surgeon, University of South Alabama Medical Center, Providence Hospital, Mobile, Alabama.

ROBERT H. WILKINS, M.D., F.A.C.S.

General Operative Technique

Professor of Neurosurgery, Duke University Medical Center. Chief of Division of Neurological Surgery, Duke University Medical Center, Durham, North Carolina.

ROBERT HOLDEN WILKINSON, JR., M.D., F.A.C.R.

Radionuclide Imaging Studies

Associate Professor of Radiology, Duke University Medical Center. Attending Staff, Durham Veterans Administration Hospital, Durham, North Carolina.

CHARLES B. WILSON, M.D., F.A.C.S.

Dural Fistulae, Chemotherapy, Sellar and Parasellar Tumors, Indications for and Results of Hypophysectomy, Stereotaxic Hypophysectomy

Professor of Neurological Surgery, Chairman of Department of Neurological Surgery, University of California, School of Medicine at San Francisco. Chief of Neurological Surgery, University Hospital, San Francisco, California.

ROBERT B. WINTER, M.D., F.A.C.S.

Scoliosis, Kyphosis, and Lordosis

Professor of Orthopedic Surgery, University of Minnesota School of Medicine. Attending Staff, University of Minnesota Hospitals, Fairview Hospital, St. Mary's Hospital, Minneapolis Children's Hospital, Minneapolis, Minnesota; Gillette Children's Hospital, St. Paul Children's Hospital, and St. Paul Ramsey Hospital, St. Paul, Minnesota.

EARL F. WOLFMAN, JR., M.D., F.A.C.S.

Nutrition and Parenteral Therapy

Professor of Surgery, University of California, School of Medicine at Davis, Davis, California. Attending Surgeon, University of California Davis Medical Center at Sacramento, Sacramento, California; Consultant in Surgery, David Grant Medical Center, United States Air Force, Travis, California; Martinez Veterans Administration Hospital, Martinez, California.

R. LEWIS WRIGHT, M.D., F.A.C.S.

Infections of Spine

Attending Neurological Surgeon, St. Mary's Hospital and Stuart Circle Hospital, Richmond, Virginia.

FARIVAR YAGHMAI, M.D., F.C.A.P.

Intracerebral and Intracerebellar Hemorrhage

Associate Professor of Pathology (Neuropathology), Medical College of Georgia. Attending Staff, Eugene Talmadge Memorial Hospital; Consulting Staff, University Hospital, Veterans Administration Hospital, Dwight David Eisenhower Army Medical Center, Augusta, Georgia, Milledgeville Central State Hospital, Milledgeville, Georgia.

M. GAZI YAŞARGIL, M.D.

Aneurysms of Anterior Circulation

Professor of Neurological Surgery, Chairman of Department of Neurological Surgery, University of Zurich, Chief of Neurological Surgery, Clinic Hospital, Zurich, Switzerland.

JULIAN R. YOUMANS, M.D., Ph.D., F.A.C.S.

Diagnostic Biopsy, Cerebral Death, Cerebral Blood Flow, Trauma to Carotid Arteries, Glial and Neuronal Tumors, Lymphomas, Sarcomas and Vascular Tumors, Tumors of Disordered Embryogenesis, Peripheral and Sympathetic Nerve Tumors, Parasitic and Fungal Infections.

Professor of Neurological Surgery, University of California, School of Medicine at Davis, Davis, California. Attending Neurological Surgeon, University of California Davis Medical Center at Sacramento, Sacramento, California; Consultant in Neurological Surgery, United States Air Force Medical Center, Travis Air Force Base, California; Veterans Administration Hospital, Martinez, California.

HAROLD FRANCIS YOUNG, M.D.

Head Injury in Adults

Professor of Neurological Surgery, Vice-Chairman of Department of Neurological Surgery, Medical College of Virginia, Commonwealth University. Chief of Neurological Surgery, McGuire Veterans Administration Hospital, Richmond, Virginia; Attending Neurological Surgeon, Medical College of Virginia Hospitals, Richmond, Virginia.

RONALD F. YOUNG, M.D.

Cephalic Pain

Associate Professor of Neurological Surgery, University of California, School of Medicine at Los Angeles. Chief of Division of Neurological Surgery, Harbor General Hospital, Torrance, California; Attending Neurological Surgeon, University of California Hospital, Los Angeles, California.

LAWRENCE W. ZINGESSER, M.D.

Encephalography

Clinical Professor of Radiology, New York Medical College. Chief of Neuroradiology, St. Vincent's Hospital and Medical Center, New York, New York.

Preface to the Second Edition

The enthusiastic reception of the first edition of *Neurological Surgery* in all areas of the world indicated the need for such a publication. The second edition is intended to fulfill that need in a more complete manner. The discussions of the earlier edition have been expanded and updated. Many new topics are included, among them: computed tomography, diagnostic biopsy for neurological disease, spinal angiography, ultrasound application in neurological surgery, cerebral death, cerebral metabolism, neuroendocrinology, pulmonary care of the comatose patient, interventional neuroradiology, genetic aspects of neurological anomalies, craniofacial congenital malformations, pathophysiology and clinical evaluation of cerebral ischemic vascular disease, extracranial to intracranial arterial anastomosis for intracranial ischemic disease, operative management of intracranial arterial occlusions and acute ischemic stroke, neurosurgical aspects of scoliosis and kyphosis and lordosis, craniofacial neoplasia, pseudotumor cerebri, tumors of the glomus jugulare, intracerebral electrical stimulation for the relief of chronic pain, management of chronic pain refractory to specific therapy, and cranial rhizopathies.

I would like to thank the users of the first edition, especially those who made helpful comments concerning it. Also my appreciation is due to Jack Hanley, Albert Meier, Suzanne Boyd, Herbert Powell, Grace Gulezian, and the others of the staff at the W. B. Saunders Company who have worked to make the second edition a publication of quality. In particular, Ruth Barker, a patient and gracious lady, has worked tirelessly and with dedication as the manuscript editor. To her I owe a special thanks for all that she has done.

Handling the reams of correspondence, manuscripts, galley proofs, page proofs, and other items related to publishing *Neurological Surgery* requires many hours of secretarial work. Anna Mary Griffin, Georgene Pucci, and the other members of the Department of Neurological Surgery at Davis merit special recognition for helping to complete this work. Lastly, I would like to thank my fellow contributors to these volumes.

JULIAN R. YOUMANS

Preface to the First Edition

Like other medical sciences, neurological surgery has undergone rapid changes in recent years. New techniques and entire areas of new knowledge have been developed. The knowledge that a competent neurosurgeon must master has increased vastly. As a result, no individual or small group can be expert in all areas. The only means of making a book authoritative in every area, and especially in the paraneurosurgical areas in which a neurosurgeon must be knowledgeable, is to use multiple authors from all over the world. The concept of *Neurological Surgery* came with the recognition of this problem and the need for a comprehensive reference volume that would include the more usual areas of concern to a neurosurgeon and also the allied areas in which he must be informed if he is going to give his patients the best care that is possible.

Neurological Surgery is intended for use by the surgeon in practice, the trainee who is beginning to assume responsibility for patient care, and the allied specialist who works with neurosurgical patients. Emphasis is placed on fundamental knowledge concerning etiology, pathogenesis, diagnosis, treatment, and prognosis for each disease entity of concern to the neurosurgeon. Essentials of operative technique are discussed and special techniques are evaluated and put into perspective with the more usual ones. Where appropriate, special sections or chapters are devoted to the basic aspects of neurobiology.

In addition to attempting to fill the need for a comprehensive reference source, *Neurological Surgery* has been set up so as to recognize ongoing problems and divergent views within our specialty. Wherever there are major differences in the points of view concerning methods of diagnosis or treatment, each viewpoint is presented by a recognized proponent. This approach avoids the inevitable dilution that occurs when a conflicting view is evaluated and summarized by an individual, regardless of his fairness and integrity, who does not believe in the merits of the opposing view. A perusal of the chapter titles will show numerous examples of this approach.

Many chapters are included that usually have not been present in previous texts of neurological surgery. Examples are chapters that discuss the psychological evaluation of the neurosurgical patient, neuro-otology, mechanisms of coma, hyperextension-flexion injuries of the neck, the post-traumatic syndrome, cerebral blood flow in clinical problems, the biology of brain tumors, affective disorders, the physiological and the psychiatric aspects of pain, and the principles of stereotaxic surgery. Special emphasis is given to preoperative evaluation and prevention and treatment of complications.

Like the shakedown cruise of a ship, the first edition of a text such as *Neurological Surgery* will have omissions and errors that will be revealed as the book is put to the scrutiny of those interested in our queen specialty. Mr. John Dusseau and his staff at the W. B. Saunders Company have been dedicated to producing a publication of quality, and I wish to give my wholehearted expression of appreciation to them. In particular, Mr. Raymond Kersey has given care and attention to reproducing the illustrations with accuracy and clarity, and Miss Ruth Barker has worked with enthusiasm and dedication throughout the years from inception to the publication. To her, I owe especial thanks for her patient help in the editing and indexing and otherwise shepherding of this book to publication.

A book such as *Neurological Surgery* can be produced only with capable secretarial help. Miss Georgene Pucci has been invaluable to me in handling the thousands of pages of manuscripts, galley proofs, page proofs, and correspondence. Only with assistance of the type given by Miss Barker in Philadelphia and Miss Pucci in Davis could *Neurological Surgery* have become a reality. Finally, I would like to thank the contributors to *Neurological Surgery* for their cooperation and help in achieving for our joint effort the degree of success that it may enjoy.

JULIAN R. YOUMANS

Contents

VOLUME TWO

VOLUME THREE

VOLUME FOUR

VOLUME FIVE

X. Tumors 2657

VOLUME SIX

I

HISTORY AND EXAMINATION

1

GENERAL METHODS OF CLINICAL EXAMINATION

With the continuing development of more precise technical diagnostic procedures and instrumentation, the trend over the years has been to displace the conventional methods of the history and physical examination in diagnosis and management of the sick. This trend has been especially prevalent, and perhaps more justified, in the neurological fields. The past two decades have seen phenomenal progress in the application of modern physical science and engineering to new procedures and the refinement of old ones for probing previously denied reaches of the nervous system. Certainly the caricature of the traditional neurologist with his armamentarium of forbidding tools putting the patient through bizarre gyrations and absurd postures is as anachronistic as the old country doctor. Nevertheless, he did have among his odd manipulations some procedures for eliciting useful information that retain their value in modern diagnosis and treatment. In fact, even today the neurological history and examination remain the diagnostic procedures of primary importance. No single technical procedure matches the neurological history in permitting the clinician to focus on the correct area of etiology; none, for the time and effort invested, matches the neurological examination in giving an overview of the functioning of the nervous system at the moment and its dysfunctions salient in the clinical problem at hand.

The properly conducted and evaluated history and examination permit the most productive choice of technical diagnostic procedures at the least expense, discomfort, and hazard to the patient. Recognition of the proper relationship of the history and examination to these procedures is the mark of the mature clinician. The planning of technical procedures prior to availing oneself of the information from the history and examination is rarely justified. The distinction between the technician and the physician is fundamentally determined by the rapport each establishes between himself and the patient. No better opportunity exists for the development of that rapport that is so essential to superlative care of the sick than the required hour that the physician spends listening to his patient's problem and systematically exploring its physical manifestations. In this age of technology and superspecialization, we must constantly and consciously avoid the tendency to impersonalization inherent in the system of patient care that has evolved.

In arriving at a clinical diagnosis, four essential steps are involved, in the order enumerated:

1. *Eliciting the clinical information* by conducting the history and physical examination. This is the keystone of consistently accurate diagnosis.
2. *Localizing the lesion or disease process* (i.e., establishing the anatomical diagnosis), accomplished in the first instance, and often without the necessity of additional procedures, by correlating the findings on the physical examination with one's knowledge of the anatomy and physiology of the nervous system.
3. *Arriving at an etiological diagnosis or differential diagnosis,* accomplished by correlating one's knowledge of the whereabouts of the lesion with the information elicited in the history as to the onset and subsequent course of the patient's present complaints and previous health data.
4. Utilizing additional diagnostic techni-

O. R. TALBERT

cal and laboratory procedures necessary to refine anatomical localization and etiological diagnosis and to plan management of the patient's ailment.

CONDUCTING THE HISTORY AND EXAMINATION

For an outline of the procedure for neurological history and examination, one may consult any of a number of textbooks on basic neurology. The emphasis here is to be on more general aims: the approach to the patient and the significance of individual findings.

In diagnosing the immediate neurological ailment presented by the patient, information as to his general state of health, pertinent previous illnesses, and the condition of the other organ systems is essential. The clinical data pertaining to the nervous system must be evaluated in the light of such general information about the patient. The method of obtaining it will vary with the circumstances in which the neurosurgeon practices, but it is his responsibility as a competent clinician to obtain the information in one way or another and to apply it in his undertaking of the neurosurgical diagnosis.

While the conventional separation of the history and physical examination into two distinctive exercises has value in teaching physical diagnosis to students, the experienced clinician may find it expedient to modify so pedantic an approach to his patient. The history and examination is best considered a single exercise, which Adams has cogently designated *elicitation of the clinical data*.[1]

The technique of the clinical examination will necessarily vary with the patient's general condition. The following is a suggested approach in examining the ambulatory, cooperative, and fully conscious patient.

The neurological examination virtually begins when the examiner first greets the patient; it is then that he begins making observations of the patient's speech, movements, and mannerisms that often give clues leading to the correct localization and cause of the patient's disorder. Even when the patient is incapable of providing a reliable history, it is informative to give him the opportunity and to observe his deficiencies.

At the termination of the history it is convenient to continue with questions aimed at evaluating the patient's mental function. This requires tact and a demeanor of objectivity. It is usually advisable to begin with a frank inquiry such as: "Do you feel that you have difficulty remembering things or keeping track of events?" This can be elucidated by phrasing questions that require informative answers as to the date, recent news events, and the like, which test orientation, memory, general fund of knowledge, and ability to calculate and think abstractly. This line of questioning usually will not be resented by the patient. If it is, reassurance that this is your attempt to give him a thorough examination should suffice. Resentment, of itself, may betray a lack of insight or abnormal irritability that is of diagnostic significance, and the matter should be explored further with the patient's relatives. After sufficient questioning to elicit the information sought, proceed directly with tests of language function by presenting the patient with pencil and paper and a passage to read.

For the remainder of the examination, the patient should be moved to the examining table or asked to sit on the side of the bed. He should be clad only in shorts and, in the case of a woman, a loosely fitting garment covering the bust and leaving the shoulder girdle and upper limbs bare. No elaborate collection of gadgets is necessary in the examiner's armamentarium; however, there are a few simple aids that are necessary for the neurological examination:

- An aromatic agent for testing sense of smell (tobacco, oil of peppermint, cloves)
- A sharp pin with round white head 3 to 5 mm in diameter
- Ophthalmoscope-otoscope
- Near vision testing card with graduated print size
- Tuning fork, C–256
- Tongue blade
- Cotton wisp or cotton tip applicator
- Reflex hammer
- Two stoppered test tubes

The patient should be seated comfortably on the table or bed, legs dangling freely. The first step in the examination proper is to direct attention to the body part to which the patient has referred complaints. This is reassuring and logical to the patient, and frequently will uncover diagnostic information from the start.

One should then return to an orderly procedure of examination, beginning with the eyes. Holding the index finger approximately 18 inches in front of his eyes, have him follow the moving finger to either side, upward and downward. Observe the pupils, lid and brow movements, and the details of ocular movements, which are elaborated upon in Chapter 17. Terminate by having the patient converge vision on the finger as it is moved in toward the nose, observing the pupillary constriction of convergence-accommodation.

Next, with the ophthalmoscope, examine the fundus, paying particular attention to the optic discs and maculae. With the otoscope light, test the pupillary light reflex in each eye separately. While this light is handy, examine the oropharynx, using a tongue blade to elicit the gag reflex on each side and observing for abnormality of pharynx and palate movements. Have the patient protrude the tongue for inspection. Finally, attach the ear speculum and inspect the auditory canals before dispensing with this instrument.

Returning to the eyes, test visual acuity of each eye separately with the near vision card. If the patient uses corrective glasses he should wear them for this test. Using the white pinhead or the "three-stage confrontation technique" described in Chapter 17, test the visual fields quadrant by quadrant in each eye. While the pin is handy, test pain sensation over both sides of the face.

Have the patient close the eyes and test smell sensation, each nostril separately, by passing the test object (peppermint, cloves, or tobacco) under the nose and asking for perception of the odor.

Have the patient whistle to observe function of the orbicularis oris muscle. This often provokes a spontaneous smile, offering the opportunity to observe emotional facial movements. Palpate the masseter and temporalis muscles bilaterally while the patient repetitively clenches the teeth. Test hearing by rubbing the thumb against the fingers near each of the patient's ears. The more precise hearing tests described in Chapter 18 may be used when hearing deficit is elicited. Palpate the sternocleidomastoid muscle on either side with the patient's head turned to the opposite side; then inspect the upper borders of the trapezius muscles and test them for strength by having the patient shrug his shoulders.

Examine the neck by having the patient extend his head, then flex it, touching the chin on the chest. Look for limitation of neck motion or pain on motion.

Now, have the patient sit erect, close his eyes, and extend his arms straight forward, palms downward and fingers spread apart. While this posture is maintained for 90 seconds, a number of valuable observations can be made. Tremors and other abnormal involuntary movements are readily evident during maintenance of this posture. It also affords an excellent opportunity to inspect the musculature of trunk and upper limbs for evidence of atrophy. Inspect the shoulder girdle front and rear. Look for abnormal curvature of the spine and other trunk deformities. Keep an eye on the arms to see if one or the other sags to betray a motor weakness or wavers about to betray a deficit in coordination or position sense. Proprioceptive sensation and cerebellar function can then be tested further by having the patient touch the tip of each index finger to his nose while the eyes remain closed, then with the eyes open.

Next, have the patient rest his arms in his lap. Move each arm passively, feeling for alteration of muscle tone. With his arms symmetrically relaxed in his lap and his legs dangling freely, test the tendon reflexes in all four limbs, comparing the two sides.

Now, have the patient lie supine on the examining table. Test the plantar, cremasteric, and cutaneous abdominal reflexes. Test sensory function, beginning with position sensibility, light touch, and the discriminatory (cortical) sensibilities. Testing for light touch with the cotton wisp should include the extremities and trunk, the corneal reflexes, and the face. Pinprick, being the most unpleasant, is usually best reserved until last. The detail to which sensory testing is carried will vary depending on the nature of the individual problem. Minimum testing should, however, include proprioceptive (vibratory and position), cutaneous (light touch and pain), and discriminatory (or "cortical") modalities. Suspicion of a cerebral lesion will require detailed testing of the discriminatory modalities, whereas information regarding the proprioceptive and cutaneous modalities will be more helpful when disease at lower levels is suspected.

The patient is queried regarding disturbance of sphincter function. Rectal examination for sphincter tone should be done if there is a history of incontinence or if one suspects spinal cord disease.

Finally, the examination should always be terminated by having the patient stand and walk. Observation of gait, posture, swinging of the arms while walking, heel-to-toe (tandem) walking, change of direction in walking, and ability to stand on a narrow base provides evaluation of motor and cerebellar functions that cannot be obtained as readily or reliably by any other technique. Having the patient sit in a low chair and rise, squat and rise, and flex the trunk from the erect posture are easy methods of evaluating strength and function of pelvic girdle and lower limb musculature and motility of the lower spine.

This technique of examination, while lengthy in description, can be carried out within a period of 15 or 20 minutes after brief experience. More prolonged examination at the initial exercise is not likely to be profitable because of fatigue on the part of both patient and examiner. When a particular system or function requires more meticulous evaluation than is afforded by the procedure described, it is best carried out in subsequent examinations.

LOCALIZING THE LESION (ANATOMICAL DIAGNOSIS)

From the body of clinical information obtained from the history and examination, one should next attempt to define the location of the lesion or disease process affecting the nervous system. Rarely can this be done on the basis of one individual finding. Accurate anatomical localization nearly always requires consideration of the *totality of physical findings* rather than any single one.

The combination of multiple findings will sometimes constitute one of three syndromes of impairment: *a syndrome of a specific function,* mediated by a structurally distinct and functionally related system of neurons; *a syndrome of a lesion in a restricted region or level of the nervous system,* sometimes impairing multiple functions; or *a syndrome of diffuse disease* of the nervous system. It is a helpful step in diagnosis to consider whether the aggregate of findings constitutes a pattern signifying one of these three categories of localization.

Syndromes of Specific Functions

Upper Motor Neuron Paralysis

The "upper motor neuron" system is more a physiological than an anatomical entity. Originally, it was defined anatomically as identical with the pyramidal (corticospinal) tract, which was thought to arise from the Betz cells in the precentral gyrus of each frontal lobe and to form the pyramids on the ventral surface of the medulla oblongata. The signs ascribed to injury to this tract were, therefore, called pyramidal signs. Subsequent investigations have led to the recognition that this concept of the pyramidal tract was inadequate, and some observers have maintained that individual components of this syndrome are due to injury to the extrapyramidal neuronal system rather than the pyramidal. Much of the controversy that has ensued is of little consequence in clinical diagnosis, but one area of disagreement seems to involve different usage of terms that denote the clinical state of muscle tone. The terms "spasticity" and "rigidity" have quite separate and distinct meanings to most clinicians, whereas they seem to be used interchangeably by some writers.

Clinically, it is both useful and conventional to regard spasticity as synonymous with the "clasp-knife" phenomenon (lengthening reaction). It is a state of altered tone of skeletal muscle that is elicited most readily when the involved limb is passively moved suddenly. At the beginning and through the initial phase of the movement there is a palpable resistance of the muscle being lengthened, then toward the end of the movement there is an abrupt disappearance of the muscle resistance and the limb gives readily to the movement. Its resemblance to the "catch" and "give" of a spring-loaded knife being closed is the source of the term "clasp-knife reaction." This disorder of muscle tone is to be distinguished from *rigidity,* which is described later.

While the older concept of the pyramidal tract is no longer adequate, there is a system of neurons in each cerebral hemisphere that gives rise to the corticospinal and corticobulbar pathways, transmitting impulses directly—i.e., without synaptic interruption—to its target cells contralaterally in brain stem and anterior gray column of spinal cord. A convenient term by which this system can be designated is "upper motor neuron." The term "pyramidal tract" is so entrenched in clinical parlance, however, that its use is likely to continue. When this system is damaged anywhere along its course, from cerebral cortex through the internal capsule and brain stem to the termination of its axons along the lateral white columns of the spinal cord, there results a syndrome of altered motor function consisting of the following elements:

1. Motor paralysis or paresis affecting functionally related groups of muscles rather than individual muscles, which may be transient and impairs mostly discrete movements of the distal limb segments.
2. Clasp-knife phenomenon (spasticity in the clinical sense) in the involved limb or limbs (except during the stage of "neuronal shock" in the early days or weeks following acute lesions).
3. Hyperactive tendon reflexes in the involved limb or limbs (except during the stage of "neuronal shock" following acute lesions).
4. Loss of the cutaneous abdominal and cremasteric reflexes on the paretic side.
5. Babinski's toe sign (extensor plantar response) on the paretic side.
6. Lack of atrophy of the involved muscles, except late from disuse, and absence of fasciculations.

A stage of "neuronal shock" that often follows acute lesions of this system may cause an initial phase of hypotonia of the muscles and areflexia in the involved limb or limbs instead of the characteristic clasp-knife phenomenon and hyperreflexia. During this phase Babinski's sign may be the only indication of the syndrome to distinguish it from that of lower motor neuron paralysis. When the lesion is a progressive one, the other signs gradually appear. Lesions that affect both this system and the extrapyramidal system at cerebral hemisphere, brain stem, or spinal cord levels will produce rigidity accompanying, and perhaps overshadowing, the clasp-knife reaction in the involved parts.

Lower Motor Neuron Paralysis

The concept of the "lower motor neuron" is likewise a physiological one; however, its anatomy is more precise. The term refers to the aggregate of the neurons of the motor nuclei of the cranial nerves and the anterior gray horn (column) of the spinal cord, each of which, along with the group of somatic muscle fibers innervated by it, constitutes a motor unit. Each neuron of the system is the final common pathway whereby all the multiple influences of the nervous system on motor function are integrated and transmitted to the effector muscle. At the spinal level the aggregate of lower motor neurons at a given spinal cord segment constitutes the efferent limb of the spinal reflex arc. A lesion affecting this system, anywhere from the parent neurons of the anterior horn (column) along their axons coursing through anterior spinal roots, spinal nerves, plexus, peripheral nerves or their synaptic junction with the muscle (motor end-plate), produces a motor syndrome consisting of the following:

1. Motor paralysis of the individual muscle or group of muscles innervated by them, the degree of paralysis varying, depending on the proportion of total motor supply impaired.
2. Persisting loss of muscle tone (flaccidity or hypotonia).
3. Diminution or absence of tendon reflexes in the involved limb or limbs.
4. Muscle atrophy that begins early, is marked, and increases for the duration of the lesion.
5. No Babinski sign or other pathological reflex.
6. Muscle fasciculations in some cases.

Since it is the final pathway, the manifestations of lower motor neuron involvement will predominate when the lesion involves it along with other pathways that influence it. Thus when both upper and lower motor neuron supplies to a limb are completely interrupted, the findings will be those of lower motor neuron paralysis; however, when the involvement of the lower motor neuron is only partial, one may find manifestations of both in the same limb. If motor paralysis is accompanied by sensory deficit in the same part, the lesion must be in a mixed nerve bundle in which motor and sensory axons coexist (both anterior and posterior roots, spinal nerve, plexus, or proximal part of peripheral nerve); if not, the lesion must be in anterior gray horn of spinal cord, or anterior root or roots, or distal enough in peripheral nerve to involve only a motor branch.

The cranial nerves present a unique situation with regard to differentiation of upper and lower motor neuron involvement and presence or absence of accompanying sensory deficits. Those that receive supranuclear (corticobulbar) influence from both sides (upper half of the face, pharynx, larynx, tongue, and some of the respiratory muscles) will show little or no paralysis from a unilateral upper motor neuron lesion, except transiently following an acute lesion. Since the only other manifestation of upper neuron paralysis testable in the cranial nerves is the jaw jerk, this can be an important reflex to test in determining the level in the neuraxis of an upper neuron lesion. In some of the cranial nerves (e.g., the fifth and seventh) the arrangement and type of sensory nerve fibers related to the motor fibers is peculiar to the individual nerve. One may consult a textbook of neuroanatomy for the anatomical details.

The Extrapyramidal Syndrome

The older anatomical concept of the extrapyramidal system has, like that of the pyramidal system, undergone modification in recent years; however, as a physiological or functional entity—or more exactly, a system the dysfunction of which is manifested by a consistent set of clinical findings—it has retained its identity over the years. The basal ganglia are still accepted as the anatomical "core" of this system. These have extensive connections with the cerebral cortex, primarily the premotor area of the frontal lobe. They are also interconnected with one another and with parts of the thalamus and hypothalamus, olivary nuclei, and brain stem reticular formation. Unlike the direct corticospinal-corticobulbar system, the extrapyramidal system is a multisynaptic system of neurons with short-chain axons and feedbacks that indirectly project to the lower motor neuron system by several scattered pathways descending the brain stem and the spinal cord; these, for the most part, cross to the side opposite from their origin at multiple levels. Their clinical manifestations are, therefore, like the corticospinal-corticobulbar system, mainly contralateral.

The cardinal clinical findings indicating involvement of the extrapyramidal system are:

1. Rigidity, a type of increased tone of skeletal musculature in which resistance to passive movement of the limb remains constant throughout the range of the movement and is present regardless of the speed at which the limb is moved. It may be of either the plastic (lead-pipe) or the cogwheel variety.

2. Hyperkinesias (dyskinesias), which are abnormal involuntary movements of several varieties including tremor at rest, chorea ("St. Vitus dance"), athetosis, and ballismus (usually occurring unilaterally as hemiballismus).

3. Bradykinesia (hypokinesia) consisting of both a paucity of spontaneous movements and slowness (inhibition) of volitional movements. Spontaneous movements that become impaired include: "automatic movements," which are carried out as accompaniments of volitional movements (e.g., swinging of arms while walking, or expressional facial movements during conversation); and the several components of a complexity of simultaneously performed movements (e.g., walking, talking, and gesticulating simultaneously).

4. Dystonia, an alteration of posture of the body or its parts due to imbalance of tone in antagonist muscle groups that ordinarily maintain the trunk and appendages in their normal posture. Such abnormal postures are mobile, develop during volitional motor activity, and tend to melt away with cessation of activity. Later ones, especially those that are maintained for long periods at a time, such as flexion of the trunk in parkinsonism, tend to become fixed.

5. Tendon reflexes that are normal or slightly hyperactive; no Babinski sign or other pathological reflexes present.

The extrapyramidal syndrome is most frequently encountered with nonsurgical diseases, parkinsonism being the most common. It sometimes occurs, however, in pure form with focal lesions situated deep in the cerebral hemisphere; and extrapyramidal manifestations are frequently seen in conjunction with upper motor neuron ones when lesions in the central nervous system involve both systems. An important fact in neurosurgical diagnosis is that *unilateral extrapyramidal signs do not necessarily signify a focal operable lesion*. More often than not, the progressive diseases of this system such as parkinsonism begin unilaterally.

Rarely does one encounter all the extrapyramidal manifestations in the same patient. The hyperkinesias, other than tremor, and the bradykinesias especially are unlikely to occur together. In fact, there is some clinical and biochemical evidence that the two are inversely related. Although rigidity is characteristic of the syndrome, chorea may actually be accompanied by hypotonia and laxity of the limbs instead.

Ataxia

The syndromes of the cerebellum are described later in this chapter. Ataxia (incoordination) is a cardinal manifestation of involvement of the cerebellum or its connecting pathways in the brain stem; however, ataxia is not necessarily of cerebellar origin. It may occur as a major manifestation in any of the following four situations:

1. Cerebellar ataxia (discussed later) including the flocculonodular (midline) syndrome and the lateral (cerebellar hemisphere) syndrome.
2. Frontal lobe ataxia (also discussed later).
3. Proprioceptive sensory ataxia in which there is loss of sense of position in one or more extremities from a lesion involving the posterior white columns of spinal cord or the proprioceptive fibers in the peripheral nervous system. In impairment of proprioceptive sensation, the defect is compensated for by substituting visual and tactile information. Ataxia characteristically develops in the part deprived of sense of position when the eyes are closed and tactile clues to the body are removed. The entire syndrome thus consists of: positive Romberg sign, loss of proprioceptive (position and vibratory) sensation, and ataxia.
4. Vestibular (labyrinthine) ataxia in which a lesion involves the labyrinth in the inner ear, the vestibular component of the eighth cranial nerve peripherally, or the vestibular nuclei and pathways within the brain stem. The syndrome consists of the combination of vertigo, nausea and vomiting, horizontal or rotary nystagmus, and a reeling type of ataxia. It is sometimes also referred to as "vertiginous ataxia" because of the prominence of vertigo. In view of the interconnections between the vestibular nuclei in the brain stem and the midline cerebellar structures, this form of ataxia may be difficult to distinguish from the midline cerebellar syndrome; indeed, the two may coexist by simultaneous involvement of both structures by a properly situated lesion in the posterior cranial fossa.

The finding and differentiation of these disorders of specific functions of the nervous system usually permits only an approximate anatomical diagnosis. Most of the syndromes just described could indicate a lesion at any of several levels. The location of a lesion can be determined more precisely by attempting to define the level or *region* to which the combination of abnormal findings points. This approach is discussed next.

Localization of Lesions by Regions

There is a priority of specificity for regional localization among individual clinical findings and syndromes. Some findings (e.g., aphasia) are highly specific indicators of the region involved, whereas others, as just discussed, are specific for particular neuronal systems or pathways traversing more than one region (e.g., upper motor neuron paralysis). By combining these two types of findings it is possible to arrive at an accurate anatomical localization and often simultaneously to determine the cause. The five major regional levels into which most syndromes of focal neurological deficit may be localized readily are the *supratentorial intracranial, the infratentorial intracranial (posterior cranial fossa), the spinal canal, the peripheral nervous system, and the skeletal musculature*. These are discussed in order.

Manifestations of Supratentorial Intracranial Lesions

Lesions localized to the anterior or middle cranial fossa are manifest neurologically by signs of cerebral, visual, olfactory, or endocrine dysfunction, depending on the precise location and nature of the lesion. Cerebral manifestations include motor, sensory, or certain mental disturbances, which may present as isolated findings but more often as symptom-complexes (syndromes), each of which has its value in anatomical diagnosis. Either irritative or destructive (deficit-producing) cerebral manifestations or both may constitute such a syndrome. The most useful of these syndromes are considered individually.

Epileptic Seizures

Epileptic attacks physiologically are irritative phenomena in which abnormal synchronous activation of aggregates of cerebral neurons occurs, usually originating in a restricted area of brain. They manifest themselves in various patterns of clinical change in the victim, depending primarily upon the function normally subserved by the originally activated cellular aggregate, its anatomical relation to other functional areas of the nervous system, and the facility and speed with which the discharge is propagated within the nervous system. Epilepsy may be divided into two categories clinically: *generalized* or diffuse seizures and *focal* seizures. The first category includes "grand mal" and "petit mal" seizures believed to arise from deep within the central brain—Penfield's centrencephalic system—and propagated rapidly to activate cerebral neurons widely. These types, beginning in childhood or adolescence, recurring over a period of months or years, and constituting the patient's only neurological abnormality ("idiopathic epilepsy"), seldom are a problem for the neurosurgeon. However, two precautions need to be taken into account here. In the first place, seizures that at first blush may seem to be of grand mal type may be revealed on further information to have additional features clearly signifying that they, in fact, have a focal onset followed by rapid spread to generalized activation. This is especially true of those attacks the very onset of which is missed by the witness-historian, those occurring during sleep, and those in which amnesia for the onset prohibits the patient's recalling the initial focal phenomena. Secondly, not all brief attacks or those in which loss of consciousness is dubious constitute petit mal epilepsy.

Focal epilepsy is the category of seizures of major importance in neurosurgical diagnosis. Seizures of this category may be regarded as invariably arising in a focus of cerebral cortex and therefore always indicating that their causative lesion is within the cranial cavity above the tentorium. They may occur alone or in company with other neurological signs that serve to further localize the lesion. An individual focal seizure may remain focal in its clinical manifestations throughout the duration of the attack (even for long spans of time in occasional cases, i.e., epilepsia partialis continua), or it may spread with varying rapidity and over varying extent of the brain with attendant progressing somatic manifestations (jacksonian march), or it may abruptly proceed from its focal manifestations to a generalized convulsion closely simulating grand mal epilepsy.

The specific patterns of clinical events signifying focal seizures are of almost infinite diversity.[10] *Any paroxysmal experience that can be ascribed, on either experimental or clinical grounds, to synchronous activation of neurons in any focal area of brain should be regarded as potentially signifying a focal seizure.* The potential is enhanced if the experience recurs wholly or in part as a stereotyped pattern and if it is brief in duration. While the two generally recognized characteristics of epilepsy are abnormal or inappropriate motor activity and impairment of consciousness, neither of these is indispensable to the diagnosis of focal epilepsy. Depending on the nature of brain function to which the activated neuronal focus contributes, the clinical manifestations of a focal seizure may be motor, sensory, or mental.[10,14] In the history, one must inquire as to subjective experiences and, *specifically, whether emotional or sensory experiences occur in association with attacks.* Not only is the patient unlikely to realize that such experiences constitute a part of his seizure, but also he may decline to divulge voluntarily bizarre sensations that he fears constitute a threat to mental integrity. Both the patient and witnesses to his attacks should provide a precise and complete chronological account of each event leading up to, comprising, and immediately following his attack.

Dementia

The syndrome of dementia is frequently the earliest and at times the only manifestation of an intracranial lesion. Dementia implies deterioration in those specific intellectual spheres dependent upon brain function in a person whose performance in these spheres was previously normal. Deterioration of (1) memory (especially that for recent events), (2) orientation in time and immediate environment, (3) ability to think abstractly, and (4) fund of general information are the cardinal manifestations to be sought. Other manifestations of altered mentation such as depression, loss of insight and judgment, visual or auditory hallucinations, delusions, personality change, and impairment of concentration may occur as components of the total syndrome; but they are not primary manifestations of dementia or necessarily indicators of organic brain disease. Nevertheless, the history of even subtle and nonspecific changes in the individual's behavior such as irritability, change in sleep habits, loss of interest and initiative at work or recreation, and unaccustomed errors in intellectual performances should alert one to the possibility of early dementia and lead one to search for loss of capacity in those specific spheres indicative of organic disease. Dementia often is a manifestation of medical diseases such as hypothyroidism, syphilis, or arteriosclerosis. Of interest in neurosurgical diagnosis, however, is the fact that the identical syndrome may herald intracranial tumor, subdural hematoma, and other neurosurgical lesions, whether it occurs alone or in company with other neurological findings. When other findings occur they may be focal and lateralized or they may be nonfocal ones such as grasp reflex or snout reflex, postural tremor or generalized seizures. Dementia of moderate or advanced degree, alone or in association with other neurological abnormalities, can usually be diagnosed by "bedside" tests of recent memory, orientation, ability to keep in mind and carry out a problem such as serial subtractions of 7 from 100, and knowledge of events expected of the patient's level of education and experience. Formal psychometric testing by a trained psychologist may be necessary to diagnose milder degrees.

Aphasia and Agnosia

Syndromes of disordered language (aphasia, agnosia) constitute a highly specific diagnostic finding. They signify a focal lesion involving the dominant cerebral hemisphere, which is the left hemisphere in virtually all right-handed and about half of left-handed persons. Language is a specialized intellectual function that is in essence the use of a system of symbols consisting of words and groups of words that convey meanings. The use of language is a dual process consisting of the reception and recognition of word symbols on the one hand and expression of them on the other. The entire process is dependent upon such a restricted mass of brain for its essential function that it may be profoundly impaired by a lesion sufficiently small to spare all other mental faculties. Aphasia is the term used to denote the selective loss of ability to comprehend or meaningfully to execute language in the absence of generalized mental impairment or motor impairment sufficient to account for the loss. Agnosia denotes the loss of ability to recognize or to appreciate the significance of stimuli although the perception of them is intact. Verbal agnosia is the specific agnosia for word symbols that pertains to language disorders. The diagnosis of aphasia and its use as a sign of a focal intracranial lesion rests primarily on evaluation of spoken language. Impairment of spoken language is usually accompanied by impairment of ability to write (agraphia) or to read (alexia). Mild degrees of aphasia (dysphasia), often manifested by only occasional misuse of a word in the course of conversation, are of as important localizing value as more severe disturbances. Furthermore, in the individual's language armamentarium there exists a hierarchy of vulnerability that becomes manifest when speech is progressively or only partially impaired: primitive and emotional speech (e.g., exclamations, swearing) and speech that is automatic by virtue of having been learned early or repeated often (e.g., salutations, the alphabet, childhood prayers and poems, the names of the months) are least vulnerable and remain relatively intact; propositional or symbolic speech, i.e., that which conveys ideas rather than feeling, is more vulnerable and is impaired to some degree in virtually all dysphasics; polyglots lose use of recently learned tongues more readily than their native and longer-used tongue. In order to elicit milder degrees of dysphasia, therefore, it is necessary to engage the patient in sufficiently extensive conversation involving propositional speech and to maintain a keen ear for recurrent mispronunciations or tendency to stereotyped responses. This can usually be accomplished during the course of taking the patient's history. Additional testing by having the patient name objects shown him, read aloud a passage from the newspaper, write a sentence to dictation, and carry out a complicated oral command will provide confirmatory evidence of a disturbance of language in the suspected case.

Two syndromes of aphasia can be recognized clinically, of which one indicates a lesion anteriorly and the other indicates a lesion posteriorly in the dominant cerebral hemisphere. Although neither is often seen in pure form, one or the other pattern will be predominant in individual cases frequently enough to help in localization.

1. *Expressive (motor) aphasia* is characterized by impairment of ability to say what one wishes to say, whether it be expressing oneself, reading aloud, or repeating what is said to him. The patient usually is alert and gives the appearance of being mentally clear. He is able to comprehend all or most of what is said to him and what he reads, but cannot execute spoken language normally. He usually cannot write without making errors in the formation of letters or spelling of words that were normally at his command. He may be able to identify objects by pantomime or circumlocution, but not call their names; parts of an object (e.g., heel, lace, sole) may be more difficult to name than the whole object (shoe). The

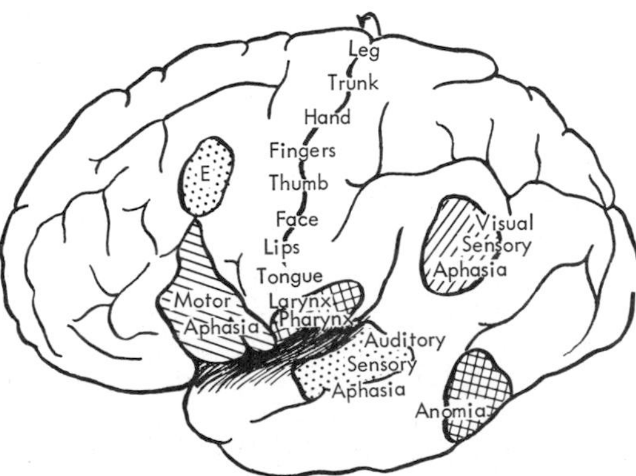

Figure 1–1 Convex surface of the left cerebral hemisphere showing the areas of major importance in disturbance of language. E, Exner's "writing center," injury to which causes dysgraphia. Both the auditory and visual areas of sensory aphasia must be involved to produce the total picture of sensory (Wernicke's) aphasia. Anomia depends on involvement of the inferior temporal area when it accompanies sensory aphasia.

mild expressive dysphasic may be able to use words or short phrases appropriately, but fail in attempts at more sustained expression. The severely aphasic may be unable to utter a word or may be reduced to emotional speech or to simple "yes" or "no" responses inappropriately used. The patient is aware of his language deficit and manifests exasperation at his inadequacy. The lesion causing this type of aphasia is almost always located in or upon the convex surface of the dominant (usually left) frontal lobe just anterior to the inferior extent of the fissure of Rolando, occasionally to the subjacent insular cortex and external capsule (Fig. 1–1). It is often accompanied by right hemiplegia (left hemiplegia in left-handed persons).

2. *Receptive (sensory or Wernicke's) aphasia* is more variable in the details of language deficit present, but most often consists of: inability to comprehend spoken language (auditory verbal agnosia), inability to comprehend written language (visual verbal agnosia), and inability to write (agraphia).

The patient is able to speak and often talks profusely, but after the first sentence or two, what he says becomes progressively unrelated to what has been said to him. Being unable to comprehend the meaning of his own words, he tends to talk in disjointed sentences and phrases (with good pronunciation and articulation) similar to those typical of the looseness of association of ideas in schizophrenia. Unlike the motor aphasic, the sensory aphasic is unaware of his language dysfunction; therefore he becomes annoyed at those speaking to him rather than at himself. The irrelevant voluble speech and annoyed behavior of the sensory aphasic may give the impression that he is mentally disturbed or hostile. For this reason, it is important to avoid mistaking his aphasic condition for the erratic behavior of the manic or the schizophrenic. *This type of aphasia results from a focal lesion involving the posterior superior portion of the convex surface of the dominant temporal lobe, called Wernicke's area* (see Fig. 1–1).

Aphasia must be differentiated from more diffuse disorder of mental function. Deterioration of language not infrequently occurs as a part of the total picture in dementia, in which case it is of dubious localizing value. Aphasia must also be differentiated from other disorders of speech mediated at a lower level: (1) dysarthria is impairment of the articulation of words resulting from motor impairment of the muscles of the lips, tongue, and pharynx involved in speaking; (2) dysphonia is loss of voice or hoarseness due to motor impairment of laryngeal muscles; (3) mutism is a nonspecific loss of speech or refusal to speak that is usually a hysterical manifestation or part of the deaf-mute state. Akinetic mutism is the clinical state in which there is loss of power or ability to speak along with generalized severe loss of motor power.

The Frontal Lobe

The most conspicuous clinical manifestations of frontal lobe lesions are motor ones (Fig. 1–2). Contralateral "upper motor neuron paralysis" results from involvement of the motor and premotor frontal areas or the axons projecting from these areas to form the corticobulbar-corticospinal tract. When the premotor area is involved, the sucking and grasp reflexes and groping response are present contralaterally. A premotor lesion that involves the projection pathways to and from the cerebellum may produce ataxia and tremor of the contralateral limbs ("frontal lobe ataxia") simulating the lateral cerebellar syndrome. Extrapyramidal signs and, when bilateral, inability to stand or walk (astasia-abasia) may be produced. These premotor signs are more prominent in widespread bilateral involvement or with a midline interhemispheric lesion than with unilateral involvement. Interference with turning of the eyes to the contralateral side (paralysis of conjugate gaze) results from involvement of a restricted cortical region immediately anterior to the premotor cortex. Motor (expressive) aphasia resulting from involvement of the posterior inferior area on the convex surface of the frontal cortex of the dominant hemisphere is described in the previous section.

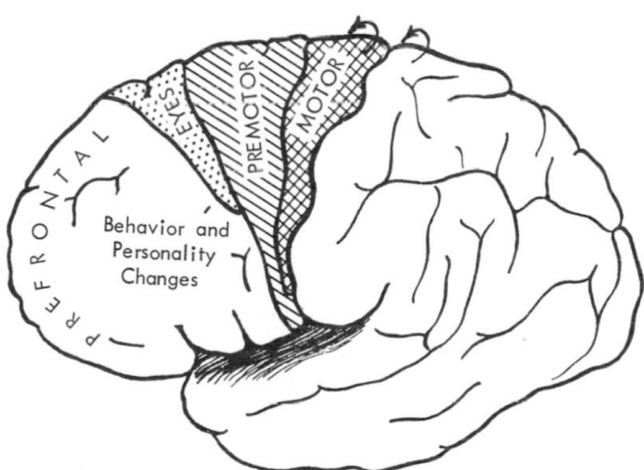

Figure 1–2 Lateral surface of the left cerebral hemisphere showing the areas of the frontal lobe related to the clinical signs described in the text. *Eyes,* the frontal motor eye field, associated with conjugate deviation of the eyes. The arrows at the top indicate extension of the precentral and postcentral gyri onto the medial cortical surface, forming the *paracentral lobule* illustrated in Figure 1–3.

THE FRONTAL LOBE SYNDROME. Anterior to these areas related to motor functions lies the prefrontal area, an extensive area of the frontal lobe in the human brain that distinguishes it grossly from the brain of lower animals (see Fig. 1–2). Disturbance of this portion of the frontal lobes results in an array of changes in mentation and personality that have been designated collectively as the frontal lobe syndrome. Historically, this syndrome is identified with the case of Phineas Gage reported by Harlow in 1848.[4] Gage, a 25-year-old railroad worker, survived for 13 years following extensive injury to both frontal lobes from a dynamite explosion that drove an iron tamping rod through his skull. Prior to the injury he had been a reverent, industrious, steady provider. Upon recovery, and thereafter for the rest of his life, he remained an irreverent, profane, impulsive vagrant.

In more recent years, study of patients following frontal lobe excision for tumors and patients subjected to prefrontal leukotomy in the treatment of mental illness has served to define the syndrome more precisely. The changes are most pronounced with bilateral prefrontal involvement; but they occur to a lesser extent with unilateral involvement, especially if it is in the dominant hemisphere. The syndrome consists in essence of loss of those traits of behavior, emotional restraint, and intelligence that characterize man's higher cultural development and is marked by (1) lack of emotional restraint, which may take the form of restless impulsiveness, inappropriate joking, childish excitement, outbursts of temper, facetiousness, social indiscretions, or loss of sexual inhibitions; (2) impairment of certain intellectual functions: distractibility and inability to concentrate, loss of initiative, mental torpor, impairment of recent memory (usually mild), difficulty adapting to new tasks, and impairment of abstract reasoning; and (3) dulling of certain neurotic traits such as worry, rigidity, compulsiveness, and anxiety. Concern over persistent pain is also reduced.

Since cultural development varies widely among normal people, one must take into account the individual's previous personality, educational accomplishments, and behavior patterns in diagnosing the frontal lobe syndrome. In equivocal cases, search for accompanying premotor changes such as the primitive snout or grasp reflexes will often help in the diagnosis. These will only be found if the causative lesion extends sufficiently far back in the frontal lobe to involve those areas concerned with motor functions. The intellectual changes found in the frontal lobe syndrome are the same as some of those constituting the syndrome of dementia, but the latter encompasses additional features not found in disease limited to the frontal lobes.

The Temporal Lobe

From the standpoint of clinical diagnosis, the temporal lobes, with the exception of Wernicke's area in the dominant hemisphere, have been regarded traditionally as "silent areas" because lesions involving these areas often must reach sufficient proportion to produce increased intracranial pressure or encroachment on adjacent structures before becoming manifest clinically.

Lesions involving the deep white matter of the temporal lobe, however, will encroach on the lower fibers of the optic radiation (Meyer's loop), resulting in a contralateral homonymous upper-quadrant anopsia—the so-called "pie in the sky" visual field defect. *This important finding may be the only clinical evidence of a temporal lobe lesion* and is one of which the patient is usually unaware (see Chapter 17).

The cortical projection areas for hearing and labyrinthine function are located on the superior surface of the temporal lobe. Although dizziness, tinnitus, and transient impairment of ability to localize sound have been reported in some instances of temporal lobe lesions, there usually is no defect in these functions because they are bilaterally represented at cortical level and, therefore, remain intact unless there is bilateral involvement.

PSYCHOMOTOR EPILEPSY. This is also called "partial complex epilepsy" and "temporal lobe epilepsy." "Psychomotor epilepsy" is a clinically descriptive term introduced by Gibbs and Lennox in 1937 to denote seizures that were associated with a common electroencephalographic pattern but with a wide variety of individual clinical patterns. The clinical patterns include: dreamy states, sensory illusions or hallucinations (olfactory, visual, auditory), automatisms (complex and purposeful but inappropriate motor acts such as smacking of lips, or disrobing), emotional experiences, and amnesia for events during part or all of the attack.

Seizures of this type have been found frequently related to abnormal electroencephalographic changes localized to one or both temporal lobes and, less frequently, to focal lesions in the same location. Accordingly, in recent years it has become common practice to use the terms "psychomotor epilepsy" and "temporal lobe epilepsy" synonymously on the assumption that such seizures are indicative of temporal lobe lesions. While the correlation is sufficiently frequent to be clinically useful, exceptions are also frequent.[9] Repeated instances are reported in which the lesion causing psychomotor attacks is found remote from the temporal lobe, usually involving components of the limbic system other than those within the temporal lobe.

In summary, aside from the signs of increased intracranial pressure when the lesion is of sufficient size, the usual clinical manifestations of a lesion in the dominant temporal lobe are: sensory (receptive) aphasia; contralateral "pie in the sky" homonymous visual field defect; or certain patterns of psychomotor epileptic seizures. In the nondominant temporal lobe, the only likely localizing manifestations are the contralateral visual field defect or psychomotor type of seizures.

The Limbic System

Although functionally separable to a great extent, the limbic system and the temporal lobe should be considered together because they overlap anatomically. The limbic lobe consists of cortex and subcortical structures that form a rim (limbus = bor-

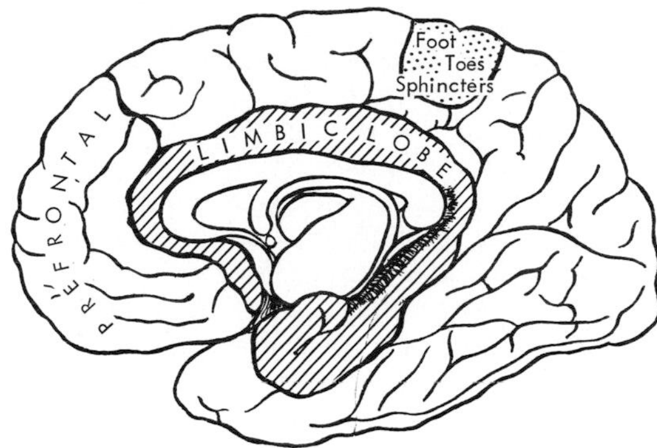

Figure 1–3 Medial surface of the cerebral hemisphere showing the cortical areas constituting the *limbic lobe*. The remainder of the limbic system lies subcortical to the area outlined. Also shown is the *paracentral lobule* (*dotted*), the extension of the precentral and postcentral gyri onto the medial surface of the hemisphere.

der) surrounding the opening of the lateral ventricle on the medial surface of each cerebral hemisphere (Fig. 1–3). On the surface it includes the septal region and part of the orbital cortex on the inferomedial surface of the frontal lobe, the cingulate gyrus, isthmus, hippocampal gyrus, uncus, and primary olfactory cortex. Its subjacent structures include the cingulum and septal nuclei, the hippocampal formation lying deep to the hippocampal gyrus, and the amygdala. These structures are richly interconnected with one another and with the mamillary bodies, the olfactory tract, the diencephalon, and the upper reticular formation of the midbrain to form the limbic system. This system constitutes the anatomical and physiological substrate for those cerebral functions having to do with visceral activity, with emotions, and with memory.

Since the limbic lobe anatomically includes almost the entire inferomedial aspect of the temporal lobe, the question of which lobe to assign a given clinical manifestation topographically would seem optional. However, the divergence of function and of structural connections of the two probably accounts largely for discrepancies not infrequently encountered in anatomical localization of lesions manifested by visceral, emotional, or memory changes. As already suggested, psychomotor seizures in many instances signify disturbance in the limbic system rather than in the temporal lobe proper.

THE KLÜVER-BUCY SYNDROME. In 1937, Klüver and Bucy reported a striking syndrome in the monkey following bilateral removal of the limbic components of the temporal lobes. It consisted of visual agnosia, compulsive oral exploration of objects, excessive attention to and reaction to visual stimuli (hypermetamorphosis), change from aggressiveness to emotional passivity, loss of fear, increased sexual activity, and bulimia. Essentially the same syndrome has been reproduced in man, as reported by Terzian and Ore.[12]

The essential features of the syndrome in man are emotional changes (poverty of feeling and docile behavior), profound loss of memory and recognition, indiscriminate hypersexuality (self-abuse, exhibitionism, heterosexual or homosexual behavior), excessive eating (bulimia), and excessive attentiveness to visual stimuli (hypermetamorphosis). It is a profoundly disabling syndrome that renders the person permanently ineffectual socially. The accumulated evidence to date indicates that its cause is the destruction, bilaterally, of the components of the limbic system located in the inferomedial part of the temporal lobes (hippocampus, uncus, and amygdaloid nucleus). The syndrome or components of it are most likely to be encountered clinically following severe head injury, or conceivably with a midline lesion in or near the third ventricle or interpeduncular space of sufficient size to encroach upon the medial aspect of both temporal lobes. It may also be caused inadvertently by a unilateral temporal lobectomy that includes the limbic structures if the patient has pre-existing unrecognized damage to the limbic lobe on the opposite side.

Current knowledge permits only limited and fragmentary correlation of clinical signs and symptoms with the highly complex limbic system otherwise. One should suspect disease involving it when disturbance of visceral functions, emotions, or memory is encountered as a part of any cerebral syndrome. Malamud has summarized the manifestations of tumors involving the system.[8]

The Parietal Lobe

The cortex of the parietal lobes, in addition to being the end-station for sensory impulses from the homolateral thalamus, is essential to the individual's orientation and awareness of the parts of his own body, his orientation in space, and his awareness of the spatial relationship of objects in his immediate environment. Lesions that irritate the parietal cortex are manifested clinically by focal sensory epileptic seizures. These may consist of primitive sensations such as tingling, or of more elaborate sensory experiences such as a feeling that a limb is disproportionate to the rest of the body in size, shape, or position. Such sensory phenomena may constitute the entire seizure or may be the aura for a generalized seizure.

THE PARIETAL LOBE SYNDROME. Destructive lesions limited to parietal cortex cause selective impairment of sensory discrimination rather than the primitive cutaneous sensations of pain, temperature, and touch. These discriminatory sensations, collectively referred to as cortical sensation, include: sense of position of body parts, ability to correctly localize a cutaneous stimulus without the aid of vision, ability to identify objects by feel (stereognosis), and two-point tactile discrimination. Along with deficit in these there may be the phenomenon of sensory extinction in which, when bilateral simultaneous cutaneous stimuli are presented, the patient fails to appreciate the stimulus applied to the affected side. In addition to cortical sensory deficit, there may be motor weakness in the same parts. The patient may have one or more of the following manifestations of body disorientation or neglect contralateral to the lesion: inability to recognize or locate a part (autotopagnosia), unawareness or denial of the motor or sensory defect in the involved part (anosognosia), or neglect of the involved side of the body in dressing and grooming himself. He may also manifest disorientation in external space by neglect of that part of the environment contralateral to his lesion. When asked to describe the details of a composite diagram shown him or draw a symmetrical diagram such as a clock face, he is likely to neglect that side of the picture or drawing contralateral to his lesion while attending adequately to the half homolateral to the lesion. When the lesion extends to involve the white matter deep to parietal cortex, there may be an associated contralateral homonymous visual field defect due to encroachment on the optic radiations passing through this area en route to the calcarine cortex (see Chapter 17). In summary, the parietal lobe syndrome includes sensory deficit of cortical type contralateral to the lesion, contralateral hemiparesis (sometimes), neglect of body parts contralateral to the lesion, neglect of external space contralateral to the lesion, and, sometimes, contralateral homonymous visual field defect.

It is characteristic of this syndrome that its component manifestations tend to fluctuate from one examination to the next and from day to day; therefore, more than one examination of sensory functions is often necessary to demonstrate fully its manifestations in the individual patient. When the lesion is on the dominant side, all or a part of the Gerstmann syndrome may also be present. This and the accompaniment of sensory aphasia make demonstration of many of the parietal manifestations difficult or impossible in dominant hemisphere lesions.

GERSTMANN'S SYNDROME.[3] This is a symptom complex somewhat related to sensory aphasia in that it includes impairment in the use of mathematical symbols, the inability to calculate (acalculia). Impairment of ability to perform mathematical calculations is likely to be encountered as a relatively early manifestation of mental deterioration from any cause, and is thus of less value as a localizing sign than aphasia. It occurs in the absence of general deterioration of mental function, however, as a component of the Gerstmann syndrome, which consists also of finger-agnosia (inability to identify, name, or select the individual fingers of either of one's own hands or those of others), right-left disorientation, and agraphia. *This syndrome signifies a focal lesion localized to the junctional area of cortex between the parietal and occipital lobes of the dominant cerebral hemisphere.*

The syndrome varies in its components in individual cases and is rarely encountered in pure and complete form. It may be accompanied by components of parietal lobe syndrome, by components of sensory aphasia in addition to agraphia, by homonymous hemianopia and other occipital lobe manifestations. In the presence of severe aphasia it is often impossible to demonstrate because of inability to communicate with the patient. Because of the rarity of the syndrome and its variability from case to case, some have questioned its validity and usefulness in clinical diagnosis.[2]

Other Syndromes of the Intracranial Cavity

There are several syndromes of importance in diagnosis of intracranial lesions that do not lend themselves to classification with the lobes of the cerebral hemispheres or with specific cerebral functions. They may indicate a lesion involving multiple cerebral areas or one located within a restricted area but manifesting itself by encroachment upon contiguous but functionally separate structures in the intracranial cavity. Some permit no more precise localization than to indicate that the causative lesion is somewhere within the cranial vault. Other syndromes are quite precise in pointing to the site of the lesion even though they signify involvement of multiple structures.

THE SYNDROME OF INCREASED INTRACRANIAL PRESSURE. Headache, mental torpor, vomiting, bilateral papilledema, and sometimes unilateral or bilateral sixth (abducens) cranial nerve palsy constitute a syndrome resulting from crowding of the structures within the bony confines of the cranial cavity. Of these, papilledema, with or without headache, is the most reliable and sometimes the only manifestation. The syndrome may result from a diffuse intracranial disorder such as meningitis or bilateral subdural hematomas or may be due to a focal intracranial lesion at or anywhere above the foramen magnum. Nevertheless, this syndrome is a very reliable indicator of disease within these confines, whether it occurs alone or in company with other neurological findings. For a comprehensive discussion of increased intracranial pressure see Chapter 24.

THE FOSTER KENNEDY SYNDROME. This syndrome, as originally defined, consisted of "true retrobulbar neuritis with the formation of a central scotoma and primary optic atrophy on the side of the lesion, together with concomitant papilledema in the opposite eye."[6] These findings, along with anosmia on the same side as the optic atrophy, were described in cases proved to have a mass lesion of the inferior part of the frontal lobe on that side. Optic atrophy with more variable involvement of the visual field in the eye homolateral to the lesion is more likely than central scotoma alone. Subsequent experience has related this syndrome to tumors of the sphenoidal ridge or olfactory groove in the floor of the anterior cranial fossa as well as lesions within the frontal lobe. Homolateral exophthalmos may accompany the ocular findings of the syndrome when the causative lesion encroaches on the bony orbit. Anosmia may be absent when the lesion is more laterally placed, or it may be present bilaterally if the lesion extends across the midline of the floor of the anterior fossa. Lesions other than tumor or abscess may cause the syndrome, including vascular abnormalities and local arachnoiditis. It is a rare syndrome, occurring in only a small percentage (1.5 per cent in one reported survey) of cases of mass lesion in the anterior cranial fossa.[13] Nevertheless, when encountered, it is of value in defining the locus of disease in an otherwise often "silent area" of brain.

PARASAGITTAL LESIONS. Lesions situated in the interhemispheric fissure may be manifest clinically by signs implicating the paracentral lobule unilaterally or bilaterally (Figs. 1–3 and 1–4). These signs include (1) paresis in the lower extremities (paraplegia), usually beginning in one foot and progressively spreading in that limb and then to the opposite member, (2) focal motor or sensory seizures beginning in the foot, (3) incontinence of urine or feces, and (4) mental changes of the frontal lobe syndrome.

The tendon reflexes may be normal, hypoactive, or hyperactive, and the Babinski sign may or may not be present early in the course. In the early stages, weakness limited to the distal parts of one lower extremity may simulate peroneal nerve palsy. Babinski's sign or hyperactive ankle jerk, if present, will permit easy differentiation. When both lower extremities are involved, and especially when this is accompanied by sphincter incontinence, the syndrome may simulate spinal cord disease. The paraplegia with parasagittal lesions is, however, almost always asymmetrical and almost never as pronounced, even in advanced stages, as with cord lesions. Furthermore, accompanying focal seizures and mental changes, when present, will define the correct regional level of the causative lesion. The most common parasagittal lesion causing this syndrome is meningioma arising on one side of the falx cerebri and producing its earliest signs in the contralateral lower extremity. Thrombosis of the superior sag-

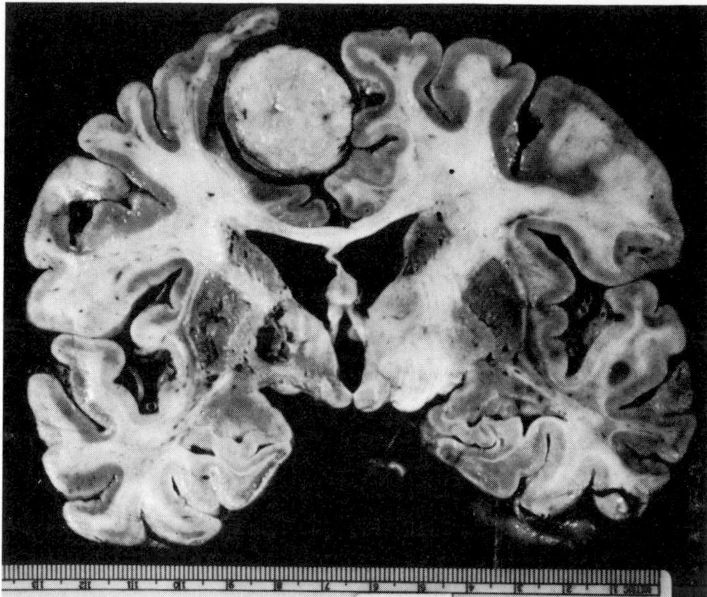

Figure 1–4 Parasagittal meningioma compressing both cerebral hemispheres.

ittal sinus may cause a similar clinical pattern, but is of more abrupt onset with more rapid development of the total deficit.

PERISELLAR LESIONS. Lesions arising in or around the sella turcica manifest themselves by (1) endocrine dysfunctions, (2) visual loss due to involvement of the optic nerves and chiasm, (3) hypothalamic signs, and (4) increased intracranial pressure due to protrusion of the lesion into the floor of the third ventricle.

The most readily recognized endocrinopathy is diabetes insipidus resulting from involvement of the pituitary stalk and posterior hypothalamus. Other alterations of endocrine function are more subtle and depend upon the degree to which the pituitary is involved and the age of the patient. They may be those of either hypofunction or hyperfunction, depending upon the nature of the lesion, and they usually require ancillary laboratory studies for their diagnosis and identification. The neurosurgeon will be more likely to encounter patients with lesions of this region because of the neurological manifestations.

The earliest neurological abnormality usually is bitemporal visual field defect due to encroachment on the midportion of the optic chiasm. At this stage it is usually asymptomatic and will be found only by special attempt on the part of the examiner. Later, progression to more extensive encroachment on optic chiasm or optic nerves results in subjective impairment of vision. The patterns of visual loss from lesions in this location are discussed in Chapter 17.

The disturbances of hypothalamic function may include alterations of sleep pattern, eating habits (with resultant cachexia or adiposity), temperature regulation and other autonomic functions, and metabolism.

The signs and symptoms of increased intracranial pressure are likely to occur early in the clinical course of suprasellar lesions with headache and papilledema as the initial findings in some instances. Even in these instances, however, careful testing will often reveal the characteristic abnormality in the visual fields. Anosmia, unilateral or bilateral, may be found if the lesion extends forward along the base of the brain. "Uncinate fits," focal seizures initiated by hallucinations of smell or taste, may occur when the lesion encroaches on posterior orbital surface of the frontal lobe or medial temporal lobe cortex.

SYNDROMES OF THE INTRACRANIAL VENOUS SINUSES. The venous sinuses within the cranial cavity are channels formed between layers of the dura mater. The veins draining the brain and other structures in and around the cranial cavity empty into them; thus they constitute the main avenue for venous drainage from the contents of the cranial cavity. They may become occluded by thrombosis from cachexia or blood dyscrasias, trauma, or spread of nearby inflammatory or neoplastic disease. Those in which occlusion is most likely to produce a recognizable intracranial syndrome are the superior sagittal, the cavernous, and the lateral sinuses. Isolated occlusion of the smaller dural sinuses is rare and their manifestations are usually obscured by those implicating these three major sinuses.

Superior sagittal sinus. The superior sagittal sinus is situated in the midsagittal plane of the intracranial cavity along the superior border of the falx cerebri. It receives the veins that drain most of the convexity of both cerebral hemispheres. It also receives the cerebrospinal fluid through the arachnoidal villi located in recesses along its walls. Occlusion causes symptoms and signs of increased intracranial pressure, seizures (generalized or jacksonian), edema of forehead and scalp (especially in children), engorgement of scalp veins (especially in children), and spastic paralysis that is most marked in the lower extremities. When the clot begins in or extends into tributary veins over the cortical surface of the brain, various focal signs may appear, depending on the area of brain drained by the occluded veins. Thus there may result hemiplegia rather than paraplegia, parietal lobe signs, aphasia, homonymous hemianopia, and the like.

Cavernous sinuses. The cavernous sinuses are situated on each lateral wall of the sella turcica. The lateral wall of each sinus is formed by a layer of dura mater extending posteriorly from the superior orbital fissure to the anterior surface of the petrous bone. The two sinuses are connected by narrow channels across the anterior and posterior margins of the sella turcica. Each cavernous sinus receives venous drainage from the upper face as well as intracranially. Through each sinus pass: the internal carotid artery on its medial wall; and, from above downward, the third, fourth, and sixth cranial nerves, and the first (ophthalmic) and second (maxillary) divisions of the fifth cranial nerve on its lateral wall. The syndrome of the cavernous sinus varies in its details, depending on which of these structures are involved. The complete syndrome consists of homolateral proptosis, chemosis, and papilledema; dilated retinal veins and retinal hemorrhage; paralysis of the homolateral third, fourth, and sixth, and the ophthalmic division of the fifth cranial nerves; pain in the eye and upper face; and normal or slightly impaired vision homolaterally. Even with unilateral lesions the syndrome may be bilateral, owing to communication between the two sinuses. Infection spreading along draining veins from the face is a common cause, in which case the signs of general septicemia are often superimposed. Aneurysm of the intracavernous portion of the carotid artery or traumatic carotid-cavernous fistula may cause the syndrome in part, accompanied by bruit and visible pulsations of the homolateral eye. Tumor in or adjacent to the sinus may produce a part or all of the syndrome, usually more gradual in its development than with the other causes.

Lateral sinuses. The lateral sinuses pass laterally and forward on either side along the line of attachment of the tentorium cerebelli to the wall of the cranial vault from the torcular Herophili near the internal occipital protuberance to the internal jugular foramen on each side. Anteriorly the sinus assumes a tortuous course on the inner wall of the mastoid bone just before emptying into the internal jugular vein. This recurving mastoid portion is designated separately by some as the *sigmoid sinus.* The lateral sinuses are usually asymmetrical, one (usually the right) being a direct continuation of all the sinuses that converge at the torcular Herophili and thus the channel through which most venous drainage from the brain ultimately leaves the cranial vault. The most common cause of lateral sinus occlusion is spread of inflammation from otitis or mastoiditis. In addition to the local signs of ear infection and systemic signs of septicemia (chills, fever, and malaise), the most constant neurological manifestations are those of increased intracranial pressure. Focal brain signs are rare, but seizures of generalized or jacksonian type sometimes occur. There may be tenderness and swelling in the mastoid region, the superficial mastoid veins, and along the course of the internal jugular vein in the neck.

The syndromes of the individual cerebral arteries are not discussed here. They rarely are of concern in neurosurgical diagnosis, and their detailed description can be found in most textbooks of clinical neurology.

Manifestations of Posterior Cranial Fossa Lesions

The posterior cranial fossa contains the brain stem, through which traverse the sensory and motor "long tracts"; cranial nerves III through XII from their nuclear origins within the brain stem to their points of exit through their respective foramina in the base of the skull; the cerebellum and its peduncles; and the caudal termination of the ventricular system, including its communication with the subarachnoid space. The cardinal manifestations of lesions localized to this region result from involvement of these structures singly or in combinations. They are: "crossed paralysis"; multiple cranial nerve palsies alone (III through XII); cerebellar signs alone; or any combination of cranial nerve palsies (III through XII), cerebellar signs, and long tract signs.

"Crossed paralysis," also called alternating hemiplegia, is the term used to designate sensory or motor paralysis that involves one or more cranial nerves on one side (homolateral to the lesion) and the limbs on the opposite side. *This finding is pathognomonic of posterior fossa localization.* In crossed motor paralysis, the cranial nerve palsy will be of the lower motor neuron type, while the limb paralysis will be of the upper motor neuron type owing to involvement of the motor tracts coursing through the brain stem. In addition to crossed hemiplegia, paralysis of one or more cranial nerves also occurs in association with disturbances of other motor functions. The following syndromes will permit precise localization of the level of the lesion within the posterior fossa.

THIRD (OCULOMOTOR) NERVE PALSY ASSOCIATED WITH DISTURBANCE OF MOTOR TRACTS. The signs of third cranial nerve palsy are described in Chapter 17. Unilateral palsy of this nerve combined with crossed hemiplegia results from involvement of the basis pedunculi and third nerve on the ventral surface of the midbrain (Weber-Leyden syndrome). *This combination is, however, more often encountered as a complication of an expanding lesion of one cerebral hemisphere when the expansion causes the medial aspect of the temporal lobe to herniate through the tentorial notch and compress the third nerve.* Dilation of the pupil or ptosis of the eyelid homolateral to the herniation is the earliest, and sometimes only, sign of third nerve involvement in this critical situation in which only slight increase in the herniation may result in compression of the midbrain with serious threat to life.

Unilateral involvement of third nerve and red nucleus, when the lesion encroaches on the tegmentum of the midbrain, results in homolateral third nerve palsy and contralateral choreiform movements, tremor, and sometimes ataxia (Benedikt's syndrome). The lesion may also involve the sensory tracts in the midbrain tegmentum, adding contralateral hemianesthesia to the findings.

Unilateral involvement of third nerve and superior cerebellar peduncle by a dorsal tegmental lesion of midbrain results in the combination of third nerve palsy and cerebellar ataxia, both homolateral to the lesion (Nothnagel's syndrome).

Unilateral involvement of the third, fourth, and sixth cranial nerves and the ophthalmic division of the fifth nerve (syndrome of Foix) by a lesion in or near the cavernous sinus has already been described.

SIXTH (ABDUCENS) AND SEVENTH (FACIAL) NERVE PALSY ASSOCIATED WITH DISTURBANCE OF MOTOR TRACTS. Unilateral involvement of these two cranial nerves and the corticospinal tract in one side of the pons causes the combination of paralysis of abduction of the eye and facial paralysis homolateral to the lesion and contralateral hemiplegia (Millard-Gubler syndrome). Sometimes the facial nerve is spared, resulting in paralysis of abduction of the eye and hemiplegia alone (Raymond-Cestan syndrome). A lesion in the vicinity of the sixth nerve may extend far enough laterally to involve the para-abducens area, resulting in paralysis of conjugate gaze toward the side of the lesion in addition to the other signs (Foville's syndrome). In such a case, not only will the eye on the side of the lesion be medially rotated and unable to abduct, but the opposite eye also will not rotate medially on attempting gaze to the side of the lesion. It will rotate medially on convergence.

It is well to remember that unilateral or

bilateral sixth nerve palsy may occur as a part of the syndrome of increased intracranial pressure; therefore when papilledema accompanies sixth nerve palsy it does not necessarily signify a brain stem or posterior fossa lesion.

Paralysis of the facial nerve alone (Bell's palsy) may be due to a lesion within the posterior fossa or along the course of the nerve through the facial canal within the petrous bone. If the lesion is within the posterior fossa it is likely to involve also the acoustic (tinnitus and hearing loss) and vestibular (vertigo and nystagmus) functions of the eighth cranial nerve and some dysfunction of the fifth (trigeminal) cranial nerve (e.g., unilateral loss of the corneal reflex or hemifacial numbness along with facial paralysis). This combination is characteristic of tumors in the cerebellopontine angle. Homolateral cerebellar ataxia and horizontal nystagmus usually accompany the cranial nerve involvements in this situation. As the lesion enlarges to encroach further on posterior fossa structures there will be involvement of additional cranial nerves and long tracts and ultimately increased intracranial pressure.

Occasionally an inflammatory or neoplastic process involving the facial nerve or its nucleus will irritate rather than paralyze it, resulting in unilateral facial spasms or contraction. This finding, when combined with contralateral hemiplegia (Brissaud's syndrome), signifies a lesion of the posterior fossa homolateral to the facial involvement.

The syndrome of the lateral medulla oblongata (Wallenberg's syndrome) results from involvement of the nucleus ambiguus of the tenth (vagus) cranial nerve, descending root and tract of the trigeminal nerve, vestibular nuclei, inferior cerebellar peduncle and cerebellar hemisphere, and spinothalamic tract. The resulting signs are: homolateral palatal paralysis causing dysphagia and dysarthria, loss of pain and thermal sensation on the face, and cerebellar signs; and contralateral loss of pain and thermal sensation of trunk and limbs. Horizontal nystagmus and homolateral Horner's syndrome (due to involvement of the descending sympathetic fibers coursing through the tegmentum of the brain stem) are also found with the complete syndrome.

The syndrome of the lateral pontine tegmentum is similar to the lateral medulla oblongata syndrome except that the main sensory nucleus of the trigeminal nerve and the nuclei of the seventh and eighth nerves are involved, while the descending trigeminal root and tract and nucleus ambiguus are spared. The resulting signs are: deafness, facial paralysis, loss of facial tactile sensation, Horner's syndrome, and cerebellar signs, all homolateral to the lesion, and contralateral hemianesthesia to pain and temperature, which may involve the face as well as the trunk and limbs. Horizontal nystagmus occurs also.

Also closely resembling the syndrome of the lateral medulla is that in which the lesion extends more medially and ventrally to involve the medial lemniscus, the nucleus of the twelfth (hypoglossal) cranial nerve, and the pyramid. In addition to, or instead of, loss of pain and temperature sensation, there will be loss of proprioceptive and tactile sensation and hemiplegia contralateral to the lesion. Homolateral atrophy and paralysis of the tongue and sometimes of the upper part of the trapezius muscle (eleventh nerve) will also occur (syndromes of Cestan-Chenais and of Babinski-Nageotte). These various syndromes of the caudal part of the posterior fossa, including those described later implicating the bulbar (lower) cranial nerves, vary from case to case and by eponymic designation owing to slight variations in the extent of the lesion in this compact and neurologically critical region.

SYNDROMES OF THE LOWER (BULBAR) CRANIAL NERVES. The ninth (glossopharyngeal), tenth (vagus), and eleventh (spinal) accessory) cranial nerves exit from the cranial cavity through the jugular foramen. The twelfth (hypoglossal) nerve exits through the immediately adjacent hypoglossal foramen situated at the lip of the foramen magnum. As would be expected, therefore, a lesion in this vicinity of the posterior fossa or retropharyngeal space will produce varying combinations of involvement of these nerves. In the syndrome of the jugular foramen (Vernet's syndrome), there is paralysis of the ninth, tenth, and eleventh cranial nerves. These, along with paralysis of the twelfth nerve (syndrome of Villaret), occur with a retropharyngeal lesion invading the posterior fossa. In some instances, involvement of two or more of these nerves in other combinations is encountered (Jackson's vagoaccessory hypoglossal paralysis, Schmidt's vagoaccessory syndrome, Tapia's vagohypoglossal palsy).

Cerebellar Signs

Although not solely a motor structure, the cerebellum is important in diagnosis for its effect on motor function. It is discussed here because the clinical manifestations of its dysfunction usually indicate disease in the posterior fossa. There are two fairly distinct syndromes of cerebellar dysfunction, differing in the major connections of its component parts that are affected.

1. The flocculonodular or midline syndrome occurs when the lesion affects chiefly the flocculus, the nodulus, and the posterior vermis. These structures receive their afferent stimuli primarily from the vestibular apparatus in the brain stem. The primary clinical sign is disturbance of equilibrium manifested mostly in the axial musculature of the trunk and lower extremities (truncal ataxia). The patient stands or walks with feet apart, thus broadening his base to compensate for the loss of equilibrium. He reels or staggers on attempting to walk. When he sits without support to his body, he often assumes the "tripod" position of propping on his hands to prevent wavering of his trunk and head (titubation). Use of the individual limbs is affected little if any in performing volitional movements, and there is no lateralization. Speech is dysarthric. Horizontal nystagmus is often present. The entire syndrome resembles vestibular disturbance in many respects.

2. The cerebellar hemisphere (lateral cerebellar) syndrome occurs when there is a laterally placed lesion affecting one cerebellar hemisphere. It is characterized predominantly by disturbance of coordination of the limbs homolateral to the lesion in executing volitional movements and consists of (1) decomposition of volitional movements, (2) tremor during performance of movements (intention tremor), (3) hypotonia of the involved limbs, and (4) instability of the limb on attempting to maintain a posture against gravity.

Decomposition of movement consists of loss of proper integration of contraction of agonist and synergist muscles with relaxation of antagonists. As a result, a movement such as touching the nose with the fingertip is broken down ("decomposed") into the various components of movement at the individual joints rather than occurring as a smoothly integrated whole movement. Furthermore, each individual component may be ill-timed or ill-measured so as to cause overshooting or undershooting of its goal.

Hypotonia is a kind of mild flaccidity of the limb so that it is hyperextendible or hyperflexible to passive movement at the joints.

The characteristic *cerebellar tremor* is that which occurs only when the limb is brought into action to perform a movement. It often has a tendency to increase in a crescendo manner as the target is approached, therefore is sometimes referred to as terminal tremor. A postural tremor is sometimes present in addition when an attempt is made to maintain an antigravity posture with the limb.

It is well to remember that, owing to the major efferent connections from each cerebellar hemisphere via the superior cerebellar peduncle to the premotor cortex of the opposite cerebral hemisphere, the lateral cerebellar syndrome may be closely simulated by a lesion in the frontal lobe (frontal lobe ataxia). The signs are homolateral to lesions of cerebellar hemisphere or superior cerebellar peduncle but contralateral to lesions in the frontal lobe. Furthermore, in the latter there are likely to be other manifestations of frontal lobe disturbance associated with the cerebellar signs.

The reflex postural changes that characterize posterior fossa lesions involving the brain stem are almost always associated with impaired consciousness, as discussed in Chapter 3. Increased intracranial pressure may accompany any of the foregoing manifestations of posterior fossa disease when the lesion encroaches upon the aqueduct of Sylvius or fourth ventricle or interferes with egress of cerebrospinal fluid via the foramina of Luschka and Magendie.

Manifestations of Lesions of the Spinal Canal

Precise localization of lesions within the spinal canal depends upon knowledge of the details of cross-sectional and longitudinal anatomy of the spinal cord, the spinal roots and nerves within the canal, and the meninges. This is found in any of the textbooks of neuroanatomy. The primary purposes here are to define those syndromes that are of help to the examiner in localizing disease within the spinal canal and to point out some limitations of the clinical method of examination alone in regional diagnosis at this level of the nervous system. Only those anatomical features of special usefulness in clinical diagnosis are reviewed.

The spinal cord extends from the foramen magnum of the skull, where it is continuous with the medulla oblongata, to the interspace between the first and second lumbar vertebrae, where it ends. Lesions of the spinal canal caudal to the first lumbar vertebra, therefore, will produce only signs of involvement of the spinal roots constituting the cauda equina and not signs of spinal cord involvement. (The cauda equina syndrome is discussed later.)

There are usually 31 pairs of spinal nerves (8 cervical, 12 thoracic, 5 lumbar, 5 sacral, and 1 coccygeal), each formed by a dorsal root entering and a ventral root leaving the spinal cord at as many segments. The first cervical (C1) pair of spinal nerves leaves the spinal canal above the first cervical vertebra (atlas); the others leave through the intervertebral foramina between the vertebrae. There being eight pairs of cervical nerves and only seven cervical vertebrae, the nerves C2 through C7 leave via the foramina above their corresponding vertebrae, and the C8 nerves leave via the foramina below the C7 vertebra. From the first thoracic (T1) pair down, the remaining spinal nerves leave the canal through the foramina immediately below their corresponding vertebrae. Owing to the discrepancy between the length of the spinal cord and that of the spinal canal, the segments of the spinal cord (each represented by a pair of spinal nerves) do not coincide in horizontal plane with their corresponding vertebrae (Fig. 1–5). Therefore care must be taken in describing the location of a lesion in the spinal canal to specify whether one is designating the spinal cord segment or the vertebral level of the lesion.

Each segment of the spinal cord has its topographical zone of representation on the skin (dermatome) from which it receives the cutaneous sensations of pain, temperature, and touch. Figures 1–6 to 1–8 show the two dermatomal maps most widely accepted. Because of overlap of nerve supply

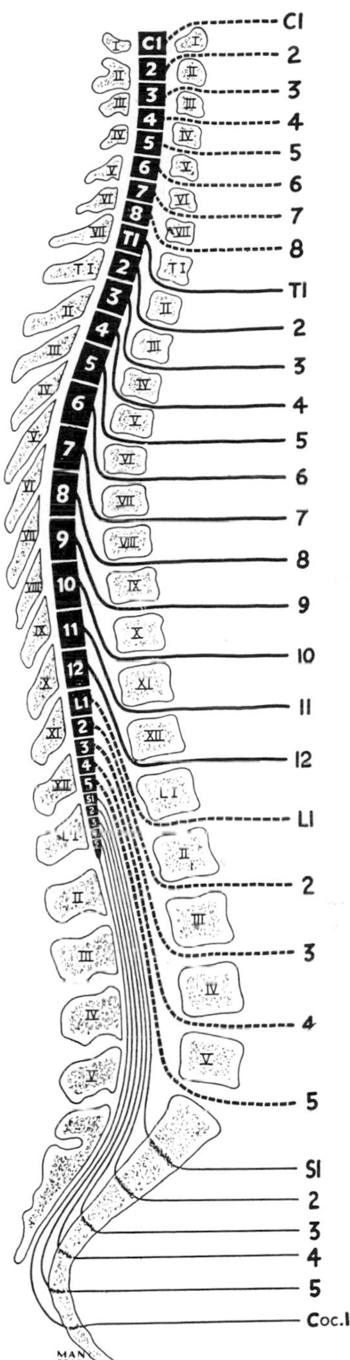

Figure 1–5 Illustration of the relationship of the spinal cord and spinal nerve segments to the vertebrae. The bodies and spinous processes of the vertebrae are indicated by Roman numerals and the spinal segments and nerves by Arabic numbers. (From Haymaker, W., and Woodhall, B.: Peripheral Nerve Injuries. 2nd Ed. Philadelphia, W. B. Saunders Co., 1953, p. 32. Reprinted by permission.)

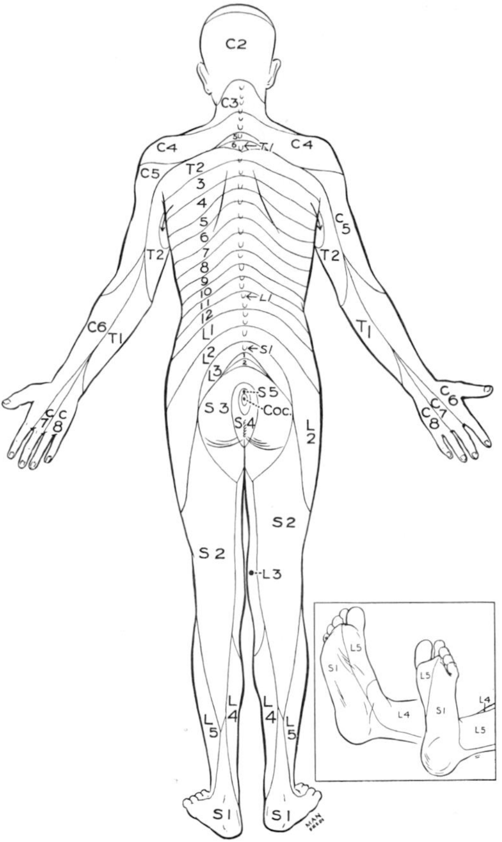

Figure 1-6 Posterior view of the dermatome patterns. (From Haymaker, W., and Woodhall, B.: Peripheral Nerve Injuries. 2nd Ed. Philadelphia, W. B. Saunders Co., 1953, p. 26—after Foerster, 1933. Reprinted by permission.)

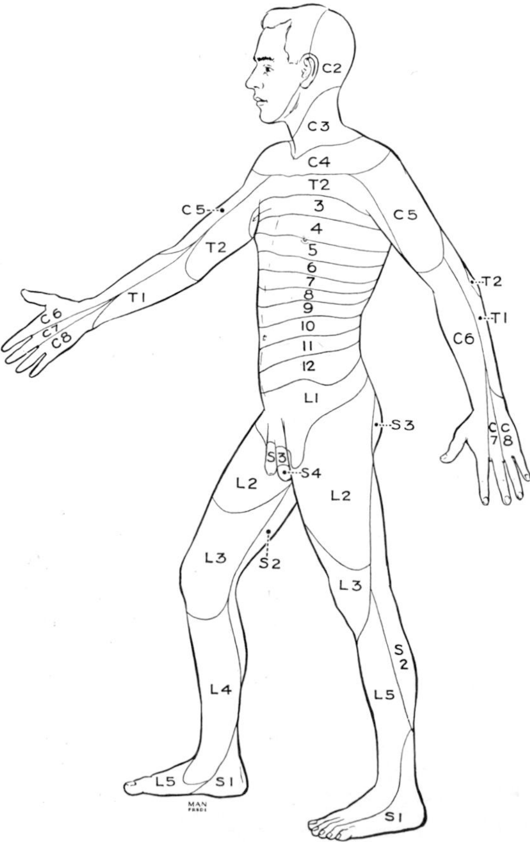

Figure 1-7 Lateral view of dermatome patterns. (From Haymaker, W., and Woodhall, B.: Peripheral Nerve Injuries. 2nd Ed. Philadelphia, W. B. Saunders Co., 1953, p. 27—after Foerster, 1933. Reprinted by permission.)

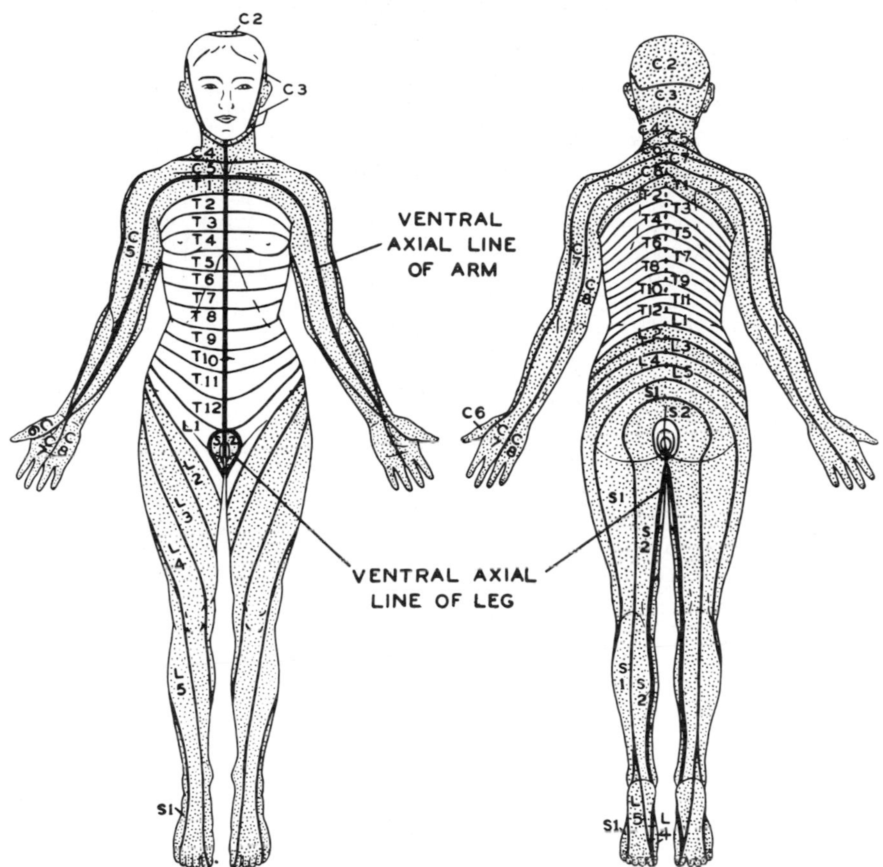

Figure 1–8 Anterior and posterior views of the dermatome patterns. (From Keegan, J. J., and Garett, F. D.: Anat. Rec., *102*:411, 1948. Reprinted by permission.)

between adjacent dermatomes, no demonstrable sensory deficit can be found unless two or more adjacent posterior roots or spinal nerves are interrupted; however, irritation of a single root or nerve will cause pain or paresthesias in that dermatome.

Within the spinal cord the structural and functional components of greatest diagnostic usefulness are: (1) the descending motor tracts in the posterior part of each lateral white column, chiefly the lateral corticospinal tract, (2) the ascending fasciculus gracilis and fasciculus cuneatus in each posterior white column, conveying proprioceptive (position and vibratory) sensation to higher centers, (3) the ascending lateral spinothalamic tract in the anterior part of each lateral white column, conveying cutaneous pain and temperature sensation to higher centers, (4) the autonomic suprasegmental descending fibers in each lateral white column and autonomic cell groups of the intermediate gray column in the thoracic segments, which give rise to preganglionic sympathetic fibers, and (5) the cervical and lumbar enlargements of the spinal cord in which the innervation and reflex arcs of the upper and lower extremities respectively are concentrated.

The Long Tracts

In addition to the corticospinal (pyramidal) fiber tract, which arises from axons in the cerebral cortex, the lateral white columns carry other descending crossed axons arising at subcortical and brain stem levels and collectively referred to as extrapyramidal pathways. All these descending pyramidal and extrapyramidal axons exert influence on the lower motor neurons of the anterior gray columns. Interruption of the lateral corticospinal tract produces the syndrome of "upper motor neuron" paralysis

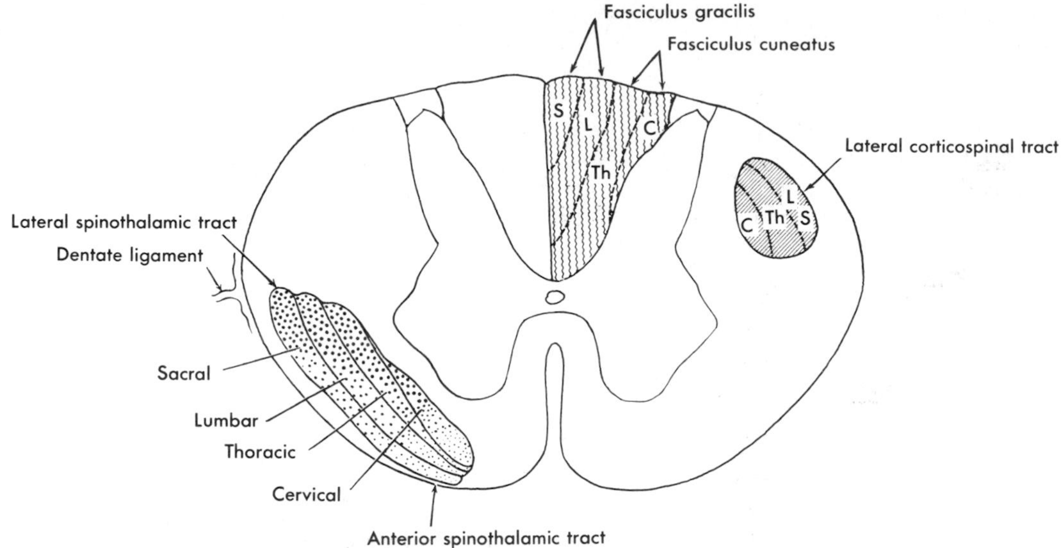

Figure 1–9 Laminar arrangement of the axons from successive spinal cord segments in the lateral spinothalamic tract (*left*). Laminar separation of the fibers mediating temperature (*large dots*), pain (*medium dots*), and light touch (*small dots*) within the tract is also illustrated. Similar laminations for the ascending proprioceptive (posterior column) and descending lateral corticospinal tract are shown on the right. (From Haymaker, W.: Bing's Local Diagnosis in Neurological Diseases. 15th Ed. St. Louis, C. V. Mosby Co., 1969, p. 8. Reprinted by permission.)

below the level of the lesion. Involvement of the extrapyramidal axons, which travel nearby, is usual, producing varying degrees of rigidity in addition to the upper motor neuron signs.

Both the lateral corticospinal tract (descending) and the fasciculi gracilis and cuneatus (ascending) undergo decussation approximately at the level of the foramen magnum of the skull in the caudal end of the medulla oblongata; therefore lesions within the spinal canal that unilaterally impair the functions mediated by these tracts will produce signs homolaterally, whereas those above the foramen magnum produce the same signs contralaterally. The lateral spinothalamic tract, on the other hand, arises as a crossed tract within the spinal cord; therefore a lesion involving it on one side either within the spinal canal or above the foramen magnum will produce deficit of pain and temperature sensation contralaterally below the level of the lesion.

The fibers of the lateral spinothalamic tract conveying impulses from the sacral segments run most laterally (i.e., peripherally) in the tract, and those joining it at successively higher levels are added on medially. Thus, it is laminated in terms of topographical cutaneous representation with the sacral dermatomes represented nearest the periphery of the spinal cord, the cervical dermatomes represented nearest the center, and the lumbar and thoracic in between (Fig. 1–9). A lesion located laterally in the spinal canal anywhere above the level of entry of the sacral segments to the tract (approximately the first lumbar vertebra) may encroach upon the spinal cord in such a way as to interfere with pain and temperature sensation of the sacral region only. For this reason in the early stages of a progressing lesion, a "sensory level" on the trunk is not reliable in indicating the level of the lesion, although it is a reliable indication that the lesion is in the spinal canal. An intramedullary spinal cord lesion, on the other hand, may encroach on only the most medial fibers of the tract to produce loss of pain and temperature sensation limited to a few segments with sparing of these sensations both above and below. This finding, referred to as a suspended sensory level or segmental sensory loss, constitutes a helpful diagnostic sign indicating that the causative lesion is most likely within the parenchyma of the spinal cord. Similar laminar arrangements of fibers in the other tracts and in the cell groups within the gray matter of the cord also exist, but they are less useful diagnostically.

Disturbance of Autonomic Function

The entirety of the paravertebral sympathetic chains receive their preganglionic nerve supply from cells in the intermediate gray columns from the T1 through L2 segments of the spinal cord whose axons leave the canal via the spinal nerves corresponding to these cord segments. These preganglionic neurons are under the control of the higher centers (cerebral cortex, hypothalamus, and brain stem reticular formation) via axons passing through the brain stem and into the spinal cord in the lateral white columns on the same side, where they form a diffuse pathway extending down to the upper lumbar cord segments. Lesions at the cervical and upper thoracic levels of the canal are likely to affect these structures, producing alterations of vasomotor activity, sweating, and respiration. Orthostatic hypotension resulting from interruption of the descending central axons controlling vasopressor and cardiac reflexes may occur with lesions above the T7 segment. Respiratory disturbances may occur with lesions at the upper cervical levels because of disturbance of innervation of intercostal and bronchial muscles as well as phrenic nerve paralysis. Alterations of sweating may occur with lesions that involve either the descending central axons or the preganglionic cell column down to the L2 cord segment. Horner's syndrome may occur homolateral to a lesion at or above the T1 segment.

Disturbance of the urethral and rectal sphincters, when of neurogenic origin, is usually indicative of a lesion in the spinal canal. The urethral sphincter receives its motor supply from neurons in the S2, S3, and S4 segments of the spinal cord. These neurons are under suprasegmental control of axons from the paracentral lobule of the frontal lobe, descending in the lateral white columns in close proximity to the lateral corticospinal tract. Different patterns of urinary dysfunction may occur, depending on the level at which the lesion occurs. *The uninhibited neurogenic bladder,* characterized by urinary frequency and urgency progressing to automatic micturition with a contracted bladder, is the type usually seen in parasagittal lesions of the frontal lobes. *The automatic (reflex) bladder,* characterized initially by urinary retention that progresses to overflow incontinence and then to automatic intermittent emptying, occurs with bilateral interruption of the suprasegmental axons traveling with the lateral corticospinal tracts at any level above the S1 spinal cord segment. Incomplete or early lesions may produce the uninhibited bladder pattern instead. *The autonomous neurogenic bladder,* characterized by dribbling incontinence without automatic emptying contractions of the detrusor muscle, results from lesions at the sacral segments of the spinal cord or involving the spinal roots from them that supply the bladder and its sphincters.

Disturbances of sexual function often accompany or precede impaired bladder function with lesions in the spinal canal. Priapism and frequent reflex ejaculation are the usual disturbances with lesions involving the spinal cord above the sacral segments, and especially those above the lower thoracic segments. Ability for normal erection may be retained. Lesions involving the lower sacral (S3, S4, and S5) segments of the cord or the nerve roots therefrom in the cauda equina usually cause total impotence with loss of ability for erection and ejaculation.

The suprasegmental *control of the rectal sphincter* is mediated by the same pathways as that for the external urethral sphincter. Its peripheral innervation is via the S3, S4, and S5 spinal cord segments. Lesions above these segments, involving the suprasegmental pathways, cause constipation associated with a spastic sphincter. Lesions of the sacral segments of spinal cord or the nerve roots from them may result in loss of sphincter tone with fecal incontinence.

The Cervical and Lumbar Enlargements

Lesions at the level of the spinal canal corresponding to the cervical enlargement of the spinal cord (C4 through T1) are likely to involve the peripheral sensory, motor, and autonomic nerve supply of one or both upper extremities and, in addition, the tracts to and from higher centers influencing the spinal segments below. Therefore, it is characteristic of lesions here to produce: "lower motor neuron" (flaccid) paralysis and segmental sensory loss in upper extremities associated with "upper motor neuron" (spastic) paralysis in one or both lower extremities, sensory loss over the trunk and lower extremities that follows one or another pattern of sensory tract involvement, and sphincter disturbance. When the lesion is limited to the middle or lower levels of the enlargement, sparing the descending motor tracts and peripheral innervation of the upper cervical segments, it is not unusual to find components of both upper motor neuron and lower motor neuron types of motor impairment (e.g., atrophy and fasciculations accompanied by hyperactive tendon reflexes) in the upper extremities, resembling the clinical picture of amyotrophic lateral sclerosis. The anterior horn cells in the cervical enlargement that give rise to the peripheral motor innervation of each upper extremity are grouped in a laminar arrangement from medial to lateral so that functionally related muscle groups may be selectively involved while other motor supply to the extremity is spared. The cells located most laterally give motor supply to the muscles of the hands and fingers; those most medial supply the shoulder girdle muscles. It is possible, therefore, for a lesion at the cervical enlargement to encroach on the anterior horn in such a way as to involve, for example, only those motor neurons to the hand and fingers, giving a distribution of motor loss that resembles ulnar nerve paralysis. In some instances, these patterns of loss make it extremely difficult to determine by clinical examination alone whether the lesion involves the spinal cord, the spinal roots from the cervical segments, the brachial plexus, or the individual peripheral nerves of the upper extremity.

Lesions involving the lumbar enlargement (L1 through S2 segments) of the spinal cord are likely to impair the peripheral motor, sensory, and autonomic innervation to the lower extremities. The motor loss will be of the lower motor neuron type and may be difficult to differentiate from that resulting from involvement of spinal nerves of the cauda equina or the peripheral nerves. Loss of cutaneous sensation to pain and temperature in the saddle area of the trunk with varying extension of the loss onto the lower extremities may occur. Disturbance of sphincter function is also likely. Examination for sensory loss in the saddle area and sphincter disturbance is important in the correct localization of lesions at this level.

The Cauda Equina Syndrome

Lesions within the spinal canal below the level of the first lumbar vertebra will not produce findings referable to the spinal cord tracts, since the spinal cord ends here. The findings will be limited to those of involvement of the lumbar and sacral spinal nerve roots making up the cauda equina. Motor loss will be of the lower motor neuron type limited to one or both lower extremities. Sensory loss is limited to the lower extremities and the saddle area. Impairment of sphincter control is likely and will be of the sacral segmental type (i.e., fecal incontinence with loss of tone of the anal sphincter and urinary incontinence indicative of the autonomous bladder). Loss of sensation of the urge to void or to defecate is also likely. As already noted, it may be impossible to differentiate between lesions in this level of the spinal canal and those of the lower segments of the spinal cord on the basis of the clinical findings alone. Myelography and other ancillary techniques are usually required. Since the cauda equina is constituted of nerve roots that are peripheral nerves, both structurally and functionally, the prognosis for return of function following removal of the lesion is good in contradistinction to the poor prognosis when the lesion involves the spinal cord.

The foregoing discussion of manifestations of spinal canal disease has dealt mostly with the localization of lesions in terms of the longitudinal plane of the structures within the spinal cord. Localization in terms of the transverse (cross-sectional) plane is of equal importance. The following syndromes indicate the transverse extent to lesions at the particular level of their maximum encroachment upon the spinal cord whether they are of considerable longitudinal extent (e.g., tumor) or sharply localized (e.g., knife wounds). Etiologically, they may be produced by operatively remediable lesions, but frequently they result from inoperable neurological diseases such as multiple sclerosis, amyotrophic lateral sclerosis, and syringomyelia.

Transection of the Spinal Cord ("Transverse Myelitis")

The manifestations of interruption of the continuity of the spinal cord in its cross-sectional plane will vary depending on several factors: the speed with which the interruption occurs, the length of time elapsed between the occurrence of the insult and the examination of the patient, whether the transection is complete or incomplete, the level of the spinal cord involved, and the cause. Sudden complete transection results immediately in spinal shock: flaccid total paralysis of all skeletal musculature and loss of all spinal reflexes below the segmental level of the lesion, loss of all cutaneous and proprioceptive sensation at and below the segmental level of the lesion, and transient urinary and fecal retention. Transection within the upper three cervical segments is usually incompatible with life because of the accompanying loss of vital functions (respiratory and vasomotor control, regulation of body temperature). Transection below the T2 spinal segment will spare the upper extremities, but vasomotor instability, especially orthostatic hypotension, is likely with transection at any level above the midthoracic segments. The latter is important to remember when transporting such patients. Bilateral Horner's syndrome will be produced by lesions at or above the T1 segment.

Spinal shock persists for one to six weeks in those who survive. Spinal reflexes then begin to return and become increasingly active over the ensuing weeks. Reflex bladder emptying develops. Clonus develops. The Babinski sign appears bilaterally. Flexor spasms begin to appear in response to cutaneous stimulation and become increasingly active on the slightest stimulation. A mass reflex response, consisting of bouts of profuse sweating and flushing, wide fluctuations in blood pressure, reflex voiding, and massive reflex contraction of the trunk and limbs below the lesion may develop in response to cutaneous stimulation. Within 6 to 12 months after the insult, extensor spasms in the limbs begin to occur, and for an indefinite period of time thereafter, reflex movements of alternating flexor spasms and extensor spasms may appear, sometimes resembling stepping movements of the lower limbs. Extensor spasms usually predominate as time passes, and ultimately sustained extensor rigidity of the lower extremities (paraplegia-in-extension) prevails. In some cases, the increased tone in flexor muscle groups rather than extensors predominates, resulting in sustained flexion posture of the lower limbs (paraplegia-in-flexion). Earlier reports based on study of paraplegics in World War I suggested that paraplegia-in-extension resulted with complete transections, and paraplegia-in-flexion resulted when the transection was incomplete; however, subsequent studies since the advent of antibiotics and other improvements in the care of such patients have led to modification of this concept. The indications are that the difference is more likely due to the *level* of the transection: transection at the cervical levels is more likely to result in paraplegia-in-extension, whereas that at midthoracic levels is more likely to result in paraplegia-in-flexion.

When the transection occurs suddenly, but is incomplete, there may be a transient period of spinal shock due to the concussive effects of the causative lesion on the spinal cord. This state will soon become clinically evident, sometimes within hours or several days, by the finding of some degree of return of the motor and sensory function originally lost. The prognosis for recovery in such cases is improved, although it may take weeks or months to assess it.

When gradual transverse encroachment on the spinal cord occurs, as in compression by tumor, the clinical manifestations of spinal shock usually do not appear. Instead, there develop a gradual upper motor neuron type of paralysis and progressing sensory loss below the lesion.

The Brown-Séquard Syndrome

Transverse hemisection of the spinal cord, interruption of the lateral half of the spinal cord on either side above the lumbar segments, results in homolateral upper motor neuron paralysis, vasomotor paralysis and loss of position and vibratory sensation below the level of the lesion, and contralateral loss of pain and temperature sensation below the level of the lesion. At times there may be a narrow band of hyperesthesia just above the level of analgesia bilaterally or homolateral to the lesion, presumably owing to irritation of the dorsal root at the site of the lesion.

This syndrome rarely occurs in pure form clinically. Acute lesions (e.g., stab wound or fracture of the spine) will usually involve less or more than this precise transverse area. Slower lesions (e.g., encroaching tumor) will present clinical signs of the incomplete syndrome before the entire syndrome develops. The essential feature of greatest diagnostic usefulness is the homolateral spastic weakness in association with a contralateral cutaneous sensory level on the trunk. As has been pointed out already, the level on the trunk below which cutaneous sensation is lost is not a reliable indication of the level of the lesion; therefore precise localization usually requires myelography unless the site is evident on inspection (e.g., stab wound).

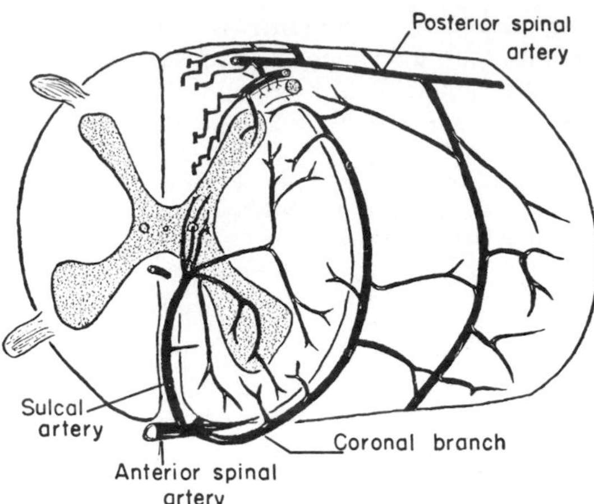

Figure 1–10 Diagram showing blood supply to spinal cord in cross-sectional plane. The illustration is that of one side of the cord, illustrating that the major supply to the areas of the lateral spinothalamic and lateral corticospinal tracts as well as the anterior two thirds of gray matter receive their major supply from the anterior spinal artery. (From Peele, T. L.: The Neuroanatomic Basis for Clinical Neurology. 2nd Ed. New York, McGraw-Hill Book Co., Inc., 1961, p. 112——after Herren and Alexander. Reprinted by permission.)

The Anterior Spinal Artery Syndrome

The arterial supply to the spinal cord is via the single anterior spinal artery, which runs in the anterior median fissure and supplies approximately the anterior two thirds of the cord bilaterally, and the paired posterior spinal arteries, each supplying half of the posterior one third. These arteries receive reinforcing blood supply at multiple segments along the canal by anastomoses from the intercostal and lumbar arteries. Anastomoses at the cervical and upper thoracic level with the thyroid artery, at the lower thoracic level, and at the upper lumbar level are especially large and are essential to maintenance of adequate supply of blood to the spinal cord throughout its length. Infarction of the spinal cord may result not only from thrombosis of its nutrient arteries, but also from lesions that occlude any of these crucial reinforcing arteries outside the spinal canal or along the nerve roots with which they enter the canal. The blood supply to any level of the cord may also be interrupted by compression of the artery by an expanding lesion such as tumor in the spinal canal. The arterial syndrome most readily recognizable clinically is that of the anterior spinal artery. Compromise of blood flow through it results in infarction or ischemia of motor cells in the anterior gray horns, the lateral spinothalamic tracts in the anterior portion of the lateral white columns, and the descending motor tracts more posteriorly in the lateral white columns (Fig. 1–10). In the thoracic and cervical segments, the autonomic pathways will also be involved. The posterior white columns are spared. Thus there results bilateral motor paralysis and cutaneous sensory loss below the level of infarction and bilateral sparing of proprioceptive (position and vibratory) sensation. Infarction involving the segments carrying the autonomic suprasegmental tracts and the preganglionic sympathetic fibers will produce autonomic signs in addition.

Central Lesions of Spinal Cord

Just anterior to the central canal in the anterior commissure, the axons from the second-order neurons of the dorsal gray horns conveying pain and temperature entering each segment of the cord cross to the opposite side to form the lateral spinothalamic tract. As has already been noted, these fibers form the most centrally (medially) placed axons within the tract as they join at successively higher levels. A lesion in the vicinity of the central canal will involve these crossing sensory fibers and may also encroach upon the medial aspect of the tract on one or both sides. The result will be a segmental sensory loss (suspended sensory level) over both sides, the extent of which will depend on the longitudinal extent of the lesion along the cord and the transverse extent of its encroachment on the lateral spinothalamic tracts. A dissociation of pain and temperature perception may also occur, since the fibers conveying thermal sensation are grouped dorsolaterally in the lateral spinothalamic tract while pain fibers are grouped anteromedially (see Fig. 1–9). The extent of the segment of sensory loss will likely differ on the two sides, especially when the lesion is asymmetrical in its transverse encroachment on the tracts. A syrinx of the cord is the lesion with which this sensory pattern is most often associated, but it may also occur with hematomyelia or with intramedullary tumors.

Manifestations of Peripheral Nerve Lesions

In terms of its gross anatomy, the peripheral nervous system consists of all the mixed nerves located outside the bony enclosures housing the central nervous system and carrying the motor, sensory, and autonomic innervation of all the deep and superficial somatic structures of the head, trunk, and limbs. From the standpoint of histological structure and potential disturbance of function, however, it should be considered as extending from the point at which the segmental nerve roots enter and leave the spinal cord to the distal terminations of its constituent axons. The clinical manifestations of its involvement by disease or injury are fundamentally the same, regardless of the point along this extent at which the involvement occurs; only the pattern of distribution of the disturbed function differs, depending on the changes in distribution of the constituent axons in their course from the spinal cord to the structures that they innervate. These axons vary in size and in thickness of their myelin sheaths in relation to the type of impulse that they transmit and the speed of transmission. Their susceptibility to some noxious agents also differs in relation to these same structural factors. *Unlike the axons within the central nervous system, those constituting the peripheral nervous system are capable of regeneration after destruction.* Factors influencing regeneration and restoration of function following peripheral nerve injuries are considered in Chapter 75.

The paired spinal nerves representing each spinal cord segment are formed by junction of their respective dorsal (posterior) and ventral (anterior) nerve roots at the intervertebral foramen from which they exit from the spinal canal. The axons constituting the ventral roots arise from parent motor neurons in the anterior gray column of the spinal cord; at the T1 through L3 segments they are accompanied by the axons of the preganglionic sympathetic neurons situated in the intermediate gray column bound for the paravertebral chain of sympathetic ganglia (white rami communicantes). Just distal to each paravertebral ganglion, the gray rami communicantes—the axons arising from postganglionic neurons within the ganglion—rejoin the nerve to reach their peripheral distribution. The axons constituting the dorsal spinal roots arise from parent sensory neurons located in the dorsal root ganglion at each segment. It will be remembered that the dorsal and ventral roots arising from the lower thoracic, the lumbar, and the sacral segments and forming the cauda equina travel for a considerable distance down the spinal canal before reaching their respective intervertebral foramina where they join. The meninges (dura and arachnoid) covering the spinal cord form a root sleeve around each pair of nerve roots extending to the intervertebral foramen where they end by fusing with the periosteum of the foramen and the connective tissue sheath of each spinal nerve.

The spinal nerves of the T2 through T12 segments continue peripherally as the intercostal nerves. Those from the C1 through C4 segments form the cervical plexus. Those of the segments C5 through T1 undergo redistribution of their constituent axons to form the brachial plexus, from which arise the peripheral nerves innervating the upper extremity and shoulder girdle. Those of the L1 through L4 segments form the lumbar plexus, and those from the L4 through S4 segments form the sacral plexus. (Because of the variation in overlap

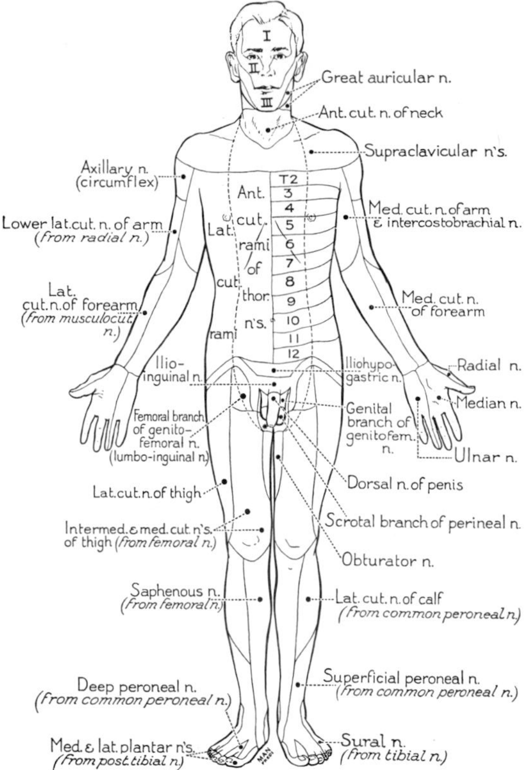

Figure 1–11 The cutaneous territories of the individual peripheral nerves viewed anteriorly. This and Figures 1–12 and 1–13 can be compared with Figures 1–6, 1–7, and 1–8, which show the *dermatomes of the spinal cord segments,* to differentiate between central and peripheral lesions. The numbers on the trunk indicate the zones supplied by each of the intercostal nerves. The asterisk beneath the scrotum indicates the territory of the posterior cutaneous nerve of the thigh as viewed anteriorly. (From Haymaker, W., and Woodhall, B.: Peripheral Nerve Injuries. 2nd Ed. Philadelphia, W. B. Saunders Co., 1953, p. 43. Reprinted by permission.)

between the two, it is clinically useful to consider these together as the lumbosacral plexus, from which arise the peripheral nerves innervating the lower extremity and pelvic girdle.) In this process of redistribution of axons from spinal nerves to plexus to peripheral nerves, an individual peripheral nerve ends up with axons arising from several spinal cord segments, and the axons constituting a single spinal nerve root may be distributed in more than one peripheral nerve.

Each peripheral nerve has its territory of cutaneous sensory supply and its somatic motor supply, just as each spinal segment has. As a result of the redistribution of the sensory axons from spinal segmental roots to peripheral nerves, the peripheral nerve territories differ substantially from the dermatome pattern shown in Figures 1–6 to 1–8. Figures 1–11, 1–12, and 1–13 map the cutaneous territories of the individual peripheral nerves. Since there is considerable overlap between adjacent peripheral nerve territories, the actual area of sensory deficit on the skin is usually less extensive when a single peripheral nerve is interrupted than that shown. It is useful, therefore, especially in the cutaneous nerve supply to the extremities, to define those zones of autonomous supply characteristic of each peripheral nerve. In examining the patient with a cutaneous sensory deficit, a helpful technique is to begin testing within the area of definite sensory loss and work out radially from this focus in mapping the entire area of deficit.

The peripheral nerves are mixed nerves in that they include axons conveying motor, sensory, and autonomic impulses. Therefore, lesions that affect them might produce disturbance of any or all of these functions, depending on the level at which they are affected. As a nerve courses peripherally, its component axons separate off into more specialized branches; therefore, the more proximally it is affected, the more likely one is to find disturbance of all three functions in its territory of supply. The general manifestations of peripheral nerve lesions are (1) motor paralysis of lower motor neuron type only; (2) sensory changes, which may consist of deficit of pain, temperature, touch, position, or vibratory sensations alone or in combinations, and subjective sensations of numbness, dysesthesias, paresthesias, or pain; (3) decrease or absence of tendon reflexes, but sparing of cutaneous reflexes and absence of pathological reflexes (e.g., Babinski sign, flexor spasms); and (4) autonomic and trophic changes consisting of edema, peripheral vasomotor instability (flushing or pallor), thick or shiny skin with regional loss of cutaneous hair, and trophic ulcers.

The patterns of distribution that these manifestations may take are (1) individual spinal root syndromes, (2) plexus syndromes, (3) mononeuropathy, in which an isolated peripheral nerve is paralyzed in part or in its entirety, (4) polyneuropathy, in which multiple adjacent peripheral nerves are involved simultaneously in a

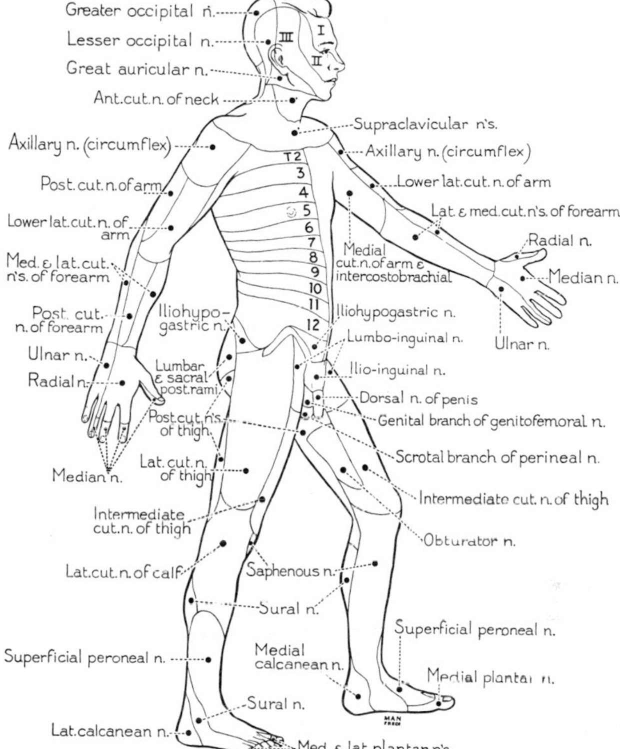

Figure 1–12 Lateral view of the cutaneous territories of the peripheral nerves. (From Haymaker, W., and Woodhall, B.: Peripheral Nerve Injuries. 2nd Ed. Philadelphia, W. B. Saunders Co., 1953, p. 42. Reprinted by permission.)

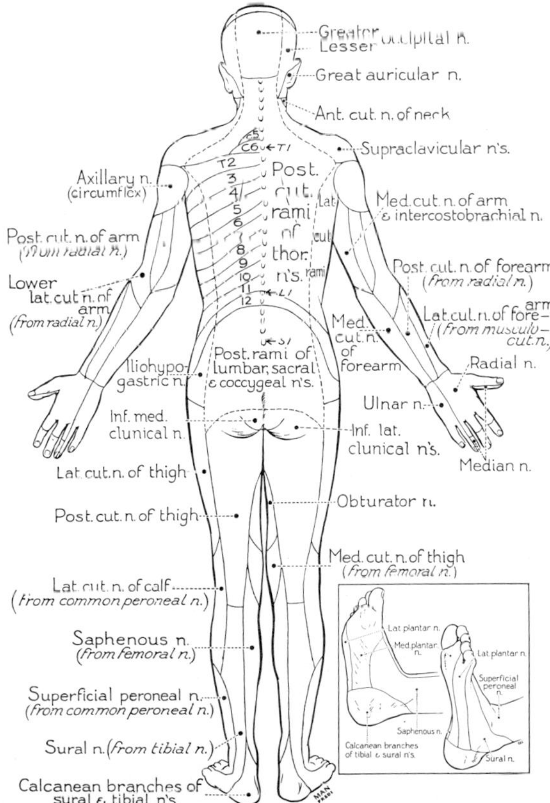

Figure 1–13 Posterior view of the cutaneous territory of the peripheral nerves. (From Haymaker, W., and Woodhall, B.: Peripheral Nerve Injuries. 2nd Ed. Philadelphia, W. B. Saunders Co. Reprinted by permission.)

bilaterally symmetrical pattern, and (5) mononeuropathy multiplex (rare), in which two or more individual peripheral nerves are paralyzed simultaneously.

Those that are of primary concern in neurosurgical diagnosis are the syndromes of the spinal roots and plexuses and the mononeuropathies.

Polyneuropathy is invariably due to medical diseases of toxic, metabolic, or inflammatory etiology and is only of concern to the neurosurgeon in that its manifestations may sometimes simulate certain neurosurgical lesions. It consists of bilaterally symmetrical distribution of flaccid weakness (diplegia), diminution or loss of tendon reflexes, sensory deficit, and autonomic changes that involve the extremities earliest and often exclusively. It may involve the lower extremities alone, the upper extremities alone, or occasionally the face alone (facial diplegia). The motor and sensory manifestations generally begin in the distal parts of the involved extremities; they may remain limited to this distal distribution or progressively ascend the extremities. The trunk musculature becomes involved only late in the course of the disease if at all, even when all four extremities are severely involved. One never finds a sensory level on the trunk. There rarely is any impairment of sphincter function, although the occasional patient may void in bed if too weak to get out of bed. This syndrome may on occasion be difficult to diagnose because it simulates transverse myelitis or a lesion of the cauda equina. Table 1–1 lists the features that distinguish the two. In rapidly progressive cases of either, the distinction may be clouded, but rarely should it be necessary to subject the patient with rapidly advancing polyneuropathy to the hazard of myelography or other technical procedures to establish the correct diagnosis.

TABLE 1–1 CLINICAL MANIFESTATIONS OF SPINAL CORD, PERIPHERAL NERVE, AND SKELETAL MUSCLE DISEASES

CLINICAL MANIFESTATIONS	SPINAL CORD LESIONS (*Myelopathies*)	PERIPHERAL NERVE LESIONS (*Neuropathies*)	MUSCLE DISEASE (*Myopathies*)
Motor	Upper or lower motor neuron type weakness, depending on acuity and "age" of the lesion and its location in relation to cord segments *Trunk and limb(s) below the lesion affected* Atrophy from disuse only	Lower motor neuron (flaccid) weakness only Predominantly in extremities; tends to involve distal limb segments more than proximal Atrophy early	Flaccid weakness only Tends to involve trunk and proximal limb segments earliest
Sensory	Cutaneous "sensory level" or "suspended sensory level" on trunk Sensory dissociation, if present, usually in terms of cord tracts	Rarely involves trunk; tends to begin distally in limbs and ascend limbs or follows distribution of a peripheral nerve supply Dissociation, if present, may be of any combination of modalities	None
Reflexes	Hyperactive tendon reflexes below lesion except during "spinal shock" with acute lesions At level of lesion, if limb segments are involved, hyporeflexia or areflexia persists or both hyper- and hyporeflexia occur in same limb(s) *Pathological reflexes* (Babinski sign, spontaneous flexor or extensor spasms) below lesion likely Cutaneous reflexes lost below lesion	Hyporeflexia or areflexia found early and persists No pathological reflexes Cutaneous reflexes spared unless their effector muscles are completely paralyzed	Tendon reflexes normal early, become progressively hypoactive as disease advances Cutaneous reflexes spared No pathological reflexes
Sphincters	External urethral and anal sphincters often impaired	Sphincters very rarely involved	No sphincter disturbance

The syndromes of the individual nerves are described in Chapters 75 and 76. The manifestations of disorders involving the major nerve plexuses and the individual peripheral nerves are also described in detail in the excellent monograph *Peripheral Nerve Injuries,* by Haymaker and Woodhall.[5]

Manifestations of Disorders of Skeletal Musculature

These disorders are rarely of concern in neurosurgical diagnosis. They are manifested clinically by muscular wasting and weakness, impairment of tendon reflexes, and sometimes muscular pains. They may in some instances simulate lesions of the peripheral nervous system or the spinal canal in which only motor function is disturbed. Usually they can be readily distinguished from such lesions by the following cardinal features that characterize the primary myopathies:

1. Motor loss is of the flaccid type. It is generally of bilaterally symmetrical distribution and may be generalized or restricted to certain muscle groups. It tends to predominate in the muscles of the trunk, the limb girdles, and the proximal parts of the limbs. Pseudohypertrophy of involved muscles, i.e., hypertrophy in which the muscles appear larger than normal but are markedly weakened, is sometimes seen.
2. The tendon reflexes are diminished or occasionally absent as in lower motor neuron paralysis, but they tend to be preserved longer than in lower motor neuron involvement with comparable degrees of weakness and wasting. The cutaneous reflexes are preserved, and pathological reflexes do not appear.
3. Sensation is preserved in all modalities.
4. The sphincters are spared.

Table 1–1 lists the clinical findings that differentiate primary diseases of somatic musculature from polyneuropathy and spinal cord lesions.

THE ETIOLOGICAL DIAGNOSIS

The final step in neurosurgical diagnosis by the clinical method is determination of the cause of the lesion. Sometimes this will have already been accomplished in the process of localizing the lesion and simultaneously considering salient items of information obtained in the process. Nevertheless, it is advisable as a conscious step in the diagnostic process to consider all the causes that are reasonably possible; the most likely is not always the correct one. Ancillary techniques are frequently required for refinement of diagnosis and planning management; the more thoroughly one has considered the etiological possibilities, the more judicious will be his choice of procedures and their priority.

The etiology of the neurosurgical diseases is considered in detail in subsequent chapters. The purpose here is not to preview these, but to provide the neurosurgeon with a "vest pocket" mental picture of the spectrum of diseases of the nervous system and their temporal profiles that he may find useful in the examining room with his patient. Of course, not all of them are generally considered "surgical diseases," whatever the implications of such a classification; but the neurosurgeon as a diagnostician is required to have a working knowledge of all categories of disease that may affect the nervous system if he is to fulfill his role as a physician and diagnostician as well as a surgical technician.

The following is an outline of the categories of nervous system diseases and a capsule condensation of their salient distinguishing features. It will be seen readily that *the determination of etiology depends primarily on adequate and accurate history* from the patient and relatives or other witnesses to his illness, whereas *anatomical localization depends primarily on the abnormal findings elicited by examination* of the patient.

Developmental Defects

Developmental defects are usually present from birth or become recognized very early in life. The clinical course of deficits in function produced by most of them is usually static (i.e., nonprogressive) or very slowly progressive over a period of years with modifications imposed by overall development of the nervous system in early life and its deterioration in later life. An exception to this general rule is that group of developmental anomalies in which rapid progression of deficit results from increasing pressure on neural structures (e.g., craniostenosis or congenital hydrocephalus).

Neoplasms

Neoplasms vary in age of onset depending on the type of tumor. Their onset is generally insidious (except when heralded by a sudden event such as an epileptic seizure), and the course of the symptoms produced is usually cumulative and progressive over a period of months or very few years. The rate of progression of symptoms within this range will vary, depending on the location of the lesion and its degree of malignancy. Metastatic lesions to the nervous system not infrequently produce symptoms antecedent to those in the primary site.

Vascular Diseases

Vascular diseases predominantly occur in middle and late adult life with the exception of congenital vascular anomalies and the (rare) inflammatory vascular diseases, which may become clinically manifest at any age. The clinical onset of vascular diseases is nearly always sudden with progression to maximal deficit in minutes to hours (occasionally a few days), followed by a plateau of static (nonprogressive) deficit, then improvement in function if the patient survives the earlier phases. Within this general time range the onset and course vary in details, depending on whether the lesion is a hemorrhage or an occlusion. In some instances the symptoms will occur intermittently over a period of days, weeks, or months, simulating demyelinative disease or occasionally a neoplastic growth. Differentiation from demyelinative disease can usually be made on the basis of the age of the patient at the time of initial symptoms and the recurrence of essentially the same manifestations with each episode. The occasional slowly progressing course seen in patients with occlusive arterial disease in the sixth decade or later can be very difficult to differentiate from the course of intracranial neoplasm; such cases usually require ancillary techniques for clarification of the diagnosis.

Demyelinative Disease

Demyelinative disease is a pathological category peculiar to the nervous system, resulting from the destruction of the myelin sheaths of axons in the central nervous system (brain, brain stem, cerebellum, and spinal cord). *Multiple sclerosis* is the most common disease in this group. The onset of its symptoms usually takes place during adolescence or early adult life, rarely after the third decade. It tends to occur in one or more acute or subacute episodes, each of which evolves to maximal deficit over a period of from 12 hours to several days, followed by a plateau of deficit, then gradual complete or partial subsidence. Successive attacks may be spaced weeks, months, or years apart, each differing in signs of localization but similar in temporal profile. Often an individual episode will subside only partially, leaving a background of permanent residual deficit upon which the deficits of subsequent attacks are superimposed. *Thus, the long-term clinical course is usually one of progressive accumulation of permanent deficit upon which are superimposed acute transient exacerbations of variable abnormal signs* indicative of involvement, successively, of different motor and sensory tracts up and down the neuraxis. Mental and emotional changes become a prominent part of the picture, usually in the later stages, because of the predilection of the cerebral lesions to cluster around the ventricular walls. Optic or retrobulbar neuritis, acute cerebellar or brain stem syndromes (or both), and acute partial or complete transverse syndromes of the spinal cord are the common forms that individual attacks tend to take. In an individual case the course may be fulminant to total disability or death within a few months, whereas in another case the attacks may be years apart and disabling residua minimal.

Acute postinfectious or postvaccinal encephalomyelitis, another fairly common demyelinative syndrome, differs from multiple sclerosis in that it usually occurs as a single acute episode with simultaneous involvement of multiple levels of the neuraxis. It most often occurs in children following immunization with certain vaccines or during the early convalescent phase of an acute exanthematous infection, usually heralded by a secondary rise in temperature, impairment of consciousness, and seizures. Its course varies from a few days to several weeks with gradual recovery to varying degrees of normalcy.

The diffuse cerebral scleroses are the other likely form that demyelinative disease takes. The onset and course vary widely depending on which of the two major types—inflammatory (exogenous, myelinoclastic) or degenerative (leukodystrophic)—occurs. The former is exemplified by Schilder's disease, which runs a rapid course of a few weeks to three years from onset to death. It is characterized by successive episodes of deficit corresponding to lesions in varying areas of white matter of the cerebral hemispheres (hallucinations and mental changes, motor or sensory hemiplegias, loss of vision, and convulsive seizures). It occurs most often in childhood or adolescence, but may begin in the third and fourth decades. The degenerative forms of cerebral sclerosis are more insidious in onset and progress over a period of several years with the development of a combination of corticospinal, extrapyramidal, mental, and cerebellar manifestations. Some types begin in early childhood and are familial; others begin in the later decades of life. *Both the inflammatory and degenerative forms of diffuse cerebral sclerosis are of importance to the neurosurgeon in that their clinical manifestations and course may closely simulate brain tumor, including the development of papilledema and other signs of increased intracranial pressure.*

Infections

Infections of the nervous system have some important differences in clinical manifestations from infections elsewhere in the body. They may take any one or a combination of three forms:

Abscess, focal infection, behaves as an expanding intracranial lesion just as a tumor does and often runs a similar course in time. It frequently is not accompanied by the usual systemic symptoms of abscess elsewhere (fever, leukocytosis). A history or findings of a source of infection (e.g., paranasal sinuses, ear, lung, antecedent head trauma) is the most helpful information in differentiating it from neoplasm.

Meningitis, a diffuse infection of meninges, may run an acute or chronic course, depending on the infectious agent. In addition to initial signs of meningeal irritation (headache, stiff neck), the chronic forms or the more prolonged acute cases may produce "neighborhood reaction" in the cortical surfaces of brain (meningoencephalitis) and surface blood vessels or multiple cranial nerve palsies. The diagnosis usually rests on examination of the cerebrospinal fluid.

Encephalitis, a direct infection of brain parenchyma, is most often of viral etiology. Its course is acute or subacute with signs indicative of diffuse cerebral or brain stem involvement.

Degenerative Disease

Degenerative diseases of the nervous system usually occur in adult life, have an insidious onset, and run a progressive course of several to many years. Some may simulate neoplasm in time course and in their early manifestations. They differ from neoplasm in clinical manifestations in that they are generally systems diseases—i.e., limited to one or a combination of two neuronal systems subserving a specific function—throughout their course, whereas neoplasm is a regional lesion. Familial incidence is not uncommon, a point of some help in the early differential diagnosis when present. The degenerative diseases often are manifest unilaterally at their outset, but eventually develop bilaterally as they progress.

Trauma

Traumatic lesions are usually self-evident by the history, but the delayed effects of trauma may present a diagnostic problem when the onset of their symptoms is remote, when the trauma may have been too trivial for the patient to mention, or when the history is inadequate.

Metabolic and Toxic Diseases

Metabolic and toxic diseases are mostly secondary to systemic diseases such as diabetes, thyroid dysfunction, or poisoning.

Some are limited to the nervous system; several of those diseases previously classified as degenerative are now regarded as metabolic with the discovery of a causative metabolic defect, and others are likely to be so reclassified in the future. The onset of metabolic or toxic syndromes of the nervous system may occur at any age, and their course may be episodic, progressive, or one of a single acute and self-limited episode, depending on the causative disturbance. The manifestations are generally diffuse and bilateral, but sometimes (e.g., in diabetic neuropathy) are localized or limited in distribution. The diagnosis usually rests on a history of antecedent systemic metabolic disorder and laboratory studies.

Recurrent Episodic Syndromes

Recurrent episodic syndromes of the nervous system may be encountered as part of many diseases, or some may occur in the absence of known underlying cause. They are more properly regarded as syndromes than diseases. Even when their underlying causative disease is known, they often must be managed per se when the cause cannot be removed. The more common of these are: epilepsy, narcolepsy-cataplexy syndromes, headaches of certain categories (migraine, muscle-contraction, or tension headaches), recurrent syncope, and Ménière's syndrome.

It is emphasized that these are general characteristics of each of the categories of disease, to which many exceptions may be found. They are intended only as "handles" that one may find helpful in attempting to arrive quickly at a working diagnosis, or more likely a differential diagnosis, in the individual case—a most important step for the mature diagnostician in planning the subsequent diagnostic and therapeutic management of his patient.

REFERENCES

1. Adams, R. D.: The clincal method of neurology: Comments and suggestions. Med. Clin. N. Amer., *36*:1393, 1952.
2. Benton, A. L.: The fiction of the "Gerstmann syndrome." J. Neurol. Neurosurg. Psychiat., *24*:176–181, 1961.
3. Gerstmann, J.: Syndrome of finger agnosia, disorientation for right and left, agraphia and acalculia. Local diagnostic value. Arch. Neurol. Psychiat., *44*:398–408, 1940.
4. Harlow, J. M.: Passage of an iron rod through the head. Boston Med. Surg. J., *39*:389, 1848.
5. Haymaker, W., and Woodhall, B.: Peripheral Nerve Injuries. 2nd Ed. Philadelphia, W. B. Saunders Co., 1953.
6. Kennedy, F.: Retrobulbar neuritis as an exact diagnostic sign of certain tumors and abscesses in the frontal lobes. Amer. J. Med. Sci., *142*:355–368, 1911.
7. Kuhn, R. A.: Functional capacity of the isolated human spinal cord. Brain, *73*:1–51, 1950.
8. Malamud, N.: Psychiatric disorder with intracranial tumors of the limbic system. Arch. Neurol., *17*:113–123, 1967.
9. Schneider, R. C., Crosby, E. C., and Farhat, S. M.: Extratemporal lesions triggering the temporal lobe syndrome. The role of association bundles. J. Neurosurg., *22*:246–263, 1965.
10. Talbert, O. R., and Clark, R. M.: Clinical manifestations of focal epilepsy. Southern Med. J., *61*:363–369, 1968.
11. Tarlov, I. M., and Herz, E.: Spinal cord compression studies. IV. Outlook with complete paralysis in man. Arch. Neurol. Psychiat., *72*:43–59, 1954.
12. Terzian, H., and Ore, G. D.: Syndrome of Klüver and Bucy reproduced in man by bilateral removal of the temporal lobes. Neurology, *5*:373–380, 1955.
13. von Wowern, F.: Foster Kennedy syndrome: Evaluation of its diagnostic value. Acta Neurol. Scand., *43*:205–214, 1967.
14. Williams, D.: The structure of emotions reflected in epileptic experiences. Brain, *79*:29–67, 1956.

2

CLINICAL EXAMINATION IN INFANCY AND CHILDHOOD

Adherence to the basic principles of physical diagnosis, specifically, obtaining a careful complete history and performing a thorough physical and neurological examination, is mandatory if one is to evaluate neurological problems in children adequately. Certain problems are, however, inherent in pediatrics. If the patient is an infant or a young child, the historical data must be obtained from the parents or some other person. The physical and neurological examinations are often hampered by the child's inability to cooperate. The systematic approach to the neurological examination that is so effectively used in adults and older children will often evoke a completely negativistic attitude in the small child. A complete examination can usually be accomplished, even in the newborn, but only if the examiner displays infinite patience and is willing to spend the time necessary to achieve that goal. The rewards of such an examination are, however, well worth the effort.

HISTORY

Present Illness

The history should begin with a description of the present illness, and a concerted effort should be made to determine the specific area of concern. A chronological progression of the disease process including onset and specific symptoms should be recorded. It is often best to allow the parents to relate the problem in their own words. Precise data can be elicited by pertinent questions posed by the examiner. In children it is essential to determine whether there has been loss of previously acquired function or whether the process is a static one. If the history clearly delineates a continued loss of previously acquired function, one can be fairly certain that the disease is progressive. On the other hand, if there has been a steady acquisition of developmental skills from birth, the disease in all probability is static. It is noteworthy that in children certain neurological signs and symptoms do not become manifest clinically until the nervous system has matured to a certain point. Athetosis, which may be the result of an intrauterine or neonatal insult, will not be clinically apparent until the child is over one year of age and usually does not appear before the age of 18 months. In the young child the insult to the nervous system often precedes the onset of the first symptom by months or years. It is therefore necessary to obtain a complete account of events earlier in the child's life.

Past History

Prenatal History

The child's development begins at the time of conception, and any factor affecting the mother's health during pregnancy may be of major significance. The mother's general state of health during the pregnancy, her age at the time of conception, and the number and outcome of previous pregnancies are all of importance in assessing the

G. R. HOGAN AND N. J. RYAN

risk to the infant. The developing fetus is at greatest risk during the first trimester. The mother should be questioned very specifically about bleeding, infections, drug ingestion (including tobacco and alcohol), and trauma during this period. The deleterious effects of maternal rubella, toxoplasmosis, and cytomegalovirus infection are well documented. The tragedy of thalidomide emphasizes the risk inherent in the use of drugs during the early stages of pregnancy. Syphilis and diabetes mellitus are frequently associated with the birth of defective babies. Toxemia of pregnancy, which, unfortunately, is still prevalent in the southeastern United States, subjects the infant to significant risk of intrauterine growth retardation, hypoglycemia, prolonged intrauterine hypoxia, and hyperviscosity (high hematocrit) syndromes. An assessment of fetal movement in utero can be of diagnostic significance (Werdnig-Hoffmann disease). An observant multiparous woman can accurately detect excessive or weak movement in utero. A change in the activity pattern of the fetus may herald the onset of a disease process.

Birth History

A careful documentation of the events surrounding the birth of the infant is an essential part of the pediatric patient's history. The duration of the various stages of labor, the type of delivery, the place of delivery (home or hospital), and the person in attendance (physician or midwife) may prove to be significant. The condition of the infant at birth is of utmost importance. Factors of vital interest are weight, maturity, Apgar score, difficulties of respiration, and type of resuscitation.

Neonatal History

The condition of the infant in the immediate neonatal period should be ascertained if possible. One should question the parents about the presence of conditions that are known to be frequently associated with neurological abnormalities. These conditions include respiratory distress, apneic episodes, seizures, jaundice, cyanosis, bleeding, feeding difficulties, infections, hypoglycemia, and high hematocrit. The low-birth-weight infant and the one who is large for gestational age are both at risk for hypoglycemia and hyperviscosity. The infant's head circumference at birth is of major importance.

Developmental History

The age at which the child reaches his developmental milestones serves as our best index to his neurological maturation. Adequate evaluation of development, however, includes an examination of four basic fields of behavior that represent different areas of growth. These four major fields, as delineated by Gesell, are: motor behavior, adaptive behavior, language behavior, and personal-social behavior.[4]

Motor behavior includes both gross control and fine coordinated movements. The gross motor capacities of the child to be evaluated are such types of bodily control as postural reaction, head control, sitting, standing, crawling, and walking. Fine motor coordination is determined by the child's approach to an object, his grasp, his use of his fingers, and his manipulation of the object. Adaptive behavior involves sensorimotor adjustments to objects and situations, the coordination of hand and eye in manipulation and reaching for objects, the ability to utilize motor skills in the solution of simple problems (e.g., putting a pellet in a bottle). Language behavior includes both visible and audible forms of communication. Personal and social behavior comprises the child's reaction to his environment. Function in this area is, of course, dependent to a large extent on cultural factors, but its attainment is dependent upon neuromotor maturity.

The scope of this chapter precludes a comprehensive review of normal growth and development, but a summary of the developmental milestones in infants and children is presented in Table 2–1. For a complete review of growth and development the reader is referred to the work of Gesell and Amatruda and Illingworth.[4,6]

After the age of 5 years the standard tests such as the Stanford-Binet test and the Wechsler Intelligence Scale for Children offer a more precise estimate of the child's developmental level.

Review of Systems

The review of systems often uncovers symptoms referrable to other organ systems that may be pertinent to the neurological disease. One should ask specifically for any history of central nervous system infection, head trauma, seizures, visual problems, emotional disorders, headache, intercurrent infections, drug ingestion (including prescribed medication), and immunizations.

Family History

The family history should include the age and general health of the parents, the age and sex of the siblings, the educational level of parents and siblings, and any specific school problem (such as dyslexia) in other family members. Also, the history of psychiatric or neurological disorders in the family, familial diseases, genetic abnormalities, or consanguinity should be noted.

NEUROLOGICAL EXAMINATION

The neurological examination is just one aspect of the physical examination, and its value can be ascertained only in relation to the complete examination of the child. The examination should begin with an evaluation of the general state of the patient. This should include the level of responsiveness, the ability to cooperate, and the presence of obvious abnormalities. The method by which this is accomplished will of course be dictated by the condition and reaction of the patient, which in most instances is directly related to his age. Though the actual method of the examination for key age groups will differ considerably, the general overall evaluation is essentially the same for all age groups. Measurements of height, weight, and head circumference are taken and recorded. The general body proportions and nutritional state are noted. The child is observed for asymmetry of size of the extremities (hemihypertrophy or hemiatrophy) and for disproportion between length of extremities and trunk. The skin and hair should be examined for appearance, color, texture, and the presence or absence of associated lesions. A search should be made for the flame nevus of Sturge-Weber, the café-au-lait spots and subcutaneous nodules of neurofibromatosis, the shagreen patch and ash leaf lesions (white spots) of tuberous sclerosis. The spine should be inspected and palpated for evidence of trauma or congenital defects. A tuft of hair or a flame nevus over the spine may be indicative of an underlying defect. The sacral dimple, if not associated with a tuft of hair, is usually benign but should be examined carefully to determine if a sinus tract is present. Deformity of the foot or leg or asymmetry of the buttocks or both should alert one to the possibility of an abnormality of the spine. The head should be examined for contour, evidence of bleeding into the scalp, scalp defects, vascular lesions, or nodules in the skin. The head should be palpated for evidence of cephalhematoma, premature closure of the sutures, widened sutures, masses protruding through the sutures, and size and tenseness of the fontanel (Fig. 2–1). The fontanel should be examined with the child in an upright position and when he is quiet. It is important to listen over the mastoids, temporal regions, and orbits for intracranial bruits. Most generalized intracranial bruits are benign. Transillumination of the head should be carried out in all infants with small heads or large heads and in those whose neurological examinations arouse suspicion. There are great rewards and some pitfalls with this simple but highly productive procedure. Hydranencephalus produces a through-and-through transillumination, and if the light is held over the occipital region there may be a red reflex in the eyes as well as a general glow to the head. In hydrocephalus, if the distance between the pia and the ventricles is 1 cm or less, the head will transilluminate posteriorly. With a subdural collection of fluid, transillumination with the light held just above the ear will be positive across the coronal sutures and will extend upward to the sagittal sinus. If the examination is carried out while the child has a caput succedaneum or an intravenous fluid infiltration of the scalp, the transillumination may be falsely positive. On the other hand, there may be falsely negative transillumination if the examiner has not allowed adequate time for dark adaptation or if the fluid is purulent or contains a significant amount of blood. For transillumination of the head the authors prefer the flashlight technique described by Dodge and Porter.[3]

Once the general evaluation has been done to determine gross anomalies of skele-

TABLE 2–1 NORMAL DEVELOPMENT*

	NEONATAL PERIOD
Motor	Flexion posture with the arms adducted at the shoulder and flexed at the elbows, wrists and fingers Hands fisted with thumb usually in palm When prone turns head from side to side—head lags when in ventral position
Visual	Fixes and follows through about 60 degrees—visual pursuit not smooth Opticokinetic response present
Reflex	Active Moro, suck, rooting, and grasp reflexes Places and steps Biceps, brachioradialis, adductor, patellar, and Achilles reflexes usually elicited with ease Plantar reflex flexor
	4 WEEKS
Motor	Position less flexed—legs extended in prone position Holds chin up in prone position and turns head from side to side Tonic neck reflex position predominates in supine position Head lags when pulled to sitting position No longer fists, and thumb is out of palm
Visual	Watches people—follows moving object Opticokinetic nystagmus can be elicited with ease
	8 WEEKS
Motor	Raises head when prone and watches moving object Maintains head in plane of body with ventral suspension Head lag when lifted to sitting position from supine position Tonic neck reflex posture still predominates in supine position
Visual	Follows moving object through 180 degrees Opticokinetic nystagmus easily elicited
Social	Smiles and coos in response to play and social contact
	12 WEEKS
Motor	When prone lifts head and chest—head above plane of body on ventral suspension Slight head lag when pulled to sitting position from supine position Head control with bobbing when in sitting position Briefly holds objects if placed in hand Reaches toward but misses objects
	12 WEEKS (*continued*)
Visual	Watches movement of own hands Follows objects in all directions Turns to object in periphery of visual field
Social	Smiles readily and makes specific sounds when stimulated and talked to Sustains social contact
	16 WEEKS
Motor	Reaches for and grasps objects and brings them to mouth Symmetrical posture with legs extended when prone No head lag when pulled to sitting position Head steady and looks around in sitting position Pushes with feet when held erect in standing position Moro reflex absent
Adaptive	Sees pellet but does not attempt to pick it up All visual responses quicker
Social	Laughs out loud—obvious pleasure to social contact Responds to sight of food
	28 WEEKS
Motor	Sits with hands supporting—stands with support—bounces when placed in a standing position
Adaptive	Reaches out for objects using one hand Transfers objects from one hand to the other Has palmar grasp and rakes at pellet Bangs objects
Language	Vowel sounds—repetitive babbles
Social	Clings to mother Responds to name Mimics Feeds self cracker
	40 WEEKS
Motor	Sits well without support Back straight Pulls to standing position Crawls using hands
Adaptive	Grasps objects with thumb and forefinger Picks up pellet with pincer movement Retrieves dropped objects
Language	Constant sounds in repetitive manner
Social	Waves bye-bye Plays peek-a-boo and pat-a-cake

* Modification of material from Gesell, A., and Amatruda, C. S.: Developmental Diagnosis. 2nd Ed. New York, Harper & Row, 1964.

TABLE 2–1 NORMAL DEVELOPMENT *(continued)*

	52 WEEKS (1 YEAR)
Motor	Walks with one hand held, walks holding onto furniture
Adaptive	Pincer movement in picking up pellet Releases object on command
Language	Two or four words with meaning Understands meaning of objects in environment
Social	Helps to dress self Plays simple games
	15 MONTHS
Motor	Walks alone but falls easily Crawls up stairs and steps
Adaptive	Makes tower of two cubes Inserts pellet in bottle Scribbles with crayon
Language	Jargon Will follow simple commands
Social	Asks for things by pointing Imitates family in play
	18 MONTHS
Motor	Runs, but stiffly Walks up and down stairs holding on Gets into and sits on small chair Throws ball Pulls toys
Adaptive	Makes tower of three cubes Dumps pellet out of bottle Imitates scribbling and vertical strokes
Language	Has average of 10 words Names pictures and points to two or three body parts Answers questions and carries out simple commands
Social	Feeds self Takes off shoes Unzips clothes
	24 MONTHS (2 YEARS)
Motor	Runs well and walks up and down stairs (two feet per step) Opens doors Bends and picks up objects without falling Climbs Kicks ball
Adaptive	Builds tower of six cubes Imitates a circle Turns pages of book one page at a time Organized play
Language	Uses two- or three-word sentences Uses pronouns (I, you, me) Asks for things by name
Social	Helps dress and undress self Feeds self (handles spoon well)
	24 MONTHS (2 YEARS) *(continued)*
	Tells stories Listens to stories with pictures Toilet training often completed
	30 MONTHS (2½ YEARS)
Motor	Jumps Walks on tip-toe
Adaptive	Holds pencil in hand Tower of eight blocks Makes vertical and horizontal strokes Can complete three-piece form board Knows one to three colors.
Language	Refers to self as I Communicates well with simple sentences
Social	Helps put toys away Tends to own toilet needs
	36 MONTHS (3 YEARS)
Motor	Rides a tricycle Walks up stairs alternating feet Stands on one foot
Adaptive	Tower of nine blocks Makes bridge with three cubes Copies a circle, imitates a cross
Language	Knows sex and age Counts three objects Says nursery rhymes Repeats three numbers
Social	Dresses self except for buttons Plays simple games with other children Dresses and undresses doll
	48 MONTHS (4 YEARS)
Motor	Hops on one foot Climbs well Throws ball overhand Uses scissors to cut out picture
Adaptive	Makes buildings out of blocks from model (bridge and gate of five cubes) Copies cross and square Draws man with two to four parts in addition to the head Can name the longer of two lines
Language	Counts three or four objects Tells fanciful stories
Social	Cooperates in play Begins social interaction and role-playing
	60 MONTHS (5 YEARS)
Motor	Skips
Adaptive	Copies triangle Knows heavier of two weights
Language	Counts up to 10 correctly Knows colors
Social	Dresses and undresses self without help Asks questions about meaning of words

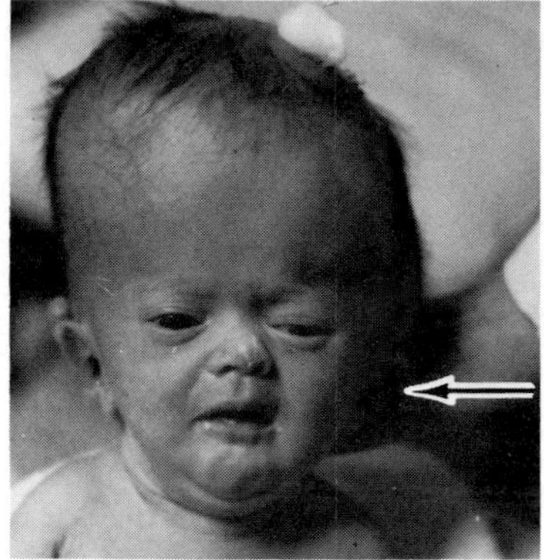
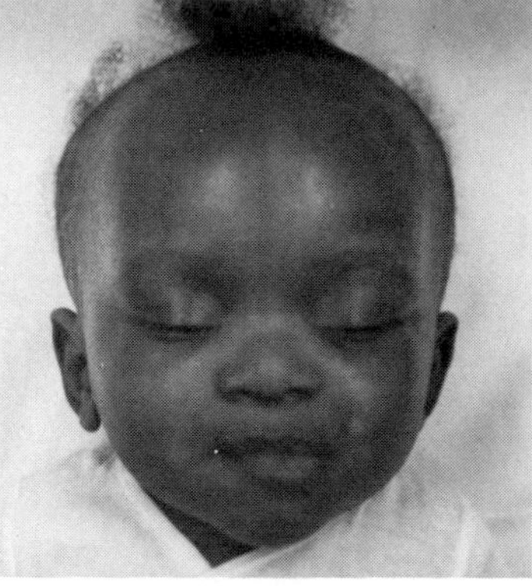
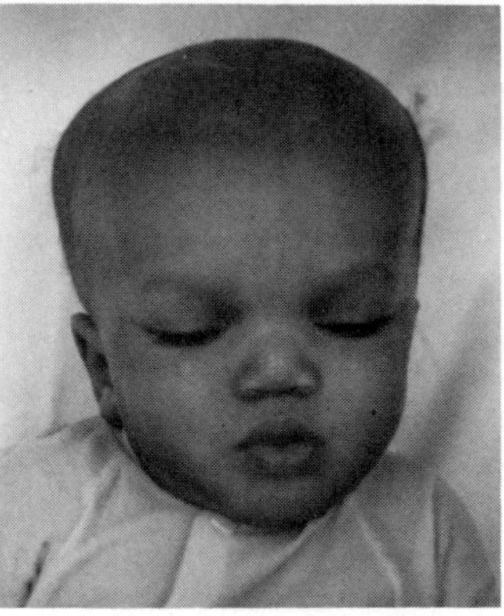

Figure 2–1 *A*. A newborn infant with congenital hydrocephalus demonstrating the marked enlargement of the head. The involvement of the base of the cranium is shown by the lateral displacement of the upper portion of the ear as a result of distortion of the petrous portion of the temporal bone (*arrow*). *B*. A 4-month-old infant with acquired hydrocephalus and enlargement of the head that is apparent above the base of the cranium. *C*. A 5-month-old infant with bilateral subdural hematoma demonstrating biparietal bossing and the "flat top" appearance associated with this lesion.

tal, vascular, and skin development, it is time for a detailed evaluation of neurological function. The method of the examination varies considerably with children at different age levels. The following methods for the examination of children at key ages are presented as a guideline; those used will, of course, vary with the neurological problem presented and the cooperation of the child.

THE NEWBORN TERM INFANT

The neurological examination is one of the most important parts of the newborn evaluation. Small portions of the examination are sometimes carried out, but frequently they are not recorded and therefore are of little use in the re-evaluation of the infant at a later examination.

There are few tests of cortical function in the newborn. The most useful parameters are visual fixing and following. It is, however, still possible to obtain enough information with a careful neurological examination to gain a basic understanding of many neurological problems in the newborn. The examination is most helpful if carried out systematically and in detail in an infant who has not been fed in the preceding hour.

For the initial phase of the examination, the infant should be completely undressed so that a general evaluation for gross abnormalities can be carried out. Careful observation of the infant for asymmetry of size or color, plethora, tachypnea, and other abnormalities of respiratory pattern is the first step. After determining that there are no gross anomalies of skeletal, vascular, or skin development, one should then turn his attention to the general alertness and posture of the infant, being especially observant of symmetry of posture, position of the head and trunk, symmetry of spontaneous movements, and general alertness.

The level of alertness in the newborn is determined by his spontaneous activity and his response to external stimulation. If the infant is stuporous, he may be briefly aroused by vigorous stimulation but will rapidly lapse back into sleep; if he is comatose, either there will be no response to stimulation or the response will be decerebrate posturing. In general the brain stem reflex level in coma corresponds to that in the older child. Therefore, in a patient with no brain stem responses, the spinal cord reflexes may reappear after a period of time without alteration in the level of consciousness.

The full-term infant is usually in a posture of flexion with the arms adducted at the shoulders and flexed at the elbows, wrists, and fingers. The thumb may be in the palm. The legs are flexed at the hips, knees, and ankles. When placed supine, the baby maintains essentially the same posture. This flexion posture is normal for the first few weeks of life. The infant then begins to extend, and the thumbs are no longer in the palms. Deviation from this flexion posture occurs with hypotonia. Conditions that produce hypotonia in the newborn include excessive sedation, hypoxia, hypoglycemia, injury to the spinal cord, Werdnig-Hoffmann disease, neonatal myasthenia gravis, and myotonic dystrophy. With injury to the spinal cord, the infant is usually initially flaccid, and bladder function is decreased or absent, a factor that can be helpful in separating this from other causes of hypotonia that may present with a similar clinical picture. The hypotonia may be associated with other physical findings that are diagnostic, as in mongolism. Altered states of consciousness will also be associated with abnormal posture and tone.

After adequate observation of the infant, the next step is to make a careful inspection that will require manipulation and measurements.

The Head

The head should be observed for contour, evidence of bleeding into the scalp, scalp defects, vascular lesions, nodules in the skin, and size and tenseness of the anterior fontanel. Irregularities of bone density when present can be felt particularly in the frontal and parietal bones (lacunar skull). Cephalhematoma is confined to the area of periosteum over one bone and is not a diagnostic problem until about the third to fifth day, when the boundaries become elevated and firm in such a manner as to make the center of the hematoma feel like a depressed fracture. The most difficult problem with cephalhematoma is in the occipital region where it is not easily distinguished from a meningocele or encephalocele. The cephalhematoma will not vary in tenseness with a Valsalva maneuver that accompanies crying. In addition, there is no underlying bone defect, and the area usually does not transilluminate.

The head circumference should be measured with a firm cloth tape or metal tape. Paper tapes vary as much as 1 cm in the first 36 cm and are not as accurate because they are difficult to place and read. Occipitofrontal measurement of the head may vary by 1 to 2.5 cm over the first three to four days of life as the molded head assumes a more normal contour. It is the measurement taken at the time of discharge from the hospital following birth that is most helpful in determining the rate of head growth early in life. The infant with a large head at birth is at risk for hydrocephalus, hydranencephalus, megalencephalus, and agenesis of the corpus callosum. Those with small heads (below 31 cm) should be investigated for congenital infections, microcephalus, polymicrogyria, trisomy 18 or 13–15, and other syndromes associated with small heads. Auscultation of the head is absolutely mandatory in an infant with high-output cardiac failure. In infancy an intracranial arteriovenous malformation may present as high-output failure associated with an intracranial bruit. Most generalized intracranial bruits at this age are benign, however.

Transillumination of the head should be carried out in each newborn at risk for central nervous system problems. This is done in a dark room after the examiner has had time to adapt to the dark. A glow of more than 1 cm around a flashlight equipped with a rubber cuff is considered abnormal.

The Cranial Nerves

The cranial nerve examination is carried out in the same fashion as in the older child except that in general the olfactory nerve is not tested, since the validity of the methods used is in doubt.

Cranial Nerve II (Optic)

The term infant is able to fix on an object and follow it through about 60 degrees. The preferred test objects are a face and a red ball. The newborn is myopic; therefore, the object should be placed within 10 to 12 inches of the baby's eyes and moved from side to side. Pursuit is not smooth, and at intervals the eyes are not completely conjugate. Visual fields can be judged by observing the child turn to a light in the periphery of his visual field. Funduscopic examination is best accomplished by positioning the baby so that his head is slightly elevated. The ophthalmoscope should be set at minus 4 to 6 diopters in order to obtain the best view of the posterior fundus. The optic disc in the newborn has a grayish-white appearance. This normal color of the disc at birth can present a problem if there is a suspicion of optic atrophy. The diagnosis of optic atrophy in the newborn is dependent upon the entire funduscopic picture, including size of the disc, size and number of vessels, macular changes, and appearance of the retina in general. Optic atrophy in the newborn is usually associated with intracranial disease. Wandering nystagmus may not be present at birth, but will develop within a few weeks in the blind infant. If there is blindness, the infant will have no fixing and following response and no opticokinetic nystagmus. He may, however, blink at a bright light. Retinal hemorrhages are reported to occur in 8 to 52 per cent of newborns.[9] The incidence, in the experience of the authors, has been closer to 5 per cent and lacks good correlation with known complications of labor and delivery. Other retinal lesions that can be of diagnostic help include the chorioretinitis of toxoplasmosis, cytomegalic inclusion disease, rubella, and syphilis. At times the lesions of cytomegalic inclusion disease and toxoplasmosis can be confused, but destructive lesions with palisading are characteristic of toxoplasmosis. In the older literature, the lesions of toxoplasmosis and cytomegalic inclusion disease were referred to as "acquired coloboma," and these have been confused with true coloboma of the retina and choroid. When the macula alone is involved, however, the lesion is most likely to represent a congenital infection.[11]

Cranial Nerves III, IV, and VI (Oculomotor, Trochlear, and Abducens)

It is sometimes difficult to find the newborn with both eyes open and looking about at the time of examination. Since the doll's head movements of the eyes are normally present in the awake state at this age, however, it is possible, by posturing the infant, to have him open both eyes without distress. Frequently the pupil and iris are so similar in color that it is not easy to determine the size and equality of the pupils with accuracy, but there should be a definite response to light. It is important to compare the eyes for size of the globes, corneae, and palpebral fissures, and for ptosis and proptosis. Full range of movement of the eyes can be achieved with the doll's head maneuver. Eye movements, whether of the doll's head type or fixing and following, are not smooth in the newborn. Nystagmus with or without elicited eye movement is abnormal in the newborn, and if spontaneous, it suggests seizure activity.

An early clue to a Horner's syndrome may be a failure of eye opening on the side of the lesion. It should lead to a careful re-evaluation of pupil size and equality. A dilated pupil in the newborn may be secondary to direct trauma, eye drops, seizure activity, or on rare occasions, to transtentorial herniation.

Cranial Nerve V (Trigeminal)

To judge masseter strength in the newborn, the examiner can place a finger in the infant's mouth and determine the power of the biting portion of the suck. Pterygoids are judged by noting any deviation of the mandible when the mouth is opened to accept a nipple or to cry. The corneal reflex has not proved to be a reliable test of sensation in the newborn, but pinprick on the face will elicit a grimacing movement that begins on the side stimulated and may then become bilateral. If there is weakness on the side of the face under examination, then observe the opposite side of the face for the response.

Cranial Nerve VII (Facial)

Facial symmetry should be looked for with the patient at rest as well as with movement of the face. If there has been a forceps delivery, it is important to observe facial movements immediately after birth. Most mild injuries to the facial nerve will immediately produce some weakness of facial muscles that becomes more marked for a time and then clears. If the entire nerve or nucleus is involved, the infant cannot wrinkle the forehead or close the eyes well when crying, and the mouth will appear to "draw" to the normal side because the angle of the mouth cannot be moved laterally on the affected side. Absence of the triangularis oris muscle, which depresses the angle of the mouth, must be distinguished from lower facial weakness. In facial weakness of central origin (cortical or corticobulbar) the upper part of the face is less likely to be involved or may be less severely involved. Usually the infant sucks ineffectively and drools excessively. At times the weakness may be bilateral and not immediately recognized. Another clue to facial weakness is the ease with which the eyes can be held open for the funduscopic examination. Exposure keratitis secondary to inadequate closure of the eye is, of course, a serious complication of facial weakness.

Although it is clear that the newborn has an awareness of taste, we do not test this regularly as part of the neurological examination.

Cranial Nerve VIII (Vestibulocochlear)

Hearing is best tested in the awake newborn by introducing a single loud noise. This will frequently result in a Moro response or at least a sudden change in behavior. It is important to prevent the possibility of the startle being caused by a proprioceptive stimulus such as banging on the crib. If the initial response is not definite, it is best to proceed with the examination and then return to this area after a few minutes in order to insure that there has been no habituation to interfere with the infant's later response. If a proper response is not achieved, then the examination of the vestibular portion of the nerve becomes more critical. To observe the oculovestibular response, the examiner holds the infant upright at arm's length and spins around once or twice. The normal response is deviation of the eyes in the direction opposite the spin. In infants with congenital hearing defects this response is often lost, and the response to ice water in the ear may be minimal as well.[7]

Cranial Nerves IX and X (Glossopharyngeal and Vagus)

These nerves are tested together. An attempt to visualize the uvula usually produces a gag reflex in the newborn. At this time it is possible to visualize the active contraction of the soft palate and pharyngeal muscles. If there is weakness of the palate, the uvula deviates to the normal side. When evaluating the newborn's cry for hoarseness, it is important to know whether the infant required an endotracheal tube at the time of resuscitation. Endotracheal intubation may produce transient hoarseness secondary to direct trauma to the vocal cords. The newborn frequently regurgitates fluids through the nose, but this is usually the result of poor coordination of nasopharyngeal closure with vomiting rather than palatine weakness.

Cranial Nerve XI (Spinal Accessory)

The sternocleidomastoid muscle is best visualized by having the infant supine with his head extended over the edge of the table. Turning the head well to either side will display the bulk of the muscle so that any evidence of shortening or hematoma can be observed. The strength of the muscle is determined by the infant's attempts to right the head.

Cranial Nerve XII (Hypoglossal)

The tongue should be observed for atrophy and fasciculations. The crying normal newborn has gross fasciculations of the tongue. Fasciculations are significant only if the infant is at rest or asleep and the tongue has a "bag of worms" type of spontaneous movement. Atrophy is suspected when there are furrows in the tongue or when the tongue seems quite narrow for the size of the mouth. Power is best tested by noting the pull on the nipple or on the examiner's finger when it is introduced into the baby's mouth. Fasciculations of the tongue are seen at birth in infants with Werdnig-Hoffmann disease, but usually not for weeks or months in Pompe's disease. Atrophy of the tongue very strongly suggests the Möbius syndrome and should cause one to be extremely careful in the evaluation of other motor cranial nerve functions—especially nerves VI and VII.

Motor Evaluation

Observation of the infant's resting posture and spontaneous activity will be of help in directing attention to a specific asymmetry or abnormal posture. The term infant's posture of flexion persists even in sleep and is normal for the first two to three weeks of life (Figure 2–2). The hypotonic infant lies in a typical frog-leg posture—arms abducted at the shoulders and flexed at the elbows with the hands open and the palms up. The hips are similarly abducted, knees flexed, and ankles plantar flexed. The

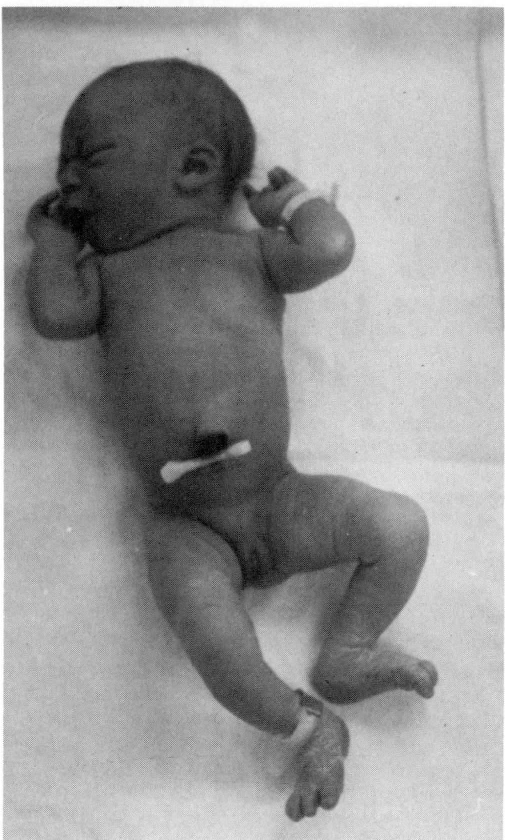

Figure 2–2 The normal flexed posture of the newborn infant at rest.

anterior-posterior diameter of the chest is decreased, and respirations may be diaphragmatic with little intercostal movement. The muscles of the face may also be lax; if the face is involved in the flaccidity, then one has to think of intracranial, metabolic, or other causes of generalized hypotonia. In the infant with a spinal cord injury, the cranial nerves will be spared unless there is marked hypoxia or superimposed intracranial injury. If the hypotonia is mild, it may be recognized as less flexion than usual for the infant, less resistance to passive movement, and more head lag when the infant is lifted by the hands into a sitting posture. If this procedure does not delineate the hypotonia, then the posture of the infant's head as he is placed back on the bed is of help. Normally, as the vertex of the head touches the bed, the infant will flex the head so as to assume a posture in which the weight of the head rests on the inion and occipital region. If tone is reduced, the infant may not be able to carry out this flexion maneuver and will be forced into a very awkward position with the head resting on the vertex. The hypotonic infant or the infant with reduced spontaneous activity should always be observed closely while at rest or asleep for fine "tremor"-type movements of the fingers and toes. These are characteristically seen in anterior horn cell disease and represent fasciculations. These movements are usually associated with a reduced muscle mass and weakness as well as hypotonia. Percussion myotonia is best demonstrated in the thenar muscles, mentalis muscle, and tongue. Because of the amount of fat present at this age it is difficult to demonstrate myotonia in other muscle groups.

Asymmetrical decrease in tone may represent peripheral nerve (brachial plexus) injury or recent hemiparesis.

Increased tone may be present shortly after birth as a result of hypoxia or intracranial bleeding. On occasion, it may be associated with hypocalcemia or hypoglycemia. The increased tone seen in the dysmature, particularly the postmature, newborn frequently is also associated with limitation of passive extension of the joints. This is usually a transient condition, and the origin of the increased tone is not understood. Decreased tone in the newborn is obvious; determination of increased tone can be a more difficult problem. To evaluate the upper extremities it is helpful to shake the wrist while holding the infant by the proximal forearm. This allows one to evaluate tone without evoking a flexion response to extension of the forearm. The same method can be used in the lower extremities. Increased tone should be suspected if the infant moves as a block with no head lag or extension at the elbows or knees when an attempt is made to pull him up with a traction grasp.

In the evaluation of tone, a comparison should be made between the two sides of the body and between the upper and lower extremities. Checking for tone in the newborn should be done with the infant's head in the midline position so as to avoid eliciting a tonic neck response.

Swallowing will be influenced by either increased or decreased tone as well as by problems of coordination of the movements of swallowing, as for example, in dysautonomia.

Strength is best evaluated by the infant's

spontaneous movements against gravity and his response to painful stimulation. The force of the infant's cry and the vigor of activity and resistance to unnatural postures or painful procedures are also helpful. In the newborn, strength cannot be tested as specifically as it can in the older child.

The normal newborn has rather smooth movements of opening and closing the hand, moving the hand to the face, and kicking spontaneously. At times any attempt at spontaneous movement will set off a series of pendular movements in a direction that may be perpendicular to the direction of his intended activity. These movements are most often seen in hypoxic infants and represent injury to the cerebellum and cerebellar connections; they are easily distinguished from the more rapid "jittery" movements seen in infants with mild hypoxia, hypocalcemia, hypoglycemia, and subarachnoid hemorrhage as well as some in whom the causes are unknown. Seizure activity must be considered as a possible cause of this movement. It can, however, be ruled out easily by supporting the extremity, whereupon the activity will cease, or by noting that the movement is of equal intensity in both directions, whereas seizure activity usually has a positive movement of flexion and extension by relaxation. The very weak newborn will sometimes make circular movements of the wrists and ankles when he cries or is excited—which has no meaning except to alert the examiner to the infant's proximal weakness.

Should arachnoschisis, meningocele, or myelomeningocele be present, a detailed description of the lesion (including its location and size, leakage, and the location of the neural ribbon or nerve roots as well as any motor and sensory deficits) should be recorded.

Brachial plexus injuries occur with some regularity and usually result from excessive traction either on the head with the shoulders in a fixed position, as in a vertex delivery, or on the body in an effort to deliver an after-coming head in the breech position. The most common injuries are the Erb's palsy or upper plexus injury (primarily C5–C6) and the complete plexus injury. Klumpke palsy (C7–T1) is less common.

The resting posture of the arm is a clue to the brachial plexus injury. The arm is usually extended and pronated. If the palsy is of the Erb type, the infant may move the fingers but does not flex or abduct the arm. The biceps reflex also will be absent. At times the diaphragm will be paralyzed on the affected side. Fracture of the clavicle or humerus may also be present and should be checked for prior to excessive manipulation. If the humerus is fractured, the possibility of radial nerve palsy must be considered as an additional problem. If Erb's palsy is bilateral, then spinal cord injury must be seriously considered and spine films obtained prior to flexion and extension of the neck on the rare chance that there may be dislocation of the cervical spine.

Klumpke's palsy, or lower brachial plexus injury, is rarely seen without Erb's palsy. The infant with the Klumpke type of paralysis has no flexion and only minimal extension of the fingers. This is noted by the lack of a grasp and avoidance response in that hand.[10] The avoidance response is produced by stroking the dorsum of the hand, causing reflex extension of the fingers. Horner's syndrome may also be present. Occasionally brachial plexus injuries are bilateral.

The developmental reflexes used to evaluate the newborn are best described as "primitive," since they do not require functional brain above the diencephalon and probably not above the mesencephalon.[8] They are, nevertheless, important. Although many developmental reflexes have been described, it is unlikely that all of them can be elicited in an infant at any one time. It is better to use six to eight developmental reflexes that usually are present in newborns and evaluate them consistently. The authors use the following ones:

The Moro reflex is easily elicited by placing one hand under the infant's shoulders and the other under his head, then suddenly dropping the head by several inches. The response consists of abduction and extension of the arms with extension of at least the third, fourth, and fifth fingers followed by adduction and flexion of the upper extremities. The infant appears startled and may cry. At times the lower extremities are extended. An asymmetry of response would suggest hemiparesis, brachial plexus injury, or fracture of the humerus or clavi-

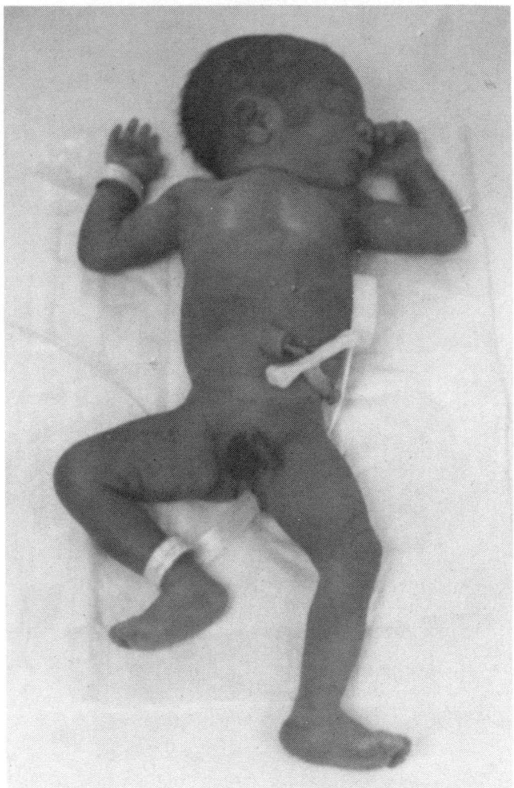

Figure 2–3 A normal term infant demonstrating an incomplete tonic neck reflex.

cle. If the infant is suspected of having a spinal cord injury, however, the neck should not be hyperextended and the reflex should be obtained by using other stimuli such as sound.

The tonic neck reflex frequently is incomplete or absent in normal infants. It is most helpful when abnormal. The response is obtained by turning the head to the side—the arm and leg on the side to which the chin is turned will extend with increased tone (Fig. 2–3). The arm and leg on the side of the occiput will flex with a decrease in tone. After a few seconds, the infant should be able to break the posture even if the head is not allowed to return to the midline.

The stepping reflex is easy to observe. The infant is held upright as his weight is applied to the foot in contact with the bed; the leg extends and the other leg flexes; then the series is reversed. The hypertonic baby will hold both legs in extension, and the hypotonic infant will not bear weight. This type of reflex stepping disappears at about 3 to 4 months of age.

The placing response is demonstrated when pressure is applied in a proximal to distal direction over the dorsum of the foot with the infant held upright. This action results in reflex placement of the foot on the stimulus object. The response should be equal bilaterally (Fig. 2–4).

Truncal incurvation (*Galant reflex*) is easily obtained if the infant is held with the anterior chest wall in the palm of the examiner's hand and firm pressure, as with the

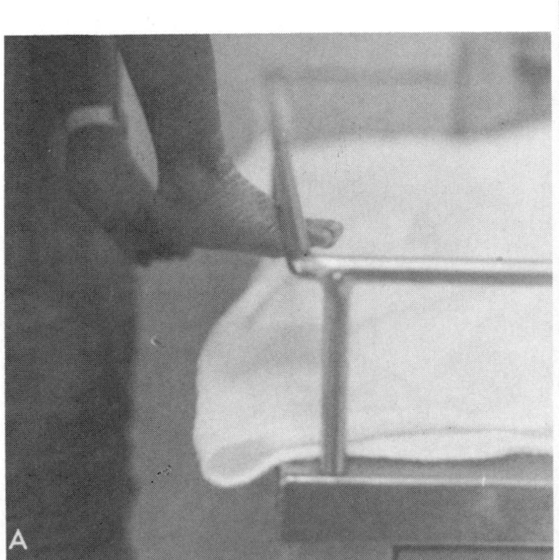

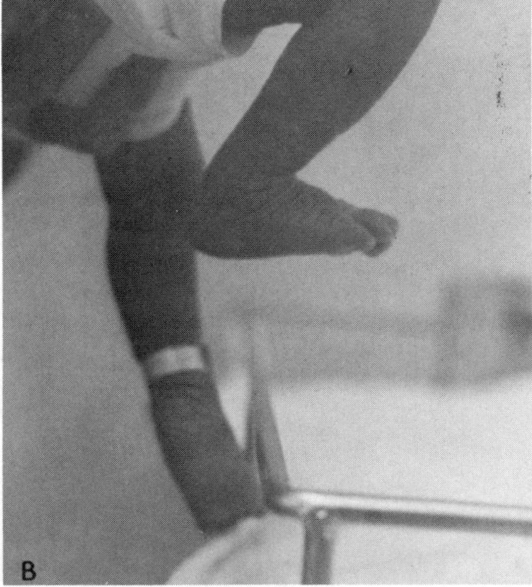

Figure 2–4 *A*. The dorsum of the newborn infant's foot is being stimulated by touch at onset of the placing reflex. *B*. Final phase of flexion of the leg in the placing reflex.

thumb, is applied along the paraspinal region of the thoracolumbar area. There is flexion of the pelvis to the side of the stimulus and there may be extension of the leg on the same side. An asymmetrical response must be evaluated in terms of any known motor or sensory deficits.

Palmar grasp is present in the newborn and is stimulated by applying pressure to the palm of the hand, which results in flexion of the fingers and a firm grasp on the object. If traction is then applied, it is possible to lift the infant from the bed, i.e., traction grasp. If there is a cervical spinal cord injury, lower brachial plexus injury, or hypotonia, this reflex is lost.

The plantar grasp is similar to the palmar grasp. A firm stimulus, the thumb, is applied to the sole of the foot just proximal to the toes, causing flexion of the toes around the stimulus object. The "tonic" plantar grasp response may be spontaneous, is seen in infants with hypertonia, particularly that secondary to hypoxia, and is not normal. Absence of the plantar grasp reflex is seen in infants with spinal cord injuries and in hypotonic infants.

The rooting reflex is elicited by touch to the cheek. The head turns to the side of the stimulus and the mouth moves in an attempt to capture the stimulus. This reflex will be weak or not present in the infant who has just been fed or in whom alertness is decreased for other reasons such as bulbar involvement, hypotonia, or hypertonia.

An adequate number of deep tendon reflexes can be obtained with ease in the newborn. Of these we usually record the biceps, brachioradialis, adductor, patellar, and Achilles reflexes. Reflexes are frequently excessively brisk in the crying infant; if the infant is sleeping or quiet, they should be normal. Sustained ankle clonus is common in the crying newborn, but when the child is at rest it is not normally present. Reflexes should be recorded in tabular form so that there is no confusion about which have been tested and their evaluation.

The plantar response in the newborn is one of flexion.[5] It is important to have the infant awake, the head in the midline, and the legs extended. The first movement of the great toe from its neutral position will be one of plantar flexion when a firm stimulus is applied to the lateral surface of the heel (Fig. 2–5). It is important to be aware of the normal response. An upgoing toe in the newborn implies brain stem or spinal cord involvement primarily. The plantar response does not correlate with hypoxia, hemorrhage, or trauma to the hemisphere in this age group.

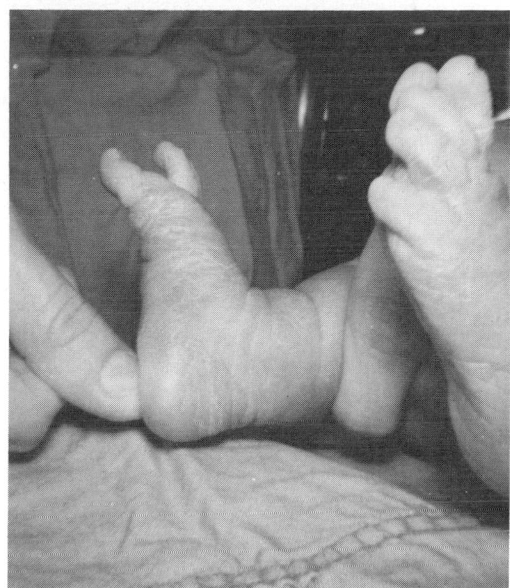

Figure 2–5 The foot of a newborn as pressure is applied to the lateral portion of the heel, demonstrating that the first movement of the great toe is in plantar flexion, the normal response in a newborn.

Sensory Evaluation

The newborn response to pain can be evaluated only when the baby is awake and relatively quiet. It must be remembered that the response to pain is much slower and less well localized in the newborn than in the older infant. Usually it is easier to interpret the response if a single stimulus is applied for a prolonged period of time—for seconds or until there is a response. The response will vary from a change in respiratory pattern or a change in heart rate, color, or level of alertness to withdrawal of the stimulated part. This method is most successful in delineating a sensory level, as in myelomeningocele. A less exact response can be obtained by a series of rapid stimuli using summation to get a more general response.

THE YOUNG CHILD (THE FIRST TWO YEARS)

The neurological examination of the young child presents the greatest difficulty to those physicians who deal primarily with adults and older children, but in some instances presents a real challenge even to the most experienced pediatrician. The manner in which the young child is first approached often means the difference between success and failure of the examination. The child is not a small adult, cannot be approached as such, often finds the situation frightening, and at this age does not respond to assurances that the examination is not painful. He is most secure in the mother's lap, and fortunately, most of the examination can be accomplished while the mother is holding him. The neurological examination of the young child consists first of clinical observation and second of specific manipulation. Observation of the child at play yields valuable information, and in addition, the use of simple toys will contribute significantly to the successful completion of the examination. Those parts of the examination that require physical manipulation and are likely to be painful or frightening should be deferred until the end.

Evaluation of the child should begin during the history taking session with observation of the child at spontaneous play. One can assess the infant's level of alertness, spontaneous movement, facial expression, efforts of vocalization, and response to his surroundings. Gross physical deformities are usually also evident. The examination itself should begin with the child sitting in the mother's lap. The examiner should make an effort to gain the child's interest and cooperation. This is best accomplished by quietly talking to him, gently touching or patting him, and engaging him in simple play.

Cranial Nerve Evaluation

Most of the cranial nerve examination can be accomplished by observation. A bright object (red ball or block) is brought into the child's field of vision and moved through the various sectors of the visual field. The child should fix on the object and follow its movement (Fig. 2–6). This enables one to test vision (cranial nerve II) and to observe extraocular movement (cranial nerves III, IV, VI). With this simple maneuver one can also check for nystagmus, strabismus, and other involuntary movement of the eyes. Failure of the infant to fix and follow indicates blindness or intellectual dullness. The opticokinetic nystagmus response should be checked by moving an opticokinetic strip slowly before the child's eyes. Failure to respond suggests blindness or lack of attention. Response in one direction only, if the child is fixing on the strip, is suggestive of a visual field defect (Fig. 2–7). One cannot easily test each eye separately in this age group, but the visual fields can be tested grossly. An object is brought from behind the child's head into the peripheral visual field. The child will turn his head toward the object as it is picked up in the periphery. Each side should be tested. A true estimate of visual acuity is difficult to ascertain in the young child. If the child can pick up a small crumb or object from the table or floor, however, it is obvious that his vision is reasonably good. A light should be directed into each eye and moved back and forth between the two eyes to determine pupillary response and to assess the size and shape of the pupils (cranial nerve III). While these maneuvers are being done the child will usually respond by smiling and laughing or by whimpering and crying, thereby allowing one to observe movement of the facial musculature (cranial nerve VII) and providing an opportunity to judge the strength and symmetry of the facial muscles. The strength of the masseter muscles (cranial nerve V) can be determined by the force of

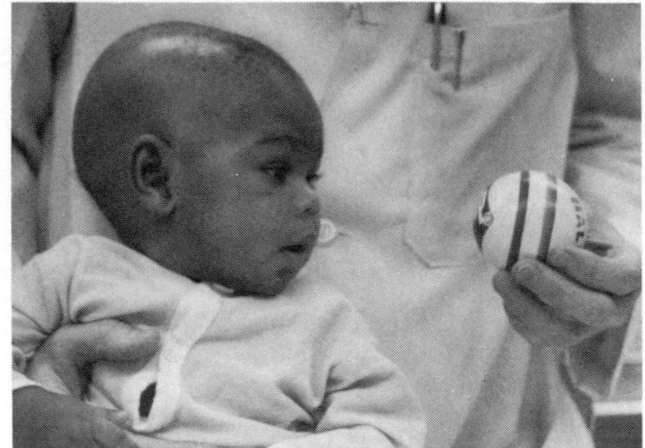

Figure 2–6 A 6-month-old infant turning his head and eyes to look at a brightly colored ball brought into his peripheral visual field.

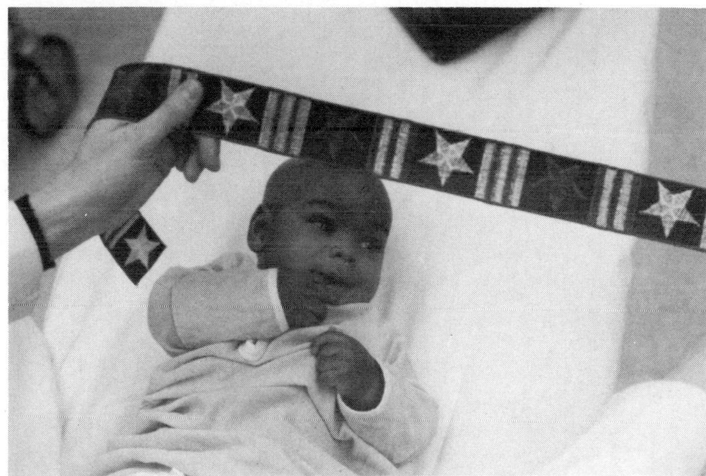

Figure 2–7 A 6-month-old infant attentively watching the opticokinetic strip and demonstrating an appropriate nystagmoid response.

the infant's suck on a pacifier, bottle, or the examiner's finger. Drooling and tongue thrusting are obvious if present. Hearing (cranial nerve VIII) can be tested grossly with the use of a bell, clacker, or tuning fork. The child must be quiet when the auditory stimulus is presented. Usually, he will turn or tilt the head to the side of the sound. He may respond by becoming very quiet, then smile and reach for the object producing the sound. Failure to respond to auditory stimuli or to the examiner's voice is usually indicative of some degree of hearing loss or of intellectual impairment. The young child will often imitate the examiner by protruding the tongue or, if he will not respond to the examiner, can usually be coaxed to stick his tongue out to lick a lollipop. This allows one to evaluate the tongue for deviation, atrophy, and the presence of fasciculations (cranial nerve XII). The remainder of the cranial nerves must be evaluated by direct manipulation of the patient.

Motor and Sensory Evaluation

The value of observation of the spontaneous movement of the infant and young child cannot be overemphasized. Gross defects of movement and coordination in carrying out simple and skilled motor tasks are easily detected and can be evaluated before the child realizes that he is being examined. This part of the examination is usually best done with the child on the floor between the mother and the examiner. The child is offered toys of different colors, sizes, and shapes, and is observed at play. His developmental milestones can be determined by his mastery of motor skills. It is of course necessary that the child's motor ability be evaluated in reference to what is average for his particular age; a summary of developmental milestones at specific ages is presented in Table 2–1.

Evaluation of the motor system requires a determination of muscle mass, tone, and power, and includes tests of coordination. In the young child it is almost impossible to test individual muscles, but observation of the child's spontaneous movement will provide information concerning weakness, spasticity, and incoordination. Spontaneous movements of the extremities are a good guide to muscle strength. Decreased movement of an extremity associated with persistent fisting, flexion posture of the arm, and palmar thumb position are all suggestive of infantile hemiparesis (Fig. 2–8). The child should be observed for hand preference. If hand preference is developed before 18 months of age, then one must strongly suspect weakness or spasticity of the opposite limb.

Muscle tone, the resistance of muscle to passive stretch, should be tested. The child must be relaxed before a true estimate of muscle tone can be made. The muscles most affected by spasticity are the flexors of the upper extremities, the adductors and flexors of the hips, the extensors of the knees, and the plantar flexors of the feet. Passive dorsiflexion of the feet at the ankles or gentle abduction of the legs at the hips meets with firm resistance if spasticity is

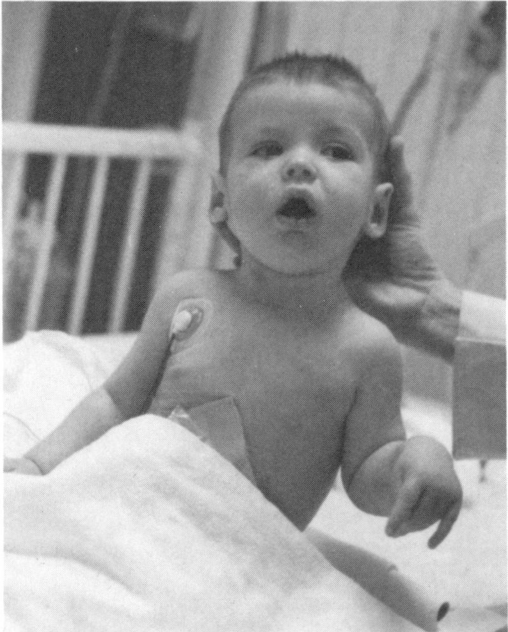

Figure 2–8 An 11-month-old infant with a left hemiparesis demonstrating flexion of the left arm at the elbow and wrist and a palmar thumb.

present. With continued steady pressure the resisting muscles give way in a clasp-knife reaction. With rigidity, the resistance to passive movement is constant throughout a full range of movement. Spasticity of the adductors of the hips results in scissoring of the lower extremities (crossing of the legs). Persistent toe walking suggests spasticity or a contracture of the Achilles tendons. Decreased resistance is characteristic of the hypotonic or floppy infant. The child lies in a frog-leg position with arms abducted at the shoulder and flexed at the elbows, the hands open with the palms up. The legs are abducted at the hips, the knees flexed, and the ankles plantar flexed. The extremities are easily extended and flexed. Head control is very poor, and when the child is held under the arms and lifted, he tends to slip through the examiner's fingers. In the evaluation of tone, a comparison should be made between the two sides of the body and between the upper and lower extremities.

Muscle mass is very difficult to evaluate in the young child because of the large amount of subcutaneous fat. An obvious asymmetry of muscle would be of concern. Excessive muscle mass is best noted in the thenar eminence, the anterior compartment of the lower leg, and the gastrocnemius or other muscles not obscured by fat. At any age, however, when muscle weakness is associated with atrophy and fasciculation, disease of the lower motor neuron is present.

Tests of coordination requiring rapid alternating movements and complicated movements are of little value in this age group. The child should be observed while reaching for an object. This will bring out dystonic and athetoid movements. The child often will refuse to do finger-to-nose or heel-to-shin tests, but he will usually reach for and touch the end of a pen light (Fig. 2–9). The intention tremor of cerebellar origin is characterized by an accentuation of the tremor as the patient approaches the target. An essential or action tremor, which is believed to be the result of dysfunction of the red nucleus and its connections, has the same amplitude of excursion throughout the action being performed. All tremors and involuntary movements, unless severe, disappear with sleep except for myoclonic jerks and clonic seizures. The persistence of involuntary movement during sleep may in some instances be an important diagnostic point.

The deep tendon reflexes are elicited in the usual manner, but in order to elicit them in a child the patient must be relaxed. Per-

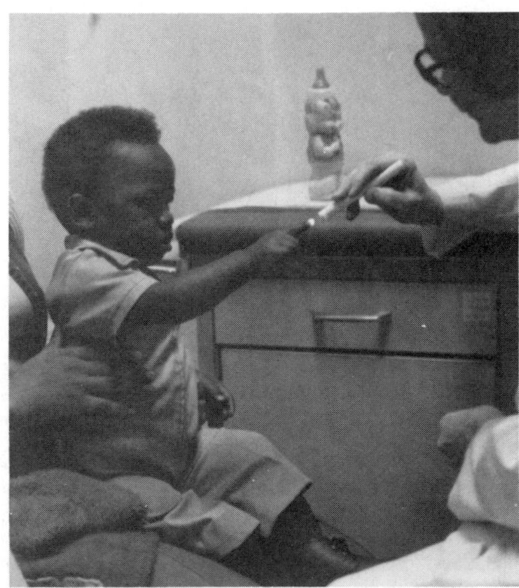

Figure 2–9 A 1-year-old child "turning off" the pen light with his index finger.

sistent absence of the deep tendon reflexes suggests anterior horn cell disease or peripheral neuropathy. Hyperactive deep tendon reflexes generally suggest upper motor neuron disease, especially if they are unilateral. The plantar reflex in children is normally flexor; an extensor plantar response in an awake child, if the test is properly performed, is abnormal. Ankle clonus after 2 months of age is abnormal in the resting infant.

A complete sensory examination is impossible in this age group. One must rely on the child's facial expression or withdrawal from touch or pinprick. The child of 1 to 2 years will often become upset when he sees the examiner with a pin. He will, however, use the pin himself with the examiner watching.

Examination of the heart, lungs, and abdomen is best accomplished while the child is sitting quietly in the mother's lap. A careful abdominal examination is necessary to evaluate hepatomegaly or splenomegaly, both of which often are present in the storage diseases. A thorough general evaluation of the child's state of nutrition, body proportions, head, skin, and extremities should be done. The specific areas of concern have been delineated previously.

The examination of the eyes, ears, nose, and throat is deferred until last. The eyes should be assessed for size and shape, epicanthus, proptosis, ptosis, cataracts, and abnormality of iris and sclera. Funduscopic examination is an essential part of the neurological evaluation. The fundi should be examined for vascular lesions, colobomas, tumors, hemorrhage, and degenerative changes. The optic discs should be examined for color, disc margin, evidence of papilledema, and abnormal masses such as the mulberry lesion of tuberous sclerosis. Examination of the fundi offers one the opportunity to check the child's ability to close his eyes tightly. The oropharynx should be examined for shape of palate and symmetry of palatal movement. The gag reflex (cranial nerves IX, X) is usually elicited with ease in the young child. The sternocleidomastoid muscle strength (cranial nerve XI) can be determined by the force with which the child moves his head from side to side in order to resist examination.

The examination ends with transillumination of the head in all children under one year of age and in older children if indicated. The method of transillumination was described earlier in the section on the neurological examination.

A complete neurological evaluation of the young child *can* be accomplished. The systematic approach, however, cannot be utilized. The examination is done in steps with no logical sequence, and the exact method is dictated by the age and the cooperation of the patient.

THE OLDER CHILD (TWO TO SIX YEARS)

The neurological examination of the older child can be done in a more systematic and formal manner. Observation and game-playing are still utilized to some degree, and the exact method of examination is, of course, determined by the attitude of the patient. The methods previously described for evaluating the younger child may be necessary in some instances, but as a general rule the child of 2 to 6 years will cooperate if examined in a relaxed and pleasant environment.

A general statement about the patient's level of responsiveness and his ability to cooperate should be recorded. Does he answer questions appropriate for his age? Examples would be questions about the patient's age and sex and the names of siblings. Is his speech understandable? Does he sit quietly in his mother's lap or a chair, or is he in constant motion? Observe parent-child interaction. Is the parent in control or is the child in control? Observe for obvious physical abnormalities, such as tics, nystagmus, facial asymmetry, abnormal movements, or seizure activity. Comment on the size (by measurement) and contour of the head.

Cranial Nerves

Cranial Nerve I (Olfactory)

The sense of smell is tested by presenting to the child certain pleasant odors such as peppermint, vanilla, coffee. Irritants should not be used, since they stimulate the trigeminal nerve. The child does not need to identify the different odors, but he should be able to distinguish a change in the odor. Each nostril should be tested separately. The most common cause for bilateral loss of smell in children is nasal congestion due to upper respiratory infections—a unilateral loss of smell would be of greater significance. It is noteworthy that tumors and congenital anomalies in the cribriform plate region are uncommon and are unusual causes of anosmia. Loss of smell in children can, however, result from head trauma.

Cranial Nerve II (Optic)

Visual acuity can be tested in the older child with standard eye charts. Special cards using pictures of toys and common objects can be used for the preschool child. Each eye should be tested separately. Visual fields should be tested. The confrontation test is an integral part of the neurological examination. The examiner should sit or stand in front of the child and have him look at the examiner's nose or eye. The patient is asked to cover one eye gently. The examiner then holds up both hands and asks the child to point to the side on which he sees a finger move. The child's ability to see small movements in each quadrant of each field should be tested. Opticokinetic nystagmus can be tested by moving across the field of vision a piece of cloth on which a series of figures or designs is printed on a plain background (see Fig. 2–7). Normally the child fixes on each figure, follows it, and jerks his eyes back to follow the next figure. For an adequate response to occur, the child must fix on the figures and have sufficient visual acuity to follow the movement. Absence of response or an asymmetrical response, if the child fixes on the figure, is abnormal and indicates loss of visual acuity or a visual field defect. All visual field and visual acuity testing should be carried out in a well-lighted room.

The funduscopic examination is mandatory, the fundi being examined for vascular lesions, colobomas, tumors, hemorrhage, and degenerative change. The optic discs should be examined for color, disc margins, evidence of papilledema, and abnormal masses such as the mulberry lesions of tuberous sclerosis. In children the optic disc margins may be indistinct and slightly elevated. This is especially true with hyperopia. In myopia, deposits of pigment, myopic crescents, are frequently seen along the temporal margin. In early papilledema, blurring of the disc margin, earliest on the nasal side, is associated with edema and streaking of the retina, venous distention, and hyperemia of the nerve head. Elevation of the nerve head, progressive blurring of disc margins, obliteration of the optic cup, and hemorrhage and exudate are signs of advanced papilledema. Acute optic neuritis in which the nerve head itself is involved presents a picture identical to that of papilledema. Loss of visual acuity, however, occurs early with optic neuritis and does not occur until late in papilledema.

Cranial Nerves III, IV, VI (Oculomotor, Trochlear, Abducens)

Pupils are observed for size and any irregularities in shape or inequality in size, anisocoria, as well as for their reaction to light, direct or consensual, and for convergence. Dilatation and constriction of the pupils is mediated through the sympathetic and parasympathetic fibers respectively. Interruption of the sympathetic pathway results in Horner's syndrome with a constricted pupil, associated mild ptosis, and loss of sweating on the ipsilateral side of the face. Interruption of the parasympathetic fibers results in a dilated fixed pupil that either does not respond or responds poorly to light. In this case, the dilated fixed pupil is usually associated with marked ptosis and inability to move the eye in the direction mediated by the extraocular muscles innervated by the third cranial nerve. If there is unilateral blindness as the result of an optic nerve or retinal lesion, the dilated pupil fails to respond to direct light but does give a consensual response of constriction when the opposite eye is illuminated. If vision in the eye is decreased rather than lost, the pupillary response to direct light stimulation is sluggish while consensual response is fully intact. The normal eye maintains equal constriction with direct and consensual stimulation. Pupillary responses are normal in children with cortical blindness, and these children will blink at a bright light. A dilated pupil that reacts briskly in accommodation but slowly in response to a bright light is referred to as a tonic, or Adies, pupil. This can occur with absence of the ankle jerks, a combination of phenomena that is not associated with known disease. A tonic pupil is frequently associated with familial dysautonomia. A dilated, fixed pupil may result from direct trauma to the eye. A transiently dilated, unreactive pupil may accompany a seizure. The pupil on the side of the seizure discharge is most often involved. Small irregular pupils that react in accommodation but not to light are referred to as Argyll Robertson pupils. These are seen in association with juvenile paresis, tabes dorsalis, and diabetes mellitus.

Strabismus, a lack of parallelism between the visual axes at rest and in following an object, is common in children. It is especially frequent in the age group 2 to 4 years and is most often due to excessive convergence in association with hyperopia. Esotropia, turning in of one eye, results from the accommodative effort necessary to overcome the refractive error. At the onset of esotropia a bright 2-year-old may complain of diplopia for several days or a week until the vision in the "squinted" eye is suppressed. The esotropia at first is intermittent, but may become constant with resultant loss of vision in the squinting eye. In this functional type of strabismus, movements of the eyes individually are full. With paralytic strabismus, the dissociation of the eyes varies with the direction of gaze. Movement of the involved eye in the field of action of the paralyzed muscle is limited when individual muscles are tested.

The examiner must have a basic knowledge of the action of the extraocular muscles in order to do adequate testing. Cogan has published a comprehensive discussion of the function of the extraocular muscles.[1] Those muscles innervated by the oculomotor nerve include the superior, inferior, and medial recti, the inferior oblique, and the elevator of the eyelid, the levator palpebrae superioris. Lesions of the third cranial, or oculomotor, nerve produce a combination of ptosis, a large pupil that is poorly reactive to light, and an outward and downward displacement of the eye with defective adduction and elevation. The trochlear nerve innervates the superior oblique muscle. With fourth cranial, or trochlear, nerve involvement, the eye fails to move down when adducted and the head may be tilted away from the side of the paretic muscle. The sixth cranial, or abducens, nerve innervates the lateral rectus. Sixth cranial nerve palsies are probably the most common in children. The eye fails to abduct, and the patient often rotates the head in the direction of the paralyzed muscle. Weakness of the extraocular movements occurs in pontine glioma, cavernous sinus thrombosis, brain stem encephalitis, myasthenia gravis, and ocular myopathy. Increased intracranial pressure often produces unilateral or bilateral sixth nerve palsy.

Abnormal eye movements can result from cerebral hemisphere or brain stem disease. With destructive lesions of the cerebral hemisphere, the eyes initially deviate toward the side of the lesion, with the conjugate gaze palsy to the opposite side. With irritative lesions of the cerebral hemisphere, the eyes deviate away from the side of the lesion. In brain stem lesions, the conjugate eye movements are deviated away from the side of the lesion and the conjugate gaze toward the side of the lesion is paralyzed. To check for gaze palsy the eyes are checked for movement together, and then each eye is checked for movement separately. With gaze palsy the eyes do not move together, although when checked separately, each eye has full range of movement.

Intranuclear ophthalmoplegia is the result of dysfunction of the medial longitudinal fasciculus and in children is most often caused by brain stem tumor. Other diseases in young children that may affect this area are brain stem encephalitis, hemoglobinopathies, leukemia, and collagen vascular diseases. These lesions are characterized by pareses of the medial rectus function of the adducting eye and a monocular nystagmus in the abducting eye. If convergence is intact, the lesion is thought to be more posterior in the pons or medulla. If convergence is absent, then the lesion involves the midbrain.[1]

External ophthalmoplegia is characterized by ptosis and paralysis of all extraocular muscles. The pupillary responses remain normal. External ophthalmoplegia is most likely to occur in diseases that affect primarily the motor end-plate or muscle. Vertical gaze paralysis is always indicative of brain stem disease. Lesions in the tectal region result in paralysis of upward gaze and, in children, they usually are the result of kernicterus, pineal tumor, hydrocephalus, or other causes of increased intracranial pressure. Paralysis of downward gaze is the result of lesions in the periaqueductal region (tectum) and may be associated with failure of upward gaze, as in Parinaud's syndrome.

The patient should be checked for the presence or absence of nystagmus in the primary position and in all four directions of gaze. The direction of the nystagmus is determined by the fast component. Horizontal jerk nystagmus is usually indicative of dysfunction of the labyrinth or the central connections within the brain stem and the cerebellum. Pure vertical nystagmus is always indicative of brain stem (pons) dysfunction. Lateral nystagmus due to cerebellar disease is usually coarser and of greater amplitude when gaze is directed toward the side of the lesion. See-saw nystagmus in which the eyes alternately rise and fall is seen with lesions about the optic chiasm that are associated with bitemporal hemianopia. The nystagmus seen in the blind child consists of irregular wandering or searching eye movements of marked amplitude without a rapid jerk component. Congenital nystagmus and the nystagmus of spasmus nutans consist of to-and-fro oscillations of one or both eyes in which the fast and slow components cannot be discerned.

Cranial Nerve V (Trigeminal)

The sensory division of the fifth cranial nerve innervates the skin over the face and the anterior half of the scalp. The motor division of this nerve supplies the muscles of mastication. Check the two masseter muscles when the patient bites hard and note if they contract equally. Determine if the mandible deviates to one side when the child attempts to lower the jaw against resistance. The jaw jerk is elicited by a gentle downward tap of the reflex hammer on the examiner's finger resting on the chin. This is a stretch reflex involving the masseter muscles and is brisk or accentuated in the presence of bilateral corticobulbar disease. Unilateral dysfunction of the fifth nerve results in deviation of the jaw to the side of the lesion because of weakness of the ipsilateral pterygoid muscle. Atrophy of the temporalis muscle with hollowing of the temporal fossa associated with a constantly open mouth and malocclusion is characteristic of myotonic dystrophy. Test for loss of sensation of touch or pinprick on the face in all three divisions separately. Disturbances of sensation are manifest by numbness and paresthesia. Test the corneal reflex by touching the cornea with a wisp of cotton while the gaze is directed upward. It is best to present the stimulus from the side in order to minimize the visual cue. The most common cause of impaired sensation in the face and loss of corneal reflex in this age group is a cerebellopontine angle or brain stem tumor.

Cranial Nerve VII (Facial)

The facial nerve is divided into motor and sensory divisions. The motor division supplies the muscles of facial expression, and the sensory division innervates the taste buds over the anterior two thirds of the tongue. Note any facial asymmetry at rest and with voluntary movement such as showing the teeth and closing the eyes tightly. Can the patient frown or raise his eyebrows? Interruption or dysfunction of the nerve at the facial nucleus in the pons or in the facial nerve trunk results in a peripheral facial paralysis of the ipsilateral side of the face. The patient is unable to wrinkle the forehead, close the eye, or retract the eye on the same side as the lesion. A lesion above the pons in the upper brain stem (supranuclear) or in the cerebral hemisphere contralateral to the side of the face involved produces a central facial weakness, which is characterized by weakness of retraction of the corner of the mouth, flattening of the nasolabial fold, and widening of the palpebral fissure opposite the side of the lesion. Wrinkling of the forehead is normal.

With disease of the facial nerve and chorda tympani in the subarachnoid space or facial canal there will also be impairment of taste on the anterior two thirds of the tongue. To test for taste, the child is asked to stick out the tongue. The examiner should hold the tongue with a piece of gauze and place on it in turn solutions containing salt, sugar, vinegar, and quinine. The child should not retract the tongue into the mouth until he has made an appropriate response. One usually does not check for taste sensation unless involvement of associated cranial nerves or lesions of the brain stem are suspected.

Cranial Nerve VIII (Vestibulocochlear)

The eighth cranial nerve is composed of an auditory and a vestibular division. These nerves originate respectively in the end-organ in the cochlea and in the labyrinth and course together through the temporal bone to central nuclei in the brain stem. There are a variety of methods to assess hearing. Does the child respond to a whispered command, turn his head toward a ringing bell, and respond to a tuning fork? Check for lateralization. The older child can be checked by formal audiometric testing. Abnormality of the labyrinth results in vestibular imbalance and is characterized clinically by vertigo. Caloric testing is used in assessing vestibular function as well as for determining the brain stem function of the comatose patient. The patient should be supine with the head flexed 30 degrees. Ice water (5 to 10 ml) is instilled into the external auditory canal. In the alert patient, the response consists of coarse nystagmus away from the ear stimulated. There is no eye deviation. As the level of consciousness decreases, the response to caloric stimulation consists first of tonic deviation of the eyes to the side stimulated and nystagmus to the opposite side. With further decrease in consciousness the response consists of tonic deviation of the eyes to the side of the lesion and loss of nystagmus. With deep coma, caloric stimulation produces no deviation of the eyes or nystagmus.

Cranial Nerves IX, X (Glossopharyngeal, Vagus)

The ninth and tenth nerves are usually tested together. Examination of the palate, pharynx, and larynx is sufficient for adequate testing. Difficulty in swallowing, regurgitation of liquid through the nose, and changes in the quality of the voice are common symptoms attributable to lesion of these nerves. The palate is observed during articulation (ah). When paralyzed, the palate does not move on the affected side and the uvula deviates away from the weak side. Movement of the uvula can be misleading, however, as sometimes it is adherent to a tonsil. With palatal weakness, the voice assumes a nasal quality. The gag reflex is tested by rubbing a cotton-tipped stick or tongue blade against the posterior wall of the pharynx. The responses of the two sides should be compared. The gag reflex is normally quite variable among patients, but a striking asymmetry of response of the two sides would be of diagnostic significance. Vocal cord dysfunction should be assessed by voice tone and volume, hoarseness, stridor, and dysphonia.

Cranial Nerve XI (Spinal Accessory)

The spinal accessory nerve supplies the sternocleidomastoid and trapezius muscles. To test the sternocleidomastoid muscle have the child turn his head to either side against resistance. The trapezius muscle is tested by having the child elevate his shoulder. These maneuvers will allow for visualization and palpation of the muscles tested, thus permitting one to discern atrophy or hypertrophy as well as strength of movement.

Cranial Nerve XII (Hypoglossal)

The tongue is innervated by this nerve, and if a lesion involves the nucleus, there will be atrophy and fasciculation of the ipsilateral side of the tongue. The tongue, on protrusion, deviates to the side of the lesion. With impairment of the tongue movement, dysarthria and dysphagia ensue. The patient cannot protrude the tongue toward the unaffected side nor can he protrude the tongue against the cheek on the unaffected side. If the lesion is bilateral, movement is decreased bilaterally and the tongue is small. With supranuclear lesions there is no atrophy or fasciculation, but dysarthria and dysphagia are prominent. The tongue may be excessively large in mongolism, cretinism, Pompe's disease, and Beckwith's syndrome.

Motor Evaluation

Station and Gait

The child is asked to stand first with eyes open and then with eyes closed. If he is unsteady, check to see whether he falls consistently to one side and whether the unsteadiness is increased when the eyes are closed. Have the child walk back and forth

TABLE 2–2 CHARACTERISTIC DISORDERS OF GAIT

GAIT	CHARACTERISTICS
Hemiplegic	Circumduction of leg, stiff knee, scraping of toe with failure of dorsiflexion of the foot
Spastic paraplegic	Slow, stiff, with tilting of pelvis and delayed flexion of hips Child walks on toes
Steppage	Flapping of feet, feet lifted too high
Sensory ataxic	Wide-based, uneven stamping steps
Cerebellar	Wide-based, irregularity and deviation or staggering on turning
Hysterical	Gait inconsistent with ability to move extremities Long hesitation before moving each foot, elaborate balancing movements of trunk and arms
Waddling	Lordosis, prominent abdomen, marked shift of pelvis as weight is shifted from one leg to other, excessive arm swing Gait typical of proximal weakness of pelvic girdle as in muscle disease or hip dislocation

in the usual manner. Normally he will walk with a narrow base, with no unsteadiness, and will display symmetrical arm swing. Observe whether he reels or deviates and whether he swings his extremities naturally. Is the base wide, and does he lift his feet unusually high? To bring out disorders of gait have the child walk with eyes open and then with eyes shut, walk on a line "heel to toe," walk on toes and heels, make sudden turns, and run. Some characteristic disorders of gait are listed in Table 2–2.

Mass, Tone, and Power

Observe the bulk of the muscle and note any hypertrophy or atrophy and the presence or absence of fasciculations. Hypertrophy of the gastrocnemius and deltoids is characteristic of Duchenne's muscular dystrophy. Atrophy associated with fasciculation is characteristic of lower motor neuron disease. Muscle strength can be tested without difficulty in the older child; a good screening test includes having the patient lift his head while in a supine position, turn the head from side to side against resistance, raise his arms above his head and keep them there against resistance, walk on heels and toes, arise from a sitting position on the floor, and walk up stairs. A method for grading muscle strength is given in Table 2–3.

TABLE 2–3 GRADING OF MUSCLE STRENGTH

GRADE	CHARACTERISTIC
0	No muscular contraction
1	Trace, visible contraction without motion of joint
2	Movement but not against gravity
3	Full movement at joint against gravity, variable resistance
4	Resists opposing force of moderate strength
5	Maximal resistance

Tone is determined by evaluating the resistance of the muscle to passive movement. Spasticity has a "clasp-knife" character, resistance being greatest at the initiation of passive movement and then giving way suddenly as the movement persists. Rigidity is characterized by constant resistance throughout passive movement. Shaking the extremity is helpful in bringing out slight degrees of altered tone. Decreased muscle tone is present in anterior horn cell disease and peripheral neuropathy. Increased tone is characteristic of corticospinal tract disease and is also associated with disease of the basal ganglia.

Coordination

The child should be observed for abnormal movements and for tremors. Incoordination is best demonstrated by having the child perform the finger-to-nose test, finger-to-finger (repetitive tapping of thumb and forefinger) test, heel-to-knee-to-shin test, rapid alternating pronation-supination movements, and rapid gentle tapping of the examiner's hand. These tests are of great value in assessing cerebellar integrity. It is obvious that weakness of an extremity will produce difficulties with coordinated movements that are often mistaken for cerebellar dysfunction.

Deep Tendon Reflexes

The deep tendon reflexes are muscle stretch reflexes and are obtained by sharply tapping the tendon of the muscle to be tested. They should be examined routinely, and their status should be recorded as shown in Table 2–4.

TABLE 2–4 EVALUATION OF REFLEXES

GRADING OF REFLEXES

	Biceps	*Triceps*	*Brachioradialis*	*Patellar*	*Achilles*	*Plantar*
R	2+	2+	2+	2+	2+	↓
L	2+	2+	2+	2+	2+	↓

SEGMENTAL LEVEL OF REFLEXES*

Reflex	*Segmental Level*
Tendon reflex	
Jaw jerk	Pons; fifth nerve
Biceps	Cervical 5–6
Brachioradialis	Cervical 5–6
Triceps	Cervical 6–8
Patellar	Lumbar 3–4
Achilles	Sacral 1–2
Other reflexes usually tested	
Corneal	Pons; fifth and seventh nerves
Gag	Medulla; ninth and tenth nerves
Abdominal	Thoracic 8–12
Cremasteric	Lumbar 1–2
Plantar	Lumbar 5; Sacral 1–2

* Modification of table from Dodge, P. R., *in* Farmer, T. W., ed.: Pediatric Neurology. 2nd Ed. Hagerstown, Md., Harper & Row, 1975.

Sensory Evaluation

A complete sensory examination is impossible in a child under 4 years of age, and in this age group, one must rely on the child's facial expression or withdrawal from touch or pinprick. In the child over the age of 4 years, one can do a complete sensory examination. At 4 years old or older, the tests can disclose abnormalities of touch, pain, temperature, vibration, and position sense. Once these modalities have been determined to be intact, one can proceed to evaluate cortical sensation. Cortical tests include two-point discrimination, stereognosis, opticokinetic nystagmus, neglect, and graphesthesia.

Two-point discrimination tests reveal the patient's ability to distinguish a stimulus of one or two points close together. The minimal discernible distance between two simultaneous points is measured. The fingertips are the areas used for stimulation. Loss of two-point discrimination when tactile sensation is present is indicative of a parietal lobe disorder.

Stereognosis is the ability of the patient to recognize objects by touch. A familiar object such as a key or coin is placed in the child's hand. He is asked to identify the object by recognizing the form, shape, or texture. Astereognosis indicates parietal lobe dysfunction.

Opticokinetic nystagmus was discussed earlier in the section on cranial nerve II in the older child.

Neglect or extinction is the inability of the patient to perceive simultaneous stimuli. This is present particularly in right parietal lobe lesions.

Graphesthesia is the ability of the patient to recognize letters or numbers when they are written on the skin. The numbers or letters are usually written in the palm or on the fingertips while the patient has his eyes closed. Dysgraphesthesia also is indicative of parietal lobe dysfunction.

Mental Status

The mental status of the young child can be evaluated by his responsiveness to his surroundings and the organization of his play. Reading proficiency should be tested with standard grade-level texts and with flash cards. The child should be asked to copy designs, to trace figures, and to perform the Draw-a-Person test. Handwriting should be examined, and the child should be asked to copy key words, letters, and numbers as well as to work simple arithmetic problems. The child's language is evaluated by his ability to understand spoken and written words. Standard tests such as the Stanford-Binet, Wechsler Intelligence Scale for Children, and wide-range achievement tests should be done in the older child as indicated.

REFERENCES

1. Cogan, D. G.: Neurology of the Ocular Muscles. 2nd Ed. Springfield, Ill., Charles C Thomas, 1956.
2. Dodge, P. R.: *In* Farmer, T. W., ed.: Pediatric Neurology. 2nd Ed. Hagerstown, Md., Harper & Row, 1975.
3. Dodge, P. R., and Porter, P.: Demonstration of intracranial pathology by transillumination. Arch. Neurol., *5*:594, 1961.
4. Gesell, A., and Amatruda, C. S.: Developmental Diagnosis. 2nd Ed. New York, Hoeber, 1964.
5. Hogan, G. R., and Milligan, J. E.: The plantar reflex in the newborn. New Eng. J. Med., *285*:502, 1971.
6. Illingworth, R. S.: Development of the Infant and Young Child. 3rd Ed. Edinburgh, E & S Livingstone, Ltd., 1967.
7. Konigsmark, B. W.: Hereditary deafness in man. New Eng. J. Med., *281*:713, 1969.
8. Peiper, A.: Cerebral Function in Infancy and Childhood. New York, Consultants Bureau, 1963.
9. Schenker, J. G., and Gombos, G. M.: Retinal hemorrhages in the newborn. Obstet. Gynec., *27*:521, 1966.
10. Twitchell, T. E.: The neurological examination in infantile cerebral palsy. Develop. Med. Child Neurol., *5*:271, 1963.
11. Walsh, F. B., and Hoyt, W. F.: Clinical Neuro-Ophthalmology. Baltimore, Williams & Wilkins Co., 1969.

3

DIFFERENTIAL DIAGNOSIS OF ALTERED STATES OF CONSCIOUSNESS

Consciousness is the highest of the brain's integrative functions, and clinical evaluation of the state of consciousness is an important part of the neurological examination in all patients with disordered brain function.

Consciousness ranges in degree from *alert wakefulness* to *coma*. The former is characterized by full and appropriate responses to both internal and external stimuli, and the latter by apparently complete unresponsiveness to even the most compelling stimuli. The gradations between these extremes are also important, for even subtle changes can influence diagnosis, management, and prognosis. The following terms are often used to define intermediate stages of consciousness, though such terms are arbitrary distinctions within a continuous spectrum of failing consciousness and are not a substitute for a specific description of the clinical observations.

Lethargy is a state of reduced or clouded consciousness characterized by drowsiness, inaction, and indifference, in which responses are delayed and incomplete, and an increased stimulus may be required to evoke a response. *Obtundation* refers to duller indifference in which little more than wakefulness is maintained. *Stupor* is the state from which the subject can only be aroused by vigorous and continuous external stimulation. *Coma* means that behavioral and motor responses to stimulation are either completely lost or reduced to only rudimentary or reflex motor responses. The term "akinetic mutism" lacks a strict definition, but describes patients who lack spontaneous speech and movement despite the appearance of alertness or at least the preservation of some aspects of consciousness, e.g., sleep-like cycles.[8] In the "locked-in" syndrome, lesions in restricted descending motor pathways in the brain stem abolish almost all voluntary movements, sparing only the most rostral motor functions such as vertical eye movements or blinking, while full consciousness may be preserved.[34,36] In some closely allied states, e.g., *delirium* and *organic confusion,* consciousness is deranged as much as it is depressed, often by the same processes that may progress to cause coma.

Examples of stupor and coma as urgent

TABLE 3–1 FINAL DIAGNOSIS IN 386 PATIENTS WITH "COMA OF UNKNOWN ETIOLOGY"*

Supratentorial mass lesions		69
Epidural hematoma	2	
Subdural hematoma	21	
Intracerebral hematoma	33	
Cerebral infarct	5	
Brain tumor	5	
Brain abscess	3	
Subtentorial lesions		52
Brain stem infarct	37	
Brain stem hemorrhage	7	
Brain stem tumor	2	
Cerebellar hemorrhage	4	
Cerebellar abscess	2	
Metabolic and diffuse cerebral disorders		261
Anoxia and ischemia	51	
Concussion and postictal states	9	
Infection (meningitis and encephalitis)	11	
Subarachnoid hemorrhage	10	
Exogenous toxins	99	
Endogenous toxins and deficiencies	81	
Psychiatric disorders		4

* From Plum, F., and Posner, J. B.: Diagnosis of Stupor and Coma. 2nd Ed. Contemporary Neurology Series. Vol. 10. Philadelphia, F. A. Davis Co., 1972. Reprinted by permission.

F. PLUM AND R. W. BRENNAN

problems in diagnosis and care are common in any busy emergency room.[24] Table 3–1 itemizes the final diagnosis in 386 patients presenting with "coma of unknown etiology," and reflects the diverse diseases that can cause severe brain dysfunction and coma. That a large proportion are reversible if given appropriate medical or surgical treatment underlines the importance of rapid and accurate diagnosis.

CLINICAL EXAMINATION OF THE UNCONSCIOUS PATIENT

The emergency care of the less than fully conscious patient must combine treatment and diagnosis. The patient must be protected from further insult by insuring a patent airway and adequate ventilation, mechanical if necessary. In every case of unexplained stupor or coma, glucose (50 ml of a 50 per cent solution) should be given intravenously immediately *after* blood has been drawn for glucose determination. The treatment is innocuous, and in hypoglycemia it gives prompt protection against further and sometimes irreversible neuronal injury. Diagnosis properly begins with a careful history, but often the sum of available information from the patient, his friends, his family, or the ambulance or police personnel is either incomplete or conflicting. Hence the need for an orderly, selective physical examination that may give findings with specific diagnostic value.

The observations listed in Table 3–2 give important clues, but diagnosis depends upon the total findings. The first question is anatomical, i.e., where does the lesion causing unconsciousness lie? Can the signs be due to a single lesion? Or, do they point to multifocal or diffuse disease? Finally, and most important for management, in what direction is the process evolving?

A plan for evaluating the nervous system in the unconscious patient follows, based on changes observed in five physiological functions: the state of consciousness, the pattern of breathing, the size and reactivity of the pupils, the eye movements, and the skeletal muscle responses.

TABLE 3–2 IMPORTANT PHYSICAL SIGNS IN COMA

Vital signs	
Hypertension	Hypertensive encephalopathy; cerebral hemorrhage; subarachnoid hemorrhage
Hypotension	Inadequate cerebral perfusion secondary to myocardial infarction, hemorrhagic shock, or pulmonary infarction
Hyperthermia	CNS infection; subarachnoid hemorrhage; bacterial endocarditis; pneumonitis with hypoxia; heat stroke; pontine infarction
Hypothermia	Metabolic or toxic coma of any cause, particularly barbiturate or phenothiazine intoxication, other depressants, or insulin coma; destructive brain stem lesions; myxedema
Skin changes	
Multiple petechiae or purpura	Thrombotic thrombocytopenic purpura; meningococcemia; bacterial endocarditis; fat embolism
Cherry pink skin	Carbon monoxide poisoning
Multiple healed venipunctures	Drug addiction
Evidence of head trauma; scalp contusion, edema; blood or CSF in nares or behind tympanic membrane; subgaleal or subperiosteal blood ("raccoon eyes," Battle's sign)	Skull fractures; cerebral concussion, contusion; acute epidural or subdural hemorrhage
Nuchal rigidity	Meningitis; cerebellar tonsillar herniation; rarely, acute subarachnoid hemorrhage (in which stiff neck takes several hours to develop)

Physiology and Pathology of Consciousness

Consciousness may be thought of as having two components, one being its crude "off-on" quality, and the other its content. In general, crude "all or none" consciousness depends upon the integrity of specific areas of the upper brain stem, while the content of consciousness depends more upon the functions of the cerebral hemispheres.

Studies of patients with disease restricted to the cerebral hemispheres led Wolff to conclude that man's highest integrative abilities are lost in proportion to the amount of involved cortex.[9] Patients with moderately advanced but selective cortical disease, e.g., Alzheimer's disease, typically show a profound decline in the content of consciousness but fully retain wakefulness. More extensive or rapid losses of the functioning cortical mass blunt responsiveness, and in functional or anatomical decorticate states, only rudiments of behavioral responsiveness remain. Even then such features as intact chewing and swallowing, food preferences, and sleep-wake cycles are preserved. Such global but selective cortical lesions are rare, however, and the great bulk of unconsciousness has other causes.

Evidence that the crude element of consciousness depends heavily on brain stem structures goes as far back as clinicopathological analyses published in the late nineteenth century.[22] Many examples are now known of discrete lesions, including tumors, infarcts, and hemorrhages restricted to paramedian areas of the pons, midbrain, and hypothalamus, that abolish or reduce consciousness.[6,8,15,20,21]

Experimental studies of the brain stem reticular core have further defined much of its normal function. Magoun and Moruzzi identified an ascending reticular activating system (ARAS) within the paramedian tegmentum of the midbrain and extending to the hypothalamus and thalamus.[30] This system diffusely projects to the cerebral cortex and profoundly influences both arousal and the electroencephalographic (EEG) pattern. In experimental animals, stimulation leads to alert behavior and an activated, desynchronized electroencephalogram, while destruction causes behavioral unresponsiveness and a slow electroencephalogram. Depressant and anesthetic drugs act selectively on the ARAS, presumably because of its highly polysynaptic organization.[1]

TABLE 3–3 METABOLIC DISORDERS CAUSING COMA AND AFFECTING RESPIRATION

Hyperventilation
- Acute metabolic acidosis
  - Uremia
  - Diabetic ketoacidosis
  - Exogenous poisoning (paraldehyde, methyl alcohol, ethylene glycol)
  - Anoxic lactic acidosis
- Respiratory alkalosis
  - Hepatic encephalopathy
  - Salicylate intoxication
  - Cardiopulmonary disease
  - Central neurogenic hyperventilation

Hypoventilation
- Respiratory acidosis
  - Depressant drug poisoning
  - Pulmonary disease with CO_2 retention

Metabolic alkalosis
- Rarely causes stupor or coma except perhaps with severe hyperadrenocorticism

An earlier view held that both sleep and coma arose passively when the tonic activating influence of the ascending reticular activating system decreased, but this concept has been disproved. Recent evidence reveals that sleep is an active process, regulated by functional subunits of the reticular core. Cerebral blood flow and metabolism remain normal even in the deepest stages of sleep, or may actually increase. In coma, on the other hand, cerebral metabolism is consistently subnormal. Sleep is a highly physiological state and coma is a most unphysiological one, and there is no basis for equating the two.

Respiration

Many of the metabolic abnormalities that cause coma increase or decrease the chemical stimuli to pulmonary ventilation. Also, because damage or depression of the brain at nearly every level affects the act of breathing, appraisal of this function becomes useful in anatomical localization. Table 3–3 lists some of the metabolic influences that can cause coma and at the same time will alter an anatomically intact respiratory system. The remainder of this section describes neuroanatomical influences on breathing that aid the clinician in reaching a localizing diagnosis.

In normal awake subjects, a significant portion of the resting stimulus to pulmonary ventilation comes from nonchemical neural sources. As a result, when a neurologically intact subject is asked to hyperventilate briefly, he continues to breathe rhythmically *after* the hyperventilation at a time when carbon dioxide and oxygen stimuli are in abeyance. This altogether unconscious and automatic influence is impaired with even moderate degrees of bilateral cerebral dysfunction, and such subjects demonstrate *posthyperventilation apnea,* usually lasting 10 to 25 seconds, after taking five good deep breaths. This abnormality is useful in distinguishing a dulled or confused subject with cerebral dysfunction from one with a psychologically induced behavioral alteration.

More severe bilateral hemispheric dysfunction impairs the nonchemical influences on the act of breathing even more, and in addition, in many such patients there is an increased respiratory responsiveness to chemical stimuli. As a result, many of them develop a breathing pattern with regular oscillations between hyperpnea and apnea. This is *Cheyne-Stokes* respiration. The regular waxing and waning, being dependent on stimuli reaching the respiratory system, has a period length equal to twice the lung-to-brain circulation time.

Involvement of anatomical centers in the posterior hypothalamus and midbrain produces moderate pulmonary edema in many patients, and a pattern of hyperpnea with a low arterial carbon dioxide tension combined with a below-normal oxygen tension is the result. A less common manifestation of midbrain–upper pontine lesions in man is a true *central hyperventilation*. This condition occurs in patients with destructive depression of the paramedian tegmentum, and is marked by respiratory rates as high as 25 to 40 per minute, a low arterial blood carbon dioxide tension, and an above-normal blood oxygen tension.

Damage to or depression of the brain stem's paramedian reticulum at or below the pons produces *irregularly irregular breathing* patterns. These may take various forms including inspiratory or expiratory apneusis, cluster breathing, gasping, or long periods of ataxic irregular breathing patterns in which the timing and depth of the next breath cannot be predicted from the past pattern. All these last-mentioned abnormalities tend to be associated with abnormal blood gases and underventilation, and thus they tend to accentuate whatever neurological injury or depression is already present.

Extensive damage to or depression of the medullary reticular formation generally destroys the central control of respiration and produces severe hypoventilation or apnea.

Pupils

At rest or in reflex motion, pupil size reflects a balance between opposite tonic motor impulses. The parasympathetic system acts upon the pupilloconstrictor muscle to induce miosis, while the sympathetic system innervates the radially arranged pupillodilator fibers that produce active mydriasis.[10] The selective loss of either influence leaves the other unopposed, with corresponding changes in pupil size. The central pathways for both pupilloconstrictor and dilator effects course through the upper brain stem and are often interrupted by lesions in this area that threaten consciousness.

Lesions above the diencephalon have little effect on pupillary size or function, although sleep and cerebral depression are associated with bilateral pupilloconstriction. Stimulation of the lateral hypothalamus produces ipsilateral pupil dilatation; destruction or functional depression of the same area results in pupilloconstriction. These effects are mediated through pupillodilator pathways that descend from the hypothalamus through all levels of the brain stem to reach second-order neurons in the upper thoracic spinal cord; the pathway then travels through peripheral fibers to third-order neurons in the superior cervical ganglion, and finally through postganglionic fibers passing with branches of the internal carotid artery to the orbit.

Active pupilloconstriction results from stimulation in another diencephalic structure, the pretectum. Destruction or depression of this area may result in bilateral pupillary dilatation. The light reflex is typically impaired as well, from involvement of the afferent limb or the pretectal relay nuclei. This and perhaps other pupilloconstrictor influences play upon the Edinger-Westphal nucleus, which is interposed between the oculomotor nuclei of the paramedian midbrain.[23] Preganglionic parasympathetic fibers pass in the peripheral parts of the oculomotor nerve, to synapse in the ciliary ganglion in the orbit.

Localizing Value of Pupillary Abnormalities in Coma

The size of the normal pupil varies widely. Miosis is common in drowsiness or sleep, while mydriasis accompanies arousal, intense emotion, or the perception of pain. Patients with bilateral cerebral dysfunction commonly exhibit small pupils (2 to 3 mm) that are reactive to light and fluctuate with the state of spontaneous and reflex arousal. The pupils may undergo cyclic changes with Cheyne-Stokes respiration, dilating in hyperpnea and constricting in apnea. In such patients, the mobility and symmetry of the pupils exclude structural injury to the brain stem proper.

Miosis on the same side as a large hemispheric lesion may indicate encroachment on the more specific pupillodilator center in the ipsilateral hypothalamus, and thus herald impending transtentorial herniation.

Midbrain damage produces clear-cut pupillary signs. Tectal or pretectal lesions interrupt the light reflex, producing midposition or slightly dilated pupils (5 to 6 mm) that are round, regular, but sometimes asymmetrical and sluggish or fixed to light. Such "tectal pupils" commonly have the spontaneous movements of hippus and retain reflex dilatation to noxious body stimuli. Discrete lesions that involve the oculomotor nerve in the ventral midbrain, or in the interpeduncular fossa, produce widely dilated (8 to 9 mm) and immobile pupils. Major injury to the midbrain, as in central infarction or hemorrhage or in the compression and distortion wrought by transtentorial herniation, nearly always interrupts both sympathetic and parasympathetic pathways. The resulting pupils are in midposition (4 to 5 mm), fixed to light, and sometimes irregular and slightly asymmetrical; such pupils may still dilate slightly in response to noxious stimuli delivered to neck or trunk (the ciliospinal reflex).[2]

Several patterns of pupillary response may occur in combination; supratentorial mass lesions, such as epidural hematomas situated laterally, may compress the ipsilateral oculomotor nerve and produce a dilated fixed pupil as a prelude to the more typical changes of transtentorial herniation.[35,40]

Pontine lesions involving the tegmentum may interrupt descending sympathetic pathways and produce small pupils on one or both sides. The acute and extensive damage of pontine hemorrhage produces pinpoint pupils (1 to 2 mm), which may lose their light reaction at least transiently.[39]

Laterally placed lesions of the medulla cause a mild Horner's syndrome, with slight ptosis and pupillary constriction, on the homolateral side, but consciousness is not impaired.

In most metabolic encephalopathies, including sedative poisoning, the pupils are small but symmetrical, regular, and fully reactive to light. In extreme cases, as with unremitting anoxia or very severe metabolic or drug depressions, the pupillary light reflex may be lost terminally. The exceptions to this rule include poisoning from glutethimide or from tricyclic antidepressants in which the anticholinergic effect of the drugs can result in fixed wide pupils (5 to 8 mm) with only moderately severe central nervous system depression. In narcotic intoxication, pupils are intensely miotic (1 to 2 mm), but reactive, and dilate in response to topical nalorphine solution.

Ocular Movements

Both voluntary and reflex conjugate movements of the eyes depend on mechanisms represented at several levels of the neuraxis. Oculomotor abnormalities in stuporous or comatose patients give clinically useful information concerning the site of the lesion that is depressing consciousness.[43]

Supranuclear fibers from voluntary or reflex conjugate gaze centers in the cerebral hemispheres descend through or medial to the internal capsule into the brain stem, decussate, and pass down the contralateral pontine paramedial tegmentum to synapse near the abducens nucleus in the low pons.[3,11] Fibers controlling conjugate vertical gaze and originating in the cerebrum travel through the regions of the pretectal and posterior commissural nuclei to reach the oculomotor nuclei bilaterally. *Internuclear fibers* connecting the oculomotor, trochlear, and abducens nuclei course in the median longitudinal fasciculus (MLF) just ventral to the periaqueductal gray matter of the midbrain and pons. This pathway decussates in the pons just rostral to the abducens nucleus. It serves to coordinate ipsilateral lateral rectus and contralateral medial rectus muscle action initiated through supranuclear conjugate gaze mechanisms. The *labyrinthine-vestibular system* also influences conjugate eye movements. Fibers from the semicircular canals, otoliths, and the fastigial nucleus of the cerebellum synapse in the vestibular nuclei, from which second-order fibers traverse the median longitudinal fasciculus to the ocular motor nuclei. Fibers conveying proprioception from the upper cervical segments probably reach the ocular motor nuclei through the caudal continuation of the median longitudinal fasciculus, which descends into the spinal cord as far as C2 or C3.

In stuporous or comatose patients, reflex eye movements may be elicited to test the integrity of many of the foregoing pathways.[25,33] The *oculocephalic reflex* or "doll's eyes" phenomenon is demonstrated by observing the eyes as the head is briefly rotated and held at the extreme position. A positive response to side-to-side movement is transient conjugate deviation of the eyes opposite to the direction of head movement (e.g., if the head is rotated to the right, the eyes deviate to the left). Vertical reflex movements may be sought by brisk flexion and extension of the head and the neck. A positive response is deviation of the eyes upward on flexion, downward on extension. The stimulus for the oculocephalic reflex involves either the labyrinthine vestibular system or proprioceptive afferents from the neck, or possibly both.[19] The *oculovestibular reflex* refers to reflex conjugate eye movements or nystagmus or both induced by caloric stimulation of the labyrinth. The head is elevated 30 degrees above the horizontal so that the lateral semicircular canal is vertical, a position in which stimulation can provoke a maximal response. A soft catheter is placed in the external canal near the tympanic membrane, and a small volume of ice water is slowly syringed into the canal of the unresponsive patient until either horizontal nystagmus or tonic ocular deviation occurs; 1 ml is usually sufficient, and volumes of more than 20 ml are rarely necessary. To test for vertical eye movements, one can irrigate both auditory canals simultaneously with ice water. In a comatose patient with intact brain stem vestibular-oculomotor connections, the eyes deviate downward. With the lateral canal inverted (head 60 degrees below horizontal), the same maneuver elicits upward eye movement.

In most patients in coma, the reflex eye movements in response to caloric stimulation and to passive head turning relate to each other as if the two stimuli differed only in degree, the first being the stronger. In the oculovestibular reflex, an induced convection current in the labyrinthine endolymph of the lateral canal alters the balance in the paired vestibular systems to produce tonic conjugate eye deviation toward the same side with cold stimuli, or to the opposite side with warm stimuli.[42] In the oculocephalic reflex, the relative currents generated by inertia of the endolymph as the head is moved stimulate the receptors of both lateral canals to produce similar but less pronounced effects. In addition, stimuli from proprioceptors in the upper cervical segments also play a role, so some patients with pontine lesions may lose the caloric response but retain the oculocephalic response.

In awake alert patients the eyes are directed straight ahead at rest. Oculocephalic responses cannot normally be elicited, and caloric stimulation yields nystagmus rather than sustained deviation.

In coma due to bilateral hemispheral depression, the eyes are directed straight ahead. For the first 24 hours or so after onset of asymmetrical or unilateral cerebral dysfunction the eyes typically deviate to the side of the lesion, occasionally with some nystagmus to that side. In patients with moderate bilateral cerebral depression, as in metabolic stupor or coma, labyrinthine stimuli cause tonic eye movements rather than nystagmus, since the quick or eye-centering phase depends on interaction between the oculovestibular system and the cerebrum and disappears as cerebral influences are reduced. In such patients, oculocephalic reflexes may be of wide amplitude and easily elicited, and tonic caloric responses may be sustained for several minutes, as if released from suprasegmental inhibition.[5] Such hyperactive responses are characteristic of patients who have diffuse cortical dysfunction from anoxia, hypoglycemia, or hepatic coma.

With coma from brain stem lesions, reflex eye movements are depressed, or otherwise abnormal. With midbrain or pontine lesions involving the median longitudinal fasciculus, the eye on the side of the lesion fails to adduct on reflex movements. Lateral pontine lesions cause the eyes to deviate conjugately away from the side of the lesion, and reflex movements toward that side are often blocked at the midline. Skew deviation, or vertical strabismus, appears with dorsolateral pontine lesions or with lesions in the median longitudinal fasciculus. It may be brought out with reflex lateral eye movements to one or both sides. Extensive pontine lesions may block reflex eye movements in all planes, while midbrain-pretectal lesions may selectively impair vertical movements alone. "Ocular bobbing'' is intermittent brisk downward movement of one or both eyes followed by a slower return to the primary position. Whether ocular bobbing occurs spontaneously or in response to caloric stimulation, the implication is the same: extensive pontine destruction in almost all cases.[17] Ocular bobbing should not be confused with the occasional finding of slow, sustained downward eye movement following unilateral caloric stimulation, as seen in sedative drug poisoning. The latter phenomenon lacks a rapid phase, always has a lateral component, and most importantly has no localizing significance and no diagnostic or prognostic meaning.[38]

Motor Function

Though motor functions depend on brain structures that are different from those that serve consciousness, motor abnormalities in patients with depressed consciousness can give further clues to the location of the disturbance and its nature.

Paratonic rigidity is a nonspecific but early sign of subcortical hemispheric motor dysfunction. It represents an abnormal increase in resistance to passive movement, but unlike spasticity or plasticity, it is intermittent; when present, it is independent of the initial position of the extremity. The resistance often has a reactive or overactive quality suggesting that the patient is voluntarily opposing every effort of the examiner to move him. Ranging in degree from slight failure to relax to intense rigidity of the entire body, paratonia is common in states of diffuse cerebral dysfunction, e.g., widespread forebrain degenerative disease or metabolic disturbances.

Motor and sensory function in patients with depressed consciousness can be estimated by applying noxious stimuli to different parts of the body and observing the response. *Appropriate responses* in a patient with acute brain dysfunction imply that both motor and sensory pathways are at least partly intact. *Inappropriate responses* are stereotypes of movement and posture in response to noxious stimuli whose pattern depends on the level of injury. *Decorticate response* consists of flexion of the arm, wrist, and fingers with adduction in the upper extremity, and extension, internal rotation, and plantar flexion in the lower extremity. The response is typically seen with disease processes that depress or destroy frontal cerebral cortex or its descending connections in internal capsule, or rostral cerebral penduncle. *Decerebrate responses* when fully developed consist of opisthotonus, adduction and extension and hyperpronation of the arms, and extension and plantar flexion of the lower extremities. The response requires at least partial and bilateral separation of midbrain and pontine structures from hemispheral influence, and is elicited commonly in conditions that destroy or depress the upper brain stem.

SUPRATENTORIAL LESIONS CAUSING COMA

Two main types of supratentorial processes can depress or abolish consciousness: localized hemispheral lesions that produce a deep destructive or mass effect because they either extend directly into deeper midline diencephalic structures or secondarily compress them, and lesions that produce diffuse bilateral impairment of either the cortical mantle or its underlying white matter but spare the brain stem. These latter usually have a metabolic origin and are discussed separately.

Anatomical Considerations

Because its confines are inelastic, the intracranial volume is essentially fixed. A progressive mass lesion must enlarge at the expense of one or more of the normal intracranial components—brain, blood, or cerebrospinal fluid. Accommodative mechanisms are limited and cannot indefinitely make room for a continually expanding process. At some point, the contents of the supratentorial space will herniate through the tentorial notch, molding and distorting the involved tissues and eventually producing hemorrhage and necrosis of the impacted area.[16,26] The dividing line between survival and death with supratentorial masses is drawn at the point at which irreversible tentorial herniation can be prevented.

TABLE 3–4 SYNDROMES OF TRANSTENTORIAL HERNIATION

Level	*Consciousness*	*Respiration*	*Pupils*	*Oculocephalic Reflex*	*Motor Response*
SYNDROME I (Central Compression and Herniation)					
Early diencephalic	Dull	Eupnea, yawns, sighs	Small, reactive	Intermittent or hyperactive	Hemiplegia, bilateral Babinski, moderate bilateral paratonia
Late diencephalic	Stupor	CSR*	Small, reactive	Hyperactive	Hemiplegia, bilateral, Babinski, decorticate pain response
Midbrain	Coma	CSR→CNH†	Midposition, fixed	Disconjugate or sluggish	Decerebrate responses
Upper pontine	Coma	CNH	Midposition, fixed	Sluggish	Less decerebrate
Lower pontine	Coma	Eupneic or ataxic	Midposition, fixed	0	Flaccid, bilateral Babinski
SYNDROME II (Lateral Compression and Herniation)					
Early diencephalic	Drowsy	Eupnea	One dilated or normal	Intact if obtainable	Developing unilateral changes
Late diencephalic	Stupor	Eupnea→CSR or CNH	One dilated→ fixed	III Nerve Palsy	Decorticate→ decerebrate
Midbrain	Coma	CNH	Dilated, fixed	Disconjugate	Decerebrate
Upper pontine	Coma	CNH	Midposition, fixed	Sluggish	Less decerebrate
Lower pontine	Coma	Eupneic or ataxic	Midposition, fixed	0	Flaccid, bilateral Babinski

* CSR, Cheyne-Stokes respiration.
† CNH, Central neurogenic hyperventilation.

Pathogenesis

As a hemispheral mass lesion enlarges and induces brain swelling, there is a compensatory shift in the medial and deep structures of the hemisphere. One of two main syndromes of transtentorial herniation evolves, depending on the location of the lesion and, hence, on the direction of the displacing force. Central diencephalic compression produces signs reflecting bilateral and generally symmetrical failure of the diencephalon, then the midbrain, pons, and finally the medulla in progressive rostrocaudal fashion (syndrome I, Table 3–4). In laterally placed lesions, the earliest signs may reflect herniation of the uncus and other structures of the medial temporal lobe over the adjacent lip of the tentorial notch and onto the ipsilateral third nerve (syndrome II). If herniation continues, signs of progressive descending brain stem failure appear soon after.[12,31]

The course of the transtentorial herniation syndrome is usually measured in hours or even days, but very rapidly evolving masses, e.g., epidural hematoma, may cause coma from irreversible brain stem injury within an hour. More indolent lesions may cause gradual, stepwise, or even fluctuating signs of incipient herniation. Cerebral hemorrhage with intraventricular rupture produces exceptionally rapid brain stem dysfunction, and frequently there are signs of medullary failure while higher functions are still preserved.[32]

SUBTENTORIAL LESIONS CAUSING COMA

Patients with destructive subtentorial lesions, e.g., primary hemorrhage or infarction of the midbrain or pons, often lose consciousness immediately, or as soon as the activating systems in the median tegmentum are involved.[27] Such lesions always give unequivocal localizing signs, and the anatomical diagnosis is not often in doubt. In further contrast to the brain stem injury caused by supratentorial masses, functions rostral to the lesion are preserved. Metabolic depression may mimic structural lesions of the brain stem, but pupillary light reflexes are spared, and ocular and motor signs are symmetrical in metabolic brain disease.

Expanding lesions in the posterior fossa influence consciousness as they directly compress the brain stem; in certain cases, upward transtentorial herniation may also play a role.[14] Herniation of the cerebellar tonsils through the foramen magnum distorts the medulla, and respiratory failure is the terminal event. One type of expanding lesion, acute cerebellar hemorrhage, is sufficiently common to warrant specific mention. As in all forms of parenchymal brain bleeding, risk factors such as pre-existing hypertension or bleeding disorder will be present in the majority. Sudden headache and repeated vomiting are always present at the outset, but symptoms specific for a posterior fossa lesion are less common. As the hematoma enlarges, signs of acute cerebellar dysfunction can usually be elicited, including dysarthria, dysmetria of extremity movements, and conjugate deviation of the eyes away from the side of the involved cerebellar hemisphere. Further expansion of the mass must result in compression or distortion of the underlying pons and medulla, and with it, progressive depression of consciousness, loss of reflex eye movements, and respiratory failure. Since the higher brain stem is intact, pupils are typically small and reactive, a point against a transtentorial herniation. Hemiparesis and hemiplegia are notably absent, an important contrast to the pattern seen with putamenal hemorrhage or primary pontine hemorrhage. In patients with very rapidly expanding cerebellar hematoma, consciousness may be lost in the first few hours and all such clinical findings of localizing value may be erased. More often, loss of consciousness progresses gradually, and an accurate clinical diagnosis can be arrived at and confirmed by radiographic procedures if time permits. Such confirmation will always be beneficial, but in those patients whose clinical condition is deteriorating rapidly, the risks involved in delaying operative treatment may sometimes outweigh the benefits of radiological documentation. The best predictors of operative outcome in acute cerebellar hemorrhage are clinical ones, particularly those findings that reflect the functional integrity of the brain stem itself: the level of consciousness, the pattern of respiration, and the presence or absence of reflex eye movements.[7,18]

METABOLIC CAUSES OF STUPOR AND COMA

Metabolic encephalopathy occurs when noncerebral diseases secondarily interfere with brain metabolism in any of several ways. Some examples may be given. In hypoxia and in hypoglycemia, extrinsic brain energy sources are insufficient, and rapid irreversible catabolic changes occur.[37,44] In electrolyte imbalances, e.g., hyponatremia or water intoxication, neuronal excitability is altered.[41] Changes in the brain's acid-base or osmotic milieu may also depress function. Uremia and hepatic failure are complex states in which cerebral function often suffers; presumably, some endogenous toxin is at fault.[4,29] Depressant drugs or other exogenous toxins are common causes of metabolic depression, sometimes to the point of profound coma.

Patients with mild metabolic encephalopathy are confused and disoriented, have mild blunting of alertness, and may show perceptual disturbances in the form of illusions or visual hallucinations. Tremor, asterixis ("flap"), or myoclonic movements are common. Diffuse and symmetrical motor abnormalities are seen, including paratonia and snouting and grasp reflexes. As the disease progresses, stupor and finally coma ensue. The pattern of respiration and motor responses varies with the stage of progression. The pupils are small, but symmetrical, and light reflexes are preserved. Oculocephalic and oculovestibular reflexes remain brisk and conjugate, except in sedative intoxication, when they are depressed or absent even in light coma.

The findings in metabolic encephalopathy bespeak widespread but selective action on brain functions, with cerebral functions being involved before those of lower structures. In certain cases, the findings suggest partial dysfunction affecting many levels of the neuraxis simultaneously, while the integrity of other functions originating at the same level is spared. Another point of difference from coma based on structural lesions is the rarity of asymmetrical or focal signs in metabolic encephalopathy. Finally, the electroencephalogram shows generalized symmetrical slowing without focal abnormality.

In certain other diseases, coma may arise from a combination of structural and metabolic effects. Coma in subarachnoid hemorrhage may come from mechanical effects, e.g., an associated hematoma acting as a supratentorial or subtentorial mass, or from some toxic metabolic action of blood products. In severe bacterial meningitis or in viral meningoencephalitis, cerebral edema is often found and may be of itself a cause of diffuse cerebral dysfunction and coma. In these several conditions, careful examination of the cerebrospinal fluid almost always gives unequivocal diagnostic information.[13]

EPISODIC UNCONSCIOUSNESS

Some common and important neurological problems present as brief and fully reversible episodes of altered consciousness. According to the classification proposed by Lee and Plum, the causes may be assigned to five major groups: failure of systemic circulation, as in vasodepressor syncope or cardiac arrhythmia; systemic disorders impairing cerebral metabolism, as in hypoglycemia; cerebral arterial insufficiency due to structural or functional changes in the brain vasculature; primary neurological disorders, e.g., epilepsy or concussion; and other causes, e.g., psychogenic unresponsiveness.[28] Unless the episode has been witnessed by the physician, the etiological diagnosis must depend heavily on a detailed history centered on what the circumstances were, what the patient felt, and what observers, if any, may have noted.

This group of disorders is peripheral to neurosurgical practice, but recurrent episodes of unconsciousness warrant close attention, for their causes can sometimes produce irreversible neurological injury as well.

REFERENCES

1. Arduini, A., and Arduini, M. G.: Effects of drugs and metabolic alterations on brain stem arousal mechanisms. J. Pharmacol. Exp. Ther., *110*:76–85, 1954.
2. Arieff, A. J., and Pyzik, S. W.: The ciliospinal reflex in injuries of the cervical spinal cord in man.

A.M.A. Arch. Neurol. Psychiat., *70*:621–629, 1953.

3. Bender, M., ed.: The Oculomotor System, New York, Harper & Row, 1964.
4. Bessman, S. P., and Bessman, A. N.: The cerebral and peripheral uptake of ammonia in liver disease with an hypothesis of hepatic coma. J. Clin. Invest., *34*:622–628, 1955.
5. Blegvad, B.: Caloric vestibular reaction in unconscious patients. Arch. Otolaryng., *75*:506–514, 1962.
6. Brain, R.: The physiological basis of consciousness. Brain, *81*:426–455, 1958.
7. Brennan, R. W., and Bergland, R. M.: Acute cerebellar hemorrhage: Analysis of clinical findings and outcome in 12 cases. Neurology (Minneap.), *27*:527–532, 1977.
8. Cairns, H.: Disturbances of consciousness with lesions of the brain stem and diencephalon. Brain, *75*:109–146, 1952.
9. Chapman, L. F., and Wolff, H. G.: The cerebral hemispheres and the highest integrative functions of man. Arch. Neurol., *1*:357–424, 1959.
10. Cogan, D. G.: Neurology of the Ocular Muscles. Ed. 2. Springfield, Ill., Charles C Thomas, 1956.
11. Crosby, E. C.: Relations of brain centers to normal and abnormal eye movements in the horizontal plane. J. Comp. Neurol., *99*:437–479, 1953.
12. Cushing, H.: Concerning a definite regulatory mechanism of the vaso-motor centre which controls blood pressure during cerebral compression. Bull. Hopkins Hosp., *12*:290–292, 1901.
13. Dodge, P. R., and Swartz, M. N.: Bacterial meningitis: II. Special neurologic problems, postmeningitic complications and clinicopathological correlations. New Eng. J. Med., *272*:954–960, 1965.
14. Ecker, A.: Upward transtentorial herniation of the brainstem and cerebellum due to tumor of the posterior fossa. J. Neurosurg., *5*:51–61, 1948.
15. von Economo, C.: Sleep as a problem of localization. J. Nerv. Ment. Dis., *71*:249–259, 1930.
16. Finney, L. A., and Walker, A. E.: Transtentorial Herniation. Springfield, Ill., Charles C Thomas, 1962.
17. Fisher, C. M.: Ocular bobbing. Arch. Neurol., *11*:543–546, 1964.
18. Fisher, C. M.: The neurologic examination of the comatose patient. Acta Neurol. Scand., *45*:suppl. 36, 1969.
19. Ford, F. R., and Walsh, F. B.: Tonic deviations of the eyes produced by movements of the head. Arch. Ophthal., *23*:1274–1284, 1940.
20. French, J. D.: Brain lesions with prolonged unconsciousness. A.M.A. Arch. Neurol. Psychiat., *68*:727–740, 1952.
21. Fulton, J. F., and Bailey, P.: Tumors in the region of the third ventricle: Their diagnosis and relation to pathological sleep, J. Nerv. Ment. Dis., *69*:1–25, 145–164, 261–277, 1929.
22. Gayet, M.: Affection encephalique (encephalite diffuse probable). Arch. Physiol. Norm. Path. 2^e ser. *2*:341–351. 1875.
23. Harris, A. J., Hodes, R., and Magoun, H. W.: The afferent path of the pupillodilator reflex in the cat. J. Neurophysiol., *7*:231–243, 1944.
24. Holcomb, B.: Causes and diagnosis of various forms of coma. J.A.M.A., *77*:2112–2114, 1921.
25. Holmes, G.: The cerebral integration of the ocular movements. Brit. Med. J., *2*:107–112. 1938.
26. Jefferson, G.: The tentorial pressure cone. Arch. Neurol. Psychiat., *40*:857–876, 1938.
27. Kubik, C. S., and Adams, R. D.: Occlusion of the basilar artery—a clinical and pathological study. Brain, *69*:73–121, 1946.
28. Lee, J. E., Killip, T., III, and Plum, F.: Episodic unconsciousness. *In* Barondess, J., ed.: Diagnostic Approaches to Presenting Syndromes. Baltimore, Md., Williams & Wilkins Co., 1971, pp. 133–166.
29. Locke, S., Merrill, J. P., and Tyler, H. R.: Neurologic complications of acute uremia. Arch. Int. Med., *108*:519–530, 1961.
30. Magoun, H. W.: The Waking Brain. Ed. 2. Springfield, Ill., Charles C Thomas, 1963.
31. McNealy, D. E., and Plum, F.: Brainstem dysfunction with supratentorial mass lesions. Arch. Neurol., *7*:10–32, 1962.
32. Meyers, R.: Systemic, vascular and respiratory effects of experimentally induced alterations in intraventricular pressure. J. Neuropath. Exp. Neurol., *1*:241–264, 1942.
33. Nathanson, M., and Bergman, P. S.: Newer methods of evaluation of patients with altered states of consciousness. Med. Clin. N. Amer., *42*:701–710, 1958.
34. Nordgren, R. E., Markesbery, W. R., Fukuda, K., and Reeves, A. G.: Seven cases of cerebromedullospinal disconnection: The "locked-in" syndrome. Neurology (Minneap.), *21*:1140–1148, 1971.
35. Pevehouse, B. C., Bloom, W. H., and McKissock, W.: Ophthalmologic aspects of diagnosis and localization of subdural hematomas. Neurology (Minneap.), *10*:1037–1041, 1960.
36. Plum, F., and Posner, J. B.: Diagnosis of Stupor and Coma. 2nd Ed. Contemporary Neurology Series, Vol. 10, Philadelphia, F. A. Davis Co., 1972.
37. Richardson, J. C., Chambers, R. A., and Heywood, P. M.: Encephalopathies of anoxia and hypoglycemia. Arch. Neurol., *1*:178–190, 1959.
38. Simon, R. P.: Delayed forced down gaze during oculovestibular testing in sedative drug-induced coma. Neurology (Minneap.), *27*:346, 1977.
39. Steegman, A. T.: Primary pontile hemorrhage. J. Nerv. Ment. Dis., *114*:35–65, 1951.
40. Sunderland, S., and Bradley, K. C.: Disturbances of oculomotor function accompanying extradural haemorrhage. J. Neurol. Neurosurg. Psychiat., *16*:35–46, 1953.
41. Swanson, A. G., and Iseri, O. A.: Acute encephalopathy due to water intoxication. New Eng. J. Med., *258*:831–834, 1958.
42. Szentagothai, J.: The elementary vestibulo-ocular reflex arc. J. Neurophysiol., *13*:395–407, 1950.
43. Walsh, F. B.: Clinical Neuro-ophthalmology. Ed. 2. Baltimore, Williams & Wilkins Co., 1957.
44. Weinberger, L. M., Gibbon, M. H., and Gibbon, J. H., Jr.: Temporary arrest of the circulation to the central nervous system: I. Physiologic effects. Arch. Neurol. Psychiat., *43*:615–634, 1940.

II

DIAGNOSTIC PROCEDURES

4

RADIOLOGY OF THE SKULL

A vast amount of radiological information relating to the skull has accumulated over the past 75 years.[1,8,11,14,15] In this chapter the approach to the skull is within the context of the present-day diagnostic armamentarium available for the neurological work-up of patients.

Prior to the availability of radioactive brain scanning and at a time when angiography carried a high rate of morbidity, extreme efforts were made to extract every possible clue from examination of the plain skull film. Many radiological features of the skull that were once considered to be diagnostic of general or specific problems have since been found to have no practical value in the management of the patient. It is no longer necessary, however, as it was in the past, to agonize over the meaning of certain findings in the plain skull film. Today brain scanning, low-risk angiography, and pneumography will resolve the questionable findings in the plain film studies. Thus, a more objective interpretation of the plain skull roentgenogram is possible.

The following work plan for the evaluation of a radiological finding stresses the relative value of various skull features and lists certain structures that should be looked for in the various skull projections.

The questions that should be asked in the evaluation of skull roentgenograms are:

Is the finding an artifact?

Is it a normal variation or a pathological finding?

Is the pathological finding a manifestation of systemic disease, a primary skull condition, or a manifestation of intracranial disease?

A sequential exploration of these questions will avoid many pitfalls.

EXTRACALVARIAL STRUCTURES SIMULATING LESIONS

It is imperative to consider the possibility of extracalvarial structures or objects simulating intracranial lesions. A dense external occipital protuberance, electroencephalogram paste, sebaceous cyst, hair braids, a glass eye, and gravel or sand in the hair or scalp are some structures or objects that will simulate intracranial densities (Fig. 4–1). An ulcerated scalp neoplasm may simulate a lytic skull lesion. Air in a gaping scalp wound may simulate a fracture (Fig. 4–1*E*).

PSEUDOLESIONS

The following features are occasionally misinterpreted as abnormal.

Apparent Suprasellar and Sellar Calcification

Normal calvarial densities, carotid siphon calcifications, or ligamentous calcifications may simulate sellar and suprasellar calcified masses (Fig. 4–2). Stereoscopic lateral radiographs are of great help, and multiple projections or laminagraphy may establish the true situation.

Dural plaques of calcification may be diagnosed by demonstrating that the calcification is adjacent to the inner surface of the vault or in the falx. Calcification of the carotid siphon is manifested by curved linear streaks of calcification parallel to one another, superimposed on the sella, and they usually occupy the cavernous portion of the carotid siphon. The superior wall of the ca-

M. M. SCHECHTER

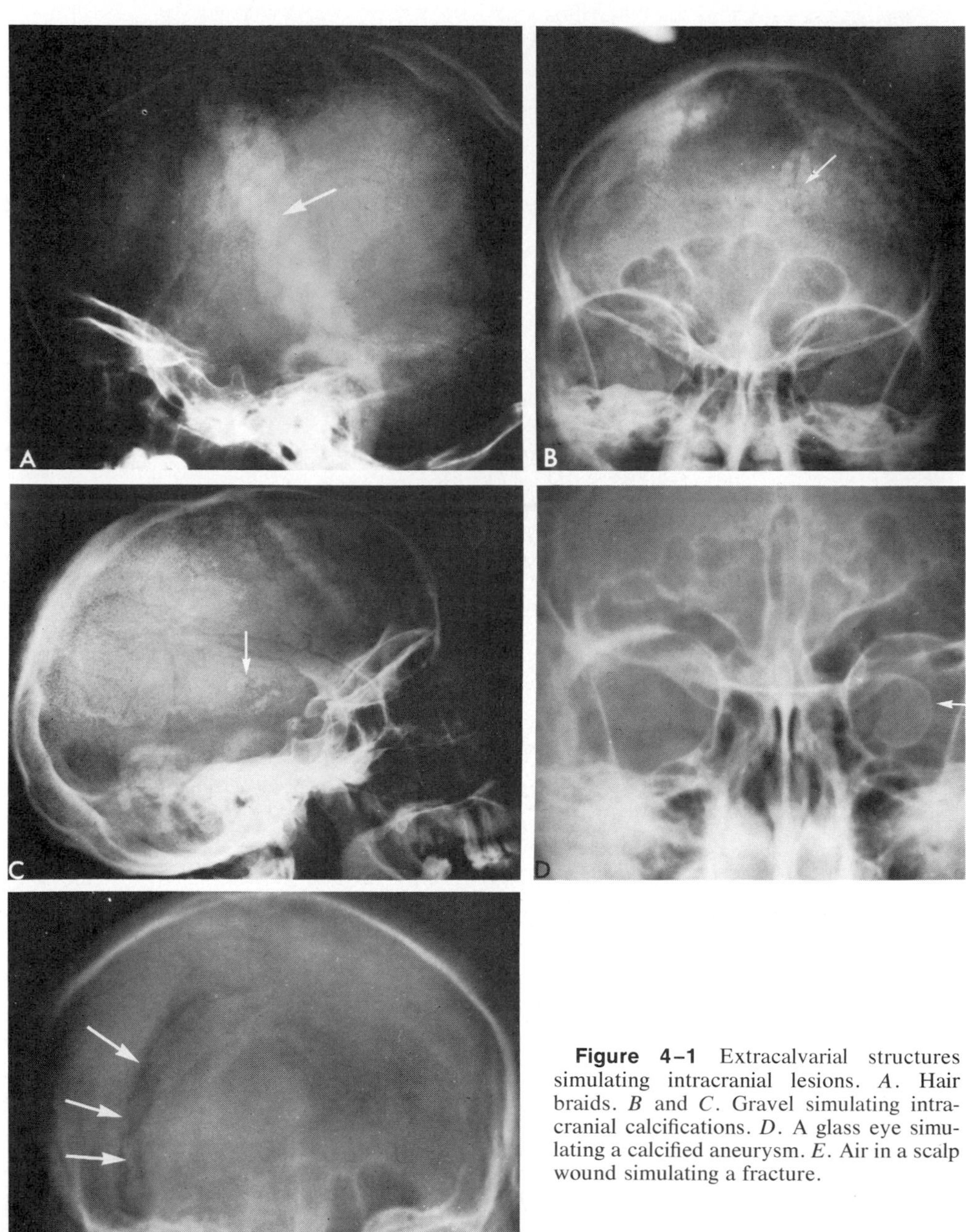

Figure 4–1 Extracalvarial structures simulating intracranial lesions. *A*. Hair braids. *B* and *C*. Gravel simulating intracranial calcifications. *D*. A glass eye simulating a calcified aneurysm. *E*. Air in a scalp wound simulating a fracture.

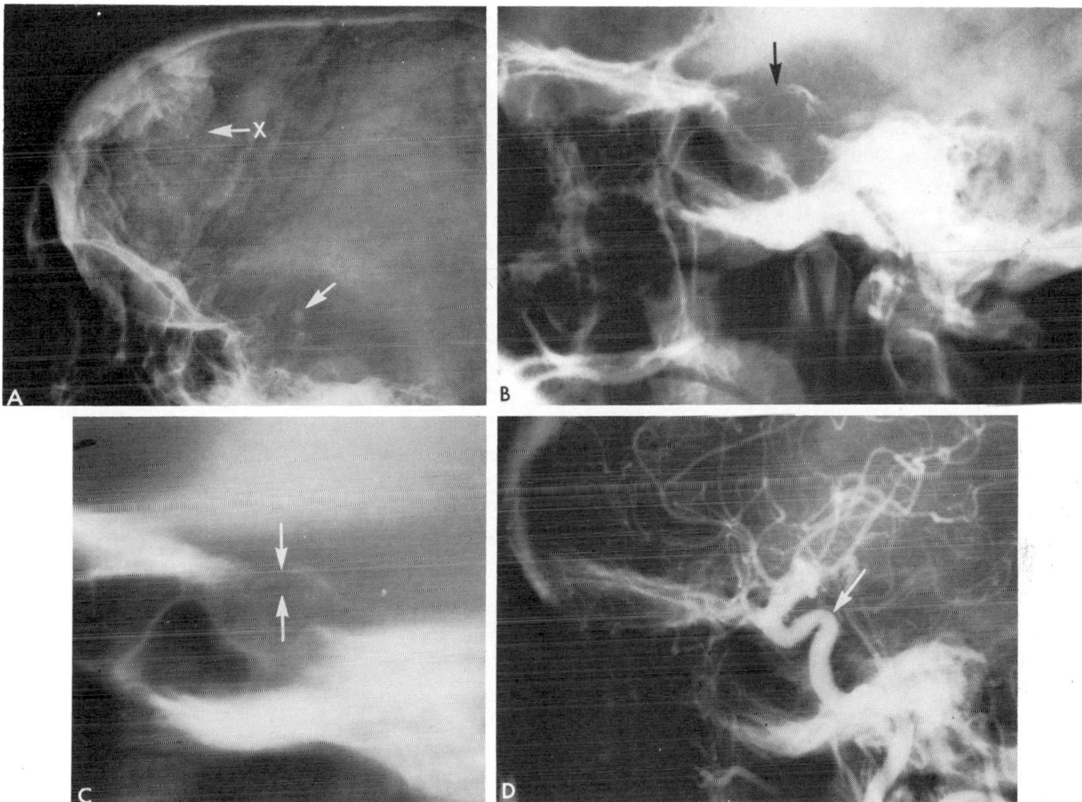

Figure 4–2 *A*. Calvarial densities (*arrows*) simulating sellar and suprasellar calcification. Note hyperostosis frontalis interna (X). *B*. Carotid siphon calcification (*arrow*) in lateral view. *C*. Carotid siphon calcification laminagram. Note the two parallel lines of calcification. *D*. Carotid siphon calcification confirmed by angiography.

rotid siphon is usually more densely calcified (Fig. 4–2). This calcification may be recognized in the anteroposterior projection, in which it shows through the ethmoid air sinus, but tomography in the coronal plane will usually demonstrate it to better advantage. Even after most extensive and meticulous studies one may have to resort to angiography to make a final diagnosis.

Absence of Greater and Lesser Sphenoidal Wings

There may be great variation in the bony density and configuration of these structures. Asymmetry is more the rule than the exception.

The bone of the wings of the sphenoid is at times so thin that routine radiographs may suggest their absence (Fig. 4–3). This presents a problem that becomes more difficult in cases of asymmetry in which there is an apparent unilateral absence of the sphenoidal wings. When there is a clinical suspicion of a lesion related to this area, the problem is further compounded and the result may be unnecessary specialized radiological work-ups. Rischbieth and Bull illustrated the normal asymmetry of the superior orbital fissure.[12] Because of its extreme variability, a diagnosis of abnormality should not be based on a single projection. The greater sphenoidal wing frequently is not seen in the Caldwell projection. If the structures are not recognized in the base projection, stereoscopic and laminagraphic examinations may be critical. Extension of the sphenoidal sinus into the greater sphenoidal wing should not be mistaken for erosion or dysplasia (Fig. 4–3).[9]

"Eroded" Foramen Ovale and Foramen Spinosum

In spite of their notoriety, the diagnostic value of these two foramina is extremely limited and they should be evaluated with much caution.

Developmental variations are frequent. The posterior wall of the foramen spinosum is the last to ossify and frequently remains unossified. The foramina spinosum and ovale may ossify as a single structure. The walls of the foramina may slant. The overlying nasopharyngeal soft tissue structures may obscure the anatomy. All these factors plus the direction of the radiographic beam may contribute to the appearance of indistinct canals (Fig. 4–3*B*). There is poor correlation between the caliber of the middle meningeal artery and the size of the foramen spinosum. Lesions involving these foramina are usually related to fifth nerve and nasopharyngeal tumors (see Fig. 4–35). The diagnositc value of these foramina in meningiomas is limited.

"Widened" Coronal Suture

The diagnosis of early changes of sutural diastasis is difficult, particularly in the very young in whom ossification is incomplete. The coronal suture is more difficult to evaluate than the others. The superior segment of the coronal suture may remain open during childhood. Frequently this presents a problem in children who are being evaluated for a possible intracranial lesion. The suture will be interpreted as widened or normal, depending upon the clinical convictions of the physician who is making the evaluation. Because of the normal variations in closure of the coronal suture, care should be taken not to base a diagnosis of increased intracranial pressure solely on the appearance of this structure (Fig. 4–3).

The "J" Sella

The terms "J sella" and "omega sella" are widely used in the literature and in the everyday evaluation of infant skull roentgenograms. Although these terms are frequently used by radiologists and neurosurgeons, there has always been considerable disagreement as to the diagnostic value of the findings. This unsatisfactory situation resulted from the previous lack of basic correlative anatomical-radiological information about the sphenoid during infancy, information that is now available from studies correlating the developmental anatomy of the sella with its radiological manifestations.[5,6] With this information, pathological changes can be differentiated from normal growth patterns. A review of the normal

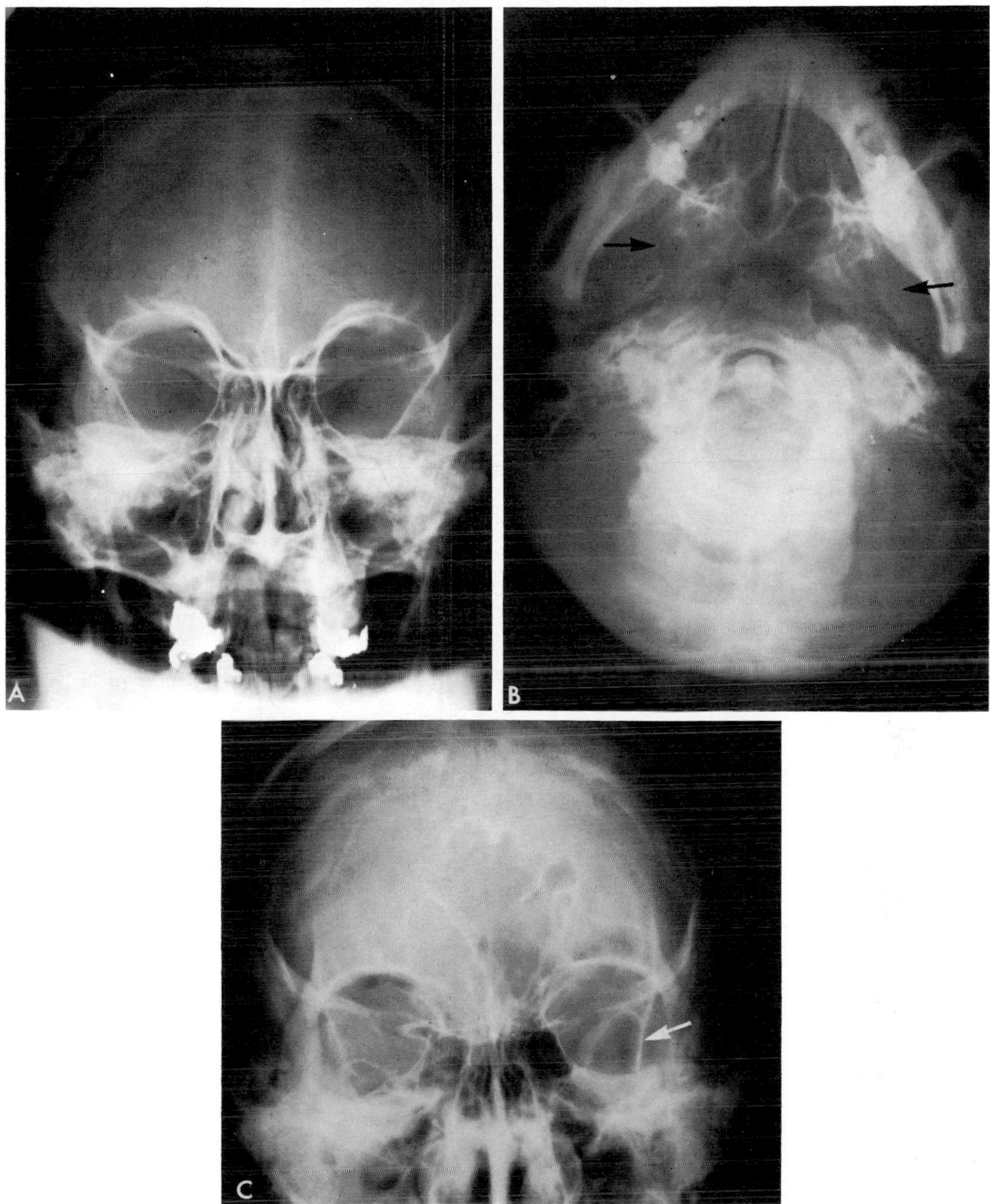

Figure 4–3 Normal structures suggesting abnormalities. *A*. Thin greater sphenoidal wing suggesting its absence. *B*. Indistinct foramen ovale and foramen spinosum. *C*. Huge sphenoid sinus simulating an eroded greater sphenoidal wing.

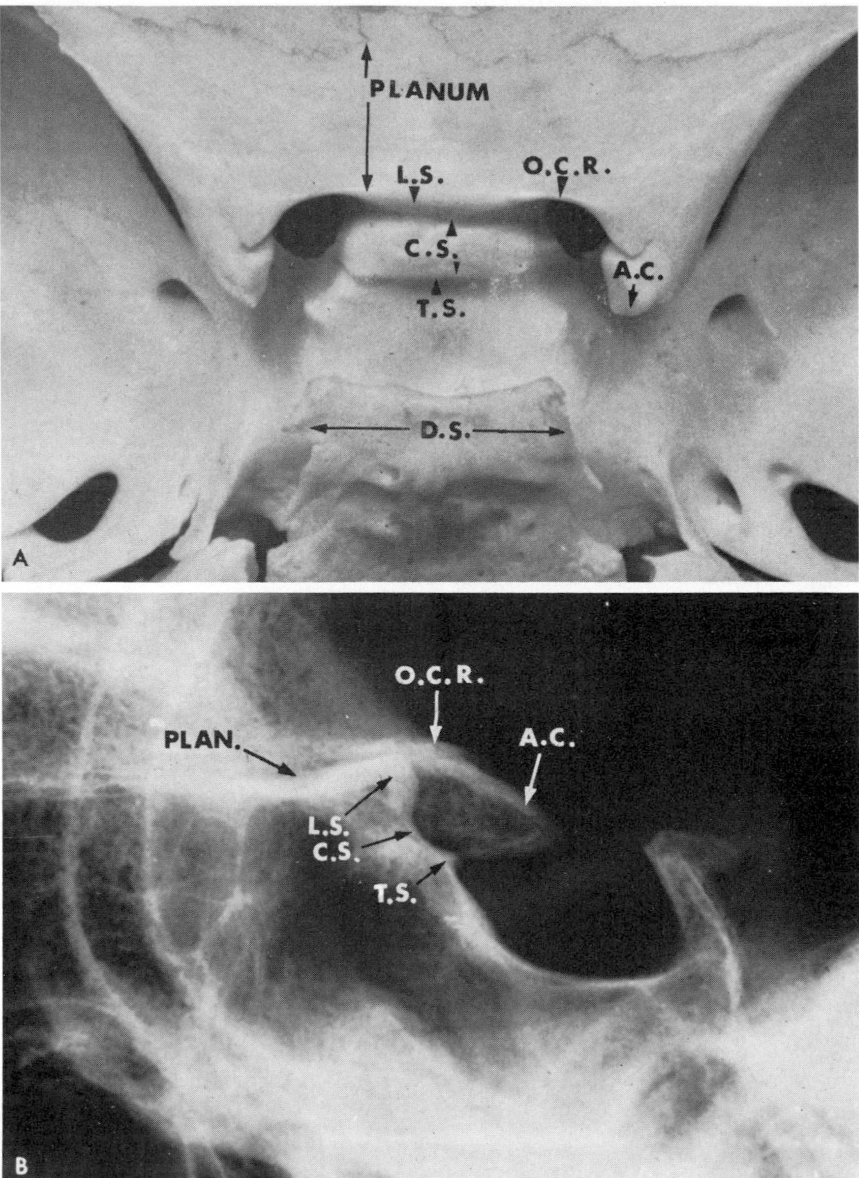

Figure 4–4 Normal adult sphenoid. *A*. Superior aspect of sphenoid bone specimen. *B*. Lateral skull roentgenogram. Note that the optic canal roof (O.C.R.) is not a prominent structure in the lateral skull roentgenogram. A.C., anterior clinoid process; C.S., chiasmatic sulcus; D.S., dorsum sellae; L.S., limbus sphenoidale; PLAN., planum sphenoidale; T.S., tuberculum sellae. (From Kier, E. L.: The infantile sella turcica: new radiologic and anatomic concepts based on a developmental study of the sphenoid bone. Amer. J. Roentgen., *102*:747–767, 1968. Reprinted by permission.)

adult sphenoid anatomy is necessary to understand the developmental changes (Fig. 4–4). An important feature of the developing sphenoid is that the planum sphenoidale is not present at birth. Prior to the formation of the planum, an elongated sulcus chiasmatis should not be mistaken for an abnormal feature.

The normally prominent roof of the optic canal during early infancy should not be mistaken for the planum sphenoidale (Fig. 4–5). This mistake accounts for many of the normal infants who have been presented in the literature as showing "abnormal excavation" of the sulcus chiasmatis. In effect, very few pathological conditions represent true abnormalities of the tuberculum sellae, sulcus chiasmatis, planum sphenoidale, and optic canal roof. Craniopharyngiomas in infancy are almost invariably associated with sellar abnormalities. Sellar abnormalities in optic gliomas are inconstant and depend upon whether the optic nerve is involved and whether the

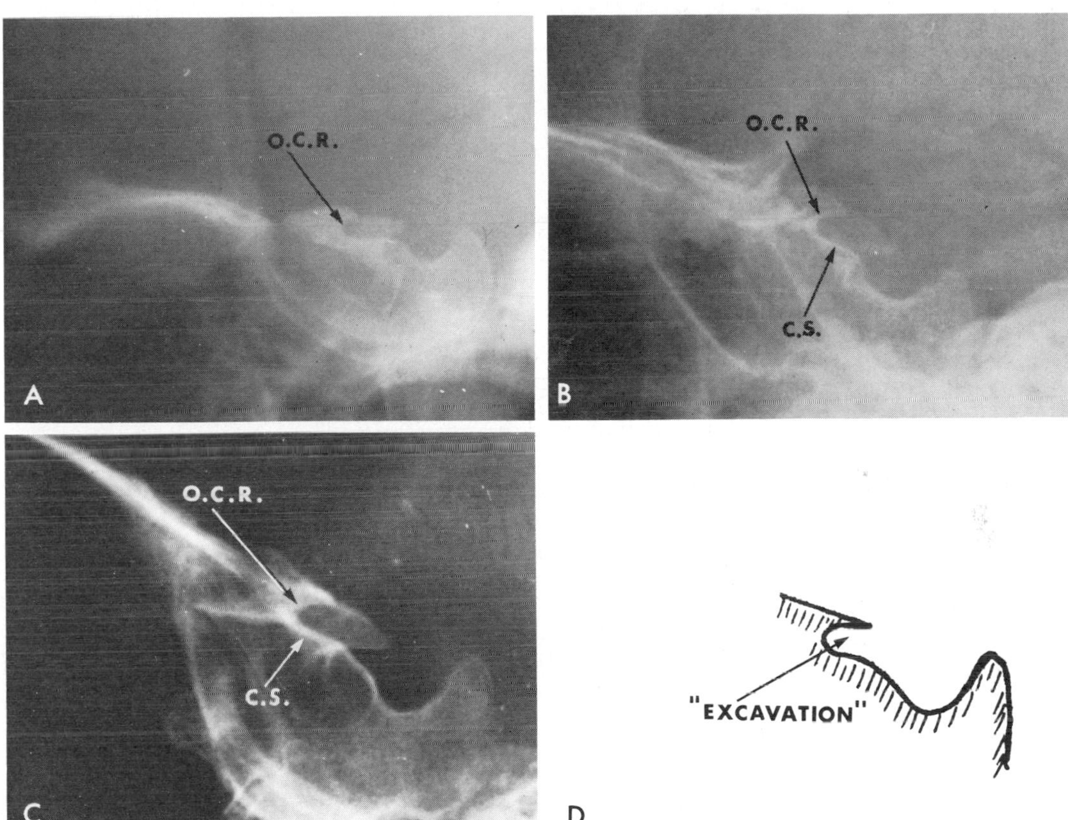

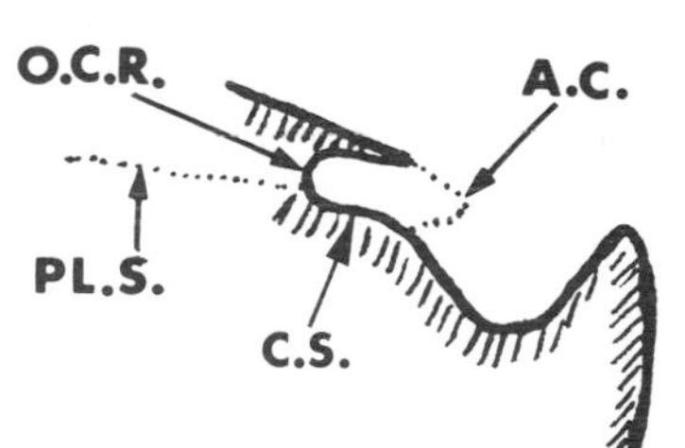

Figure 4–5 Elucidation of the mythical "excavation." *B* and *C*. Children with normal presellar sphenoids. These are similar to the cases presented in the literature as showing "excavation under the anterior clinoid process." *D*. Tracing similar to the ones presented in the literature to illustrate the "abnormal excavation." Note that the so-called excavation is a roentgenological illusion resulting from the prominence of the optic canal roof (O.C.R.) during infancy. The laterally positioned optic canal roof forms the superior component of the so-called excavation and projects as a dense white line that appears to be continuous with the normal and midline chiasmatic sulcus (C.S.). *E*. Tracing demonstrating the correct anatomical components of the "excavation." A.C., anterior clinoid process; PL.S., planum sphenoidale. Cases such as these have resulted in the loss of the diagnostic value of this term. (From Kier, E. L.: The infantile sella turcica: new radiologic and anatomic concepts based on a developmental study of the sphenoid bone. Amer. J. Roentgen., *102*:747–767, 1968. Reprinted by permission.)

chiasm is pre-fixed or post-fixed. Sellar changes due to posterior fossa masses are very rare. The terms "J sella" and "omega sella" and the like are diagnostically meaningless, harmful to the objective assessment of the sphenoid in infancy, and should be discarded.

The "Enlarged" Optic Canal

The radiological evaluation of the optic canal is difficult because of the direction of its axis and its complex three-dimensional architecture. A review of the normal anatomy is appropriate at this time. The term "foramen" should not be used, as it is actually a canal with two openings (Fig. 4–6). An obviously enlarged canal presents no diagnostic difficulty (Fig. 4–7). Figures for its normal dimensions are available.[14] A difference between the transverse diameters of the two canals of over 25 to 30 per cent as an indicator of disease is an easy figure to remember.[3]

Mistaking a normal variation for a pathological condition has not been infrequent in the past. This resulted from the previous lack of information about the changing features of the infantile optic canal, information that has now been provided by study of the development of the canal, correlating its radiological and anatomical features.[6] The optic canal roof was found to be a very prominent structure during early infancy. The optic canal floor develops slowly and demonstrates many developmental variations. Normal variations such as vertical optic canal, asymmetry, absence of the floor of the cranial opening of the canal, and the vertically large orbital opening of the canal in childhood should not be mistaken for pathological features (Figs. 4–8 and 4–9). The transverse diameter of the canal is a more reliable index of abnormality than the vertical diameter. The roof of the optic

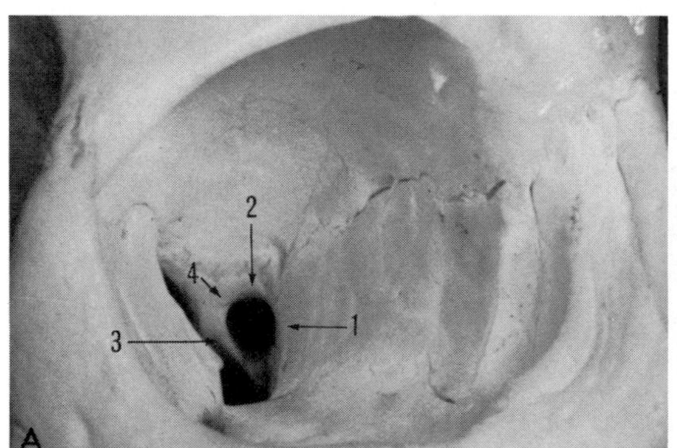

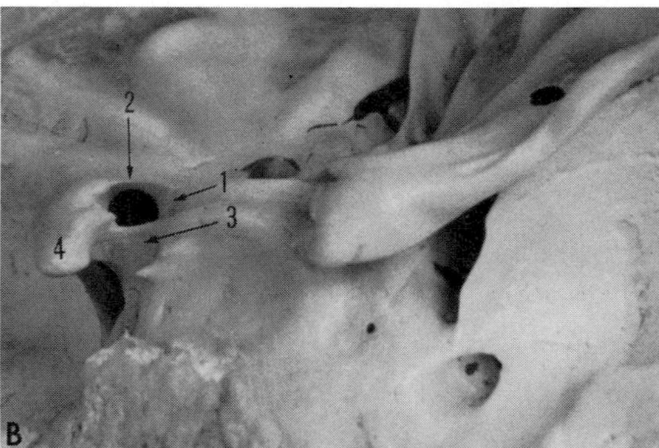

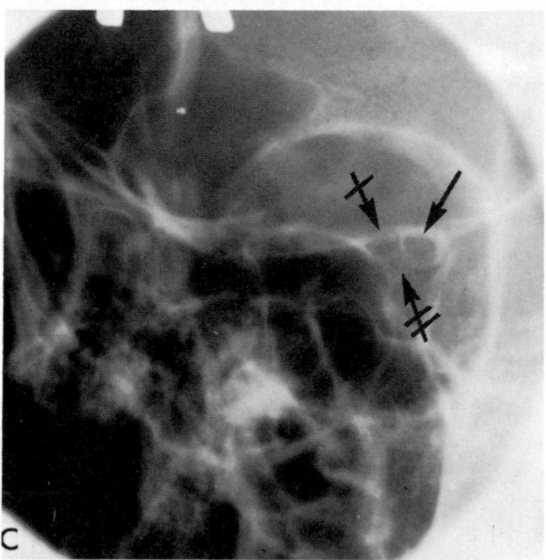

Figure 4–6 Normal adult optic canal. *A*. View of apex of orbit showing the orbital opening. *B*. View of the cranial opening within the skull. Note that cranial opening has its long diameter in the horizontal plane and the orbital opening has its long diameter in the vertical plane. The canal walls are formed by the lateral wall of the sphenoid sinus (1), the lesser sphenoid wing (2), the optic strut (3), and the anterior clinoid processes (4). The optic strut separates the superior orbital fissure from the optic canal. *C*. A pneumatized anterior clinoid process (*arrow*) should not be mistaken for the optic canal (*arrow with single crossed shaft*). Note the optic strut (*arrow with double crossed shaft*) separating the superior orbital fissure from the optic canal. (From Kier, E. L.: Embryology of the normal optic canal and its anomalies; an anatomic and roentgenographic study. Invest. Radiol., *1*:346–362, 1966. *A* and *B* reprinted by permission.)

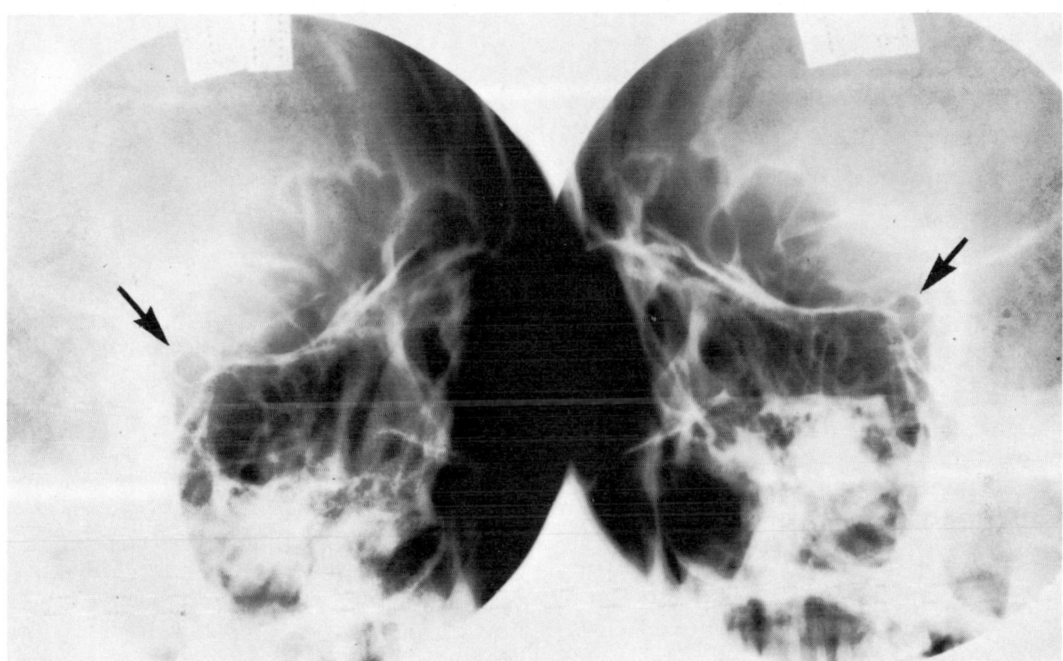

Figure 4–7 Case with optic canal enlargement secondary to optic glioma. Note the difference in size between the two sides.

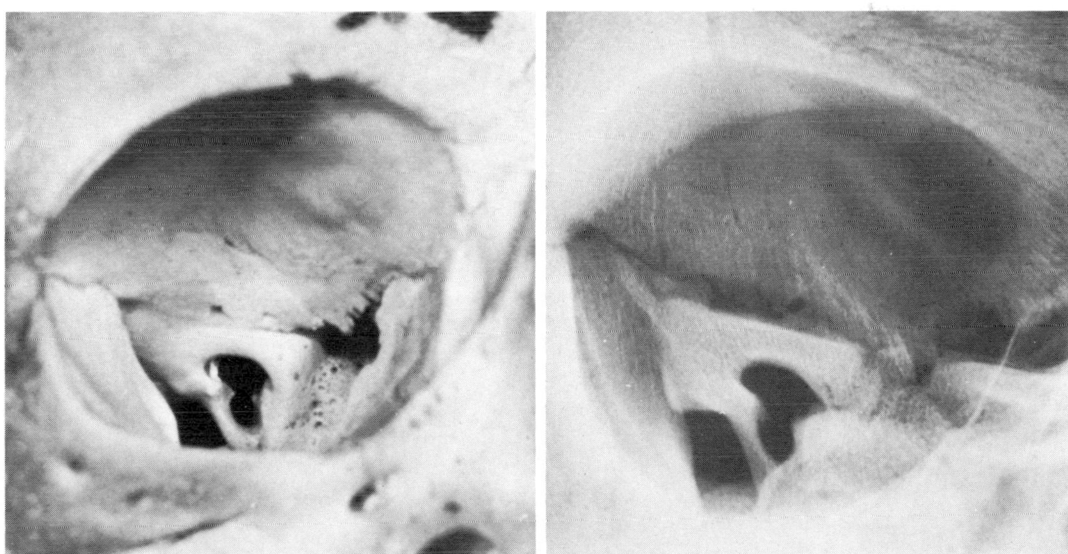

Figure 4–8 Optic canal anomalies. The fetal "keyhole" configuration of the optic canal may persist through childhood. The configuration in childhood should not be mistaken for erosion of the floor or an enlarged canal in the vertical diameter. (From Kier, E. L.: Embryology of the normal optic canal and its anomalies; an anatomic and roentgenographic study. Invest. Radiol., *1*:346–362, 1966. Reprinted by permission.)

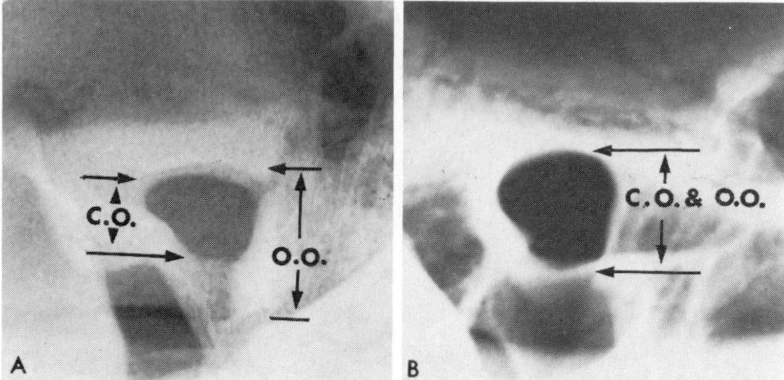

Figure 4–9 The difference between infantile and adult optic canals. *A*. In the child the vertical diameter of the orbital opening (O.O.) is much larger than the vertical diameter of the cranial opening (C.O.). *B*. In the adult the two openings are about equal. This should be considered in the stereoscopic and laminagraphic evaluation of the infantile optic canal. (From Kier, E. L.: Embryology of the normal optic canal and its anomalies; an anatomic and roentgenographic study. Invest. Radiol., *1*:346–362, 1966. Reprinted by permission.)

canal may be normally so thin as to not be demonstrated radiographically.

Sphenoid "Meningioma"

Normal densities at the junction of the greater and lesser sphenoidal wings should not be mistaken for hyperostosis resulting from a sphenoid meningioma (Fig. 4–10).

"Fractures"

Among the structures that should not be mistaken for fractures are: the metopic suture of the frontal bone, the vascular grooves on the cranial bones, and the inner table suture lines.

The frontal bone ossifies from two centers. Usually ossification is complete at birth; occasionally the two ossification centers do not unite at all or unite late in childhood. The nonunion will result in a transitory or permanent frontal (metopic) suture (Fig. 4–11*A*). Vertical midline fractures of the frontal bone are rare. Furthermore, digitations will be recognized in a careful perusal of the area in question, and perisutural densities are present. Caffey has documented other infantile sutures and synchondroses that should not be mistaken for fractures. These include wormian bones, the mendosal suture, and other occipital bone changes (Fig. 4–11*C*).[2]

A recurrent problem in trauma to the back of the head in childhood is the presence of a linear lucency extending through

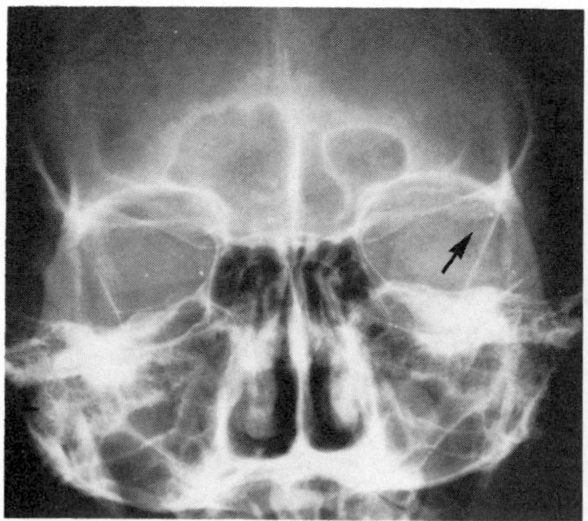

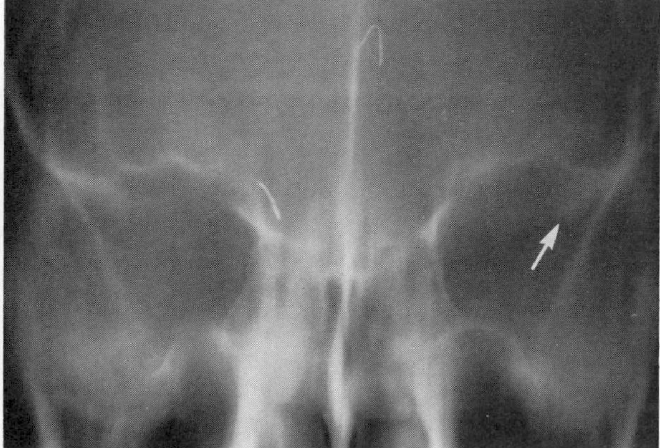

Figure 4–10 Normal sphenoidal densities (*arrows*) at the junction of the greater and lesser sphenoidal wings.

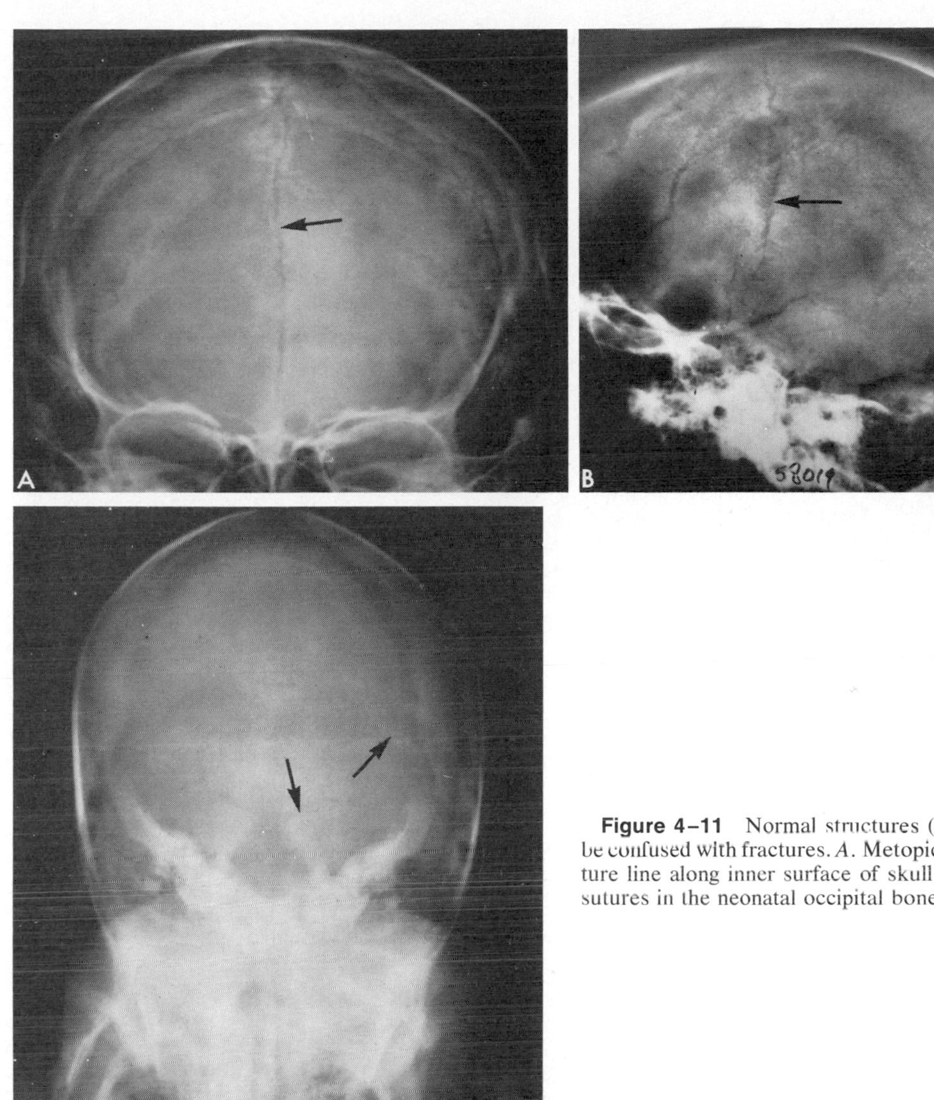

Figure 4–11 Normal structures (*arrows*) not to be confused with fractures. *A*. Metopic suture. *B*. Suture line along inner surface of skull. *C*. The many sutures in the neonatal occipital bone.

the occipital bone to the foramen magnum. Embryological studies show no suture formation simulating this lucency. These lines, therefore, usually constitute fractures.

Grooving of the external surface of the frontal bone and the external surface of the temporal squama is produced by the supraorbital artery (a branch of the ophthalmic artery) and by the middle temporal artery (a branch of the superficial temporal artery) respectively. When the markings are bilateral they tend to be symmetrical, and the question of a fracture should hardly arise.

The inner table of a suture line has a linear appearance and might be mistaken for a fracture. The outer table, however, has interdigitations and if these are recognized a mistaken diagnosis will not be made (Fig. 4–11*B*).

The grooves for the middle meningeal artery are slightly tortuous, taper gradually, and have branches. Middle meningeal vascular grooves do not cross one another. Occasionally the two borders of the groove have slightly sclerotic margins. The shadow they cast is usually not as dense as that of a

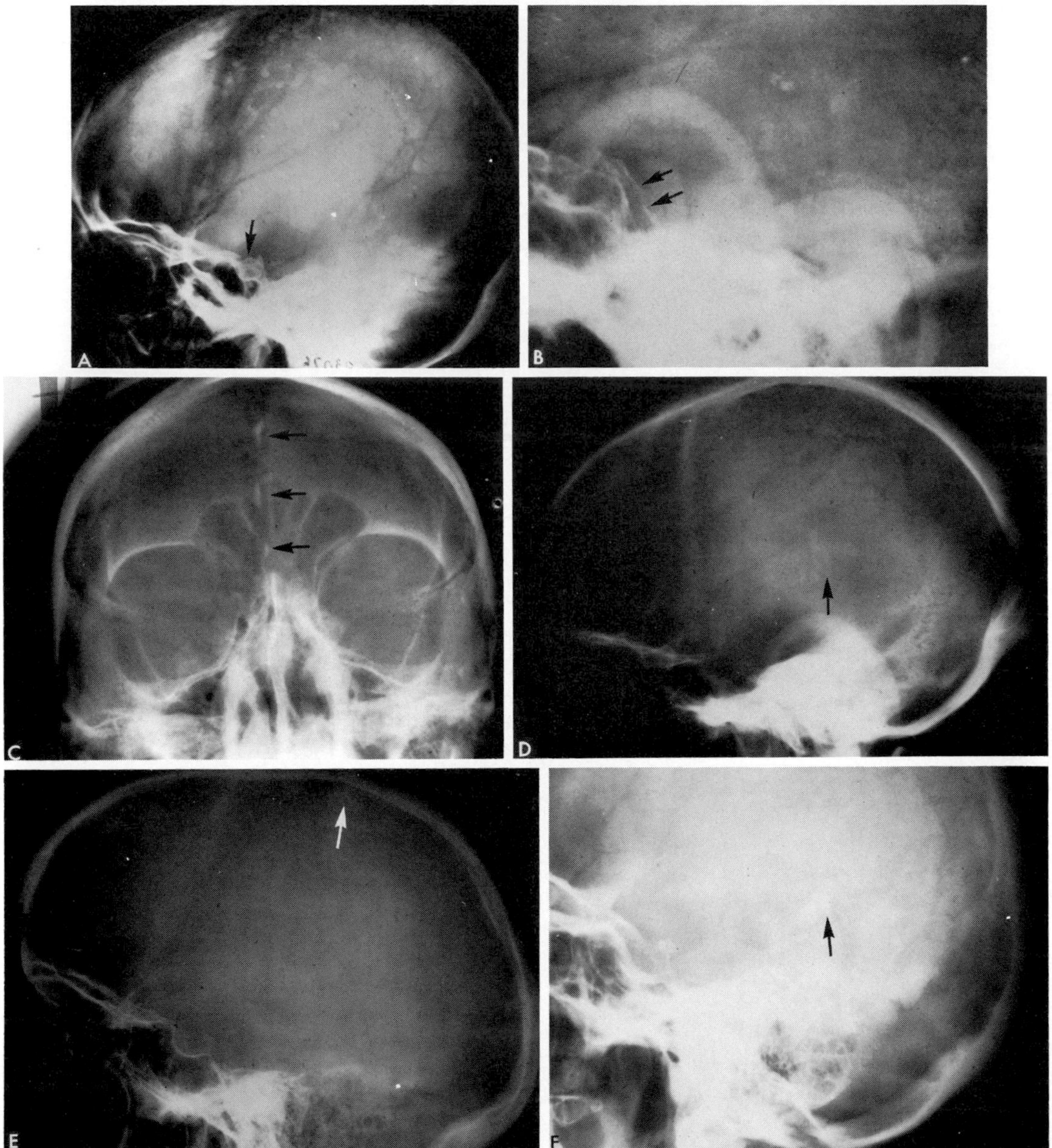

Figure 4–12 Normal intracranial calcification. *A*. Bridged sella. *B*. Petroclinoid ligament. *C*. Falx. *D*. Glomus of choroid plexus. *E*. Pacchionian granulations. *F*. Calcification in tentorium.

fracture since they do not involve the entire thickness of the skull.

Calcified "Lesions"

The following structures may be calcified and should not be interpreted as pathological: the dura including the falx and the tentorium, the petroclinoid and interclinoid ligaments, the carotid siphon, the pineal gland, the choroid plexus, the habenular commissure, and pacchionian granulations (Fig. 4–12).

Reference already has been made to dural calcification and calcification in the carotid siphon. The most characteristic changes of dural calcification relate to the regions where it encompasses the sagittal sinus and where it joins the tentorium. The Y-shaped streaks of calcification in the region of the sinus are characteristic (Fig. 4–12). In the anteroposterior projection, calcification of the point where the falx meets the tentorium may be mistaken for pineal calcification. When the streak of calcification exhibits an inverted V shape, the situation is obvious, but when the calcification is more marked in one lateral leaf of the tentorium it may be mistaken for a displaced pineal gland.

The frequently calcified petroclinoid ligament should not be mistaken for a retrosellar or clivus lesion. The calcification is distinguished by its attachment to the posterior clinoid processes and by the way it extends obliquely downward toward the apices of the petrous pyramids (Fig. 4–12*B*).

The most common site of calcification in the choroid plexus is the glomus, which is situated in the trigone of the lateral ventricle. When both are symmetrically calcified there is usually no problem of mistaken diagnosis. When one calcifies or one calcifies asymmetrically it may be mistaken for a tumor or for a displaced pineal gland. Calcification of the glomus is usually more extensive than that of the pineal and is usually situated behind and below the pineal calcification (Fig. 4–12*D*).

Pacchionian granulations, when calcified, may be recognized as small densities lying just to the side of the sagittal sinus (Fig. 4–12*E*).

The calcified pineal is discussed later in this chapter.

PROBLEM STRUCTURES

The following questions present an almost daily radiological dilemma. Are the vascular markings abnormally increased? Are the convolutional markings abnormal? Is the skull lucency abnormal? Can the pineal body be evaluated in a rotated skull film?

Vascular Markings

There are numerous vascular markings on the inner and outer tables of the skull and also between the two tables. These include dural sinuses, dural veins, diploic veins, and arterial grooves. The extremely wide range of normal venous vascular markings limits the diagnostic value of these structures. The recognition, if possible, of a hypertrophied arterial channel may suggest the presence of a meningioma or a tumor that has invaded the dura, or an arteriovenous malformation. The meningeal vascular grooves accommodate arteries and veins. The channels transmitting mainly arteries may be distinguished from those transmitting veins because the margins are straighter and more regular than those of the veins. A large groove with regular margins that transports an artery and that enlarges as it courses distally is usually associated with a meningioma (Fig. 4–13). Other grooves may be seen to converge toward the area where the meningioma has its attachment. Thus the problem is: first, to distinguish between an arterial groove and a venous groove; and second, to decide if the arterial groove is normal or abnormal. Fortunately the availability of brain scanning greatly helps to resolve this problem. The majority of lesions producing increased vascular markings will also produce positive brain scans.

Convolutional Markings

Experience confirms the statement that convolutional markings as a single finding

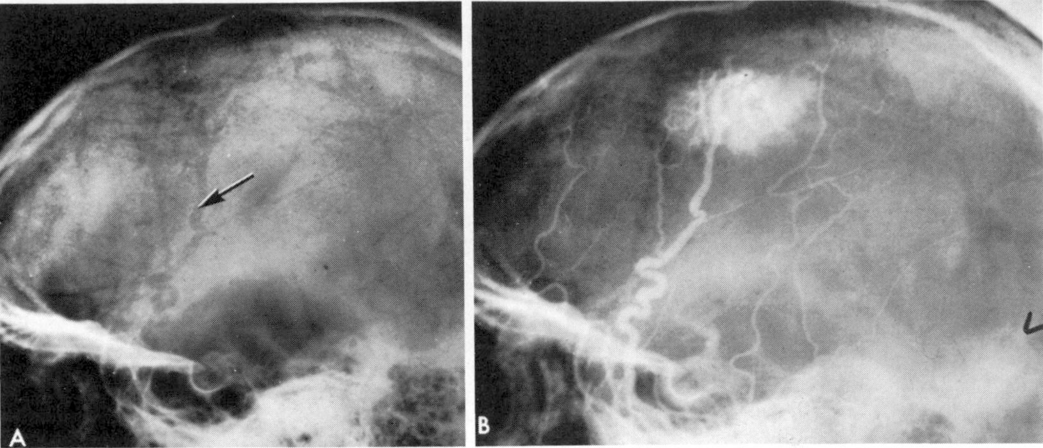

Figure 4–13 *A*. Unilaterally enlarged meningeal groove (*arrow*). *B*. External carotid angiogram demonstrates an enlarged middle meningeal artery within the groove and supplying a meningioma.

are of no significance.[15] In the presence of long-standing raised intracranial pressure, digital markings are usually accompanied by other more diagnostic changes such as an eroded sella.

Skull Lucencies

Benign-appearing skull lucencies are an extremely frequent radiological diagnostic dilemma. A large number of undiagnosable cases remains even after the exclusion of obvious lesions such as pacchionian granulations, venous lakes, emissary veins, parietal foramina, epidermoids, and hemangiomas. These problem cases are extremely vexing and cannot be resolved except by periodic follow-up to determine if they change in appearance, and by specialized contrast studies.

The Pineal in Rotated Films

An experimental study with a pineal model has demonstrated that the normal pineal body in the rotated skull films stays within its range of normal variation (2 to 3 mm) in both anteroposterior and posteroanterior projections.[7] This is related to the center of rotation of the skull on the spine. The pineal is located near the axis of rotation of the skull on the spinal column.

The pineal is also at the center of an imaginary circle formed by the middle and posterior fossae. As a result of these relationships, it remains in the midline in rotated skull films. In extremely rotated skull films the pineal should be correlated with the occipital bone and greater sphenoidal wing, which respectively form the posterior and anterior margins of the imaginary circle.

THE PATHOLOGICAL SKULL

Once an artifact is excluded and it is determined that the finding is of pathological significance, the sequential exploration continues. Then the question must be asked: Is the pathological finding a manifestation of systemic disease, a primary skull condition, or a manifestation of intracranial disease?

In an evaluation of the pathological changes, certain features are of importance, and usually one or more of these will be present.

The Sella Turcica

Changes in the sella may be due to raised intracranial pressure, lesions in adjacent structures, or intrasellar lesions. Definite signs of sellar abnormality are a complete or partial absence of the dorsum sellae and posterior clinoid processes, the floor of the sella, the tuberculum sellae, and the anterior clinoids. A single structure may be involved or the complete sella may be destroyed. In the senile skull these structures

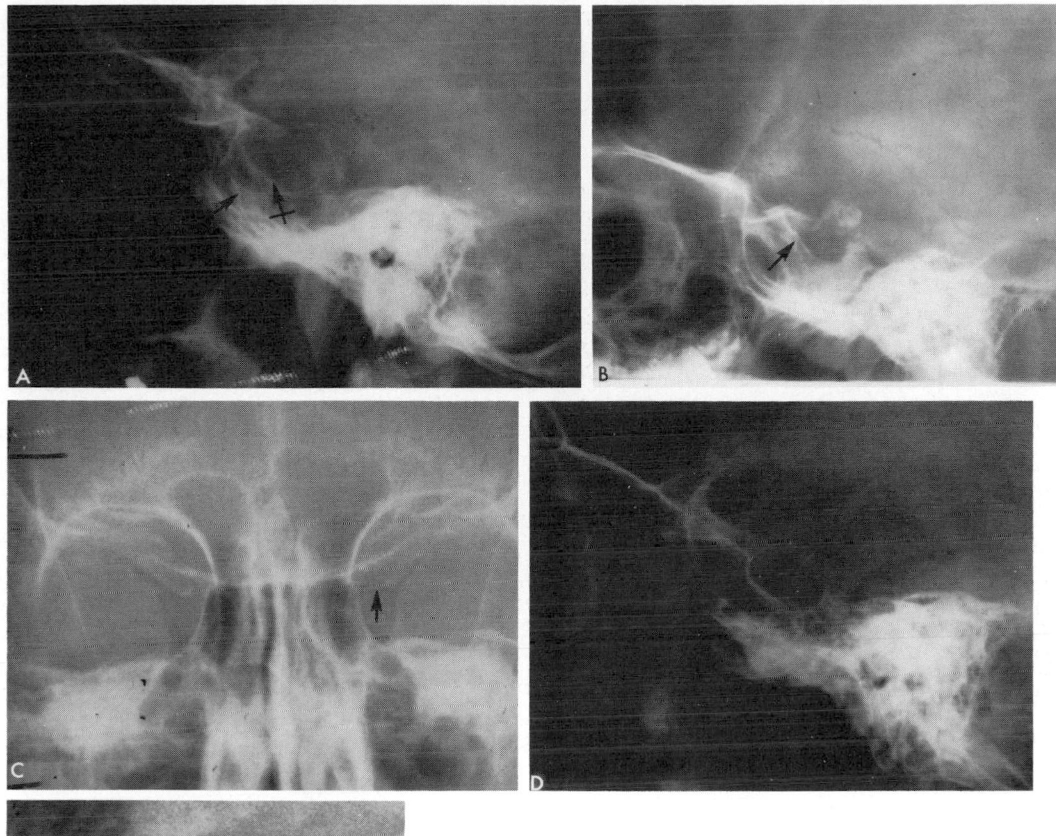

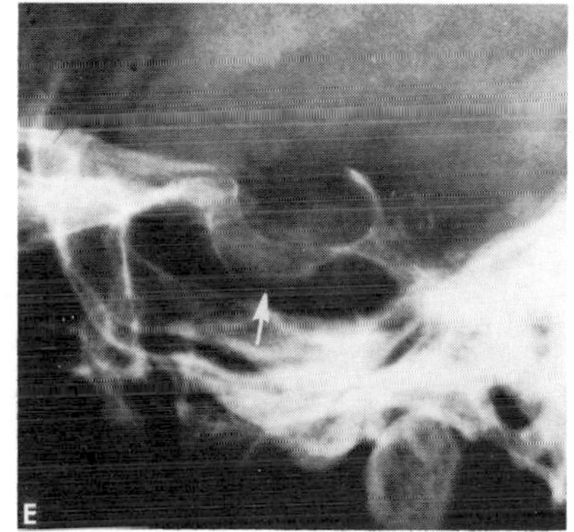

Figure 4–14 Sellae. *A*. Absence of floor. Anterior part of floor of sella is destroyed. The line (*crossed arrow*) is in the lateral skull wall. *B*. Erosion of tuberculum sellae by craniopharyngioma. *C*. Absence of anterior clinoid processes secondary to chromophobe adenoma. *D*. Senile sella showing demineralized dorsum. *E*. Double sella floor secondary to chromophobe adenoma.

may be indistinct, and caution should be exercised in not overinterpreting their absence (Fig. 4–14). A large pituitary adenoma, craniopharyngioma, carotid aneurysm, chordoma, metastatic deposit, and nasopharyngeal tumor may cause total destruction of the sella.

Intrasellar and suprasellar calcifications, craniopharyngiomas, chordomas, meningiomas, aneurysms, and teratomas may show intracranial calcification (see discussion of calcification later in this chapter).

Hyperostosis definitely indicates sellar abnormality. Meningiomas may arise from the clinoid processes, planum sphenoidale, diaphragma sellae, or tuberculum sellae (Figs. 4–15 to 4–19). The area of tumor attachment may show marked bone thickening. A particular type of hyperostosis, the blistering effect of the planum sphenoidale is considered almost pathognomonic for this condition.

Various estimations of the size of the sella in the lateral projection have been de-

Text continued on page 95.

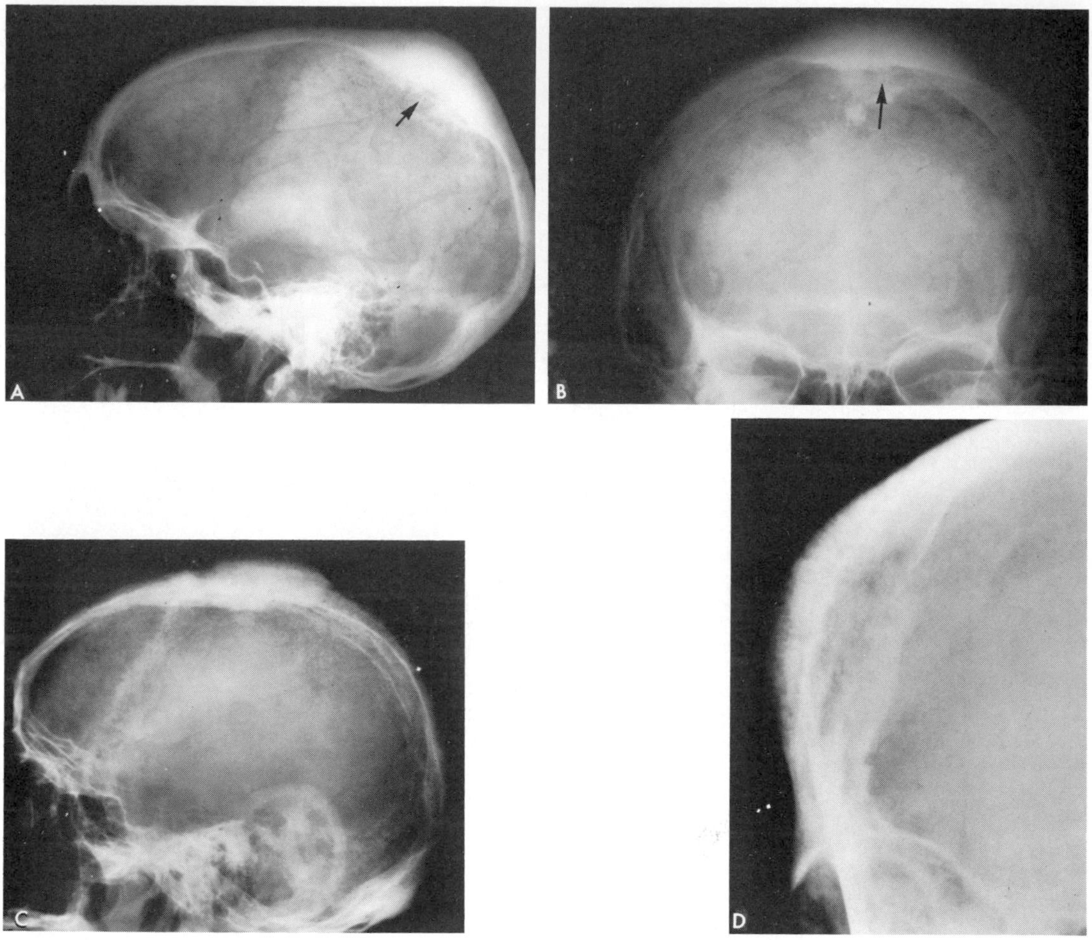

Figure 4–15 Hyperostosis in meningiomas. *A*. Convexity meningioma. *B*. Convexity meningioma. *C*. Parasagittal meningioma. *D*. Frontal meningioma with sunburst appearance, widening of diploë, and extension through the inner table.

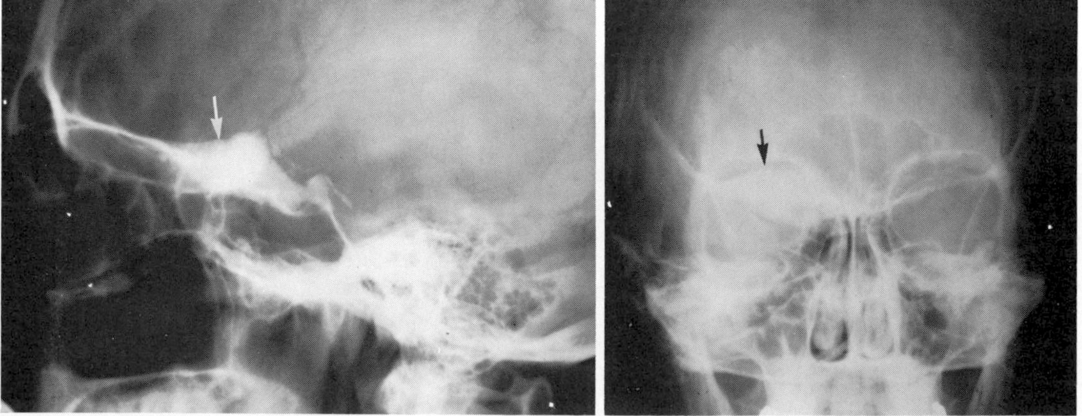

Figure 4–16 Meningioma of lesser sphenoid wing.

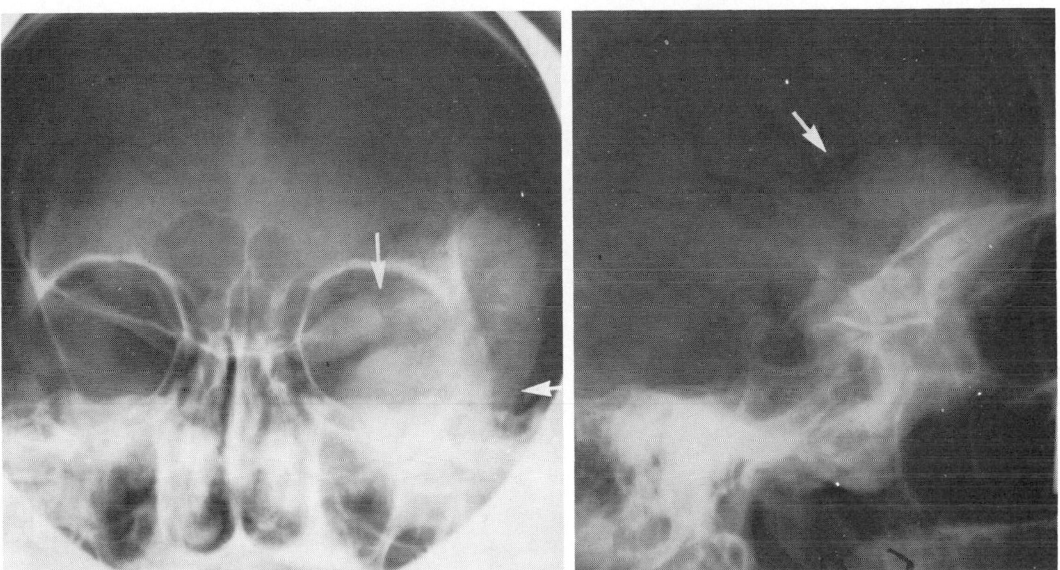

Figure 4–17 Meningioma of greater and lesser wing of the sphenoid bone.

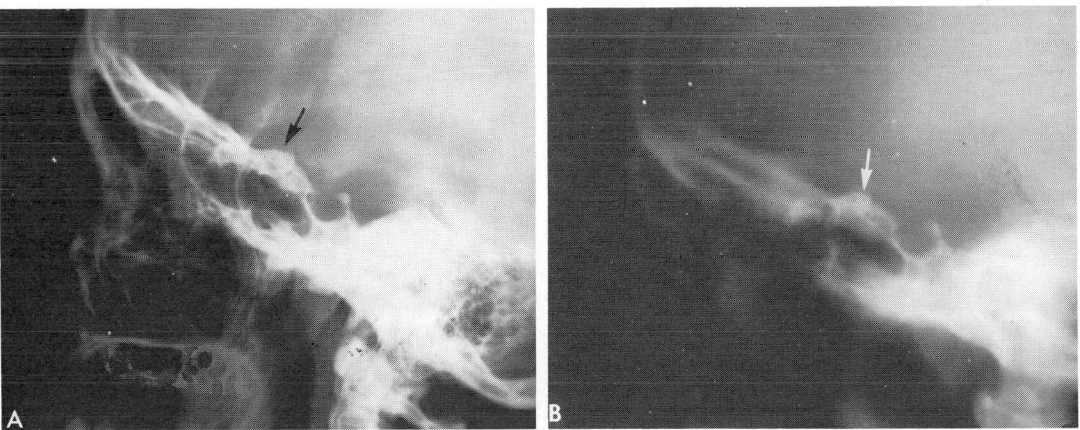

Figure 4–18 Meningioma of planum sphenoidale. *A*. Lateral view. *B*. Tomogram.

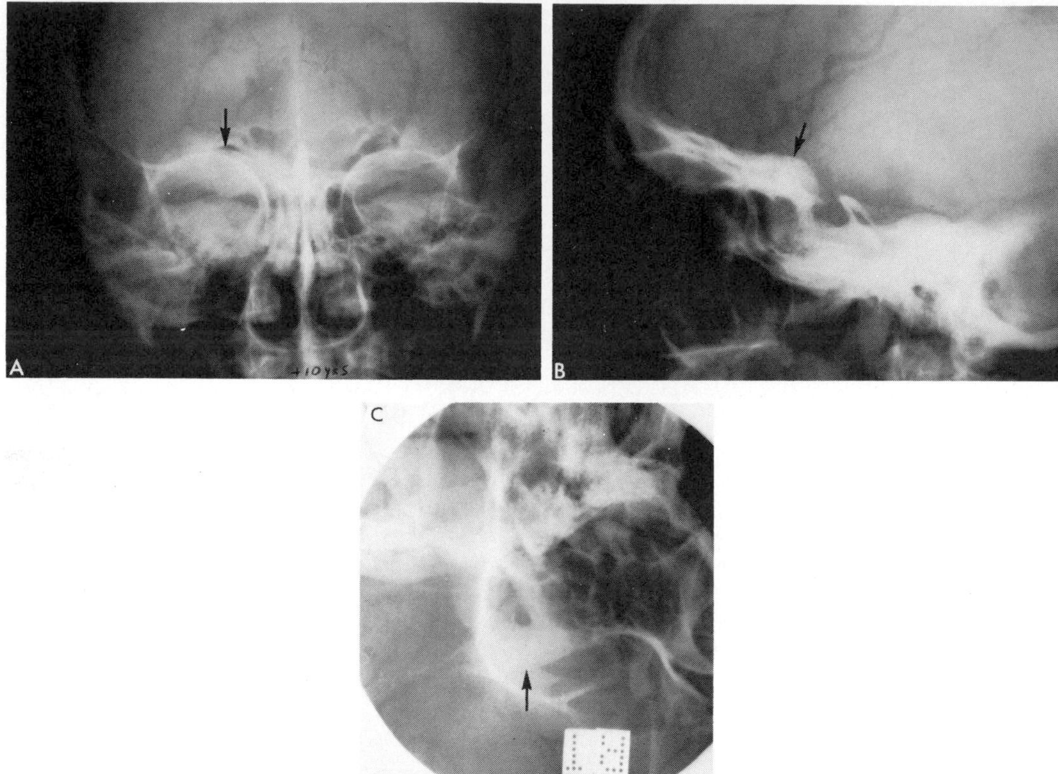

Figure 4–19 Sphenoid meningioma surrounding optic canal. *A*. Anteroposterior view. *B*. Lateral view. *C*. Optic canal view.

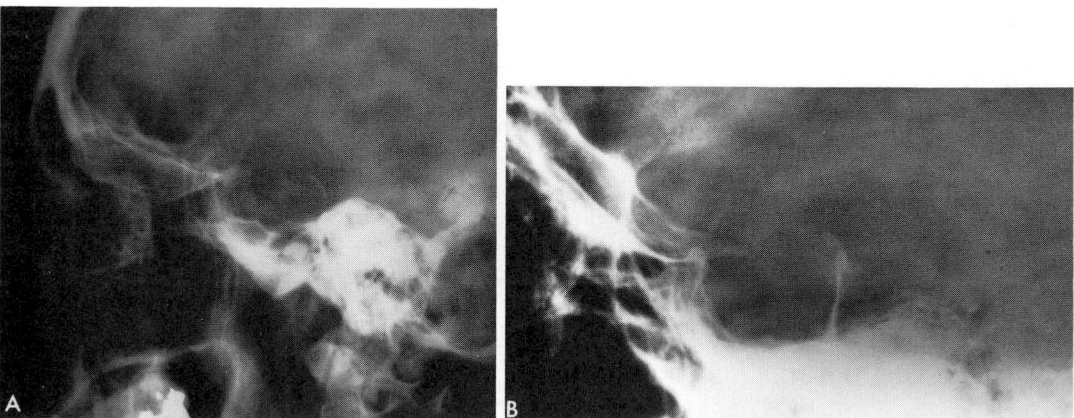

Figure 4–20 *A*. Chromophobe adenoma demonstrating an enlarged sella, absence of floor of sella, anterior clinoid processes tipped up, destruction of tuberculum sellae, displaced dorsum sellae, and "floating" posterior clinoid processes. *B*. Chromophobe adenoma. Note large sella, destruction of floor, pointed anterior clinoid process, and thinning of posteriorly displaced dorsum sellae.

TABLE 4–1 DISTINCTION BETWEEN INTRASELLAR AND EXTRASELLAR LESIONS

INTRASELLAR LESIONS	EXTRASELLAR LESIONS
Sella ballooned	Sella enlarged, not ballooned
Anterior clinoids undermined	No undermining
Double floor	Usually single floor
Posterior clinoids preserved	Posterior clinoids usually destroyed
Posterior clinoids floating	No sloping of dorsum sellae
Dorsum sellae sloping backward	

scribed. Any sella with a depth of over 15 mm and an anteroposterior diameter of over 20 mm is definitely abnormal.

Certain changes in the sella have been referred to in the past as definite signs of abnormality. The signs listed as follows are now considered questionable, since they have not proved to have consistent diagnostic value. They are: (1) sloping floor (double floor), (2) depth of 13 to 15 mm and anteroposterior diameter of 17 to 20 mm, (3) pointed anterior clinoids, and (4) a demineralized dorsum and floor. The J-shaped sella has been covered earlier in this chapter.

The distinction between an intrasellar lesion and an extrasellar lesion may be assessed as shown in Table 4–1.

Displaced Physiological Calcifications

The best known method for evaluating pineal position in the lateral projection is the Vastine-Kinney method.[16] The method described by Oon is simple, reliable, and easy to master.[10] Pineal displacements are usually to the side and downward. Upward displacements are unusual.

The calcified glomus, shown in Figure 4–21, has been discussed earlier in this chapter.

Trauma

The vault may be fractured and there may be a tear in the membranous coverings of the brain. When the fracture line passes through a nasal sinus or through the mastoid air cells, cerebrospinal fluid may escape into the sinuses and mastoid spaces with rhinorrhea and otorrhea resulting. Air may pass from these structures into the subarachnoid spaces and into the ventricles. Blood may also enter the sinuses, which then become radiopaque. A fluid level may be present in the sinuses (Figs. 4–21 and 4–22).

Fractures may be linear, depressed, diastatic, and comminuted (Figs. 4–23 and 4–24). The fracture line may further involve an air sinus or may traverse a middle meningeal artery or a dural sinus. The indriven spicule may tear a dural sinus or damage brain cortex. The foramina of the skull have an area of thick bone surrounding them, and it can be readily understood how fracture lines take a zigzag course following the lines of least resistance.

The radiological evidence of a skull fracture is the fracture line and displacement of bone. Infants may, however, have fractures without evidence of a fracture line, since the soft skull may indent like a ping-pong ball. Loose skin folds in the neonate should not be mistaken for fracture lines. Fracture lines appear as dark radiolucent shadows when the x-ray beam passes directly through the plane of the fracture. If the ray passes a little obliquely to the fracture plane, the margins of the fracture will be less sharp and may even appear wider apart. The fracture may not be recognized at all if the x-ray beam meets the fracture plane at right angles. The fracture line is usually sharper on the side closest to the film. This may be an important lateralizing sign when the fracture cannot be recognized in other projections. In depressed fractures the fragments may overlap. Overlapping of the margins will cause them to appear more dense radiologically. Without overlap of the margins or turning of a fragment so as to increase its density, depression of a fracture may be missed unless tangential views are taken.

A cephalhematoma, in the chronic stage, may calcify and appear as a dense mass attached to the outer table of the skull. The sutures limit its extent (Fig. 4–25).

The dura may tear during skull trauma, and gradually the edges of the fracture may

Text continued on page 100.

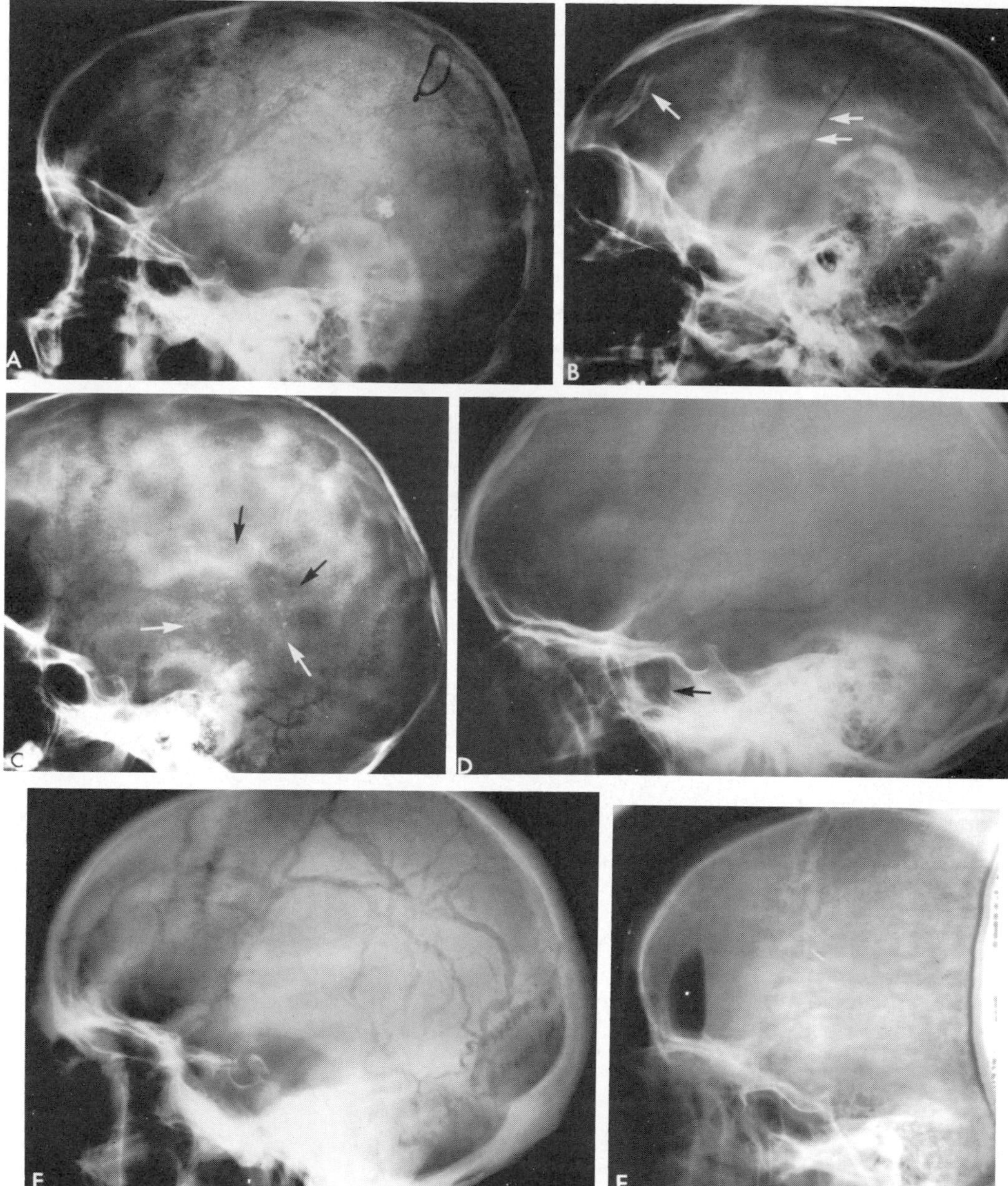

Figure 4–21 Abnormal features on lateral studies. *A*. Displaced calcified glomus of choroid secondary to a mass lesion. *B*. Depressed fracture (*single arrow*). Linear fracture (*double arrow*). *C*. Fine calcifications secondary to ependymoma. *D*. Fluid level in sphenoid sinus secondary to trauma. *E*. Opaque sphenoid secondary to nasopharyngeal carcinoma. Note vascularity of skull. *F*. Unsuspected air-fluid level in frontal brain abscess. Gas-forming organism.

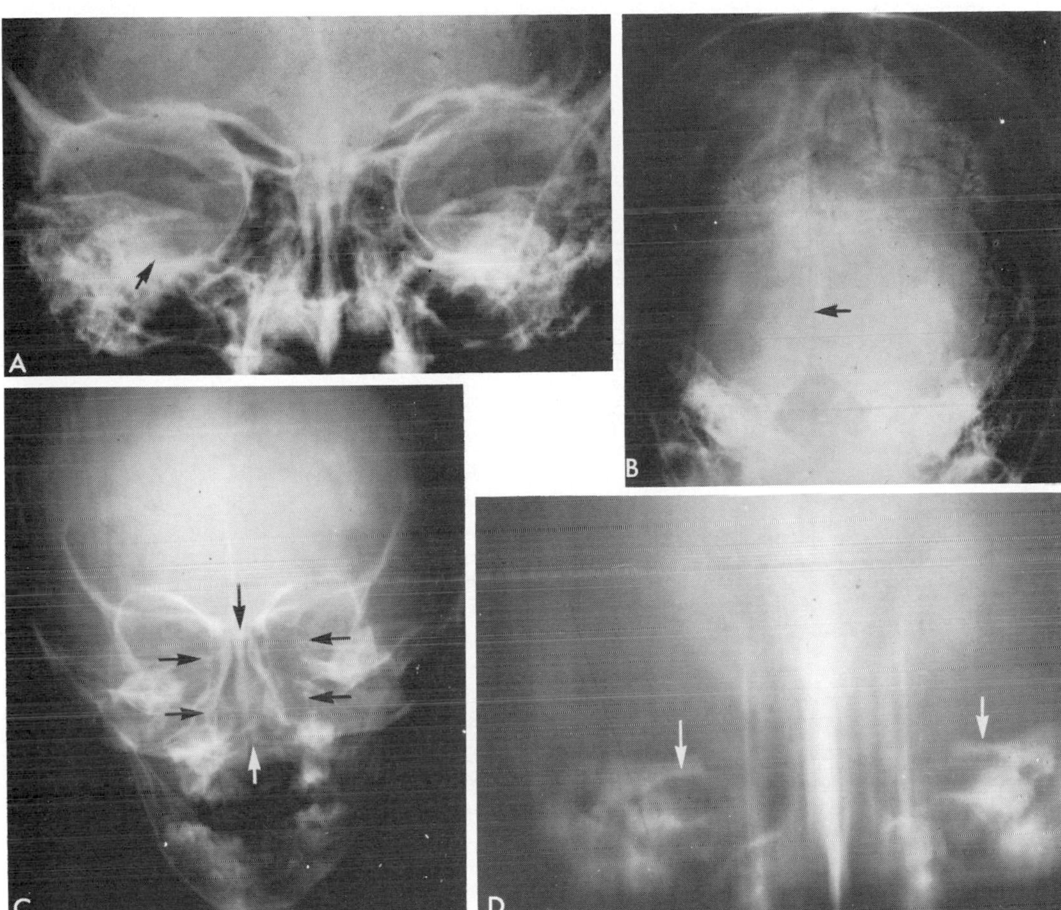

Figure 4–22 Abnormal features on anteroposterior, posteroanterior, and Towne's projections. *A*. Widened internal auditory meatus secondary to acoustic tumor. *B*. Occipital fracture. *C*. Absence of body of sphenoid secondary to nasopharyngeal tumor. Note the bony void in the center of the face in the region of the nose. *D*. Laminagram of petrous bones of a patient with von Recklinghausen's disease with widening of both auditory canals.

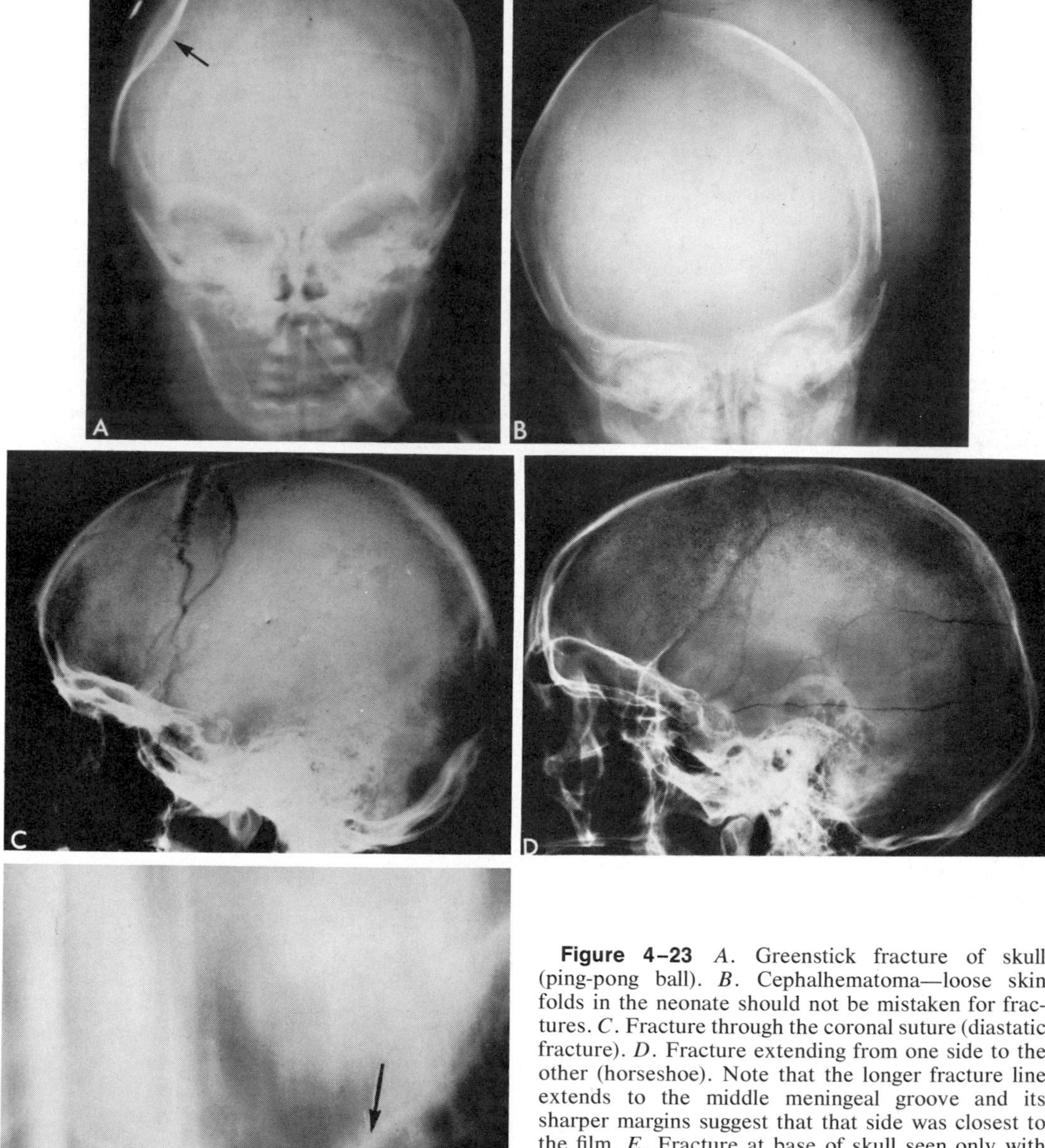

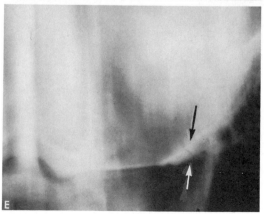

Figure 4–23 *A*. Greenstick fracture of skull (ping-pong ball). *B*. Cephalhematoma—loose skin folds in the neonate should not be mistaken for fractures. *C*. Fracture through the coronal suture (diastatic fracture). *D*. Fracture extending from one side to the other (horseshoe). Note that the longer fracture line extends to the middle meningeal groove and its sharper margins suggest that that side was closest to the film. *E*. Fracture at base of skull seen only with laminagraphy.

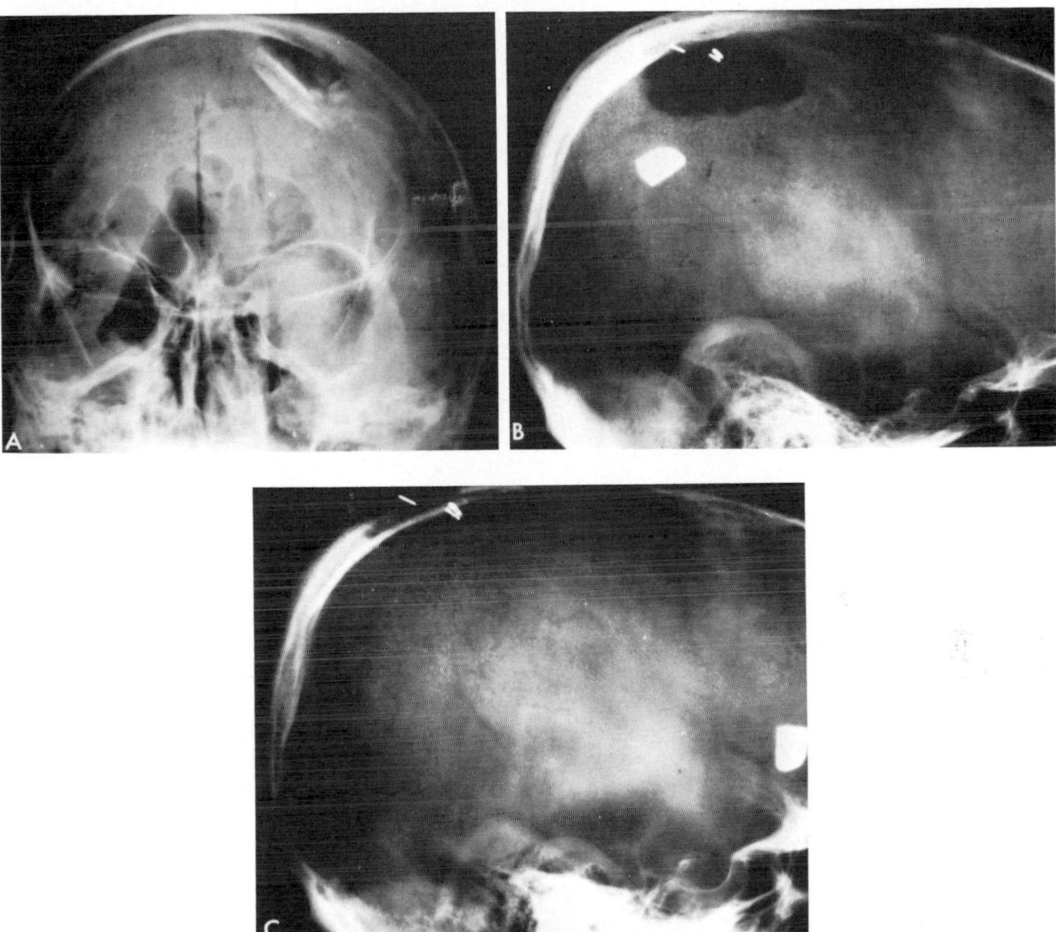

Figure 4–24 *A*. Depressed comminuted fracture. A tear in the coverings of the brain has allowed air to enter the ventricular system. *B* and *C*. Bullet in brain. Brow-up and brow-down films reveal movement of missile, suggesting its location within a ventricle.

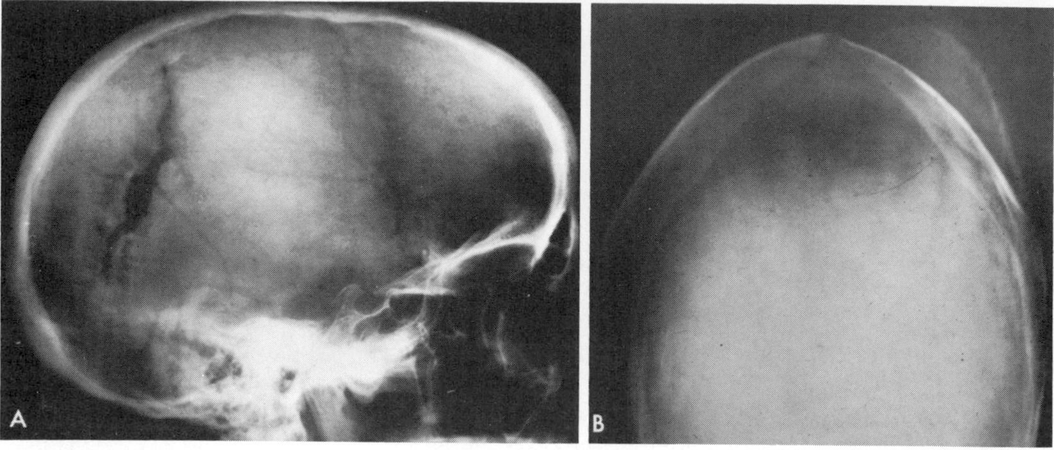

Figure 4–25 *A*. Growth fracture in an adult. Note scalloped margins. *B*. Calcified cephalhematoma.

become scalloped while the gap grows larger (Fig. 4–25). These changes result in the so-called growth fracture or leptomeningeal fracture and may present as a lytic lesion.

Calcification

Physiological calcification has already been discussed. There are also many conditions that may produce pathological intracranial calcification (Fig. 4–26). Because of the large number of conditions that may produce it and the difficulty of establishing the nature of the intracranial calcification, the causes are divided into focal and diffuse as shown in Table 4–2.

Curvilinear calcification at the base of the skull usually suggests an aneurysm, and multiple linear shadows in parallel pairs may suggest an arteriovenous malformation. Sturge-Weber calcification is usually related to the occipital area and has a classic appearance (Fig. 4–27).

The calcification of tumors is usually not characteristic except for lipomas of the corpus callosum, in which two large vertical curvilinear streaks outline the tumor. Teratomas are usually in the midline and may have teeth in them. Other calcifications may be topographically related to particular structures such as the pineal gland, the choroid plexus, the great vein of Galen, the wall of the ventricle, and the basal ganglia, in which case their location is suggestive of their etiology (Fig. 4–28).

Lytic and Hyperostotic Lesions

The lesions may be single or multiple (Table 4–3). A few of these conditions have characteristic changes such as those in Paget's disease, in which a diffuse area of lysis occurs and basilar invagination is marked. The epidermoid has a sclerotic margin, and the eosinophilic granuloma has sharp, punched-out margins without sclero-

TABLE 4–2 CAUSES OF INTRACRANIAL CALCIFICATION

FOCAL CALCIFICATION	DIFFUSE CALCIFICATION
Arteriovenous malformation	Tuberous sclerosis
Aneurysm	Encephalitides
Tumor	Viral
Sturge-Weber syndrome	Parasitic
Chronic subdural hematoma	Endocrine disorder
Teratoma	Tuberculoma
	Tuberculous meningitis

TABLE 4–3 LYTIC AND HYPEROSTOTIC LESIONS

SINGLE LESIONS	MULTIPLE LESIONS
Surgical defect	Pacchionian granulations
Osteoporosis circumscripta	Paget's disease
Meningioma	Persistent parietal foramina
Osteomyelitis	Radiation necrosis
Metastatic disease	Osteomyelitis
Solitary myeloma	Metastatic disease
Epidermoid	Multiple myeloma
Eosinophilic granuloma	
Hemangioma	

Text continued on page 105.

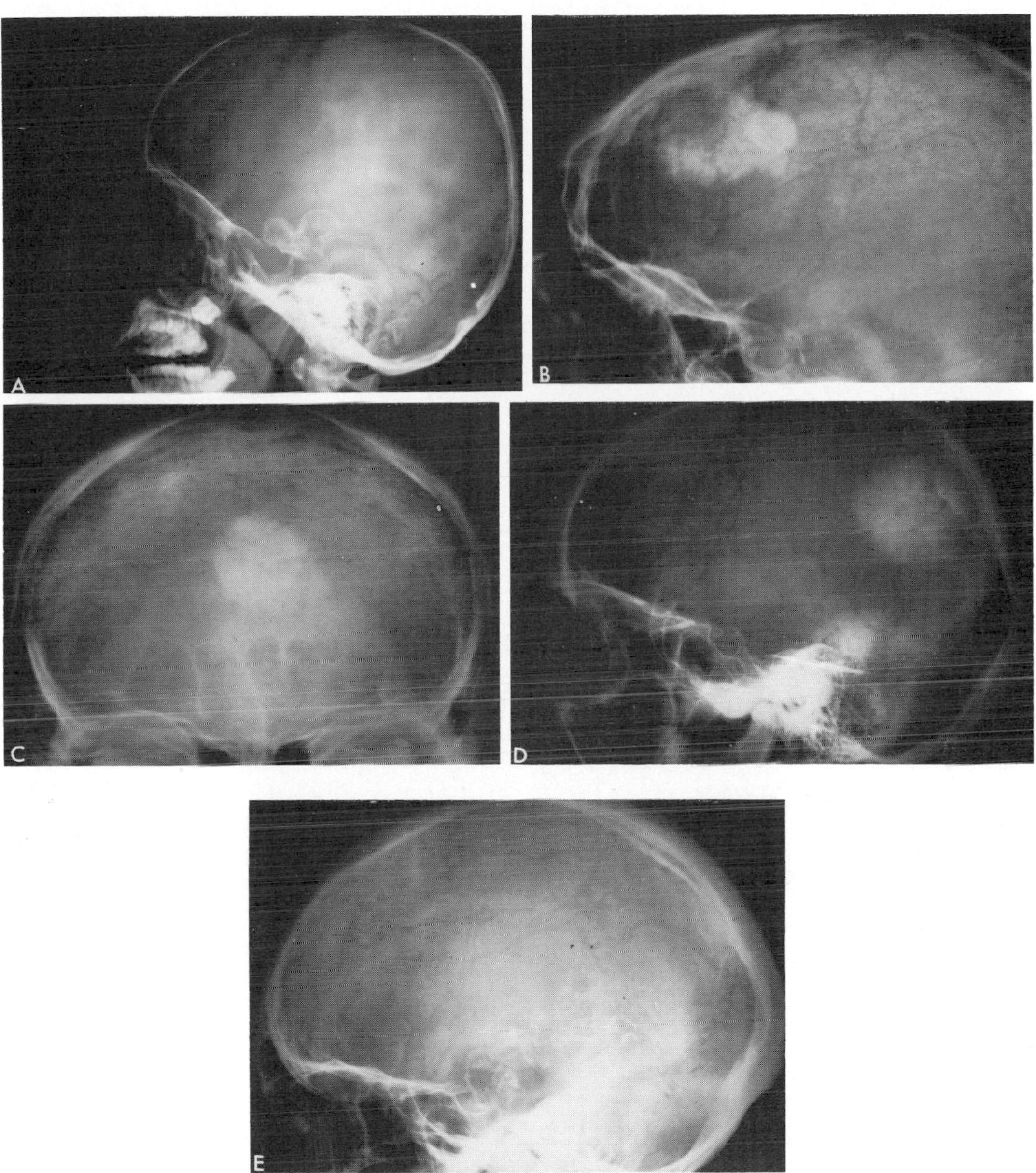

Figure 4–26 *A*. Calcification within a craniopharyngioma. *B* and *C*. Calcification in a falx meningioma. *D*. Calcified convexity meningioma. *E*. Oliogodendroglioma. Note bands of calcification.

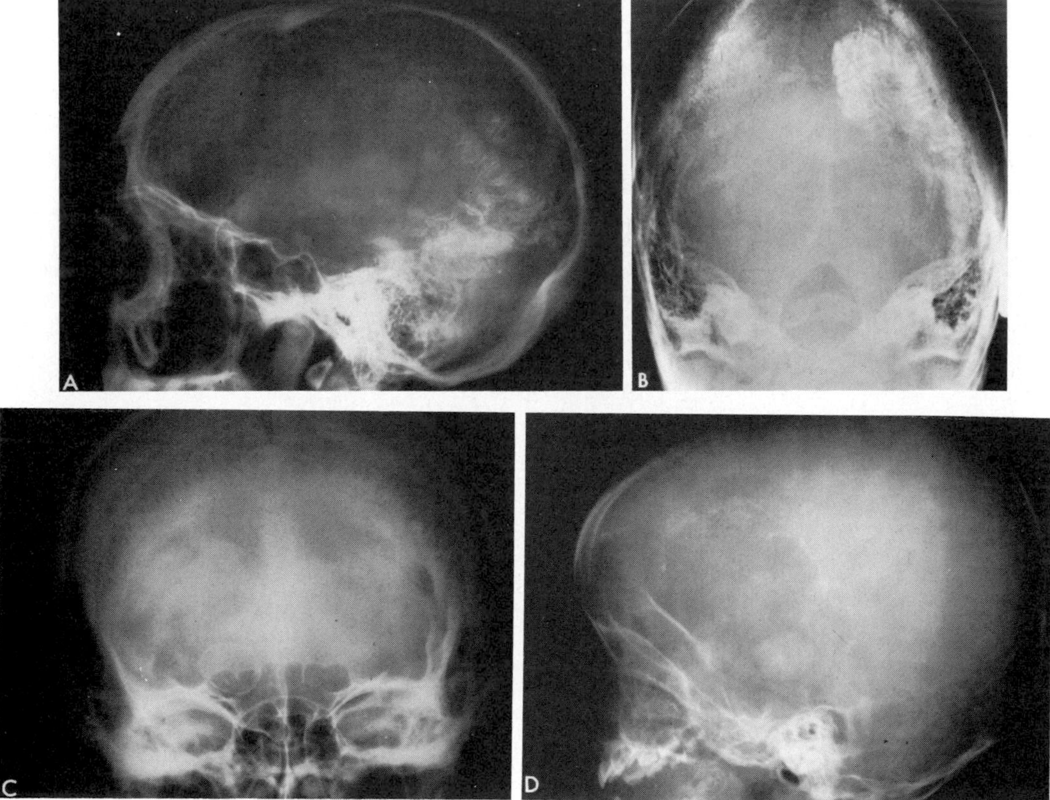

Figure 4–27 *A*. Sturge-Weber syndrome. Note classic unilateral occipital areas of linear calcifications paralleling one another. *B*. Sturge-Weber calcification in the anteroposterior projection. *C*. Calcification in the wall of an aneurysm. *D*. A large lucent lesion representing the fatty tissue of an intracerebral teratoma. The margins are calcified. The presence of a tooth was confirmed at operation.

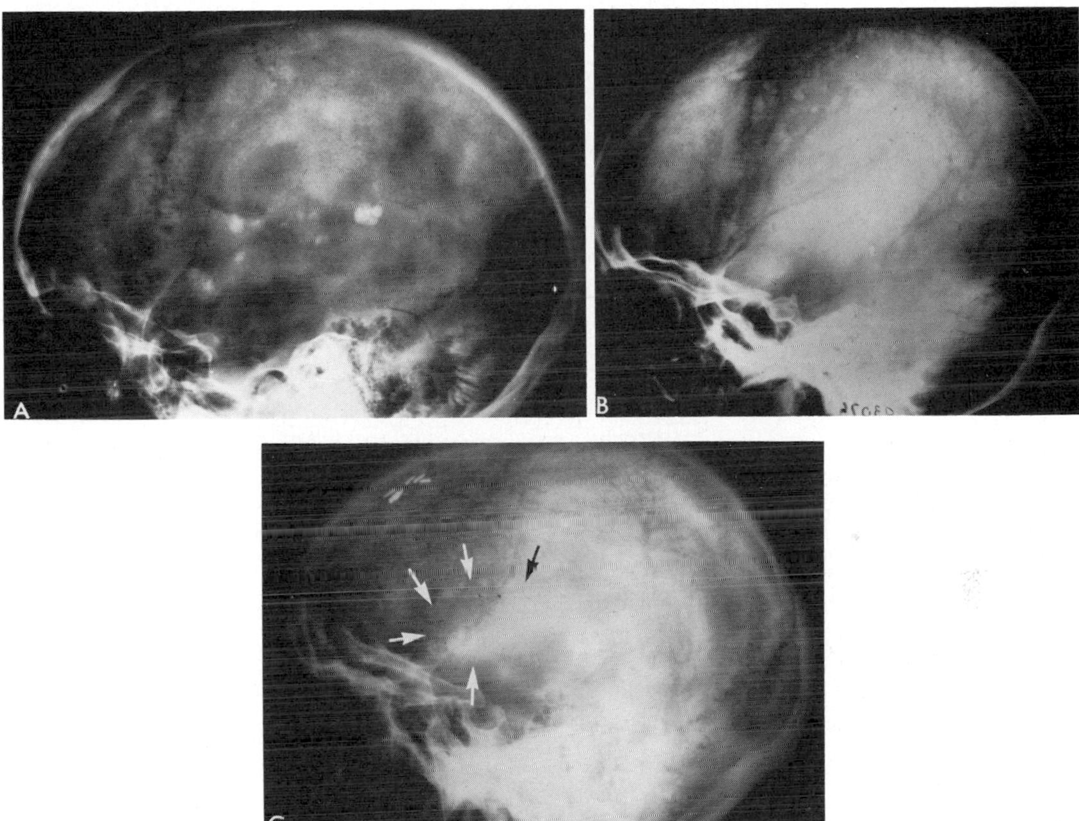

Figure 4–28 *A*. Tuberous sclerosis. Scattered areas of dense calcification in the paraventricular areas. *B*. Toxoplasmosis. Pleomorphic and disseminated areas of calcification. *C*. Basal ganglia calcification. Note the typical distribution in the head of the caudate nucleus and the lentiform nucleus.

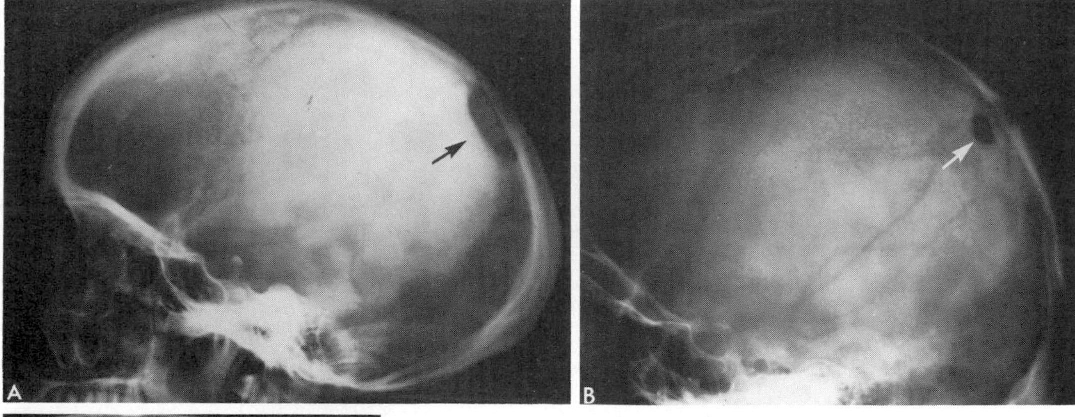

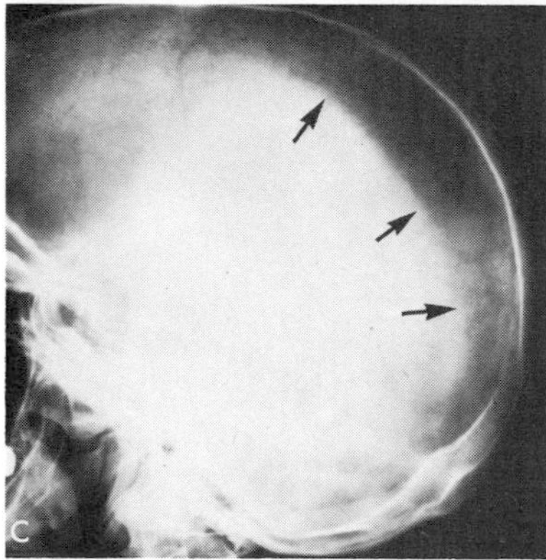

Figure 4–29 *A* and *B*. Parietal foramina are usually situated in upper part of parietal bone, 1 to 2 inches above the lambda, and are bilateral. Similar but more extensive changes are seen in parietal thinning, *C*.

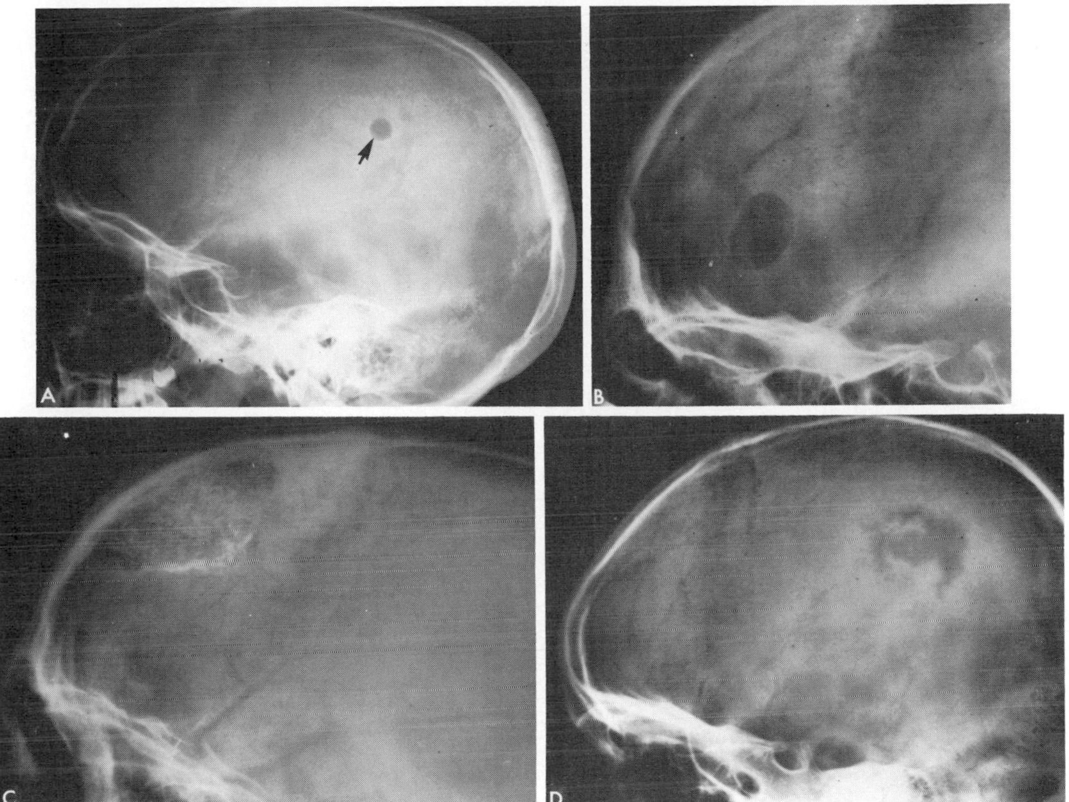

Figure 4–30 *A*. Epidermoid. There is a smooth sclerotic margin around the translucency. *B*. Eosinophilic granuloma. Note the sharp punched-out appearance without a sclerotic margin. *C*. Hemangioma. This expands the table of the skull and has a soap-bubble appearance. *D*. Osteomyelitis has an irregular lytic area with a "moth-eaten" appearance. A similar appearance may be seen in syphilis, tuberculosis, and focal radiation necrosis.

sis. The hemangioma expands the tables of bone and has a soap-bubble appearance (Fig. 4–30).

The hyperostotic lesions are usually meningiomas (shown in Figs. 4–15, 4–16, 4–17, 4–18, and 4–19) and fibrous dysplasia (Fig. 4–32). Fibrous dysplasia is usually associated with a young age group and may be confined to the base of the skull. Meningiomas tend to occur at a later age and favor females. Various bone changes are described in meningiomas, ranging from diffuse hyperostosis of bone to the sunburst appearance of spicules laid down vertically to the skull surface. Meningiomas occasionally produce lytic lesions of bone.

Certain basic projections are taken in the evaluation of the skull. Each projection may show particular structures to better advantage. Occasionally specialized projections may be taken to outline areas such as the petrous pyramid, the optic canals, and the foramina at the base of the skull. Specific features are best seen in each of the various projections. The frontal view is most useful to study the position of the pineal gland. If the pineal gland is not recognized in the lateral projection it will not be visible in the anterior projection. The sphenoid wings, the orbital fissures, the internal auditory meatuses, and the anterior clinoids, however, are seen to better advantage in this projection.

Special oblique views are necessary for visualization of the optic canals. Laminagraphy is essential for the evaluation of the components of the optic canal such as the cranial and orbital openings, roof, floor, and optic strut. Because of marked normal variability in its vertical diameter, the horizontal diameter of the canal should be used for assessment of pathological enlargement. A difference of at least 25 per cent of this measurement between the two sides is

Text continued on page 110.

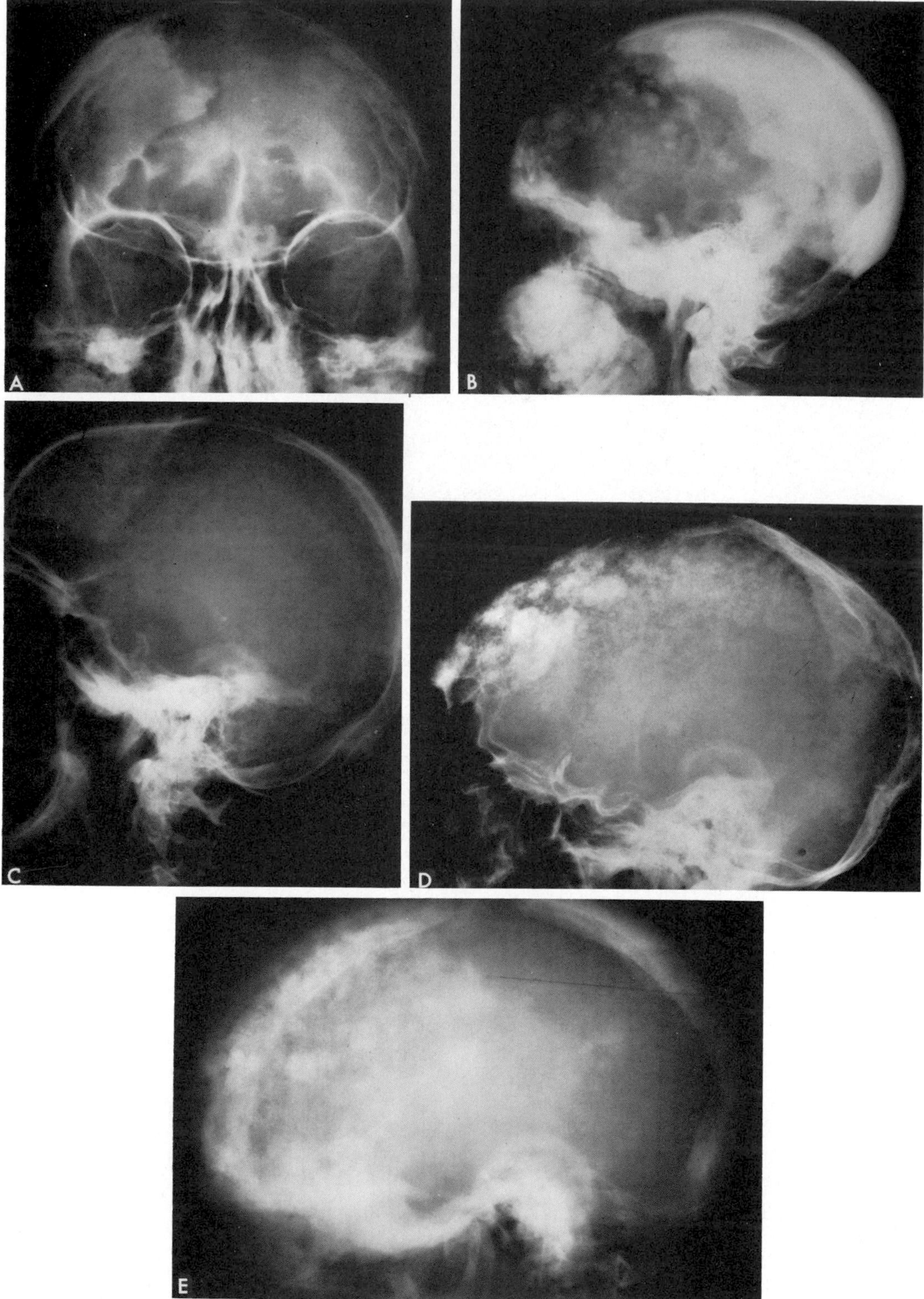

Figure 4–31 *A*. Osteoporosis circumscripta involving mainly frontal bone; *B*, involving multiple bones; and *C*, involving frontal and temporal area. *D*. Paget's disease with widened separation of tables of the skull and a mixture of translucent and dense paths. Note the basilar invagination. *E*. Paget's disease with extreme basilar invagination.

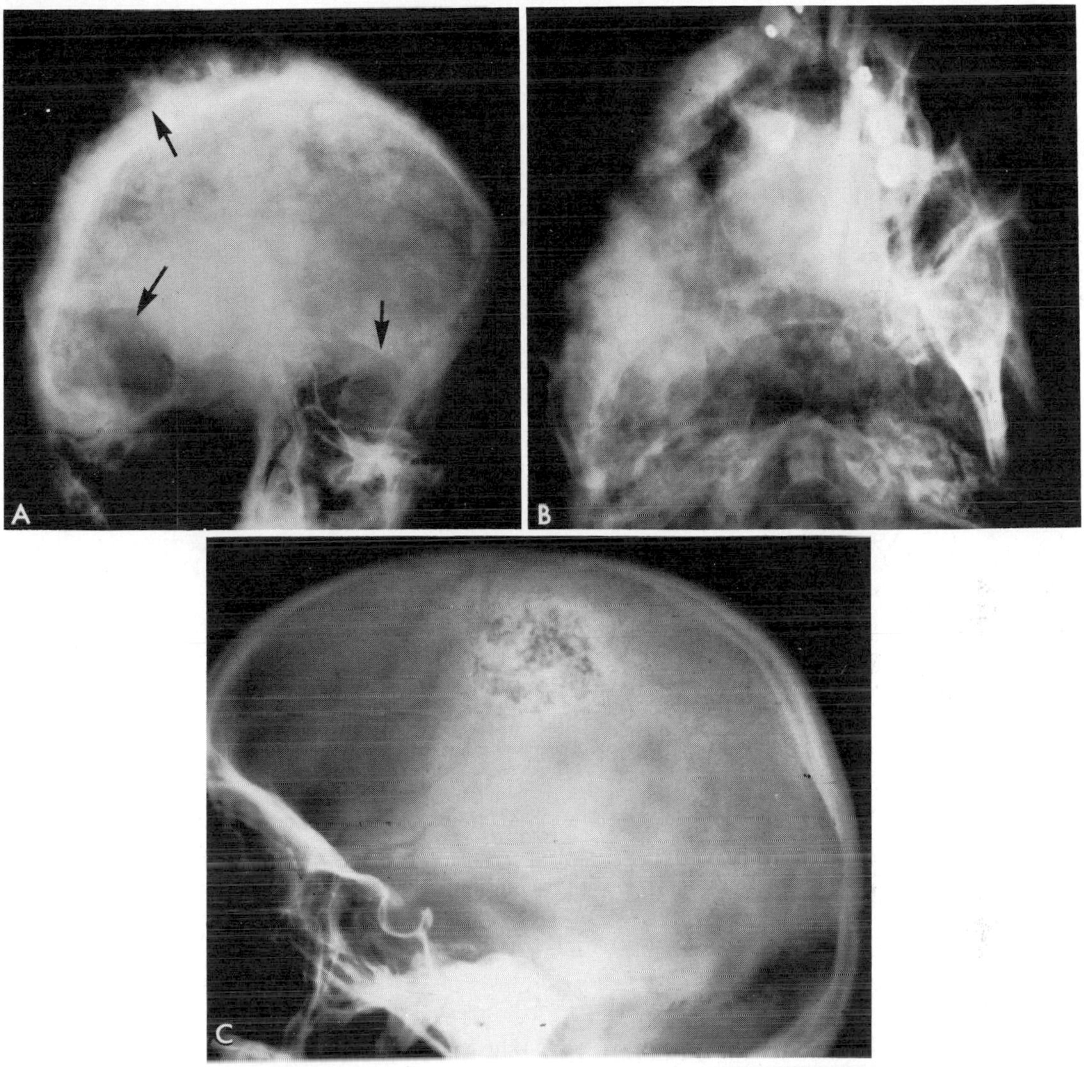

Figure 4–32 *A*. Fibrous dysplasia. Mixture of lucencies and sclerosis resembling Paget's disease, but areas of sclerosis are better defined and more homogenous. The blister type of expansion of the vertex is typical of this condition. Arrows point to "blistering" and to orbits. *B*. In base view note that the disease is more extensive on the right side. *C*. Localized form of fibrous dysplasia.

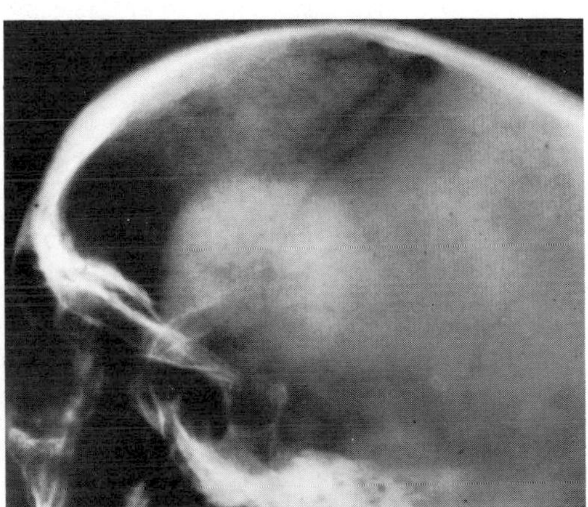

Figure 4–33 Osteoma of parietal region. This affects the outer table. Specialized views differentiate this from a meningioma, which usually affects the inner table.

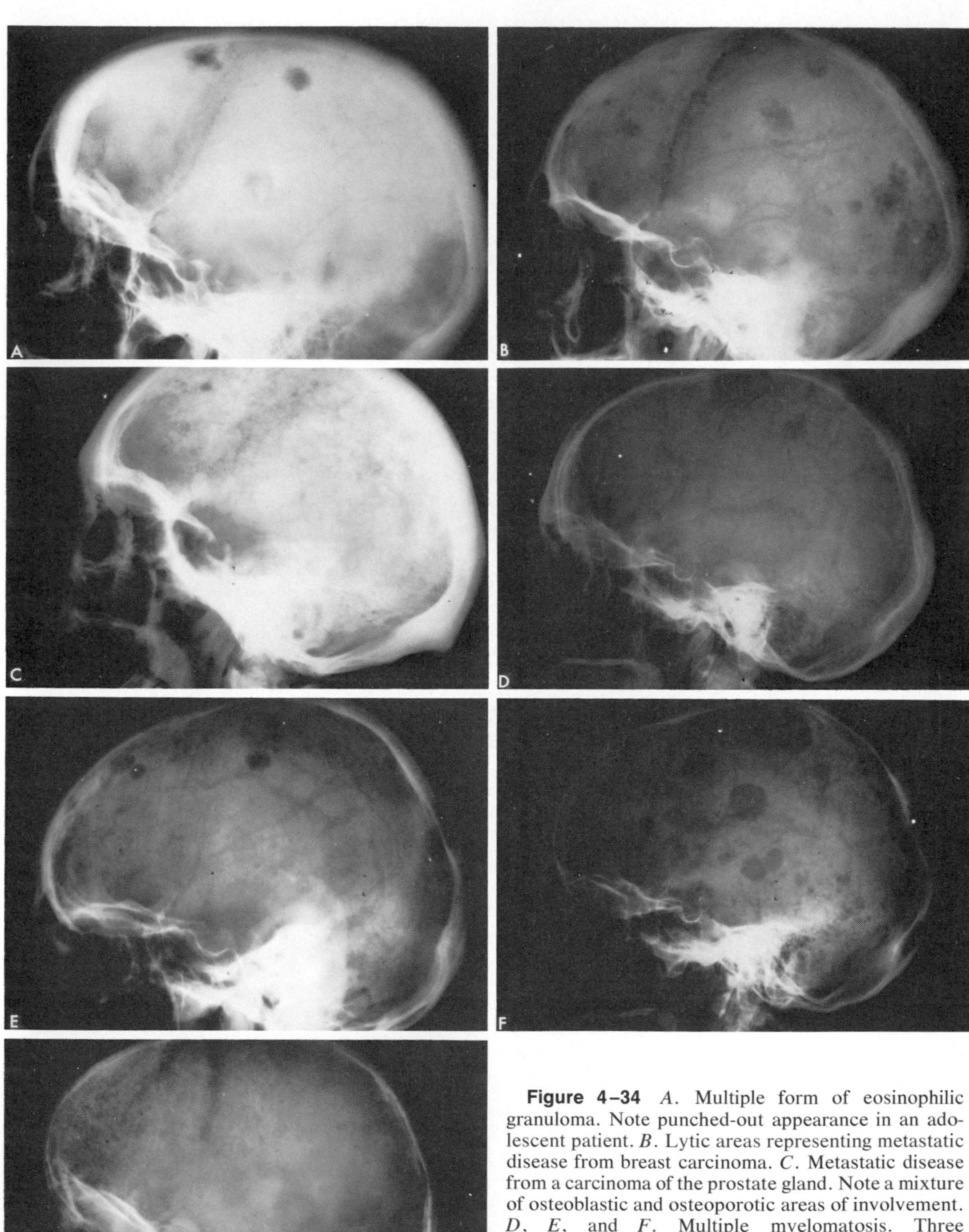

Figure 4–34 *A*. Multiple form of eosinophilic granuloma. Note punched-out appearance in an adolescent patient. *B*. Lytic areas representing metastatic disease from breast carcinoma. *C*. Metastatic disease from a carcinoma of the prostate gland. Note a mixture of osteoblastic and osteoporotic areas of involvement. *D*, *E*, and *F*. Multiple myelomatosis. Three progressive stages of the disease. *G*. Neuroblastoma. Note the widened suture. The tumor involves the skull and meninges and infiltrates the suture lines.

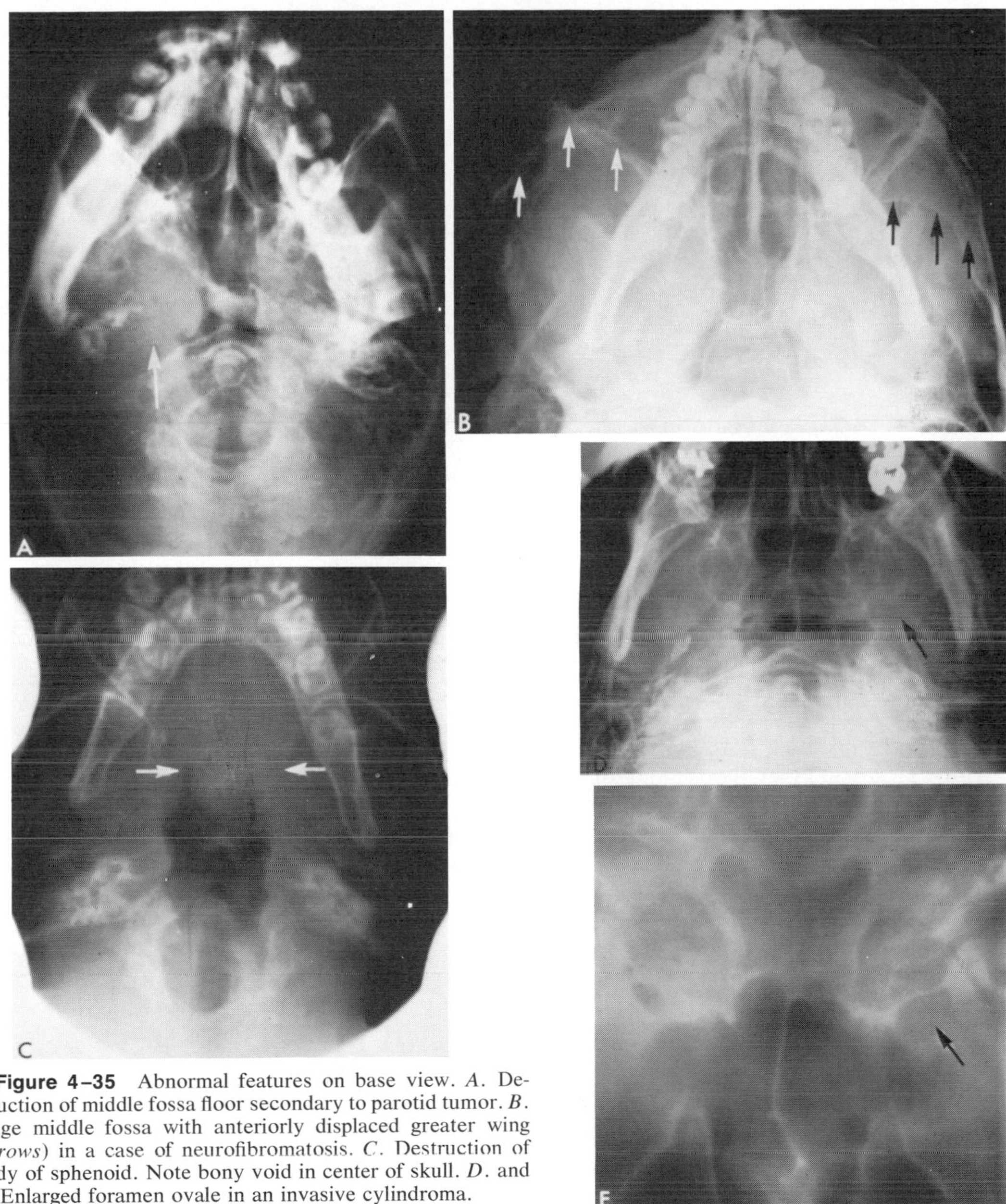

Figure 4–35 Abnormal features on base view. *A*. Destruction of middle fossa floor secondary to parotid tumor. *B*. Huge middle fossa with anteriorly displaced greater wing (*arrows*) in a case of neurofibromatosis. *C*. Destruction of body of sphenoid. Note bony void in center of skull. *D*. and *E*. Enlarged foramen ovale in an invasive cylindroma.

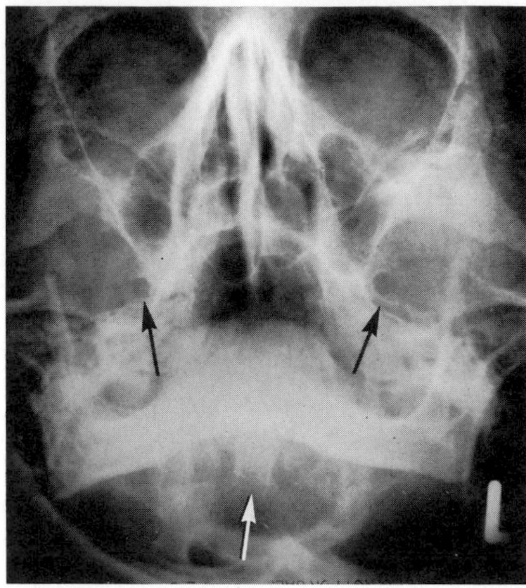

Figure 4–36 Special view for foramen ovale. This is an extended Water's view, useful for visualization of the odontoid through the foramen magnum.

an indication of an expanding lesion in this area. A pneumatized anterior clinoid should not be mistaken for the optic canal (see Fig. 4–6).

Laminagraphy is also essential for the evaluation of the internal auditory canal and its components such as the posterior wall of the meatus and the crista falciformis. Because of frequent asymmetry between the two sides, the height of the canal is not a reliable indicator of pathological change. Because of earlier diagnosis today, the percentage of abnormalities of the petrous bone recognized in the routine x-ray studies is diminishing.

The base view is useful for study of the basal foramina, the greater sphenoidal wing, the pterygoid plates, and the body of the sphenoid. (The evaluation of the foramen ovale and foramen spinosum was dealt with earlier in the chapter.) This projection is particularly useful for visualization of the jugular foramen when lesions of this region such as glomus jugulare tumors are suspected.

REFERENCES

1. duBoulay, G. H.: Principles of X-Ray Diagnosis of the Skull. London, Butterworth & Co., 1965.
2. Caffey, J.: Pediatric X-Ray Diagnosis. 5th Ed. Chicago, Year Book Medical Publishers, 1967.
3. Farberov, B. J.: Roentgenological diagnostics of the foramen opticum. Acta Radiol., *18*:594, 1937.
4. Kier, E. L.: Embryology of the normal optic canal and its anomalies; an anatomic and roentgenographic study. Invest. Radiol., *1*:346, 1966.
5. Kier, E. L.: The infantile sella turcica; new radiologic and anatomic concepts based on a developmental study of the sphenoid bone. Amer. J. Roentgen., *102*:747, 1968.
6. Kier, E. L.: 'J' and 'omega' shape of sella turcica; anatomic clarification of radiologic misconceptions. Acta Radiol., *9*:91, 1969.
7. Kier, E. L., and Schechter, M. M.: Criteria for Interpreting Rotated Neuroradiologic Studies. In preparation.
8. Kohler, A.: Borderlands of the Normal and Early Pathologic in Skeletal Roentgenology. 10th Ed. New York, Grune and Stratton, 1956.
9. Morley, T. P., and Wortzman, G.: The importance of the lateral extensions of the sphenoidal sinus in post-traumatic cerebrospinal rhinorrhea and meningitis. Clinical and radiologic aspects. J. Neurosurg., *22*:326, 1965.
10. Oon, C. L.: New method of pineal localization. Amer. J. Roentgen., *92*:1242–1248, 1964.
11. Pendergrass, E. P., Schaeffer, J. P., and Hodes, P.J.: The Head and Neck in Roentgen Diagnosis. 2nd Ed. Springfield, Ill., Charles C Thomas, 1956.
12. Rischbieth, R. H. C., and Bull, J. W. D.: The significance of enlargement of the superior orbital (sphenoidal) fissure. Brit. J. Radiol., *31*: 125–135, 1958.
13. Schechter, M. M., and Elkin, M.: The role of radiology in the management of head trauma. *In* Feiring, E., ed.: Injuries of the Brain and Spinal Cord and Their Coverings. 5th Ed. New York, Springer Publishing Co., 1974, pp. 336–398.
14. Schinz, H. R., ed.: Roentgen Diagnosis. Vol. III. New York and London, Grune & Stratton, 1969.
15. Taveras, J. M., and Wood. E. H.: Diagnostic Neuroradiology. Baltimore, Md., Williams & Wilkins Co., 1964.
16. Vastine, J. A., and Kinney, K. K.: The pineal shadow as an aid in the localization of brain tumors. Amer. J. Roentgen., *17*:320, 1927.

5

COMPUTED TOMOGRAPHY

The clinical use of computed axial tomography (CAT), or computed tomography (CT), began in 1972 when Hounsfield of EMI Ltd. developed the first CT brain scanner, which was installed at Atkinson Morley's Hospital in Wimbledon, United Kingdom.[2,28] Since then, wide experience in the use of this instrument has been accumulated. Its great detective capacity and diagnostic accuracy have been accepted as fact, and it has had a major effect on clinical medicine, especially neurosurgery. Undoubtedly, future technological achievements and clinical experience will continue to improve the capabilities of these devices.

Computed tomographic scanning is performed by a device utilizing one or more x-ray tubes that, during the scan, face one or more scintillation crystals or other types of radiation detectors. The detector signals are digitized and assembled into one or more computers, which by varying methods regenerate a display composed of small picture points (pixels) in a larger matrix of variable size by assigning an anatomically accurate x-ray attenuation coefficient to each pixel. Each pixel, when assigned this coefficient or its relative, a CT number, is then displayed, with brightness modulation related to the pixel values, on a cathode ray tube, now usually a television monitor. The displayed image may be photographed on Polaroid or standard x-ray film.

All scanners rotate around the body part to be examined, e.g., the head, and initially reconstruct the images in the same plane as that in which they were taken. That is, if the head is imaged in an axial plane, an axial slice is generated. Coronal sections may be obtained by varying the head position in relation to the gantry of the unit so that the tube-detector system rotates coronally, but most scanners are also able to rearrange axially produced images into coronal and sagittal planar images.[25,38,50] The image represents a section, or "slice," whose thickness depends upon the collimation of the x-ray tube and varies between 2.0 and 15 mm.

CT scan times vary from two seconds to four minutes per slice or pair of slices. As a rule, the shorter the scan time, the more complex and expensive the equipment. Reduction in scan time, however, decreases motion artifact, which may improve image quality and allow more accurate diagnosis.

The data display systems are scaled so that a CT number of zero is related to the absorption coefficient of water. Any material denser than water will be more absorptive and therefore have a higher absorption coefficient and, thus, a higher CT numerical value. For practical purposes, only fat and air are less absorptive than water, and both have CT numbers lower than zero, i.e., negative numbers. Incidentally, the numbers used as reference vary from machine to machine, and some of the numerical systems have changed with time. For instance, the EMI scale originally used (E) was doubled with the newer head units, and therefore, each E value is now equivalent to two units on the newer Hounsfield (H) scale. One must be aware of the scale used in his own institution. Formulae are available to convert all CT numbers to the Hounsfield values.

Regardless of the system used, cerebrospinal fluid values are slightly higher than those of water, about 3 to 8 H, and normal tissue ranges from 25 to approximately 35 or 40 H. In the usual display mode, the higher the CT number, the "whiter" or "denser" the image of the object or tissue, although, of course, this may be reversed by changing

D. O. DAVIS AND A. KOBRINE

the polarity of the display system, whether it be film or an electronic display. So, in general, one sees "white" bones, "black" cerebrospinal fluid, and a range of grays in between with the image contrast dependent upon the window level settings utilized. For further discussion of this topic, pertinent works listed in the references should be consulted.[8,9,29,47,54]

The phenomenal success of computed tomography is based on the fact that, in contradistinction to earlier doctrine, the x-ray linear attenuation coefficients of many "soft" tissues in the body differ. In the past, on the basis of standard radiographic techniques, all "soft" tissues were believed to be equally absorptive. These tissues may, however, be separated by CT scanning. Cerebrospinal fluid, blood, brain parenchyma, and blood clot, for example, may contrast with one another because of their absorption differences. These absorption differences are brought out better by computed tomography than by standard radiography because the image produced is of a thin section, there is minimal x-ray scatter, and multiple x-ray projections are used.

While the brain was the first organ to be examined extensively, the new scanners allow excellent evaluation of the base of the skull, the sinuses, the spine, and other body structures. In none of these areas, however, is the clinical impact of CT scanning as noteworthy as it has been in study of the brain. Its importance in investigating problems of the brain lies in the fact that heretofore it has been difficult to evaluate the brain adequately by other than invasive techniques and also in the distinct symmetry and predictability of the calvarial contents, which is not found elsewhere in the body. This latter aspect makes it relatively easy to distinguish normal anatomy from abnormality.

Depending on the mode of operation, the radiation dosage varies between 2 and 10 rads. Dosage through the slice is heterogeneous and considerably less at most points than the maximum dosages, which are those usually quoted. It is a general rule that the higher the radiation dosage, the better the image quality. Evolution of the technology may lead to more flexible modes wherein screening of minimally symptomatic patients may be accomplished with less radiation, and visualized abnormalities may be evaluated with a more definitive mode utilizing a higher radiation flux in which the dosages are higher. This type of flexibility will come about if clinical users indicate the need for it and help to guide the manufacturers in the direction that new advances should take.

GENERAL CONSIDERATIONS

The use of computed tomography is mandatory in the evaluation of most neurologically symptomatic patients. While there has been criticism of the technique by various agencies and individuals, all who work in this field realize that it has contributed to the diagnosis of their patients' problems and to the patients' ultimate well-being.

It is imperative that clinical findings and the question to be resolved be known before the scan is begun. The examination should be tailored to the need. Clinical findings will dictate at what angle to the base the scan is performed. They will dictate whether contrast enhancement is immediately preferred, or whether unenhanced computed tomography, either alone or as the preliminary study is indicated. If the problem is in the sellar or orbital areas, noncontrast computed tomography of those areas alone may be a sufficient preliminary study. In patients who have had head trauma or operation or possible hemorrhage, a precontrast scan should always be performed and may be sufficient, especially for the short term. All patients with cerebral hemispheric lesions should have a scan that encompasses the entire cerebrum to the highest point of the convexity. If a posterior fossa lesion is suggested, the foramen magnum should be seen and contrast medium should be infused.

It is also important that the scans be performed under direct supervision of a radiologist who is interested in the neurological field. Judgment of when a study is complete requires understanding of the clinical problem. This is especially true in the case of the acutely ill, agitated patient for whom too long an examination, with or without heavy sedation, may be dangerous, but for whom a prematurely terminated examination is equally dangerous.

A special problem arises in the evaluation of the pediatric patient. While anesthesia is required infrequently, some of these patients, especially those aged 18 months to four years and those who are mentally retarded, may require quite heavy sedation. Sedation usually is accomplished with chloral hydrate in fairly large doses, if necessary up to 1500 to 1800 mg in the active child weighing 50 to 60 pounds. If this is not sufficient, a sedative "cocktail" consisting of 25 mg of meperidine (Demerol) and 6.5 mg each of promethazine (Phenergan) and chlorpromazine (Thorazine) per milliliter is given intramuscularly. The usual dose is 1 ml per 40 lb body weight, but in the agitated retarded child, especially one receiving extensive medication, the cocktail is utilized at a dosage of 1 ml per 20 pounds. Both during and after the study, these patients need constant attention, which requires a physician in attendance. They must be monitored very carefully.

In the adult patient requiring sedation, intravenous diazepam (Valium) is utilized in the usual dosage range; occasionally up to 30 mg may be given before appropriate sedation occurs. While it is unfortunate that these high dosages are occasionally required, the image degradation that is seen when the patient moves, even slightly, is so great that significant lesions may be totally overlooked. Faster scanners help, but the patient must be motionless during any scan.

CLINICAL CONSIDERATIONS

Computed tomography is useful in two areas. The first is *detection*. It is the authors' opinion that any focal symptoms or signs that may be referable to the brain deserve a CT scan and probably deserve contrast-enhanced computed tomography (CECT) in which iodinated contrast material is injected intravenously prior to the scan, often after a precontrast, or "baseline," study has been made. A possible exception is the symptom of headache only. In the case of headache without other findings the yield of abnormalities detected by computed tomography is small, although if there are any accompanying symptoms or signs the yield becomes quite impressive. In the authors' experience with CT scans for headache alone, a positive yield of abnormalities was found in 8 per cent. In contrast, the yield of abnormalities from CT scans performed on patients in coma was 68 per cent. These percentages represent the highest and lowest yields for various indications. Therefore, while the screening of asymptomatic patients is not recommended, in view of the superb diagnostic capability of computed tomography, the evaluation of all symptomatic patients is extremely useful.

Concomitantly, the infrequency of false negative results in CT scanning, especially when contrast enhancement is used, has obviated the need for the performance of angiography and pneumoencephalography in many of these patients, sparing them the risk and expense of the other procedures.

The detection of a brain lesion usually results from observation of several phenomena on the scan. First, there is usually evidence of a mass effect within the brain, with resultant deformity of the ventricular system. Second, even if there is no deformity, the presence of hypoabsorptive (hypodense) brain edema causes a "lucency" in the brain parenchyma, allowing identification of a lesion. Third, rarely, calcification may be present within a lesion and may well be shown as hyperdensity by the superior contrast sensitivity of CT scans even though it is too faint to be identified on plain x-ray films of the skull.

Finally, the use of contrast enhancement, that is, computed tomography after injection of contrast medium, may markedly aid in the detection of many lesions, especially in the posterior fossa, where mass effect and edema may be more difficult to evaluate.[43]

CT scanning is also vitally important in the *analysis* of brain masses, First, it may definitively localize the lesion in the midst of a mass effect. Additionally, the pattern and degree of contrast enhancement may significantly aid in the characterization of the lesion. For instance, one can be fairly accurate in separating low-grade from high-grade astrocytomas.

Malignant Intraparenchymal Brain Masses

The glial tumors are the most common primary lesions in this category, and depending upon the clinical utilization of com-

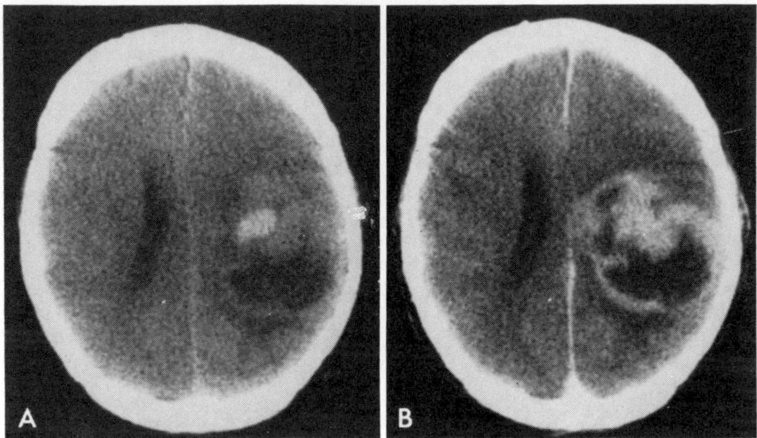

Figure 5–1 Glioblastoma. *A*. There is a mixed hyper- and hypodense lesion in the right parietal region, with a hypodense necrotic zone posteriorly and a sharply defined radiodensity anteriorly that represents a small hemorrhage into the tumor. *B*. Contrast-enhanced scan showing enhancement of a rind and nodule of tissue surrounding the necrotic zone.

puted tomography, metastatic brain tumors are also relatively common. Pathologically, these tumors range from slowly growing, less invasive, less irritating lesions to rapidly growing, markedly irritating, highly malignant tumors.

Because of the mass effect, whether due to the tumor or to its accompanying edema, these lesions are usually easily discerned on the noncontrast CT scan. Displacement or deformity of the ventricular system, the degree of which is related to both the tumor's mass and its distance from the ventricular system, is usually the tip-off to the presence of the lesion. The actual location may be identified by visualizing either a nodular mass or hypodense edema, or both. If no edema is present, the nodular portion of the tumor may be isodense with the surrounding brain and not shown by computed tomography or even, rarely, by contrast enhancement. Specifically, those lesions with only slightly increased density and bulk, less edema, and less contrast enhancement are more likely to be lower-grade lesions; those with large mass effects, a great deal of edema, extensive lucency, and extensive enhancement tend to be the more malignant or higher-grade astrocytomas. The higher-grade astrocytomas often show an area of central lucency that may be only slightly more dense than cerebrospinal fluid.[56] This area is occasionally cystic, but quite frequently represents necrosis (Fig. 5–1). Seepage of contrast material into this area has been reported on occasion when delayed scans were utilized.[39] The peripheral nodular enhancement seen with contrast is caused by leakage of the iodinated contrast material through the damaged blood-brain barrier, similar to the leakage of isotope in a positive radionuclide scan.[22]

While most low-grade astrocytomas are either slightly dense or isodense with nor-

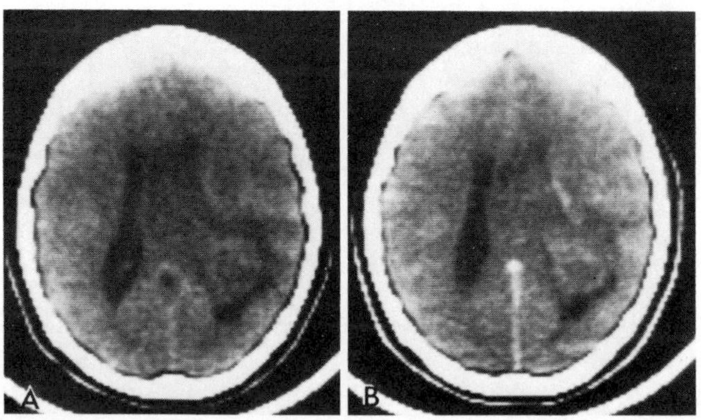

Figure 5–2 Astrocytoma. *A*. Massive isodense tumor within the body of the right lateral ventricle distends the ventricle and displaces the midline to the left. *B*. Contrast-enhanced computed tomography shows very faint enhancement of most of the tumor and more striking enhancement of nodular portions in the atrium of the lateral ventricle.

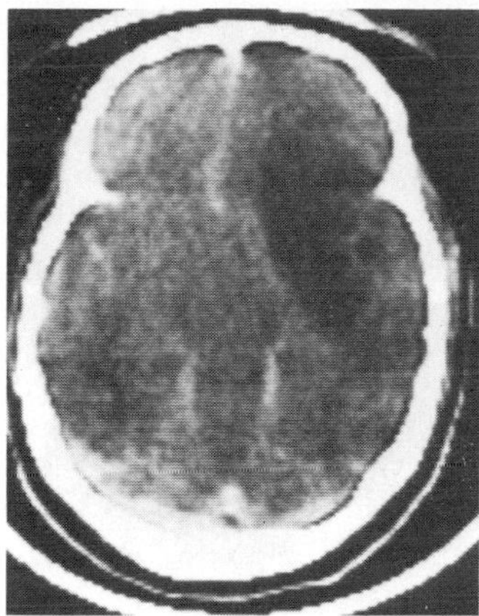

Figure 5–3 Astrocytoma, grade I. Contrast failed to enhance a sharply defined lucent zone in the right frontotemporal region, which was a grade I astrocytoma. The hypodense tumor is indistinguishable from edema or even an old hematoma. The tumor was solid.

mal brain tissue, rarely they may present as a sharply defined lucent zone that closely resembles a cyst (Figs. 5–2 and 5–3). At operation, however, the lesion proves not to be cystic. Such lesions are not visualized on radionuclide scans, and, of course, being avascular, are not defined on angiograms. Truly cystic lesions are also fairly common, with or without significant mass effect and enhancement (Fig. 5–4).

In the higher-grade lesions the intensity of enhancement by contrast suggests that many lesions should be revealed as "vascular" at angiography. Most are not. All lesions that "stain" on angiography, however, are enhanced by contrast. While some localizing information similar to that obtained from ventriculography may be gained from the ventricular deformity that is present, coronal and sagittal sections would be more helpful. Fortunately, since the actual site of the lesion is usually shown by either edema or contrast enhancement or both, it is usually not necessary to rely on indirect signs as much as one does with angiography or encephalography.

The character and location of the lesion and the type of contrast enhancement may help separate neoplasm from abscess or infarction.

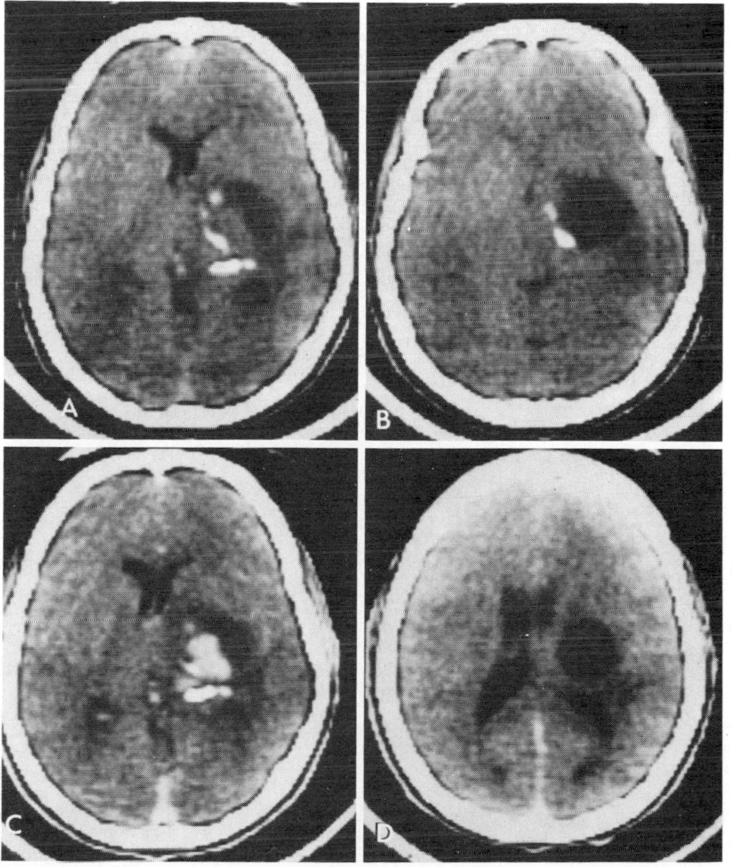

Figure 5–4 Cystic astrocytoma. *A*. Computed tomography shows markedly radiodense calcific zones interspersed with soft tissue in a nodule surrounded by a fluid-containing structure. *B*. Lower section reveals minimal edema laterally in the temporal lobe and a sharply defined cyst with adjacent calcification. *C*. Contrast enhancement reveals the nodule and the extent of the midline displacement. *D*. A significant amount of the tumor mass, impinging upon the lateral ventricle, is not enhanced.

Metastatic Tumors

Although these tumors are often multiple, when single they may be exceptionally difficult to characterize definitely. Their presentation on computed tomography runs the gamut from homogeneous nodules to rindlike borders around a cystic core. It is generally impossible to separate the single lesions from astrocytomas (Fig. 5–5). Obviously, clinical data are helpful, but biopsy may be required for definitive evaluation.

Multiple lesions, of course, tend to suggest metastatic tumor, assuming that one can exclude nonmalignant disease (Fig. 5–6). CT scanning tends to identify more lesions than are shown by radionuclide scanning, but the two modalities may be complementary in the evaluation of patients with possible or presumed metastatic disease of the brain.[5]

Certain lesions, such as medulloblastomas, pinealomas, ependyomas, and "ectopic pinealomas" or suprasellar dysgerminomas, usually tend to spread through the cerebrospinal fluid spaces (Fig. 5–7).[1] Often presenting with nodules located variously in the cisterns, fissures, and sulci, these lesions may grow into the ventricles in sheets, subsequently appearing as a ventricular "cast."

Lymphomas appear as slightly dense or isodense masses, without surrounding edema, and are enhanced considerably with contrast.[48,55] Except for their peripheral location they are indistinguishable from other malignant brain lesions (Fig. 5–8).

Abscess

As might be expected, most brain abscesses cause a great deal of edema and often show significant mass effect.[37] Both of these findings, however, may be absent. On occasion, an intracranial abscess or abscesses may be invisible on plain computed tomography and require contrast enhancement for their demonstration. On enhancement, abscesses may be homogeneous and nodular, or more often, a rim may be enhanced, suggesting a cavity within the cen-

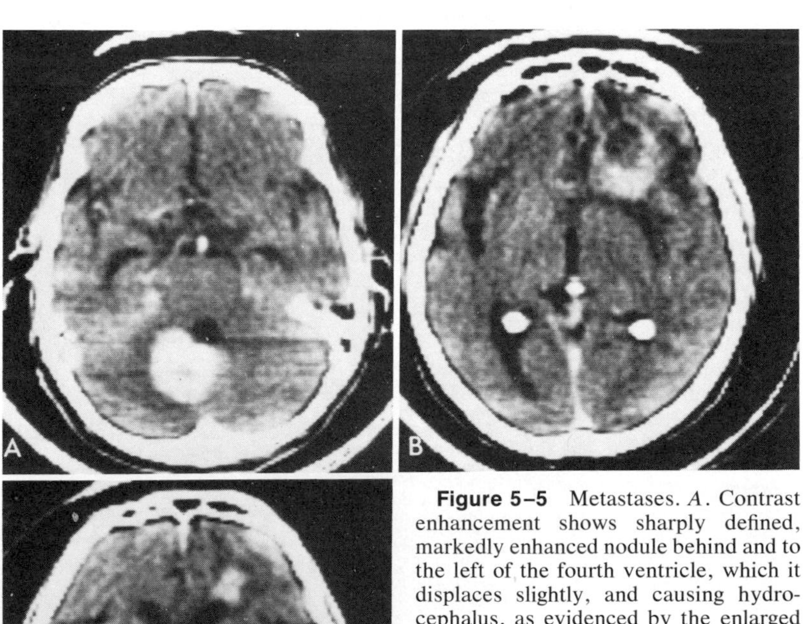

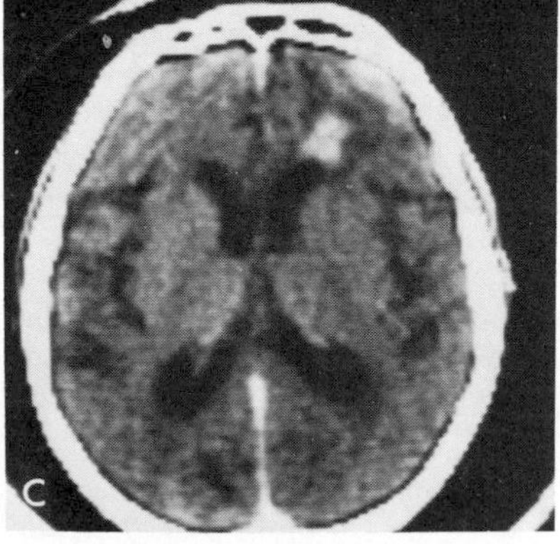

Figure 5–5 Metastases. *A*. Contrast enhancement shows sharply defined, markedly enhanced nodule behind and to the left of the fourth ventricle, which it displaces slightly, and causing hydrocephalus, as evidenced by the enlarged temporal horns. There is a faint central lucency. No other lesions were visualized. *B*. Large, multinodular metastasis in the right frontal region, with central lucency and surrounding brain edema. *C*. Marked shrinkage of the tumor and reduction of the ventricular deformity are seen two months after radiation therapy. Some edema is still present around the periphery of the tumor.

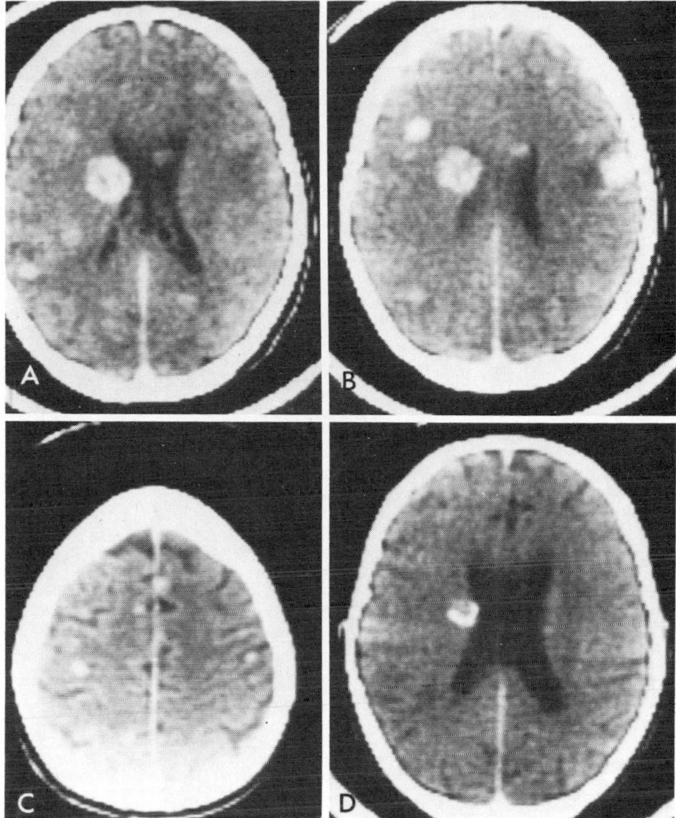

Figure 5–6 *A*, *B*, and *C*. Multiple enhanced metastatic nodules from carcinoma of the lung. *D*. Four months after radiation and chemotherapy the size of the main nodule is markedly reduced and most of the other nodules have disappeared. There is calcification in the visible nodule, as evidenced by the markedly hyperdense semilunar collection on its posterior aspect. Primary neoplasm was in the lung.

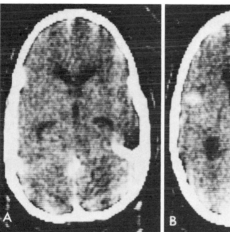

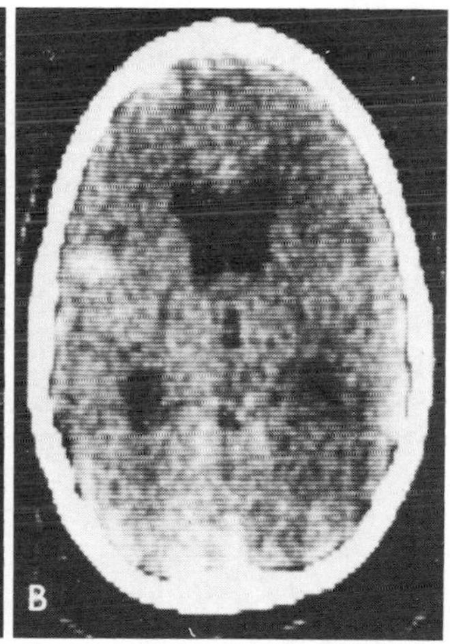

Figure 5–7 Medulloblastoma. *A*. Computed tomography shows calcified density in the posterior fossa, at the site of a previously diagnosed medulloblastoma that was treated with radiation and chemotherapy. Mild hydrocephalus is evidenced by the temporal horn enlargement. *B*. Contrast enhancement of a metastatic nodule, invisible on a noncontrast scan, representing metastasis to the sylvian fissure.

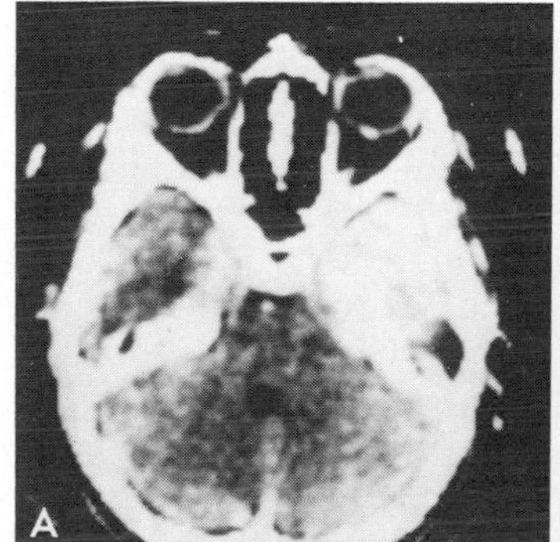

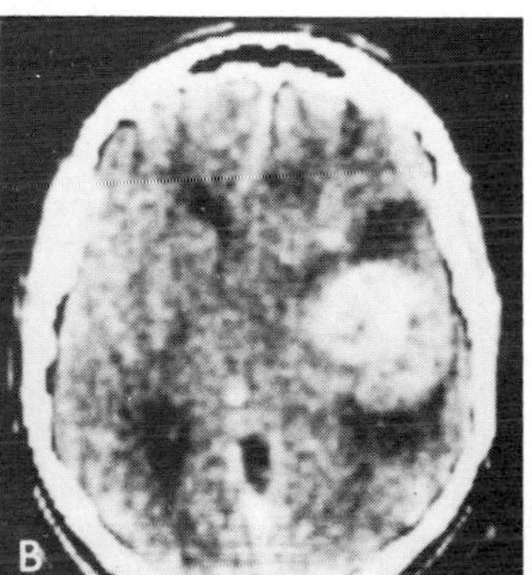

Figure 5–8 Lymphoma. *A*. Contrast enhancement shows homogeneously radiodense tumor low in the middle fossa, extending medially to the sella. *B*. Higher section shows the superior extent of the lesion into the temporal lobe. The lesion arose from the floor of the middle fossa and markedly elevated the temporal lobe, but was extra-axial.

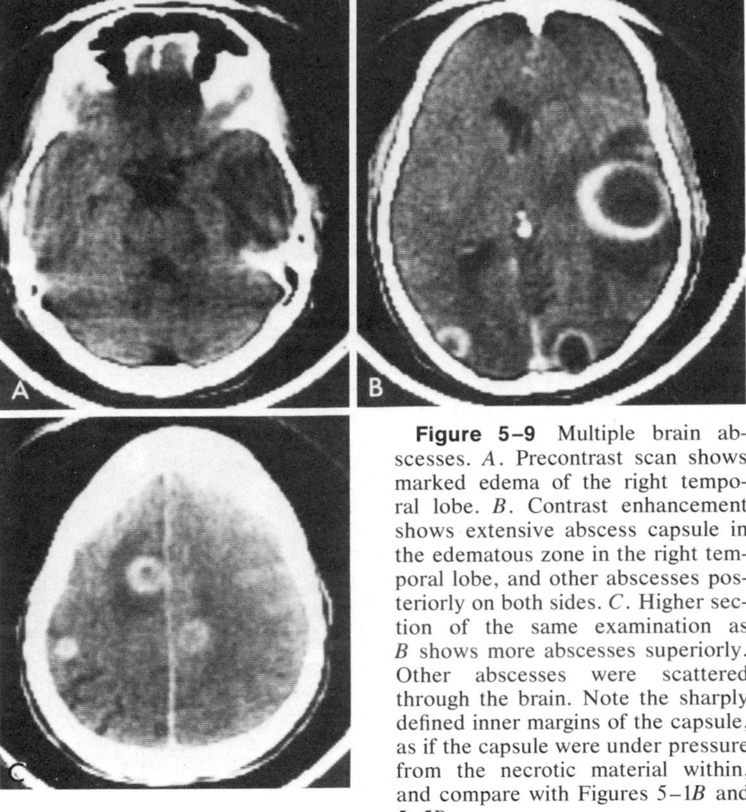

Figure 5–9 Multiple brain abscesses. *A*. Precontrast scan shows marked edema of the right temporal lobe. *B*. Contrast enhancement shows extensive abscess capsule in the edematous zone in the right temporal lobe, and other abscesses posteriorly on both sides. *C*. Higher section of the same examination as *B* shows more abscesses superiorly. Other abscesses were scattered through the brain. Note the sharply defined inner margins of the capsule, as if the capsule were under pressure from the necrotic material within, and compare with Figures 5–1*B* and 5–5*B*.

tral portion of the mass (Fig. 5–9). In the authors' experience, the innermost portion of the enhanced rim is smoother and usually under more "tension" than the lucent central defect seen in many high-grade gliomas. Metastatic lesions and, rarely, cystic meningiomas may, however, closely mimic the classic computed tomographic findings of abscess. It is often difficult to be certain about the diagnosis.

Cerebral Infarction

Most cerebral infarctions present clinically in a fashion that leads to correct diagnosis, but their patterns on computed tomography may be quite variable. First, the scan is normal after a transient ischemic attack (TIA); since there is insufficient damage to leave any residual clinical changes, one would not expect enough damage to allow their identification. Of those patients who suffer a reversible ischemic neurological deficit (RIND) or an acute stroke, about 25 or 30 per cent may show computed tomographic findings in the first four or five days, but if contrast-enhanced computed tomography is performed, this percentage is increased.

The hallmark of the acute stroke is a hypodense or radiolucent zone in the brain parenchyma.[33] It usually appears within four to seven days, although a more massive clinical stroke may be visualized immediately or within a few hours of the ictus (Fig. 5–10). Depending on the area involved and the severity of the stroke, some mass effect may be present, and midline shift or ventricular deformity may be apparent. Some infarctions that are invisible on plain CT scans may be visualized by contrast enhancement, presumably because of leakage of contrast medium through the blood-brain barrier (Figs. 5–11 and 5–12). On the other hand, some strokes, faintly visualized as a lucency on plain or precontrast computed tomography, may be rendered invisible by the injection of contrast material. Presumably there is

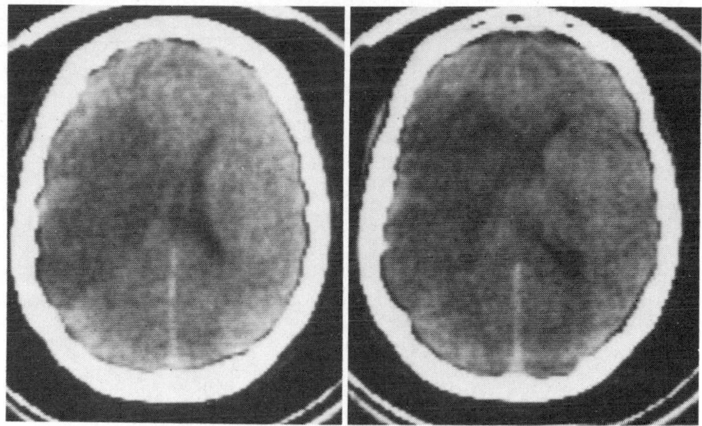

Figure 5–10 Massive acute cerebral infarction. There are a massive edematous zone in the left middle cerebral artery territory and a marked midline shift. Note the similarity in the hypodensity to the low-grade glioma shown in Figure 5–3. The edema of infarction is, however, usually slightly less hypodense than that of low-grade glioma or hematoma.

enough iodine leakage to nullify the decreased absorbency of the edematous tissue.

Some strokes on the surface of the brain, which are invisible by computed tomography, may show a positive radionuclide scan. Lesions that are more deeply placed within the brain, especially in the region of the internal capsule, usually can be visualized, especially if serial scans are performed. Incidentally, the character of the contrast enhancement in some of the deeper infarctions, especially those in the region of the putamen and caudate nucleus, may suggest an infiltrating glioma. This finding may be a diagnostic problem in the younger individual in whom strokes are considered to be unlikely clinically. Angiography may be helpful in the patient whose CT findings are suggestive of glioma, but if the clinical findings are suggestive of stroke, the prudent course is to delay fur-

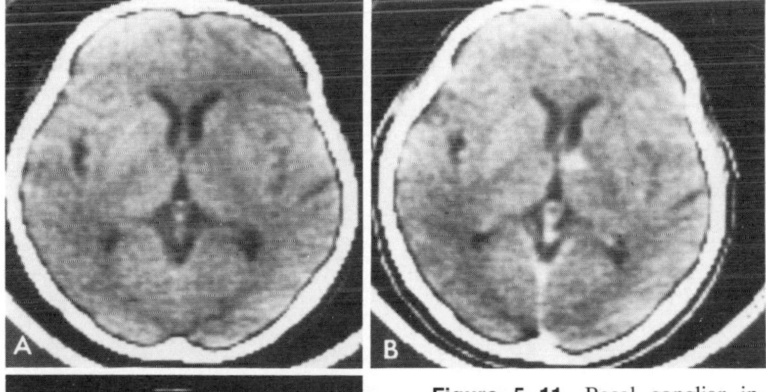

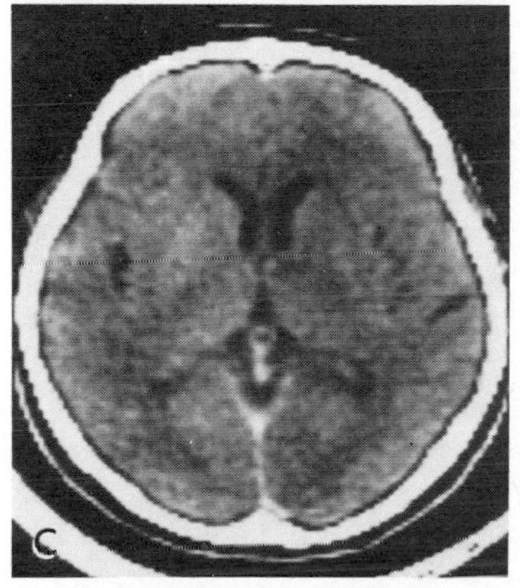

Figure 5–11 Basal gangliar infarction. *A*. CT scan of patient with acute left-sided symptoms shows no diagnosable abnormality. *B*. Contrast enhancement at the same time as *A* shows angular, sharply defined, homogeneous enhancement in the anterior thalamic region adjacent to the third ventricle. Clinical symptoms suggest an acute infarction, but the location is unusual. *C*. Contrast-enhanced scan two months later shows no enhancement, but there is a small elliptical hypodense zone in the site of the previous enhancement.

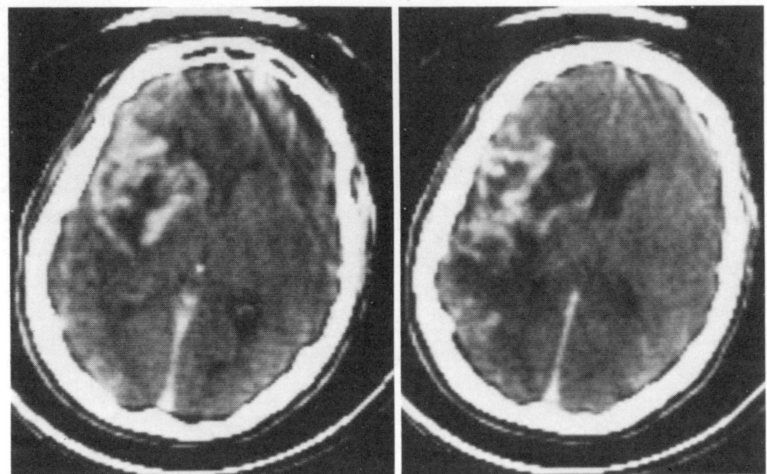

Figure 5–12 Subacute cerebral infarction. Contrast-enhanced computed tomography performed one week after infarction shown in Figure 5–10 shows extensive irregular enhancement of the infarcted zone, which, in view of the edema and contralateral shift, could easily be misdiagnosed as an enhanced astrocytoma.

ther evaluation for a week or two. Clinical improvement or rapid change in the appearance of the CT scan suggests infarction.

The contrast enhancement seen with infarction may not be distinguishable from that seen in tumor or even in arteriovenous malformation.[59] In general, however, enhancement patterns in infarction are more homogeneous and regular than those in tumor. Also, although an arteriovenous malformation may be suggested by the postcontrast study, review of a precontrast study will usually show isodensity or slight hyperdensity in the malformation, while in infarction, hypodensity (lucency) is more likely. Additionally, although the patient with an infarction may improve clinically, the contrast enhancement may be present for as long as nine months (most enhancement decreases in 8 to 12 weeks).

Chronic infarcts tend to be extremely hypodense. In fact, the CT values in these lesions often are similar to those of cerebrospinal fluid. Presumably, this indicates a cystic area of encephalomalacia, partially or completely fluid filled. If the encephalomalacia is extensive, there may be enlargement of the ipsilateral ventricle and a midline shift toward the lesion. Extensive regional cortical sulcal enlargement may also be present (Fig. 5–13).

Occasionally, a new infarct may occur in a previously infarcted region, resulting in mixed findings on computed tomography. Also some infarctions are hemorrhagic, which may additionally confuse the picture.

Since most strokes are obvious clinically, one of the major indications for computed tomography in these patients is concern about hemorrhage. This concern is especially pertinent if anticoagulation is contemplated.

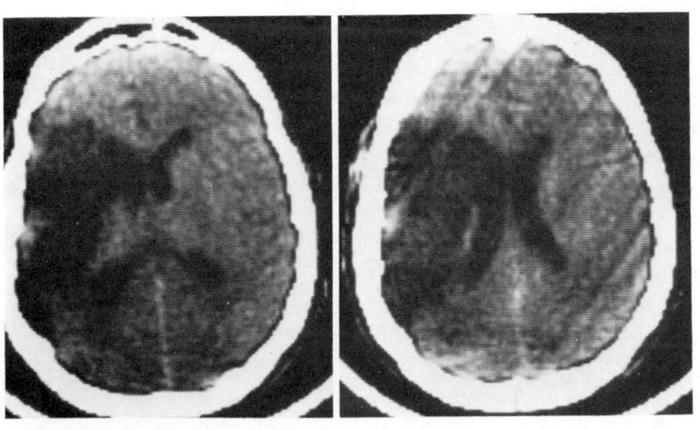

Figure 5–13 Cerebral infarction. Scans taken five months after those shown in Figures 5–10 and 5–12. The septum pellucidum has returned to the midline, and the ipsilateral ventricle has dilated. The residual hypodense zone in the left middle cerebral artery territory is much more lucent now, indicating chronic encephalomalacic changes.

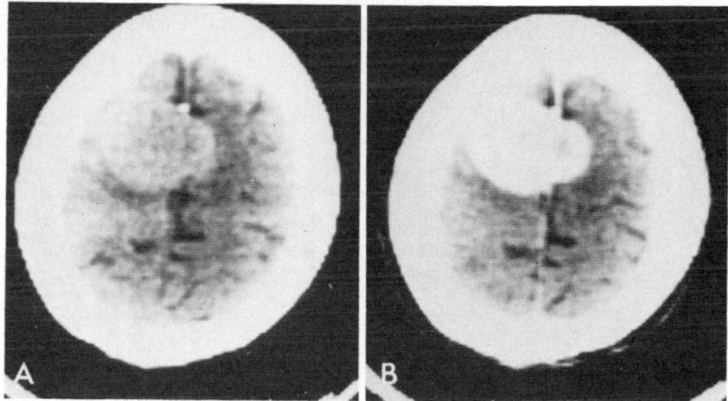

Figure 5–14 Meningioma. *A*. Computed tomography shows dense mass arising in the parasagittal region of the left side and extending across the midline to the right. The radiodensity is secondary to moderately heavy calcific deposits within the meningioma. *B*. Marked contrast enhancement of the meningioma.

Extra-Axial Brain Masses

Meningioma

These tumors frequently are diffusely calcified, albeit too faintly for visualization by plain skull films (Fig. 5–14). Computed tomography will, however, reveal quite small amounts of calcification, which present as faint blushes of homogeneous density with CT numbers in the range of 30 to 59 H.[41] More densely calcified lesions stand out as hyperdense areas, resembling bone, with CT numbers over 150 to 200 H.[12]

The numbers themselves reflect the fact that when more calcium is present there is increased absorption of x-ray, and thus a higher CT number. While it would seem that detailed evaluation of the CT number of a lesion would be helpful, there is a great deal of overlap. Thus, the main clinical use of CT number evaluation is to separate blood clot from calcification. If the CT values of a density are below 105 H, yet still hyperdense, either calcification or blood may be present. Clinical judgment usually allows separation of the two.

Meningiomas may present, as is well known, anywhere along the calvarium or base. If basilar they are difficult to separate from acoustic neuroma, aneurysm, and pituitary adenoma. Midline floor lesions may cause extensive bifrontal edema and be mistaken for demyelination (Fig. 5–15).

Meningiomas along the cerebral convexity, with or without mass effect, edema, and calcification, are more easily identified. Rarely these tumors may be cystic, in which case the differential diagnosis may be more difficult. In the more obvious surface lesion, angiography may be dispensed with unless the tumor is near a major dural venous sinus. All basal lesions should, however, be evaluated by angiography.

Noncalcified meningiomas may be isodense with the surrounding brain. If no edema is present, they may be invisible by computed tomography. All meningiomas except the heavily calcified lesions are enhanced after contrast injection. Because of their variable clinical presentation and variable appearance without contrast, it is necessary to perform contrast-enhanced scans in essentially every patient who could have a brain tumor.

It is easy to justify injection of a contrast medium into any patient with focal signs

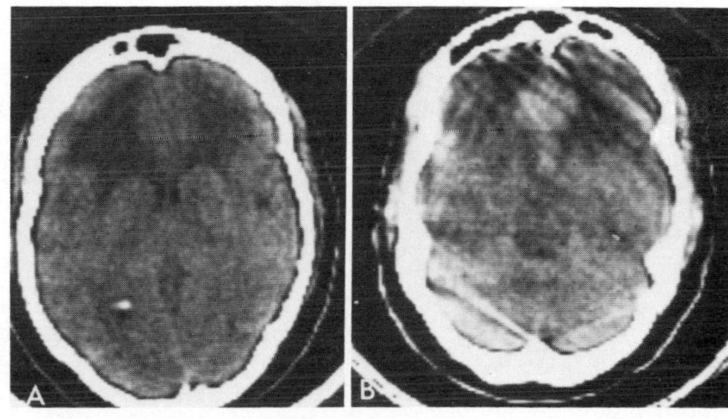

Figure 5–15 Calcified meningioma. *A*. Precontrast scan reveals butterfly lucencies involving the frontal lobes bilaterally, with an isodense zone in the midline. *B*. Contrast enhancement of the isodense zone seen on the previous scan. This represented a midline meningioma rising from the floor of the anterior fossa, involving the undersurface of both frontal lobes, and causing extensive edema, which resulted in the butterfly pattern seen on the baseline scan.

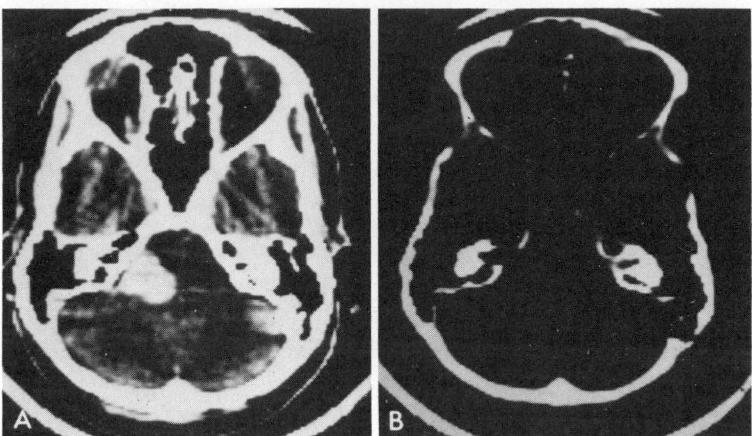

Figure 5–16 Acoustic neuroma. *A*. Contrast-enhanced computed tomography reveals a sharply defined nodule in the left cerebellopontine angle cistern, arising from the posterior aspect of the petrous pyramid and extending into the cerebellum and pons. *B*. View of the petrous bones reveals enlargement of the left internal auditory canal, confirming that the tumor seen in *A* is an acoustic neuroma.

and symptoms, or any patient with late-onset seizures. The question of whether contrast agents should be employed in all patients with headaches prior to CT scan is more difficult to answer. Probably it should be done, but the chance of allergic reaction to the contrast medium is a serious consideration. The authors use contrast agents in patients with focal headaches or repeated headaches occurring in the same area, but not in patients whose headaches carry the obvious clinical diagnosis of migraine. This technique not only helps to avoid missing meningiomas but also helps to show other lesions that may be invisible on nonenhanced scans, e.g., acoustic neuroma, arteriovenous malformation, venous angioma, and occasionally a clinically unsuspected isodense subdural hematoma, among others (the latter three may present with nondescript, nonfocal signs).

Acoustic Neuroma

The acoustic neruroma is a special case. While meningiomas in the cerebellopontine angle tend to be calcified, albeit sometimes faintly, acoustic neuromas "never" calcify. At least 50 per cent of acoustic neuromas are invisible on the plain CT scan. While edema, a cyst, or displacement of the fourth ventricle may help to identify some, in many others there will be no indirect signs.[24] Unless contrast material is used, the tumor will be missed.[15] Contrast enhancement diagnoses essentially all acoustic neuromas larger than 1.25 cm (Fig. 5–16). Although the spatial resolution of CT scanners is about 1 or 1.5 mm, computed tomography is not 100 per cent accurate in the diagnosis of acoustic neuromas smaller than 1 or 1.25 cm. While the authors have shown lesions as small as 6 mm (extracanalicular), larger ones may be missed even when appropriate imaging is done. In part, these larger tumors are missed because of the adverse effect of the adjacent very dense petrous bone on images of the cerebellopontine angle and brain stem.

The acoustic neuromas and other extra-axial masses tend to have broad bases adjacent to bone (Figs. 5–17 and 5–18). This finding is a good indication that the lesion is extra-axial in origin.[31] Usually it is easy to discern in angle masses, since they arise from the posterior aspect of the petrous pyramid and thus are in profile on the axial

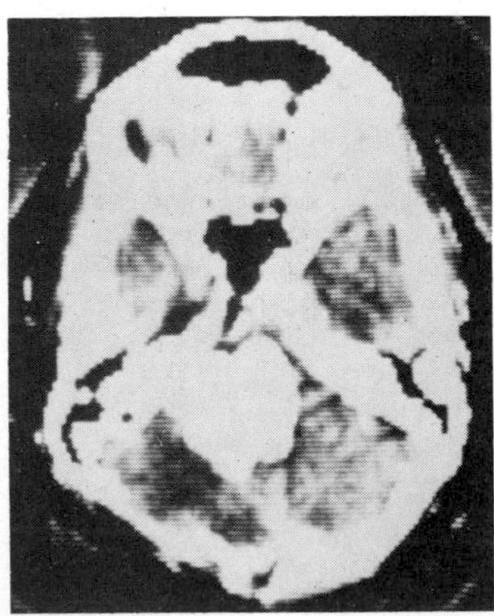

Figure 5–17 Massively radiodense tumor in the cerebellopontine angle and floor of the posterior fossa on the left side was a recurrent meningioma.

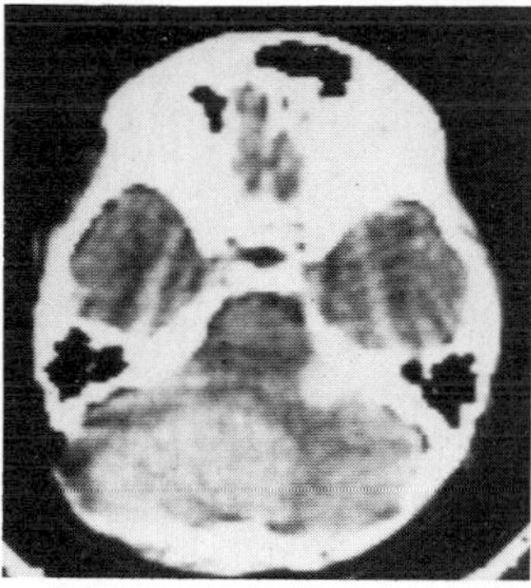

Figure 5–18 Neurofibromatosis. Computed tomography reveals a huge contrast-enhanced mass in the left side of the posterior fossa, indenting the cerebellum, representing a huge meningioma, and two radiodense nodules in the cerebellopontine angle cisterns bilaterally, which represent bilateral acoustic neuromas.

scan. If, however, the lesion arises from a base whose orientation is perpendicular to the alignment of the slice, one may not get this perspective. This is particularly bothersome in lesions arising from the floor of the anterior and middle fossae.

A recently developed technique, CT air cisternography, may reveal an "empty" or patulous internal auditory canal or a small, otherwise invisible eighth nerve tumor. Air (3 to 6 cc) is instilled via a lumbar puncture and placed in the appropriate angle cistern. CT scans of the area will reveal a tumor or normal filling of the canal. This procedure is benign and may be performed on an outpatient basis.

Vascular Lesions

Arteriovenous Malformations

Arteriovenous malformations may be difficult to diagnose by computed tomography.[40] About 25 per cent of them have varying amounts of irregularly distributed and irregularly absorptive calcification. Additionally, blood is denser than brain tissue, which may allow visualization of large blood pools in certain malformations.[32] In other words, an arteriovenous malformation may be strongly or slightly hyperdense. Occasionally zones of focal encephalomalacia are adjacent to a vascular malformation, producing a lucent zone, which may prompt further investigation. For practical purposes, however, an arteriovenous malformation is best diagnosed by contrast-enhanced computed tomography. The hallmark of an arteriovenous malformation is an extensive irregular zone of opacification, often with enlarged linear densities that represent dilated arteries or veins (Fig. 5–19). If hemorrhage has occurred, clot may be identified, or subarachnoid hemorrhage may be seen. If an intraparenchymal brain hemorrhage that the patient may survive is visualized and angiography is not performed, contrast enhancement should be employed to rule out an underlying vascular abnormality after the clot resorbs or decreases in density.

Aneurysms

Like arteriovenous malformations, aneurysms may, on occasion, be hyperdense because of calcification. Aneurysms smaller than approximately 1.5 to 2.0 cm can not be visualized reliably, even with contrast enhancement. Giant aneurysms are well shown, however. They are often hyperdense because of the intrinsic intraluminal blood pool, as discussed earlier, and if not filled with clot, are usually homogeneously opacified on contrast-enhanced computed tomography (Fig. 5–20). A giant,

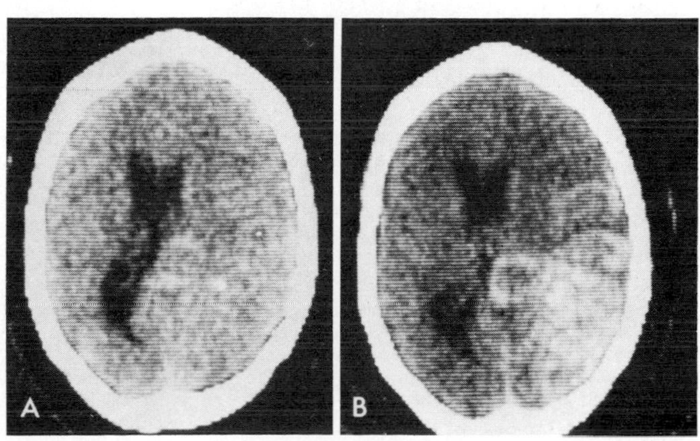

Figure 5–19 Arteriovenous malformation. *A*. Precontrast scan shows irregular mottled density at the parieto-occipital zone on the right. These densities represent blood pooling and some calcification within the malformation. *B*. Massive contrast enhancement of the parieto-occipital zone and large sinuous channels that represent tortuous draining veins.

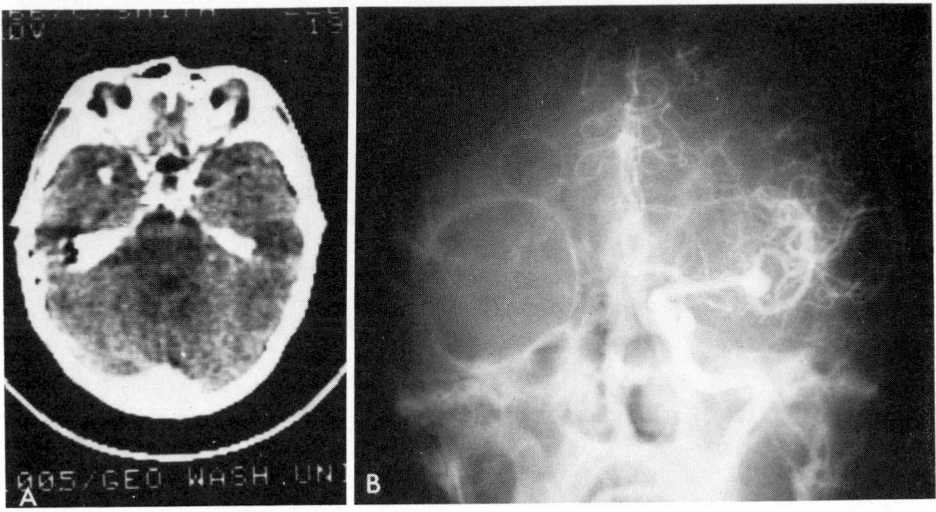

Figure 5–20 Aneurysm. *A*. Contrast-enhanced computed tomography shows radiodensity in the course of the middle cerebral artery on the left side, representing an aneurysm. *B*. Angiogram of the same patient.

clot-filled aneurysm has a characteristic enhancement pattern wherein an inner rim of the mass is enhanced, leaving the central, and often the peripheral, rim unchanged (Fig. 5–21). If an aneurysm is located near the sella, it may be mistakenly diagnosed as a craniopharyngioma. Any calcified lesion near the base of the brain that shows enhancement should be evaluated with angiography prior to operation.[46]

Spontaneous Subarachnoid Hemorrhage

Computed tomography is exceedingly useful in the evaluation of a ruptured aneurysm or arteriovenous malformation. Subarachnoid hemorrhage can be visualized approximately 90 per cent of the time (Fig. 5–22). If clinical suspicion of hemorrhage is not verified by the scan, then lumbar puncture is still indicated. Contrast-enhanced computed tomography should not be the primary procedure in subarachnoid hemorrhage, since the enhancement pattern of granulomatous meningitis may mimic the subarachnoid density seen in subarachnoid hemorrhage. If there is a small intraparenchymal clot, usually one can surmise the location of the bleeding aneurysm, especially in the patient with multiple aneurysms (Fig. 5–23). Additionally, angiography may be better planned if the clot location is known.[14,52] An intraparenchymal hematoma may be localized prior to operation. As already mentioned, most patients, especially those without preceding head trauma and those who are young, should have angiography prior to operation, since an underlying vascular lesion may be present. Of course, this may not be possible in some emergency situations.

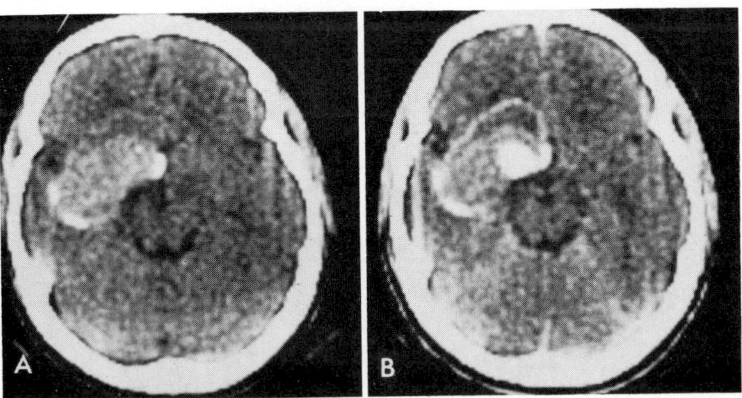

Figure 5–21 Giant aneurysm. *A*. Computed tomography shows huge sausage-shaped radiodensity extending laterally from the midline into the sylvian fissure and temporal lobe, which represented a clot-filled aneurysm with some calcification in its walls. *B*. Rimlike contrast enhancement around the periphery of the lesion, which is relatively characteristic of these lesions. There is also a sharply defined zone medially that represents contrast material in the lumen of the aneurysm.

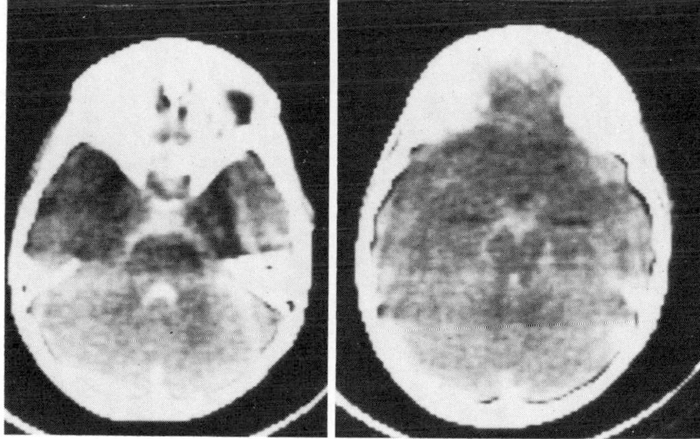

Figure 5–22 Subarachnoid hemorrhage. Computed tomographic scans showing radiodensity in the fourth ventricle and prepontine and perimesencephalic cisterns, representing acute subarachnoid hemorrhage in those zones.

Computed tomography can show intraventricular blood after a hemorrhage. If there is a significant amount of blood, it may be necessary to institute ventricular drainage. Following this, the size and clot content of the ventricles can be serially evaluated. If a patient does not improve appropriately after a subarachnoid hemorrhage, CT scanning may demonstrate enlargement of the ventricles, indicating obstructive hydrocephalus, which may respond to a ventricular shunt.

Head Trauma

Computed tomographic findings in head trauma will, of course, vary with the nature and severity of the injury.[17] Often, no abnormality will be found in a patient with clinical concussion, which indicates appropriate treatment and also, usually, a good prognosis. If the patient's condition deteriorates or does not improve as expected, repeat scans may be advisable to rule out delayed hematoma formation.

Skull Fractures

It is more efficient to evaluate for skull fracture by routine radiography, but with appropriate manipulation of the window level and window width, a CT scan may show a fracture. Calvarial fractures are identified as abrupt lucent breaks in the integrity of the bone. These must be separated from normal sutures. Correlation with skull films, of course, solves this problem. Occasionally, basal skull fractures are better visualized on computed tomography than on routine radiography.[11] Depressed fracture may be best shown by this technique (Fig. 5–24).

Vasomotor Paralysis

Acute head trauma may paralyze the cerebrovascular perfusion bed, allowing it to dilate, which increases intracerebral blood volume. If focal, this may displace normal structures and cause a contralateral midline shift. Computed tomography may demonstrate this displacement and also

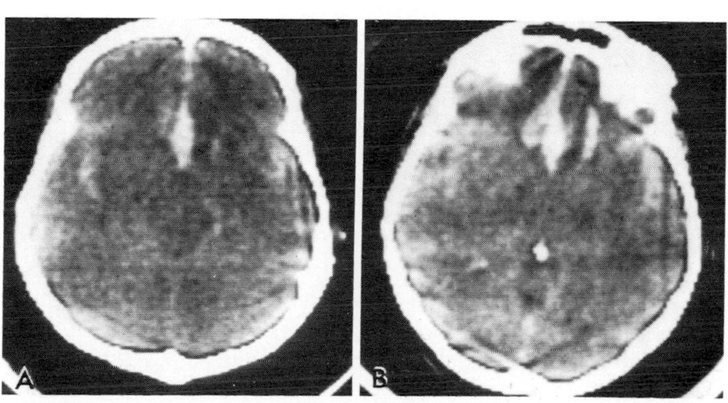

Figure 5–23 Subarachnoid hemorrhage. *A*. Computed tomography shows subarachnoid hemorrhage in the sylvian and perimesencephalic region. A sharply defined area of increased radiodensity in the midline, median hemispheric fissure, represents a small clot, indicating that the hemorrhage is due to a ruptured anterior communicating artery aneurysm. *B*. The patient's clinical condition worsened, and rescan shows marked enlargement of the clot, indicating recurrent hemorrhage of the aneurysm.

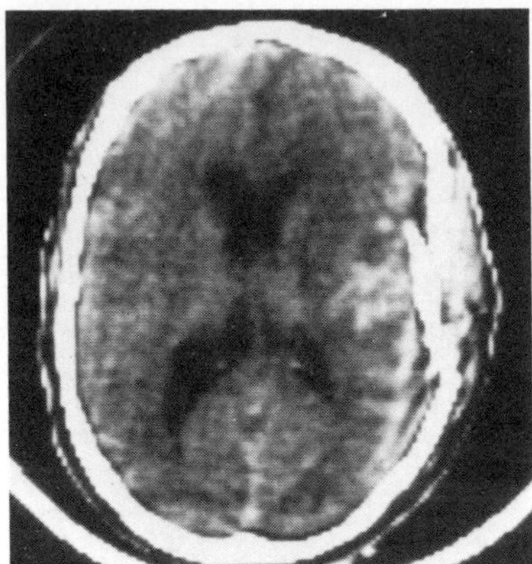

Figure 5–24 Depressed skull fracture. A depressed fracture fragment on the right impinges upon the brain surface and is associated with intraparenchymal and probably subarachnoid hemorrhage.

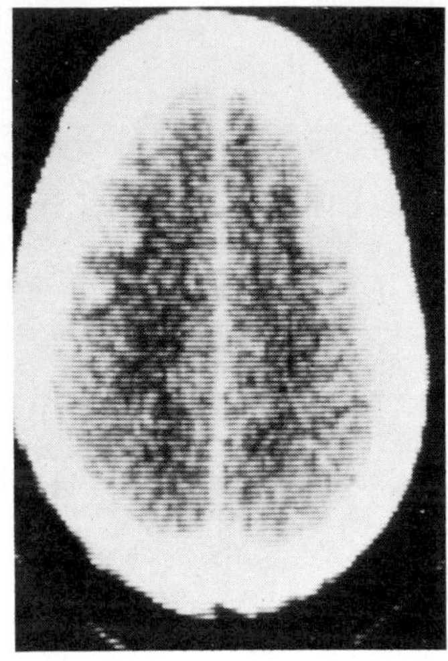

Figure 5–25 Cerebral contusions. Computed tomography reveals multiple radiodense zones bilaterally in the cortical region representing bilateral brain contusions resulting from recent head trauma.

may show a focal or regional increase in intensity because of the increased blood pool that is present in the damaged area. This density will be considerably less than that of an acute blood clot.

Contusion

Intraparenchymal hemorrhage due to brain contusion usually is visible as a sharply defined increased density similar to that of hematoma. Multiple contused zones may present as multiple but separate lesions (Fig. 5–25). These lesions usually are superficial in the posterofrontal or parietal region, but may extend deeply into the white matter. Deep extension is especially common in the frontal and temporal lobes.

In general, the more severe the clinical findings, the more edema and clot are present. The brain may be pulped. Pulping, or extensive contusion, consists of a variable mixture of edema, necrosis, and hemorrhage, the last probably secondary to brain laceration. These severe contusions. or pulped brain, may involve any area but are frequently located in the frontal or temporal poles and may involve one or more regions.

With bilateral masses or generalized edema, the lateral ventricles may be in normal position but slitlike. If the ventricles are elongated and narrow, and outlined completely on one section, one should suspect compression due to bilateral mass effect. Extensive generalized edema, evenly distributed, may be difficult to diagnose on computed tomography, since no focal lucent zone is present.

Herniation

If there is transfalcine herniation, there may be a midline shift. This displacement is no different from that seen with other lesions, nor is the ventricular deformity different. Other brain herniations are often present, and they may be difficult to diagnose by computed tomography. Cerebellar or tonsillar herniation is usually not visualized. Uncal or hippocampal herniation may be suspected when, along with a significant midline shift, there is obliteration of the cisterns around the brain stem and also of the cisterns over the suprasellar region. Occasionally, the medial aspect of the ipsilateral temporal lobe will seem to be markedly displaced medially. Dilatation of the contralateral ventricle, especially its temporal horn, may also be a hallmark of transtentorial hippocampal herniation, presumably owing to obstruction of the foramen of Monro or the third ventricle or both by the pressure caused by the shifted brain.[53]

Computed tomography usually does not demonstrate intra-axial hemorrhages in the brain stem. Presumably these hemorrhages, shown at postmortem examination, are too small to be resolved definitively with the present equipment. Future improvements in technology may well lead to an improvement in the demonstration of these lesions.

Epidural and Subdural Hematomas

The computed tomographic hallmark of an extra-axial hematoma is a sharply defined radiodensity along the outer surface of the brain, adjacent to the inner table of the skull (Fig. 5–26). Usually it is possible to separate epidural hematomas from subdural hematomas, even immediately. An epidural hematoma is generally lens-shaped in the axial view, similar to the classic angiographic appearance of a chronic subdural hematoma. Small epidural hematomas are usually easily visualized, but occasionally one may not be definitely identified as an epidural lesion, although in general, lesions of short length are epidural. The diffuse nature of the subdural hematoma usually leads to a more extensive abnormality as seen on the scan, at least in those that become clinically apparent.[21]

Subdural hematomas, also radiodense immediately, are usually distributed along the surface of the brain (Fig. 5–27). They may be quite large, extending from the frontal to the occipital poles. The inner margin usually parallels the outer margin, whereas in the epidural hematoma, the inner margin is usually straight or curved in the opposite direction from the outer margin. The inner margin of the subdural hematoma may dissect into the brain fissures on the surface, which does not happen with an epidural hematoma.

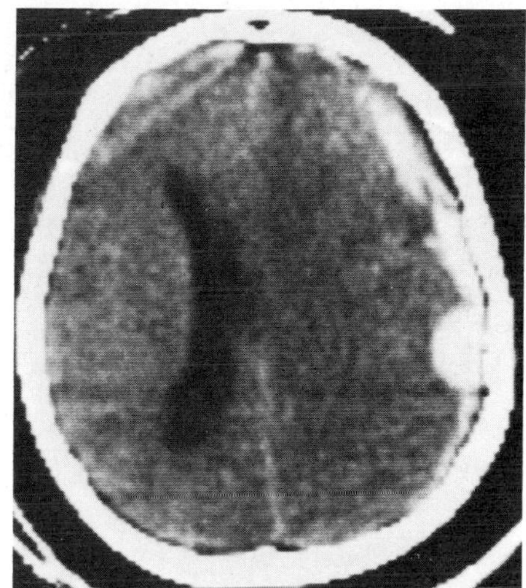

Figure 5–27 Subdural hematoma. A radiodense subdural hematoma on the right side causes some brain edema and shift of the ventricles to the left. Note its length in relation to its thickness, as compared with Figure 5–26. Also, notice that the inner margin of the hematoma is parallel to the calvarial surface, just opposite to the findings in Figure 5–26.

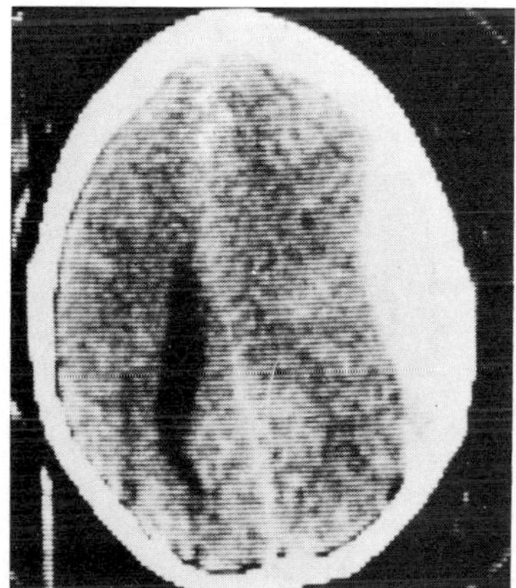

Figure 5–26 Acute epidural hematoma is revealed by a sharply defined elliptical density in the right calvarial region.

Acute subdural and epidural hematoma densities are indistinguishable; that is, both are quite hyperdense, with numbers ranging from 75 to 105 H. The reason for the density is not totally understood. Undoubtedly, it represents, at least partially, the result of plasma loss that leaves a higher than normal concentration of radiodense protein and iron.

The authors have seen one isodense acute epidural hematoma. Probably it was isodense because the blood was not clotted at the time of the first CT scan, taken shortly after injury. Two days later, the lesion was radiodense, presumably because of clot formation. Another possibility is that a cerebrospinal fluid leak into the hematoma had diluted the blood so that its density was equivalent to that of the adjacent brain tissue.

Occasionally, in conjunction with a supratentorial low convexity hematoma, blood may dissect beneath the temporal lobe and loculate on the tentorium, presenting as a density that, in the axial projection, resembles an intra-axial posterior temporal tumor (Fig. 5–28). Coronal CT sections may help to resolve this uncertainty by localizing the loculated clot adjacent to the

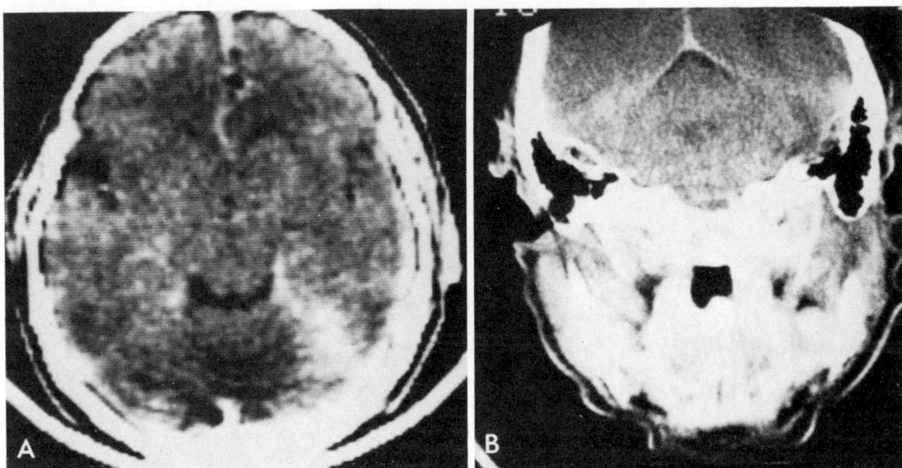

Figure 5–28 Tentorial subdural hematoma. *A*. A radiodense zone on the right side in the posterior temporal region might represent an enhanced tumor. This was also seen on the baseline study, and did not change with contrast injection. *B*. The coronal section reveals that the density on the right is immediately adjacent to the tentorium. Review of *A* reveals a thin subdural hematoma on the right side; the density above the tentorium represents extension of the subdural hematoma into the subtemporal space posteriorly.

tentorium, which when correlated with the other findings and clinical status may lead to the correct diagnosis.

It is also likely that the routine use of coronal scans will diminish the number of misdiagnoses in isodense or thin superior convexity subdural hematomas, which may be difficult to diagnose by axial scans. This is especially true when the lesions are bilateral, have balancing mass effects, and do not significantly displace the ventricles. If clinical findings suggest possible surface lesions, radionuclide scanning may be useful to detect the presence of a chronic subdural hematoma.

As clot resorption takes place, the clot radiodensity may decrease so that in three or four weeks the lesion may become isodense with the brain and thus difficult to visualize on computed tomography (Fig. 5–29). Further resorption leads to hygroma, with CT values similar to that of cerebrospinal fluid, that is, hypodense with relation to the brain (Fig. 5–30). Epidural hematomas are usually removed immediately, but if not, they should follow a time and density course similar to that of the subdural hematoma.[6]

One third to one half of isodense subdural and epidural clots will show postcontrast enhancement of their edges. Membrane enhancement explains visualization of the subdural clot. Enhancement of the adjacent damaged brain surface or dura may explain the visualization of the margin of the subacute epidural hematoma. Where there is new hemorrhage into an old subacute or chronic subdural hematoma, layering of the new blood may occur, making the dependent portion of the hematoma cavity radiodense while the upper portion remains radiolucent. On occasion, it may be useful to confirm this by positioning the patient in a decubitus or prone position so that the lateral or frontal portions of the head are de-

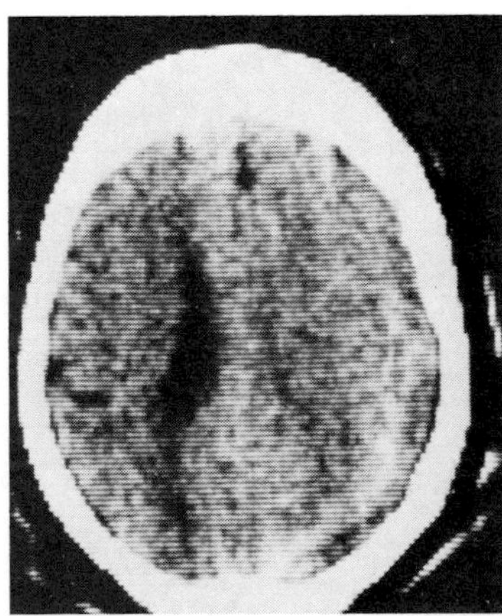

Figure 5–29 Subdural hematoma. A hematoma on the right side is largely isodense, with some radiodensity posteriorly that represents either calcification or possibly some more recent hemorrhage. Note the shift of the midline structures.

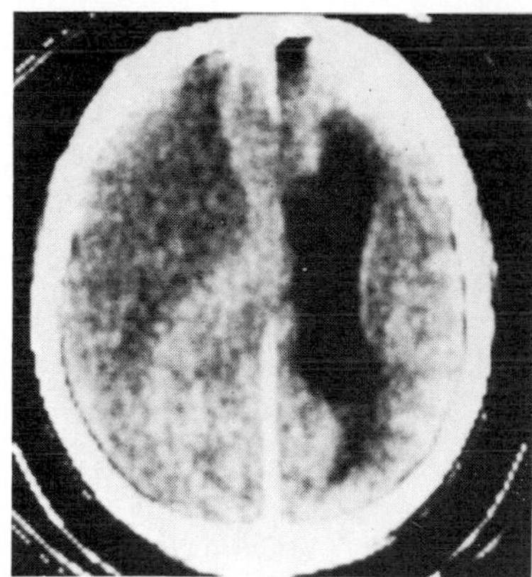

Figure 5–30 Subdural hematoma. Extensive hygroma on the left side represents an old subdural hematoma with massive displacement of the midline to the right side.

pendent and different layering is visualized.

In a patient with severe brain injury, it is common to see blood in the subarachnoid space, indicating that subarachnoid hemorrhage is also present.

Intra-Axial Hematoma

Sharply defined areas of radiodensity in the brain parenchyma may result from head trauma, but most frequently they are seen after spontaneous or hypertensive hemorrhage, especially in the basal gangliar region (Fig. 5–31). These hemorrhages have the same density characteristics as extra-axial clot; that is, they are quite dense at first but may resorb to a point of isodensity with the brain.[58] Eventually, they may become radiolucent. Thus, a radiolucency in the brain parenchyma with an accompanying mass effect may well be due, albeit rarely, to an old hematoma. Some low-grade gliomas also are radiolucent, however. When contrast material is injected, development of a ring of density around the lucency tends to support the diagnosis of subacute or chronic hematoma, since the low-grade gliomas usually are not significantly opacified by the contrast agent.[60]

Contrast enhancement frequently produces an enhanced ring of density around the dense hematoma, undoubtedly identifying the area of acutely damaged, but presumably viable, brain tissue around the clot (Fig. 5–32). Occasionally chronic hematomas calcify. While this finding causes no diagnostic difficulty when the hematoma is extra-axial, in an intra-axial one it may mimic a calcified malignant brain tumor.

Posterior Fossa Hematoma

While not intrinsically different from supratentorial clots, posterior fossa hematomas may be more difficult to diagnose because of the greater bone artifact in the posterior fossa. Additionally, after the injection of iodinated contrast material intravenously, extensive opacification of the lateral dural venous sinuses on one or both sides may lead one to suspect a low-lying extra-axial mass such as a posterior fossa subdural hematoma. Obviously clinical correlation will help, but occasionally angiography may be necessary for further evaluation.

Enlarged Ventricles

Hydrocephalus

Computed tomography is quite useful in the evaluation and follow-up of the pediatric patient with an enlarged, or too rapidly

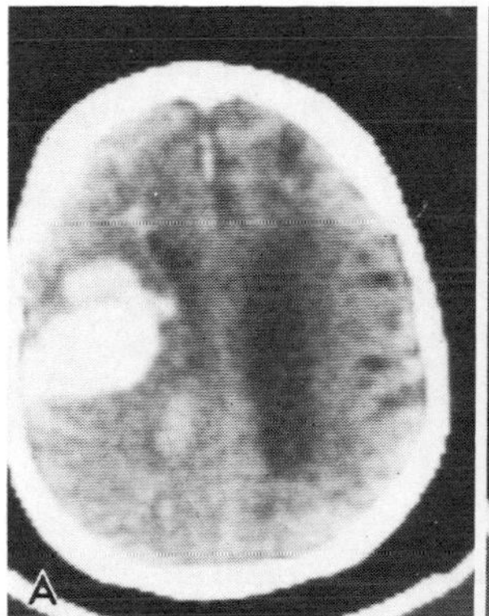

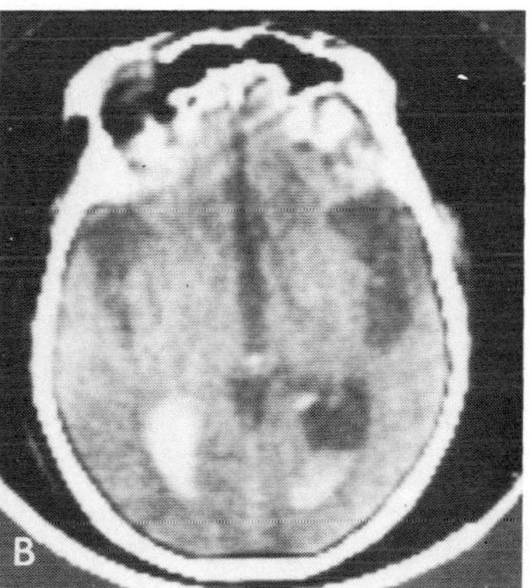

Figure 5–31 Intraparenchymal and intraventricular hemorrhage. *A*. The sharply defined homogeneous density in the left temporoparietal region represents an acute intraparenchymal hemorrhage. *B*. Note the pooling of fresh blood in the lateral ventricles.

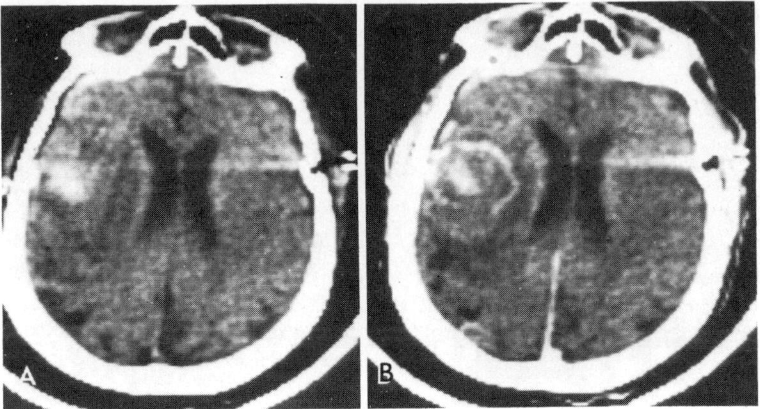

Figure 5–32 Hematoma. *A*. CT scan shows radiodense hematoma in the frontal parietal region with surrounding edematous zone and slight shift of the ventricles to the right. *B*. Contrast enhancement reveals "ring" around the periphery of the hematoma.

enlarging, head. Patients who have a cranial measurement over the ninety-eighth percentile should have a CT scan. Some of these patients will be found to have hydrocephalus, but in many the ventricles are normal or only slightly enlarged, which excludes the diagnosis of hydrocephalus. These patients are considered to have megaencephaly or other cerebral dysgenetic problems that do not require definitive treatment but may be usefully followed by serial CT scans.[34] In many of these patients, one may see rather extensive enlargement of the posterior portion of the ventricular system, especially in the region of the atria, which most likely is due to the dysgenesis and does not represent hydrocephalus. In most of these patients, no further radiological work-up need be performed.

Enlargement of the ventricular system is common in adults. It may be difficult to establish its cause, especially when one tries to differentiate atrophy or hypoplasia from true obstructive hydrocephalus. Ventricular size can be definitively evaluated on CT scans by various computer programs or measurements that allow comparison with known normal standards.[27] In general, however, with some experience, it is possible to identify ventricular enlargement visually. The diagnosis of hydrocephalus is not difficult if the enlargement is massive or if there is an obvious cause for it, e.g., an obstructing lesion (Figs. 5–33 and 5–34). The hallmark of true obstructive hydrocephalus is a relatively symmetrical and smooth enlargement of the ventricular system, usually including enlargement of the third and possibly the fourth ventricles, depending on the site of the obstruction.

Enlargement of the temporal horns is the most useful sign for determining whether obstruction is present. While it is not unusual to see one or both temporal horns enlarged in a patient who otherwise is normal or has some temporal lobe atrophy, the presence of bilateral *symmetrical* temporal horn enlargement, consistent with the amount of enlargement in the rest of the lateral ventricular system, strongly supports the diagnosis of obstructive hydrocephalus. Obviously, if the obstructing lesion is distal in the ventricular system, third or fourth ventricular enlargement is diagnostically helpful. Massive enlargement of the anterior third ventricle with impingement on the sella turcica is another useful hallmark, as is posteriorly convex bulging of the posterior third ventricle.

If hydrocephalus is present, and no cause is apparent on computed tomography, contrast enhancement should be performed, since occasionally lesions, especially in the posterior fossa, may not be shown otherwise.

Lucency in the periventricular white matter is frequently seen in patients with acute or chronic hydrocephalus. The cause for this lucency is not known, but it may represent either transependymal transudation of the cerebrospinal fluid, demyelination, or other damage to the white matter or its substrate as a result of the increased ventricular pressure.

Patients with obstructive hydrocephalus

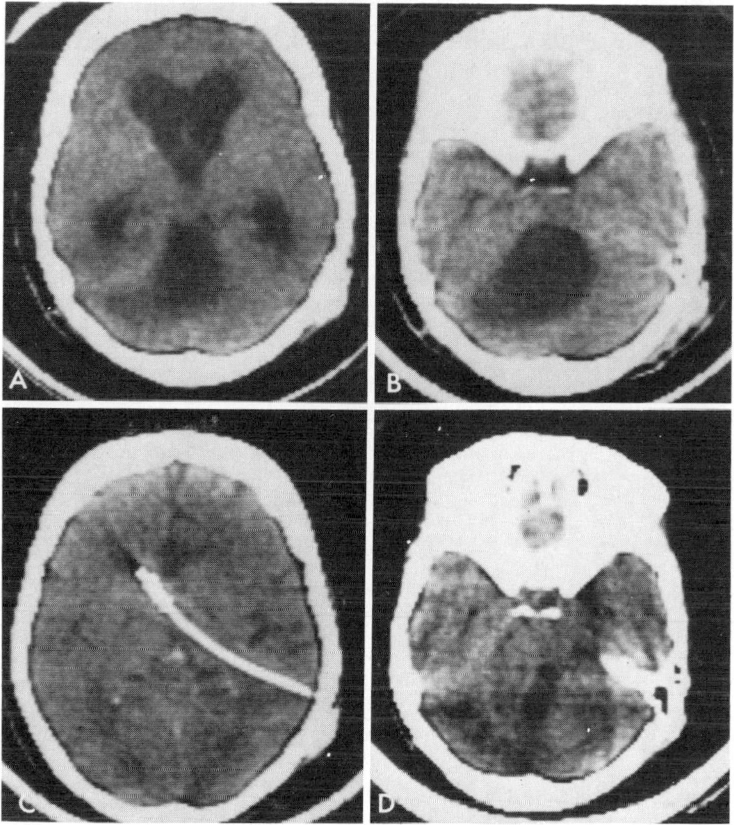

Figure 5–33 Hydrocephalus. *A*. Dilated third and lateral ventricles, and markedly enlarged temporal horns, consistent with the ventricular body enlargement, indicate massive hydrocephalus. *B*. A lower section reveals a sharply defined massively dilated fourth ventricle. *C*. After a ventricular shunt procedure, the ventricles seem to have essentially disappeared, indicating that the shunt is effective. *D*. Postshunt scan of the posterior fossa shows marked reduction in size of the cystic fourth ventricle, confirming that the ventricular pathways are communicating and that the shunt is effective.

are often definitively treated by ventricular shunt or drainage without other diagnostic evaluation, especially if the obstructive lesion is detected on computed tomography, e.g., a posterior fossa tumor. On the other hand, in those patients in whom the diagnosis cannot be made unequivocally, other studies may be necessary. In patients with

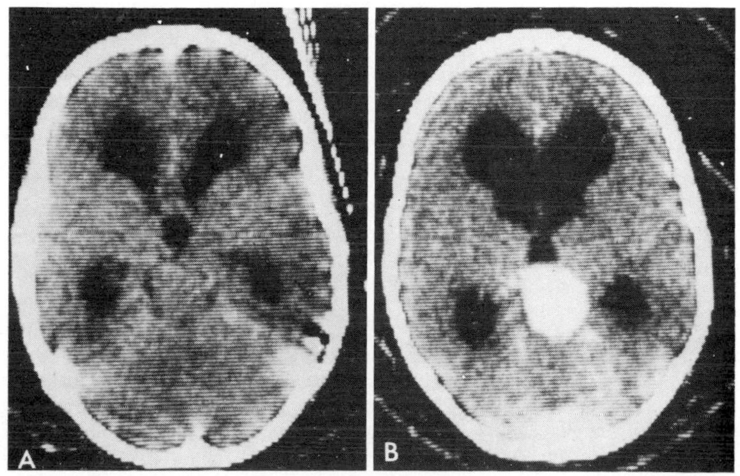

Figure 5–34 Hydrocephalus. *A*. Marked enlargement of the frontal and temporal horns and the third ventricle indicates hydrocephalus. *B*. Contrast enhancement reveals a sharply defined mass indenting the posterior third ventricle, which is the cause of the ventricular pathway obstruction. This was a vein of Galen aneurysm.

obstructive communicating or normal-pressure hydrocephalus due to obstruction in the subarachnoid pathways adjacent to or proximal to the absorption areas on the hemispheric convexities, it may be useful to perform isotope cisternography to evaluate the direction of cerebrospinal fluid transit or flow. If the intrathecal isotope progresses swiftly into the ventricular system and remains there for 24 to 48 hours, the diagnosis of obstructive communicating hydrocephalus is well established. On the other hand, if part of the isotope goes into the ventricular system and part progresses around the surface of the brain (mixed cisternographic findings), a definite diagnosis of hydrocephalus cannot be made. Incidentally, if at the time of cisternography, 4 to 6 cc of air instilled and directed to the ventricular system flows freely into the ventricles, there is no internal obstruction, something that cannot be deduced from a "normal" isotope cisternogram.

Cerebral Atrophy

Atrophy, or brain shrinkage, as evidenced by ventricular and sulcal enlargement, is common with increasing age and is often clinically silent. In fact, Gado and coworkers have suggested that the ventricular and sulcal enlargement seen with increasing age be considered "involution" rather than atrophy.[22] However, it is not uncommon in an older individual to visualize ventricles that are the same size as those usually seen in patients in the second and third decades, which may indicate that the enlarged ventricles and sulci seen in the older age groups are actually abnormal, albeit common. Whatever the cause, the fact is that enlargement of the ventricles and sulci is commonly seen without clinical symptoms, and it should be understood that such changes do not imply clinical dementia.

The criteria for the computed tomographic diagnosis of atrophy or involution include enlargement, to a greater or lesser degree, of the ventricles and sulci (Fig. 5–35). Many of these patients, especially if the sulcal enlargement is on the mid and high convexity, may well be asymptomatic, but frequently those with sulcal enlargement on the lower convexity are clinically symptomatic, e.g., if not demented, at least forgetful. The extent of abnormality visualized in the atrophic brain may be surprising when compared with the paucity of clinical findings. It is the authors' belief that these patients are probably more susceptible to prolonged permanent residua after small vascular or other insults than those with a more normal brain.

As noted, it may be quite difficult to separate the patients with cerebral atrophy from those who have normal-pressure hydrocephalus. It has been fashionable to conclude that enlargement of the sulci on the surface of the brain tends to exclude normal-pressure hydrocephalus and lack of such enlargement tends to support that diagnosis. Both tendencies are correct, but they are not diagnostically useful, since some patients with normal-pressure hydrocephalus may have large sulci, and many patients with ventricles enlarged because of severe shrinkage, especially shrinkage due to hypoxia or vascular changes, may not show significant enlargement of the sulci.

It is quite helpful to use computed tomography to follow the effect of ventricular shunting or drainage procedures. Rather rapid reduction of the ventricular size may take place after shunting (see Fig. 5–33). Occasionally a postshunt scan will show extensive subdural hygroma, unilateral or bilateral, especially in patients with longstanding hydrocephalus. On the other hand, marked reduction of ventricular size, to the point of essential invisibility, may indicate shunt dependency. If the ventricles do not shrink, the shunt may be nonfunctional, but additional investigation is needed to assess this problem definitively.

Patients whose condition has clinically improved and stabilized after a shunting procedure for a chronic lesion should have a repeat scan as a baseline for comparison in case future deterioration occurs.

Inflammatory Disease of the Brain

As noted earlier, cerebral abscess often presents with mass effect due to the abscess and edema, and often is enhanced after the injection of contrast material.

Encephalitis

While some patients with encephalitis undoubtedly show no abnormality, patients

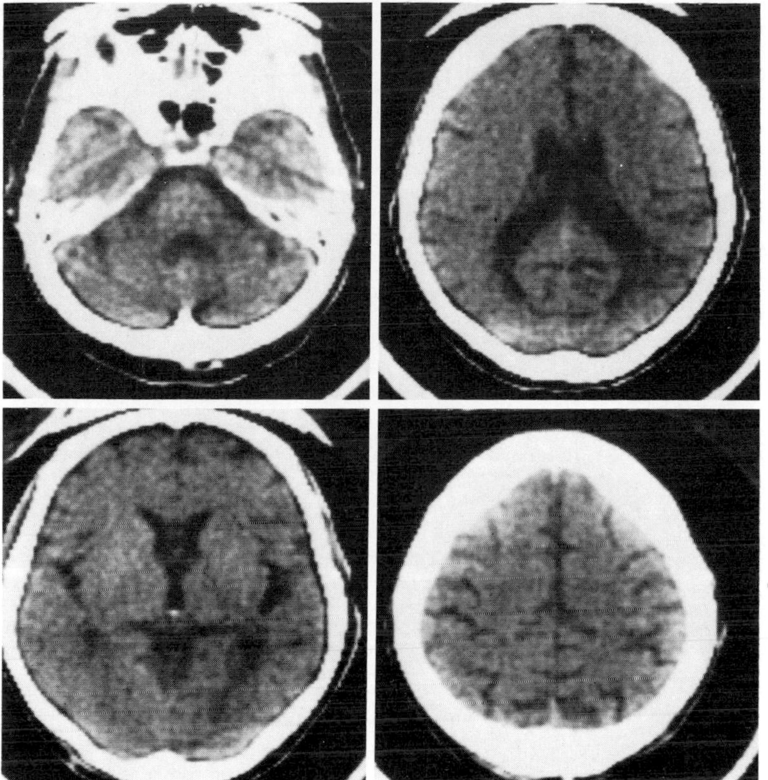

Figure 5–35 Cerebral atrophy. Enlargement of the fourth, third, and lateral ventricles, with marked enlargement of the prepontine and cerebellopontine angle cisterns, and the insular and convexity sulci, indicates generalized brain shrinkage. There was no temporal horn enlargement.

with severe encephalitis may show a variety of changes. There may be focal or generalized areas of parenchymal lucency with or without mass effect, although focal mass effect is uncommon. Ventricular narrowing secondary to generalized edema may be present, and there may be heterogeneous and irregular areas of enhancement. In herpes simplex encephalitis, extensive lucency of the temporal and deep frontal areas may occur, focally or symmetrically, unilaterally or bilaterally.[18,57] It is impossible to identify the cause of encephalitis by CT scanning (Fig. 5–36).

Meningitis

Meningitis is usually not diagnosed by computed tomography. When there is cerebrospinal fluid pathway obstruction secondary to the meningitic component, hydrocephalus, which often involves the entire ventricular system, may be shown. In granulomatous meningitis, contrast infusion may cause significant enhancement of a great deal of the meninges, a picture that may mimic the findings seen on plain computed tomography in patients who have had extensive subarachnoid hemorrhage.[19]

Post-Therapeutic Computed Tomography

Computed tomography allows quick evaluation of the brain after operation and may be useful when expected recovery does not occur or complications ensue.[36] Hemorrhage, hematoma, or hydrocephalus may be present and easily visualized (Fig. 5–37). Since many of the postoperative complications are secondary to hemorrhage, it is imperative that one perform a baseline CT scan without contrast, since enhancement by the iodinated contrast material might lead to the suspicion of a clot where none was present.

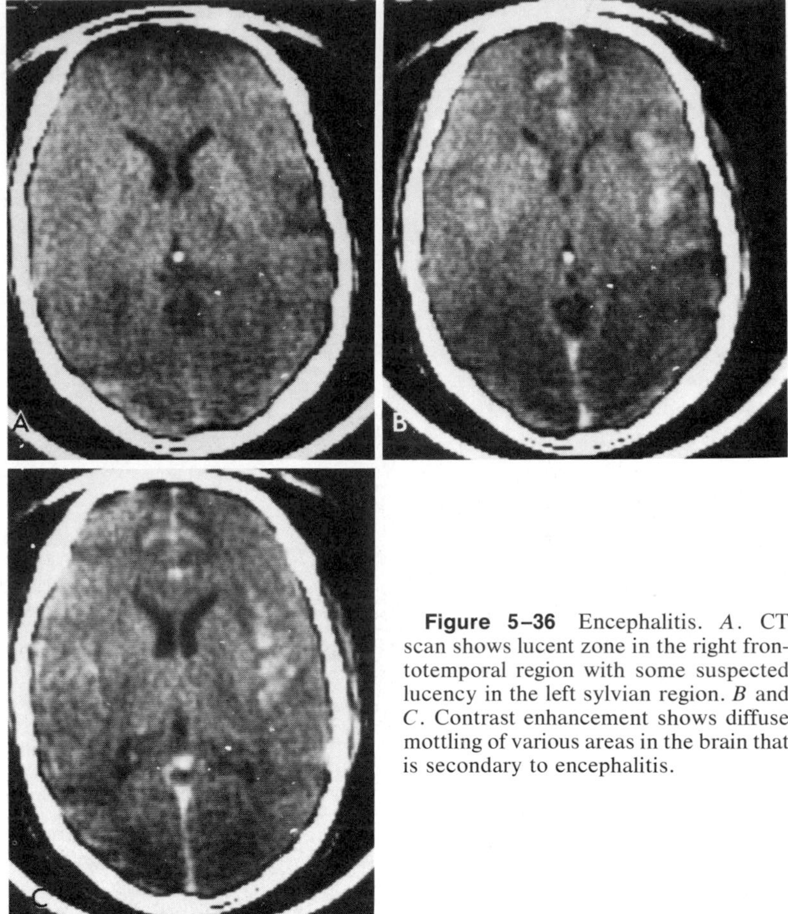

Figure 5–36 Encephalitis. *A*. CT scan shows lucent zone in the right frontotemporal region with some suspected lucency in the left sylvian region. *B* and *C*. Contrast enhancement shows diffuse mottling of various areas in the brain that is secondary to encephalitis.

After brain operations, contrast-enhanced computed tomography will often show an irregular enfolded zone of enhancement in the periphery of the operative site, presumably the zone of blood-brain barrier breakdown at the margin of the procedure. This peripheral enhancement diminishes with time and usually disappears in a few months (Fig. 5–38).

In those patients who have had an operation for aneurysm, clinical worsening may indicate either hemorrhage, infarction, or edema secondary to spasm. Edema, as mentioned before, presents as a lucent

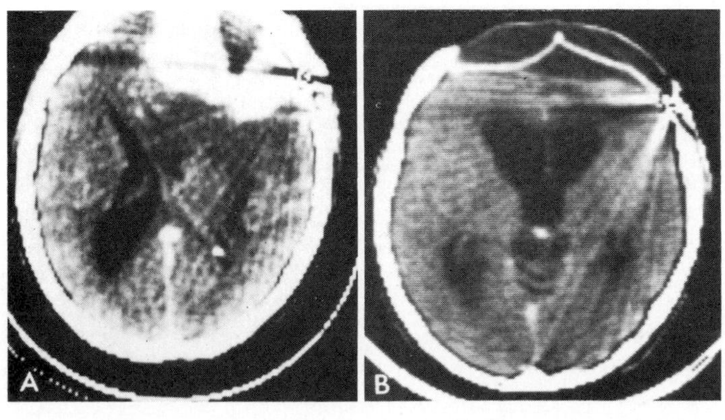

Figure 5–37 Postoperative hydrocephalus. *A*. Contrast-enhanced scan after first operation and before second operation shows huge right frontal meningioma indenting the brain and compressing and displacing the ventricular system. *B*. Repeat scan four months after operation reveals postoperative changes and massive hydrocephalus. Shunting was then performed without further examination and symptoms were relieved.

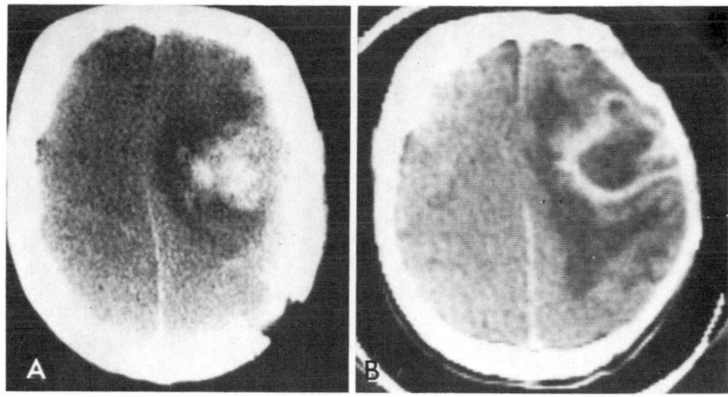

Figure 5–38 Change following operation. *A*. CT scan reveals hemorrhage in the right posterior frontoparietal area. The hematoma was evacuated. *B*. Contrast enhancement reveals scalloped radiodense "rind" surrounding the operative site. This is a common finding after operation and presumably represents the margin of the procedure. Involution of this abnormality occurs with time, but it may be seen up to six months after operation.

zone, while hemorrhage presents as a typical radiodense mass if it is intraparenchymal, or diffusely if in the subarachnoid space.

After radiation therapy, the tumor mass effect can be followed for regression or resolution. If there is considerable improvement followed in 12 to 18 months by worsening, rescans may show extensive zones of lucency and contrast enhancement that may be reminiscent of recurrent tumor. In some of these cases, the findings are indistinguishable from those of tumor but are due to radiation necrosis. Obviously, if the location of the lesion is remote from the original tumor site, or if there are multiple lesions, it is more likely to be necrosis than recurrence. If the lesion is in the same area as the previous tumor, however, it may be difficult to separate one from the other.

Necrosis usually appears on the CT scan as extensive edema of white matter, either focally or generally, depending on the radiation dose and pattern, and also may show markedly dense areas of contrast enhancement (Fig. 5–39). If these are irregular and scattered, the diagnosis of necrosis seems to be more tenable. Serial scans may help solve this difficulty.[7]

Cysts

Cysts are characterized by sharply defined margins and, usually, hypodense (lucent) contents, with the exception of the colloid cyst, which is most frequently radiodense (40 to 60 H), although an occasional lucent colloid cyst has been reported.[49] Additionally, also infrequently, minimal contrast enhancement in colloid cyst has been reported. The cause for this is unknown. Colloid cysts are located at the junction of the lateral ventricles with the

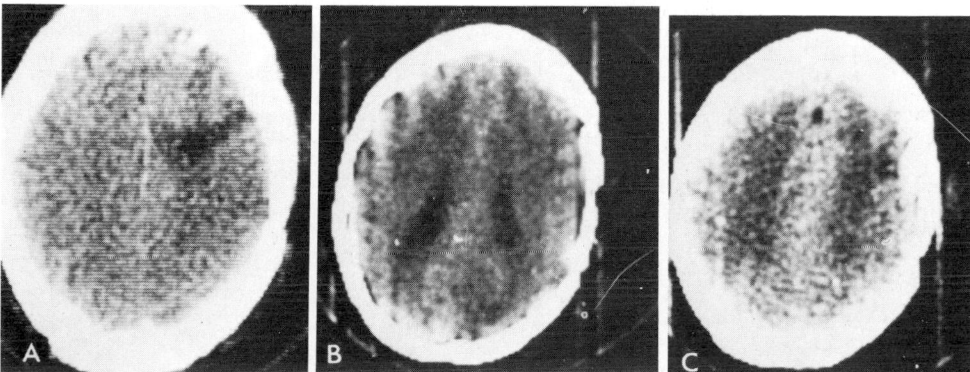

Figure 5–39 Radiation necrosis. *A*. Postoperative contrast-enhanced scan showing residual encephalomalacic zone presumably due to the previous operation for a glioma in the median frontal lobe on the right side. Patient received radiation therapy utilizing fast neutrons. *B* and *C*. CT scans taken two years after *A* reveal a diffuse white matter lucency bilaterally, indicating a leukoencephalopathy or dysmyelination presumably due to the radiation. Patient underwent reoperation and was found to be free of tumor but succumbed to postoperative complications.

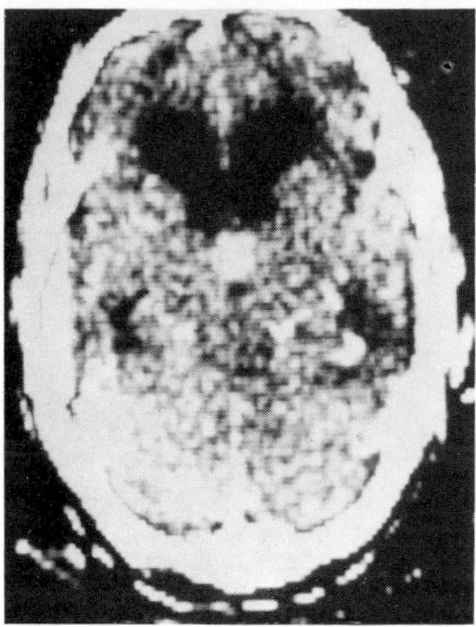

Figure 5–40 Colloid cyst. A sharply defined radiodense mass in the foramen of Monro with accompanying hydrocephalus was proved to be a colloid cyst. This represents the classic CT pattern for colloid cyst.

third ventricle at the foramen of Monro and frequently cause some obstructive hydrocephalus (Fig. 5–40).[23] Some colloid cysts, however, are nonobstructive and present as incidental findings on CT scans.

Arachnoid cysts are usually located at the periphery of the brain or in the sylvian fissure, occasionally in the sellar region (Fig. 5–41). They usually contain fluid of the density of cerebrospinal fluid (0 to 8 H) and may or may not be space-occupying, depending on the length of time that they have been present. Huge extra-axial arachnoid cysts may surround the cerebellum and cause minimal mass effect, although occasionally they lead to hydrocephalus.[4]

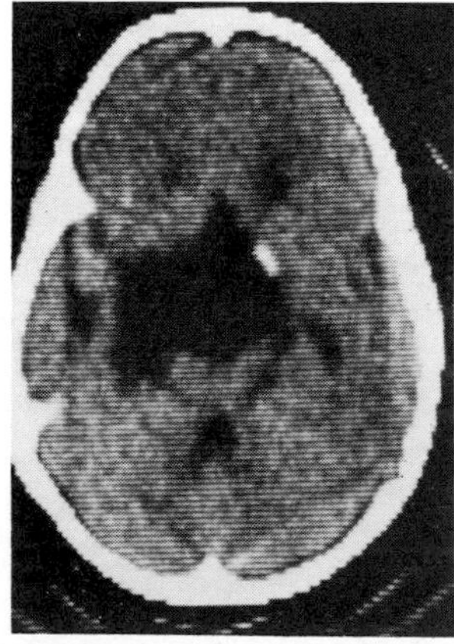

Figure 5–41 Arachnoid cyst. A sharply defined and markedly hypodense zone in the suprasellar area, displacing the temporal lobes laterally and the brain stem posteriorly, was found at operation to be an arachnoid cyst. The cause of the radiodensity in the right lateral portion of the scan, presumably representing calcification, was not determined.

Epidermoid cysts may have similar CT values, depending on their intracystic contents. Some epidermoid cysts have CT numbers ranging slightly below zero H. True epidermoids with fatty contents, or lipomas, have a cystic appearance, often being sharply defined and quite radiolucent, but the CT values may range down to minus 100 H.

Sellar and Juxtasellar Lesions

To evaluate the sella, CT planes should be at a zero-degree angle to the canthomeatal line. This angle gives a better view of the sella and its temporal, orbital, and brain stem relationships. It doesn't allow quite as good a view of the suprasellar cistern, which is better shown if the angle of the plane is 20 degrees to the canthomeatal line.

The authors always perform baseline CT scanning of the sellar area, followed by contrast-enhanced computed tomography of the sella and entire brain in those patients who have clinical findings referable to the sellar area.

Empty Sella Turcica

The CT scan is quite sensitive in the evaluation of the enlarged sella.[3] Most large

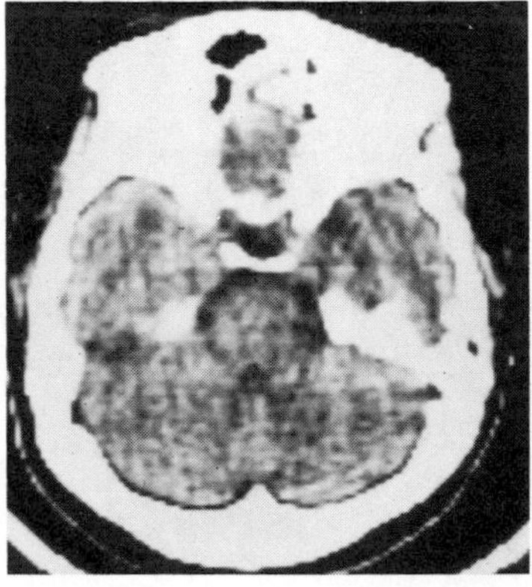

Figure 5–42 Empty sella. Radiolucency of the density of cerebrospinal fluid is seen filling the enlarged sella. This is consistent with an empty sella, which was proved at pneumoencephalography.

sellas are due to the "empty sella" phenomenon, that is, remodeling of the sella secondary to intrasellar projection of the cerebrospinal fluid–containing subarachnoid space.[51] In this condition, at computed tomography, the sella is seen to be filled with tissue of a low density compatible with cerebrospinal fluid (Fig. 5–42).[43] Rarely, an intrasellar cyst may cause similar findings and may not be separable from empty sella on axial scans. Coronal scans, either direct or computer reassembled, may help to differentiate them. In fact, it is in this area that coronal scans are most useful. Intrathecal metrizamide, maneuvered into the sellar region, may reveal sellar penetration, allowing a definitive diagnosis.

Pituitary Adenoma

The sella is usually enlarged by macroadenoma, and tissue present within it may be enhanced by contrast (Fig. 5–43).[41] Plain computed tomography may show obliteration or partial filling of the pentagon-shaped suprasellar cistern. Failure to visualize the cistern, however, does not necessarily indicate the presence of a mass, as it may not be seen in younger individuals, especially on scans at zero degrees to the baseline.

Suprasellar extension of the adenoma may be isodense, or slightly hyperdense, and is usually markedly enhanced by contrast (Fig. 5–44). The suprasellar extension may be slight or massive, and coronal sections may be useful to evaluate its superior extent definitively. Lateral extension may also occur, and on occasion, retrosellar extension may be discerned.[10,42]

Microadenomas may not be detected by CT scanning. Since these lesions are usually too small to be shown by pneumoencephalography, this is not surprising. Care should be taken not to confuse the frequent normal enhancement of the pituitary stalk with a

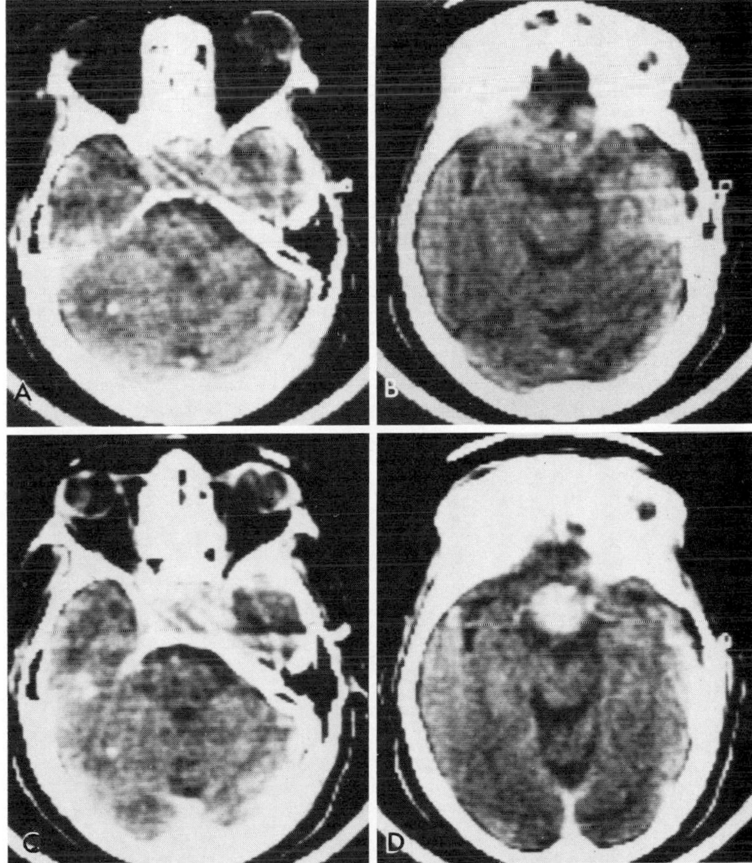

Figure 5–43 Large pituitary adenoma. *A*. CT scan showing marked enlargement of the sella, which is eroded anteriorly and posteriorly by a minimally hyperdense mass. *B*. The suprasellar cistern is filled with an isodense nodule, representing suprasellar extension. *C*. Marked contrast enhancement of the intrasellar component of the chromophobe adenoma. *D*. Similar enhancement in the suprasellar area.

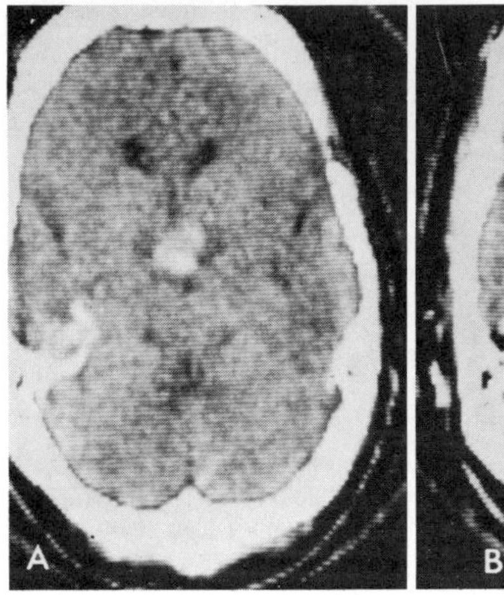

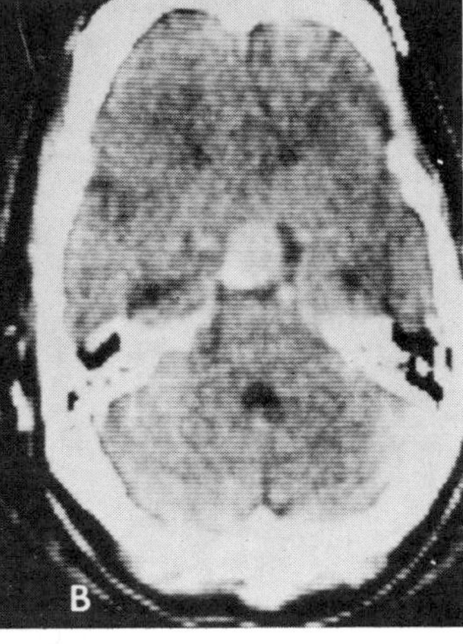

Figure 5–44 Hyperdense pituitary adenoma. *A*. CT scan revealing hyperdense nodule in the suprasellar space, representing a chromophobe adenoma that is undoubtedly diffusely and moderately calcified. *B*. Contrast enhancement of the nodule. This could not be distinguished from meningioma or aneurysm.

small adenoma. The newer scanners are able to show microadenomas in some patients.

Meningioma

These may arise in various sites and often are faintly or densely calcified. If noncalcified and suprasellar, they may not be distinguishable from chromophobe adenoma (Fig. 5–45).

Craniopharyngioma

Often calcified, these lesions may be solid or cystic, or contain enough fat (cholesterol) within them to show CT values well below zero (Fig. 5–46). If the latter occurs, the diagnosis is assured.[20] The solid, isodense portion of the tumor may be enhanced markedly, leading to confusion with pituitary adenoma. If the sella is small, however, the latter diagnosis is unlikely.

Aneurysm

Presenting in the usual fashion, that is, as slightly hyperdense lesions with or without calcification, these may be extremely difficult to diagnose definitively, although they may be suggested (Fig. 5–47). Because of this, it is prudent to perform angiography in all patients who present with lesions adjacent to, especially above, the sella. Once again, the presence of a normal sella in

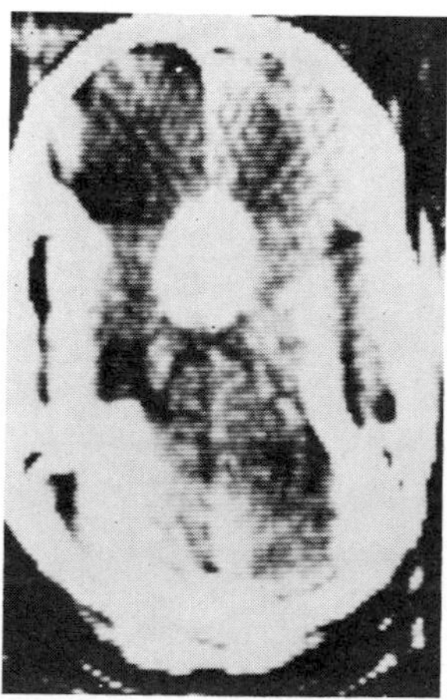

Figure 5–45 Tuberculum-planum meningioma. Contrast enhancement reveals a large basilar mass in the midline and over the sella turcica, which represented a very large meningioma in this region. Without further procedures, this cannot be totally distinguished from a huge suprasellar aneurysm.

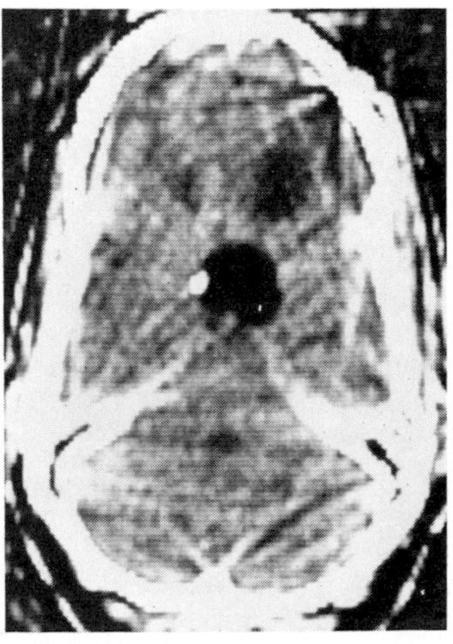

Figure 5–46 Craniopharyngioma. There is a radiolucent zone over the sella turcica, associated with a small fleck of calcium. The CT values of the radiolucency were well below zero, indicating a high fat content, allowing the diagnosis of craniopharyngioma.

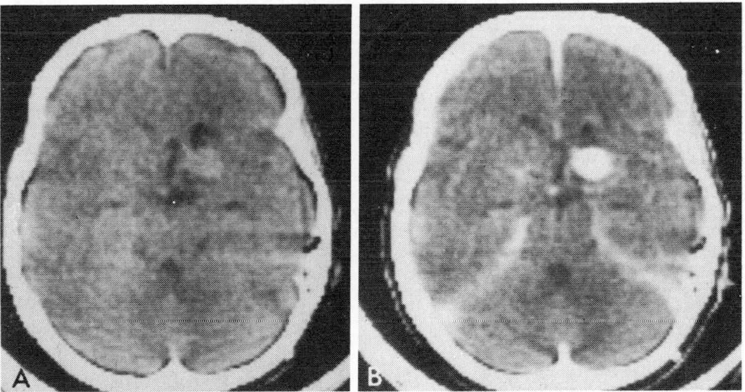

Figure 5–47 Aneurysm. *A*. Before contrast enhancement a mildly radiodense nodule is seen in the right suprasellar area. *B*. The nodule is homogeneously enhanced after the infusion of contrast material. The mildly hyperdense precontrast finding is undoubtedly a mixture of some calcification and increased density in the blood due to the blood collection in the lumen of the aneurysm. The blood pool is markedly enhanced after iodine infusion.

these patients tends to exclude the diagnosis of pituitary adenoma.

Other Lesions

Optic gliomas, teratomas, and hypothalamic astrocytomas present as suprasellar masses, often showing significant enhancement. The first of these may be diagnosed by their extension along one or both optic nerves and the consequent enlargement. These masses, however, may be difficult to separate from each other and from some of the previously discussed lesions by computed tomography alone. In other words, computed tomography is a superb device for detecting and localizing these masses, but it may not allow their definitive histological identification.

Finally, invasive lesions arising in or near the base of the skull may be shown on computed tomography, usually with a soft-tissue mass in the sphenoid sinuses, possibly extending into the skull, and often showing contrast enhancement.[44] Lymphoma, nasopharyngeal or sinus carcinoma, and metastatic disease are the most common entities, although rhabdomyosarcoma and nasopharyngeal angiofibroma may present in similar fashion.

COMPUTED TOMOGRAPHY OF THE SPINE

Computed tomography of the spine is in the early stages of development.[13,16,26,30] The examination must be performed on a scanner that encompasses the whole body, although some information about the upper cervical spine and craniovertebral junction may be gleaned from examinations performed on the head scanners. At the present time spinal computed tomography seems to be useful in evaluating several problem areas: spinal tumors, spinal stenosis, and fractures of the spinal column. Herniated discs are being shown with increasing frequency, and computed tomography will probably be the examination of choice for this diagnosis in the future.

Tumors

Computed tomography may be profitably used to evaluate vertebral body or neural arch tumors, to analyze the extent of involvement of paraspinal and intraspinal areas, and to help plan operative or radiation treatment.[45] It has not been highly useful, at least until now, as a detection device, since most lesions are more easily and more cheaply shown by regular radiographic or radionuclide studies. The extent of an intraspinal mass such as a neurofibroma may be well shown, especially if it extends laterally through the intervertebral foramen (Fig. 5–48).

Lipomas also can be shown nicely by this method, but other solid intraspinal lesions are not well delineated. The use of intrathecal aqueous contrast media may significantly improve the efficacy of computed to-

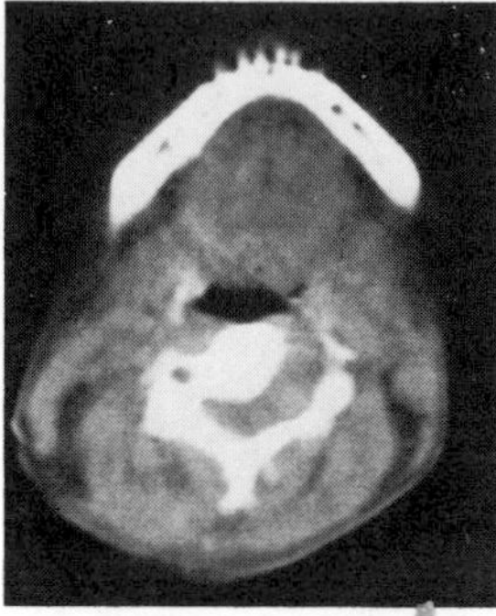

Figure 5–48 Neurofibroma of cervical spinal cord. Note the enlarged foramen extending anterolaterally on the right, which represented erosion of the foramen by a large neurofibroma. A faintly enhanced nodule at the spinal origin of this erosion represented the intraspinal portion of the tumor.

mography in this area, but whether this examination will replace myelography remains to be seen.

Syringomyelia (hydromyelia) may be identified on occasion, especially if the central cavity is large enough. Intravenous contrast enhancement may improve this study, as will the use of metrizamide. Failure to detect a solid tumor in the spinal canal, however, in no way excludes its presence.

Recently, computed tomography was used in the evaluation of 36 spinal neoplasms.[35] Eleven of nineteen intraspinal tumors were shown, as were all of the paraspinal masses. Most intramedullary tumors were not shown. The use of higher resolution scanners promises to improve the diagnostic capabilities of computed tomography in this area.

Spinal Stenosis

This problem is one of the areas in which computed tomography is most promising. Occasionally difficult to diagnose on plain lumbar spine films, the stenotic canal causes increased sensitivity to small disc herniations, and many, if not appreciated, continue to cause significant clinical problems even after a single appropriate laminectomy has been done.

Stenosis may be diagnosed by comparing the canal height, intrapedicular distance, interfacet distance, and pedicle height with normal measurements. The configuration of the canal is also quite important. The normal canal is capacious and circular or bell-shaped. The stenotic canal is quite small and has a flattened triangular shape due to reduction in the anteroposterior diameter and ''overgrowth'' of the facets and lamina (Fig. 5–49).

Fracture

Most spinal fractures will be shown on regular radiographs. Some may be discerned only on the CT scan. Most useful is the analysis of the displacement of fragments, especially into the spinal canal or

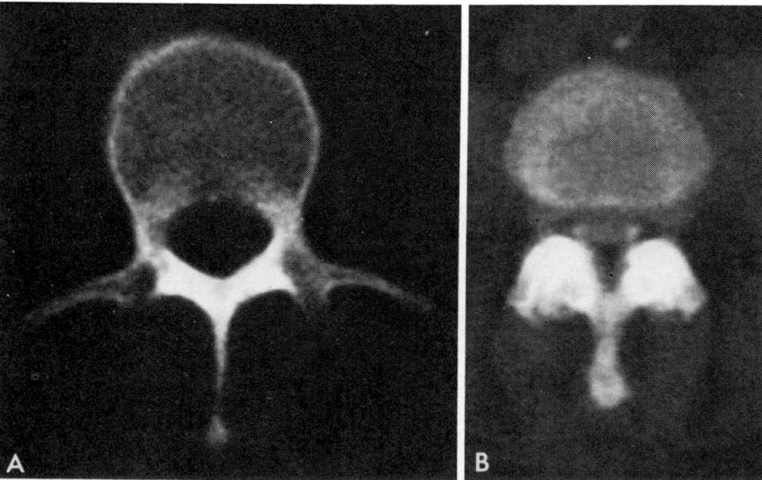

Figure 5–49 *A* CT scan of normal lumbar vertebral body. Note the size of the spinal canal. *B*. Metrizamide instillation into the thecal space reveals a markedly constricted canal (intrathecal space is opacified), mostly occupied by fatty tissue. The spinal stenosis extended from the third through the fifth lumbar segments.

nerve root canal, so that the operative intervention can be complete.

Sophisticated computer techniques that automate measurement of the vertebral region and also allow for coronal or sagittal rearrangement and three-dimensional viewing of the spine and its contents are under development. If these techniques are successful and made widely available, the use of computed tomography of the spinal area will increase with time to a point at which myelography will follow pneumoencephalography into history.

REFERENCES

1. Aimmerman, R. A., Bilaniuk, L. T., and Pahlajani, H.: Spectrum of medulloblastomas demonstrated by computed tomography. Radiology, *126*:137–141, 1978.
2. Ambrose, J.: Computerized transverse axial scanning (tomography). Part 2. Clinical application. Brit. J. Radiol., *46*:1023–1047, 1973.
3. Bafraktari, X., Bergstrom, M., Kerstin, B., Goulatia, R., Greitz, T., and Grepe, A.: Diagnosis of intrasellar cisternal herniation (empty sella) by computer assisted tomography. J. Comput. Assist. Tomog., *1*:1:105–116, 1977.
4. Banna, M.: Arachnoid cysts on computed tomography. Amer. J. Roentgen., *127*:979–982, 1976.
5. Bardfeld, P. A., Passalaqua, A. M., Braunstein, P., Raghavendra, B. N., Leeds, N. E., and Kricheff, I. I.: A comparison of radionuclide scanning and computed tomography in metastatic lesions of the brain. J. Comput. Assist. Tomog., *1*:3:315–318, 1977.
6. Bergstrom, M., Ericson, K., Levander, B., Svendsen, P., and Larsson, S.: Variation with time of the attenuation values of intracranial hematomas. J. Comput. Assist. Tomog., *1*:1:57–63, 1977.
7. Brismar, J., Roberson, G. H., and Davis, K. R.: Radiation necrosis of the brain. Neuroradiological considerations with computed tomography. Neuroradiology, *12*:109–113, 1976.
8. Brooks, R. A., and Di Chiro, G.: Slice geometry in computer assisted tomography. J. Comput. Assist. Tomog., *1*:2:191–199, 1977.
9. Chesler, D. A., Riederer, S. J., and Pelc, N. J.: Noise due to counting statistics in computed x-ray tomography. J. Comput. Assist. Tomog., *1*:1:64–74, 1977.
10. Citrin, C. M., and Davis, D. O.: Computerized tomography in evaluation of pituitary adenomas. Invest. Radiol., *12*:27, 1977.
11. Claussen, C. D., Lohkamp, F. W., and Krastel, A.: Computed tomography of trauma involving brain and facial skull (craniofacial injuries). J. Comput. Assist. Tomog., *1*:472–481, 1977.
12. Claveria, L., Sutton, D., and Tress, B. M.: The radiological diagnosis of meningiomas, the impact of EMI scanning. Brit. J. Radiol., *50*:15–22, 1977.
13. Coin, C. G., Chan, Y. S., Keranen, V., and Pennink, M.: Computed assisted myelography in disk disease. J. Comput. Assist. Tomog., *1*:398–404, 1977.
14. Davis, K. R., New P. F. J., Ojemann, R. G., et al.: Computed tomographic evaluation of hemorrhage secondary to intracranial aneurysm. Amer. J. Roentgen., *127*:143, 1976.
15. Davis, K. R., Parker, S. W., New, P. J., Roberson, G. H., Taveras, J. M., Ojemann, R. J., and Weiss, A. D.: Computed tomography of acoustic neuroma. Radiology, *124*:66–81, 1977.
16. Di Chiro, G., and Schellinger, D.: Computed tomography of spinal cord after lumbar intrathecal introduction of metrizamide (computer-assisted myelography). Radiology, *120*:101–104, 1976.
17. Dublin, A. B., French, B. N., and Rennick, J. M.: Computed tomography in head trauma. Radiology, *122*:365–169, 1977.
18. Dublin, A. B., and Merten, D. F.: Computed tomography in the evaluation of herpes simplex encephalitis. Radiology, *125*:133–134, 1977.
19. Enzmann, D. R., Norman, D., Mani, J., and Newton, T. H.: Computed tomography of granulomatous basal arachnoiditis. Radiology, *120*: 341–344, 1976.
20. Fitz, C. R., Wortzman, G., Harwood-Nash, D. C., Holgate, R. C., Barry, J. F., and Boldt, D. W.: Computed tomography in craniopharyngiomas. Radiology, *127*:687–691, 1978.
21. French, B. N., and Dublin, A. B.: The value of computerized tomography in the management of 1000 consecutive head injuries. Surg. Neurol., *7*:171–183, 1977.
22. Gado, M. H., Phelps, M. E., and Coleman, R. E.: An extravascular component of contrast enhancement in cranial computed tomography. Part I. The tissue blood ratio of contrast enhancement. Radiology, *117*:589–593, 1975.
23. Guner, M., Shaw, M. D., Turner, J. W., et al.: Computed tomography in the diagnosis of colloid cyst. Surg. Neurol., *6*:345–348, 1976.
24. Gyldensted, C., Lester, J., and Thomsen, J.: Computer tomography in the diagnosis of cerebellopontine angle tumors. Neuroradiology, *11*:191–197, 1976.
25. Hammerschlag, S. B., Wolpert, S. M., and Carter, B. L.: Computed coronal tomography. Radiology, *120*:219–220, 1976.
26. Hammerschlag, S. B., Wolpert, S. M., and Carter, B. L.: Computed tomography of the spinal canal. Radiology, *121*:361, 1976.
27. Hanson, J., Levander, B., and Lilliequist, B.: Size of the intracerebral ventricles as measured with computer tomography, encephalography and echoventriculography. Acta Radiol. (suppl.) (Stockholm), *346*:98–106, 1975.
28. Hounsfield, G. N.: Computerized transverse axial scanning (tomography). I. Description of system. Brit. J. Radiol., *46*:1016–1022, 1973.
29. Hounsfield, G. N.: Picture quality of computed tomography. Amer. J. Roentgen., *127*:3–9, 1976.
30. James, H. E., and Oliff, M.: Computed tomography in spinal dysraphism. J. Comput. Assist. Tomog., *1*:391–397, 1977.
31. Kendall, B., and Symon, L.: Investigation of patients presenting with cerebellopontine angle syndromes. Neuroradiology, *13*:65–84, 1977.
32. Kendall, B. E., and Claveria, L. E.: The use of computed axial tomography (CAT) for the diag-

nosis and management of intracranial angiomas. Neuroradiology, *12*:141–160, 1976.

33. Kinkel, W. R., and Jacobs, L.: Computerized axial transverse tomography in cerebrovascular disease. Neurology (Minneap.), *26*:924–930, 1976.
34. Lee, B. C. P., and Gawler, J.: Tuberous sclerosis. Comparison of computed tomography and conventional neuroradiology. Radiology, *127*:403–407, 1978.
35. Lee, B. C. P., Kazam, E., and Newman, A. D.: Computed tomography of the spine and spinal cord. Radiology, *128*:95–102, 1978.
36. Lin, J. P., Pay, N. Naidich, T. P., et al.: Computed tomography in the postoperative care of neurosurgical patients. Neuroradiology, *12*: 185–189, 1977.
37. Lott, T., El Gammal, T., Dasilva, R., et al.: Evaluation of brain and epidural abscesses by computed tomography. Radiology, *122*:371, 1977.
38. Maravilla, K. R.: Computer reconstructed sagittal and coronal computed tomography head scans: Clinical applications. J. Comput. Assist. Tomog., *2*:189–198, 1978.
39. Messina, A. V., Potts, D. G., Rottenberg, D., et al.: Computed tomography: Demonstration of contrast medium within cystic tumors. Radiology, *120*:345–347, 1976.
40. Michels, L. G., Bentson, J. R., and Winter, J.: Computed tomography of cerebral venous angiomas. J. Comput. Assist. Tomog., *1*:149–154, 1977.
41. Naidich, T. P., Lin, J. P., Leeds, N. E., et al.: Computed tomography in the diagnosis of extraaxial posterior fossa masses. Radiology, *120*:333–345, 1976.
42. Naidich, T. P., Pinto, R. S., Kushner, M. J., et al.: Evaluation of sellar and parasellar masses by computed tomography. Radiology, *120*:91–99, 1976.
43. Naidich, T. P., Pudlowski, R. M., Leeds, N. E., Naidich, J. B., Chisolm, A. J., and Rifkin, M. D.: The normal contrast-enhanced computed axial tomogram of the brain. J. Comput. Assist. Tomog., *1*:16–29, 1977.
44. Nakagawa, H., and Wolf, B.: Delineation of lesions of the base of the skull by computed tomography. Radiology, *124*:75–80, 1977.
45. Nakagawa, H. Huang, Y. P., Malis, L. I., and Wolf, B. S.: Computed tomography of intraspinal and paraspinal neoplasms. J. Comput. Assist. Tomog., *1*:377–390, 1977.
46. Peterson, N. T., Duchesneau, P. M., Westbrook, E. L., et al.: Basilar artery ectasia demonstrated by computed tomography. Radiology, *122*:713, 1977.
47. Phelps, M. E., Hoffman, E. J., and Ter-Pogossian, M. M.: Attenuation coefficients of various body tissues, fluids and lesions at photon energies of 18 to 136 keV. Radiology, *117*:573–583, 1975.
48. Radvany, J., and Levine, H.: Computed tomography in the diagnosis of primary lymphoma of the central nervous system. J. Comput. Assist. Tomog., *2*:215–217, 1978.
49. Ramsey, R. G., and Huckman, M. S.: Computed tomography of porencephaly and other cerebrospinal fluid-containing lesions. Radiology, *123*:73–77, 1977.
50. Rosenbaum, H. E.: Three dimensional computerized tomographic scans of brain. A new approach to intracranial diagnosis. Arch. Neurol., *34*:386–387, 1977.
51. Rozario, R., Hammerschlag, S. B., Post, K. D., et al.: Diagnosis of empty sella with CT scan. Neuroradiology, *13*:85–88, 1977.
52. Scotti, G., Ethier, R., Melancon, D., et al.: Computed tomography in the evaluation of intracranial aneurysms and subarachnoid hemorrhage. Radiology, *123*:85–90, 1977.
53. Stovring, J.: Contralateral temporal horn widening in unilateral supratentorial mass lesions: A diagnostic sign indicating tentorial herniation. J. Comput. Assist. Tomog., *1*:319–323, 1977.
54. Ter-Pogossian, M. M.: Computerized cranial tomography: Equipment and physics. Seminars Roentgen., *12*:13–25, 1977.
55. Tadmor, R., Davis, K. R., Roberson, G. H., and Kleinman, G. M.: Computed tomography in primary malignant lymphoma of the brain. J. Comput. Assist. Tomog., *2*:135–140, 1978.
56. Thomson, J. L.: Computerized axial tomography and the diagnosis of glioma: A study of 100 consecutive histologically proven cases. Clin. Radiol., *27*:431–441, 1976.
57. Thomson, J. L.: Computed axial tomography in acute herpes simplex encephalitis. Brit. J. Radiol., *49*:86–87, 1976.
58. Walshe, T. J., Davis, K. R., and Fisher, C. M.: Thalamic hemorrhage: A computed tomographic-clinical correlation. Neurology (Minneap.), *27*:217–722, 1977.
59. Wing, S. D., Norman, D., Pollock, J. A., et al.: Contrast enhancement of cerebral infarcts in computed tomography. Radiology, *121*:89, 1976.
60. Zimmerman, R. D., Leeds, N. E., and Naidich, T. P.: Ring blush associated with intracerebral hematoma. Radiology, *122*:707–711, 1977.

6

RADIONUCLIDE IMAGING STUDIES

In the past three decades, intracranial disease detection by means of radiopharmaceuticals and radiation-detecting instruments has gained prominence as a reliable contributor to the practice of neurological surgery.

The increasing sophistication of nuclear medicine and specifically "nuclear imaging" has carried with it a growing terminology applied to the instrumentation, radiopharmaceutical tracers, and procedures used. This has created an expanding vocabulary. In the interest of brevity and common understanding, the term "brain scan" is used to refer to radionuclide brain imaging and applies to the images obtained with either stationary scintillation cameras or rectilinear moving detectors. The scans produced by brain imaging or cranial computer assisted tomographic scanners that employ a small beam of x-rays, discussed in the preceding chapter, are called "CT scans."

HISTORICAL BACKGROUND

Several early radioactive tracer studies were developed as analogues of stable element dye compounds used for various clinical laboratory tests. An example is diiodofluorescein labeled with ^{131}iodine, reported by Moore in 1948 as a radionuclide tracer for brain tumor localization.[143] This development followed the observation that sodium fluorescein when administered intravenously exhibited a consistent affinity for brain tumors.[142] Erickson and co-workers and Selverstone and Solomon, in the same year, reported studies of brain tumor concentration of ^{32}phosphorus.[64,185] Chou and associates, in 1951, reported ^{131}iodine-labeled human serum albumin as a suitable agent for tumor localization.[29]

Historically there have been parallel areas of investigation contributing to the present state of brain imaging with radionuclides. These areas are instrumentation and radiopharmaceutical development. The technique for detection and localization involved point counting with a Geiger-Müller tube positioned at symmetrically located points over the calvarium. Later scintillation detectors with their greater sensitivity for gamma emissions were introduced. When these scintillation detectors were coupled to rectilinear scanning mechanisms, by Cassen and associates, the brain scan as a cartographic display came into being.[27] Much of the success of this mechanized scanning technique is owed to the use of the heavy shielding, collimators, and spectrometers reported by Allen and Risser, Francis and co-workers, and Shy and co-workers.[4,77,186] Concurrently, positron emitters, such as ^{74}arsenic and ^{64}copper were used to advantage with coincidence counting techniques.[23,229]

Subsequent instrument developments in 1955, 1956, and 1959 were photorecording modifications for scan data presentation on film.[17,105,118] Three other notable imaging devices for radioactivity distribution recording were developed in this period. These were the scintillation camera, which was invented by Anger in 1957; the autofluoroscope which Bender and Blau invented in 1960; and the Ter-Pogossian camera, developed in 1963.[6,7,18,205]

A continuing search for radionuclide tracers with greater tumor affinity led to the development of ^{203}mercury-labeled chlormerodrin by Blau and Bender in 1963.[19] The low-energy, shorter half-life radiopharma-

R. H. WILKINSON, JR., AND J. K. GOODRICH

ceutical, ^{197}mercury-labeled chlormerodrin, introduced clinically by Sodee in 1963, served as a widely used brain scanning agent until the development of ^{99m}technetium sodium pertechnetate by Harper and associates in 1964.[97,188] In 1967 Stern and co-workers reported ^{133m}indium (a daughter product of ^{133}tin) chelated to form ^{133m}indium diethylenetriamine pentaacetic acid (DTPA) as a suitable agent for brain scanning.[192] ^{99m}Technetium chelated to DTPA was recommended for brain scanning.[181] ^{169}Ytterbium chelated with DTPA was described by Hosain and co-workers in 1968.[106] Edwards and Hayes at Oak Ridge Institute of Nuclear Studies reported an affinity of ^{67}gallium citrate for soft-tissue tumors, including brain tumors.[61,62]

INDICATIONS FOR BRAIN SCAN

The brain scan as a diagnostic screening procedure should be considered when a careful neurological history and physical examination lead the clinician to suspect intracranial disease. As a screening effort, the scan has proved useful in patients with primary or metastatic neoplasms, cerebral vascular accidents, inflammatory lesions, and head trauma.

As a more definitive study, the brain scan often serves to detail the size and location of various intracranial lesions. This is a particularly useful aid in selecting the optimal neuroradiographic procedures to follow. In some instances, e.g., multiple metastatic lesions, the scan has obviated the need for further diagnostic studies. Furthermore, the scan may assist in determining the feasibility of operative intervention. The brain scan provides the radiation therapist with a means for selecting the size and position of his external beam treatment portals. As a follow-up examination, the brain scan serves as an innocuous study suited to outpatient care. Here it is especially useful in determining recurrence of brain tumors, resolution of intracranial abscesses, and appearance of new foci of metastatic disease.

Table 6–1 lists the most common indications for a brain scan.

TABLE 6–1 INDICATIONS FOR BRAIN SCANNING

Brain tumor
Primary neoplasm
Metastatic foci
Cerebrovascular disease
Arteriovenous malformations
Intracranial hemorrhage
Cerebral ischemia
Cerebral infarction
Hematoma: subdural, epidural, or intracerebral
Venous sinus thrombosis
Cerebral contusion
Inflammatory cerebral disease
Meningitis
Cerebritis
Abscess
Other benign (intracranial) disorders
Hydrocephalus
Porencephaly
Cysts

RADIOPHARMACEUTICAL TRACERS

The first radionuclide tracer, ^{131}I diiodofluorescein, was introduced for brain tumor localization in 1948.[143] Since this initial work, a multitude of radiopharmaceuticals have been applied to brain scanning and studying cerebral perfusion. The agents that have proved effective enough to warrant the Food and Drug Administration approval for use are ^{131}iodine-labeled human serum albumin, chlormerodrin labeled with ^{203}mercury or ^{197}mercury, ^{99m}technetium pertechnetate, ^{99m}technetium-labeled DTPA, ^{99m}technetium glucoheptonate, and ^{133}xenon.*

^{131}Iodine human serum albumin has a significantly prolonged biological retention within tumors as compared with normal cerebral tissue. In order to obtain a favorable tumor to nontumor activity ratio, a delay of at least 24 hours was required prior to scanning.[186] This proved to be a clinical disadvantage that was compounded by the long imaging period necessitated by the small allowable tracer dose.

^{203}Mercury-labeled chlormerodrin, while displaying a favorable tumor to nontumor concentration ratio, carried a renal cortical irradiation dose that was reported as high as 75 rads per millicurie. Its counterpart, ^{197}mercury-labeled chlormerodrin, delivered

* Abbreviated summary of approved radiopharmaceutical drug products. September 1, 1978, supplied by Food and Drug Administration, Department of Health, Education, and Welfare, Rockville, Maryland.

a considerably smaller renal irradiation dose of approximately 5 rads per millicurie. This tracer had a weaker gamma emission, which somewhat reduced the definition of lesions by its scatter within the calvarium. ^{203}Mercury-labeled chlormerodrin has been restricted by the Nuclear Regulatory Commission to the investigation of suspected deep-seated intracranial lesions.

^{99m}Technetium sodium pertechnetate is one of the most frequently employed radionuclide cerebral imaging tracers in use today. Those features that have led to its popularity are: (1) its simple elution from the sterile ^{99}molybdenum-^{99m}technetium generator; (2) its short half-life, which permits administration of a larger dose and hence a greater photon density in imaging; (3) its relatively low patient exposure dosage; and (4) its ready incorporation into various compounds whose characteristics permit the imaging of other organs.

Several investigators, including Di Chiro and co-workers, have reported that some brain lesions that were not demonstrated by ^{99m}technetium pertechnetate were identified when other tracers were employed.[56]

Use of ^{99m}technetium-labeled human serum albumin gives the combination of the favorable biological properties of ^{131}iodine human serum albumin with the markedly superior photon density of the short half-life tracer, ^{99m}technetium pertechnetate. ^{99m}Technetium human serum albumin may be readily prepared in the licensee's radiopharmacy by using commercially available kits. This radiopharmaceutical, however, images the normal vasculature more prominently than other tracers and is not generally employed.

The short-lived tracer, ^{113m}indium, when chelated with diethylenetriamine pentaacetic acid (DTPA) has been shown to be effective as a brain scan agent.[192] Its significant attribute by comparison with ^{99m}technetium pertechnetate is its lack of concentration in choroid plexus and salivary glands. Although millicurie doses equal to those of ^{99m}technetium provide high photon yields for scanning, the nearly threefold greater gamma energy necessitates scan detector collimation that reduces detector efficiency for collimator assemblies of equal resolution. The ^{113m}indium DTPA must be formulated in the licensee's radiopharmacy. The present Nuclear Regulatory Commission regulations limit the use of ^{113m}indium DTPA to broadly licensed institutions, and it is not a practical tracer for those with access to ^{99m}technetium radiopharmaceuticals.

A limited number of investigators have reported using intra-arterially injected ^{131}iodine-labeled macroaggregated human serum albumin for the detection of intracerebral lesions.[113,114,147,179] These investigators cited as the tracer's advantages that it provides better posterior fossa disease detection and more rapid imaging capability. The reported and potential complications as well as the necessity for arterial puncture appear to outweigh these advantages.[114]

The availability of ^{99m}technetium DTPA has gained proponents for its use in brain imaging. Some investigators have reported this agent to be superior to ^{99m}technetium pertechnetate in the detection of cerebral infarcts and neoplasms.[182] This tracer has the advantage of not concentrating in the choroid plexus and salivary glands, and it clears rapidly from the vascular spaces by glomerular filtration.[98]

^{169}Ytterbium DTPA has been proposed not only for radionuclide cisternography, but also for brain imaging.[106] In the presence of impaired renal function, the radiation exposure dose may be excessive. The 32-day physical half-life of ^{169}ytterbium together with the renal excretion of ^{169}ytterbium DTPA may make it undesirable in the incontinent patient.

The recent development of ^{99m}technetium glucoheptonate as a brain scanning agent has led several groups of investigators to advocate this radiopharmaceutical over ^{99m}technetium pertechnetate. There is no choroid plexus tracer concentration. An overall higher percentage of cerebral neoplasms and cerebral infarctions have been detected with this agent than have been reported with ^{99m}technetium pertechnetate.[173,198] Tanasescu and co-workers report overall tumor detection at 94 per cent.[198] This is in contrast to 82 to 90 per cent detection with ^{99m}technetium pertechnetate, as reported in previous series. One group has reported better detection of cerebral neoplasms but comparable results in cerebral infarcts.[121]

^{57}Cobalt-labeled bleomycin has been reported as superior to ^{99m}technetium pertechnetate by one group in the detection of neoplasms.[128]

Although chiefly used in the detection of soft-tissue metastases or septic lesions, ^{67}gallium citrate has been shown to concentrate in various cerebral abnormalities, including neoplasms, infarcts, and abscesses.[110,214,215] Its nonspecificity, the need for a two- to three-day delay between injection and imaging, and relatively longer imaging period are the reasons for its nonacceptance as a routine imaging agent. Waxman and co-workers have felt that it was at least equal to and in some instances superior to ^{99m}technetium pertechnetate in the detection of cerebral neoplasms.[215]

Attempts at more definitive brain lesion diagnosis have employed multiple tracers administered serially. From a practical standpoint, use of multiple tracers can add only a small improvement in the overall accuracy of disease detection when compared with ^{99m}technetium tracer agents used alone. Repeat brain scans using an alternate tracer may provide desirable information in circumstances in which neuroradiographic procedures are limited or delayed. Currently there is an imaging delay of two to four hours following injection of ^{99m}technetium tracer agents. Gates and co-workers, Ramsey and Quinn, and Meisell and co-workers report an increase in positive results as well as better definition of initially equivocal lesions.[81,134,170] Patton and Christenson report that in four series in which brain scanning was initiated at less than one hour following tracer injection, 84 per cent of tumors were detected.[159] In a compilation of six series in which the period between administration of the tracer and brain scanning exceeded one hour, however, the detection of 85 per cent of tumors was reported.[159]

Table 6–2 reviews the salient features of radionuclide tracers employed for brain scanning.

The question of how the commonly employed radiopharmaceuticals accumulate in or about neoplastic lesions has not been fully resolved. The generally accepted explanation for the appearance of radioactive tracers within the majority of cerebral lesions has been ascribed to a breakdown in the "blood-brain barrier." A precise and basic understanding of the "blood-brain barrier" remains to be elucidated. Bakay has reviewed the complex and oftentimes conflicting opinions and data relevant to this subject.[11,12] He classified the evidence into the following categories: (1) blood content of tumor tissue, (2) permeability of central nervous system membrane by passive diffusion or active carrier transport or both, (3) pinocytosis, (4) neoplastic blood vessel structure, (5) extracellular space, (6) peritumoral or tumoral edema or both, and (7) cellular metabolism. It would appear that more than one of these factors are involved in the accumulation and retention of tracer. Furthermore, the factors involved may vary with the tracer employed. At present, there is no tracer that will localize within a tumor to a greater degree than it will in certain organs elsewhere in the body, e.g., blood.[62] Thus the relative paucity of activity in normal brain tissue makes the "increased" level of tracer activity within the neoplasm a "positive" area. Tator has pointed out that the phrase "absence of blood-brain barrier" should replace the phrase "breakdown in the blood-brain barrier" in the case of meningiomas and acoustic neuromas because these are areas in tissue that do not have a blood-brain barrier.[12] A more detailed discussion and references on this subject are to be found in the work of Bakay.[11,12]

Quantitative regional assessments of cerebral blood flow following administration of diffusible or nondiffusible radiopharmaceuticals have been employed largely on an investigational basis. Holman states, "although the quantification of cerebral blood flow has been valuable in elucidating the parameters of cerebrovascular hemodynamics, these techniques appear limited as clinical tools."[102]

INSTRUMENTATION

The instrumentation for radionuclide portrayal of intracranial disease may be classified as moving detector and stationary detector imaging devices. Moving detectors, stationary detectors, and tomographic imaging devices are mechanically and electronically linked to recording devices. These produce images of the tracer distribution in the field under study. The recording may be portrayed on photographic or radiographic film, polaroid film, or on computer-type recording material (e.g., tape, disc). Any combination of these records may be produced. The degree of tracer concentration may be illustrated pictorially by a black or white "dot" presentation in which either the number of "dots" or the shade of gray of each "dot" reflects the level of tracer activity. Multiple color renditions arranged according to activity levels as perceived by the detector have also been used.

Single moving detector "scanners" were superseded by dual moving detector scanners. The latter permit the simultaneous recording of opposing projections. Currently the dual moving detector scanners have ceased to be commercially produced and commercial production has been directed to scintillation camera–type imaging devices.

The stationary scintillation detector assembly portrays activity distribution patterns from any particular area of the body. A field size of up to 16 inches in diameter is currently available. The image is displayed on an oscilloscope or television monitor, which may be photographed for permanent record. Computer or video tape recording may also be used. The capability of this scintillation camera to record rapidly changing sequential events such as the passage of the radiopharmaceutical through the cerebral circulation following bolus injection sets it apart from the rectilinear scanner. The resulting serial images provide a gross low-resolution "angiogram."

With the advent of sophisticated data retrieval instruments, kinetic recordings may be quantitated for region-to-region comparison. Commercially available tomographic instruments provide detailed study of the radionuclide distribution in the head. Work is currently under way to perfect emission-computed axial tomographic instruments designed to image positron- or gamma-emitting radionuclides.[162]

SCANNING TECHNIQUE

The variety of commercial instruments for brain scanning prevents a detailed discussion of scanning technique. Certain basic tenets should be observed, however. These are: (1) careful daily calibration of the instrument, (2) proper detector collimator selection according to tracer and desired image detail, (3) premedication as indicated for sedation or when certain tracers are employed (see Table 6–2), (4) attention to proper patient position and comfortable immobilization, and (5) the use of a standardized photorecording technique that depicts as much information as is available from the count rates that are present.

Serial imaging of the passage of the tracer through the cerebral circulation is accomplished following rapid injection of a small-volume bolus into an antecubital vein. This may be accomplished by either the saline flush technique or by preinjection blood pressure cuff occlusion with rapid release technique.[120,151] Recording by scintillation camera may be made from the anterior, vertex, or posterior projection.

Routine static brain scans employ anterior, posterior, and both lateral projections. In some institutions, the vertex projection is included. Special views involving oblique positioning may be of assistance. Use of the pinhole collimator or "converging" collimator may be helpful in better delineating the posterior fossa.

NORMAL BRAIN SCAN

The normal appearance of the ^{99m}technetium pertechnetate brain scan is portrayed in Figure 6–1. Rectilinear scans as well as images recorded by stationary detectors may be considered to present the cranial vault delineated in the sagittal and coronal planes. Detailed descriptions of normal anatomy may be found in several articles and texts.[156,210,217]

Brain scanning using the tracer ^{99m}technetium pertechnetate produces an image of tracer concentration within the choroid plexus in a significant number of cases. This choroidal concentration can be blocked effectively by oral premedication with 0.2 to 1 gm of sodium or potassium perchlorate.[107,108,224,227] Atropine sulfate in doses up to 1 gm administered intramuscularly or intravenously have been advocated in selected cases to decrease the naso- and oropharyngeal activity.[103] Choroid plexus blockade with Lugol's solution may be used, but is reported to be less effective.[227]

Figure 6–1 illustrates rectilinear scanner images obtained after sodium perchlorate

TABLE 6–2 RADIOPHARMACEUTICALS FOR BRAIN SCANNING AND CISTERNOGRAPHY

RADIO-PHARMA-CEUTICALS	PHYSICAL HALF-LIFE	PRINCIPAL GAMMA ENERGY (KEV)	ROUTE OF AD-MINIS-TRATION	DOSAGE	PREMEDI-CATION	INTERVAL UNTIL EXAMINA-TION TIME	LENGTH OF EXAMINA-TION	TOTAL BODY DOSE (RADS PER MILLICURIE)	TARGET ORGAN AND DOSE (RADS PER MILLI-CURIE)
^{203}Hg Chlor-merodrin	45.7 d	280	IV	10 μc/kg max. 750 μc	Mercuhydrin 1 ml IM	1–3 hr	3–4 hr	0.46	Kidney 75
^{197}Hg Chlor-merodrin	67 hr	72 (mean)	IV	14 μc/kg max. 1 mc	Mercuhydrin 1 ml IM	1–24 hr	3–4 hr	0.1	Kidney 10
^{99m}Tc pertech-netate	6.13 hr	140	IV	7.5–25 mc	Lugol's solu-tion or per-chlorate or nothing	30 min–4 hr	45–60 min	.02	Large bowel 0.5
^{113m}In DTPA	1.7 hr	393	IV	10–15 mc	None	None	1½ hr	0.015	Bladder 0.5
^{99m}Tc Human serum	6.13 hr	140	IV	10 mc (brain scan)	None	30 min–24 hr	1½ hr	0.01	Blood 0.04
albumin			SF	2 mc (cister-nography)		4,24,48 hr			
^{99m}Tc DTPA	6.13 hr	140	IV	15–20 mc	None	60–90 min	45–60 min	0.05	0.015
^{99m}Tc Gluco-heptonate	6.13 hr	140	IV	10–15 mc	None	1–4 hr	45–60 min	0.01	Bladder 0.8
^{169}Yb DTPA	32 d	63	IV	10 mc (brain scan)	None	30–90 min	60 min	0.02	Bladder 0.3
		177	SF	0.5 mc (cister-nography)		4,24,48 hr	30 min/da	—	Spinal cord 8.0
^{111}In DTPA	2.8 d	198 173 247	SF	0.5 mc	None	4,24,48 hr	30 min/da		Spinal cord 5.0

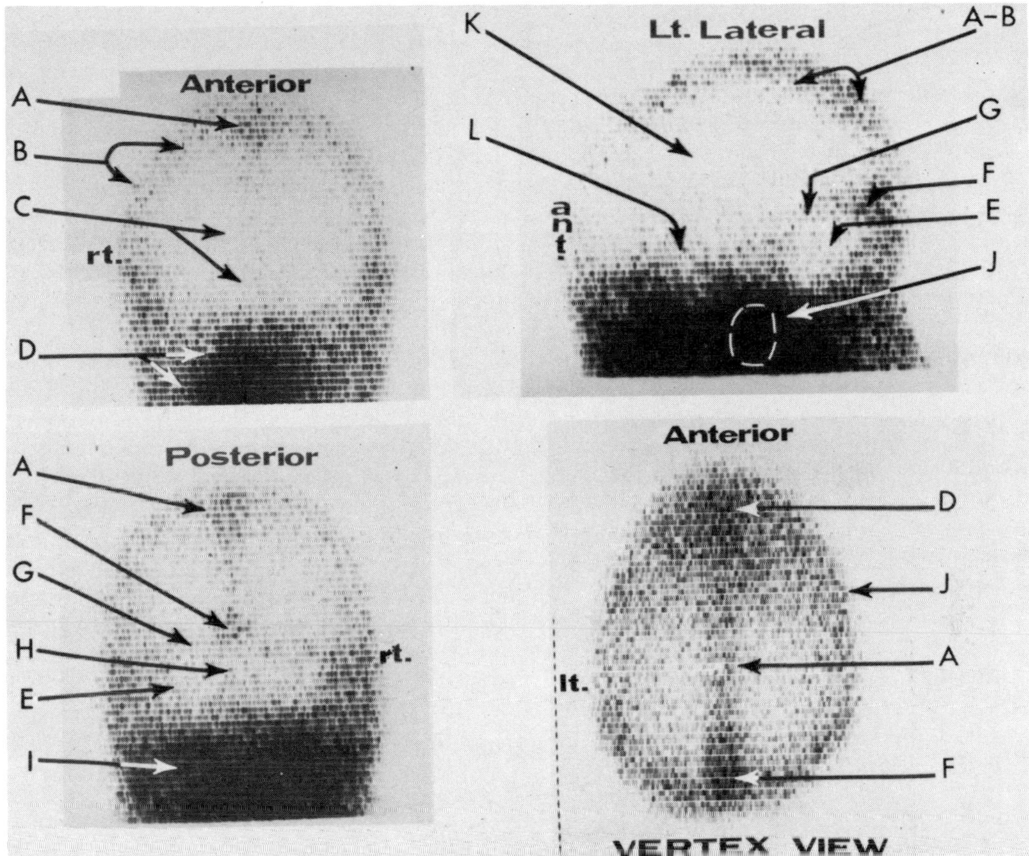

Figure 6–1 Normal ^{99m}technetium pertechnetate brain scan anatomy. Superior sagittal sinus, A; scalp, diploë, and meningeal vascularity, B; midline vasculature, C; oronasopharynx, D; posterior fossa, E; torcular Herophili, F; transverse sinus, G; straight sinus, H; nuchal vascularity, I; parotid gland, J; hemisphere, K; and sella turcica, L.

premedication. Frequent normal scan variations are: unilateral dominance of the transverse sinus on posterior and lateral views, and peripheral frontal tracer concentration adjacent to the superior sagittal sinus, which are attributable to prominent irregular venous drainage pathways; and vascular activity at the periphery of the cranium, which overlies the sellar region on the lateral view.

^{99m}Technetium pertechnetate ion contained in saliva, gastric contents, and tears may, on occasion, produce a false focus of activity by surface contamination.

APPEARANCE OF DISEASE

Static and Dynamic Images

The brain diseased by tumor or vascular insult may be expected to evidence the abnormality by retention of an appropriate radionuclide tracer. The resulting concentration of radioactivity is relatively higher in diseased tissue than in surrounding normal brain. The *static image* recording technique is designed to display this activity differential. There are, however, uncommon lesions that may be detected by the converse. Cysts, for example, having little or no vascularity to allow tracer entry may present as areas of reduced tracer concentration by comparison with activity in a contralateral hemispheric region.[140]

Several factors may affect the detectable concentration of tracer activity, including tumor cell structure and location, size of the lesion, duration of symptoms, and the like. Typically, grade III and grade IV astrocytomas and meningiomas are seen as dense tracer concentrations. Metastatic lesions are distinctive when multiple, but the tracer levels in the individual lesions may range from barely perceptible to dense concentrations. Cerebrovascular lesions are occasionally definable by the anatomical distribution of the greater tracer concentration in the region of the vessel system involved. This appearance may be mimicked by a neoplasm. Thus, a specific lesion diagnosis cannot be made with absolute certainty on the basis of the scan appearance alone.

A normal cerebral vascular pattern on the *dynamic study* includes relatively equivalent tracer activity bilaterally in the carotid artery regions and bilaterally symmetrical appearance and distribution of the tracer in the cerebral hemispheres.[36]

Abnormal patterns may be characterized as early or delayed appearance of tracer, increased or decreased tracer activity in the carotid arteries and cerebral hemispheres, or both. A detailed categorization of these patterns has been compiled by Cowan.[36]

Neoplastic Lesions

Although the positive brain scan does not dictate the specific nature of intracranial disease, there are often salient features that may serve as clinical clues. They are: (1) tracer concentration in the lesion in relation to adjacent normal activity levels, (2) configuration of the abnormal focus, (3) definition of lesion margins, (4) location within the cranial vault, and (5) multiplicity of foci. From a practical standpoint, the positive brain scan may be considered as a confirmation of the clinical suspicion of disease and direct the selection of subsequent neuroradiographic studies.

Table 6–3 presents a collation of 21 clinical series reporting radionuclide brain scan results in confirmed intracranial neoplastic disease.

The detection of intracranial disease by brain scanning is more than 90 per cent successful for meningiomas; astrocytomas, grades III and IV; and medulloblastomas (Figs. 6–2 and 6–3). The brain scan feature common in the majority of these lesions is the tumor tracer concentration, which equals or is greater than the activity in the scalp, superior sagittal sinus, or retro-orbital pool areas. Occasionally in large lesions, central necrosis may produce a

TABLE 6–3 COMPILATION OF REPORTED BRAIN SCAN RESULTS IN NEOPLASTIC LESIONS

NEOPLASM	AUTHORS (See References)	NUMBER OF CASES REPORTED	INCIDENCE OF ALL TUMORS (PER CENT)	NUMBER OF POSITIVE CASES	PER CENT OF POSITIVE CASES
All gliomas	1, 20, 24, 26, 44, 59, 67, 91, 92, 101, 116, 124, 144, 148, 153, 155, 169, 180, 213, 225	1269	40.9	1075	84.7
Astrocytomas Grades I and II	20, 24, 26, 44, 59, 67, 91, 92, 101, 116, 124, 144, 153, 155, 169, 180, 213	438	14.1	324	74.0
Grades III and IV	20, 24, 26, 44, 59, 67, 81, 91, 92 101, 116, 124, 144, 148, 153, 155, 169, 180, 213, 225	713	23.0	659	92.4
Ependymomas	1, 20, 24, 44, 59, 81, 91, 92, 101, 225	41	1.3	35	85.4
Oligodendrogliomas	1, 44, 59, 67, 91, 153, 180, 183, 213, 225	85	2.7	75	88.4
Medulloblastomas	1, 24, 91, 92, 124, 153, 180, 225	40	1.3	38	95
Other gliomas	20, 24, 59, 91, 92, 148, 153, 169, 180, 213	40	1.3	28	70
Meningiomas	1, 20, 24, 26, 44, 59, 81, 91, 92, 101, 116, 122, 124, 144, 148, 153, 155, 169, 180, 213, 225	478	15.4	454	94.9
Craniopharyngiomas	1, 20, 26, 44, 81, 91, 92, 101, 116, 153, 155, 169	28	0.9	19	67.8
Pituitary adenomas	1, 20, 26, 44, 81, 91, 92, 101, 153, 155, 169, 213, 225	132	4.2	70	53.0
Acoustic neuromas	1, 20, 24, 81, 91, 92, 101, 116, 124, 153, 155, 169, 213, 225	91	2.9	67	73.6
Metastases	1, 20, 24, 26, 44, 59, 91, 92, 101, 116, 124, 144, 148, 153, 155, 169, 180, 213	769	24.8	650	84.5
Miscellaneous tumors	1, 24, 26, 81, 91, 92, 101, 148, 153, 155, 169, 180, 213, 225	247	8.0	155	62.8
Total		3102		2574	83.0

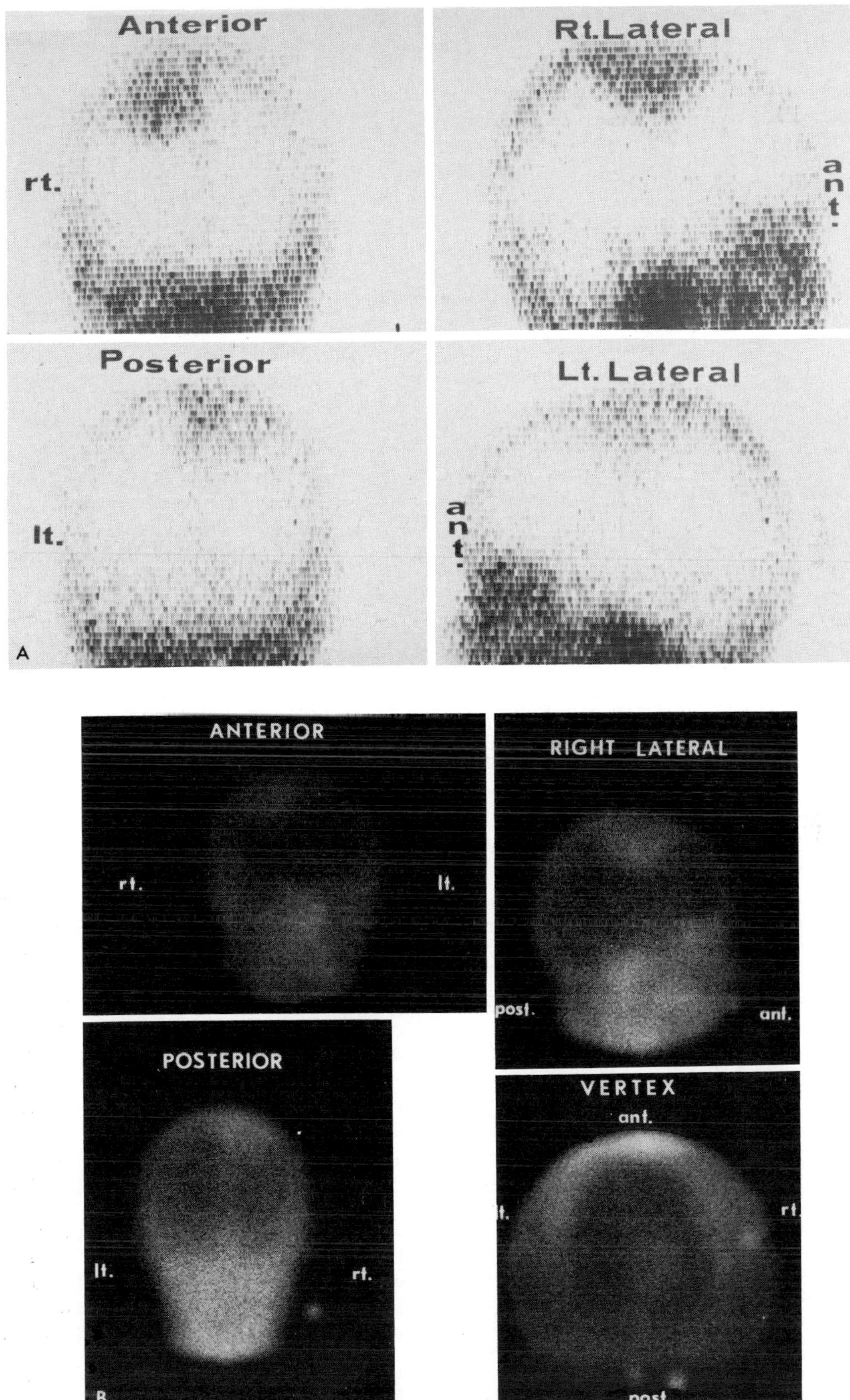

Figure 6–2 *A*. Right parasagittal meningioma recorded by rectilinear scanner. *B*. The same meningioma recorded by scintillation camera. Note vertex view at lower right.

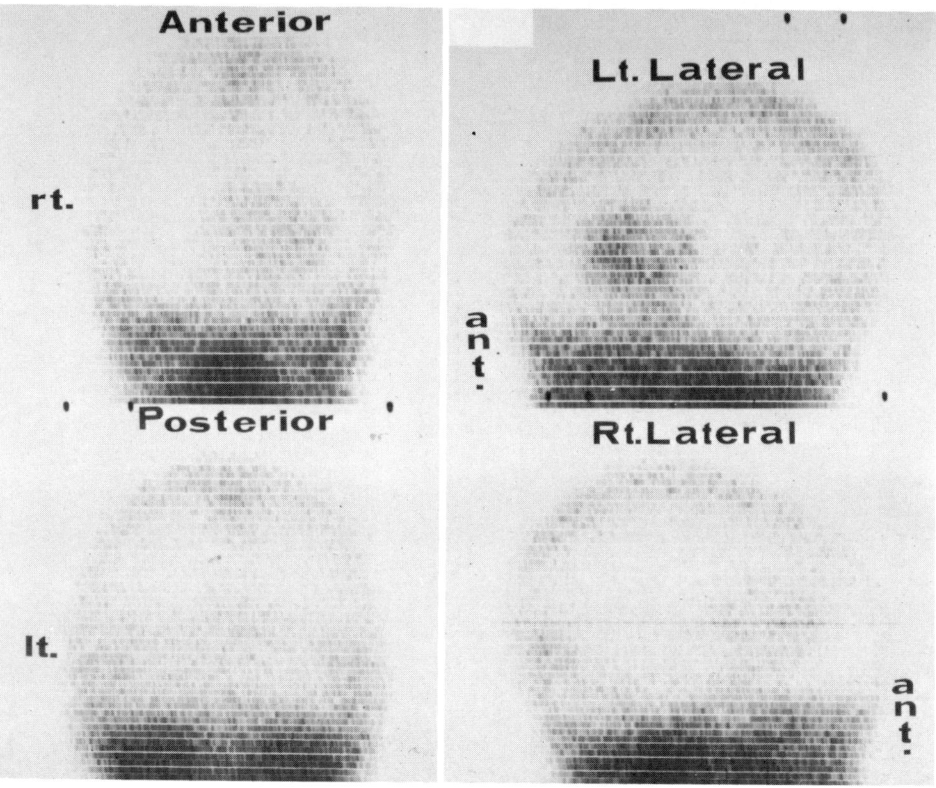

Figure 6–3 Astrocytoma, grade IV (glioblastoma multiforme). Note central clear zone in the lesion (the "doughnut sign").

"doughnut" configuration of lower central activity surrounded by higher peripheral activity levels in the lesion (see Fig. 6–3). This central defect of tracer concentration may also be found on occasion in intracerebral abscess, cerebral infarction, cerebral hemorrhage, subdural hematoma, and skull lesions.[199] In contrast to astrocytomas of grades III and IV, astrocytomas of grades I and II have been demonstrated in 74 per cent of the proved cases as shown in Table 6–3.

More than 80 per cent of metastatic lesions and oligodendrogliomas and ependymomas have been reported to be detectable by scanning.[42,144] The tracer concentrations in metastases are variable. The presence of multiple foci of abnormal tracer activity is strongly suggestive of metastatic disease when a primary neoplasm has been discovered (Fig. 6–4). In patients with established extracranial primary carcinoma, caution must be exercised in ascribing a solitary lesion on brain scan as reflecting a metastasis.[171] The relative incidence of detected metastatic brain lesions correlated with the origin of the primary carcinoma has been compiled.[221] The multiplicity of lesions seen on occasion with arteriovenous malformations and other vascular abnormalities as well as with cerebral abscesses may mimic the brain scan appearance of metastatic disease.

There has been some variation in reported identification of acoustic neuromas by scanning (Fig. 6–5). Failure to detect these tumors when they are small may be attributed to their proximity to the parotid gland and other physiological pools of activity at the base of the calvarium. DeLand and Wagner reported the successful identification of 12 of 14 (86 per cent) proved cases, and Ostertag and co-workers reported 33 of 36 (92 per cent) proved cases.[48,151] This accuracy is not reflected by the 91 acoustic neuromas reported in Table 6–3.

Pituitary adenomas, illustrated in Figure 6–6, craniopharyngiomas, and occasionally meningiomas, are the midline sellar, supra-

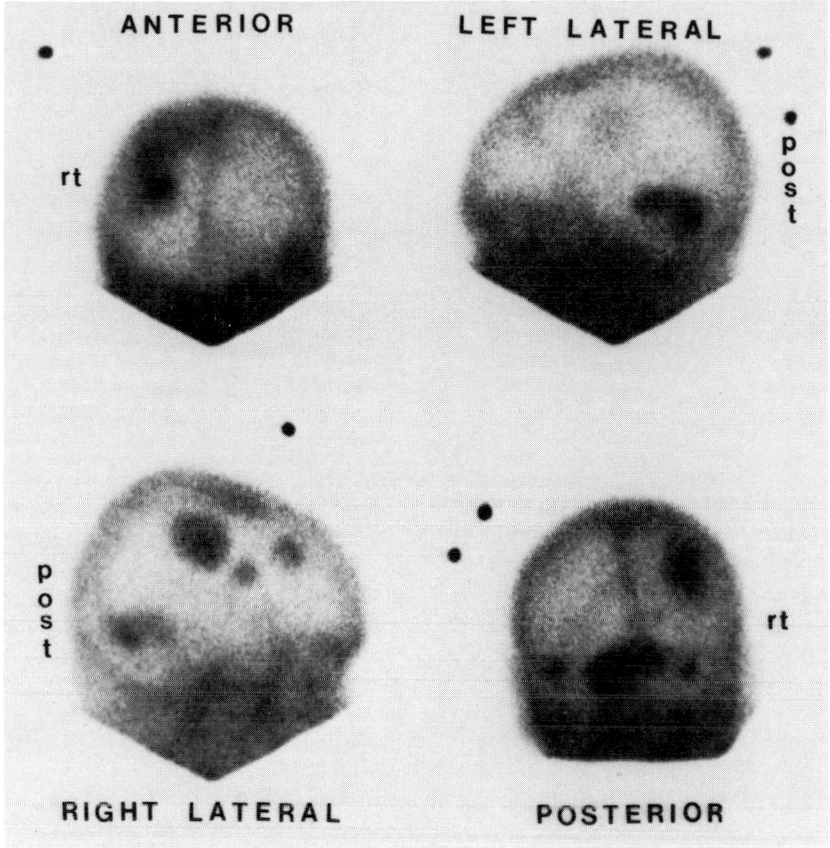

Figure 6–4 Intracerebral metastases.

sellar, or parasellar tumors detected by scanning. Here too, the proximity of these lesions to physiological pools of tracer activity may render them more difficult to discern by scanning.

The miscellaneous group in Table 6–3 encompasses the incidence of the less frequently encountered neoplasms. Examples of these include hemangioblastoma, pinealoma, and sarcoma.

The value of the radionuclide cerebral dynamic study, together with static brain scan, in the detection of cerebral neoplasms has been evaluated (Table 6–4). In the pre-

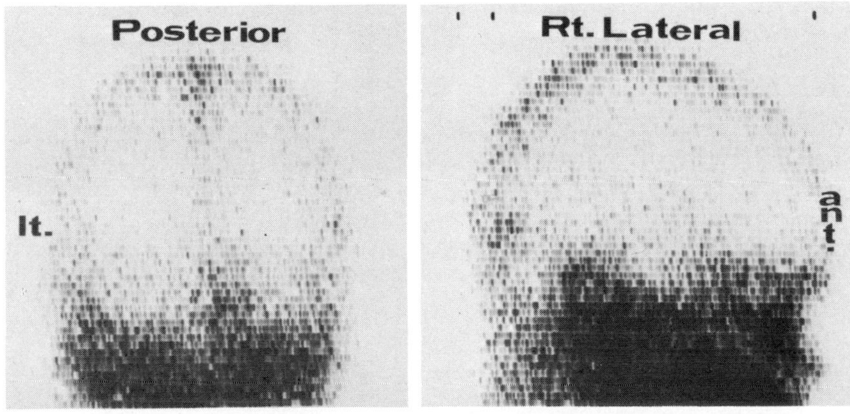

Figure 6–5 Acoustic neuroma.

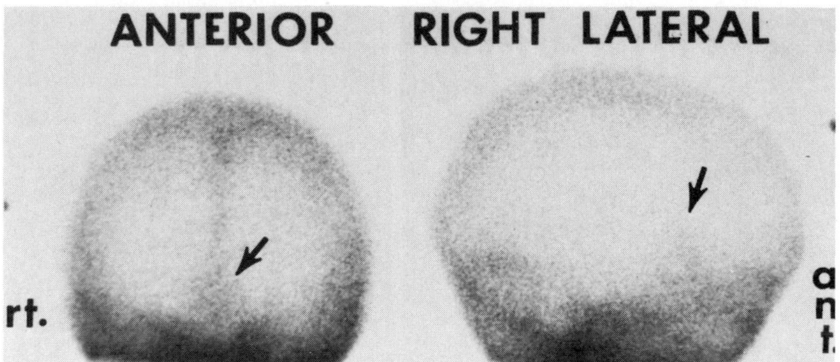

Figure 6–6 Chromophobe adenoma.

operative patient there has been no evidence to indicate that a neoplasm will be detected on the dynamic study that is not seen on the subsequent static images.[42,144] While an isolated case is possible, these series suggest that this would be an infrequent occurrence. Although the meningioma carries a higher incidence of abnormal dynamic studies as compared with other neoplasms in the preoperative patient, its scan occurrence is not sufficient to differentiate it from other neoplasms with absolute certainty.

Post-Treatment Brain Scanning

Patients who have received operative or radiation therapy for a brain tumor may be followed by brain scanning at appropriate intervals.[73,220] These intervals may be governed by the post-treatment clinical course. In each case an early post-treatment baseline scan is desirable. This is particularly true following craniotomy, when postoperative tissue changes will result in a positive tracer uptake. The abnormal appearance due to the operation may persist for months or years. Thus the baseline study will serve for comparison with subsequent scans searching for recurrence of disease.

Table 6–4 indicates that recurrence of neoplasm can be detected by dynamic and static brain imaging. One report has suggested that the dynamic study may be more sensitive than the static study in detecting recurrent anaplastic gliomas. False positive and negative scans, as judged by clinical follow-up, do occur, however.[228]

Detection of cerebral neoplasms by brain scanning can be significantly impaired by the administration of corticosteroids (e.g., dexamethasone) as early as 18 hours after initiation of the medication.[72,129,193]

Nonneoplastic Disease

The brain scan appearance in nonneoplastic disease is similar to that described for neoplasms. In some instances, factors such as the contour of the abnormal tracer concentration, the position of the lesion, or

TABLE 6–4 COMBINED DYNAMIC AND STATIC BRAIN SCANNING IN CEREBRAL NEOPLASMS

			POSITIVE		BRAIN SCAN	
			Dynamic Study		*Static Study*	
NEOPLASM	AUTHORS (See References)	TOTAL NUMBER OF PATIENTS	*Number*	*Per Cent*	*Number*	*Per Cent*
Astrocytomas	42	8	0	0	7	88
Glioblastoma	42, 144	46	8	17	39	85
Meningioma	42, 144	28	15	54	25	89
Metastatic	42, 144	73	6	8	66	90
Low-grade glioma	144	15	1	7	7	47
Miscellaneous	42	16	3	18	10	62
Postoperative	42, 228	33	28	85	22	67

TABLE 6–5 COMPILATION OF REPORTED BRAIN SCAN RESULTS IN NONNEOPLASTIC LESIONS

LESION	AUTHORS (See References)	NUMBER OF CASES REPORTED	NUMBER OF POSITIVE CASES*	PERCENTAGE OF POSITIVE CASES
Cerebral infarction	8, 31, 69, 70, 122, 146, 154, 223, 225	486	255	46.7
Arteriovenous malformation	31, 39, 59, 94, 112, 119, 122, 145, 154, 208, 212, 225	217	176	81.8
Intracerebral hematoma	31, 59, 145, 154, 223	34	24	70.5
Cerebral abscess	43, 46, 59, 76, 89, 111, 122, 130, 154, 195, 223, 225	91	88	96.7
Epidural and subdural hematoma and abscesses	22, 31, 34, 41, 59, 85, 86, 104, 145, 154, 209, 223, 225	410	349	85.1

* All equivocal cases were recorded as negative.

combined dynamic and static images coupled with other clinical data may narrow the differential diagnosis, e.g., cerebrovascular accident.[39] Reports of scanning results in nonneoplastic disease from 31 series have been summarized in Table 6–5.

Cerebrovascular Accidents

Cerebrovascular accidents have been reported to demonstrate a correlation between positive scan results and the time that has elapsed between the onset of clinical symptoms and patient imaging. Table 6–6 summarizes this correlation. The static brain scan image of a cerebrovascular accident may reveal a lesion clearly within the distribution of a specific intracerebral artery (Fig. 6–7). This is not always the case, however, and multiple areas of cerebral infarction may be found. If scans of suspected cerebrovascular accidents are negative in the first 10 days, they may be repeated in the second to fourth week after the onset of symptoms to improve the probability of lesion detection. Moses and Tow and their co-workers have reported their series of serially scanned cerebrovascular accident patients.[146,207] In their series the cerebral hemorrhage patients showed earlier positive scan findings and had a higher overall percentage of positive studies than those patients who had cerebral thrombosis. Serial scans may differentiate cerebrovascular accidents from tumor because the scan image of a cerebrovascular accident should return to normal by three months in contrast to that of a tumor, which will remain abnormal. This presumes of course, that a second cerebrovascular insult has not occurred in the interval.

Radionuclide dynamic imaging has added significantly to the detection of cerebrovascular disease. Cowan has reported a compilation of four series that employ the dynamic study to detect carotid artery stenosis. Although the numbers are relatively small, abnormal radionuclide dynamic studies reflected a poor yield if there was less than 80 per cent stenosis.[38] As might be expected bilateral disease was more difficult to define.

TABLE 6–6 PERCENTAGE OF POSITIVE BRAIN SCANS AT WEEKLY INTERVALS AFTER CEREBRAL VASCULAR ACCIDENTS

	1ST WEEK	2ND WEEK	3RD WEEK	4TH WEEK	COMBINED 5TH–12TH WEEKS	AFTER 12 WEEKS
Authors (see references)	8, 88, 93, 141, 207, 218	8, 88, 93, 141, 207, 218	8, 88, 93	88, 93, 141, 207	88, 154	88, 145, 154
Total number of cases	310	218	84	27	47	30
Number of positive cases*	123	110	57	16	20	0
Percentage	39.6	50.4	67.8	59	42.5	0

* All equivocal cases were recorded as negative.

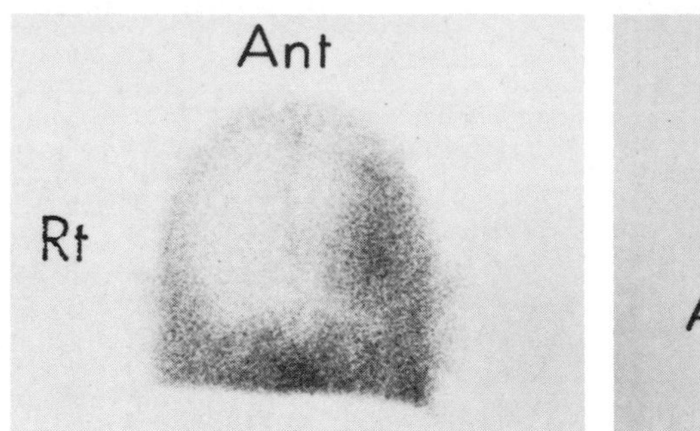

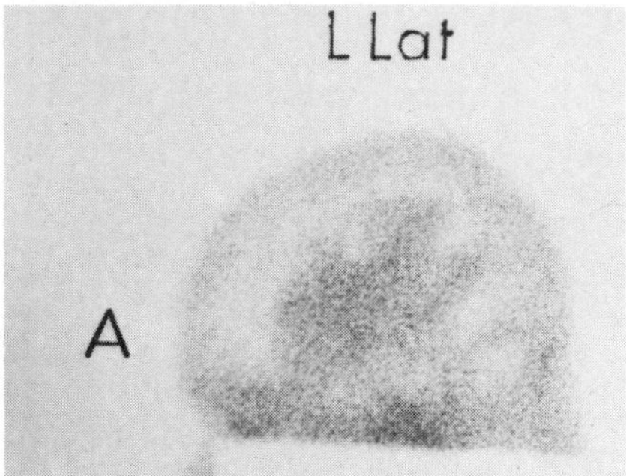

Figure 6–7 "Static" images 15 days after a cerebrovascular accident involving left middle cerebral artery.

Table 6–7 demonstrates the greater sensitivity of the dynamic brain imaging study as compared with the static brain scan in detecting cerebrovascular disease. These studies revealed, however, that the overall detection of cerebrovascular disease is enhanced by combining the dynamic and static brain imaging studies.

The majority of cerebrovascular accidents when presenting an abnormal perfusion pattern on the dynamic study will display delayed or decreased (or both) tracer activity in the early phase of hemispheric perfusion. This may or may not be followed by a brief period of relatively greater hemispheric tracer activity in the abnormal region. On occasion one may see increased hemispheric perfusion in the early phase, which has been termed "the hot stroke" phenomenon.[38,187,231] This has been described as reflecting the "luxury perfusion" phenomenon and is more often found in an embolic cerebrovascular accident.[187,231] This early hemispheric "hyperperfusion" phenomenon is not exclusively associated with cerebrovascular accidents but may be seen in other conditions (e.g., seizures, meningioma).[37]

Transient ischemic attacks have also been evaluated with the dynamic and static brain imaging studies. As would be expected, the dynamic study is more sensitive, but in comparative studies using contrast arteriography, there are both false positive and false negative scans (see Table 6–7).[129,146]

In an evaluation of 44 patients with cerebrovascular accidents in which ^{99m}Tc glucoheptonate was used, Tanasescu and coworkers have reported abnormal static brain scans in 62 per cent of the patients, and when these were combined with the dynamic study, the detection rate was 90 per cent.[198] ^{99m}Technetium polyphosphate and ^{99m}technetium diphosphonate have been reported to be superior to ^{99m}technetium pertechnetate in defining cerebral infarcts.[68,219]

Figure 6–8 illustrates an abnormal dynamic brain imaging study in a patient with a cerebrovascular accident. The delayed static brain images were normal. Figure 6–9 shows abnormal dynamic and static brain imaging studies in a patient with a cerebrovascular accident. The dynamic study illustrates the so-called "hot stroke" phenomenon.

Intracranial Hematomas

Experience has shown the brain scan to be a significant detector for subdural hema-

TABLE 6–7 EVALUATION OF DYNAMIC AND STATIC BRAIN IMAGING IN CEREBRAL VASCULAR DISEASE

	TRANSIENT ISCHEMIC ATTACKS	CEREBROVASCULAR ACCIDENT		
		Acute/Subacute	*Chronic*	*Combined Acute/Subacute and Chronic*
Authors (see references)	42, 70, 144, 146, 178	70, 146, 178	70, 146	42, 69, 70, 146, 178
Dynamic	35 of 133 (26%)	103 of 175 (59%)	24 of 50 (48%)	264 of 523 (50%)
Scan	4 of 133 (3%)	68 of 175 (39%)	7 of 50 (14%)	143 of 523 (27%)

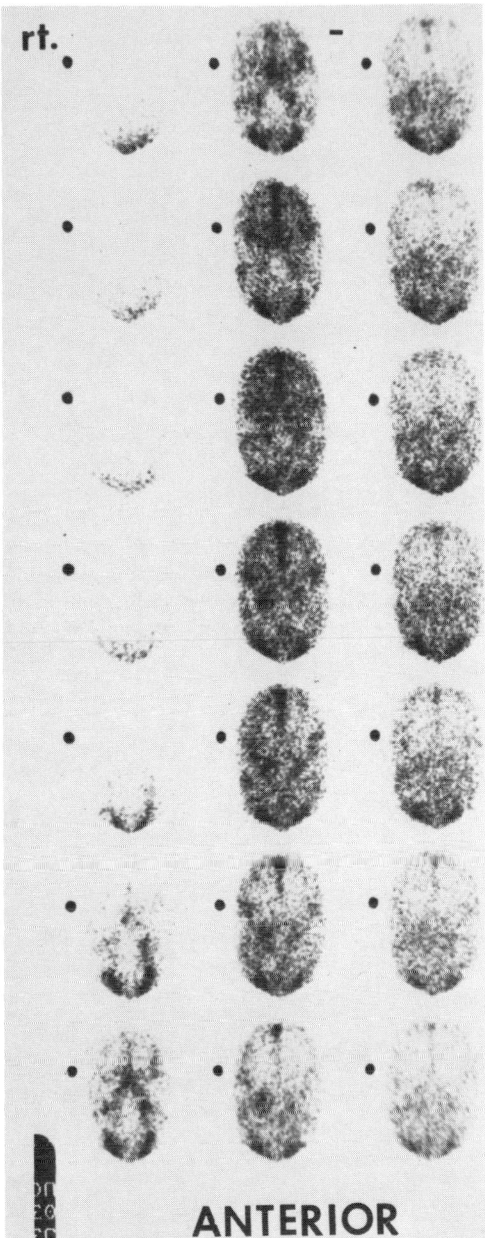

Figure 6–8 Cerebrovascular accident. The dynamic study demonstrates delayed perfusion to the right hemisphere with transient greater perfusion in later sequences. The delayed static images were normal.

tomas. Epidural hematomas may also be detected. The unilateral hematoma presents as a tracer collection that widens the convexity tracer activity of the brain scan image on the anterior or posterior projection or both (Fig. 6–10). A classification of subdural hematoma brain imaging patterns has been proposed.[197] Cowan has tabulated five series that report the sensitivity of the dynamic study in the presence of subdural hematomas. An overall detection rate of 83 per cent is recorded, with the majority of the investigators reporting 100 per cent detection.[40] "False positive" dynamic studies do occur, largely as a consequence of the abnormality being secondary to pathological changes other than a subdural or epidural hematoma. When correlated with the static images and the clinical history, however, this should be less of a problem. Bilateral subdural hematomas are a more difficult problem because identification often depends on comparison of opposing convexities of the cranial image. The anterior and posterior scan views for static and dynamic studies are the projections most likely to demonstrate the existence of a subdural hematoma. The lateral static views may show a diffuse increase of tracer activity over the brain or may give no evidence of any abnormality. The crescent appearance of peripherally increased cranial tracer activity was originally believed to be pathognomonic of subdural hematoma. This is not true. Heiser and associates reported also finding this pattern in cerebrovascular accident, craniotomy defect, granulomatous pachymeningitis, meningioma, metastatic breast lesion, extracranial trauma, and other lesions.[100]

Concentration of radiopharmaceuticals in subdural hematomas has been reported to occur in greater concentration in either the subdural membrane or within the fluid.* Detection on the static brain scan images is apparently improved by delaying imaging and by the existence of the subdural membrane.[9,41]

The interval that elapses between the traumatic incident and the delayed brain imaging appears to have an effect upon the reliability of detection of a subdural hematoma. In one series only half the lesions were detected within the first 10 days but 86 per cent of the hematomas were observed after a 10-day interval.[40] These studies, however, were not performed with delayed images nor did they include a dynamic study. Epidural hematomas and subdural collections in children have demonstrated abnormal studies.[34,40,85]

* See references 9, 57, 87, 133, 222, 232.

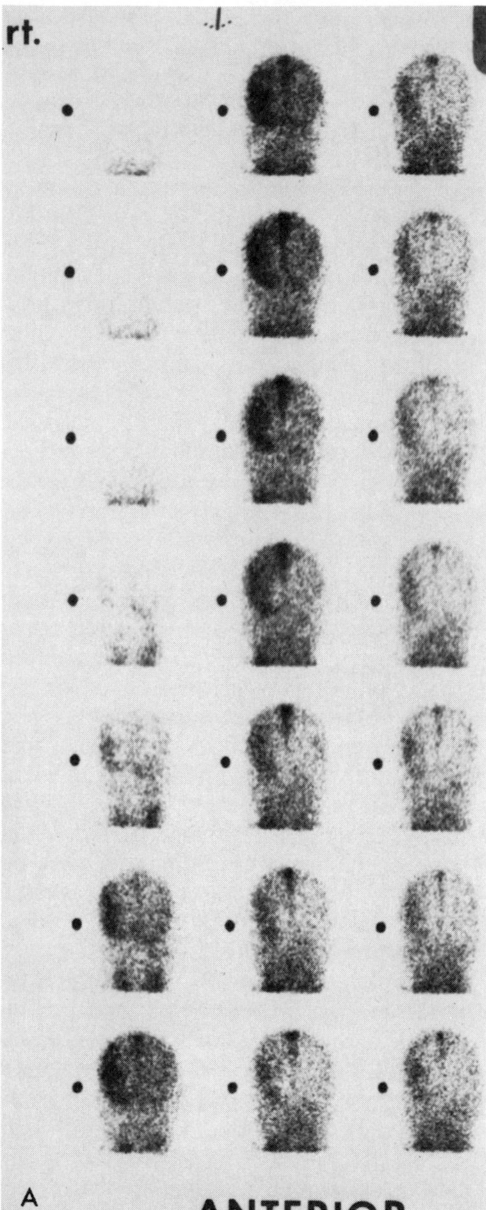

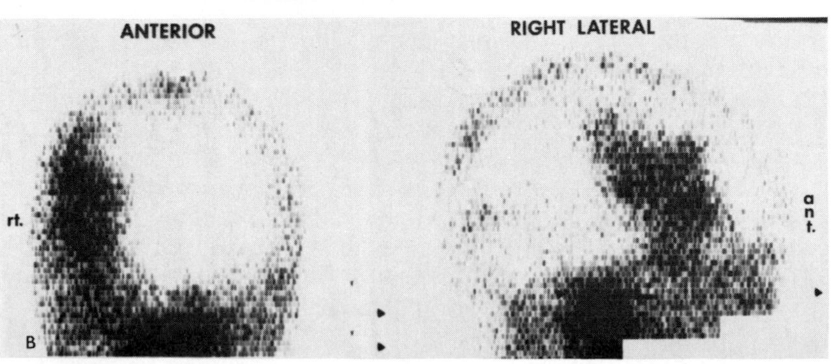

Figure 6–9 Cerebrovascular accident, ''hot stroke'' phenomenon. *A*. The dynamic study shows ''hyperfusion'' on right. *B*. The delayed static images reveal abnormal tracer activity in the right cerebral artery distribution.

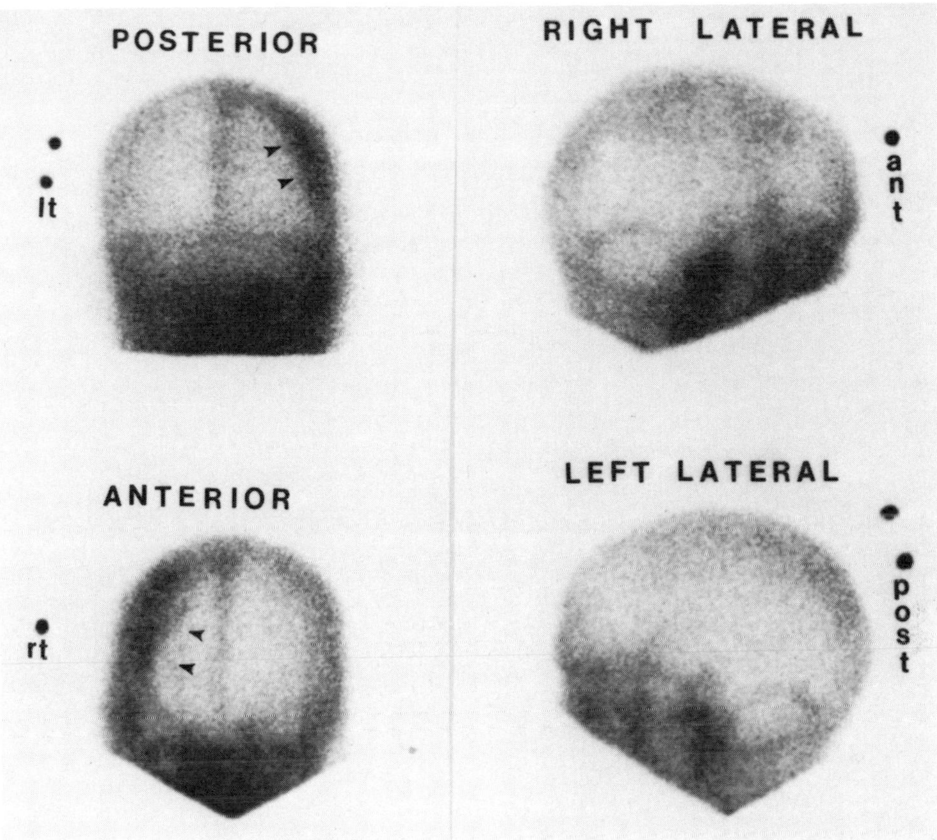

Figure 6–10 Right subdural hematoma. Note widened convexity border identified by arrows.

Intracerebral hematomas may also be identified by scanning. These lesions are indistinguishable from neoplasms and most cerebrovascular accidents. Sugitani and coworkers have experimentally shown that the maximum distribution of ^{99m}technetium pertechnetate in cerebral hematomas is greatest during the first through the third week.[183]

Intracerebral Inflammatory Disease

Intracerebral abscesses may be detected by static brain scanning with a high degree of sensitivity (see Table 6–5). In the light of a clinically suspected cerebral inflammatory process and the presence of a focal area of abnormal tracer activity, the clinician may be tempted to assign these findings solely to abscess. It should be remembered, however, that both cerebritis and meningitis may present a similar picture. Thus, neuroradiographic studies are of significant value in the determination of the presence of a mass lesion effect accompanying the formation of an abscess. The scan appearance of meningitis and cerebritis is often that of a diffuse irregular tracer retention; however, this may appear focal.[82] A subdural empyema cannot be distinguished from the subdural hematoma by radionuclide scan alone. Further, the clinician should be alert to the appearance of peripheral tracer activity that may accompany a diagnostic fontanelle tap in children.

Arteriovenous Malformation

Approximately 81 per cent of all intracerebral arteriovenous malformations can be detected by static brain imaging (see Table 6–5). In contrast to other tumors, an arteriovenous malformation may be detected on an early postinjection (''no delay'') study as well as or better than on a ''delayed'' study.[25,165,184] Static brain scan images of an arteriovenous malformation are shown in Figure 6–11.

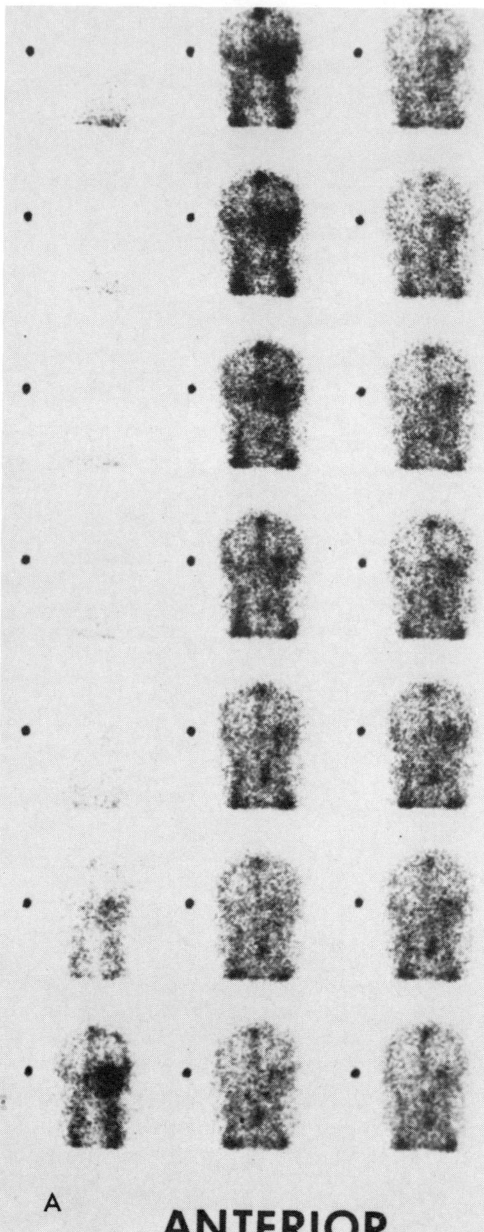

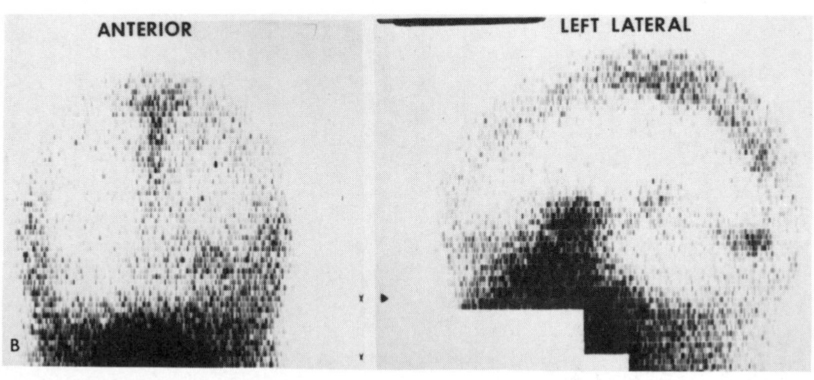

Figure 6–11 Arteriovenous malformation. *A*. The dynamic study shows the characteristic perfusion pattern. *B*. The delayed static images are also normal.

The dynamic brain imaging study increases the specificity of radionuclide brain imaging in arteriovenous malformations. Characteristically, there is a variable fading of the tracer activity in later dynamic sequence images (Fig. 9–11).[132,177] This is not pathognomonic, however, and on occasion may be seen with other entities (e.g., aneurysm, glioblastoma multiforme).[37,208]

Trauma

Trauma producing scalp contusion or laceration, skull fracture, or cerebral contusion generally will yield a positive scan image. The scan may not allow clear differentiation of these entities, however. Coincident skull fracture and cerebral contusion cannot be separately identified unless there is contrecoup contusion. Cerebral contusions generally present as relatively localized areas of tracer activity. The positive scan in cerebral contusion occurs early after trauma and may be expected to resolve in 6 to 10 weeks, according to Gilson and Gargano.[87] Intracerebral hematomas and contusions are indistinguishable by scanning. Appropriate interpretation of the brain scan in cases of trauma may be made only after review of the skull x-rays and examination of the patient's scalp for signs of topical damage.

Skull Lesions

Positive brain scans have been reported to occur in lesions of the skull. The skull lesions that may produce positive scans include primary bone neoplasms, metastases, Paget's disease, hyperostosis frontalis interna, cholesteatoma, dermoid cysts, fibrous dysplasia, hemangiomas, fractures, inflammatory lesions, and craniotomy defects.[131]

Tow and Wagner reported the relative tracer activity of bone lesions and brain tumors using ^{85}strontium or ^{87m}strontium and ^{99m}technetium in laboratory animals and humans.[206] They determined that it might be possible to distinguish peripheral intracerebral lesions from skull lesions by this technique. A combination of ^{99m}technetium pertechnetate, ^{99m}technetium phosphate complex, and ^{67}gallium citrate brain imaging examinations have been reported to show promise in differentiating craniotomy defects from recurrent cerebral neoplasms.[110,216] This has not become a standard procedure, however. It must be kept in mind that the ^{99m}technetium phosphate complexes can concentrate in intracerebral neoplasms and infarcts as well as in skull lesions.[68]

It is obvious that skull radiographs are useful in the interpretation of all brain scans and in particular those of patients who have had trauma to or operations on the head.

BRAIN SCANNING AFTER CAROTID ARTERIOGRAPHY

Several authors indicated that cerebral arteriography might produce a false positive brain scan.[16,123,189] Subsequently, Heinz and co-workers reported 10 cases of brain scans performed before and after arteriography with no apparent false positive scan results.[99] They concluded that careful arteriographic technique would prevent a false positive radionuclide brain study. Anderson and Siemsen reviewed a series of 116 scans and found nothing to indicate angiographically induced positive scans.[5] Planiol did not observe any adverse effects on the brain scan following cerebral arteriography in 800 cases.[164] The same result may be expected from any radiographic procedure involving the intravenous injection of an iodinated contrast material.

BRAIN SCANNING IN CHILDREN

With the advent of shorter-lived, lower-energy gamma-emitting radiopharmaceuticals, the reluctance to use radionuclide brain scanning in children has been reduced. The brain scan has become an accepted diagnostic procedure in the appropriate clinical setting.

The overall reliability of radionuclide brain scanning in the detection of cerebral neoplasms in children is similar to that in adults. Table 6–8 tabulates several representative series. Conway has presented an extensive tabulated survey of the literature up to 1972.[32] Supratentorial lesions for which the rate of detection is relatively high

TABLE 6–8 COMPILATION OF REPORTED PEDIATRIC BRAIN SCAN RESULTS IN NEOPLASTIC LESIONS

LESION	AUTHORS (See References)	NUMBER OF CASES REPORTED	NUMBER OF POSITIVE CASES	PERCENTAGE OF POSITIVE CASES
Supratentorial				
Optic glioma	33	10	10	100
Glioblastoma	33, 130, 138	11	11	100
Astrocytoma	33, 83, 137	32	27	84
"Glioma"*	83	15	13	87
Ependymoma	33, 83, 130, 138	21	21	100
Craniopharyngioma	33, 83, 130, 138	22	11	50
Pinealoma	33, 130, 138	5	3	60
Other	33, 83, 130, 138	41	33	80
Metastases	33, 83, 138	11	11	100
Infratentorial				
Medulloblastoma	33, 83, 130, 138	48	43	90
Cerebellar astrocytoma	33, 130, 138	54	52	96
Brain stem glioma	33, 130, 138	15	6	40
Ependymoma	33, 138	6	5	83
Other	138	2	0	0
Subtotal-Infratentorial		125	106	85
Subtotal-Supratentorial		168	140	83
Total		293	246	84

* These did not include astrocytomas or ependymomas.

are optic gliomas, glioblastomas, astrocytomas, ependymomas, and metastases. Craniopharyngiomas and pinealomas are less reliably detected. Among the infratentorial lesions, medulloblastomas, cerebellar astrocytomas, and ependymomas are detected with a relatively high degree of accuracy. Unfortunately, less than half of brain stem gliomas are detected.

The combined series of Conway and Vollert and of Gilday and co-workers, in which the static brain scan was used to detect pediatric subdural fluid collections, reveal 86 of 105 cases of bilateral dural fluid collections being defined (82 per cent). Sixty-one of sixty-seven unilateral dural fluid collections were demonstrated by brain scanning (91 per cent).[34,86] Gilday and associates report an overall correct diagnosis rate of 94 per cent and a false positive rate of 10 per cent.[86] A point to be stressed is that sterile subdural effusions are seldom positive on the brain scan whereas those secondary to meningitis are frequently demonstrated.

Although seen less frequently than in adults, cerebrovascular accidents in children present an appearance on the dynamic and static images similar to that seen in adults. Arteriovenous malformations also have dynamic and static patterns essentially the same as adults.

Cerebral inflammatory disease patterns on the radionuclide brain scan in the child range from focal lesions to diffuse areas of increased cerebral tracer activity. Gilday characterized these patterns in 48 cases from a series of 1150 brain scan studies gathered over a 20-month period.[82] The patterns were defined as: (1) diffuse increase in radionuclide activity throughout the brain (e.g., diffuse encephalitis), (2) peripheral increase in radionuclide activity (e.g., meningitis); (3) focal increase of radionuclide activity (e.g., focal encephalitis), or cerebral abscess, and (4) increased radionuclide activity outlining the lateral ventricles (e.g., ventriculitis).

In summary, the authors believe that the judicious use of brain scanning in children with neurological defects has been shown to have diagnostic value. The request for the pediatric brain scan should be made with an appreciation of the radiation exposure attendant to these studies. Kereikes and co-workers have calculated the radiation dose to target organs and whole body for the newborn, several pediatric age groups, and the adult.[181] Use of the radionuclide brain scan in the pediatric population should be balanced against the advantages of performing a CT scan.

RADIONUCLIDE DYNAMIC IMAGING

With the development of stationary imaging devices such as the Anger scintillation camera, the Autofluoroscope, and the Ter-Pogossian camera, the ability to take rapid-sequence serial images of the transit pattern of a radiopharmaceutical through an organ or region became a reality.[7,18,205] Several groups reported recording the vascular flow pattern in cerebral studies. The diagnostic value of this procedure in the occlusion of the carotid or major cerebral arteries has been amply shown by many investigators and is discussed in a previous section.[71,167,175,176] A vascular occlusion results in decreased tracer perfusion in the region of the affected vessel or vessels. The striking feature has been that in vascular occlusion, the dynamic studies were frequently positive when the routine scans were negative (cf. Fig. 6–11). The dynamic study was shown to have clinical importance in a cerebrovascular accident in the early postocclusive period when the static cerebral scan is ordinarily negative. Maynard and associates have noted decreased tracer activity in some instances in which there was tumor displacement of normal vessels.[132] This might simulate a lesion secondary to cerebrovascular occlusion. As noted earlier, the arteriovenous malformations usually show increased tracer activity early in the arterial phase, but lose activity in the late venous phase.[132,177] Meningiomas and astrocytomas of grade III and grade IV may produce a prompt "blush" of tracer activity that persists throughout the study. Investigative work in the quantification of cerebral blood flow studies offers further expansion of the intracerebral use of radionuclide tracers. These studies have been well summarized by Ronai.[174]

RADIONUCLIDE CEREBROSPINAL FLUID STUDIES

Early studies applying radionuclides to elucidate the physiology of the cerebrospinal fluid were reported by several groups. Sweet and co-workers counted serial samples of cerebrospinal fluid, blood, and urine following the intrathecal injection of the radionuclide tracer.[196] Chou and French employed external counting to determine the rates of diffusion, absorption, and clearance of intrathecally injected ^{131}iodine-labeled human serum albumin.[28] Crow and associates reported localizing cerebrospinal fluid fistulae by counting the radioactivity on cotton wool pledgets placed in the nasopharynx after injection of ^{24}sodium into the cisterna magna.[45] A further review of the early development of the intrathecal use of radionuclides may be found in articles by di Chiro and co-workers.[55,57]

Di Chiro and Tator and their colleagues have detailed the course of normal flow of cerebrospinal fluid labeled with ^{131}iodine-labeled human serum albumin.[55,202] When the labeled tracer was injected into the lumbar subarachnoid space it was carried to the basal cisternae within two hours. At six hours, the tracer was seen in the sylvian cisternae and along the interhemispheric fissure. Within 24 hours the tracer accumulated along the superior sagittal sinus, and at 48 hours most of the radioactivity had disappeared. In normal subjects, no significant radioactivity was recorded in the ventricular system.

When ^{131}iodine-labeled human serum albumin was injected into the cisterna magna, the majority of the tracer passed around the medulla to the cisterna medullaris and up into the cisterna pontis. Some of the tracer descended into the spinal subarachnoid space. Usually all basal cisternae could be identified by scanning the tracer within one hour after injection. Within four hours the sylvian cisternae, the cisterna lamina terminalis, and the callosal cisternae could be recorded by scanning. At 24 hours the tracer had collected over the cerebral hemispheres in the parasagittal areas and in the interhemispheric fissure.

Several authors have reported the use of ^{131}iodine-labeled human serum albumin as a variation of the myelogram.[14,15] This myeloscintigram, however, lacks the image detail of the radiographic myelogram with air or opaque contrast material and is of limited value.

Until recently a widely used radioactive tracer agent for cisternography or ventriculography was human serum albumin labeled with high concentrations of ^{131}iodine. This tracer necessitated a high specific activity in the order of 50 to 100 μc of ^{131}iodine per milligram of albumin. Material with high specific activity was recommended by di Chiro in order to reduce the incidence of aseptic meningitis. The initial two cases of aseptic meningitis reported in the literature occurred after intrathecal injection of 27 mg of albumin in one case and 100 to 130 mg of albumin in the other case.[50,150] These cases prompted di Chiro to recommend doses of albumin on the order of 4 mg or less for intrathecal injection.[52] Oldham and Staab reported two cases of aseptic meningitis following the intrathecal injection of less than 2 mg of ^{131}iodine-labeled human serum albumin.[152]

Subsequently, the use of ^{111}indium DTPA in cisternography resulted in the report of aseptic meningitis.[109] Endotoxin detected by the Limulus test but not by the standard USP rabbit test for pyrogens was discovered in several commercial lots of ^{131}I HSA and ^{111}In DTPA that had been administered to patients who had then developed adverse reactions. These investigators recommended the use of both tests for intrathecally injected radiopharmaceuticals.[65]

Other radiopharmaceuticals have been employed in the study of cerebrospinal fluid distribution. These include ^{99m}technetium-labeled human serum albumin and ^{169}ytterbium DTPA (see Table 6–2).

The more common clinical applications of radionuclide cerebrospinal fluid studies include cerebrospinal fluid leak detection and localization, evaluation of communicating and noncommunicating hydrocephalus, and evaluation of shunt patency.

Radionuclide Otorrhea and Rhinorrhea Study

The cerebrospinal fluid leak study was developed as a parallel technique to dye studies using indigo carmine. Localization of cerebrospinal fluid leaks relied on the staining of cotton pledgets carefully placed at the orifices of the paranasal sinuses and near the cribriform plate. In the case of the radionuclide study, a radiopharmaceutical is substituted for the dye. The radiopharmaceutical is injected in the lumbar subarachnoid space following placement of the pledgets. Appropriate positioning is important to encourage leakage and reduce cross contamination. In the authors' experience a clearly positive radionuclide cerebrospinal fluid leak study has required cotton pledgets from a particular area to have several-fold greater count rate when compared with the other pledgets. It should be noted that some radioactivity will appear on all pledgets because of the free unbound tracer ions and the release of tracer ions from the albumin label. They subsequently appear in the nasal secretions and blood, and may simulate abnormal tracer accumulation.

In addition to counting the cotton pledgets, serial image recording of the cerebrospinal fluid leak may be of value. Rectilinear scans or scintillation camera images, in the authors' experience, have recorded gross leaks (Fig. 6–12). Small and intermittent leaks were more difficult or impossible to localize by the imaging technique. Di Chiro and Ashburn and their co-workers have published interesting illustrations of cerebrospinal fluid leaks demonstrated by the scintillation camera.[10,58] Recently "controlled overpressure" cisternography has been advocated in the detection of otorrhea and rhinorrhea.[127] This involves the infusion of artificial cerebrospinal fluid to increase pressure and thereby enhance leakage. An editorial commentary has emphasized the hazards of this procedure and suggested that modification of the procedure be considered.[74]

Radionuclide Cisternography and Ventriculography Study

The radionuclide cisternogram of the patient with the normal-pressure hydrocephalus may be performed by lumbar intrathecal injection or by the direct instillation of the tracer into the cisterna magna. The scan image may record tracer activity in the dilated ventricles within the first 24 hours. Subsequent 48-hour and 72-hour scans in normal-pressure communicating hydrocephalus will generally not show any evidence of the radioactivity distributed over the superior cortical surface and in the area of the superior sagittal sinus. While pneumoencephalography may show patency of the subarachnoid space, it does not depend on the active circulation of the spinal fluid. The radionuclide tracer, however, must be distributed by active cerebrospinal fluid flow.[203] Hence, the radionuclide cisternogram may be considered a relatively sensitive test for distinguishing normal-pressure hydrocephalus from other forms of hydrocephalus. While the criteria are not universally accepted, the majority of authorities

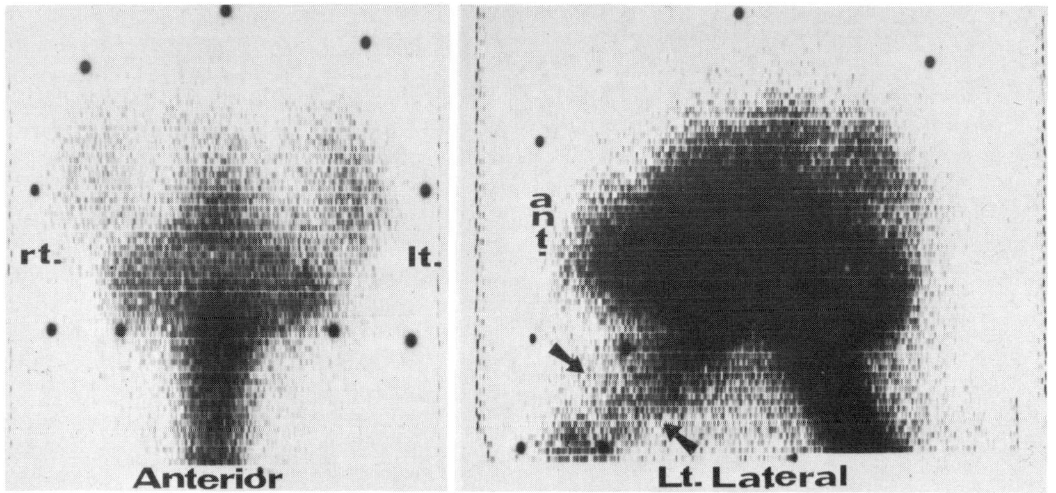

Figure 6–12 Anterior and left lateral scans following intrathecal injection of 1 mc ^{99m}technetium human serum albumin. Arrows identify the cerebrospinal fluid leak arising from the middle fossa.

would agree that the presence of persistent ventricular tracer activity and delay or absence of passage of the tracer over the convexities for 24 and 48 hours constitutes the appearance of normal-pressure hydrocephalus by radionuclide imaging.[13,158,190,200] There would appear to be gradations in these scan patterns that may or may not reflect the presence and severity of normal-pressure hydrocephalus. The complementary use of pneumoencephalography or CT scanning or both with the radionuclide study has been discussed in several reports.[13,107,190] One group has felt that the radionuclide study alone provided reliable information when the characteristic patterns of normal pressure hydrocephalus were present.[13] Early work suggested that the more characteristic the radionuclide imaging pattern for normal-pressure hydrocephalus, the better the chance for successful response to shunting.[190,200] It was cautioned that a normal study did not exclude the possibility for the surgically successful treatment of hydrocephalus.[200] Recent investigators have cast doubt as to the prognostic value of the radionuclide imaging study in those patients who should undergo or have undergone a shunt procedure.[107,197] An example of normal pressure hydrocephalus is illustrated in Figure 6–13.

Radionuclide ventriculography performed by instilling the radiopharmaceutical directly into the ventricle has assisted in the evaluation of shunt patency and in the identification of a spontaneous cerebrospinal fluid shunt.[54] Evaluation of the hydrocephalic child by intrathecal tracer injection and scanning has been reported as a useful procedure.[125] Harbert has summarized the literature pertaining to radionuclide cisternography in shunt procedures in the pediatric age group.[95]

COMPUTED TOMOGRAPHY AND RADIONUCLIDE BRAIN IMAGING

The development of computed tomography (CT brain scan) has resulted in a major advance in the diagnosis of neurological disease. Rapid technological advances in this instrumentation in terms of time of imaging, levels of radiation exposure and the information provided made its comparison with radionuclide brain imaging (RN brain scan) as an initial neurodiagnostic procedure mandatory. In a recent series of articles the merits of both procedures have been weighed. Evans and Jost indicate that in terms of cost effectiveness and diagnostic efficacy, in most cases the CT scan is preferable to the RN brain scan where both modalities are available.[65] Anderson and co-workers report that with the exception of arteriovenous malformations, computed tomography detects an equal or better percentage of brain tumors. In a compilation of reports, they found an overall detection

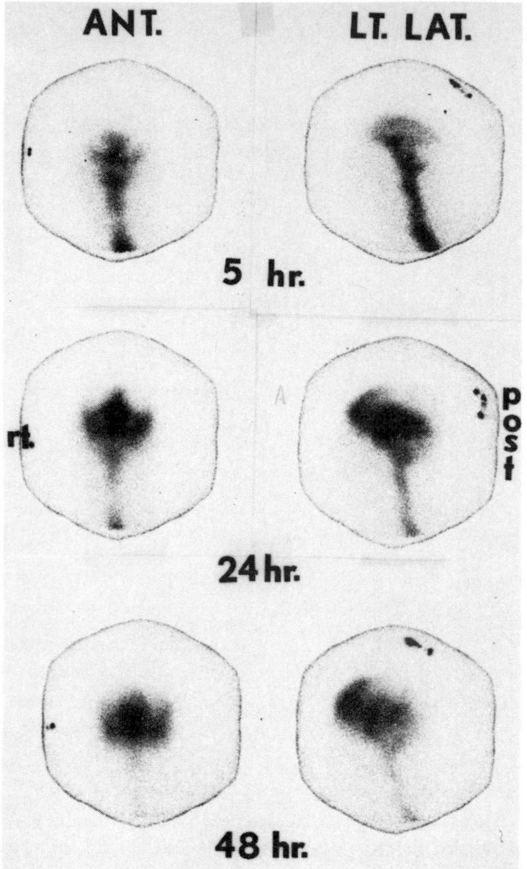

Figure 6–13 ^{169}Ytterbium DTPA cisternogram study in a patient with normal-pressure hydrocephalus.

rate of 93 per cent for the CT scan as compared with 85 per cent for the RN brain scan.[3] In the same issue, Fordham emphasized the complementary nature of these two procedures.[75]

Table 6–9 summarizes reports that have compared cranial computed tomography with radionuclide brain imaging. As already noted, with exception of the arteriovenous malformation, the CT scan is equal to or superior to RN brain scanning in the detection of neoplasms. The lower percentage of detection in inflammatory disease does not reflect the greater specificity of the CT scan. Table 6–9 and Table 6–10 reflect a compilation of several series evaluating CT and RN brain scanning in cerebral infarction. The two studies may be considered complementary. At least one author feels the radionuclide study should precede computed tomography in the evaluation of cerebrovascular disease.[117] Intracerebral hemorrhage, however, is apparently better defined by CT scanning.[146]

It is clearly evident that CT scanning has affected and will significantly affect the overall number of radionuclide brain scanning studies performed. Whether emission cranial computed tomography will be shown to be a clinical advance is, at the time this is written, debatable and unproved. Its ultimate value may rest with the development of more disease specific radiopharmaceuticals. The understandable and justified enthusiasm for the CT scan should not obscure the value and complementary nature of radionuclide brain imaging study as a scanning procedure. The financial considerations, as well as the logistics of handling large numbers of patients requiring neuroradiological work-up, must be weighed. This is particularly true in small community hospitals. The untoward reactions associated with the intravenous injection of radiopaque contrast material must be balanced against the disadvantages of the administration of radioactive materials. Radionuclide brain imaging will assume a less prominent role in the work-up of the patient with defined neurological problems but will be of value as a complementary study and as a reliable screening procedure.

Harbert and his associates note that in their institution, for detection of hydrocephalus, computed tomography has replaced the radionuclide cisternogram. In pediatric age groups, the CT scan is the initial procedure.[96] This is likewise true in most cases of adult dementia, although there are certain clinical circumstances pointing to the desirability of radionuclide cisternography.[79] Indeed, shunt patency and cerebrospinal fluid flow dynamics in both the adult and pediatric age groups are, at the time this is written, better defined by the radionuclide study.

CONCLUSION

In recent years remarkable advances have been made in the radiological approaches to the detection of intracranial disease. Significant improvements in the technology of radionuclide brain scanning have been brought about through developments in radiopharmaceuticals and in imaging instrumentation and the applications of

TABLE 6–9 COMPILATION OF STUDIES COMPARING COMPUTED CRANIAL TOMOGRAPHY AND RADIONUCLIDE BRAIN IMAGING

LESION	AUTHORS (See References)	COMPUTED TOMOGRAPHY			RADIONUCLIDE BRAIN IMAGING		
		Total Number of Cases	*Number of Positive Cases*	*Percentage of Positive Cases*	*Total Number of Cases*	*Number of Positive Cases*	*Percentage of Positive Cases*
Neoplasm							
Gliomas	78, 157, 160	61	58	95	61	51	84
Meningiomas	78, 157, 160	25	25	100	24	24	100
Metastases	47, 78, 157, 160	152	139	91.4	152*	133*	87.5
					149†	133†	89.3
Sellar and parasellar tumors	78, 149, 157, 172	41	37	90.2	36	21	60
Location of neoplasm							
Supratentorial	30, 157	122	108	88.5	122	103	84.4
Infratentorial	30, 135, 136, 157	78	58	74.3	66	47	71.2
Nonneoplastic Disease							
Epidural/subdural hematoma	2, 30, 78, 160	44	40	90.9	44	38	86.3
Cerebral contusion, hematoma	2, 30, 135	24	23	95.8	24	20	83.3
Inflammatory lesions	30, 163	20	12	60	20	17	85
Arteriovenous malformations	30, 78, 157, 160	13	10	76.9	14	12	85.7
Cerebral infarct	30, 80, 117	71	39	54.9	65	41	63.1

* Includes three cases of positive brain scan with skull metastases called negative.

† The three cases have been dropped from the total number of patients.

TABLE 6–10 TEMPORAL COMPARISON OF COMPUTED CRANIAL TOMOGRAPHY AND RADIONUCLIDE BRAIN SCANS IN CEREBRAL INFARCTION*

	CT SCANS			RN BRAIN SCANS		
	Total Number of Cases	*Total Positive Cases*	*Percentage of Positive Cases*	*Total Number of Cases*	*Total Positive Cases*	*Percentage of Positive Cases*
0 to 7 Days	30	19	63	20	33	61
7 to 21 Days	11	6	54	9	6	67
>21 Days	16	7	44	15	4	27

* See references 30, 79.

computer analysis to radiopharmaceutical kinetics and imaging. In some classifications of cerebral disease, these advances have improved the percentages of true-positive results over those reported in the first edition of this text. Tables 6–9 and 6–11 summarize several studies that have compared various diagnostic modalities in the evaluation of neurological diseases. Cranial computed tomography has, in many respects, revolutionized cerebral disease detection. The cost for such instrumentation, however, stimulated a nationwide interest in cost-benefit relationships in this sector of the medical arena. The scientific reports which have emanated from a wide distribution of this equipment throughout the United States, have shown the value of CT scan examinations (see Table 6–9). Careful comparisons of computed tomographic scans and radionuclide brain scans have been cited earlier in this chapter. It is the authors' opinion that the CT examination of the brain, including contrast enhancement, offers the most comprehensive overall initial radiological evaluation of cerebral disease. The radionuclide brain scan, including serial rapid-sequence cerebral perfusion imaging, contributes additional information and, in some instances, records disease not perceived by the CT examination. The radionuclide brain scan remains a reasonably reliable screening diagnostic procedure, particularly in those institutions not equipped or staffed for computed tomography. The combination of physical examination, comprehensive radionuclide brain imaging, and electroencephalography can continue to provide a thorough, noninvasive diagnostic neurological evaluation. Finally, the authors recognize the profound change that CT scanning has introduced into the evaluation of the patient with suspected cerebral disease but believe that this chapter should not constitute an obituary for radionuclide cerebral studies at this time.

The names of radionuclides are, at the publisher's option, expressed in the form recommended in *Words into Type*, 3rd Ed., Prentice-Hall, 1974.

TABLE 6–11 RESULTS OF SEVERAL DIAGNOSTIC TESTS FOR BRAIN TUMORS

	AUTHORS (See References)	TOTAL	POSITIVE*	PER CENT CORRECT
Radionuclide brain scans	1, 59, 91, 148, 155, 213, 225	519	432	83
Neurological examination	47	118	110	93
Skull radiographs	1, 91, 155, 213, 225	381	144	38
Carotid and brachial arteriogram	1, 59, 91, 155, 213, 225	325	277	85
Pneumoencephalogram	1, 91, 155, 225	38	32	84
Ventriculogram	1, 59, 91, 155	34	33	97
Combined pneumoencephalogram and ventriculogram	1, 59, 91, 155, 213, 225	121	106	88
Electroencephalogram	1, 91, 148, 155, 213, 225	289	222	77

* All equivocal cases were recorded as negative.

REFERENCES

1. Afifi, A. R., Morrison, R. R., Sahs, A. L., and Evans, T. C.: A comparison of chlormerodrin Hg-203 scintiencephalo-scanning with neuroradiology and electroencephalography for localization of intracranial lesions. Neurology (Minneap.), *15*:56–63, 1965.
2. Alavi, A., Uzzell, B. P., Kuhl, D. E., and Zimmerman, R. A.: Radionuclide and computerized tomography scans in evaluation of head injured patients. J. Nucl. Med., *18*:614, 1977. (Abstract)
3. Alderson, P. O., Gado, M. H., and Siegal, B. B.: Computerized cranial tomography and radionuclide imaging in the detection of intracranial mass lesions. Seminars Nucl. Med., *7*:161–173, 1977.
4. Allen, H. C., Jr., and Risser, J. R.: Simplified apparatus for brain tumor surgery. Nucleonics, *13*:28–31, 1955.
5. Anderson, W. B., and Siemsen, J. K.: Brain scanning after cerebral angiography. Radiology, *89*:492–494, 1967.
6. Anger, H. O.: The scintillation camera: A new instrument for mapping the distribution of radioactive isotopes. U.C.R.L. Report 3845, 1957.
7. Angle, H. O.: The scintillation camera with multichannel collimators. J. Nucl. Med., *5*:515–531, 1964.
8. Antunes, J. L., Schlesinger, E. B., and Michelsen, W. J.: The value of brain scanning in the management of strokes. Stroke, *6*:659–663, 1975.
9. Apfelbaum, R. I., Newman, S. A., and Zingesser, L. H.: Dynamics of technetium scanning of subdural hematomas. Radiology, *107*:571–576, 1973.
10. Ashburn, W. L., Harbert, J. C., Briner, W. H., and Di Chiro, G.: Cerebrospinal fluid rhinorrhea studies with the gamma scintillation camera. J. Nucl. Med., *9*:523–529, 1968.
11. Bakay, L.: Basic aspects of brain tumor localization by radioactive substances. J. Neurosurg., *27*:239–245, 1967.
12. Bakay, L., and Klein, D. M., eds.: Brain Tumor Scanning with Radioisotopes. Springfield, Ill., Charles C Thomas, 1969.
13. Bartelt, D., Jordan, C. E., Strecker, E.-P., and James, A. E.: Comparison of ventricular enlargement and radiopharmaceutical retention: A cisternographic-pneumoencephalographic comparison. Radiology, *116*:111–115, 1975.
14. Bauer, F. K., and Yuhl, E. T.: Myelography by means of I-131: The myeloscintigram. Neurology (Minneap.), *3*:341–346, 1953.
15. Bell, R. L.: Automatic contour myelography in infants. J. Nucl. Med., *3*:288–292, 1962.
16. Bender, M. A.: Discussion of papers: Medical Radioisotope Scanning. Vienna, Int. Atomic Energy Comm., 1959, p. 208.
17. Bender, M. A., and Blau, M.: A versatile high-contrast photoscanner for the localization of human tumors with radioisotopes. Int. J. Appl. Radiat., *4*:154, 1959.
18. Bender, M. A., and Blau, M.: Autofluoroscope: The use of nonscanning device for tumor localization with radioisotopes. J. Nucl. Med., *1*:105, 1960.
19. Blau, M., and Bender, M. A.: Clinical evaluation of Hg-203 neohydrin and I-131 albumin in brain tumor localization. J. Nucl. Med., *1*:106–107, 1960.
20. Bowallius, M., Larsson, A., Skoldborn, H., and Wickbom, I.: Brain scanning in conventional neuroradiologic methods and intracranial tumors. Acta Radiol. [Diagn.], *13*:634–642, 1972.
21. Brown, A. J., Zingesser, L., and Scheinberg, L. C.: Radioactive mercury labeled chlormerodrin scans in cerebrovascular accidents. Neurology (Minneap.), *17*:405–412, 1967.
22. Brown, R., Weber, P. M., and dos Remedios, L. V.: Dynamic static brain scintigraphy: An effective screening test for subdural hematoma. Radiology, *117*:355–360, 1975.
23. Brownell, G. L., and Sweet, W. H.: Localization of brain tumors with positron emitters. Nucleonics, *11*:40–45, 1953.
24. Bucy, P. C., and Ciric, I. S.: Brain scans in diagnosis of brain tumors scanning with chlormerodrin Hg-203 and chlormerodrin Hg-197. J.A.M.A., *191*:93–99, 1965.
25. Budabin, M.: Diagnostic value of RIHSA and chlormerodrin Hg-197 brain scanning in intracranial arteriovenous malformation. J. Nucl. Med., *8*:879–890, 1967.
26. Bull, J. W. D., and Marryat, J.: Isotope encephalography: Experience with 100 cases. Brit. Med. J., *1*:474–480, 1965.
27. Cassen, B., Curtis, L., Reed, C., and Libby, R.: Instrumentation for I-131 use in medical studies. Nucleonics, 9:46–50, 1951.
28. Chou, S. N., and French, L. A.: Systemic absorption and urinary excretion of RISA from subarachnoid space. Neurology (Minneap.), *5*:555–557, 1955.
29. Chou, S. N., Aust, J. B., Moore, G. E., and Peyton, W. T.: Radioactive iodinated human serum albumin as tracer agent for diagnosing and localizing intracranial lesions. Proc. Soc. Exp. Biol. Med., *77*:193–195, 1951.
30. Christie, J. H., Mori, H., Go, R. T., et al.: Computed tomography and radionuclide studies in the diagnosis of intracranial disease. Amer. J. Roentgen., *127*:171–174, 1976.
31. Ciric, I. S., Quinn, J. L., and Bucy, P. C.: Mercury 197 and technetium-99m brain scans in the diagnosis of non-neoplastic intracranial lesions. J. Neurosurg., *27*:119–125, 1957.
32. Conway, J. J.: Radionuclide imaging of the central nervous system in children. Radiol. Clin. N. Amer., *10*:291–312, 1972.
33. Conway, J. J., and Quinn, J. L., III: Brain imaging in pediatrics. In James, A. E., Wagner, H. N., and Cooke, R. E., eds.: Pediatric Nuclear Medicine, Philadelphia, W. B. Saunders Co., 1974, pp. 115–176.
34. Conway, J. J., and Vollert, J. U.: Accuracy of radionuclide imaging in detecting pediatric dural fluid collections. Radiology, *105*:77, 1972.
35. Cooper, J. F., and Harbert, J. C.: Endotoxin as cause of aseptic meningitis after radionuclide cisternography. J. Nucl. Med., *16*:809–813, 1975.
36. Cowan, R.: Table 6.2 Dynamic studies. Central Nervous System, Chapter 6, Section A., Nu-

clear Medicine, Vol. 1. Cleveland, CRC Press, Inc., 1977, p. 512.

37. Cowan, R.: Table 6.2.2 Abnormal cerebral dynamic patterns. Central Nervous System, Chapter 6, Section A, Nuclear Medicine, Vol. I. Cleveland, CRC Press, Inc., 1977, p. 514–517.
38. Cowan, R. J.: Table 62.3 Degree of carotid stenoses compared to dynamic study results. Central Nervous System, Chapter 6, Section A, Nuclear Medicine, Vol. I. Cleveland, CRC Press, Inc., 1977, p. 518.
39. Cowan, R. J.: Cerebral dynamic studies. Continuation Education Lectures—1972, Chapter 20. Atlanta, Southeastern Chapter, Society of Nuclear Medicine, 1972, pp. 20–1 to 20–19.
40. Cowan, R. J.: Table 6.3.2, Abnormal dynamic studies in patients with subdural hematomas (Reported series). Central Nervous System, Chapter 6, Section A., Nuclear Medicine, Vol. I. Cleveland, CRC Press, Inc., 1977, p. 544.
41. Cowan, R. J., and Maynard, C. D.: Trauma to the brain and extracranial structures. Seminars Nucl. Med., *4*:319–338, 1974.
42. Cowan, R. J., Maynard, C. D., and Meschan, I., et al.: Value of routine use of cerebral dynamic radioisotope study. Radiology, *107*:111–116, 1973.
43. Crocker, E. F., McLaughlin, A. F., Morris, J. G., et al.: Technetium brain scanning in the diagnosis and management of cerebral abscess. Amer. J. Med., *56*:192–201, 1974.
44. Cronqvist, S., Efsing, H. O., and Hughes, R.: Brain scanning in the differential diagnosis of supratentorial tumors. Acta Radiol. [Diagn.], *13*:678–692, 1972.
45. Crow, H. J., Keogh, C., and Northfield, D. W. C.: Localization of cerebrospinal fluid fistulae. Lancet, *2*:325–327, 1956.
46. Davis, D. O., and Potchen, E. J.: Brain scanning and intracranial inflammatory disease. Radiology, *95*:345–346, 1970.
47. Deck, M. D. F., Messina, A. V., and Sockett, J. O.: Computed tomography in metastatic disease of the brain. Radiology, *119*:15–120, 1976.
48. DeLand, F. H., and Wagner, H. N., Jr.: Brain scanning as a diagnostic aid in the detection of eighth nerve tumors. Radiology, *92*:571–575, 1969.
49. DeLand, F. H., Sauerbrunn, B. J. L., Boyd, C., Wilkinson, R. H., Jr., et al: Ga-citrate imaging in untreated primary lung cancer: Preliminary report of cooperative group. J. Nucl. Med., *15*:408–411, 1974.
50. Detmer, D. E., and Blacker, H. M.: A case of aseptic meningitis secondary to intrathecal injection of I-131 human serum albumin. Neurology (Minneap.), *15*:642–643, 1965.
51. Di Chiro, G.: RISA encephalography and conventional neuroradiologic methods. A comparative study, Acta Radiol. (Stockholm), suppl. 201, 1961.
52. Di Chiro, G.: Specific activity of radioiodinated human serum albumin for intrathecal injection. A correction. Neurology (Minneap.) *15*:950, 1965.
53. Di Chiro, G.: Observations on the circulation of the cerebrospinal fluid. Acta Radiol. [Diagn.], *5*:988–1002, 1966.
54. Di Chiro, G., and Grove, A. S., Jr.: Evaluation of surgical and spontaneous cerebrospinal fluid shunts by isotope scanning. J. Neurosurg., *24*:743–748, 1966.
55. Di Chiro, G., Ashburn, W. L., and Briner, W. H.: Technetium Tc-99m serum albumin for cisternography: The use of high specific activity technetium Tc-99m serum albumin as a tracer for subarachnoidal and ventricular scintiphotography. Arch. Neurol., *19*:218–227, 1968.
56. Di Chiro, G., Ashburn, W. L., and Grove, A. S., Jr.: Which radioisotope for brain scanning? Neurology (Minneap.), *18*:225–236, 1968.
57. Di Chiro, G., Reames, P. M., and Matthews, W. B., Jr.: RISA ventriculography and RISA cisternography. Neurology (Minneap.), *14*:185–191, 1964.
58. Di Chiro, G., Ommaya, A. K., Ashburn, W. L., and Briner, W. H.: Isotope cisternography in the diagnosis and followup of cerebrospinal fluid rhinorrhea. J. Neurosurg., *28*:522–529, 1968.
59. Dugger, G. S., and Pepper, F. D.: The reliability of radioisotopic encephalography. A correlation with other neuroradiological and anatomical studies. Neurology (Minneap.), *13*:1042–1053, 1963.
60. Dunbar, H. S., and Ray, B. S.: Localization of brain tumors and other intracranial lesions with radioactive iodinated human serum albumin. Surg. Gynec. Obstet., *98*:433–436, 1969.
61. Edwards, C. L., and Hayes, R. L.: Tumor scanning with ^{67}Ga citrate. J. Nucl. Med., *10*:103–105, 1969.
62. Edwards, C. L., and Hayes R. L.: Scanning malignant neoplasms with Ga-67. J.A.M.A., *212*:1182–1190, 1970.
63. Engbring, N. H.: Brain scan artifact from saliva contamination. J.A.M.A., *199*:861, 1967.
64. Erickson, T. C., Larson, F. C., and Gordon, E. S.: Uptake of radioactive phosphorus by glioblastoma multiforme and therapeutic application. Trans. Amer. Neurol. Ass., *73*:112, 1948.
65. Evans, R. G., and Jost, R. G.: The clinical efficacy and cost analysis of cranial computed tomography and the radionuclide brain scan. Seminars Nucl. Med., *7*:129–136, 1977.
66. Feindel, W., Yamamato, Y. L., McRae, D. L., and Zanelli, J.: Contour brain scanning with iodine and mercury compounds for detection of intracranial tumors. Amer. J. Roentgen., *92*:177–186, 1964.
67. Fiebach, O., Sauer, J., Otto, H., et al.: Comparative study of brain scintiphotography, cerebral angiography and pneumoencephalography in detection of gliomas. Neuroradiology, *3*:27–31, 1971.
68. Fischer, K. C., McKusick, K. I., Pendergrass, H. P., et al.: Improved brain scan specificity utilizing Tc-99m pertechnetate and Tc-99m (Sn) diphosphonate. J. Nucl. Med., *16*:705–708, 1975.
69. Fischer, R. J., and Miale, A., Jr.: Evaluation of cerebral vascular disease with radionuclide angiography. Stroke, *3*:1–9, 1972.
70. Fish, M. B., Barnes, B., and Pollycove, M.: Cranial scintiphotographic blood flow defects in arteriographically proven cerebral vascular disease. J. Nucl. Med., *14*:558–564, 1973.

71. Fish, M. B., Pollycove, M., O'Reilly, S., et al.: Vascular characterization of brain lesions by rapid sequential cranial scintiphotography. J. Nucl. Med., *9*:249–259, 1968.
72. Fletcher, J. W., George, E. A., Henry, R. E., et al.: Brain scan, Dexamethasone therapy and brain tumors. J.A.M.A., *232*:1261–1263, 1975.
73. Flipse, R. C., Vuksanovic, M., and Fonts, E. A.: Sequential brain scanning in radiation therapy of malignant tumors of the brain. Amer. J. Roentgen., *102*:88–92, 1968.
74. Foltz, E. L.: The use of controlled overpressure cisternography to localize cerebrospinal fluid rhinorrhea (Editorial). J. Nucl. Med., *18*:187, 1977.
75. Fordham, E. W.: The complementary role of computerized axial transmission tomography and radionuclide imaging of the brain. Seminars. Nucl. Med., *7*:129–136, 1977.
76. Forster, D. N. C., and Bethell, A. N.: The diagnostic value of scintillation brain scanning. Clin. Radiol., *20*:257–268, 1969.
77. Francis, J. E., Bell, P. R., and Harris, C. C.: Medical scintillation spectrometry. Nucleonics, *13*:82–88, 1955.
78. Gado, M., Coleman, R. E., and Alderson, P. O.: Clinical comparison of radionuclide brain imaging and computerized transmission tomography, I. *In* Noninvasive Brain Imaging: Computed Tomography and Radionuclides. Chapter 9. New York, Society of Nuclear Medicine, Inc., 1975, pp. 147–171.
79. Gado, M. H., Coleman, R. E., Lee, K. S., et al.: Correlation between computerized transaxial tomography and radionuclide cisternography in dementia. Neurology (Minneap.), *26*:555–560, 1976.
80. Gado, M. H., Coleman, R. E., Merlis, A. L., et al.: Comparison of computerized tomography and radionuclide imaging in "stroke." Stroke, *7*:109–113, 1976.
81. Gates, G. F., Dore, E. K., and Taplin, G. V.: Interval brain scanning with sodium pertechnetate Tc-99m for tumor detectability. J.A.M.A., *215*:85–88, 1971.
82. Gilday, D. L.: Various radionuclide patterns of cerebral inflammation in infants and children. Amer. J. Roentgen., *120*:247–253, 1974.
83. Gilday, D. L., and Ash, J.: Accuracy of brain scanning in pediatric craniocerebral neoplasms. Radiology, *117*:93–97, 1975.
84. Gilday, D. L., and Kellam, J.: In-DTPA evaluation of CSF diversionary shunts in children. J. Nucl. Med., *14*:920–923, 1973.
85. Gilday, D. L., Ash, J., and Milne, N.: Dural fluid collections in infants and children. Radiology, *114*:367–372, 1975.
86. Gilday, D. L., Coates, G., and Goldenber, D.: Subdural hematoma–what is the role of brain scanning in diagnosis? J. Nucl. Med., *14*:283–287, 1973.
87. Gilson, A. J., and Gargano, F. D.: Correlation of brain scans and angiography in intracerebral trauma. Amer. J. Roentgen., *94*:819–827, 1965.
88. Glasgow, J. L., Currier, R. D., Goodrich, J. K., and Tutor, F. T.: Brain scans of cerebral infarcts with radioactive mercury. Radiology, *88*:1086–1091, 1967.
89. Gold, L. H., and Lohen, M. K.: Retrospective evaluation of isotope images of the brain in 852 patients. Radiology, *92*:1473–1476, 1969.
90. Goodman, J. M., and Heck, L. L.: Confirmation of brain death at bedside by isotope angiography. J.A.M.A., *238*:966–968, 1977.
91. Goodrich, J. K., and Tutor, F. T.: The isotope encephalogram in brain tumor diagnosis. J. Nucl. Med., *6*:541–548, 1965.
92. Goodrich, J. K., and Wilkinson, R. H., Jr.: The effectiveness of brain scanning for detecting intracranial disease. *In* Central Nervous System Investigation with Radionuclides, Charles C Thomas, Springfield, Ill., pp. 365–374.
93. Gutterman, P., and Shenkin, H. A.: Cerebral scans in completed strokes. Value in prognosis of clinical course. J.A.M.A., *207*:145–147, 1969.
94. Handa, J.: Dynamic Aspects of Brain Scanning. Baltimore, University Park Press, 1972, p. 42.
95. Harbert, J. C.: Radionuclide techniques in the evaluation of cerebrospinal fluid shunts. Crit. Rev. Diagnostic Imaging. *9*:207–228, 1977.
96. Harbert, J. C., McCullough, D. C., and Schellinger, D.: Computed cranial tomography and radionuclide cisternography in hydrocephalus. Seminars. Nucl. Med., *7*:197–200, 1977.
97. Harper, P. V., Beck, R., Charleston, D., and Lathrop, K. A.: Optimization of a scanning method using Tc-99m. Nucleonics, *22*:50, 1964.
98. Hauser, W., Atkins, H. L., Nelson, K. G., and Richards, P.: Technetium-99m DTPA: A new radiopharmaceutical for brain and kidney scanning. Radiology, *84*:679–684, 1970.
99. Heinz, E. R., Brylski, J. R., Izenstark, J. L., and Weens, H. S.: Post-angiography isotope brain scanning: Positive or negative? Amer. J. Roentgen., *98*:336–344, 1963.
100. Heiser, W. J., Quinn, J. L., and Mollihan, W. V.: The crescent pattern of increased radioactivity in brain scanning. Radiology, *87*:483–488, 1966.
101. Holman, B. L.: The brain scan. Med. Trial Techn. Q., *21*:232–245, 1974.
102. Holman, B. L.: Concepts and clinical utility of the measurement of cerebral blood flow. Seminars Nucl. Med., *6*:233–251, 1976.
103. Holmes R. A., Herron, C. S., and Wagner, H. N., Jr.: A modified vertex view in brain scanning. Radiology, *88*:498–503, 1967.
104. Hopkins, G. B., and Kristensen, K. A. B.: Rapid sequential scintiphotography in the radionuclide detection of subdural hematoma. J. Nucl. Med., *14*:288–290, 1973.
105. Horwitz, N. H., and Lofstrom, J. E.: Photographic recording method for scintillation scanning. Nucleonics, *13*:56, 1955.
106. Hosain, F., Reba, R. C., and Wagner, H. N., Jr.: Ytterbium-169 diethylenetriaminepentaacetic acid complex. Radiology, *91*:1199–1203, 1968.
107. Jacobs, L., and Kinkel, W.: Computerized axial transverse tomography in normal pressure hydrocephalus. Neurology (Minneap.), *26*:501–507, 1976.
108. Jaskar, D. W., Griep, R. T., and Nelp, W. B.: The uptake and concentration of the pertechnetate by the choroid plexus. J. Nucl. Med., *8*:387, 1967.

109. Jayabalau, V., White, D., and Bank, M.: Adverse reactions (Aseptic meningitis) from ^{111}In-DTPA cisternographic examinations. Radiology, *115*:403–405, 1975.
110. Jones, A. E., Frankel, R. S., Di Chiro, G., and Johnston, G. S.: Brain scintigraphy with Tc-99m pertechnetate, Tc-99m polyphosphate and Ga-67 citrate. Radiology, *112*:123–129, 1974.
111. Jordan, C. E., James, A. E., Jr., and Hodges, F. J., III: Comparison of cerebral angiogram and brain radionuclide image in brain abscess. Radiology, *104*:327–331, 1972.
112. Kelly, D. L., Alexander, E., Jr., David, C. H., Jr., et al.: Intracranial arteriovenous malformations: Clinical review and evaluation of brain scans. J. Neurosurg., *31*:422–428, 1969.
113. Kennady, J. C., and Taplin, G. V.: Albumin macroaggregated for brain scanning experimental bases and safety in primates. J. Nucl. Med., *6*:566–581, 1965.
114. King, E. G., Wood, D. E., and Morley, T. P.: The use of macroaggregates of radioiodinated human serum albumin in brain scanning. Canad. Med. Ass. J., *95*:381–389, 1966.
115. Klatzman, K., Clasen, R., Klatzo, I., et al.: Edema in stroke. Stroke, *8*:512–540, 1977.
116. Klopper, J. F.: Brain scanning with Tc-99m pertechnetate. A comparative study in 2,000 cases. S. Afr. Med. J., *47*:1792, 1973.
117. Krishnamurthy, G. T., Murthy, K. N. N., Paramesh, K. et al.: Accuracy of current neurodiagnostic tests in the detection of cerebrovascular disease. J. Nucl. Med., *18*:613–614, 1977.
118. Kuhl, D. E., Chamberlain, R. H., Hale, J., and Gorson, R. O.: A high contrast photographic recorder for scintillation counter scanning. Radiology, *66*:730–739, 1956.
119. Landman, S., and Ross, P.: Radionuclides in the diagnosis of arteriovenous malformations of the brain. Radiology, *108*:635–639, 1973.
120. Lane, S. D., Patton, D. D., Staab, E. V., and Baglan, R. J.: Simple technique for rapid bolus injection. J. Nucl. Med., :118–119, 1972.
121. Leveillé, J., Pison, C., Karakand, Y., et al.: Technetium-99m glucoheptonate in brain tumor detection: An important advance in radiotracer techniques. J. Nucl. Med., *18*:957–961, 1977.
122. Lorentz, W. B., Simon, J. L., and Benua, R. S.: Brain scanning in children. J.A.M.A., *201*:5–7, 83–85, 1967.
123. McAfee, J. G.: *In* Quinn, J. L., III, ed.: Scintillation Scanning in Clinical Medicine. Philadelphia, W. B. Saunders Co., 1964.
124. McClintock, J. T., and Dalrymple, G. V.: The value of brain scans in the management of suspected intracranial lesions. J. Nucl. Med., *5*:189–192, 1964.
125. McCullough, D. C., and Leussenhop, A. J.: Evaluation of photoscanning of the diffusion of intrathecal RISA in infantile and childhood hydrocephalus. J. Neurosurg., *30*:673–678, 1969.
126. Mack, J. F., Webber, M. M., and Bennett, L. R.: Brain scanning: Normal anatomy with technetium-99m pertechnetate. J. Nucl. Med., *7*:633–640, 1966.
127. Magnaes, B, and Solheim, D.: Controlled overpressure cisternography to localize cerebrospinal fluid rhinorrhea. J. Nucl. Med., *18*:109–111, 1977.
128. Mamo, L., Nonel, J. P., Robert J., and Chai, N.: Use of radioactive bleomycin to detect malignant intracranial tumors. J. Neurosurg., *39*:735–741, 1973.
129. Marty, R., and Cain, M. L.: Effects of corticosteroid (dexamethasone) administration on the brain scan. Radiology, *107*:117–121, 1973.
130. Maynard, C. D., and Kelsey, W. M.: Brain scanning in the pediatric age group. Develop. Med. Child Neurol., *11*:69–76, 1969.
131. Maynard, C. D., Hanner, T. G., and Witcofski, R. L.: Positive brain scans due to lesions of the skull. Arch. Neurol., *18*:93–97, 1968.
132. Maynard, C. D., Witcofski, R. L., Janeway, R., and Cowan, R. J.: Radioisotope arteriography as an adjunct to the brain scan. Radiology, *92*:908–912, 1969.
133. Mealey, J., Jr., Dehner, J. R., and Reese, I. C.: Clinical comparison of two agents used in brain scanning radioiodinated serum albumin vs. chlormerodrin Hg-203. J.A.M.A., *189*:260–264, 1964.
134. Meisel, S. B., Izenstark, J. L., and Siemsen, J. K.: Comparison of accuracy between initial and delayed technetium and mercury brain scanning. Radiology, *109*:117–120, 1973.
135. Messma, A. V., Potts, G., and Sigel, R. M.: Computed tomography: Evaluation of the posterior third ventricle. Radiology, *119*:581–592, 1976.
136. Mikhael, M. A., and Mattor, A. G.: Sensitivity of radionuclide brain imaging and computerized transaxial tomography in tumors of posterior fossa. J. Nucl. Med., *18*:26–28, 1977.
137. Miller, M. S., and Simmons, G. H.: Optimization of timing and positioning of the technetium brain scan. J. Nucl. Med., *9*:429–435, 1968.
138. Mishkin, F.: Brain scanning in children. Seminars Nucl. Med., *2*:328–342, 1972.
139. Mishkin, F.: Determination of cerebral death by radionuclide angiography. Radiology, *115*:135–137, 1975.
140. Mishkin, F., and Truksa, J.: The diagnosis of intracranial cysts by means of the brain scan. Radiology, *90*:740–746, 1968.
141. Molinari, G. F., Pircher, F., and Heyman, A.: Serial brain scanning using technetium-99m in patients with cerebral infarction. Neurology (Minneap.), *17*:627–636, 1967.
142. Moore, G. E.: Fluorescein scan agent in the differentiation of normal and malignant tissues. Science, *106*:130–133, 1947.
143. Moore, G. E.: Use of radioactive diiodofluorescein in the diagnosis and localization of brain tumors. Science, *107*:569–571, 1948.
144. Moore, J. S., Jr., Kieffer, S. A., Goldberg, M. E., et al.: Intracranial tumors: Correlation of angiography with dynamic radionuclide studies. Radiology, *115*:393–398, 1975.
145. Morrison, R. T., Afifi, A. K., Van Allen, M. W., and Evans, R. C.: Scintiencephalography for the detection and localization of non-neoplastic intracranial lesions. J. Nucl. Med., *6*:7–15, 1965.
146. Moses, D. C., James, A. E., Jr., Strauss, H. W., et al.: Regional cerebral blood flow estimation in the diagnoses of cerebrovascular disease. J. Nucl. Med., *13*:135–141, 1972.
147. Murphy, E., Cervantes, Q. B., and Maass, R.: Radioalbumin macroaggregate brain scanning:

A histopathologic investigation. Amer. J. Roentgen., *102*:88–92, 1968.

148. Murphy, J. T., Gloor, P., Yamamoto, Y. L., and Feindel, W.: A comparison of electroencephalography and brain scan in supratentorial tumors. New Eng. J. Med., *276*:309–313, 1967.

149. Nadich, T. P., Pinto, R. S., Kushner, M. J., et al.: Evaluation of sellar and parasellar masses by computed tomography. Radiology, *120*:91–99, 1976.

150. Nichols, C. F.: A second case of aseptic meningitis following isotope cisternography using I-131 human serum albumin. Neurology (Minneap.), *17*:199–200, 1967.

151. Oldendorf, W. H., Kitano, M., and Shimizu, S.: Evaluation of a simple technique for abrupt intravenous injection of a radioisotope. J. Nucl. Med., *6*:205–209, 1965.

152. Oldham, R. K., and Staab, E. V.: Aseptic meningitis following the intrathecal injection of radioiodinated serum albumin. Radiology, *87*:317–321, 1970.

153. Ostertag, C., Mundinger, F., McDonnell, D., and Hoefer, T.: Detection of 247 midline and posterior fossa tumors by combined scintiscanning and digital gamma encephalography. J. Neurosurg., *39*:224–235, 1974.

154. Overton, M. C., III, Haynie, T. P., and Snodgrass, S. R.: Brain scans in non-neoplastic intracranial lesions. Scanning with chlormerodrin Hg-203 and chlormerodrin Hg-197. J.A.M.A., *191*:431–436, 1965.

155. Overton, M. C., III, Snodgrass, S. R., and Haynie, T. P.: Brain scans in neoplastic intracranial lesions. Scanning with chlormerodrin Hg-203 and chlormerodrin Hg-197. J.A.M.A., *192*:747–751, 1965.

156. Overton, M. C., III, Haynie, T. P., Otte, W. K., and Coe, J. E.: The vertex view in brain scanning. J. Nucl. Med., *6*:705–710, 1965.

157. Passalaqua, A. M., Braunstein, P., Krickeff, I., et al.: Clinical comparison of radionuclide brain imaging and computerized transmission tomography, II. *In* Noninvasive Brain Imaging: Computed Tomography and Radionuclides. New York, Society of Nuclear Medicine, Inc., 1975, Chapter 10, pp. 173–181.

158. Patten, D. H., and Benson, D. F.: Diagnosis of normal pressure hydrocephalus by RISA cisternography. J. Nucl. Med., *9*:457–461, 1968.

159. Patton, D. D., and Christenson, P. C.: Table 6.5B Sensitivity of brain scans in the detection of primary intracerebral tumors. Central Nervous System, Chapter 6, Section A, Nuclear Medicine, Volume I. Cleveland, CRC Press, Inc., 1977, p. 560.

160. Pendergrass, H. P., McKusick, K. A., New, P. F. J., et al.: Relative efficacy of radionuclide imaging and computed tomography of the brain. Radiology, *116*:363–366, 1975.

161. Perryman, C. R., Nobel, P. R., and Bragdon, F. H.: Myeloscintigraphy: A useful procedure for localization of spinal block lesions. Amer. J. Roentgen., *80*:104–111, 1958.

162. Phelps, M. E., Hoffman, E. J., Highfill, R., and Kuhl, D. E.: A new emission computed axial tomograph for positron emitters. J. Nucl. Med., *18*:603, 1977.

163. Pinsky, S., Yum, H. Y., Patel, D., et al.: Use of the radionuclide brain scan and computerized tomography for intracranial infections. J. Nucl. Med., *18*:631, 1977.

164. Planiol, T.: Discussion of papers: Medical Radioisotope Scanning. Int. Atomic Energ Comm., 1959, p. 208.

165. Planiol, T., and Akerman, M.: Gamma encephalography in supratentorial arteriovenous malformation: Study of 54 cases. Presse Méd., *73*:2205–2210, 1965.

166. Poulose, K. P., Reba, R. C., and Goodyear, M.: Gallium-67 citrate in cerebral infarction. Invest. Radiol., *11*:20–23, 1976.

167. Powell, M. R., and Anger, H. O.: Blood flow visualization with the scintillation camera. J. Nucl. Med., *7*:729–732, 1966.

168. Quinn, J. L., III.: Scintillation Scanning in Clinical Medicine. Philadelphia, W. B. Saunders Co., 1964.

169. Quinn, J. L., III, Ciric, I., and Hauser, W.: Analysis of 96 abnormal brain scans using technetium-99m (pertechnetate form). J.A.M.A., *194*:158–160, 1969.

170. Ramsey, R. G., and Quinn, J. L., III.: Comparison of accuracy between initial and delayed Tc-99m pertechnetate brain scans. J. Nucl. Med., *13*:131–134, 1972.

171. Raskind, R., Weiss, S. R., Manning, J. J., et al.: Survival after surgical excision of single metastatic brain tumors. Amer. J. Roentgen., *111*:323–328, 1971.

172. Reich, N. E., Zelch, J. V., Alfidi, R. J., et al.: Computed tomography in the detection of juxtasellar lesions. Radiology, *118*:333–335, 1976.

173. Rollo, F. D., Cavalieri, R. R., Born, M., et al.: Comparative evaluation of ^{99m}Tc GH, ^{99m}Tc O_4, and ^{99m}Tc DTPA as brain imaging agents. Radiology, *123*:379–383, 1977.

174. Ronai, P.: Chronological listing of methods of analysis of cerebral dynamic studies. Central Nervous System, Chapter 6, Table 6.2.8, Section A, Nuclear Medicine, Vol. I. Cleveland, CRC Press, Inc., 1977, pp. 524–541.

175. Rosenthall, L.: Application of the gamma ray scintillation camera to dynamic studies in man. Radiology, *86*:634–639, 1966.

176. Rosenthall, L.: Detection of altered cerebral arterial blood flow using technetium-99m pertechnetate and gamma ray scintillation camera. Radiology, *88*:713–718, 1967.

177. Rosenthall, L.: Radionuclide diagnosis of arteriovenous malformation with rapid sequence brain scans. Radiology, *91*:1185–1188, 1968.

178. Rosenthall, L., and Martin, R. H.: Cerebral transit of pertechnetate given intravenously. Radiology, *94*:521–527, 1970.

179. Rosenthall, L., Aguayo, A., and Stratford, J.: A clinical assessment of carotid and vertebral artery injection of macroaggregates of radioiodinated albumin (MARIA) for brain scanning. Radiology, *86*:499–505, 1966.

180. Rhoton, A. L., Jr., Carlsson, A. M., and Ter-Pogossian, M. M.: Brain scanning with chlormerodrin Hg-197 and chlormerodrin Hg-203. Arch. Neurol., *10*:369–375, 1964.

181. Saenger, E. L., and Kereiakes, J. G.: Radiobiology and dosimetry. *In* Nuclear Medicine in Clinical Pediatrics. New York, Society of Nuclear Medicine, Inc., 1975, pp. 209–229.

182. Sakimura, I. T., Waxman, A. D., and Siemsen, J. K.: Comparison of delayed technetium-99m

DTPA and pertechnetate camera brain imaging. J. Nucl. Med., *16*:564–565, 1975 (Abstract).

183. Schall, G. L., Heffner, R. R., and Handmaker, H.: Brain scanning in oligodendrogliomas. Radiology, *116*:367–372, 1975.
184. Schlesinger, E. B., DeBaves, S., and Taveras, J.: Localization of brain tumors using radioiodinated human serum albumin. Amer. J. Roentgen. *87*:449–462, 1967.
185. Selverstone, B., and Solomon, A. K.: Radioactive isotopes in study of intracranial tumors: Preliminary report of methods and results. Trans. Amer. Neurol. Ass., *73*:115–119, 1948.
186. Shy, G. M., Bradley, R. B., and Matthews, W. B., Jr.: External collimation detection of intracranial neoplasia with unstable nuclides. Edinburgh, E. & S. Livingstone Ltd., 1958.
187. Snow, R. M., and Keynes, J. W., Jr.: The "luxury-perfusion syndrome" following a cerebrovascular accident demonstrated by radionuclide angiography. J. Nucl. Med., *15*:907–909, 1974.
188. Sodee, D. B.: The result of 350 brain scans with radioactive mercurial diuretics. J. Nucl. Med., *4*:185, 1963.
189. Spencer, R.: Scintiscanning in space occupying lesions of the skull. Brit. J. Radiol., *38*:1–15, 1965.
190. Staab, E. V., Allen, J. H., Young, A. B., et al.: I-HSA cisternograms and pneumoencephalograms in evaluation of hydrocephalus. *In* Harber, J. C., et al., eds: Cisternography and Hydrocephalus. A Symposium. Springfield, Ill., Charles C Thomas, 1972, pp. 235–248.
191. Stein, S. C., and Langfitt, T. W.: Normal-pressure hydrocephalus: Predicting the results of cerebrospinal fluid shunting. J. Neurosurg., *41*:463–470, 1974.
192. Stern, H. S., Goodwin, D. A., Scheffel, U., and Wagner, H. N., Jr.: In-113m for blood-pool and brain scanning. Nucleonics, *25*:62–65, 1967.
193. Stetner, F. C.: Steroid effect on brain scan in a patient with cerebral metastases. J. Nucl. Med., *16*:320–321, 1975.
194. Sugitani, Y., Nakama, M., Yamauchi, Y., et al.: Neovascularization and increased uptake of Tc-99m in experimentally produced cerebral hematoma. J. Nucl. Med., *14*:912–915, 1973.
195. Sutherland, J. B., Hill, N., Banerjel, A. K., et al.: Brain scanning and brain abscess. J. Canad. Ass. Radiol., *23*:176–181, 1972.
196. Sweet, W. H., Brownell, G. L., School, J. A., et al.: The formation flow and absorption of cerebrospinal fluid: Newer concepts based on studies with isotopes. Res. Publ. Ass. Nerv. Ment. Dis., *34*:101–159, 1954.
197. Sy, W. M., Weinberger, G., Ngo, N., et al.: Imaging patterns of subdural hematomas—a proposed classification. J. Nucl. Med., *15*:693–698, 1974.
198. Tanasescu, D. E., Wolfstein, R. S., and Waxman, A. D.: Critical evaluation of Tc-99m glucoheptonate as a brain scanning agent. J. Nucl. Med., *18*:630, 1977 (Abstract).
199. Tarcan, Y. A., Fajman, W., Marc, J., et al.: "Doughnut" sign in brain scanning. Amer. J. Roentgen., *126*:842–852, 1976.
200. Tator, C. H., and Murray, S.: The value of CSF radioisotope studies in the diagnosis and management of hydrocephalus. *In* Harbert, J. C., et al., eds.: Cisternography and Hydrocephalus. A Symposium. Chapter 19, Springfield, Ill., Charles C Thomas Publisher, 1972, pp. 249–284.
201. Tator, C. H., Morley, T. P., and Olszewski, J. A.: A study of the factors responsible for the accumulation of radioactive iodinated human serum albumin (RIHSA) by intracranial tumors and other lesions. J. Neurosurg., *22*:60–76, 1965.
202. Tator, C. H., Fleming, J. F. R., Sheppard, R. H., and Turner, V. M.: Studies of cerebrospinal fluid dynamics with intrathecally administered radioidionated human serum albumin (I-131 HSA). Canad. Med. Ass. J., *97*:493–503, 1967.
203. Tator, C. H., Fleming, J. F. R., Sheppard, R. H., and Turner, V. M.: A radioisotope test for communicating hydrocephalus. J. Neurosurg., *28*:327–340, 1968.
204. Tauxe, W. N., and Thorsen, H. C.: Cerebrovascular permeability studies in cerebral neoplasms and vascular lesions: Optimal dose-to-scan interval for pertechnetate brain scanning. J. Nucl. Med., *10*:34–39, 1969.
205. Ter-Pogossian, M., Kastner, J., and Vest, T. B.: Autofluorography of the thyroid by means of image amplification. Radiology, *81*:984–988, 1963.
206. Tow, D. E., and Wagner, H. N., Jr.: Scanning for tumors of brain and bone. J.A.M.A., *199*:610–614, 1967.
207. Tow, D. E., Wagner, H. N., Jr., DeLand, F. H., and North, W. A.: Brain scanning in cerebral vascular disease. J.A.M.A., *207*:105–108, 1969.
208. Tyson, J. W., Witherspoon, L. R., Wilkinson, R. H., Jr., and Goodrich, J. K.: Accuracy of radionuclide cerebral angiograms in the detection of cerebral arteriovenous malformations. J. Nucl. Med., *15*:953–958, 1974.
209. Vaughn, R. J., Lovegrove, R. T. A., Gleay, R. F., et al.: Scintiscanning in detection and diagnoses of subdural hematoma and hygroma. Aust. New Zeal. J. Surg., *40*:343–347, 1971.
210. Wagner, H. N., Jr.: Principles of Nuclear Medicine. Philadelphia, W. B. Saunders Co., 1968.
211. Wagner, H. N., Jr.: Mechanisms of localization of radiopharmaceuticals. *In* A Comprehensive Review of Nuclear Medicine. Springfield, Ill., Charles C Thomas, 1974.
212. Waltimo, O., Eistola, P., and Vuolio, M.: Brain scanning in detection of intracranial arteriovenous malformations. Acta Neurol. Scand., *49*:434–442, 1973.
213. Wang, Y., Shea, F. J., and Rosen, J. A.: Comparison of the accuracy of brain scanning and other procedures used for brain tumor detection. Neurology (Minneap.), *15*:1117–1119, 1965.
214. Waxman, A. D., and Siemsen, J. K.: Gallium scanning in cerebral and cranial infections. Amer. J. Roentgen., *127*:309–314, 1976.
215. Waxman, A. D., Lee, G., Wolfstein, R., and Siemsen, J. K.: Differential diagnosis of brain lesions by gallium scanning. J. Nucl. Med., *14*:903–906, 1973.

216. Waxman, A. D., Siemsen, J. K., Wolfstein, R. S., et al.: Evaluation of postcraniotomy patients by radionuclide scan. J. Neurosurg., *43*:471–475, 1975.
217. Webber, M. M.: Normal brain scanning. Amer. J. Roentgen., *94*:815–818, 1965.
218. Welch, D. M., Coleman, R. E., and Hardin, W. B.: Brain scanning in cerebral vascular disease: A reappraisal. Stroke, *6*:136–144, 1975.
219. Wenzel, W. W., and Heasty, R. C.: Uptake of Tc-99m stannous polyphosphate in an area of cerebral infarction. J. Nucl. Med., *15*:207–209, 1974.
220. Wilkins, R. H., Pircher, F. J., and Odom, G. L.: The value of post-operative brain scan in patients with supratentorial intracranial tumors. J. Neurosurg., *27*:111–118, 1967.
221. Wilkinson, R. H., Jr.: Table 6.5.5 Radionuclide brain imaging in the detection of cerebral metastases. Central Nervous System, Chapter 6, Vol. I. Cleveland, CRC Press, Inc., 1977, p. 555.
222. Williams, C. M., and Garcia-Bengochea, F.: Concentration of radioactive chlormerodrin in the fluid of chronic subdural hematoma. Radiology, *84*:745–747, 1965.
223. Williams, J. L., and Beiler, D. D.: Brain scanning in non-tumorous conditions. Neurology (Minneap.), *16*:1159–1166, 1966.
224. Witcofski, R. L., Maynard, C. D., and Janeway, R.: Concentration of technetium-99m by the choroid plexus: Experimental demonstration in vivo. Arch. Neurol. (Chicago), *18*:301–303, 1968.
225. Witcofski, R. L., Maynard, C. D., and Roper, T. J.: A comparative analysis of the accuracy of the technetium-99m pertechnetate brain scan: Follow-up of 1000 patients. J. Nucl. Med., *8*:187–196, 1967.
226. Witcofski, R. L., Roper, T. J., and Maynard, C. D.: False positive brain scans for extracranial contamination with 99m technetium. J. Nucl. Med., *6*:524–527, 1965.
227. Witcofski, R. L., Janeway, R., Maynard, C. D., et al.: Visualization of the choroid plexus on the technetium-99m brain scan. Arch. Neurol. (Chicago), *16*:286–289, 1967.
228. Witherspoon, L. R., Mahaley, M. S., Jr., Leonard, J. R., et al.: Cerebral dynamic studies for early detection of recurrent anaplastic intracranial gliomas. J. Neurosurg., *43*:142–149, 1975.
229. Wrenn, F. R., Jr., Good, M. L., and Handler, P.: The use of positron-emitting radioisotopes for the localization of brain tumors. Science, *113*:525, 1951.
230. Yalag, K., and Treves, S.: Brain scanning and cerebral radioisotope angiography (CRA) in children. Pediatrics, *54*:696–703, 1974.
231. Yarnell, P., Burdeck, D., and Sanders, B.: "The hot stroke." Arch. Neurol. (Chicago), *30*:65–69, 1974.
232. Zingesser, L. H., Mandell, S., and Schecter, M. M.: The gamma encephalogram in extracerebral hematomas. Acta Radiol., *5*:972–980, 1966.

7

ECHOENCEPHALOGRAPHY

The use of ultrasound to extend man's perception is not limited to medical science. Sound above the range of human hearing is also extensively used in oceanography and the communications and metallurgic industries. The ability of bats, whales, and dolphins to generate and discriminate subtle variations in this mode is among the great wonders of nature; man's endeavors in this area are comparatively crude. Man's limitation in the use of the mode is particularly evident in its application as a diagnostic tool in neurological surgery. In the past, much research has focused on refinements in ultrasound technology in hopes of making it an energy mode by which the brain could be visualized in a two-dimensional plane. These endeavors have been damped in recent years by the introduction of computer tomography. One-dimensional sonography continues to fill a need in the management of patients with neurological disorders, but unfamiliarity with the technique has been a deterrent to its wider application.

DEFINITION OF ULTRASOUND

Sound is classified by its frequency. The range of audible sound is from 16 to 18,000 cycles per second. Infrasound has a frequency below this. Ultrasound spans a frequency of 18,000 cps to 100,000 megacycles per second. The lower spectrum of ultrasound is readily transmitted in air. Galton's whistle, which has a frequency of 24,000 cps, serves as an example. In this discussion, ultrasound in the higher frequency ranges only is considered. These frequencies vary from 1 to 10 megacycles per second. One megacycle per second is one million cycles per second, or one megahertz (MHz). The most commonly used transducer houses a crystal that vibrates at 2.25 MHz; it is the only frequency mode under discussion in this chapter. Ultrasound in the megacycle range is for practical purposes not transmissible in air but is readily conducted in solids and liquids. Hence, a coupling medium that excludes air between the crystal and the structure under examination is required in order to gain meaningful information.

HISTORICAL SURVEY

In 1917, Langevin was commissioned by the French Government to design a method of ultrasonic submarine detection.[16] With the end of World War I, interest in this investigation ceased, although significant progress had been made. World War II revived the interest, and by 1943 the SONAR (SOund Navigation And Ranging) system had been developed in several countries. Naval history records the consequences of this discovery. In the early 1940's Sokolov in Russia and Firestone in the United States developed their reflected ultrasound techniques for metal flaw detection, using very short pulses of energy.[8,22] In 1949 Bergmann published an exhaustive discussion of the physics and applications of ultrasound, listing more than two thousand references.[2]

The first attempts to adapt ultrasound for diagnostic purposes in medicine date back to 1937. The brothers Dussik in Vienna, utilizing direct transmission continuous ultrasound, attempted to outline the cerebral

P. DYCK

ventricular system. They called their technique hyperphonography and continued to develop it for more than a decade until Guettner showed that the variations in sound attenuation were largely caused by the skull, which obscured any detectable variation within the brain.[4,14]

Although the use of direct transmission ultrasound in medical diagnosis was abandoned, reflection techniques were being developed. French, Wild, and Neal, in 1950, demonstrated at autopsy that ultrasonic reflections or "echoes" were obtainable from brain tumors.[11] In 1951 they recorded similar "tumor-echoes" from the brain of a living patient at the time of craniotomy.[12]

In 1956 Leksell published a monograph that opened extensive investigation into the diagnostic applications of ultrasound.[17] He demonstrated that the midline structures of the brain reflected ultrasound and that their lateral displacement could be demonstrated in craniocerebral trauma.[18] He coined the term "echo-encephalography" to describe his technique.

Diagnostic sonography has now attained a useful role in the management of patients afflicted by neurological disorders. Assiduous attention to detail and anatomical correlation determines the reliability of the technique. The required expertise is gained only with experience and familiarity with the equipment. Therein lies the art of echoencephalography.

Conventionally, echo-ranging has been employed to demonstrate through an intact skull the position of the diencephalic midline. The thickness of the cerebral mantle can also be measured, particularly in the pediatric age group. Ultrasonic measurement of the cerebral mantle has applications in the management of infants with hydrocephalus, even though computer tomography is readily available in many hospitals; computed tomography requires anesthesia in the uncooperative patient and it is costly.

Transcalvarial sonography for the detection of intracranial neoplasms or hematomas in the adult is not consistently reliable. For this reason it has been abandoned by most investigators. Intraoperative sonography, on the other hand, remains a harmless, expeditious, and extremely valuable adjunct to the surgical management of intracranial lesions.

PHYSICAL PRINCIPLES OF ULTRASOUND

In 1880, J. and P. Curie discovered that when quartz, a natural piezoelectric crystal, was compressed, an electrical potential was generated.[3] In 1881, Lippmann reasoned that if stress applied to a piezoelectric crystal produced an electrical potential, the converse must also be true.[13,19] That is, if one applied a potential to such a crystal, the molecular lattice could be rearranged. This deformation would result in an alteration in the shape of the crystal.

It logically followed, therefore, that if one applied a high-frequency alternating electric current, the crystal would vibrate, arranging and rearranging its molecular lattice in response to polarity change. The frequency of vibration would vary with the frequency of the alternating current applied and the natural resonant frequency of the crystal. If such a vibrating crystal were placed in an appropriate conducting medium, a disturbance would be created. At megacycle frequency, this disturbance is termed ultrasound. Such ultrasound has three types of waves: surface, or Rayleigh, waves (e.g., waves on a pond); longitudinal waves; and transverse, or shear, waves. These shear waves have an up-and-down motion of particles at right angles to the direction of the force setting up the shear stress. Longitudinal waves are propagated by compression and expansion of molecules moving parallel to the direction of the wave impulse. These latter waves can be directionally beamed when the transducer dimensions are large compared with their wavelengths. These same waves are the energy source of diagnostic ultrasound.[26]

Although natural minerals such as quartz are still used as piezoelectric oscillators, medical diagnostic units almost exclusively employ manmade crystals that are composed of oxides of various metals. These materials, of which barium titanate ($BaTiO_3$) is the most widely used polycrystalline ceramic, are baked and polarized by the application of a static potential difference (e.g., 50,000-volt direct electrical current per inch). Such a crystal is now capable of converting electrical energy into mechanical energy and vice versa. It has, in other words, piezoelectric properties.

The block diagram indicates that the piezoelectric crystal housed in a transducer is connected to a sender and receiver system (Fig. 7–1). The received information is displayed on the y-axis of a cathode ray tube. An attached polaroid camera is provided to photograph and permanently record the displayed data.

The crystal in the transducer head is activated for $^{1}/_{1,000}$ of a second and this produces a pulse of ultrasound. This ultrasonic burst is transmitted to the surrounding medium, wherein it is propagated at a constant speed. When it encounters a medium of differing molecular density (e.g., brain–third ventricle interface), part of the ultrasound is reflected and returned to strike and activate the piezoelectric crystal, which is now at rest. The resulting sonic stress produces deformation of the crystal and, hence, piezoelectricity. This minute electrical potential is amplified and displayed on the y-axis of the cathode ray tube. This reflected ultrasound is said to have echoed and forms the basis of one-dimensional ultrasonography or A-scanning.

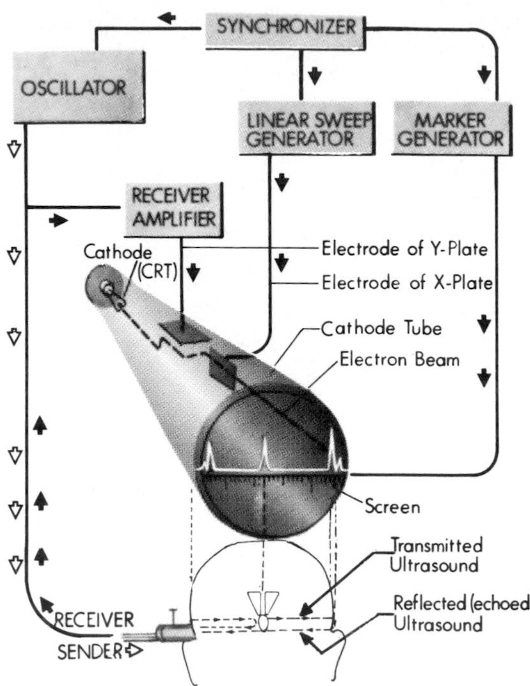

Figure 7–1 Block diagram of an echo-ranging system.

PROPERTIES OF ULTRASOUND

Most diagnostic units employ a 2.25-MHz transducer. This sound frequency will generally penetrate 17 to 18 cm of soft tissue and return recordable echoes. Higher-frequency ultrasound, having a shorter wavelength, gives better resolution of detail but poorer penetrance of tissues. For example, a 5-MHz crystal produces sound that will travel only 5 cm in soft tissues and still return meaningful echoes.

The human skull is a major obstacle to ultrasound; approximately 90 per cent of the sound energy is reflected, absorbed, and deflected by this structure, never entering the cranial cavity when the transducer is applied to the head. For this reason it is at times technically impossible to obtain satisfactory echoencephalograms with a conventional 2.25-MHz transducer. A 1-MHz crystal will usually overcome this difficulty, since it has greater penetrance of tissues.

A simple equation relates the velocity (v), the wavelength (λ), and the frequency (f) in the following manner:

$$\lambda = \frac{v}{f} \text{ or } v = \lambda f.$$

For example, at 1 MHz (f), sound would travel at a velocity (v) of 1.5 km per second in water. Consequently, the wavelength (λ) would be $1.5 \text{ km} \times 10^{-6}$, or 1.5 mm.

Sound of such frequency is poorly transmitted in air and not at all in a vacuum. It travels well in liquid and solid media because their molecules are closely packed together. The velocity of ultrasound also increases with temperature rise. At 37°C, ultrasound travels at velocities that differ according to the density of the medium in which it is transmitted (Table 7–1).[15]

TABLE 7–1 VELOCITY OF ULTRASOUND IN VARIOUS MEDIA AT 37°C

MEDIUM	METERS PER SECOND
Water	1526
Cerebrospinal fluid	1538
Blood	1548
Brain	1571
Bone	3265

DIAGNOSTIC TECHNIQUE

There are a number of diagnostic units on the market. The Echoline-20 (Smith-Kline

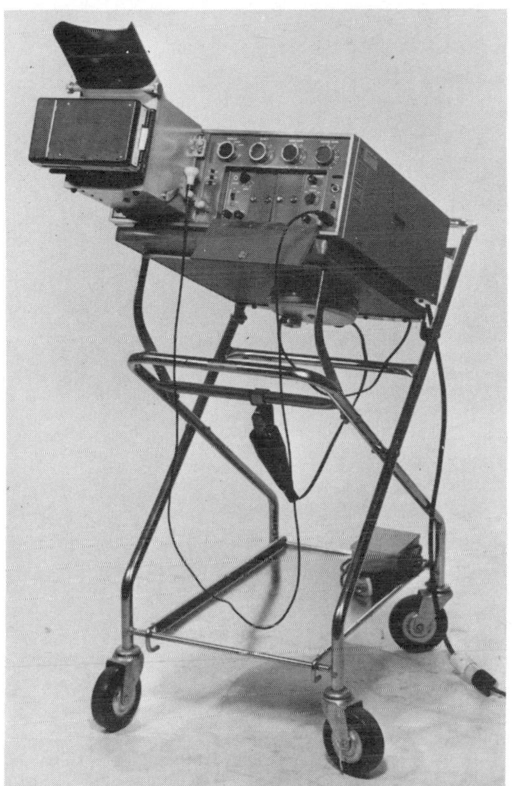

Figure 7–2 The sonographic unit discussed in this chapter. The equipment is not portable, but is transportable to the patient's bedside or the operating theater. The cart is collapsible.

Instrument Company) is used in this chapter to illustrate the technique and clinical data. This unit is not easily portable, but is transportable to the bedside or operating theater (Fig. 7–2). Routine echoencephalography is best performed with the patient lying supine and the head turned to one side.

Aquasonic, a commercially available water-soluble medium, is used to provide good contact between the transducer and scalp (Fig. 7–3). Enough contact jelly is applied, particularly in hairy areas, to exclude all air between the crystal and the anatomical structure under examination.

Having acquired a basic understanding of how ultrasound is reflected, one must gain familiarity and confidence with the equipment. This confidence comes only with experience and an understanding of the various controls on the instrument panel (Fig. 7–4). Most of these controls are self-explanatory; some warrant a few comments.

Although various operating frequencies are available, the 2.25-MHz transducer is referred to throughout this text. Higher frequencies produce better resolution but penetrate less tissue (e.g., 5 cm in soft tissues at 5 MHz). The converse is also true.

A sweep generator is used to create a linear horizontal deflection along the x-axis of the oscilloscope screen. This is electronically calibrated at 2-mm intervals. The "marker" switch controls this scale. A "depth" knob expands or contracts the scale. For general use the "reject" and "intensity" settings should remain on number 2 of the designated scale. The "near gain" adjusts the ultrasonic reverberations in the immediate vicinity of the crystal. The "coarse gain" is intended to vary the amount of echo amplification, regardless of depth of penetration. It is the most extensively used control. The module labeled "depth composition" provides a "delay"

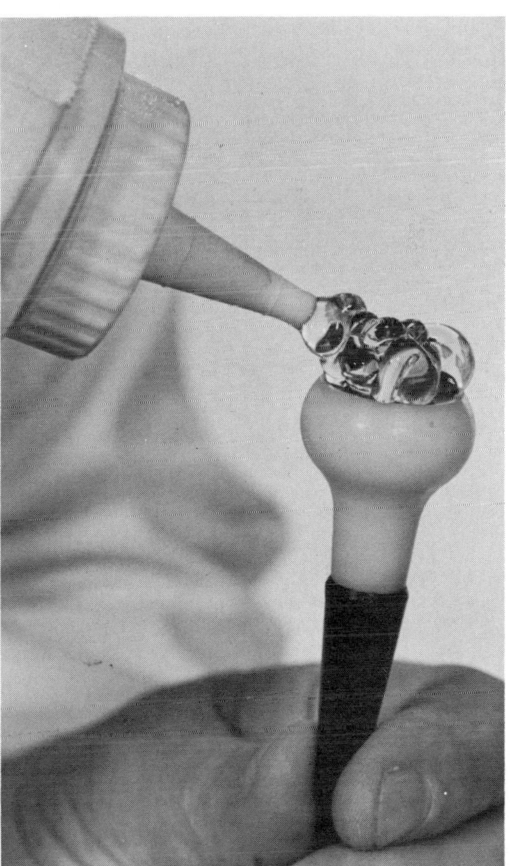

Figure 7–3 A commercially available water-soluble jelly (Aquasonic) is used to exclude air between the transducer and the patient's head.

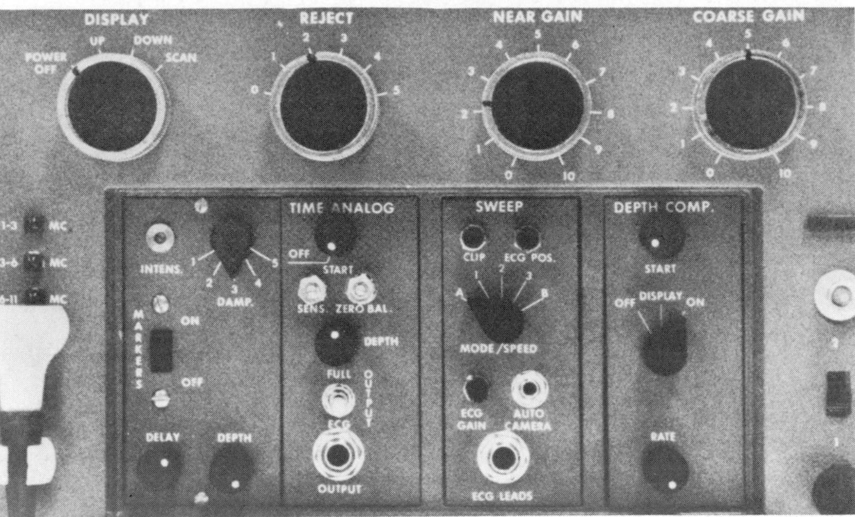

Figure 7–4 An ultrasound control panel. The "time analog" and "sweep" modules are not used during intraoperative or bedside sonography. A sweep generator creates an electronically calibrated (2-mm intervals) linear horizontal deflection along the x-axis of the oscilloscope screen. The "marker" switch controls this scale, and a "depth" knob expands or contracts it. The "reject" and "intensity" settings usually remain on number 2. The "near gain" adjusts the ultrasonic reverberations in the immediate vicinity of the crystal; the "coarse gain" varies the amount of echo amplification, regardless of depth of penetration. The "depth composition" module provides a "delay" and "sweep-gain" (rate knob) to the ultrasonic energy display, introducing increasing amplification with depth to compensate for the attenuation of ultrasound as it passes through sound-absorbing tissues so that similar structures far from and near to the transducer will display echoes of similar amplitude. The equipment is usually adjusted to record meaningful deflections on the y-axis of the cathode ray tube with the least energy possible. The "display" switch turns on the electric power and provides an upper and lower horizontal sweep. Polaroid film is used to record the oscilloscopic display. With experience, a satisfactory echoencephalogram can be obtained in one to three minutes.

and "sweep-gain" (rate knob) to the ultrasonic energy display. These controls introduce increasing amplification with depth until a maximum intensity is reached and maintained. The purpose of these functions is to compensate for the attenuation of ultrasound as it passes through sound-absorbing tissues so that similar echo-producing structures far from and near to the transducer will display echoes of similar amplitude. Many manufacturers refer to these functions as time-gain-compensation (TGC).

As a rule, the equipment is adjusted to record meaningful deflections of the y-axis of the cathode ray tube, employing the smallest amount of energy possible. The switch labeled "display" turns on the electric power and provides an upper and lower horizontal sweep. Polaroid film is used to make a permanent record of the oscilloscopic display.

With experience, a satisfactory echoencephalogram can be obtained in one to three minutes. The thickness of the cerebral mantle and the width of the third ventricle in infants are usually available in less than five minutes. Intraoperative sonography of cerebral mass lesions should not require more than 10 minutes.

THE NORMAL AND ABNORMAL ECHOENCEPHALOGRAM

A normal echoencephalogram is illustrated in Figure 7–5. By convention, the upper tracing represents echo-ranging from the right, the lower from the left, side of the head. Such ultrasonic reflections from the third ventricle are most consistently recorded when the transducer is applied to an area of the scalp as shown in Figure 7–6.

The "initial echo" represents a marker deflection and an electronic artifact known as "crystal noise." In spite of this, one can on occasion identify underlying skull echoes. The "end echo" is composed of skull and scalp reflections. The most prominent of these is the echo reflected from the brain–inner table interface. The outer skull tables also reflect ultrasound. Often a

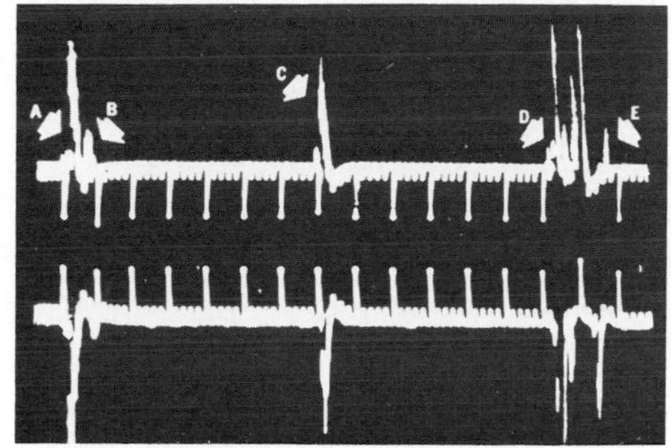

Figure 7–5 A normal echoencephalogram. The upper tracing represents echo-ranging from the right side of the head; the lower, from the left. A, initial echo; B, skull echo occasionally obtained; C, midline or diencephalic M-echo complex; D, echoes from the inner table of skull (beyond it are reflections from the outer table); E, scalp-air interface. The far-wall echoes must measure equal distances from both right and left sides.

"scalp echo" can be obtained. This latter reflection is frequently of lesser amplitude than the skull echoes; it arises from the scalp-air interface. The respective "end-echoes" from the right and the left sides must measure equal distances, or line up as it were, for proper interpretation of the "M-echo" complex.

Scalp contusion, cephalhematoma, or subgaleal hematoma will produce separation of the skull and scalp echoes. In such instances, alignment of the prominent inner skull reflections should be sought. In the presence of a subdural hematoma, there may be no "end-echo" complex obtainable when the transducer is applied contralateral to the lesion, as shown in Figure 7–7. The reason for this is that the inner hematoma membrane reflects all the useful ultrasound, leaving none to echo back from the inner table of the skull beyond it to the transducer.

Midline structures of the brain, such as the pineal gland, septum pellucidum, interhemispheric fissure, and falx cerebri, are capable of reflecting ultrasound. When a transducer is placed in the suggested position above or in front of the ear, however, the third ventricle is the source of most such midline reflections. This was shown by Ford and corroborated by the author by means of echoencepalograms made immediately before and after pneumoencephalography (Fig. 7–8).[9] Because reflections from the third ventricle resemble the letter M, they have been called "M-echoes." Closer scrutiny reveals, however, that midline reflections may be as variable as the third ventricular anatomy itself. Figure 7–9

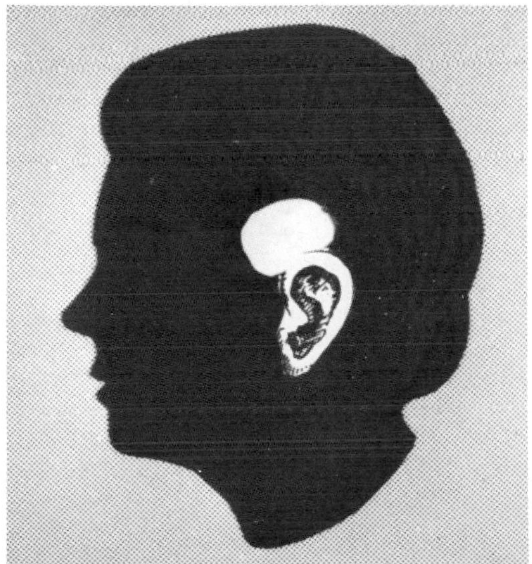

Figure 7–6 Area from which most satisfactory midline and far-wall echoes can be obtained simultaneously.

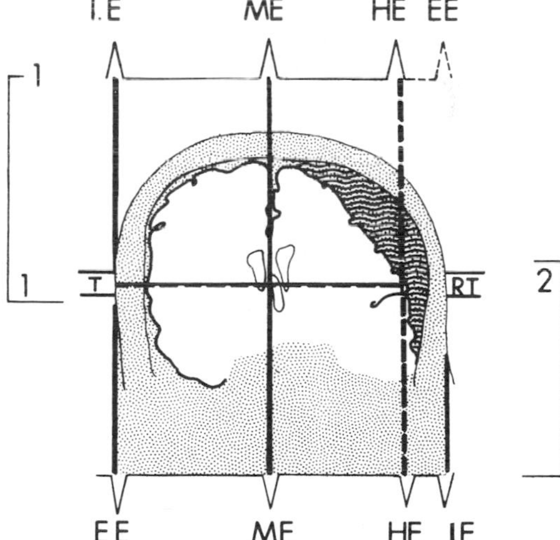

Figure 7–7 One method by which a hematoma echo (HE) is obtained. With the transducer placed on the right side (1) no end-echo (EE) is obtained. All reflecting energy is spent at the hematoma-brain interface. With the transducer on the left (2), one obtains both a hematoma echo (HE) and an initial echo (IE) on some occasions. ME, midline echo; T and RT, sites of transducer application to skull. Chronic subdural hematomas most commonly produce such findings. The third ventricle may be so deformed or tilted that it is incapable of reflecting ultrasound back to the transducer; hence no midline echo (ME) may be obtained.

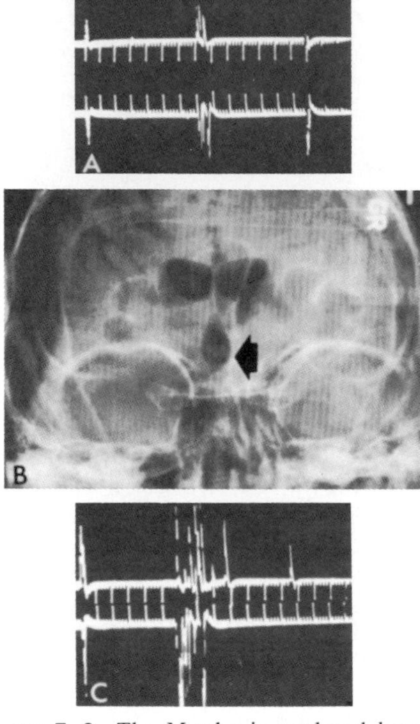

Figure 7–8 The M-echo is produced by reflections from the third ventricle. To confirm this fact, echoencephalography was performed before, *A*, and after, *C*, the instillation of 15 cc of air. Both sonography and pneumoencephalography showed the third ventricle to be 8 mm wide. After the instillation of air into the third ventricle, all ultrasound was reflected from it, as expected.

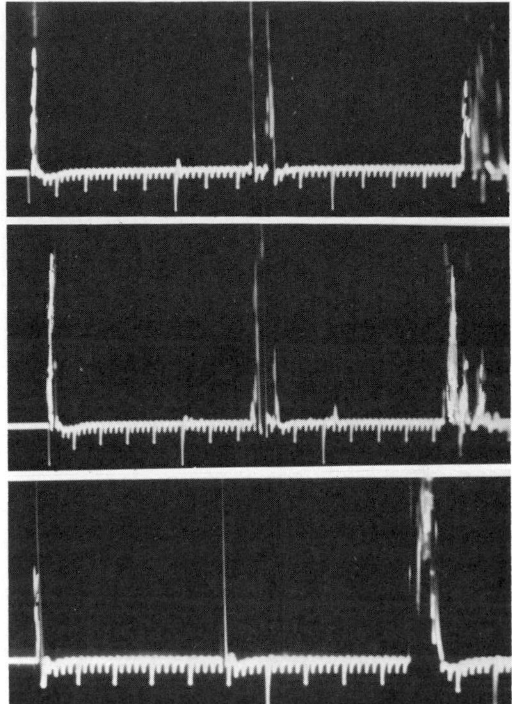

Figure 7–9 Three configurations the M-echo may assume are illustrated. The upper tracing shows a 6-mm wide third ventricle; the middle illustration, a summation of midline reflections; the lower tracing, a single reflection suggesting a narrow third ventricle. Only sonography from the right side of the head is shown.

illustrates several types of configurations of the third ventricle.

Figure 7–10 shows an echoencephalographic shift. A 6-mm displacement of the third ventricle away from the midline, produced by a mass in the left cerebral hemisphere, was responsible for this displacement. Any "M-echo" displacement of more than 3 mm is considered abnormal; in children even a 2-mm shift is probably pathological.

Distortion of the diencephalic midline is sometimes so massive that it becomes impossible to record echoes from it. This has been observed in extensive intracerebral hematomas, massive subdural collections, or ventricular casting with blood. Under these circumstances, the third ventricle is so distorted that it is physically incapable of reflecting enough appropriately directed ultrasound to record an M-echo complex. In spite of this limitation, the M-echo can be obtained in more than 90 per cent of patients by utilizing a standard 2.25-MHz transducer. If none is recorded, the 1-MHz transducer may be used. If reflections are recorded from only one wall of the third ventricle, a "false positive shift" may be obtained, as shown in Figure 7–11. The author and Zuelch have emphasized that frontopolar and occipital mass lesions may not

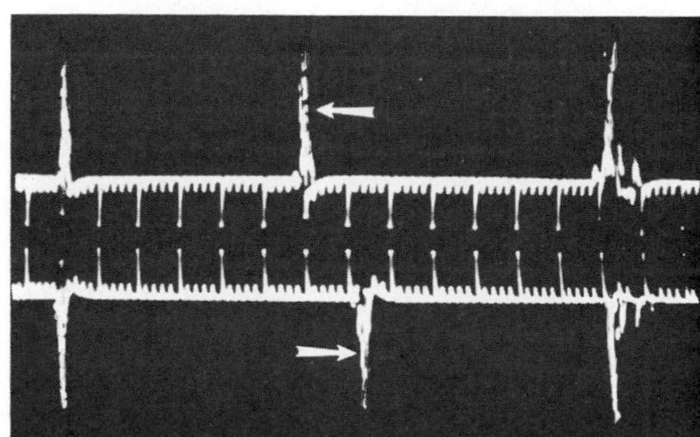

Figure 7–10 This is an abnormal echoencephalogram, showing a 6-mm left-to-right shift of the third ventricle away from the midline.

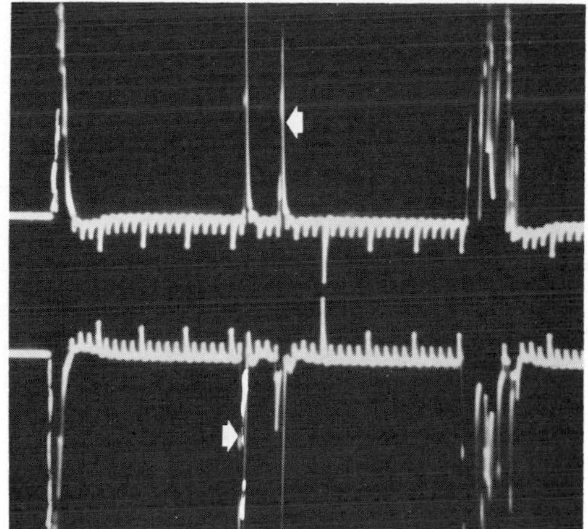

Figure 7–11 The third ventricle in this infant measured 10 mm. The arrows point to reflections from the left wall of the ventricle. If echoes from the right ventricular wall are not recorded, a so-called "false positive" shift is obtained.

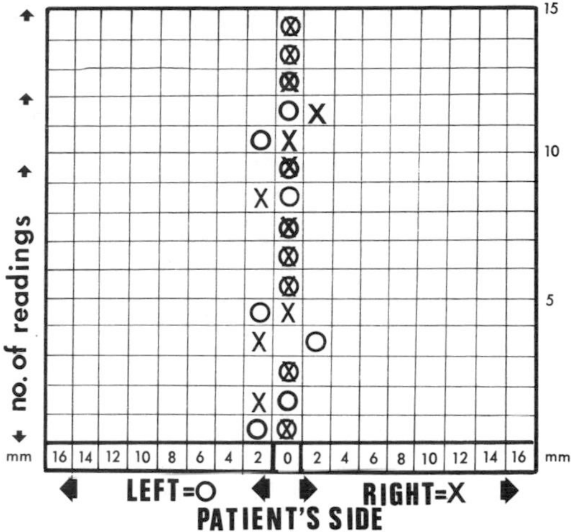

Figure 7–12 An ideal histogram from an automatic midline computer is shown. Thirty recordings are obtained, 15 from the right (X) and 15 from the left side (O) of the head.

necessarily cause a third ventricular shift.[1,27] Likewise, bilateral supratentorial mass lesions of equal size, e.g., subdural hematomas, will not produce a midline shift. It is important to remember this fact and correlate clinical with ultrasonic findings in order to arrive at a meaningful diagnostic formulation. Technicians can be taught to perform routine echoencephalography, but diagnostic sonography in its fullest sense will remain in the hands of physicians.

An automatic midline computer has been developed.* This unit has no cathode ray tube. It operates at low power and sensitivity. Thus, it records only the highest amplitude echoes that can be generated from any ultrasonic pulse. A digital clock is incorporated into the system. This clock measures the propagation time of two high-amplitude echoes from inside the skull. The propagation time of these echoes is measured and electronically adjusted. A histogram is constructed by the technician after recording 15 readings from each side of the head. An ideal histogram is shown in Figure 7–12. This portable diagnostic unit can be used only for diencephalic midline determinations.

*Diagnostic Electronics Corp., Lexington, Massachusetts.

SONOVENTRICULOGRAPHY

The human cerebral ventricles have a very complex contour; hence precise ultrasonic documentation of their shape is probably not possible. Some information, however, can be obtained. In adults, the width of the third ventricle can be measured in most instances. Should this measurement exceed 7 mm, it is considered abnormal.

Schiefer and Kazner have described a brain mantle index.[21] Under normal circumstances this index should be 2 to 2.2. That is, the thickness of the cerebral mantle in the region of the temporal horns measures about half that hemisphere's cross-section. With ventricular enlargement, the cerebral mantle thins, and thus the index increases as shown in Figure 7–13.

Ford and McRae have also shown that it is feasible to measure the posterior frontal cerebral mantle by recording echoes from the frontal horns of the ventricular system. This is accomplished by placing the transducer 4 cm above and 4 cm in front of the ear.[10]

These methods were utilized in evaluating a large number of infants with hydrocephalus. Young children are more amenable to sonoventriculography because their skulls are thinner and absorb less ultrasound. Computer tomography yields far superior information, but in order to obtain

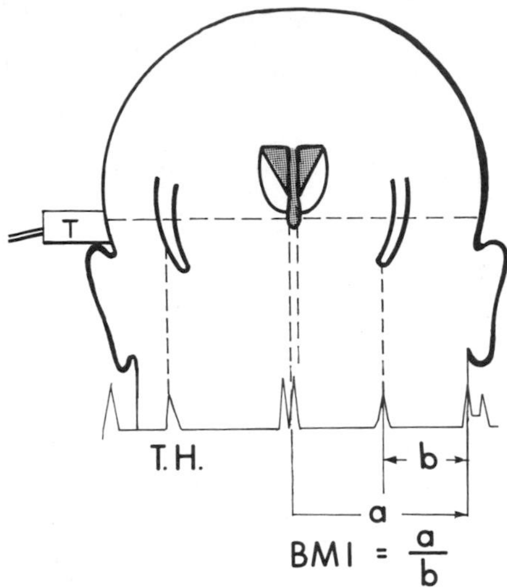

Figure 7–13 A schematic demonstration of the brain mantle index (BMI) is shown. Normally the value is 2 to 2.2. This index increases with progressive hydrocephalus. T, transducer; TH, temporal horn. (After Schiefer, W., and Kazner, E.: Klinische Echo-Encephalographie. Berlin, Heidelberg, New York, Springer-Verlag, 1967, p. 56.)

Figure 7–14 The relationship of the ventricular system to sections obtained by computed tomography.

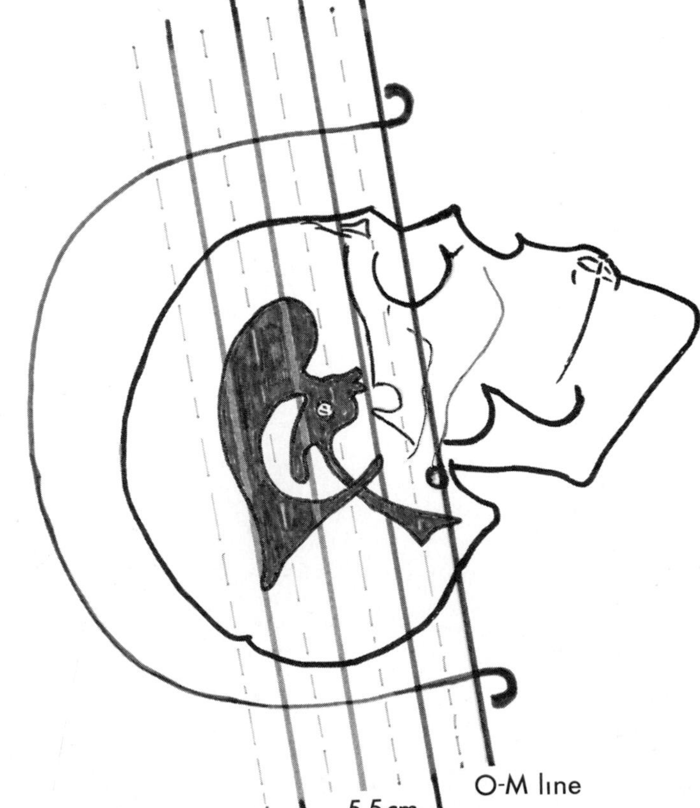

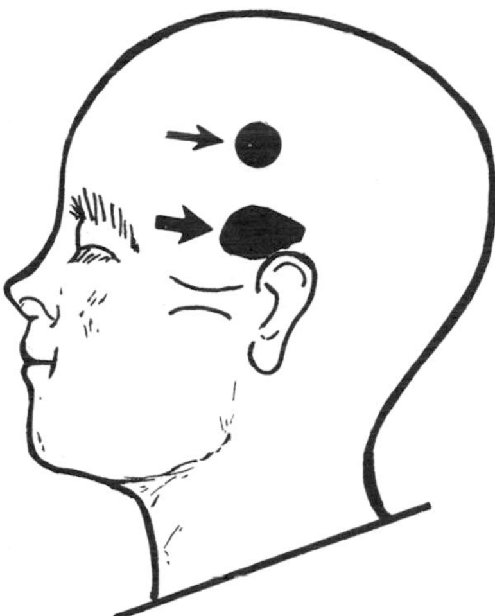

Figure 7–15 A child is best examined lying supine, the head turned to one side. The third ventricle and temporal horn echoes are obtained in the area immediately above the ear (*large arrow*). The frontal cerebral mantle thickness is measured farther above and in front of the ear (*small arrow*).

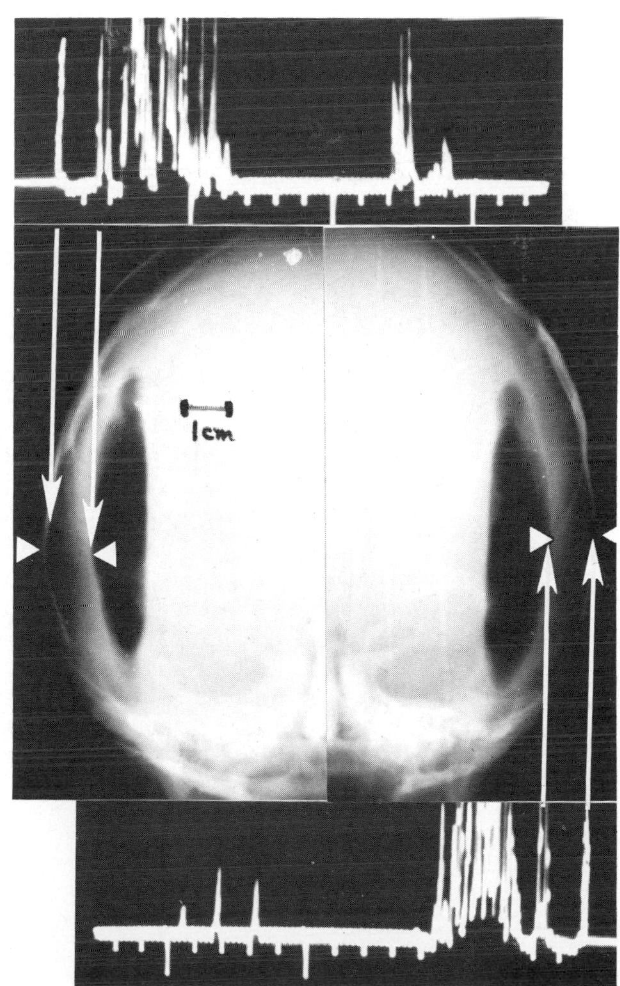

Figure 7–16 To show that a cerebral mantle may be reliably measured by transcalvarial sonography, echo-ranging was performed with air in the ventricular system. The radiographs and ultrasonic data were obtained with the child's head turned to the right, then to the left side. The so-called cerebral mantle measures the distance from the surface of the scalp to the lateral ventricular wall. The multiple echoes beyond it are reflections from air in the ventricle.

these data an infant must be anesthetized. This is not necessary with sonoventriculography, and the procedure is more expeditious and less costly.

Owing to diversion of the x-ray beam, the measurements obtained at pneumoventriculography are approximately 15 per cent larger than those recorded by ultrasonic means. Figure 7–14 shows the relationship of the x-ray tomographic sections to the ventricular system. These interrelationships must be remembered when diagnostic studies such as air contrast, x-ray tomography, and sonoventriculography are being compared.

A third ventricular width of up to 25 mm can be sonographically determined with relative certainty in most infants and children. In adults, these midline echoes are obtained slightly above the ear; in children, above and in front of the ear, as shown in Figure 7–15. Reflections from the temporal horn are frequently concurrently recorded at the time of third-ventricular sonography. Whenever these data become available, Schiefer's brain mantle index may be calculated.

In infants with hydrocephalus, the frontal brain mantle is frequently much thicker than its occipital counterpart. The Echoline-20 diagnostic unit reliably measures a cerebral mantle thickness that measures more than 1 cm, as shown in Figure 7–16. Sonoventriculography may be repeated frequently, particularly in those hydrocephalic infants in whom shunt malfunction is suspected. Caution is advised in order not to confuse echoes from the insula with those arising from the frontal horns of the ventricular system. The insular echoes are frequently more superficial. They are broader and pulsate in synchrony with the heart beat. When a shunting procedure for hydrocephalus is contemplated in an infant who has not undergone pneumoventriculography, the occipitoparietal brain mantle thickness can be sonographically determined with ease. In some instances this avoids a need for intraoperative exploratory needling with a ventricular cannula.

When serial sonoventriculography is required, echo-ranging must be performed from the same area of the scalp each time in order to derive comparable measurements.

In summary, sonoventriculography, can reliably measure the width of the third ventricle and the thickness of the cerebral mantle in any desired area, particularly in infants. Therein lies its usefulness in the management of infant hydrocephalus.

TRANSDURAL SONOGRAPHY

Despite the sophistication of other available diagnostic procedures, the neurosurgeon can benefit by an intraoperative sonographic evaluation of a mass lesion. Echo-ranging demarcates, characterizes, and determines depths of such lesions without the need for exploratory needling or cerebrotomy. Although the difference in ultrasonic velocities between brain and cerebral neoplasia is only slight (e.g., brain 1530 m per second, meningioma 1550 m per second), these differences are sufficient to provide an interface or mirror from which ultrasound can be reflected. Because of necrosis, hemorrhage, cavitation, and variable cellular density within a tumor, multiple interfaces or ultrasonic reflections are created. As a group, these reflections are called "tumor-echo complex."

Tanaka and his pupils probably have the most extensive experience with this technique.[24] The author and others have confirmed its usefulness.[7] Mueller has ingeniously refined the transdural technique. He has projected a reference grid onto the operative field. The equipment was modified so that serial photographs could be made and recorded on the same Polaroid film. This creates a two-dimensional representation of the lesion.[20]

When the calvarium, the major obstacle to ultrasound, has been removed, intraoperative sonography becomes extremely reliable. Tumor echoes can be detected in almost all cerebral neoplasms. When dealing with extra-axial lesions, ultrasound demarcates the medial extent of such neoplasms much better than does angiography. When infiltrative tumors are encountered, ultrasound locates the areas most severely involved and points to regions of cystic degeneration. The subcortical depth and medial extent of an intracerebral hematoma can be measured, and the character of the clot determined. This information is meaningful, particularly when parenchymal hematomas must be evacuated through vulnerable regions of the brain. The characteristics of the "tumor-echo complex" are determined not by the histological type but rather by the physical properties of the neoplasm.

Supratentorial Lesions

In order to avoid damage to the crystal by repeated sterilization, to prevent bacterial contamination of the operative field, and to further reduce electrical hazard, a technique has been developed to avoid direct contact between transducer and patient. Once the bone flap has been reflected, the operative field is circumferentially covered by sterile towels. Next, the dura mater is moistened and covered with a sterile plastic drape (SteriDrape). The transducer is applied to the protected operative field, and the underlying area of pathological change is mapped out. The sonographer is able to direct the transducer with one hand and manipulate the instrument controls with the other. After completion of the sonographic evaluation, the plastic drape and the surrounding towels are removed, and the surgeon changes gown and gloves and proceeds with the operation (Fig. 7–17). This technique has been used for more than a decade without wound infection or untoward side effects. Exploratory needling of the brain has become unnecessary whenever transdural sonography has been employed.

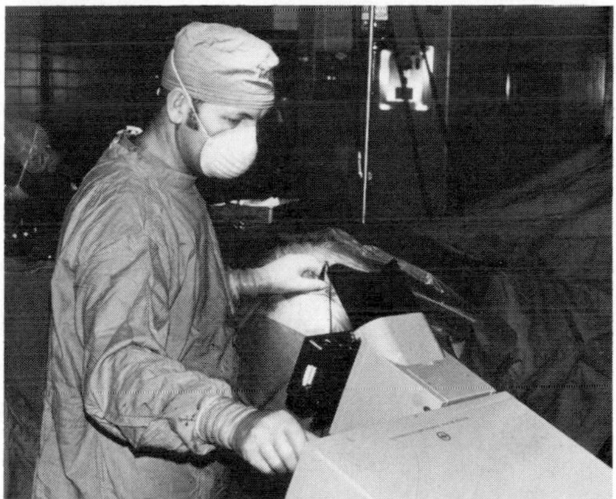

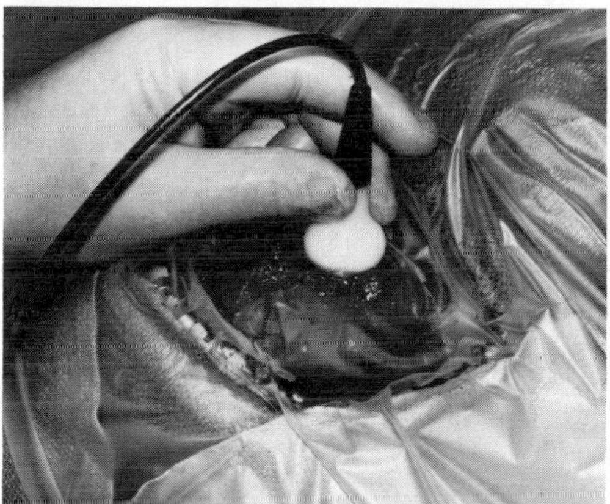

Figure 7–17 The technique of transdural sonography. The operative field has been protected by a sterile transparent drape; the underlying circumferentially placed towels are visible. The transducer head is not sterile; thus, the operator contaminates himself during sonography. At completion of sonic probing, the transparent drape is removed; gown and gloves are changed; and the operation is continued.

By their reflections of ultrasound, all cerebral lesions may be divided into solid, cystic, or a combination of the two, irrespective of their histological type. These divisions are diagramatically depicted in Figure 7–18. When the lesion has a homogeneous consistency (e.g., metastases, fibrous meningioma, or nonliquefied hematoma), frequently uniform equal amplitude reflections of ultrasound are recorded. In contrast, a glioblastoma multiforme with its variable tissue architecture produces a tumor echo complex made up of variable-intensity ultrasonic reflections. Metastatic lesions frequently develop central necrosis, and parenchymal hematomas eventually liquefy. As these changes in consistency are made, the configuration of the tumor echo complex is altered to reflect the morphological change. Because of the changing consistency, it is difficult to classify brain tumors as to their histological type on the basis of their ultrasonic properties.

Figure 7–19 shows tumor complexes of three meningiomas. Note the generally uniform, equal amplitude reflections with clear demarcation of depth and medial extent of the lesion as shown in the upper tracing and compare this to the middle echo complex, which was obtained from a patient with a fibrous medial sphenoid ridge meningioma. The tumor echo in this tracing begins at a 4-cm depth. The reflections at the 2-cm

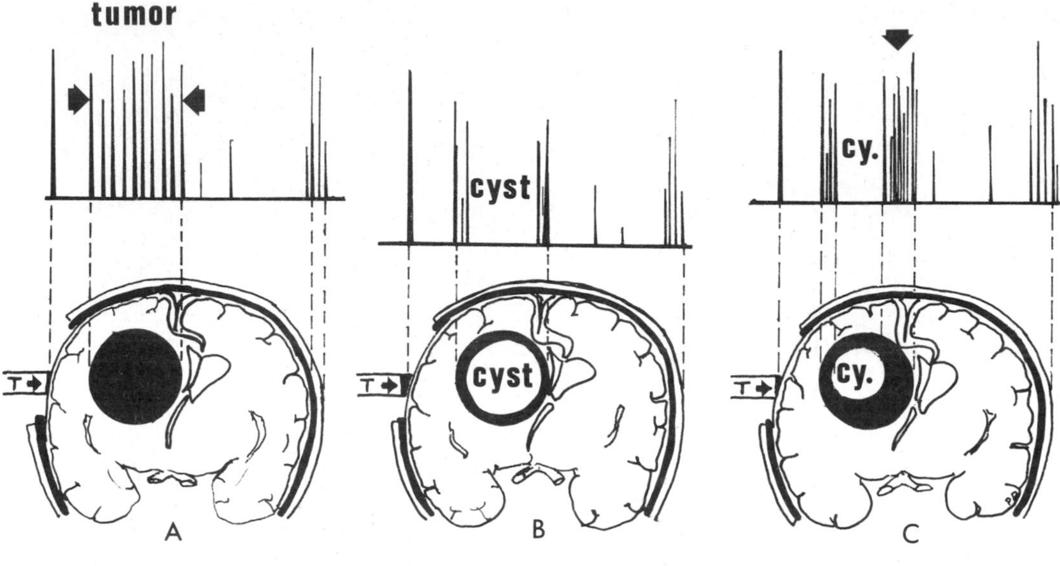

Figure 7–18 A cerebral lesion may be solid, *A*; cystic, *B*; or solid with a cystic component, *C*. Ultrasound reflects these morphological properties.

depth were produced by the insula. The lower tracing illustrates variable amplitude reflections that were recorded from a cerebellopontine angle meningioma. Part of this lesion was removed by suction; other areas had to be resected. The tumor echo suggested this possibility. Tumor echoes from six other lesions are shown in Figure 7–20. A 23-year-old man presented with progressive left-sided external ophthalmoplegia. The last of three computed tomograms suggested the presence of a lesion in the region of the left cavernous sinus. The angiographic findings were unimpressive. Transdural sonography confirmed the presence of an extensive lesion, as shown in Figure 7–21. It proved to be a chondrosarcoma. Sonography served as a useful guide to safe biopsy of this extradural lesion.

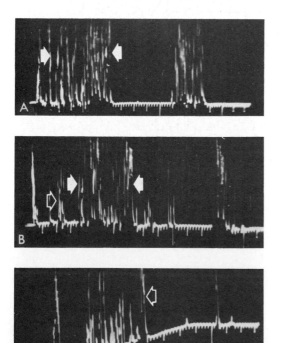

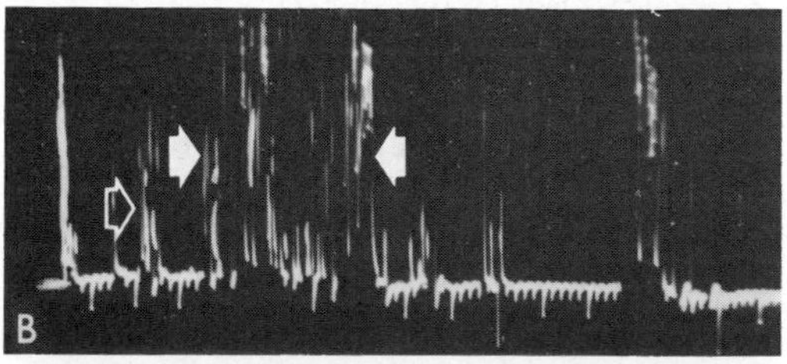

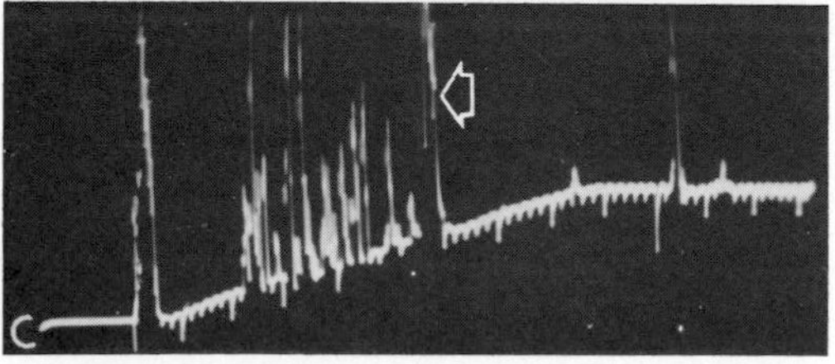

Figure 7–19 A morphologically homogeneous lesion reflects frequent similar intensity echoes. *A*. A tumor complex from a fibrous meningioma is shown, but similar configurations may be obtained from a metastic lesion, a pituitary adenoma, or a parenchymal hematoma. *B*. A middle cranial fossa meningioma with a central soft component. The open arrow points to reflections from the insula. *C*. The tracing obtained from a posterior fossa meningioma. Tentorial echoes are indicated by the open arrow.

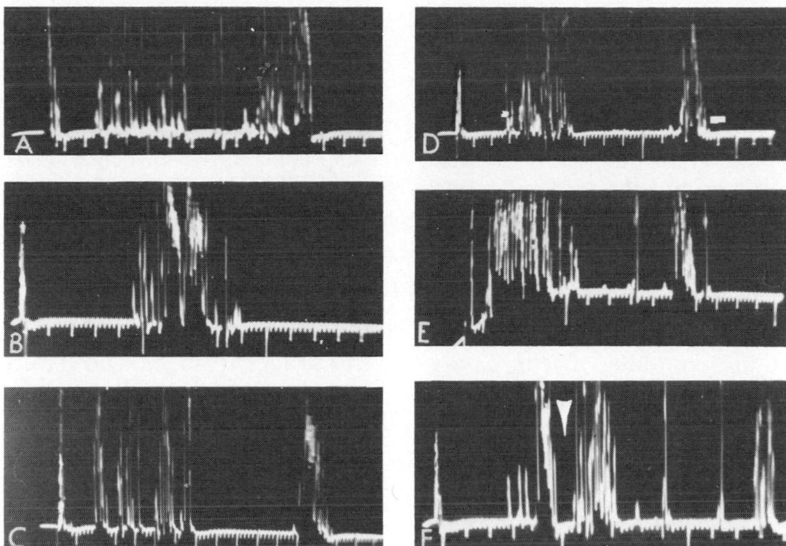

Figure 7–20 Tumor complexes of various lesions. *A*. Microglioma. *B*. Hypothalamic astrocytoma. *C*. Multicystic astrocytoma. *D*. Metastatic adenocarcinoma. *E*. Fibrous meningioma. *F*. Partially liquefied hematoma (arrow points to liquid component). The morphological rather than the histological type of the lesion determines the configuration of the tumor complex.

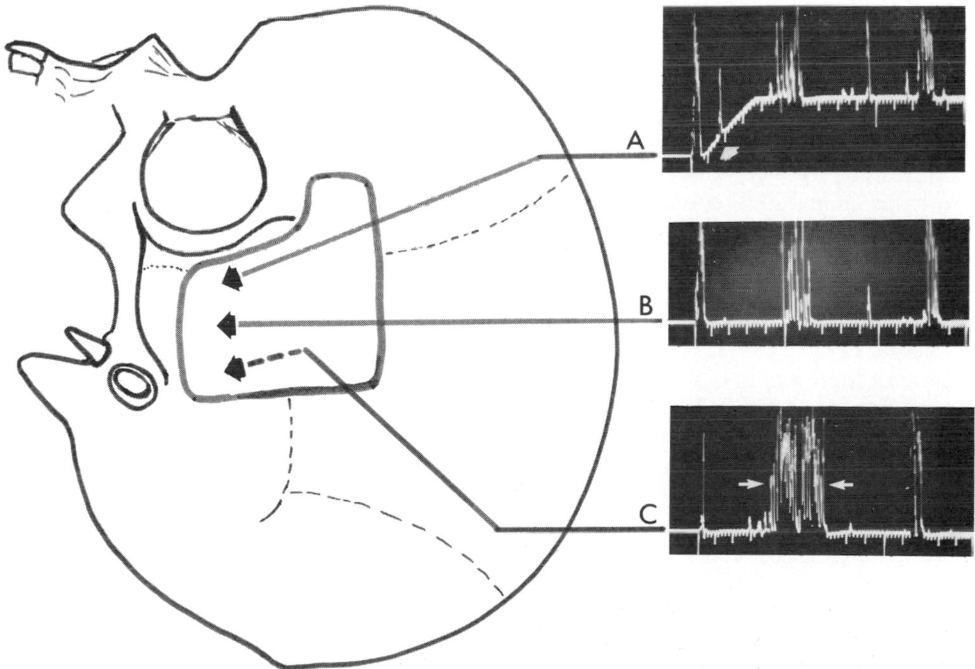

Figure 7–21 A 23-year-old man presented with complete left external ophthalmoplegia. Prominent tumor echoes were recorded, particularly in the lower tracing, *C*. Biopsy identified an extradural chondrosarcoma. The "time-gain" slope used for echo-ranging is displayed in *A* (*white arrow*).

Edematous brain produces spurious reflections of ultrasound. Pituitary adenomas, because of their uniform architecture, reflect uniform and equal-amplitude echoes. Delayed irradiation necrosis has been sonographically studied in one case. Variable amplitude and interval reflections of ultrasound were recorded. The configuration of the "echo complex," however, was indistinguishable from those obtained in patients with glioblastoma multiforme. A brain abscess reflects ultrasound from the wall, but not the contents, of the cavity. The thickness of this wall can be sonographically ascertained.

Infratentorial Lesions

Sonographic demarcation of infratentorial lesions has received less attention than that of supratentorial lesions. Tanaka has reported 20 cases in which ultrasound was intraoperatively employed.[23] Uematsu and Walker have alluded to sonographic properties of a cerebellar astrocytoma and a medulloblastoma.[25] The author has used transdural sonography to study the form and structure of 11 posterior fossa lesions. Part of this experience has been previously reported.[5,6] In spite of the addition of computer tomography to the diagnostic armamentarium of the neurosurgeon, occasions arise on which the site and structure of a posterior fossa lesion are not readily apparent. Transdural sonography in these instances obviates the utilization of more aggressive means, such as exploratory needling or incision of the cerebellar hemispheres.

Equipment identical to that used in sonography of supratentorial lesions is employed. The technique has been modified to make it more suitable to a limited operative exposure. All patients have been operated on in the sitting position. Once the posterior fossa dura mater had been exposed, the operative field was circumferentially protected by sterile towels. A large sterile drape with an adhesive undersurface was applied to these towels in order to hold them together and at the same time protect the exposed epidural space from contamination. Such a transparent drape also provides visual orientation within the operative field. Since bony exposure is limited, multiple placement of the ultrasonic transducer is frequently not possible. A sector scan can, on the other hand, be obtained by tilting the transducer in a vertical or a horizontal plane and photographically recording the data. In the sitting position, with the head tilted forward, the tentorium cerebelli acts as a prominent source of ultrasonic reflection as shown in Figure 7–22. Tilting the transducer from right to left in a horizontal plane makes possible further sonographic demarcation of infratentorial lesions without the need for multiple placement of a transducer (Fig. 7–23). Because the clivus and petrous pyramids provide prominent reflections of ultrasound, the tumor complexes of cerebellopontine angle lesions are best separated from these basal skull reflections when the ultrasonic beam is directed parallel to the posterior margins of the petrous pyramid. Assiduous anatomical correlation makes it apparent that the entire posterior fossa is amenable to sonographic probing, even though a small craniectomy. Like lesions of the cerebral hemispheres, the cerebellar lesions may be classified into cystic or solid complexes, or a combination of the two. An example of a solid lesion is shown in Figure 7–24, which demonstrates the close correlation between sonographic and x-ray tomographic data. Figure 7–25 illustrates the ultrasonic properties of a cyst. The lesion was a liquefied hematoma of the left cerebellar hemisphere. A combination of cystic and solid components is illustrated in Figure 7–26. The lesion was a hemangioblastoma with a large cystic component. The author has studied one instance of focal necrotizing encephalitis. Vertebral angiography was unremarkable, but computed tomograms suggested the presence of a vermis mass lesion. Transdural sonography yielded a group of echo reflections in this instance that were indistinguishable from those of a glioma. Exposure of the lesion revealed extensive infarction with multiple foci of hemorrhage.

In summary, transdural sonography of infratentorial lesions is of value during the operative process. It obviates or lessens the need for aggressive manipulation of or trauma to structures vital to life.

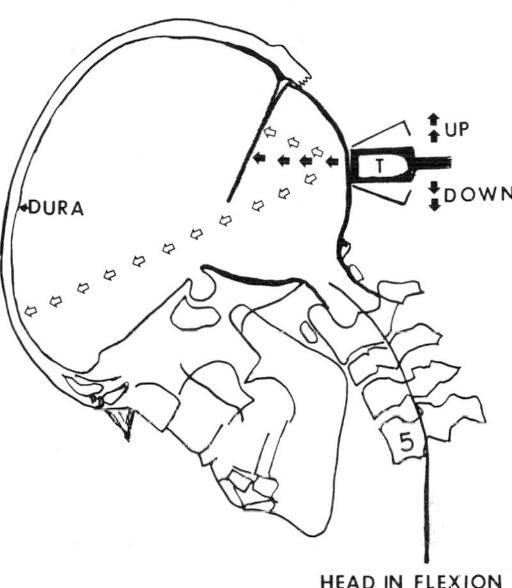

Figure 7–22 When the head is flexed forward, the tentorium cerebelli forms a prominent source of echoes. By tilting the transducer head (T) up and down, a vertical sector scan of the posterior fossa is obtained.

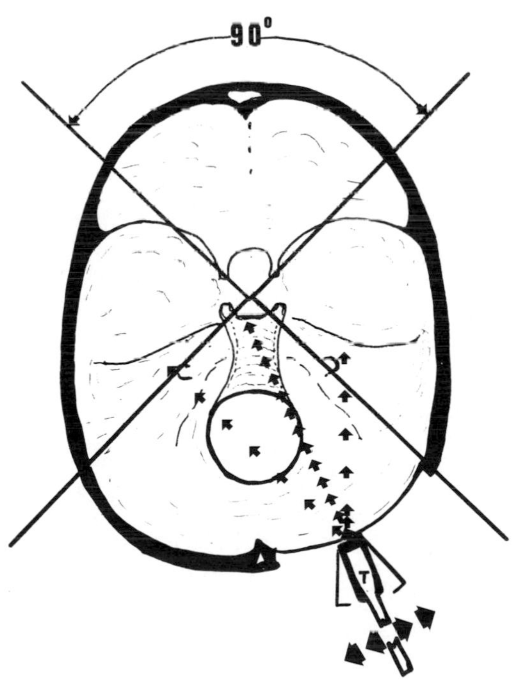

Figure 7–23 A horizontal sector scan may be obtained by recording echo complexes at frequent intervals while the transducer head (T) is being tilted from right to left.

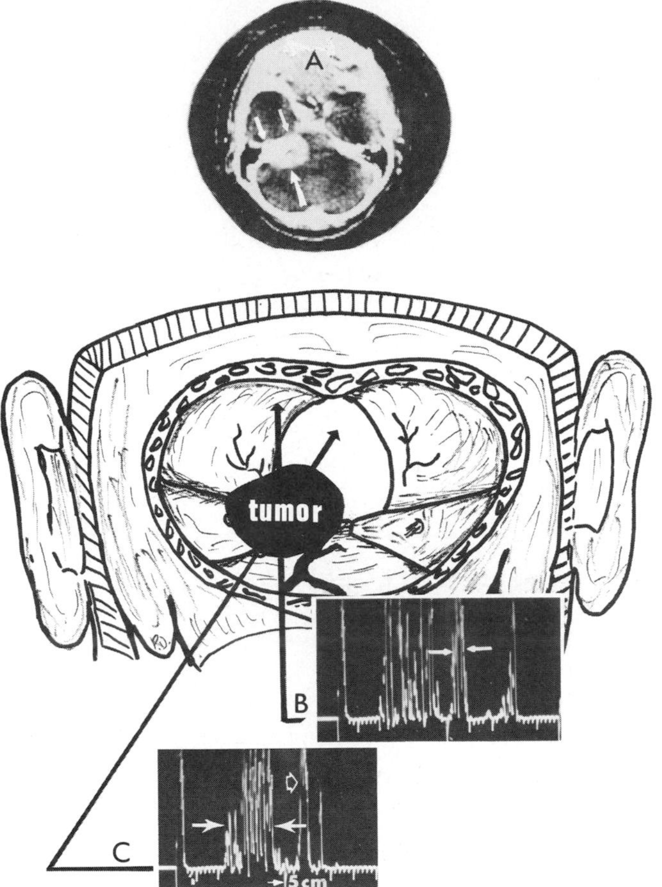

Figure 7–24 Sonographic tumor complexes from a cerebellopontine angle meningioma are shown in *B* and *C*. For correlation, a computed tomogram is shown in *A*. The arrows in *B* point to echoes reflected from the tentorium. The solid arrows indicate the tumor complex; the open arrow, the reflections from the clivus.

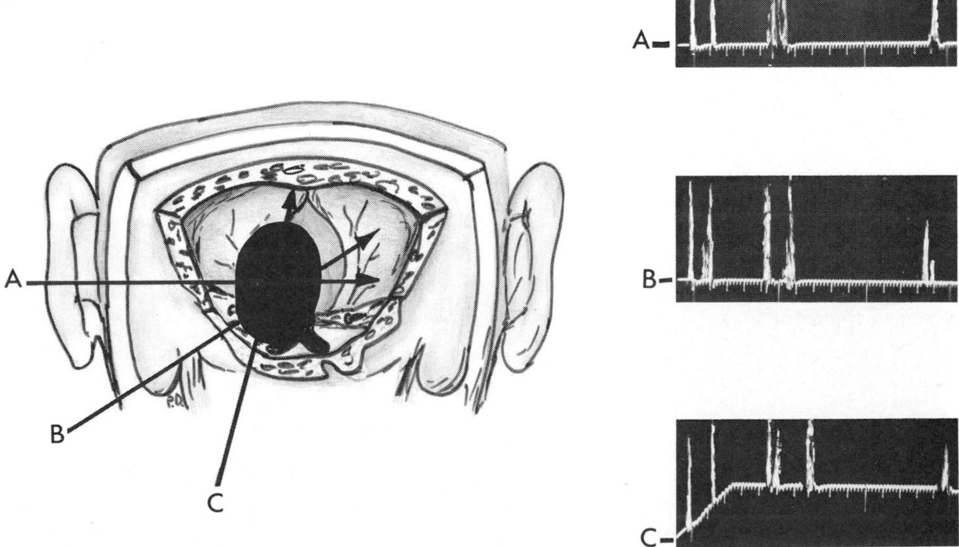

Figure 7–25 Echoes from a liquefied cerebellar hematoma. A "cyst pattern" is recorded. At operation, a hematoma cavity measuring 3 cm in diameter was encountered at a 1.5-cm depth.

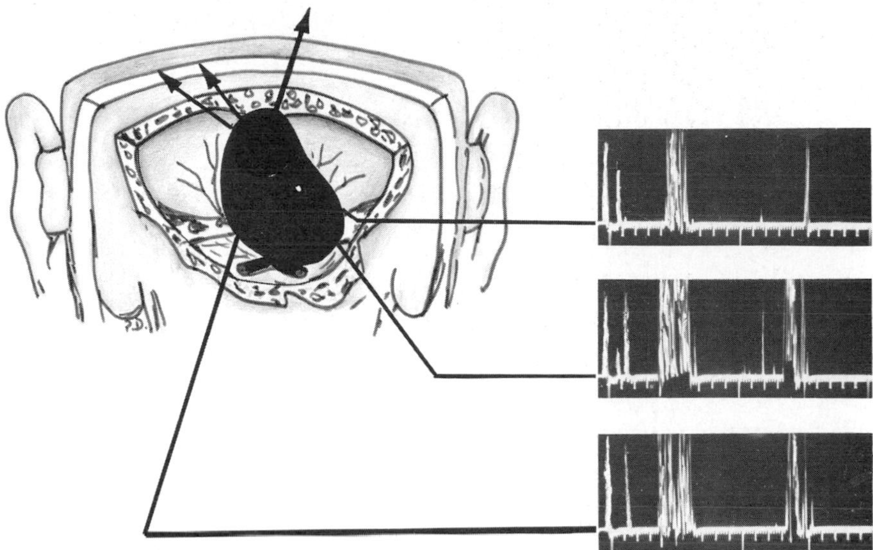

Figure 7-26 A tumor complex showing a cystic and a solid component was obtained from this large vermis hemangioblastoma. The cyst cavity was entered at a 1.5-cm depth as predicted by ultrasonography. The solid component, removed en masse, measured 3 cm in largest dimension. The sonographic and operative findings showed close correlation.

SUMMARY

Echoencephalography should be viewed as an extension of the neurological examination of a patient suspected of harboring an intracranial mass lesion that has produced a shift of the diencephalic midline structures. The A-scanning technique yields meaningful information in the assessment of hydrocephalic patients, particularly in the pediatric age group. Transdural sonography of intracranial mass lesions is a useful adjunct to the management of these lesions. The primary limitation of the technique is that experience is required in order to obtain meaningful information.

REFERENCES

1. Barrows, H. S., Dyck, P., and Kurze, T.: The diagnostic applications of ultrasound in neurological disease. The intracerebral midline. Neurology, *15*:361–365, 1965.
2. Bergmann, L.: Der Ultraschall und seine Anwendung in Wissenschaft und Technik. Stuttgart, S. Hirzel Verlag, 1949.
3. Curie, J., and Curie, P.: Dévelopement par pression de l'électricité polaire dans les cristaux hémièdres à faces inclinées. C.R. Acad. Sci., Paris, *91*:294, 1880.
4. Dussik, K. T., Dussik, F., and Wyt, L.: Auf dem Wege zur Hyperphonographie des Gehirnes. Wien. Med. Wschr., *97*:425–429, 1947.
5. Dyck, P.: Transdural sonography of posterior fossa lesions. *In* Vlieger, M. de, and Kazner, E., eds.: Handbook of Medical Ultrasound. New York, John Wiley & Sons, Inc., 1978.
6. Dyck, P., and Doyle, J. B.: Transdural echoranging of posterior fossa tumors. Second European Congress of Ultrasonics in Medicine, Munich, 1975.
7. Dyck, P., Kurze, T., and Barrows, H. S.: Intraoperative ultrasonic encephalography of cerebral mass lesions. Bull. Los Angeles Neurol. Soc., *31*:114–124, 1966.
8. Firestone, F. A.: Flaw detecting device and measuring instrument. U.S. Patent No.2280226, 1942.
9. Ford, R., and Ambrose, J.: Echoencephalography. The measurement of the position of midline structures in the skull with high frequency pulsed ultrasound. Brain, *86*:189–196, 1963.
10. Ford, R., and McRae, D. L.: Echoencephalography a standardized technic for the measurement of the width of the third and lateral ventricles. *In* Grossinan, C. C., Holmes, J., Joyner, C., and Purnell, E. W., eds.: Diagnostic Ultrasound. New York, Plenum Press, 1966, pp. 117–129.
11. French, L. A., Wild, J. J., and Neal, D.: Detection of cerebral tumors by untrasonic pulses: Pilot studies on postmortem material. Cancer, *3*:705–708, 1950.
12. French, L. A., Wild, J. J., and Neal, D.: The experimental application of ultrasonics to localization of brain tumors: Preliminary report. J. Neurosurg., *8*:198–203, 1951.
13. Gordon, D.: Ultrasound as a Diagnostic and Surgical Tool. Baltimore, Md., Williams & Wilkins Co., 1964, p.39.
14. Geuttner, W., Fielder, G., and Paetzold, J.: Ueber Ultraschallabbildungen am menschlichen Schaedel. Acustica, *2*:148–156, 1952.

15. Iizuke, J. H.: Correlation between neuroradiological and echoencephalographical findings. Symposium Neuroradiol., Paris, 1967.
16. Langevin, M. P., and Chilowsky, N. C.: Procede et appareils pour la production de signaux sousmarins dirigés et pour la localisation à distance d'obstacles sousmarins. French Patent No. 502913, 1918.
17. Leksell, L.: Echoencephalography. 1. Detection of intracranial complications following head injury. Acta Chir. Scand., *110*:301–315, 1955–56.
18. Leksell, L.: Echoencephalography. 11. Midline echo from the pineal body as an index of pineal displacement. Acta Chir. Scand., *115*:255–259. 1958.
19. Lippmann, G.: Principe de la conservation de l'électricité. Ann. Chim. Phys., *24*:145–178, 1881.
20. Mueller, H. R.:Die transdurale Echoencephalographie. Bern, Stuttgart, Vienna, Verlag Hans Huber, 1971.
21. Schiefer, W., and Kazner, E.: Klinische Echo-Encephalographie. Berlin, Heidelberg, New York, Springer-Verlag, 1967, pp. 56–63.
22. Sokolov, S. J.: Ultraacoustical methods for studying the properties of temperatured steel and the detection of internal defects in metalic goods. J. Tech. Phys. (U.S.S.R.), *11*:160, 1941.
23. Tanaka, K.: Diagnosis of Brain Disease by Ultrasound. Tokyo, Shindan-To-Chiryo Sha Co. Ltd., 1969.
24. Tanaka, K., Ito, K., and Wagni, T.: The localization of brain tumors by ultrasonic technics. A clinical review of 111 cases. J. Neurosurg., *23*:135–147, 1965.
25. Uematsu, S., and Walker, A. E.: A Manual of Echoencephalography. Baltimore, Williams & Wilkins Co., 1971.
26. White, D. N.: Elementary Acoustics. Ultrasonic Encephalography. Kingston, Ont., Hanson & Edgar Ltd., 1970, pp.9–53.
27. Zuelch, K. J.: The morphologic bases of the abnormal echoencephalogram. *In* Proceedings of International Symposium on Echoencephalography, Erlangen, 1967. New York, Springer-Verlag, 1968.

8

ELECTROENCEPHALOGRAPHY

The electroencephalogram (EEG) is best viewed as an extension of the neurological examination.[8] It records the electrical signs of neurological function, whereas the physical examination is directed to the clinical signs. In any patient, the results may be abnormal in one or both examinations or in neither, just as they may, for example, in any two subtests such as motor strength and reflexes. Conversely, the results of both examinations may be normal, even though the patient has anatomical abnormalities detectable by contrast study or by computed tomography. An intelligent integration of the results of the various tests, such as the electroencephalogram, the clinical examination, the contrast studies, and the computed tomogram, requires an understanding of the value and limitations of each test.

BASIC CONCEPTS AND DEFINITIONS

The electroencephalogram is recorded by commercially available machines that usually contain 8, 16, or even more channels, each of which functions as a voltmeter that records potential differences between electrode pairs connected to it. Because the potentials measured are in microvolts, the original signal must be amplified about a million times before the difference is large enough to drive a galvanometer, which causes an ink-writing pen to produce a fluctuating trace on paper that moves at a constant rate. The fluctuating line reflects, within the limits of the system, the temporal variability characteristics of the potential differences between two input electrodes attached to a specific location on the head and connected to that channel. In order to appreciate the spatial characteristics of one temporal pattern in one channel, however, recording must be made simultaneously from many electrode pairs at other locations—thus the need for, preferably, 16 or more channels.

Overall, electroencephalographic study involves an evaluation of the relative spatial and temporal variability characteristics within potential differences recorded between members of various electrode pairs located on the surface of the head. (When the electrode pairs are placed on the surface of the cortex, the study is called an electrocorticogram; when they are placed within the depth of the brain, the study is called a depth electroencephalogram.) Once the various types of electrographic patterns are identified, inferences can be drawn concerning the nature and location of the generators as well as the normality and abnormality of the activity. This inference must be interpreted in the context of the patient's overall clinical condition. As previously mentioned, the interpretation requires an understanding not only of the technical aspects of electroencephalography but also of neurological disease.

Abstracting the important relative spatial and temporal variability characteristics from the multichannel ink-written record by visual analysis is complex. There are, however, three basic steps.

One, a particular pattern of pen deflection in one channel identifies a particular temporal pattern of potential variability at one location. This pattern, followed from one occurrence to another on one page and then on multiple pages in one record or in sequential records, traces a picture of its short- and long-term variability and can identify temporal characteristics such as wave duration, frequency, amplitude,

F. W. SHARBROUGH AND T. M. SUNDT, JR.

phase, and form. When waves recur sequentially, the patterns they form may be sustained or intermittent.

Two, after a particular pattern has been identified in one channel, its phase, latency, and amplitude variability can be followed from one channel to another (from top to bottom on the EEG page, where a picture of its spatial variability characteristics within one vertical dimension is created). This one-dimensional picture, then, combined with a knowledge of the montage (which identifies the pairs of electrodes whose potential is being recorded in each channel) and of the electrode placement (which identifies the location of these pairs on the head), can be translated into a two-dimensional picture of the spatial and temporal variability characteristics of the activity on the surface of the head. Included are such important features as the boundary extent, peak localization, spatial contour, and synchrony of the potential within both the longitudinal and the transverse dimensions of the head. These characteristics, followed from one occurrence to another in one page, in one record, or in sequential records, form a picture of the short- and long-term variability of the potential.

Three, the relativity of the identified variability characteristics is determined by its relationship to other factors and events in the environment: the subject, the instrument, and the interface between the instrument and the subject. The reactive relationship of the potentials to preceding events is important. Such reactions are termed "activation" if the preceding event or procedure elicits or enhances a potential (normal or abnormal) and "attenuation" if the stimulus or procedure reduces the amplitude of a particular electroencephalographic activity or pattern. The activity is considered an evoked potential if the potential has a fixed latency relationship to an identifiable activating or eliciting stimulus; it is a spontaneous potential if it has no fixed latency relationship to such stimuli.

In summary, the temporal variability characteristics of the electroencephalogram are determined by the pattern of pen deflection in a channel. The spatial and temporal variability characteristics of the pattern are derived from the phase, amplitude, and latency variability of the pattern in multiple channels. The pattern's relativity is based on its relationship to other events that may be recorded directly by the pen's deflections or indirectly as a hand-written observation by a technician. The identified relativity of the spatial and temporal variability characteristics of the electroencephalographic potential allows the nature and location of its source to be inferred as well as its normality or abnormality. Integrated into the total clinical picture, this inference can be interpreted and the significance of the finding can be determined.

THE ELECTROENCEPHALOGRAPH

Interface Between Instrument and Subject—Electrodes and Electrode Placement

To record potentials from the head, small metal discs containing conducting gels are attached to the scalp with collodion. For the alternating-current recordings commonly used in electroencephalography, various metals such as gold, tin, or chlorided silver are used with a suitable electrolyte solution. The effect of electrode material on direct-current recording is discussed in detail elsewhere.[6]

Each metal disc attached to the head forms the terminal end for a flexible wire that is then connected into a jackbox and ultimately through a switching panel to the input terminals of the individual channels of the machine. After the electrodes have been applied and filled with conducting gel, interelectrode impedances are checked; impedance should not exceed 5000 ohms.[11]

In order to locate the peaks and boundaries of a temporal pattern, a sufficient number of electrodes must be placed systematically on the head. The full 21 electrodes and placements recommended by the International Federation are now considered minimal for clinical electroencephalography (Fig. 8–1).[11,17]

Besides the 21 electrodes routinely utilized in the 10–20 system, additional scalp electrodes may be added for a more refined localization, and special electrodes (e.g., sphenoidal and nasopharyngeal) may be used.[8,17] Also, operatively applied electrodes, such as those placed on the surface of the brain for electrocorticography or in the depth of the brain for depth electroencephalography, can be used. The naso-

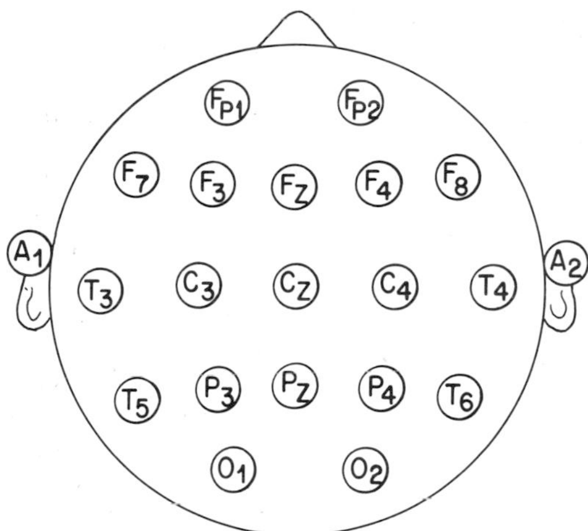

Figure 8–1 Placement and nomenclature of 19 scalp and 2 ear electrodes routinely utilized in the 10–20 system.

pharyngeal and sphenoidal electrodes are associated with artifacts and have no immediate neighboring surface electrode with which to be compared. Because of this, both their placement and interpretation require experience, and sporadic use of such electrodes may result in misdiagnosis, with extracerebral potentials being interpreted as cerebral abnormalities.

Machine Characteristics—Operational Control

All electroencephalographs are essentially voltmeters that record potential differences between members of electrode pairs connected to the two input terminals of the channel. Previously called grid 1 and grid 2 when the amplification system utilized vacuum tubes, with present-day transistor amplification systems, these terminals are called input terminal 1 and input terminal 2 or simply terminal 1 and terminal 2. Sufficiently amplified, the input potential differences are used to cause an ink-writing galvanometer to inscribe a fluctuating trace on a moving piece of paper. The accuracy of the ink-written trace as it reflects the original temporal variability characteristics of the input from the surface of the head is influenced by the character of the electrodes and the adequacy of their connection to the head and to the machine. It is also influenced by the electronic characteristics of the machine and the mechanical characteristics of the galvanometer. The machine characteristics must be modified advantageously or detrimentally, depending on use of the operational controls on the instrument. A full description of the techniques for appropriate calibration and use of operational control has been detailed elsewhere, but there are certain important general concepts.[6,17]

Sensitivity

The amplification ability of each channel of the electroencephalograph is expressed in terms of a sensitivity ratio, defined as a ratio of input in microvolts to pen response in millimeters. The standard electroencephalogram is run with a sensitivity ratio of between 5 and 10 μv per millimeter. This ratio defines the input that is needed to produce the standard pen deflection, and by definition, the numerical value of the ratio decreases as the amplification of the machine increases (because as amplification increases, less input is required to produce the same standard pen response). Although the standard sensitivity ratio is between 5 and 10 μv, the ratio should be appropriately adjusted in each individual case so that an adequate-sized pen deflection is obtained without consistently overloading the amplifier and causing flattening of the top of the waveforms at the extremes of the pen excursion (blocking), thus grossly distorting the relationship between the write-out and the temporal variability characteristics of the input. When properly calibrated, the setting on the sensitivity controls of the electroencephalograph should reflect the actual sensitivity of the machine. This must, however, be checked at the beginning and end of each record by putting in a standard signal and measuring the response.

Linear Frequency Range

Ideally, the machine should uniformly amplify all frequencies that reach its input terminals. Although the ideal is never attained, the machine amplifies all frequencies reasonably uniformly within a certain "linear frequency range" or "band width." This range is determined by the low linear frequency response setting of the amplifier, which identifies the lowest frequency at which the machine will maintain a specified percentage of its ability to amplify a reference frequency. (The exact percentage specified by the designer may vary from one machine to another but, in general, will be between 70 and 80 per cent.) Most records are routinely run with a low linear frequency response of 1 Hz. The high linear frequency setting defines the highest frequency at which the machine still maintains a specified percentage of its ability to amplify a reference frequency; the low linear frequency is determined by the time constants of the resistance-capacitance coupling of the channel to its input terminals. The time constant, the length of time that the machine can maintain at least 37 per cent of its original response to a direct-current signal, can be measured directly from the calibration signal. When the time constant is known, formulas and tables can be used for converting to the low linear frequency response.[6] The high linear frequency response is determined by the response characteristics of the amplifier and by the highest frequency response of which the recording galvanometer is capable. In conventional machines, the galvanometer does not respond well to frequencies above 70 Hz and thus sets the maximal upper limit of the machine's high linear frequency response, but the response can be further reduced by adjusting the settings on the instrument's high linear frequency control, which usually ranges as high as 70 Hz to as low as 15 Hz. Ordinarily, the high linear response is set at a maximum, but in appropriate situations, especially if there is an interest in activity in the low frequencies to the relative exclusion of high frequencies, lower settings may be used with a full understanding of how they alter the characteristics of the recording.[6] Finally, in addition to high and low linear frequency controls, most machines have a finely tuned 60-Hz notched filter that markedly attenuates signals at or close to 60 Hz, the frequency of most common external interference from various alternating-current sources in the laboratory. If 60-Hz interference cannot be eliminated by any other means, it can be reduced by these filters, but the advantages and disadvantages of their use, as well as the use of other filters, must be fully appreciated by the technician and the electroencephalographer.[6]

Polarity Conventions, Derivations, Montages, and Localizations

The study of electroencephalographic polarity conventions, derivations, and montages allows the pattern of pen deflections to be translated into a concept about the spatial variability characteristic of the potential on the surface of the head. These characteristics include the boundary extent, the peak polarity and localization, and the spatial contour of the pattern, including its symmetry about the midline. Determinations of peak localization and polarity allow inferences to be drawn about the localization of the end of the generator that is responsible for a local surface peak.

A local surface peak is defined as a point on the surface of the head that has the same relative potential sign with respect to all immediately surrounding points. The relative potential sign of one point with respect to another is defined as the sign of the potential difference between the two.

Local peaks of negativity and positivity usually identify areas on the head where the negative and positive poles of an electrical generator have their maximal effect. All generators have two poles, one relatively negative and the other relatively positive. The generators recorded by the electroencephalograph—whether they are cerebral or extracerebral—are in essence alternating-current generators, in which the negative and positive poles alternately switch locations with time. Because these cerebral potentials are produced by dendritic generators radially oriented to the surface, a surface electrode usually detects only one end of the generator (either the negative or positive pole) at one instant in time. At the same time, however, the other end of the generator may be detected by an electrode that has been passed through the cortical surface into the depth.

In order to convert pen deflection into peak localization, it must be realized that the deflection from the baseline indicates that the electrodes attached to the two input terminals of that channel have a potential difference whose numerical value can be calculated by multiplying the amplitude of the pen deflection by the sensitivity setting for that channel. Furthermore, these electrodes have opposite relative signs with respect to each other. The polarity convention is set by international agreement and specifies that the differential amplifiers in each channel be constructed so that relative negativity on terminal 1 and relative positivity on terminal 2 cause an upward deflection of the pen, while relative positivity on terminal 1 and relative negativity on terminal 2 cause a downward deflection. To relate the relative sign of an electrode attached to a particular terminal to the sign of the local peak producing the sign, it is necessary to realize that the opposite sign relationship between electrodes attached to the two input terminals of a channel may be produced by one of three possible sets of circumstances: (1) the electrode attached to the relatively negative terminal may be nearer to a local peak of negativity, (2) the electrode attached to the relatively positive terminal may be nearer to a local peak of positivity, or (3) there may be a combination of these conditions. Thus, from the pen deflection in one channel, the numerical value of the potential difference and the relative sign relationships between the two electrodes attached to that channel can be determined, although the sign and location of the local surface peak producing the potential difference cannot be identified.

Determining the sign and location of the local surface peak that produces a particular pattern of pen deflection requires the use of montages containing multiple derivations in a particular order. A derivation refers to a one-channel recording of potential differences between the members of the electrode pair connected to the input terminals of that channel, and a montage refers to a collection of derivations from multiple channels simultaneously recorded and arranged in a specified order, which determines which derivation will appear in a particular channel.

Without regard to the particular order in which derivations appear, there are two basic types of electroencephalographic montage, one referential, and one sequential and bipolar. The referential montage has two or more exploring electrodes attached to input terminal 1 on two or more channels, and their potential differences are measured with respect to one common reference electrode attached to terminal 2 in each of the channels (Fig. 8–2). The sequential bipolar montage refers to a collection of two or more channels recording from a sequence of three or more electrodes in such a way that each electrode within the sequence appears as a common electrode in two channels that usually lie adjacent to each other as shown in Figure 8–2. The common electrode appears on opposite terminals in these two channels. In the upper channel, it is applied to terminal 2 and is compared with the electrode that precedes it in the sequence and is attached to terminal 1. In the lower channel, the common electrode is connected to terminal

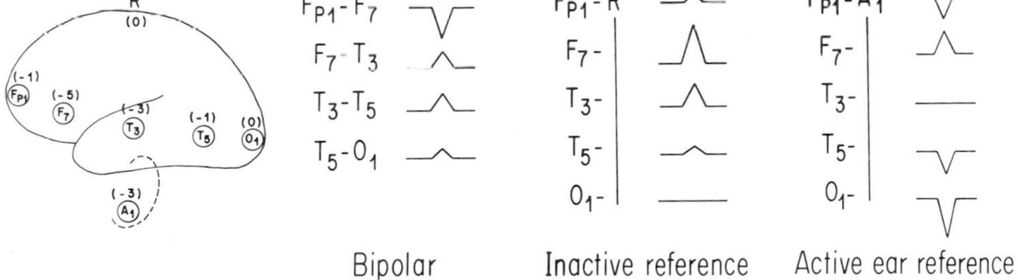

Figure 8–2 Schematic representation showing how F_7 can be identified as relatively more negative than the two electrodes (F_{P1} and T_3) that surround it in the temporal sequence from F_{P1} to O_1. With the sequential bipolar technique, this is indicated by a convergent phase reversal between the first and second channels that share F_7 as the common electrode. With an inactive reference, the pen deflection in all channels is upward, and F_7 is recognized as relatively more negative because it produces more upward pen deflection than the two electrodes that surround it. With an active reference, there is phase reversal in the referential recording, but once again, F_7 is recognized as relatively more negative because it produces more upward pen deflection than does F_{P1} (which actually produces downward pen deflection) and T_3 (which produces no pen deflection when compared with the active ear reference). To prove that F_7 is actually a surface peak of negativity, it would be necessary to prove that it is also relatively more negative than the electrodes immediately surrounding it in the transverse dimension.

1 and is compared with the electrode that follows it in the sequence and is connected to terminal 2.

Regardless of whether the basic derivations within a montage are referential or bipolar, they can be organized into a bewildering variety of different orders. To allow for relatively easy translation from a localization on the electroencephalogram to a localization on the surface of the head, however, it is recommended that standard montages be used that reflect the sequential or at least the symmetrical anatomical origins of the derivations in orderly fashion. The order in which the channels are connected should produce a record that can be read from above downward to reflect the anterior-to-posterior order of derivations originating along one longitudinal line or the left-to-right order of derivations originating along a transverse line. Derivations that originate along transverse lines may also be arranged to reflect the symmetry of their origins about the midline. In such cases, the channels are connected alternately, one to the left side and the next to the symmetrically located site on the right side, until all sites on the transverse line are covered. The derivations then reflect the left-to-right order in which they originate in the transverse dimension.

Whether sequential bipolar runs or referential runs are used, the detection of a local peak of potential activity depends on proving that one electrode simultaneously has the same relative sign with respect to the two electrodes that surround it in the longitudinal dimension and to the two other electrodes that surround it in the transverse dimension.

With sequential bipolar runs, an electrode can be identified as being over a local peak if it simultaneously produces the same type of phase reversal in both longitudinal and transverse bipolar sequences that cross through it and share it as a common electrode. Phase reversal in sequential bipolar runs refers to the simultaneous deflection of pens in opposite directions in the channels that contain a common electrode (see Fig. 8–2). When the common electrode produces a convergent phase reversal in both the longitudinal and transverse sequences, the pens in adjacent channels that share the electrode deflecting toward one another, then that electrode is over a local peak of negativity. If the common electrode produces the opposite type of phase reversal in both longitudinal and transverse sequences, it is over a local peak of positivity.

With a common reference recording, an electrode can be identified as being over a local peak of potential activity if it produces greater-amplitude pen deflection in one direction than does any of the four electrodes surrounding it in the longitudinal and transverse dimensions. This type of localization problem is easy to solve visually when the common reference is located at or outside the boundary of the potential activity being investigated and therefore is either uninvolved or relatively uninvolved by the peak of the potential. In such cases, the pen deflection in all channels is in the same direction, and the exploring electrode that produces a higher upward pen deflection than any four immediately surrounding electrodes is over a peak of negativity (as shown in Figure 8–2); the electrode that produces a greater pen deflection downward than any four immediately surrounding electrodes is over a local peak of positivity.

The problem is more complicated when the reference becomes active because it is located near the peak of a potential being studied with the exploring electrodes. In such situations, phase reversal is seen between some referential channels that contain an exploring electrode near the reference but relatively closer to the peak than the reference and other channels that contain exploring electrodes some distance from and also relatively farther from the peak than the reference (see Fig. 8–2). When such a phase reversal occurs in a referential montage, the reference electrode probably is active, but the peak is still localized under the exploring electrode that produces a pen deflection of greater amplitude in one direction than do any of the four immediately surrounding electrodes. In such cases, the activity of the reference should be checked with bipolar sequences near or through the reference or with a reference that is further removed from the suspected peak.

Finally, the most confusing situation arises when the reference is located over the peak and all exploring electrodes are less active than the reference. In such cases, the amplitudes of the pen deflections become greater the further removed and, therefore, the less active an exploring electrode is with respect to the peak. Although such a situation theoretically can be identified by careful analysis of the pen deflection within the montage, it can be detected much more easily if the referential montage is combined with sequential bipolar montages or if different references are used.

One final point to be emphasized is that, if the same sets of electrodes are used in either a sequential bipolar montage or a referential montage, they will contain equivalent information. The two montages, however, present the information in different ways. In some cases, the sequential bipolar method of presentation may be easier to interpret, and in others, the referential method may be easier. Since the entire purpose of using different montages is to make interpretation as easy as possible, both sequential bipolar and referential derivations should be used.

POTENTIALS OF EXTRACEREBRAL ORIGIN

Extracerebral potentials, often spoken of as artifact, represent electrical potentials that do not originate from the brain. There are four main sources of artifact: the environment, the subject, the instrument, and the interface between the instrument and the subject.

The most common source of environmental artifact is 60-Hz activity from the various alternating-current sources in the laboratory. Appropriate detection and elimination of such artifact is discussed elsewhere.[17] The usual source of the problem is faulty equipment, faulty grounding, or high electrode resistance. In some electrically susceptible patients, such problems may be hazardous as well as a nuisance to the recording.[2] Numerous interesting artifacts that can arise from poor electrode contact are detailed elsewhere.[6] With electrode artifact, almost any waveform can be generated, and other than experience, the most important element in recognizing electrode artifacts is a high degree of suspicion whenever a high-amplitude potential is recorded from one electrode site, with absolutely no reflection in nearby electrodes.

Much more interesting than the extracerebral potentials arising from outside the patient are those that arise from within the patient. These potentials are important because they are an almost invariable feature of the electroencephalogram, and their total absence should arouse suspicion about the technical reliability of the recording. Although usually considered only a nuisance, their appearance in the record sometimes is of diagnostic value.

Spontaneous Ocular Potentials

The source of the spontaneous ocular potential is a direct-current potential difference of 5 to 10 μv between the relatively more positive cornea and the relatively more negative retina. Being a direct-current potential, it will not be detected by the conventional alternating-current resistance-capacitance–coupled electroencephalographic amplifier unless there is movement of the eye or eyelid.[17] A blink, with mainly movement of the eyelid, enhances spread of the positive corneal-retinal potential up to the forehead, producing a positive deflection concomitant with each blink.[17] Movement of the eye in any direction induces relative positivity on the electrodes toward which it moves and relative negativity on the electrodes away from which it moves, which allows lateral eye movements in the temporal leads to be easily detected (see Fig. 8–22). Occasionally, recorded nystagmus is the only positive electroencephalographic evidence of brain stem disease. The eye movement responsible for the potentials can often be recognized by the technician. The potentials are otherwise recognized by their characteristic distribution, being maximum in the more anterior derivations and falling off exponentially in the more posterior derivations.

Evoked Retinal Potentials—the Electroretinogram

The graded electrical response of the retina to flashes of light (the electroretinogram) is uniformly detected when high amplifications (sensitivity of 1 microvolt per millimeter) are used in recordings involving suspected cerebral death. The origin of the response can easily be recognized by its characteristic one to one relationship to the photic stimulus, its location in the anterior head regions, and its unilateral attenuation when one eye is covered (Fig. 8–3). This is

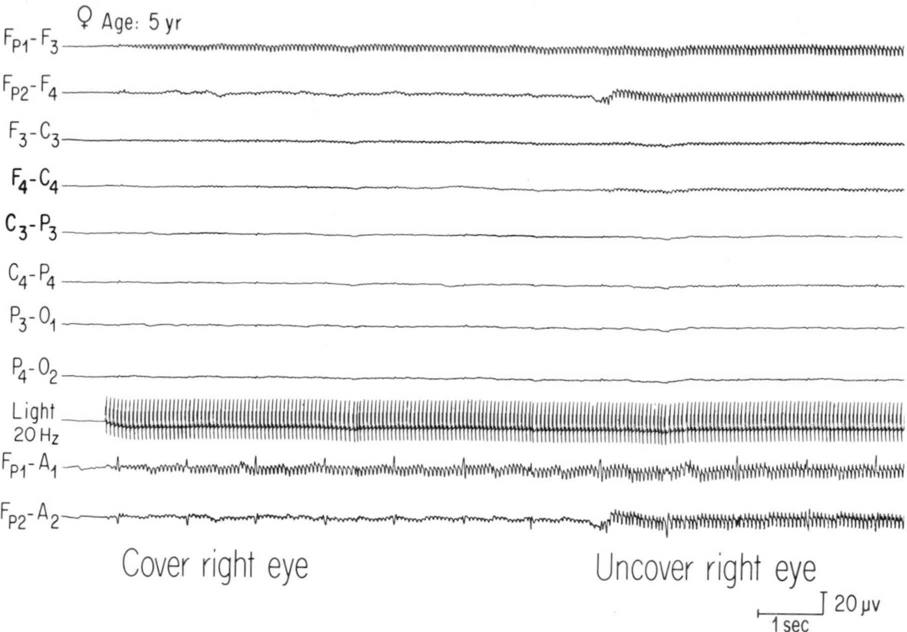

Figure 8–3 The effect on the electroretinogram of covering one eye. Electrocerebral inactivity and a well-developed electroretinogram recorded from F_{P1} and F_{P2} in response to photic stimulation are shown. In addition to its characteristic location, the attenuation of this response on the right by covering the right eye further confirms the retinal origin of the potential.

another expected extracerebral potential that is valuable in identifying the integrity of the recording system in tests for suspected cerebral death.

Myogenic Potentials

These are commonly present, and although usually only a nuisance, they may

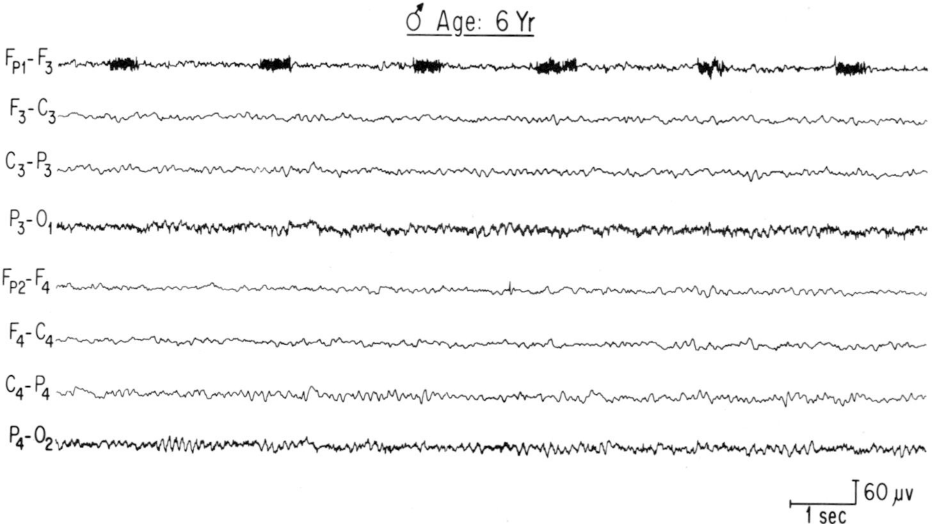

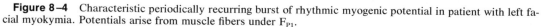

Figure 8–4 Characteristic periodically recurring burst of rhythmic myogenic potential in patient with left facial myokymia. Potentials arise from muscle fibers under F_{P1}.

be of significant diagnostic value, pointing to brain stem abnormalities or abnormalities of the cranial nerves.[25] Important diagnostic types of electromyographic activity include the rhythmic type that is characteristic of facial myokymia shown in Figure 8–4, the characteristic increasing myogenic potentials associated with hemifacial spasm, and the very rhythmic myogenic potentials associated with palatal myoclonus.

Glossokinetic Potentials

These are due to movements of the charged tongue (the tip is relatively negative and the base is relatively positive). On the basis of their association with tongue movement and a different spatial distribution, glossokinetic potentials can be differentiated from eye movement potentials and potentials of cerebral origin.

Potentials of Cardiovascular Origin

Electrocardiographic potentials often can be detected on the head, especially when high gains are used. These potentials can be of diagnostic aid because some patients may have cardiac arrhythmia that is detected only on the electroencephalogram (Fig. 8–5). Pulsation of arteries can cause a rhythmic artifact because of varying contact resistance of an electrode near the artery.

Potentials Related to Movement

Potentials related to respiratory movements are not commonly seen except at high amplification, but the detection of respiratory activity with or without special monitoring techniques sometimes identifies characteristic patterns such as Cheyne-Stokes respiration or sleep apnea. In such cases, special transducers may be helpful for detection of respiratory air flow. Rhythmic tremor may be detected for a variety of reasons, including electrode movement and movement-induced changes in capacitive or inductive coupling. Rhythmic movement-induced artifacts may be identified by the technician or by associated rhythmic myogenic potentials and, if necessary, with extracerebral electrodes or an accelerometer to monitor movement.

POTENTIALS OF CEREBRAL ORIGIN

Normal Spontaneous Potentials

The cerebral potentials recorded with scalp electrodes represent summated dendritic potentials arising from large populations of neurons—in the order of 10^5 or more.[20] Action potentials, because of their short time course, do not contribute to the activity recorded with scalp macroelectrodes. All potential generators, whether cerebral or extracerebral, behave as dipoles; that is, the generator must have two poles, one relatively negative and the other relatively positive with respect to each other. This dipolar electrical generator relationship on neurons results when synaptic activity is unevenly distributed along the apical and basilar neuronal surface. The pyramidal cells, considered to be the major contributors of these potentials, are perpendicular to the cortex. This perpendicular orientation explains why cerebral electrical generators often show opposite polarity when recorded on the surface and when recorded in the depth—the surface electrodes detect one pole and the depth electrodes detect the opposite pole.

Normal electroencephalographic patterns vary considerably with the age and the alertness of the patient. In patients between 20 and 60 years old, however, the following regional patterns are frequently seen in the normal waking state. (A particular pattern is discussed under a given region if its boundary is confined to that region or, in the case of more widespread patterns, if its peak is usually located in that region.)

Occipital Patterns

Alpha rhythm is a bilateral, symmetrical, posterior, sustained 8- to 13-Hz rhythmic pattern with recurrent peak-to-trough amplitudes usually in the 20- to 60-μv range (Fig. 8–6). When present, this rhythm is activated or accentuated during the eyes-closed, mentally relaxed waking state and is attenuated by such factors as eye open-

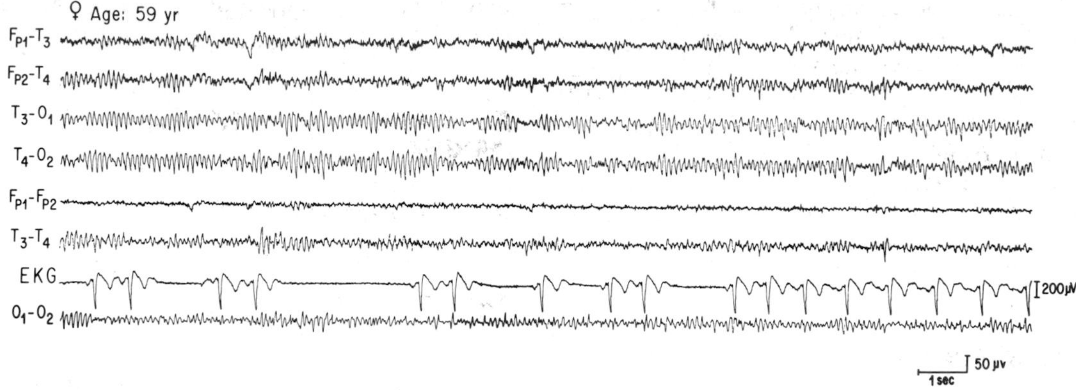

Figure 8–5 Electroencephalogram with electrocardiographic monitoring (channel 7) was the first study to demonstrate the cardiac origin of the patient's recurrent spells of a tingling sensation in the head and a feeling that she might black out. Previous prolonged cardiac monitoring had, by chance, been carried out during an asymptomatic interval.

ing, mental activity, and drowsiness. Alpha rhythm itself is defined by its location, its reactivity, and its frequency. Neuronal generators in the posterior head regions may, however, produce activity with the same distribution and same reactivity pattern but in different frequency bands, such as the beta or theta bands. This type of activity in the beta band is always normal and is called a fast alpha variant pattern. Activity in the theta frequency band—the slow alpha variant—may be normal if it is harmonically related to activity that is in the alpha frequency band and if it shows the same reactivity and spatial distribution as this harmonically related activity.[4] In an adult, however, the presence of posterior activity that is always 7 Hz or less without any associated faster frequencies is a distinctly abnormal finding.

Central Patterns

The central regions at times generate a recognizable rhythm often referred to as the mu rhythm. This type is a spontaneous bilateral but often asymmetrical and asynchronous rhythm that is usually maximal in the centroparietal area and occurs in either sustained or short trains, usually with a frequency in the alpha range. This activity is most apparent when the patient

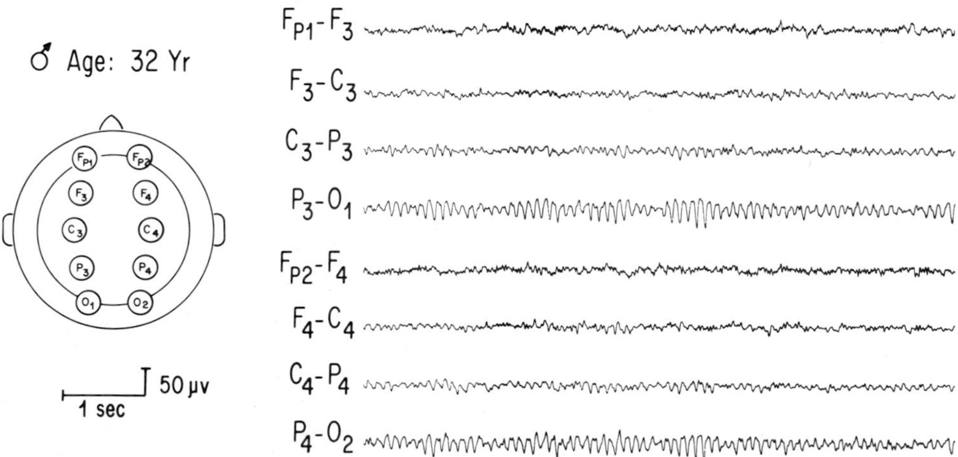

Figure 8–6 Normal alpha rhythm of adult patient during wakefulness with eyes closed is seen maximally over occipital regions (channels 4 and 8).

is relaxed and not moving any extremities or receiving somatosensory stimuli. Mu rhythm is attenuated by movement of an extremity or by somatosensory stimuli delivered to the extremities. Although it is often bilateral in response to a unilateral stimulus of movement, the attenuation may sometimes be more prominent or present only contralaterally. This type of central activity often has a distinctive morphological pattern, the so-called mu form, in which the positive phase has a round contoured peak and the negative phase has a sharp peak. This distinctive waveform accounts for the name attached to this rhythm—the mu rhythm. A central rhythmic pattern satisfying all these criteria may be present in as many as 34 per cent of normal subjects. If the distinctive mu waveform is not required, however, a central rhythm with all these reactive characteristics can be seen in a significantly higher percentage of patients. In addition to the mu rhythm, the central areas may generate an associated beta-range activity with a similar distribution and pattern of reactivity, which at times may be harmonically related to the mu rhythm in the alpha frequency range.

Frontocentral Patterns

The frontocentral regions may show activity of variable frequency. Beta-range activity, which is nonreactive to movement of an extremity, frequently is maximal in this distribution, and although beta activity may be relatively confined to this area, it frequently has a much more widespread distribution. In most normal adults, beta activity is of low voltage (less than 20 μv). Beta rhythm is usually continuous and may increase in amplitude during drowsiness, but it commonly disappears during the spindle stage of sleep. This low-amplitude, anteriorly maximal, nonreactive beta activity with its more widespread distribution may be seen in normal adults who are not receiving medication, but beta activity becomes increasingly higher in amplitude and more widespread with the use of certain sedative drugs.

Temporal Patterns

The temporal regions may show a wide variety of activity during the waking state. The posterior temporal regions usually generate the normal alpha rhythm. In addition to this more sustained activity, the temporal regions may generate asymmetrical single and serial transient waveforms that become increasingly prominent with age and drowsiness and that have to be distinguished from abnormal activity occurring in the temporal area.[16]

As subjects fall asleep, the electroencephalogram undergoes sequential alterations as the subjects pass through various stages of non-REM or slow-wave sleep that may be classified into stages of drowsiness, light sleep, and deeper sleep. In the adult, the onset of drowsiness is frequently associated with roving eye movement, which is easily detected in montages with temporal coverage. With drowsiness, the previous alpha rhythm often disappears and may be replaced by low-voltage, mixed-frequency activity or by rhythmic theta-range activity. These replacements represent normal drowsiness patterns in the occipital area. In contrast, the frontocentral beta rhythms ordinarily persist, and their amplitude may even increase during drowsiness. Single and serial slow waves of cerebral origin occurring independently in either temporal area become more prominent during drowsiness. As the patient descends further into sleep, various characteristic single and serial slow-wave components develop, as well as rhythmic faster components. During sleep, as during the waking state, a very distinctive difference exists among patterns seen in the occipital regions, the preoccipital parasagittal regions, and the temporal regions.

Occipital Sleep Patterns

During the later stages of drowsiness and light sleep, single and repetitive sharp occipitally positive transient waveforms are frequently seen, and their amplitude is usually less than 50 μv. These are called "positive occipital sharp transients of sleep," or "posts," and represent a normal phenomenon.

Preoccipital Parasagittal Sleep Patterns

The activity in the preoccipital parasagittal region during lighter and deeper levels of sleep is characterized by a mixture of slower components occurring singly, seri-

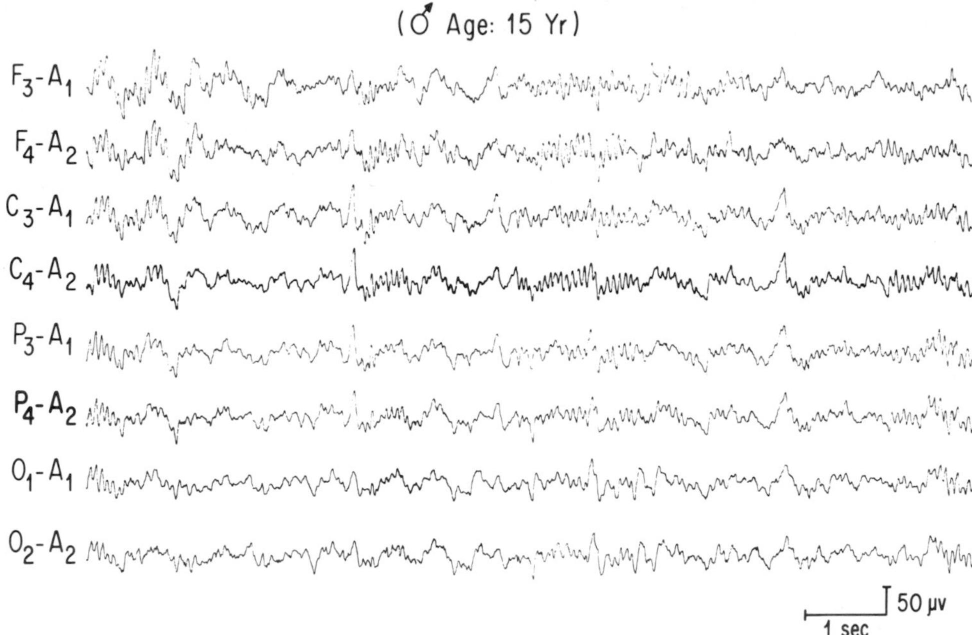

Figure 8–7 Normal electroencephalogram of 15-year-old patient during sleep shows intermittent burst of waxing and waning rhythmic 14-Hz spindles intermixed with slower and at times somewhat sharply contoured vertex waves, maximal in the centroparietal region.

ally, and maximally in the vertex regions (the vertex waves) as well as by brief, intermittent bursts of waxing and waning of 14-Hz waves also generally maximal in the central midline regions (sleep spindles) (Fig. 8–7). The slower vertex waves and the faster 14-Hz sleep spindles may occur independently or together as a complex (at which time they are termed "K-complexes"), either spontaneously or in response to stimulus. As sleep deepens, single and serial slow waves often occur with more widespread distribution, maximal in the frontal area—the so-called F-waves of sleep. In addition, as sleep deepens, the spindle activity may slow in frequency to 12 Hz and may develop a frontal maximum rather than the central maximum usually seen with the 14-Hz spindles. The other important feature as sleep deepens is the appearance of more continuous, irregular, generalized delta activity, and with deeper levels of sleep, the record is dominated by this latter pattern.

Temporal Sleep Patterns

Various nonspecific and unimportant temporal transients seen during the awake state and accentuated during drowsiness fortunately disappear during lighter and deep sleep. The posterior temporal regions in younger people, however, frequently generate a distinctive pattern consisting of intermittent bursts of arch-shaped waves with a sharply contoured positive component most commonly at a frequency of 14 or 6 Hz (or both) currently termed "the 14- and 6-Hz positive burst" and previously called "the 14- and 6-Hz positive spikes." The majority of early workers almost universally considered these abnormal, but the commonly held current opinion is that they represent an interesting type of sleep activity without any clinical significance.[8,21]

Other electrographic patterns occurring during sleep that may be confused with significant abnormalities include the so-called small sharp spikes, which in themselves are of no definite clinical significance and must be distinguished from significant spikes that have a clinical correlation with seizures, as discussed in a following section.

Abnormal Potentials

Electroencephalographic abnormalities may be conceptually divided into two general types: the distortion and ultimate dis-

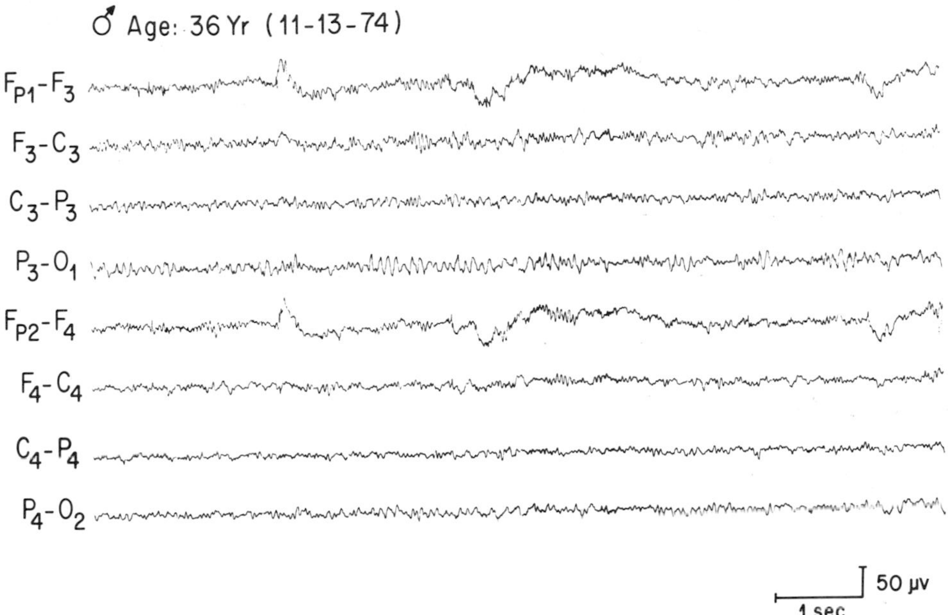

Figure 8–8 Significant asymmetry with right-sided reduction of normal components in patient with Sturge-Weber syndrome involving right side of brain. Interestingly, the patient presented only with focal seizures and was free of any interictal neurological deficit in spite of abnormality in the electroencephalogram.

appearance of rhythms, both normal and abnormal; and the appearance of abnormal rhythm, with or without significant disturbance of the normal rhythm.

Some overlap of these two types exists, inasmuch as some abnormal rhythms may be related to a distortion of previously normal rhythms. The distortion and disappearance of rhythms, as well as the appearance of abnormal rhythms, may occur in various distributions, including a regional or hemispheric distribution, a bilateral (symmetrical or asymmetrical) distribution, and a unilateral distribution.

When normal rhythms are distorted unilaterally in a regional or hemispheric distribution, the distortion produces asymmetry of amplitude, frequency, or reactivity of the rhythm. Such asymmetry, if major, is usually associated with focal cerebral disease (Fig. 8–8). The most extreme type of abnormality that can exist is the disappearance of all rhythms, normal and abnormal, in a bilateral, generalized fashion—the so-called state of electrocerebral inactivity or silence seen in cerebral death as well as in coma from some reversible causes such as drugs and, rarely, hypothermia (see Fig. 8–3).

The abnormal rhythms may be sustained, that is, present most or all of the time, or they may occur intermittently. The intermittency is characterized by the sudden appearance and disappearance of the waveform and is called a "paroxysmal abnormality." Most abnormal rhythms—whether sustained or intermittent—are nonspecific either because they do not have a distinctive pattern or because their distinctive pattern is not associated with a specific pathological condition or a specific cause (Figs. 8–8, 8–9, 8–10, and 8–11). Some patterns usually occurring paroxysmally, however, are more specific in that they have a distinctive waveform (such as a spike, spike and wave, sharp wave, a seizure pattern, or relatively specific periodic complexes) (Figs. 8–12 through 8–19). In addition to having a distinctive form, the specific patterns also have a high degree of correlation with either a specific disorder, such as epilepsy, or a relatively specific etiological condition, such as subacute sclerosing panencephalitis, Jakob-Creutzfeldt disease, or another disorder, as described in the section on encephalopathies and coma. The nonspecific abnormalities are more indicative of underlying signifi-

Text continued on page 214.

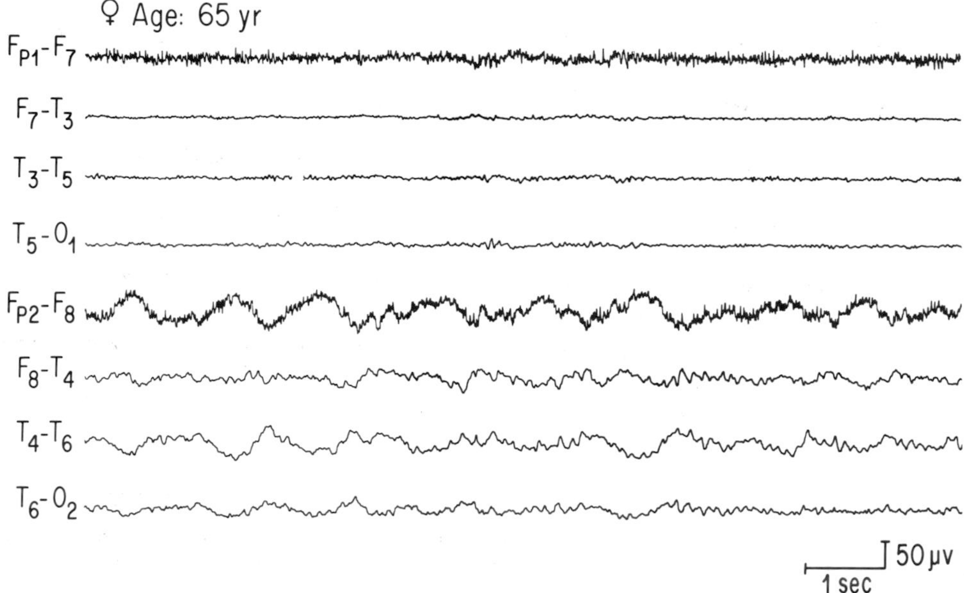

Figure 8–9 Focal sustained and irregular delta range slowing is characteristic of an underlying cerebral lesion, in this case, glioma of the right temporal lobe, although it is not specific for a particular cause. In addition to delta range slowing, background frequencies are also slowed, mainly into theta frequency range.

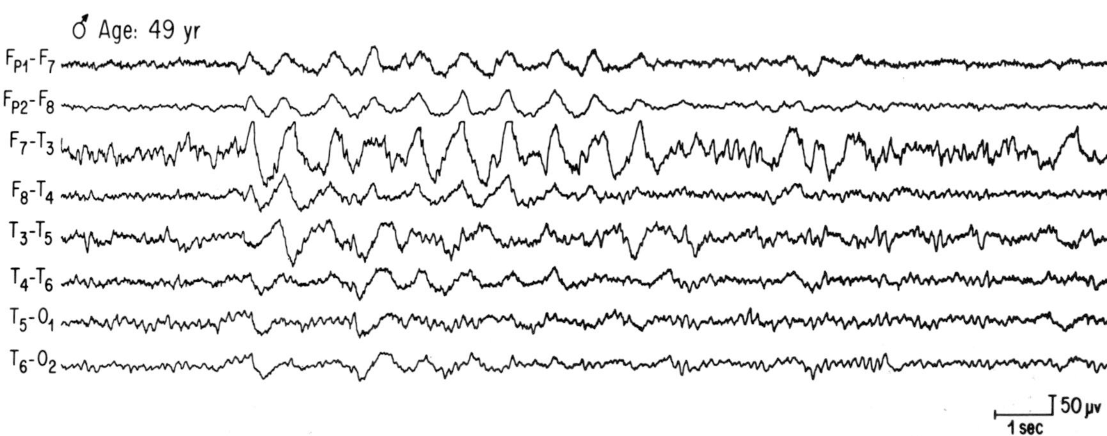

Figure 8–10 In addition to sustained irregular delta activity and slowing of background in left temporal area (see channels 3 and 5), the electroencephalogram shows bilateral high amplitude and more widespread rhythmic slowing lasting for about 10 waves. This paroxysmal rhythmic slowing (frontal intermittent rhythmic delta activity) is often called a "projected rhythm" or "rhythm at a distance" because it is often far removed from a source of focal disease. Furthermore, this type of abnormality is nonspecific, being seen in almost any type of acute disease whether it is associated with a focal cerebral lesion, as in this case of recurrent left temporal glioma, or a diffuse encephalopathy (see Fig. 8–11).

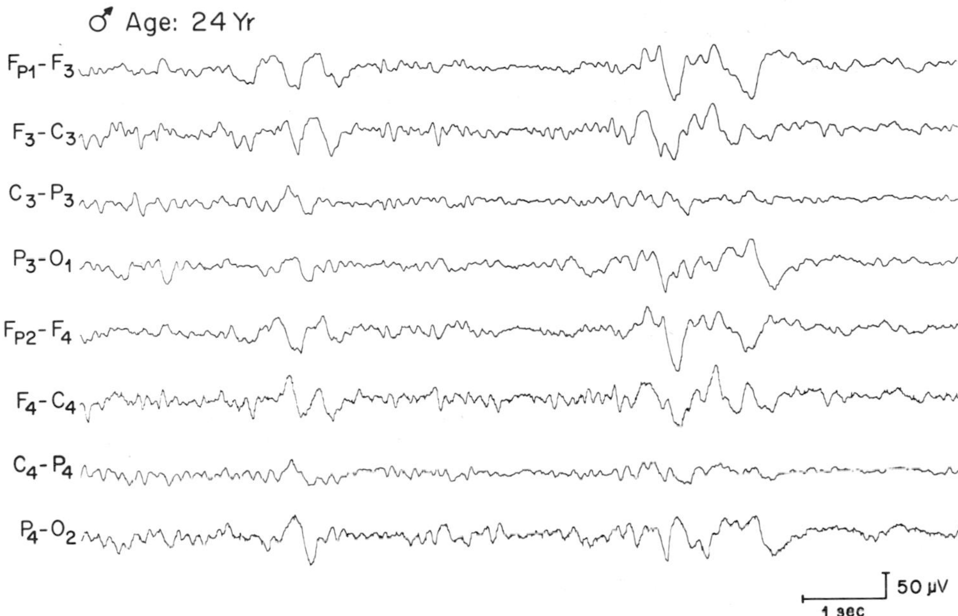

Figure 8–11 The type of persistent slowing in background into the 7-Hz range as well as low-amplitude generalized irregular delta slowing frequently seen in acute encephalopathies regardless of cause. In addition, some of these cases will show paroxysms of higher-amplitude intermittent rhythmic slowing (in this case of uremia [urea >400, mental confusion] one paroxysm begins approximately three seconds after the sample begins and another ends about three seconds before the sample ends). This type of paroxysmal rhythmic activity, as noted in Figure 8–10, is nonspecific, being seen in many acute cerebral disturbances whether of a diffuse or focal nature.

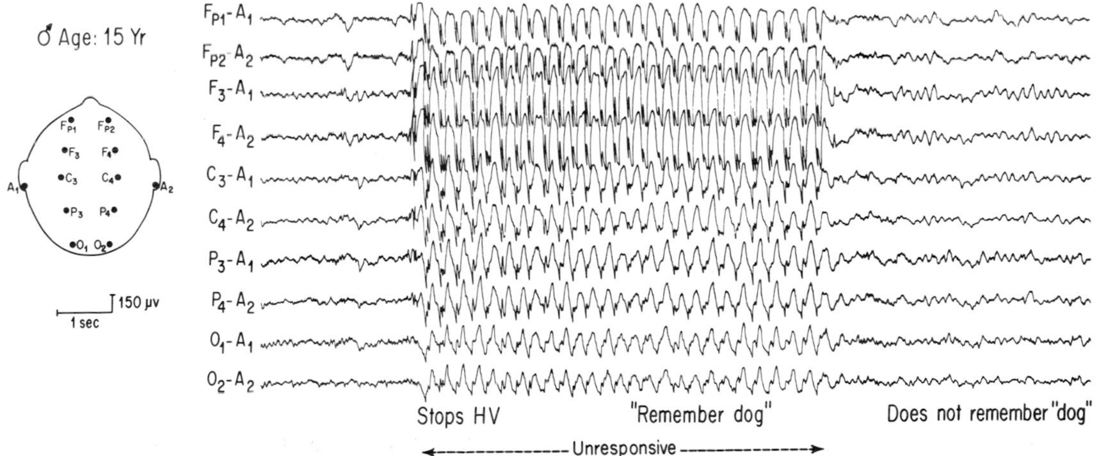

Figure 8–12 Classic nonevolving generalized three-per-second spike and wave discharge associated with typical petit mal absence. During paroxysm, patient was unresponsive and did not remember word presented to him.

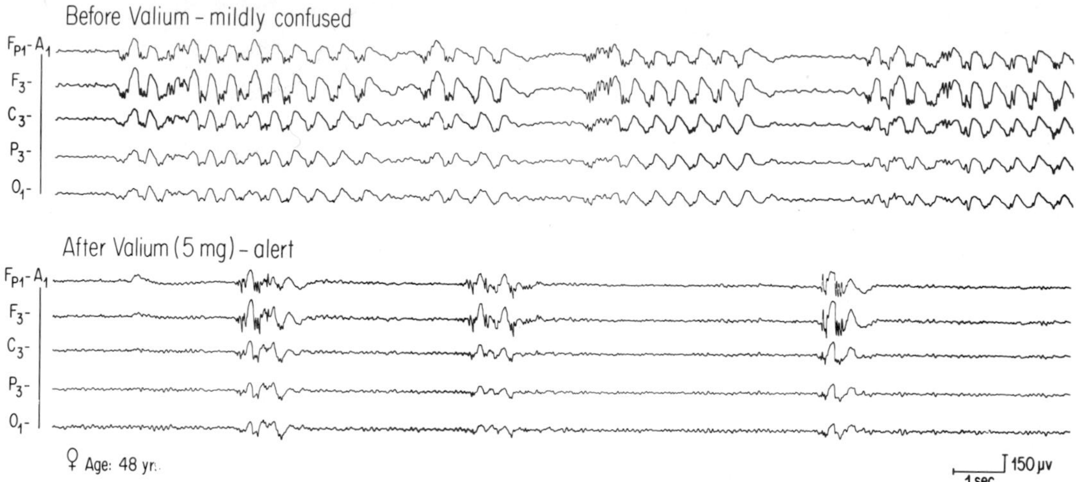

Figure 8–13 Absence status. The main difference between the nonevolving spike and wave seizure pattern associated with the absence status and the interictal spike and wave burst is primarily increased duration and persistence of the burst during the absence status.

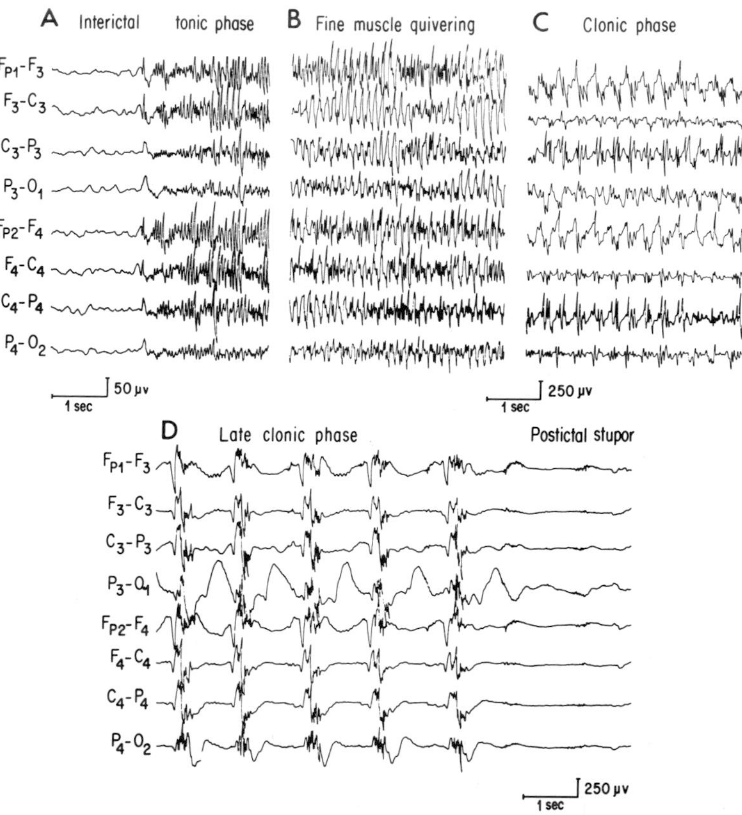

Figure 8–14 Marked evolution of electroencephalographic seizure pattern associated with typical tonic-clonic grand mal convulsion. Tonic phase is initiated by high-frequency generalized seizure discharge, *A*. As cerebral electric discharge progressively slows in frequency, tonic phase gradually gives way to low-amplitude quivering as clonic phase begins, *B*. As seizure progresses, frequency of seizure discharge slows further, and interval between clonic jerks becomes progressively longer, *C* and *D*, until seizure terminates in postictal stupor after last clonic jerk (last several segments of *D*). It is instructive to compare the marked evolution of the seizure pattern in this tonic-clonic seizure with the relative lack of evolution of the seizure pattern in the typical absence seizure (see Fig. 8–12).

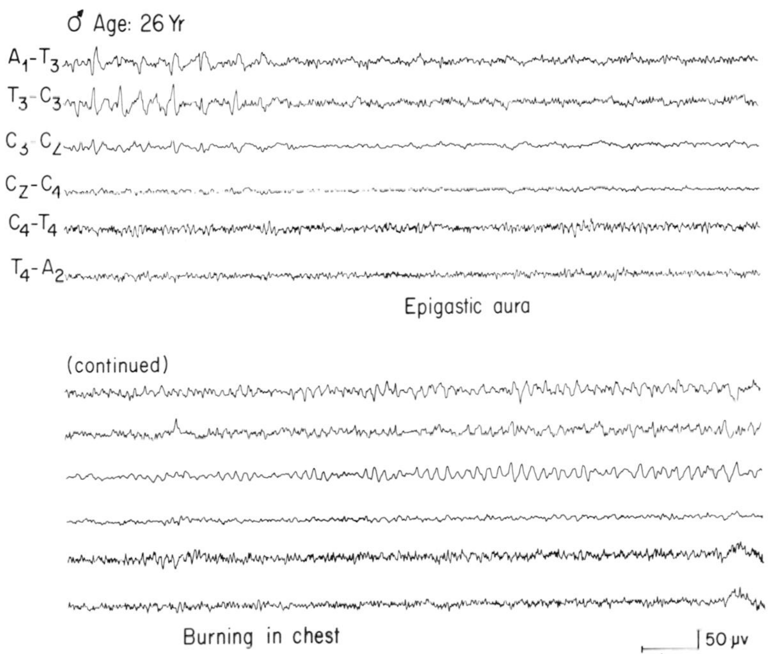

Figure 8–15 Sudden attenuation of repetitive interictal left temporal spikes (first seconds of the upper segment) at onset of patient's clinical left temporal lobe seizure, characterized by epigastric aura. It is not until later on in the seizure (when subjective symptoms of burning in chest develop) that the rhythmic evolving alpha-range seizure discharge becomes apparent at the scalp (lower segment). Note striking difference between rhythmic evolving seizure pattern associated with symptoms and interictal spike not associated with symptoms.

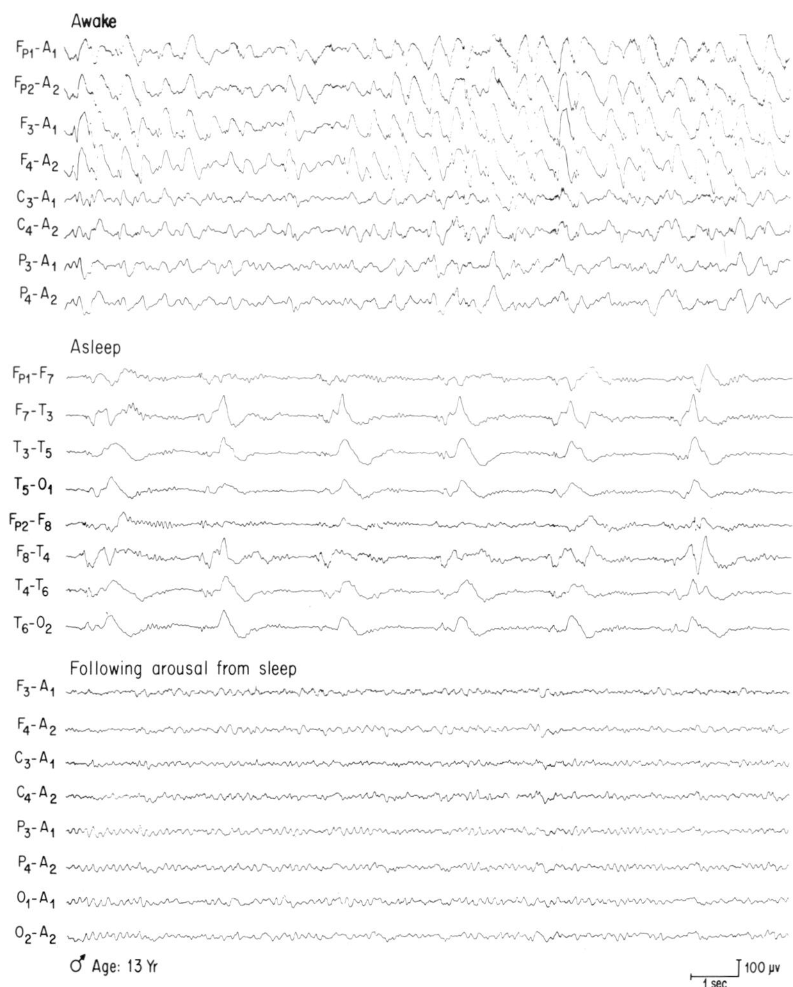

Figure 8–16 Sleep may bring out the periodically recurring stereotyped complexes characteristic of subacute sclerosing panencephalitis at a time when the waking trace fails to show them. The interval between stereotyped complexes is usually more than four seconds, although in this case, it is only three seconds.

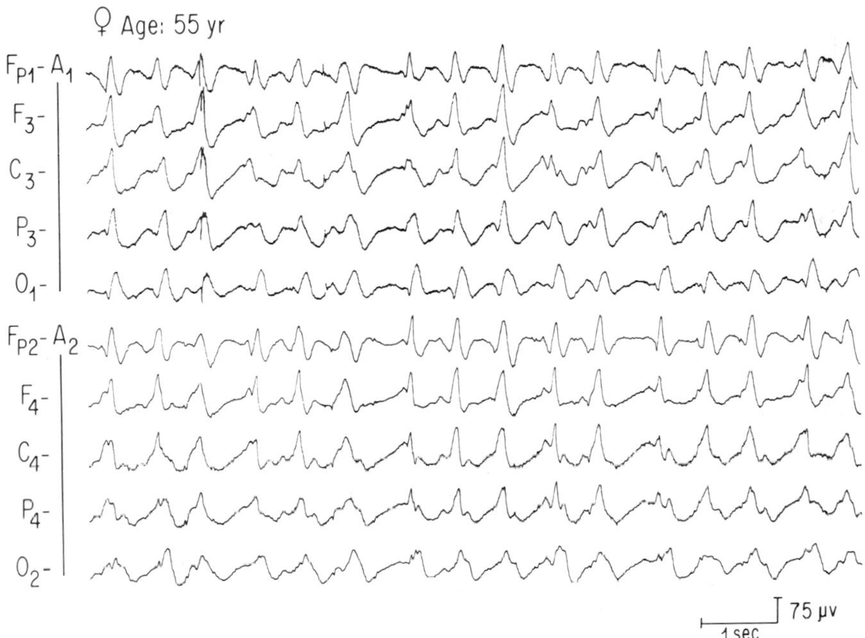

Figure 8–17 Generalized bilateral periodically recurring sharp and slow wave complexes characteristically seen in Jakob-Creutzfeldt disease, especially when the patient reaches the stage of mental deterioration with beginning myoclonic jerks. Interval between complexes in this disease is usually less than one second, as is the case here.

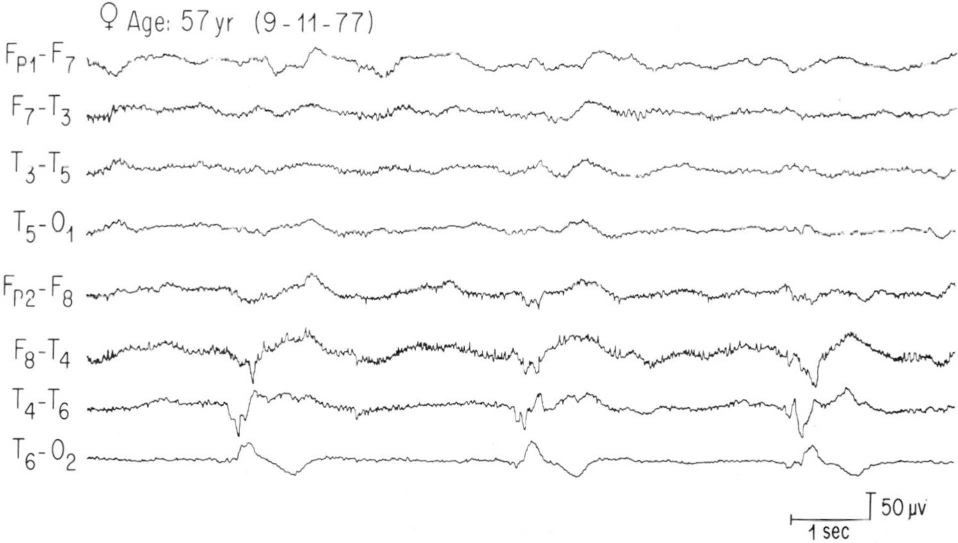

Figure 8–18 Herpes simplex encephalitis. Right-sided periodically recurring lateralized epileptiform discharges may be seen with any acute potentially epileptogenic condition involving the brain. When these complexes are seen in a patient who has a short-duration febrile illness with recent focal neurological signs, however, the possibility of herpes simplex encephalitis must be considered if focal structural disease can be excluded. A computed tomographic scan at the time of this electroencephalogram showed no abnormality. There had been fever for six days, focal signs for two days, and coma for one day.

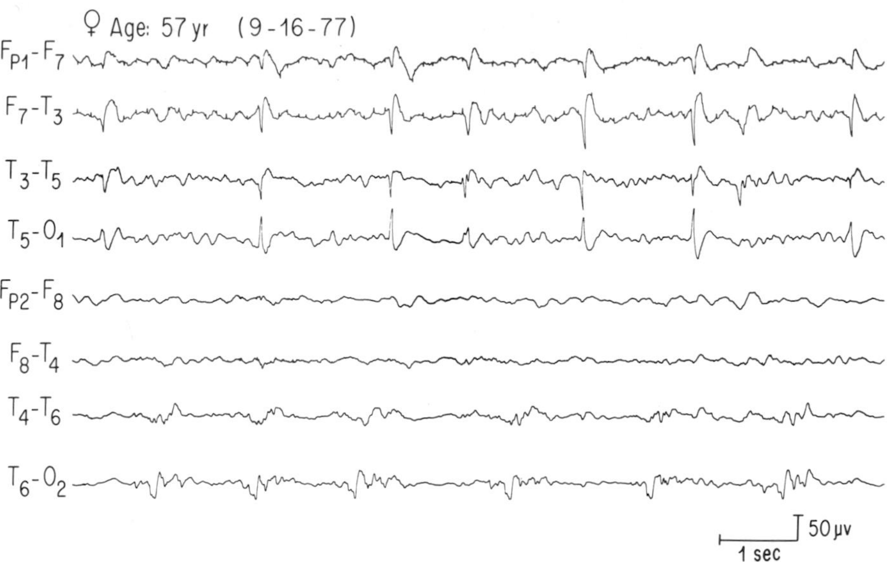

Figure 8–19 Five days after the first electroencephalogram (shown in Figure 8–18), independent periodic lateralized epileptiform discharges developed on the left at a time when the periodic epileptiform discharges on the right (see the last two channels) were becoming less prominent. These sequential findings, taken in context with the clinical history, are almost diagnostic of herpes simplex encephalitis, which was ultimately confirmed. At this time, fever had lasted 11 days, focal signs 7 days, and coma 6 days.

cant pathological change if they are more sustained and nonreactive and in the delta frequency range with an irregular waveform (see Figs. 8–9 and 8–10). Such findings, if they occur focally, are commonly associated with an underlying focal change, although they do not in themselves indicate a specific cause.

Once the abnormalities have been identified, they should be classified in terms of their degree of abnormality, their localization, and the various known types of abnormality.[8,16] Unfortunately, there is no uniform, accepted standard for classifying electroencephalographic abnormalities, and one simply has to use the system that he inherits at his local institution or design his own. Regardless of the specific system, a valid classification provides an abbreviated summary of the individual recording that is convenient for conveying the results to knowledgeable clinicians as well as subdividing the electroencephalograms into groups that are then useful for retrieval and review. Finally, a system of classification is useful for assessing the uniformity of interpretation among different readers.[8] Whatever system is used, the general concept is as follows: The so-called mildly abnormal records may be without clinical significance, both in a control group and in a disease population, although abnormality is generally more frequent in the disease population than in the control group. The percentage of abnormalities in the electroencephalogram associated with clinically significant conditions increases to the point that, by the time severe abnormalities appear, they are almost always associated with definable alteration in function.[16]

Important to remember is that patients who do not have clinically significant neurological disease may have "abnormal electroencephalographic findings." Therefore, classification is only the first step in the clinical use of electroencephalography, and the finding also must be related to the overall clinical picture. The ability to interpret the electroencephalogram meaningfully depends not only on the skill in detecting and classifying the abnormality but also on the neurological knowledge and expertise of the reader. The electroencephalogram is much like the neurological examination except that clinical abnormalities are replaced by electrical abnormalities; in each test, the abnormalities must be related to the overall clinical picture and course. For instance, a major unilateral abnormality in one hemisphere is analogous to major hemiparesis in that its significance depends on the context in which it occurs, that is, the age of the patient, how long the lesion has been present, and whether the lesion is changing or not. The electroencephalogram is also like the clinical examination in that a specific etiological diagnosis seldom can be made on the basis of findings in one examination.

To understand when the electroencephalographic, the neurological, or the radiographic examination will or will not show abnormal reactions to a pathological process, we must always consider that various diseases themselves have different dynamic spatial and temporal variability characteristics that will influence the appearance of abnormality on only one, on all, or on various combinations of these examinations.[8] The spatial characteristics that increase the likelihood of producing an abnormal electroencephalogram are involvement near the surface of the brain and involvement of wider areas. The more acute the process, the more likelihood that significant abnormalities can be detected. A process that is diffuse and infiltrating may produce major electrical abnormalities and clinical change before obvious change is visible on the radiographic examinations, including computed tomography. A lesion located far from the cortex, however, that does not produce secondary alteration in consciousness, that is small and either slowly growing or static, but that has a density different from that of normal brain usually would be easily detected on radiographic tests such as the computed tomographic scan but might be completely missed by the electroencephalogram and the clinical examination if specific pathways were not involved. Finally, if the pathological process produces epileptogenic activity, it is more likely that the electroencephalogram will detect the abnormality even when the patient shows no abnormality on neurological examination and has normal radiographic studies.

Localized brain stem lesions without secondary obstruction of the cerebrospinal fluid pathways frequently do not alter the electroencephalogram. Fortunately, with newer electrophysiological tests, such as the brain stem auditory evoked potential studies discussed later, brain stem abnormalities can be detected when the electroencephalogram is normal and at times even before signs become obvious on the clinical or radiographic examination.[23]

Reaction to Activating Procedures and Stimuli

Activating Procedures

An activating procedure is any procedure designed to enhance or elicit normal or abnormal electrical activity.[14] In electroencephalography, it is most commonly used to elicit specific epileptiform patterns or evidence of focal abnormality.

Three minutes of hyperventilation are routinely used in most patients except those who have recently suffered subarachnoid hemorrhage or who for some other reason should not be stressed. This type of hyperventilation commonly elicits three-per-second spike and wave bursts in patients with typical petit mal absence seizures. Although less frequently eliciting abnormalities in complex partial seizure disorders, hyperventilation is an effective activating procedure, even under these circumstances. With hyperventilation, a bilateral rhythmic slow response is of no diagnostic significance, and only the activation of either specific waveforms or focal abnormalities is of any clinical significance. Also, hyperventilation occasionally produces typical symptoms when the major problem is the hyperventilation syndrome.

A sleep recording is commonly used to elicit either focal or generalized spike or spike and wave discharges. The incidence of specific epileptiform activity in complex partial seizure disorders increases significantly with sleep. Depriving the patient of sleep the night before the test increases the likelihood of obtaining a sleep recording and of producing specific abnormalities. If a patient cannot fall asleep, then various forms of sedation are used routinely. In a sleep recording, it is important not to overinterpret such findings as 14- and 6-Hz positive spikes and small sharp spikes as positive evidence of an underlying seizure disorder.[21]

Brief repetitive flashes from a strobe light delivered at frequencies ranging between 1 and 30 Hz are commonly used as an activating procedure. This test is most useful in patients with generalized seizures and

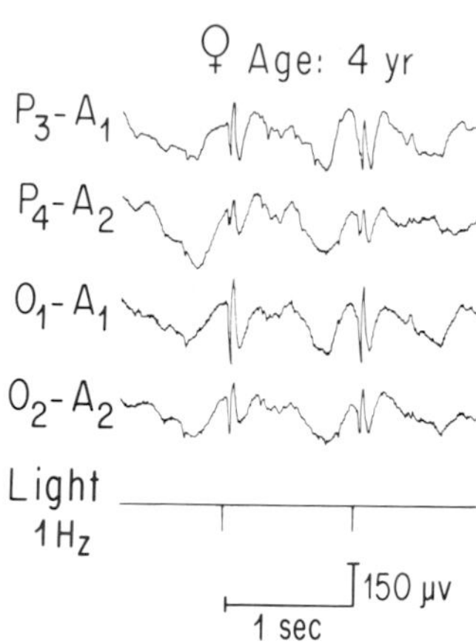

Figure 8–20 Type of high-amplitude spike discharges seen in response to a low flash stimulus that, when taken in context of the clinical history and the abnormality of the resting record, are characteristic of late infantile neuronal lipidosis of the Bielschowsky-Jansky type.

rarely evokes a focal abnormality. Occasionally, slow-frequency flashes evoke enlarged and distorted single responses that may be useful in diagnosis of late infantile cerebromacular degeneration, as described later (Fig. 8–20).[19] The activation of diffuse spike and wave discharges, which become independent of the frequency and duration of the stimulus, is called a photoparoxysmal response, and such activation is most commonly seen in patients with primary generalized epilepsy but may be seen in patients undergoing drug withdrawal or with an acute metabolic disturbance. These abnormal responses of cerebral origin must be differentiated from photomyogenic responses that are repetitive electromyographic discharges time-locked to the stimulus and emanating from the muscles of the anterior or posterior head regions.

In the epilepsies, the most important activating stimulus is the one that the patient has identified as precipitating his individual seizure. For instance, for patients who consistently report that seizures occur within the first 15 or 20 minutes after arousal, the recording should be made during that time. Otherwise, the record may be normal. Other persons who report jaw jerking or more overt seizure manifestations in response to reading should be tested while they are reading. Patients who show hand jerking in response to movement should be tested during such movements. Therefore, although there are some common general activating procedures, those used should be modified according to the patient's clinical history. Otherwise the yield of useful information on the electroencephalogram is reduced.

The intravenous administration of pentylenetetrazol (Metrazol) was formerly a common activating technique. The drug is rarely used now, however, except in an attempt to elicit the patient's characteristic seizure when he is being evaluated as a candidate for an operation. The main reason for not using Metrazol routinely is that it produces generalized convulsive seizures, even in nonepileptic persons; disagreeable subjective symptoms; and generalized nonspecific buildup, which may mask diagnostic focal abnormalities even in patients who have pre-existing focal disease.

Evoked Potentials

Evoked potentials are electrical responses that have a fixed time latency with respect to the eliciting stimuli. These evoked potentials were of interest to earlier workers, and their detection was initially limited to the larger amplitude responses that could be detected without any special technique. These include the so-called K-complexes (a mixture of vertex waves and spindles) that occur in response to stimulus during sleep, as well as epileptiform spikes that occur in response to stimulation, as illustrated in Figure 8–20, and the normal photic driving that may be considered a steady-state evoked response to repetitive flashes of light in contrast to the single transient response that occurs with a single flash. The modern study of evoked potentials did not begin again until Dawson's work in 1947.[7] Ultimately, it has culminated in the present-day computer-summated or averaged evoked potential studies. These studies are based on the phenomenon that, when activity immediately following the stimulus is summated, the evoked potentials with a fixed latency relationship to the stimulus summate much more rapidly than does the spontaneous activity that has a variable latency relationship to the stimulus.

Evoked potential studies can be used in the same way as electroencephalography is used to localize cerebral abnormalities.

Such techniques, however, like the routine electroencephalogram, require multiple channels that are not ordinarily available in evoked potential work, and therefore these studies are not commonly used to localize cerebral lesions.

Evoked potential studies, however, can be used to study conduction times within central pathways, and this measurement requires fewer channels and often reveals information not readily available by other techniques. Study of conduction time in the visual system with pattern stimulation has led to the detection of latent abnormalities in patients with optic neuropathy due to multiple sclerosis or other conditions. This technique appears to be a potentially powerful diagnostic tool and is currently under rapid development.[3]

Generally, evoked potential studies, like the electroencephalogram, sample activities that arise in the cerebral cortex (so-called near-field recording indicating that the electrical field originates in nearby generators). However, Jewett and Williston in 1971 proved that, with proper use of summating and averaging techniques, scalp electrodes could record activity originating at successive levels in the brain stem auditory pathway (potential fields originating from far-removed sources—the so-called far-field responses).[15] This activity is less than 1 μv in amplitude and occurs within the first 10 ms after stimulation. Of the first seven waves, waves 1, 2, 3, and 5 are believed to arise, respectively, from the acoustic nerve, the cochlear nucleus, the superior olive, and the inferior colliculi. The generator loci for the other waves are less well known, but wave 4 probably arises from the nuclei of the lateral lemniscus. Being remarkably constant in a normal control population and not influenced by sleep or most drugs, these waves are extremely useful in physiological studies of brain stem dysfunction. Study of the waves can detect slowing of conduction within the brain stem auditory pathway, giving evidence of brain stem abnormality in patients with multiple sclerosis and intrinsic brain stem tumors before there is clinical or roentgenographic evidence of abnormality.[23] Study of the waves also can differentiate drug coma with electrocerebral silence from postanoxic coma with electrocerebral inactivity. In the former, brain stem responses are preserved; in the latter, they are lost except for that in wave 1 (the eighth nerve potentials). In general, evoked potential studies add a new dimension to electrophysiology, just as computed tomography adds a new dimension to roentgenology. The evoked potential studies do not replace the electroencephalogram but supplement it and add to the potential power of electrophysiological studies by allowing specific sensory system and brain stem functions to be studied directly, whereas the electroencephalogram best reflects general cortical function directly and subcortical and brain stem function only indirectly.

EPILEPSY AND OTHER PAROXYSMAL CONDITIONS

An epileptic seizure is due to paroxysmal, abnormal, and excessive electrical discharge within the brain that results in sudden and usually brief subjective or objective disturbances in neurological behavior. Epilepsy refers to a chronic abnormality within the electrical organization of the brain that results in recurrent epileptic seizures.

The electroencephalogram is an important diagnostic tool in epilepsy, in both the interictal and the ictal states, because the disturbance in neurological behavior characterized as an epileptic seizure is due to abnormal and excessive electrical discharge within the brain and because epilepsy with recurrent seizures is due to a chronic abnormality within the brain's electrical organization.

There are two types of electrical abnormality that have a relatively specific association with epilepsy: interictal and ictal.[9]

The specific interictal abnormalities, often termed "epileptiform abnormalities," refer to distinctive waveforms or complexes that occur paroxysmally, have an easily identifiable form distinguishable from other background activity, and are seen in the interictal records of a significant proportion of patients suffering from epilepsy.[14] These discharges are rarely seen in records from a normal control population or in the records taken from a nonepileptic patient population. Epileptiform abnormalities include spikes or sharp waves, occurring alone or with slow waves, and occurring singly or in serial trains in a regional or generalized distribution.

Besides the interictal epileptiform abnormalities, there are ictal electrographic seizure discharges or seizure patterns, defined as a paroxysmal rhythmic discharge lasting at least several seconds, which usually evolve through several distinct stages, each of which has its own characteristic frequency, form, and distribution. The entire discharge usually begins and ends suddenly. These electroencephalographic seizure patterns are usually seen with the clinical manifestations of the epileptic seizure. The discharges may be seen without overt clinical manifestations, however, and in such cases, they are classified as subclinical or larval seizure patterns.

The electroencephalographic seizure patterns may be subdivided into the relatively nonevolving and the evolving types.[16] An example of the relatively nonevolving seizure discharge is the classic generalized three-per-second spike and wave burst associated with classic petit mal absence attacks (see Fig. 8–12). With the relatively nonevolving ictal discharge, the seizure pattern closely resembles that of the interictal epileptiform discharge. In fact, the only difference between them is that the seizure pattern tends to be more widespread, more rhythmic, and of longer duration and higher amplitude (see Fig. 8–13). Because the ictal pattern with the nonevolving discharge is so morphologically similar to the interictal pattern, however, differentiating between them is sometimes difficult.[9]

In the evolving seizure pattern of the type associated with most clinical seizures other than typical absences, there is often very little resemblance between the morphological appearance of the seizure pattern and the morphological appearance of the interictal epileptiform activity in the same patient (see Fig. 8–15). The evolving seizure pattern, especially at the scalp surface, may express itself merely in terms of attenuation of normal and abnormal interictal pattern, and the subsequent appearance of rhythmic components in one segment may more closely resemble normal rhythmic activity than the usual interictal spikes or sharp waves. The significance of the pattern is recognized by its characteristic paroxysmal onset and termination and its close association with clinical seizures. As mentioned in the original definition, no matter how a seizure pattern is morphologically defined, these patterns can occur without clinical accompaniment. Theoretically, this discrepancy happens because the seizure discharge has to reach a threshold level of intensity and extent before disturbances of clinical function are observable.

Analogies in electrocardiography can be helpful in clarifying the relationship between the interictal epileptiform discharges, which represent an abnormality of electrical organization of the brain that exists when the patient is asymptomatic, and the actual seizure discharge, which represents an excessive neuronal discharge usually associated with the clinical seizure. For example, a brief run of ventricular tachycardia may be detectable on the electrocardiogram of a patient who is totally asymptomatic, but the detection of such an abnormality means that the patient is at high risk of having more prolonged runs of ventricular tachycardia giving rise to symptoms. This relationship is analogous to the brief asymptomatic burst of spike and wave and the more prolonged, relatively nonevolving burst of spike and wave discharges in the electroencephalogram associated with clinical symptoms. In both patients, a close morphological relationship exists between the symptomatic and asymptomatic discharges, and the transition from the symptomatic to the asymptomatic seems to be related mainly to the intensity, extent, and duration of the discharge.

Electrocardiographic abnormalities seen in the asymptomatic patient—for example, multifocal premature ventricular contractions—may give rise to a morphologically different type of symptomatic electrical abnormality, that is, ventricular fibrillation. The electroencephalographic counterpart of this situation is seen when interictal spikes or sharp waves give rise to a morphologically different and evolving seizure pattern (see Figs. 8–14 and 8–15).

In both the electrocardiogram and the electroencephalogram, major abnormalities of rhythm can be found within the record of a patient who has never had symptomatic electrical disturbances of either the heart or the brain. Finally, the absence of specific abnormality, in either modality, does not exclude the possibility that the patient may have significant abnormalities of cardiac or cerebral rhythms giving rise, respectively, to symptomatic cardiac arrhythmias or to epileptic seizures.

In patients suspected of having a seizure disorder, the detection of specific interictal epileptiform discharges not only increases the likelihood that the diagnosis is correct but also may identify the specific location of the discharge. The detection of a focal epileptiform discharge may point out the possibility of previously undetected focal cerebral disease in this area or may distinguish between complex partial seizures and generalized complex absence seizures on the basis of the localization of the discharge, i.e., temporal spikes versus generalized spike and wave discharge, and thus suggest the most appropriate antiepileptic drug treatment. The presence of specific interictal epileptiform activity does not establish with certainty that the patient is having clinical seizures, because specific asymptomatic disturbances of rhythm may occur in patients in whom symptomatic disturbances of rhythm never develop. In neurology and cardiology, the electrical abnormalities always must be correlated with the clinical findings before a final diagnosis and treatment plan are reached. Furthermore, in electroencephalography, a number of patterns can be considered "pseudoepileptiform" because they bear a morphological resemblance to the epileptiform patterns of definite clinical significance. Despite this resemblance, the patterns by themselves have no relationship to conditions that neurologists and neurosurgeons consider as epilepsy. These waveforms include 14- and 6-Hz positive spikes, small sharp spikes, and six-per-second spike and wave.[8,21] Their presence in a record should not be taken as evidence that the patient has epilepsy. If these are the only patterns found, then the record probably gives no more information than does a perfectly normal record.

Just as the presence of an interictal epileptiform abnormality does not establish with certainty that the patient has epilepsy, the absence of a specific interictal abnormality in the electroencephalogram does not exclude epilepsy. The likelihood of detecting a specific epileptiform abnormality in a patient who has epilepsy increases with the duration of the recording, the use of activating procedures, and the nearness in time of the recording to a seizure. Therefore, abnormal findings are more likely to be present in records of patients who have frequent seizures than in those of patients whose seizures are infrequent. Patients who have one or more seizures per day probably will have an interictal electroencephalogram with specific epileptiform abnormality. If a patient is having one or more attacks per day with a normal tracing between attacks, then the attacks may not be of epileptic origin. If this question cannot be answered on the basis of the clinical information, recordings lasting up to eight hours or longer should be done in an attempt to register individual attacks. During a recorded epileptic attack, the electroencephalogram probably will be altered. Findings are always diagnostic in generalized epileptic convulsions, absence seizures, and almost any epileptic attack with overt alteration in the patient's consciousness (see Figs. 8–12 and 8–14). Epileptic seizures are more likely to occur without any surface change in the tracing if the patient experiences only subjective aura or some very localized motor symptoms without loss of consciousness or postictal state. In addition to identifying patients who are having epileptic seizures, the recording of attacks and the monitoring of such parameters as the electrocardiogram may help identify other organic causes for attacks, such as symptomatic cardiac arrhythmia and syncope of various origins, and may even determine whether the patient is simply having functional attacks (see Fig. 8–5).

In medically intractable epilepsy, electroencephalographic recordings are essential for identifying suitable candidates for operation, who ideally should have a single stable interictal epileptiform focus in a relatively nonessential area of the brain such as the temporal pole, the frontal pole, or any region so damaged that it no longer serves any useful physiological function. In addition to these interictal requirements, the evaluation of a potential candidate for an operation should include a recording during one or more clinical seizures in order to determine whether the seizures arise from the region of the interictal focus. Generally, the decision regarding whether the patient is a good candidate for an operation is based on surface interictal and ictal recordings with or without special electrodes. At times, long-term depth recordings may be used to establish with certainty whether the patient's seizures come from one potentially resectable focus, but fortunately this is not always necessary. The short-term use of cortical and depth recordings during resection of an epileptic focus is discussed in a following section.

So far, the discussion has concerned the use of the electroencephalogram in epilepsy in which there is a chronic abnormality within the electrical organization of the brain that gives rise to recurrent seizures. Acute focal or lateralized potentially epileptogenic abnormalities may occur in the brain during the course of any acute focal or lateralized cerebral insult, whether the insult is due to a progressive condition (such as an infection or expanding lesion) or to a transient condition (such as an acute postoperative state, an acute post-traumatic condition, or a recent vascular insult). Less commonly, such acute, potentially epileptogenic abnormalities are secondary to an acute flare-up in a focal seizure disorder. Whatever the cause, the type of electrical abnormality detected between seizure occurrences either may be nonspecific or may show some relatively characteristic findings of such acute conditions as periodic lateralized epileptiform discharges (PLEDs) or subclinical electrographic seizure pattern (see Fig. 8–18).[5] In this acute condition, the epileptogenic capacity of the condition usually diminishes as the acute phase of the disturbance subsides, whether or not there is an underlying progressive pathological process. This is important to recognize. Furthermore, during the acute phase, the patient may have major contralateral neurological deficit and disturbance of consciousness, both of which may show remarkable improvement when the epileptogenic capability of the condition subsides, so long as the causative pathological process is not progressive. In such patients, much of the original deficit, in both disturbance of consciousness and focal signs, probably was secondary to ictal and postictal effects. Also, these conditions do not necessarily result in a chronic epileptogenic abnormality within the organization of the brain, even though the underlying pathological process may go into a more chronic phase.

FOCAL CEREBRAL LESIONS

Electroencephalographic changes in the presence of focal cerebral lesions represent an electrical reaction to injury. Such reactions can be produced by trauma, vascular disease, tumors, inflammation, or any underlying pathological process. The identification of the most likely cause on the basis of the electroencephalogram, as well as on the clinical findings, is dependent primarily on the rate and rapidity of the evolution of the abnormality as determined by either sequential examinations or historical information.

One type of abnormality seen with focal lesions is the focal distortion or disappearance of normal rhythms that produces an asymmetry of amplitude, frequency, or reactivity of the rhythm. When such asymmetries are large, the abnormal hemisphere is usually easy to identify (see Fig. 8–8). If the asymmetries are slight and involve only amplitude, it may be difficult both to determine whether the abnormality is significant and to identify the abnormal side. Mild asymmetries that result in different frequencies of the background rhythm or decreased reactivity are more definitely abnormal, and the side showing the slower frequency and decreased reactivity is the abnormal one.

In addition to focal distortion of normal rhythms, there is focal appearance of abnormal rhythms, which may be specific, as described in the preceding section, or nonspecific, with either intermittent rhythmic slowing or the more continuous arrhythmic delta slowing. The more continuous and the more arrhythmic the pattern is, the more reliable the evidence of a clinically significant focal cortical abnormality (see Figs. 8–9 and 8–10). In addition to focal signs, more widespread and distant signs may appear in the electroencephalogram; these include generalized slowing of the background, usually associated with obtundation secondary to increasing pressure or brain stem compression (or both). Intermittent rhythmic activity in the delta range over the frontal regions is often spoken of as frontal intermittent rhythmic delta activity (FIRDA) (see Figs. 8–10 and 8–11). In children, similar rhythmic activity may be seen in the posterior head region.[13] Although obvious, this pattern is frequently located far from the primary focus and, therefore, has been termed "rhythms at a distance" or "projected rhythms." These patterns do not have a specific localizing value, but merely indicate that the pathological process is acute or evolving (see Fig. 8–11).

Primary abnormality of the posterior fossa and brain stem usually does not produce electroencephalographic changes until secondary obstruction develops or sufficient destruction of the brain stem occurs to alter consciousness. Generally, the disturbances are nonlocalizing and may include the frontal intermittent rhythmic delta activity. This activity, however, in the absence of focal cerebral abnormality, is not specific for a posterior fossa lesion because it can be seen in a wide variety of diffuse encephalopathies (see Fig. 8–11). In contrast to the insensitivity of the routine electroencephalogram to intrinsic brain stem lesions, the brain stem auditory evoked response may be extremely sensitive to these lesions and may show dramatically positive signs even before there is roentgenographic or clinical evidence of brain stem involvement.[23] Visual evoked potentials also may become abnormal before electroencephalographic abnormalities develop in patients who have subfrontal tumors involving mainly the optic pathways without causing major focal cerebral abnormalities.

Focal cerebral lesions are more likely to appear in the electroencephalogram before they do either on clinical examination or on roentgenographic studies if the abnormalities are potentially epileptogenic, are located in a silent area, or have infiltrated without any gross distortion in shape or density of the structure. Furthermore, dramatic changes may appear on the electroencephalogram and in the clinical examination when the changes are due to postictal disturbances, post-traumatic concussion, or inflammatory or degenerative changes that do not produce gross structural change. Serial electroencephalograms may be helpful in determining the rate (rapid, slow, or static) and direction (improving or progressing) of evolution in an underlying focus.

The first indication of a brain tumor, e.g., an infiltrating lesion in a clinically silent area that has not as yet caused significant density changes or structural distortion of the brain tissue, may be a focal abnormality in the electroencephalogram. The presence of intermittent rhythmic slow waves with focal abnormalities suggests that the lesion is either acute or progressive (see Figs. 8–10 and 8–11).

In vascular disease, major vessel ischemia and occlusion result in large focal changes, whereas small capsular infarcts usually do not alter the electroencephalogram. The tracing in transient ischemic attacks without neurological residual is frequently normal, but in the authors' experience with patients undergoing carotid endarterectomy, between 15 and 20 per cent of those who have had only transient ischemic attacks demonstrate a residual focal abnormality. Half of these abnormalities are evident during the waking trace, but the other half become evident only during anesthesia. In these cases the focus may exist in a clinically silent area, or the electrical disturbance may not be severe enough to be detectable at the clinical level. An unruptured aneurysm will not cause changes in the electroencephalogram unless it is a giant aneurysm producing a mass effect. An arteriovenous malformation may be the site of a seizure focus, but otherwise may not produce any significant abnormality if bleeding has not occurred.

Chronic widespread hemispheric disease (such as seen in Sturge-Weber syndrome or infantile hemiplegia) characteristically produces widespread voltage attenuation over the abnormal hemisphere (see Fig. 8–8). In a recent study, this electrographic accompaniment was seen in every patient with Sturge-Weber syndrome, although the same can be seen in any widespread hemispheric disease.[1]

In trauma, both focal and generalized abnormalities may be seen. The generalized abnormalities are usually associated with alteration in consciousness, including coma, which is discussed in the following section. Focal abnormalities can be produced by contusion, intracerebral hemorrhage, subdural hematoma, or a combination of these. A single finding early in the course of the disease does not allow a distinction between these possibilities. The changes on sequential electroencephalograms, however, are much more helpful in making this diagnosis.[8]

Focal inflammatory disease often produces dramatic and marked electrical change long before any obvious roentgenographic change occurs; but, unfortunately, the type of change produced is not specific enough to allow the nature of the focal inflammatory process—epidural, subdural, or intracerebral bacterial infection or a viral encephalitis—to be identified. The sequential appearance, however, of periodic lateralized epileptiform discharges—first on one side and then on the other—in the clinical picture of a patient with a recent febrile illness and acutely developing focal neurological deficit is highly suggestive of herpes simplex encephalitis (see Figs. 8–18 and 8–19).

ENCEPHALOPATHIES AND COMA

Encephalopathy is a generalized disturbance of cerebral function that impairs the waking cognitive function of the brain. Clinical signs of wakefulness without evidence of cognition imply functional integrity of the brain only up to the level of the brain stem. In this context, wakefulness is defined as a neurological state that may include cognitive function or only have the appearance of cognitive function. At a minimum, wakefulness is recognizable by lid, eye, and pupil movement and chewing, swallowing, yawning, and sighing. However, the addition of cognitive function to the minimal signs of wakefulness implies a degree of functional integrity of the brain all the way up to the cerebral hemispheres. In chronic conditions, cognitive function is often impaired without any alteration of cyclic signs of wakefulness (dementia). In the extreme states, the patient may show no signs of cognitive function, although he shows cyclic signs of apparent wakefulness (noncognitive wakefulness or chronic vegetative state). In acute encephalopathies, alteration of wakefulness often parallels alteration of cognitive function, and when the patient reaches a point at which he no longer shows either spontaneous or evoked periods of wakefulness, he is said to be in *coma*.

The electroencephalographic examination in patients with the various types of encephalopathy may be helpful in determining the nature and location of the underlying pathological process, but in general, it is most helpful in separating functional from organic conditions and, as a supplement to the clinical examination, in determining the severity and the rate and direction of evolution of the encephalopathy at the hemispheric level.

Separation of Functional from Organic Causes

The electroencephalogram is extremely helpful in separating functional from organic causes of altered consciousness, especially when the patient shows no apparent signs of awareness. In the functional condition, a normal waking organization and reactivity are recorded while the clinical examination shows no evidence of long-tract signs. Loss of consciousness due to organic causes is usually associated with marked and significant electrical changes consisting of loss of background activity and generalized slowing.

Etiological Diagnosis

The appearance of certain periodic complexes may be extremely useful in suggesting and confirming a diagnosis of slowly and rapidly progressing viral or presumed viral conditions such as subacute sclerosing panencephalitis, Jakob-Creutzfeldt disease, and herpes simplex encephalitis. In subacute sclerosing panencephalitis, the characteristic findings are those of very stereotyped, generalized, periodic discharges (see Fig. 8–16). The interval between the regularly occurring discharges is usually greater than four seconds. The discharge may appear early in the course of the disease, before the clinical diagnosis is obvious. In these earlier stages, the discharges may be more prominent during sleep than during the waking state, as shown in Figure 8–16.[26] By contrast, in Jakob-Creutzfeldt disease, the periodic complexes are usually sharp and slow wave complexes, with the interval between them usually being one second or less (see Fig. 8–17). Frequently, these complexes do not appear until later in the course of the disease when intellectual deterioration is obvious, and they often appear about the time that myoclonic jerks begin to develop. Earlier, these complexes may be less prominent in sleep than during the waking state.

The diagnosis of herpes simplex encephalitis often is suggested by sequential electroencephalograms (see Figs. 8–18 and 8–19). When the patient has an early febrile illness and later has neurological signs, and about that time, periodic lateralized epileptiform discharges appear in one hemisphere, and later independent periodic discharges appear in the other hemisphere, this sequence of conditions almost guarantees that the condition is herpes simplex encephalitis.[22] Another important diagnostic electroencephalographic feature occurs in the late infantile neuronal lipidosis of the Bielschowsky-Jansky type. As the condition progresses, there is nonspecific generalized slowing of the background as well as epileptiform discharges. The most striking feature, however, is the presence of single, high-amplitude polyphasic spike discharges in response to low flash stimuli, which Pampiglione and Harden have emphasized as an important diagnostic feature in this entity (see Fig. 8–20).[19]

Another distinctive and essentially diagnostic pattern occurs during an intermediate stage of hepatic encephalopathy. The typical electroclinical picture consists of clinical obtundation combined with reduction or loss of normal electroencephalographic background rhythms and with appearance of broad triphasic waves that are bilaterally symmetrical and synchronous with a frontal maximum. The most prominent phase of the wave is the intermediate phase of positive polarity, with a time lag from the anterior to posterior head regions. Not all triphasic waves are caused by hepatic disease, especially when they do not fulfill all the electroclinical criteria just mentioned. For example, in certain stages of Jakob-Creutzfeldt disease, the rhythmic complexes resemble those in hepatic disease, but when the overall electroclinical picture is considered, the two conditions can be easily distinguished.

The diagnosis of drug abuse and drug withdrawal often can be suggested by the electroencephalogram. In a patient who has had a recent seizure of undetermined cause, the presence of a large amount of beta activity and a photoparoxysmal response, both of which disappear when the patient is hospitalized, is strongly suggestive that the seizure is due to drug abuse or drug withdrawal.

Finally, when the patient presents in acute coma of less than 24-hour duration and the cause is not apparent, the appearance of widespread, generalized, sustained activity with a maximum in the anterior head regions—so characteristic of the anesthetic pattern—is almost diagnostic of drug-induced coma (Fig. 8–21).[8]

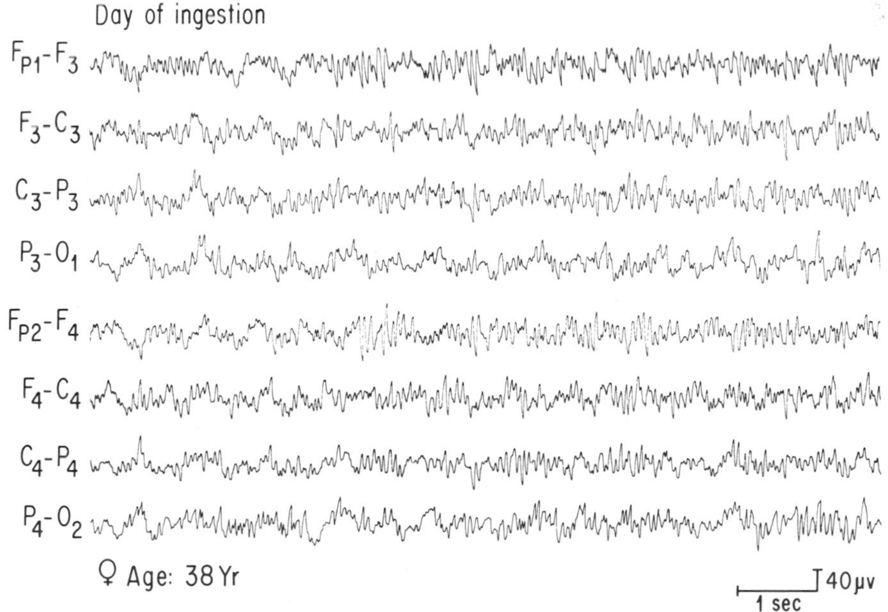

Figure 8–21 Sustained rhythmic pattern commonly seen in patients with coma due to drugs. This type of sustained rhythmicity is essentially identical to the pattern seen during anesthesia. When this pattern is seen in a patient who has suddenly lapsed into coma, it is almost diagnostic of drug-induced coma. In this case, coma followed ingestion of 1000 mg Valium.

The electroencephalogram is specifically helpful in identifying unsuspected absence seizure status as the cause of altered consciousness (see Fig. 8–13).

In addition to suggesting specific etiological factors, the electroencephalogram on occasion gives evidence of focal hemispheric abnormality that secondarily produces alteration of consciousness. In general, however, it shows mainly widespread, diffuse, nonspecific abnormalities of the sustained and paroxysmal type in association with encephalopathy due to a wide variety of causes.

Evaluation of Severity and Evolution of Hemispheric Dysfunction

Generally, the electroencephalogram is most beneficial as a supplement to the clinical measurement of the severity and rate of evolution of encephalopathy at hemispheric levels. As long as the patient retains some cognitive function, clinical evaluations are very helpful in following the status of brain dysfunction at the hemispheric level. Conditions in which cognitive function is impaired but not lost are usually reflected in electrical change that consists of a slowing in background activity as well as the appearance of generalized, irregular delta-range slowing. A consistent slowing of the background rhythm to and below 7 Hz almost always correlates with clinical evidence of intellectual impairment (see Fig. 8–11). In the very chronic, slowly progressive conditions, however, the patient may have major intellectual impairment without change in the electroencephalogram.

When the patient loses all clinical evidence of cognitive function, whether he shows signs of wakefulness (noncognitive wakefulness) or not (coma), the clinical examination merely reflects function of the brain at the stem level and provides little information about function at the cerebral cortical level. In these conditions, the electroencephalogram may be an extremely useful supplement to the clinical examination because it allows measurement of the severity of the encephalopathy at the cerebral hemispheric level. However, an isolated measure of the severity of the encephalopathy based on combined electroclinical evaluation is not enough to make a meaningful prognosis for useful recovery of intellectual function. Such a prognosis depends on knowledge of both the underlying cause and the severity of the encephalopathy. Even when the cause is known (and more so when it is not known), a reliable prognosis usually must be made on the basis of sequential records. If such sequential records show improvement, the prognosis is usually good; if they ultimately show deterioration or no change, they are usually associated with a much graver outlook.

In coma, some of the more optimistic signs include a retention of physiological patterns (especially spindles and posterior rhythms) and reactivity (Figs. 8–22 and 8–23). These findings in patients who are comatose after encephalitis, trauma, or cardiac arrest are usually associated with a good outlook for recovery of consciousness if there are no additional superimposed complications.

Evidence of severe-to-extreme encephalopathy includes the appearance of the unusually sustained, generalized rhythmic pattern, maximum in the anterior head regions and resembling the types seen in anesthesia. Periodic complexes of the type spoken of as burst suppression are another sign of severe alteration of cortical function during coma. Finally, low-amplitude patterns of less than 20 μv, if intermittent and especially if persistent, are an extremely poor prognostic sign. The ultimate in severity of electroencephalographic abnormalities during coma is the extreme of the low-amplitude pattern, that is, the absence over all head regions of identifiable electrical activity of cerebral origin, even at highest amplifications with sensitivity at 1 μv per millimeter. These represent the so-called electrocerebral inactivity (see Fig. 8–3).[12] Even the more severely abnormal patterns may, however, be associated with a chance for complete recovery, especially in drug-induced coma. The brain stem auditory evoked response is helpful in distinguishing between drug-induced electrocerebral inactivity, which shows relatively normal brain stem evoked response, and anoxia-induced electrocerebral inactivity, which shows either a marked reduction in or an absence of the brain stem auditory evoked response beyond wave 1. The presence of electrocerebral inactivity in a patient suspected of brain death is a reliable confirmatory sign

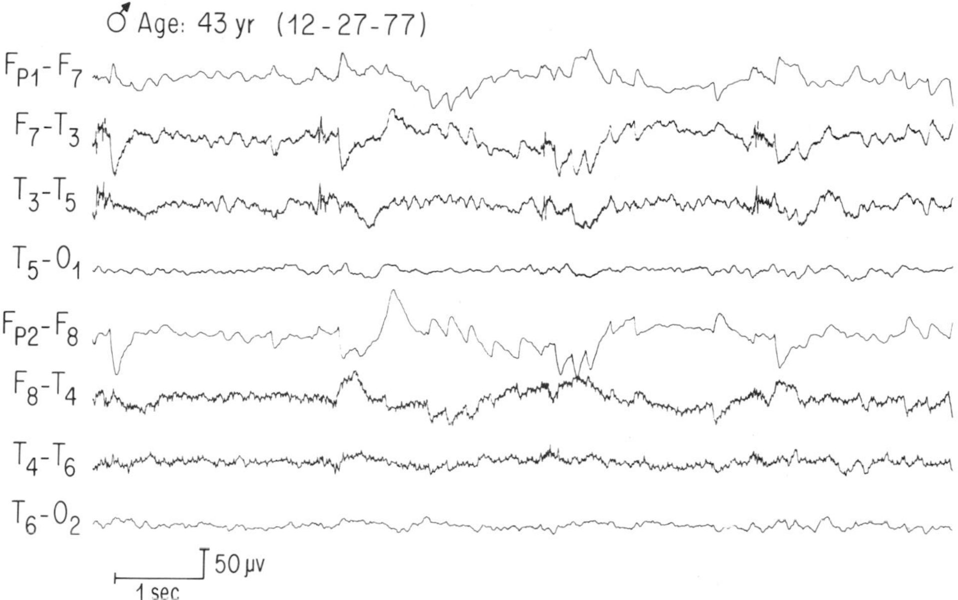

Figure 8–22 Noncognitive wakefulness in the postencephalitic state. Patient had lapsed into coma two weeks earlier during course of encephalitis with major brain stem involvement and, at the time of this electroencephalogram, was in a cycle of wakefulness but gave no evidence of consciousness or cognitive function. The tracing is markedly abnormal, but the only finding that suggests brain stem involvement is the chaotic nystagmus superimposed on the slow eye movement and seen maximally in F_7 and F_8. Because this is lateral eye movement, polarity will be positive on the side toward which the eye is moving and negative on the side away from which the eye is moving. This out-of-phase relationship can be seen for both the slow and rapid eye movements.

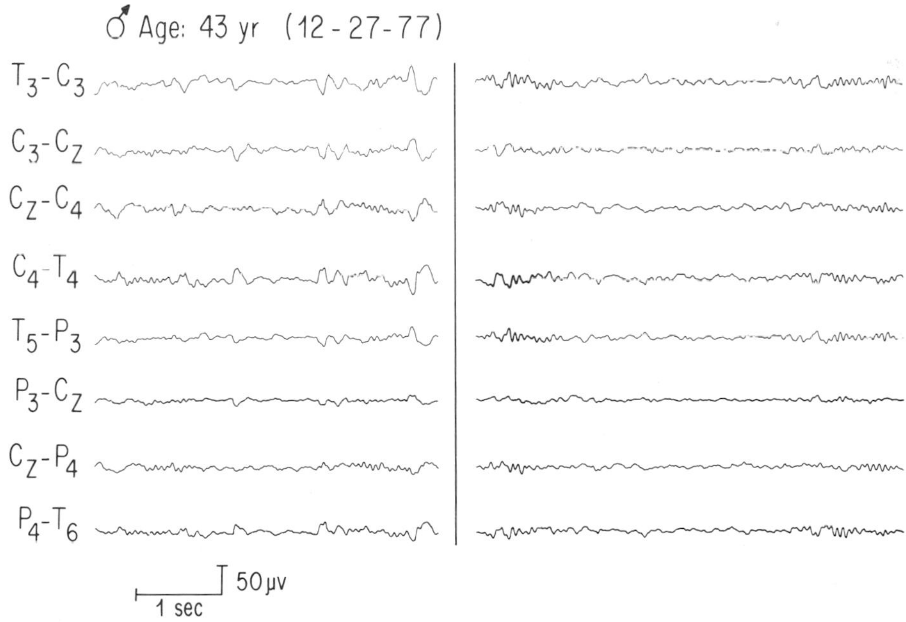

Figure 8–23 A well-developed vertex wave (*left segment*) and spindle bursts (*right segment*) in the patient whose waking record is demonstrated in Figure 8–22. Presence of preserved sleep pattern, even though patient had not recovered cognitive function since lapsing into coma two weeks earlier, was interpreted as a good prognostic sign for eventual recovery of consciousness. Patient recovered consciousness and full mental capacity over the next several weeks, although he was left with a severe motor disability secondary to brain stem dysfunction and continued to show the dramatic waking nystagmus seen in Figure 8–22.

when drugs or hypothermia can be excluded as the cause. In both the latter cases, the brain stem auditory responses are present. The converse, however, is not true; that is, the presence of some electrical activity is not necessarily an indication that the patient will survive and, in particular, will survive with useful recovery of intellectual function. In fact, certain patterns of sequential electroencephalographic evaluation over the first several days after a cardiopulmonary arrest are highly suggestive of severe, irreversible cortical damage, even though the patient is recovering sufficient brain stem function to survive in the chronic noncognitive wakeful state more or less indefinitely.[27]

INTRAOPERATIVE ELECTROENCEPHALOGRAPHIC RECORDING

Intraoperative electroencephalographic recording includes classic electrocorticography as well as short-term depth studies at the time of excision of an epileptic focus.[10] At the authors' institution, however, the most common intraoperative use of electroencephalography is for monitoring during carotid endarterectomy. In addition to the value of monitoring spontaneous activity during an operation, monitoring visual evoked response during transsphenoidal procedures has been helpful in identifying potentially reversible compression of the optic pathways.[28]

Corticography is mainly an interictal study and thus identifies the same characteristic interictal epileptiform discharges as were seen on the scalp. This identification helps determine whether the localization based on scalp recordings is correct. In addition, because the amplitude of the activity is larger on cortical recordings than on surface recordings, additional epileptiform activity not recognized at the surface may be seen—it is to be hoped, still emanating from the area of resection. Short-term depth studies (especially when the electrodes are placed in the amygdala and hippocampus) in temporal lobe resections may give evidence of a deep focus that shows more interictal activity than does the surface. These interictal recordings serve mainly as a preoperative baseline. Almost invariably, the decision to operate has been made before the craniotomy flap is turned, and the cortical recordings only confirm the accuracy of that decision. Finally, if corticography reveals the characteristic epileptiform activity persisting after the excision, it is an indication that the excision is insufficient and should be extended further if it is possible to do so with relative safety.[10] The absence of residual interictal epileptiform activity does not, however, guarantee that an adequate excision has been performed because the interictal recording is a brief one and epileptiform activity may be absent during that time. Therefore, the largest possible resection that can be done safely should be done at the very beginning of the procedure.

Since 1972, the authors have monitored more than 600 patients during endarterectomy. In addition, a lesser number of patients have been monitored during other procedures such as ligation of the carotid artery for inoperable internal carotid artery aneurysms and catheterization of the internal carotid artery for occlusion of carotid cavernous sinus fistulas.

Electroencephalographic monitoring during carotid endarterectomy is most valuable when shunting is utilized during clamping of the vessels only in patients who have ischemia at the time. Data can be supplied rapidly on whether the patient needs to have a shunt or whether the operation can be performed safely without the additional technical problem and additional risk inherent in inserting a vascular shunt.

In the uncomplicated case, the electrical changes do not develop with carotid artery clamping unless blood flow decreases below a critical level that, with halothane anesthesia and a normal Pco_2, is between 17 and 18 ml per 100 gm per minute. With enflurane, the critical range probably is lower, but this latter relationship is still under investigation. When the blood flow decreases below the critical range as the carotid artery is clamped, the typical change in the electroencephalogram is an ipsilateral attenuation of the normal anesthetic components and the appearance of abnormal slowing (which is first rhythmic and then arrhythmic), and finally (in the extreme situation) in attenuation of the abnormal slowing—the rhythmic first and then the arrhythmic (Fig. 8–24).

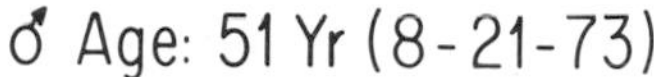

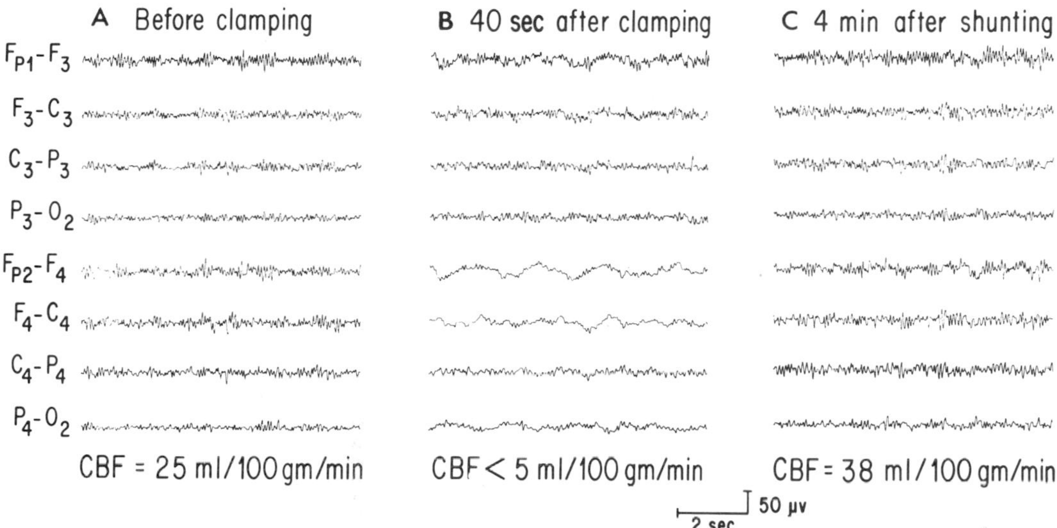

Figure 8–24 Dramatic ipsilateral attenuation of rhythmic anesthetic pattern with appearance of arrhythmic slowing when patient develops ischemia secondary to right carotid clamping, *B*, during endarterectomy. This is in marked contrast to symmetrical baseline pattern, *A*, as well as to postshunting pattern, *C*. Note: paper speed is 1.5 cm per second, which is half the usual speed of 3.0 cm per second.

The other major problem that may be detected by electroencephalographic monitoring is embolization, which may occur at any time before or during shunting or at shunt removal. Electroencephalography is the only reliable method of detecting this complication, which, in the authors' experience, is the most common cause of a new or increased neurological deficit developing during the anesthesia. Such a complication develops in approximately 1 to 2 per cent of patients, depending on the severity and the extent of the atherosclerosis involved in the artery being operated on.

During endarterectomy two other methods are commonly used to determine when a shunt is needed: the intracarotid injection of xenon for measuring blood flow and the measurement of the back pressure in the distal stump of the clamped carotid artery. Of these two methods, the distal stump pressure measurement is the simplest, but it also is the least reliable because the actual amount of blood delivered to the brain may remain constant and adequate even though the stump pressure varies considerably. For instance, pressures as low as 28 mm of mercury may give an adequate flow and there are no changes in the electroencephalogram. On the other hand, stump pressures as high as 78 mm of mercury may give an inadequate flow and electrographic changes are seen. These findings suggest that blood flow measurements are more reliable than stump pressure measurements.[18] Flow measurements, however, are influenced by Pco_2 and require special attention to technique. Furthermore, the critical flow level at which shunting is required may vary somewhat with different anesthetic agents. With halothane, a flow of 20 ml per 100 gm per minute is adequate to prevent any significant cerebral ischemia for prolonged periods. One additional difficulty is that flow monitoring is only intermittent and thus gives no evidence of problems developing in the intervals between measurements; furthermore, flow may appear normal even in the presence of massive embolization.

The adequate use of electroencephalographic monitoring during anesthesia requires awareness of the usual steady-state anesthetic pattern, which consists of sustained 8- to 14-Hz, 20- to 100-μv rhythmic activity with a widespread distribution and a preoccipital maximum (Fig. 8–25). The frequency of the sustained rhythmic pattern during anesthesia overlaps that of the waking alpha rhythm, and both are sustained

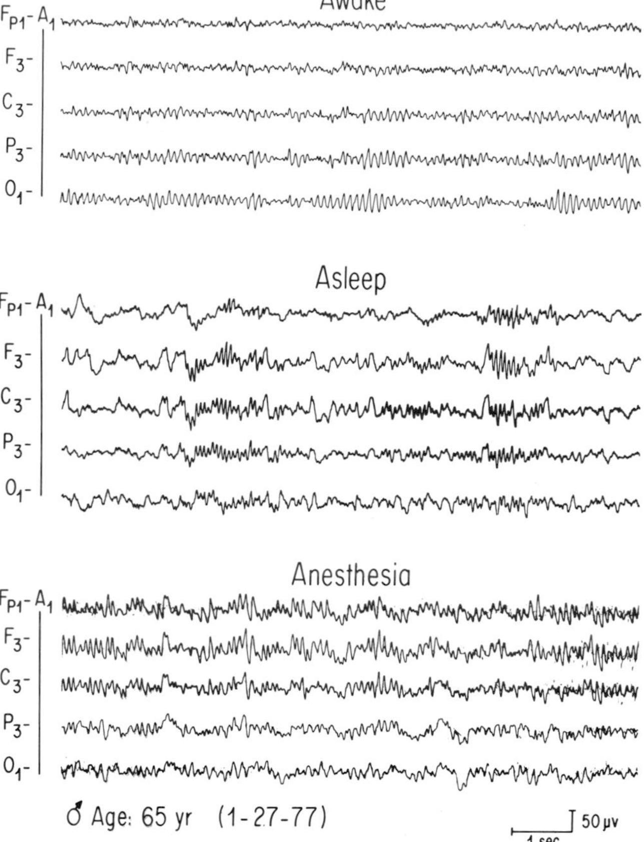

Figure 8–25 Three samples from the recording taken from the left hemisphere, demonstrating that waxing and waning rhythmic activity during sleep and anesthesia is maximally located over the anterior head regions, whereas waxing and waning alpha rhythm characteristic of the waking state is maximal and located posteriorly. In addition, the rhythmic activity of sleep occurs in intermittent bursts, whereas the rhythmic activity of both the waking state and anesthesia is more sustained.

patterns, but the rhythmic activity during anesthesia has a distinctly different distribution from that of the alpha rhythm; the spatial distribution of the anesthetic rhythm is similar to that of sleep spindles. Sleep spindles tend to occur in intermittent bursts that last only a few seconds, however, whereas rhythmic anesthetic patterns tend to occur over long sustained intervals.

In addition to the rhythmic pattern, there may be varying amounts of rhythmic frontal slow waves and generalized irregular delta slowing. In order to detect changes, the anesthetic state should be adjusted to emphasize the rhythmic patterns at the expense of the more irregular delta patterns. The rhythmic pattern tends to be most prominent when anesthesia is maintained below the minimal alveolar concentration of the anesthetic agent required to prevent movement in 50 per cent of patients with a normal or slightly high carbon dioxide tension and will be especially prominent during painful stimulation. Many factors will dramatically change the general electroencephalographic picture, including rapid changes in level of anesthesia (especially during induction and emergence), the P_{CO_2}, and the level of stimulation. Low levels of P_{CO_2} and stimulation tend to reduce the rhythmicity and increase the irregular delta activity, whereas normal to higher levels of P_{CO_2} and higher levels of stimulation have the reverse effect.

Electroencephalographic monitoring during carotid artery operations and during resection of an epileptic focus may be useful in indicating appropriate modifications of the operative strategy, either during the procedure or for future procedures. Intraoperative visual evoked studies may serve a similar role in transsphenoidal hypophysectomy, but further study is needed in this area.

SUMMARY AND CONCLUSIONS

The electroencephalogram is an electrical study of function that may add new or confirmatory information about the patient's clinical condition. Several points need emphasizing, however. First, an abnormality on the tracing may not be clinically significant but may reflect some electrical disturbance that has been present for a long time. Second, a normal electroencephalogram, just like a normal neurological examination, does not exclude significant underlying neurological disease; it must always be interpreted with the total clinical findings. Finally, although a standard approach is important, no one approach is adequate for every patient; the electroencephalogram should be modified for the clinical problem to be solved. The electroencephalographer should be actively involved in selecting special procedures for special problems, whether they be the diagnosis of sleep apnea or seizures, or under special circumstances, the monitoring of function during an operative procedure. As a dynamic tool to investigate function during the acute or evolving stages of various neurological conditions, electroencephalography is a powerful and effective study. If used only in the static phase of disease after all other tests have been performed, however, and if the interpretation is delayed and is made in the absence of any clinical input, it is seldom helpful. Generally, the electroencephalogram is useful when it is obtained early during the course of an evaluation, is done sequentially, and is done shortly after an acute, unexplained change has occurred in the neurological status of the patient.

REFERENCES

1. Brenner, R. P., and Sharbrough, F. W.: Electroencephalographic evaluation in Sturge-Weber syndrome. Neurology (Minneap.), *26*:629–632, 1976.
2. Broughton, R. J., ed.: Part A. Acquisition of bioelectrical data: Collection and amplification. *In* Rémond, A., ed.: Handbook of Electroencephalography and Clinical Neurophysiology. Vol. 3. Amsterdam, Elsevier Scientific Publishing Co., 1976.
3. Celesia, G. G., and Daly, R. F.: Visual electroencephalographic computer analysis (VECA): A new electrophysiologic test for the diagnosis of optic nerve lesions. Neurology (Minneap.), *27*:637–641, 1977.
4. Chatrian, G. E., and Lairy, G. C., eds.: Part A. The EEG of the waking adult. *In* Rémond, A., ed.: Handbook of Electroencephalography and Clinical Neurophysiology. Vol. 6. Amsterdam, Elsevier Scientific Publishing Co., 1976.
5. Cobb, W. A., ed.: Part B. EEG interpretation in clinical medicine. *In* Rémond, A., ed.: Handbook of Electroencephalography and Clinical Neurophysiology. Vol. 11. Amsterdam, Elsevier Scientific Publishing Co., 1976.
6. Cooper, R., Osselton, J. W., and Shaw, J. C.: EEG Technology. 2nd Ed. London, Butterworth & Co., Ltd., 1974, p. 60.
7. Dawson, G. D.: Cerebral responses to electrical stimulation of peripheral nerve in man. J. Neurol. Neurosurg. Psychiat., *10*:134–140, 1947.
8. Department of Neurology and Department of Physiology and Biophysics, Mayo Clinic and Mayo Foundation: Clinical Examinations in Neurology. 4th Ed. Philadelphia, W. B. Saunders Co., 1976, pp. 275–297.
9. Gastaut, H., and Tassinari, C. A., eds.: Part A. Epilepsies. *In* Rémond, A., ed.: Handbook of Electroencephalography and Clinical Neurophysiology. Vol. 13. Amsterdam, Elsevier Scientific Publishing Co., 1975.
10. Gloor, P.: Contributions of electroencephalography and electrocorticography to the neurosurgical treatment of the epilepsies. Adv. Neurol., *8*:59–105, 1975.
11. Guidelines in EEG No. 5: Provisional Recommendations for Telephone Transmission of EEGs. Willoughby, Ohio, American EEG Society, 1976.
12. Harner, R., and Naquet, R., eds.: Altered states of consciousness, coma, cerebral death. *In* Rémond, A., ed.: Handbook of Electroencephalography and Clinical Neurophysiology. Vol. 12. Amsterdam, Elsevier Scientific Publishing Co., 1975.
13. Hess, R., ed.: Part C. Brain tumors and other space occupying processes. *In* Rémond, A., ed.: Handbook of Electroencephalography and Clinical Neurophysiology. Vol. 14. Amsterdam, Elsevier Scientific Publishing Co., 1975.
14. International Federation of Societies for Electroencephalography and Clinical Neurophysiology: A glossary of terms most commonly used by clinical electroencephalographers. Electroencephalogr. Clin. Neurophysiol., *37*: 538–548, 1974.
15. Jewett, D. L., and Williston, J. S.: Auditory-evoked far fields averaged from the scalp of humans. Brain, *94*:681–696, 1971.
16. Kooi, K. A.: Fundamentals of Electroencephalography. New York, Harper & Row, 1971.
17. MacGillivray, B. B., ed.: Part C. Traditional

methods of examination in clinical EEG. *In* Rémond, A., ed.: Handbook of Electroencephalography and Clinical Neurophysiology. Vol. 3. Amsterdam, Elsevier Scientific Publishing Co., 1974.

18. McKay, R. D., Sundt, T. M., Michenfelder, J. D., Gronert, G. A., Messick, J. M., Sharbrough, F. W., and Piepgras, D. G.: Internal carotid artery stump pressure and cerebral blood flow during carotid endarterectomy: Modification by halothane, enflurane, and Innovar. Anesthesiology, *45*:390–399, 1976.
19. Pampiglione, G., and Harden, A.: Neurophysiological identification of a late infantile form of "neuronal lipidosis." J. Neurol. Neurosurg. Psychiat., *36*:68–74, 1973.
20. Pollen, D. A.: Discussion: On the generation of neocortical potentials. *In* Jasper, H. H., Ward, A. A., Jr., and Pope, A., eds.: Basic Mechanisms of the Epilepsies. Boston, Little, Brown & Co., 1969, pp. 411–420.
21. Reiher, J., and Klass, D. W.: Two common EEG patterns of doubtful clinical significance. Med. Clin. N. Amer., *52*:933–940, 1968.
22. Smith, J. B., Westmoreland, B. F., Reagan, T. J., and Sandok, B. A.: A distinctive clinical EEG profile in herpes simplex encephalitis. Mayo Clin. Proc., *50*:469–474, 1975.
23. Stockard, J. J., Stockard, J. E., and Sharbrough, F. W.: Detection and localization of occult lesions with brainstem auditory responses. Mayo Clin. Proc. *52*:761–769, 1977.
24. Sundt, T. M., Jr., Sharbrough, F. W., Trautman, J. C., and Gronert, G. A.: Monitoring techniques during carotid endarterectomy. Clin. Neurosurg., *22*:199–213, 1975.
25. Westmoreland, B. F., Espinosa, R. E., and Klass, D. W.: Significant prosopo-glossopharyngeal movements affecting the electroencephalogram. Amer. J. EEG Technol., *13*:59–70, 1973.
26. Westmoreland, B. F., Gomez, M. R., and Blume, W. T.: Activation of periodic complexes of subacute sclerosing panencephalitis by sleep. Ann. Neurol., *1*:185–187, 1977.
27. Westmoreland, B. F., Klass, D. W., Sharbrough, F. W., and Reagan, T. J.: Alpha-coma: Electroencephalographic, clinical, pathologic, and etiologic correlations. Arch. Neurol., *32*:713–718, 1975.
28. Wilson, W. B., Kirsch, W. M., Neville, H., Stears, J., Feinsod, M., and Lehman, R. A. W.: Monitoring of visual function during parasellar surgery. Surg. Neurol., *5*:323–329, 1976.

9

CEREBRAL ANGIOGRAPHY

The discovery of the x-ray beam by Röntgen in 1895 was rapidly followed by its diagnostic application to the nervous system. Walter Dandy's ingenious discovery of pneumography was inspired by Luckett's report of air within the ventricular system of a patient who had sustained serious head tramua.[30,120] It was not long before Dandy introduced air into the lumbar subarachnoid space, and so encephalography was born.[31] In 1927, Egas Moniz published a report of his first attempts at cerebral angiography in human patients.[129] The first attempt at carotid angiography, performed on a patient suffering from general paralysis of the insane, was by means of a percutaneous carotid injection of 7 cc of a 70 per cent solution of strontium bromide. The patient did not complain of any unpleasant sensations, and so it was assumed that this had been injected into the jugular vein. The radiographs, however, showed no filling of the vessels. With the second and third cases (parkinsonism), he was also unsuccessful. In the fourth case, the needle was dislodged and 10 cc of solution was extravasated into the tissues of the neck. Moniz therefore decided to modify his technique and inject into the carotid artery after operative exposure. In the fifth case, therefore, the right internal carotid artery was exposed and ligated. The artery was punctured twice and 4 cc of 70 per cent strontium bromide was injected. The patient complained of a painful sensation and became agitated. He had difficulty with speech and later stopped speaking (the first neurological complications of cerebral angiography), but was well on the third day. The radiographic exposures were made a little late and no angiogram was obtained.

In the sixth case, a 48-year-old patient with Parkinson's disease, a temporary ligature was placed on the internal carotid artery for two minutes and 13 to 14 cc of 70 per cent solution of strontium bromide was injected. The first film showed contrast filling of the middle and posterior cerebral arteries. This was the first carotid angiogram in a living patient. Unfortunately, the patient died eight hours later from thrombophlebitis. This prompted Moniz to abandon the bromides for the iodides. In 1933, Moniz and Aleves reviewed 600 carotid angiograms from their archives and also described the radiological anatomy of the carotid tree.[130]

Engeset popularized the percutaneous technique of carotid angiography, and Shimidzu also described his percutaneous technique for carotid angiography and his technique for vertebral angiography.[44,193] The older toxic contrast media have today been modified or replaced by safer solutions.

Thus angiography, a one-time hazardous technique, has passed through phases of development and has today become a simple and safe procedure. In recent years the pendulum has swung away from pneumographic studies toward angiography, and with further refinements and improvements it is anticipated that fewer air studies will be undertaken as the primary contrast diagnostic technique of choice.

ANGIOGRAPHIC TECHNIQUE

Many techniques are used today to visualize the major vessels leading to the head and their intracranial course. The choice of

M. M. SCHECHTER

technique depends, in part, on the particular problem and also upon personal preference.

The diagnostic quality of radiographs and the amount of information obtained from a cerebral angiogram are greatly enhanced if the techniques are controlled by a radiologist competent in the field and fully conversant with the problem. Joint consultations between the neurology, neurosurgery, and neuroradiology services are mandatory in deciding upon the information required and the choice of procedure.

Approaches

Carotid Angiography

To opacify the carotid tree, the following approaches may be used.

1. Direct puncture (usually performed percutaneously) of the internal carotid artery, the external carotid artery, or the common carotid artery.
2. Direct puncture of the carotid artery with catheterization of the internal carotid artery, the external carotid artery, or the common carotid artery (either anterograde or retrograde).
3. Retrograde catheterization of the carotid artery via the superficial temporal artery.
4. Selective catheterization via the femoral artery (with catheter tip in the common carotid artery on either side).
5. Segmentally selective opacification via the femoral artery (catheter tip in innominate artery), the brachial artery (with or without catheterization), or the axillary artery.
6. Nonselective opacification (aortic arch opacification) via the femoral artery (catheterization), the brachial artery (with or without catheterization), the common carotid artery (retrograde catheterization), or the axillary artery.
7. Intravenous technique.

Vertebral Angiography

To opacify the vertebral tree, the following approaches may be considered.

1. Direct vertebral artery puncture, either high cervical and occipital or mid and low cervical, with Sheldon needle and modifications with needle opening directed up or down, short-beveled needles, Cournand needle, Touhy needle, or by catheterization.
2. Selective catheterization via another vessel (accomplished either percutaneously or through open exposure) via the brachial, the femoral, the radial, or the subclavian artery.
3. Segmentally selective opacification by means of brachial artery puncture (with or without catheterization); subclavian artery puncture, either supraclavicular (with or without catheterization) or infraclavicular; axillary artery puncture with or without catheterization; radial artery puncture with open exposure and catheterization; femoral artery puncture with catheter tip in innominate or subclavian artery; retrograde carotid artery opacification with or without catheterization; or retrograde superficial temporal artery catheterization.
4. Nonselective opacification (aortic arch opacification) via the femoral artery (catheterization), the brachial artery (with or without catheterization), the common carotid artery (with catheterization), or the axillary or subclavian artery.
5. Intravenous techniques.

A few of the foregoing techniques are seldom used; only the more popular are considered here.

Equipment

Skull Unit

This is a matter of personal taste. There are quite a few skull units on the market, some of which have facilities for rotating the patient through 360 degrees.

Film Changing Equipment

A single-exposure technique should not be acceptable today. The use of biplane rapid serial angiography should be routine practice because of the advantages it affords, such as a comparison of the anterior projection and lateral projection viewed simultaneously, the early angiographic changes, and sequential changes. Simultaneous biplane angiography also eliminates one injection.

Image Intensifier

This facilitates the placement of catheters and, of course, must be available when cinematography is used.

Automatic Injectors

Most injections are made by hand unless high pressures are required. Some centers routinely use an automatic injector. The author reserves the automatic injector for catheterization techniques in which the rapid introduction of a bolus of contrast medium is necessary or chronologically comparable phase studies are to be made.

All percutaneous vertebral artery injections should be made by hand. When a needle becomes dislodged, the increased resistance to the introduction of saline or contrast medium will immediately become obvious and the injection can be terminated.

Syringes

The routine use of the following syringes will help to obviate the chance of a mistake: (1) 20-ml conventional for irrigating with saline (2) 10-ml conventional for contrast medium, (3) special long narrow (20-ml BD X2003) syringe for pressure injections of contrast media, and (4) 4-ml for local anesthetic agent.

Head Binder

A binder should be used for immobilization. This might consist of a muslin band, which is attached to two rollers on the side of the skull table, and adhesive tape passing over the forehead and over the chin to the sides of the table. Even with a cooperative patient, a head binder may help to give him an extra sense of stability.

Protection

Various types of protection have been designed. Detailed descriptions can be found in radiological texts.

Preparation and Positioning of Patient

The patient has usually fasted for six hours before the examination. Sensitivity tests to iodine compounds may be used, but are not very reliable.

Before the procedure is started, the neck should be shaved and surgically prepared with pHisoHex or Betadine. A waterproof sheet is placed over the patient's chest and abdomen, and sterile towels are draped about the operative field. After being removed from their solutions, all catheters, guides, needles, connecting tubes, and adapters are rinsed carefully in saline before use. The procedure should have already been explained to the patient and the risks discussed. The patient is warned of a possible burning sensation behind the eyes or in the jaw, teeth, tongue, and lips that may last for a few seconds. He is told not to move during the injection and is assured that the burning sensation is only momentary.

In apprehensive patients and in young children and in hospitals where excellent anesthesiology is obtainable, it may be desirable to conduct the procedures under a general anesthetic. If local anesthesia is used, pentobarbital sodium (Nembutal, 100 mg) may be given a half hour prior to the examination. All patients should receive atropine alkaloids (atropine alkaloids (atropine sulfate, 0.4 mg) intramuscularly, for protection against sinus effects, and a barbiturate (Luminal, 30 mg) in an effort to avoid reactions to the local anesthetic. Patients with head injuries should receive a minimum of premedication for fear of masking signs and symptoms.

It is necessary that the patient have an adequate airway, and apparatus for suctioning should be present in the room. Resuscitation apparatus should be immediately available, and the angiographer should be familiar with its use.

The patient usually lies in the supine position, but under very exceptional circumstances, the study may be performed with the patient in other positions. It is important that no packing be placed under the shoulders to extend the neck. Neck extension stretches muscles, ligaments, and fascial planes, rendering the vessels less palpable. The neck should be flexed with the chin brought in toward the chest. In this position the vessels will be much more easily palpable.

Projections Used

The three most useful views are the lateral, the 20-degree anteroposterior or fronto-occipital, and the half-axial or Towne's view.

For the lateral projection the film is arranged vertical to the table top, and the direction of the x-ray beam is horizontal to the table top. It is not satisfactory to turn the head to the side and use a vertical beam, as it is difficult to obtain a true lateral projection in this position. For carotid angiography the central beam is directed 2.5 cm above and 2.5 cm anterior to the external auditory meatus. For vertebral angiography the beam should be directed 2.5 cm behind the external auditory meatus (Fig. 9–1).

The 20-degree anteroposterior or fronto-occipital projection is obtained by tilting the tube (Fig. 9–2).

The half-axial or Towne's view is particularly useful in vertebral angiography because it projects the posterior cerebral arteries and superior cerebellar arteries above the petrous bone (Fig. 9–3).

Other useful projections are the 15- or 20-degree anteroposterior oblique, the true anteroposterior, the periorbital, the full axial, and the tangential views.

A 15- or 20-degree anteroposterior oblique projection with the head turned away from the side of the puncture is par-

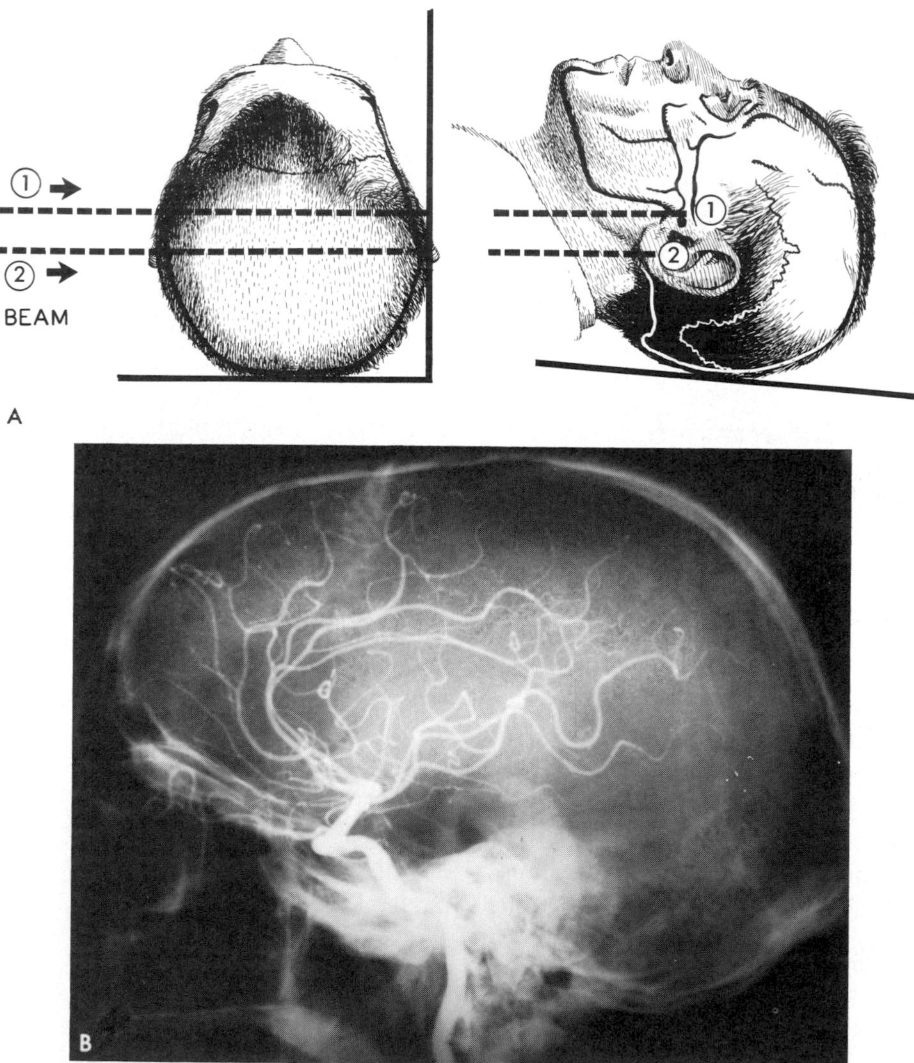

Figure 9–1 Lateral projection. *A*. The orbitomeatal line may be at right angles to the table top, and the central beam is directed 2.5 cm above and 2.5 cm in front of the external auditory meatus for carotid angiography (1). For vertebral angiography (2), the beam should be directed 2.5 cm behind the auditory meatus. *B*. Angiogram produced by this technique.

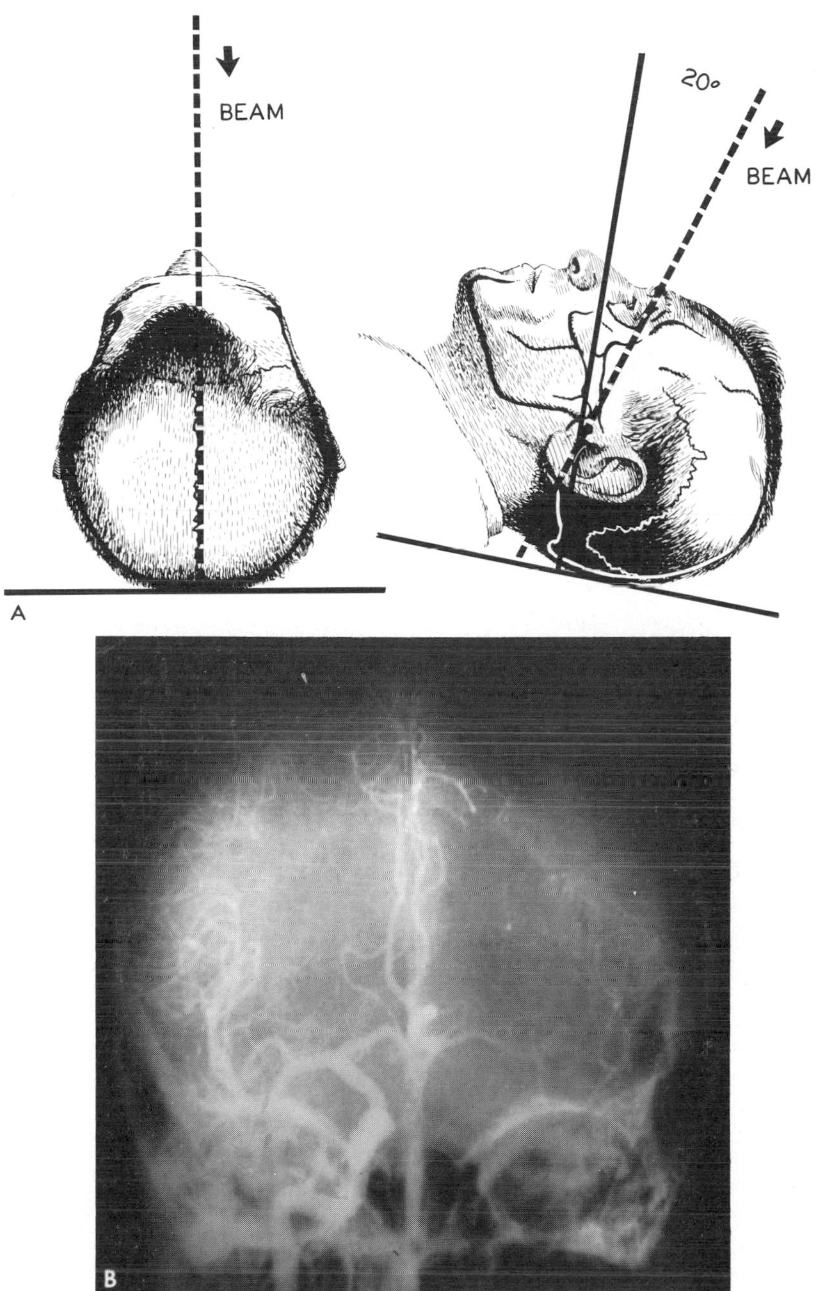

Figure 9–2 Twenty-degree fronto-occipital or anteroposterior projection. *A*. The baseline is at right angles to the table top. The central beam passes through the frontal bone and through the external auditory meatus. The central beam makes an angle of 20 degrees with the baseline. *B*. Carotid angiogram made using this technique.

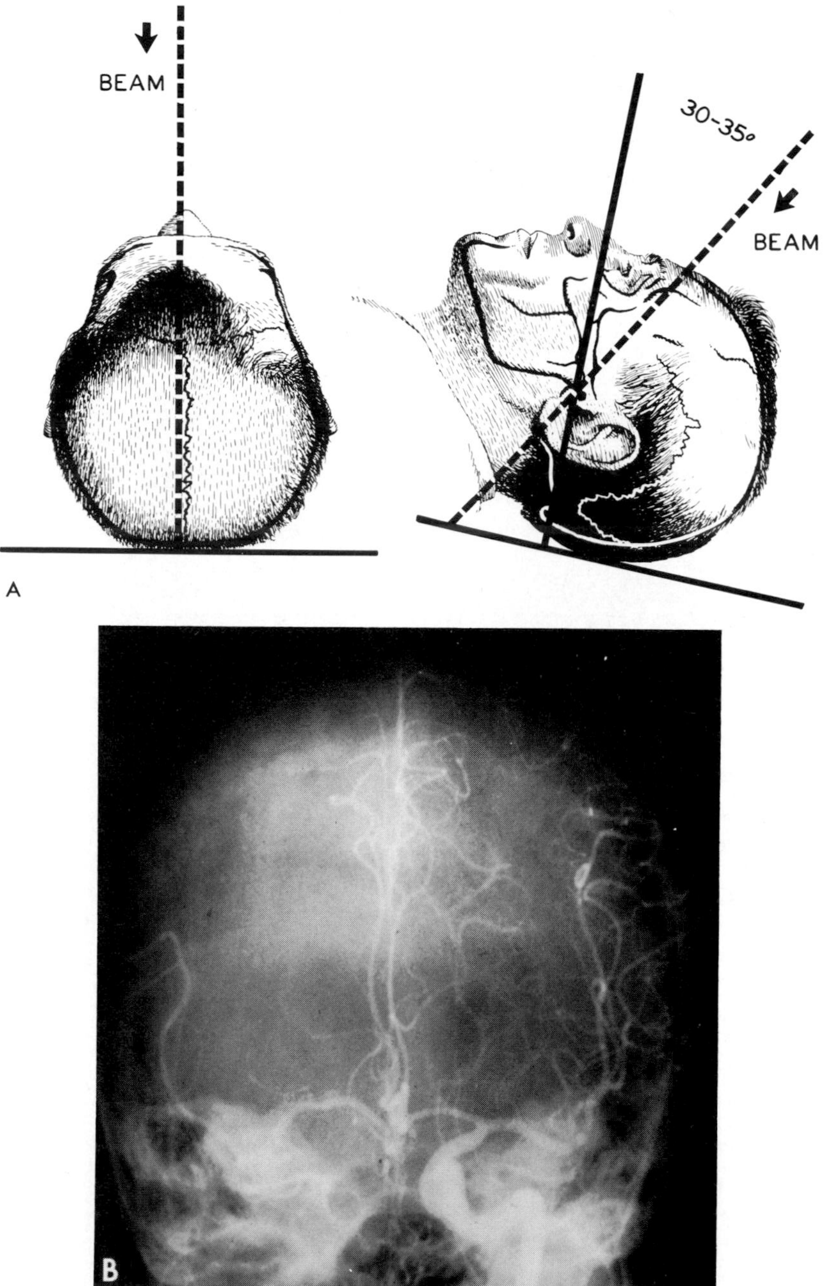

Figure 9–3 Towne's or half-axial projection. *A*. The baseline is at right angles to the table top, and the central beam passes through the external auditory meatus and makes an angle of 30 to 35 degrees with the baseline. *B*. Carotid angiogram made in this position—contralateral carotid compression has resulted in filling of branches of opposite carotid artery.

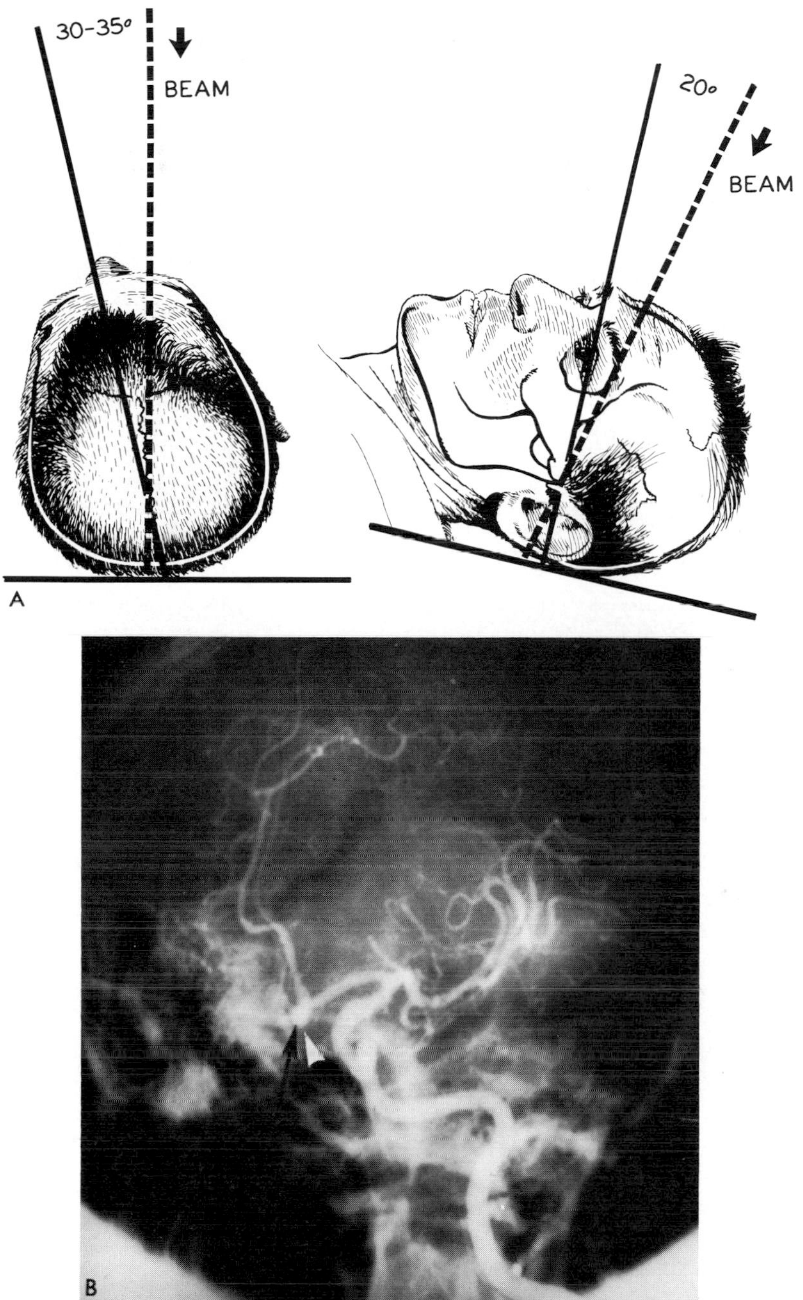

Figure 9–4 Fronto-occipital oblique or anteroposterior oblique projection. *A*. The orbitomeatal line is at right angles to the film. The head is rotated 30 to 35 degrees away from the injected side. The central beam passes through the frontal bone toward the feet and is centered 4 cm lateral to the glabella and 2 cm above the superior margin of the orbit. The central beam makes an angle of 20 degrees with the orbitomeatal line. *B*. Carotid angiogram made in this position. Note aneurysm of anterior communicating artery (*arrows*) shown in this projection.

ticularly useful for the region of the anterior communicating artery and also to outline the deep dural sinuses and veins during the venous phase of the study (Fig. 9–4). The beam is directed 20 degrees caudally, and the head is turned through 30 to 35 degrees. The opposite oblique view may also be used.

A true anteroposterior view is shown in Figure 9–5.

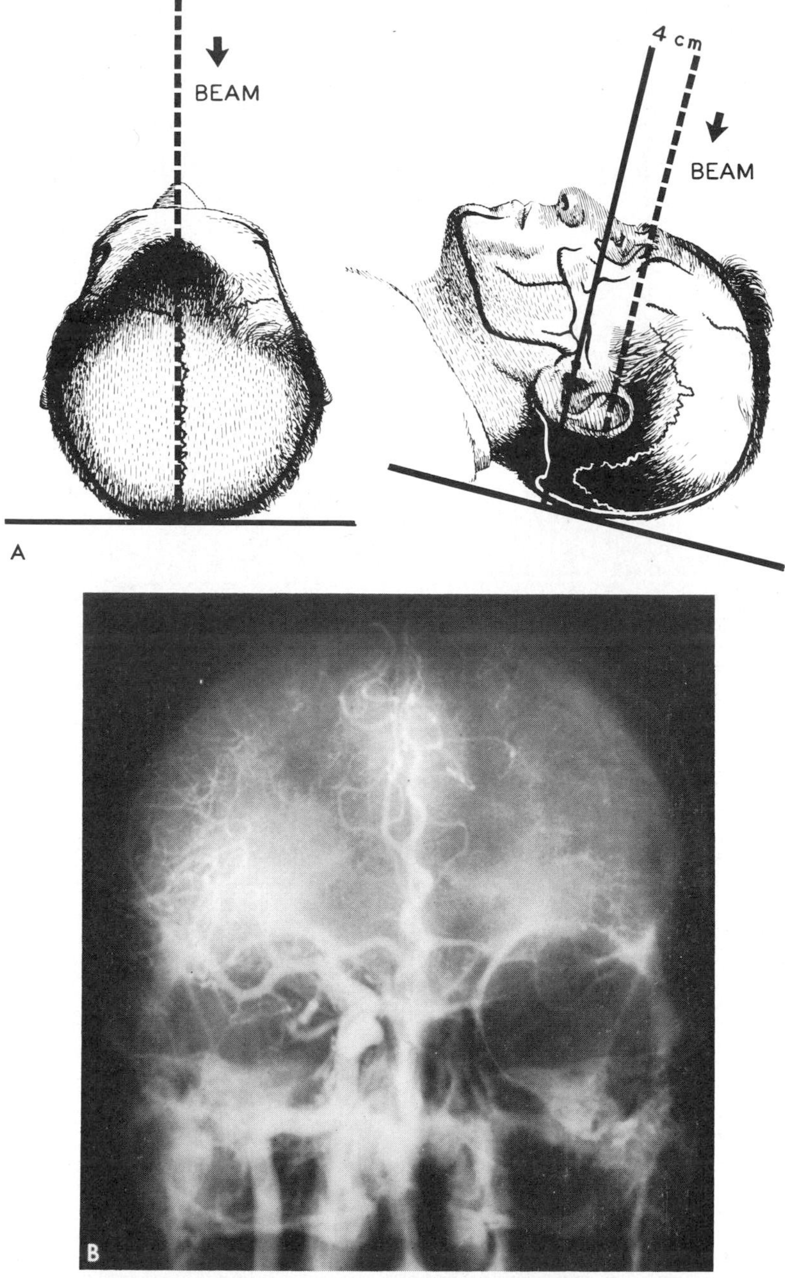

Figure 9–5 Anteroposterior projection. *A*. The orbitomeatal line is at right angles to the film, and the central beam is directed 4 cm above the superior margin of the orbit and parallel to the orbitomeatal line. *B*. Carotid angiogram made in this position.

The perorbital view for the trifurcation of the middle cerebral artery is particularly useful in examining the first part of the middle cerebral artery. Here the head is turned 10 degrees toward the side injected. The x-ray beam is vertical and is directed through the center of the orbit (Fig. 9–6).

The full axial (submentovertical) view is useful in investigating aneurysms in the region of the anterior communicating artery and the middle cerebral artery (Fig. 9–7).

The tangential view, with the head turned about 20 degrees away from or toward the side injected, may sometimes show a subdural hematoma to better advantage (Fig. 9–8).

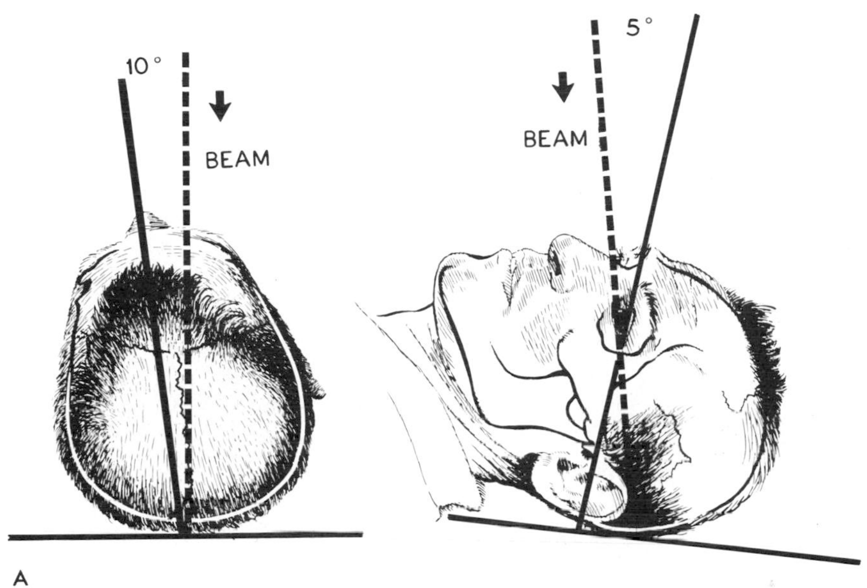

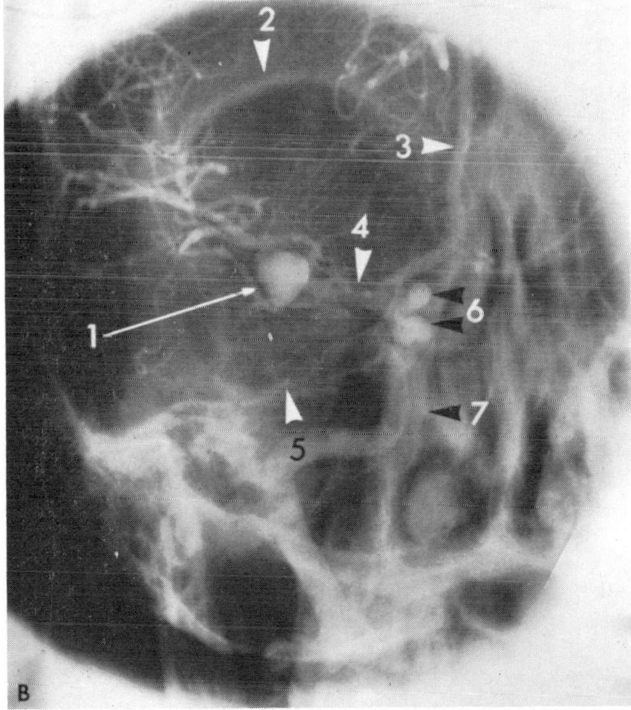

Figure 9–6 Perorbital projection. *A*. The orbitomeatal line is at right angles to the table top. The head is displaced and rotated 10 degrees toward the injected side. The central beam is tilted upward 5 degrees through the center of the orbit. *B*. Carotid angiogram made in this position: (1) aneurysm of middle cerebral artery, (2) superior margin of orbit, (3) anterior cerebral artery, (4) middle cerebral artery, (5) inferior margin of orbit, (6) carotid siphon, (7) intracavernous portion of carotid artery.

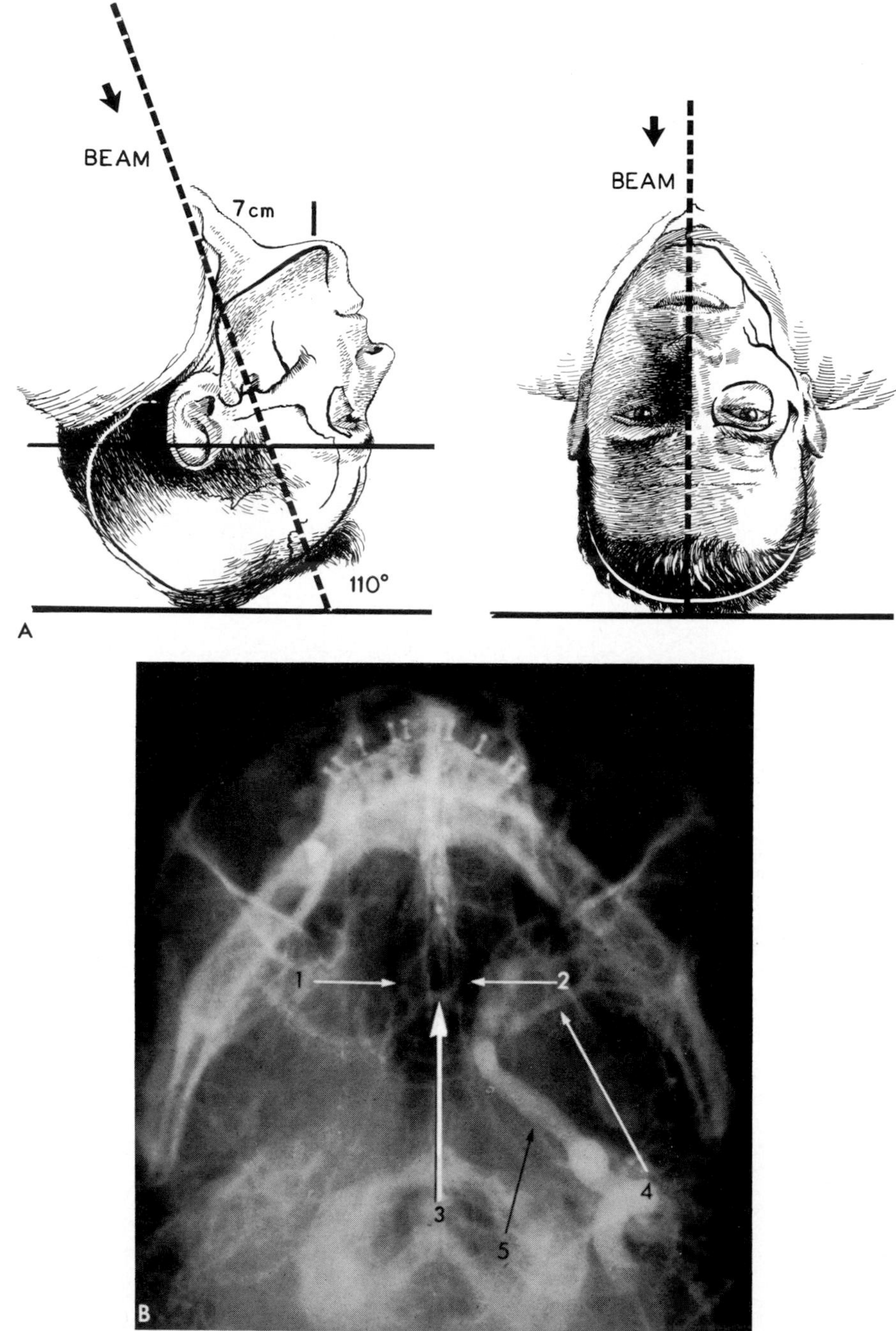

Figure 9–7 Submentovertical (full axial) projection. *A*. The degree of extension of the neck will vary with each patient. The central beam is directed midway between the angles of the jaw and about 7 cm behind the symphysis mentis. The angle between the baseline and the central beam should be 110 degrees. *B*. Carotid angiogram made in this position. Although other projections suggested aneurysm in the region of the anterior communicating artery, this projection cleared this region. (1 and 2) Anterior cerebral arteries, (3) anterior communicating artery, (4) middle cerebral artery, (5) internal carotid artery.

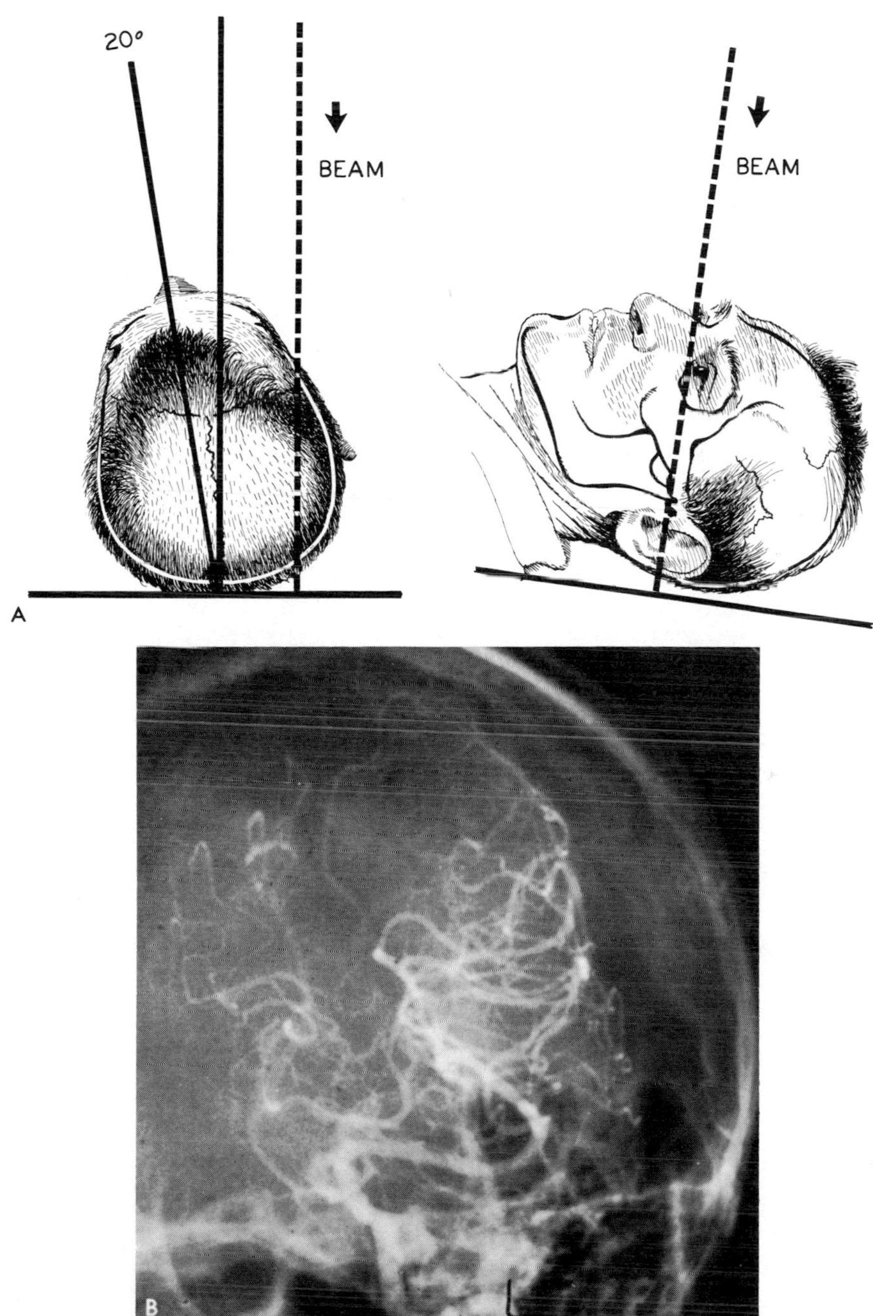

Figure 9–8 Tangential projection. The head is displaced so that the involved side is over the center of the film. *A*. The head is turned away 20 degrees from the injected side, and the central beam is directed at a tangent to the parietal region and at right angles to the film. *B*. For subdural hematomas situated in the frontal region; the head is rotated 10 degrees toward the injected side.

Time Interval Between Films

This will vary from case to case. Usually two films per second for a total of six seconds is recommended, but with a rapid circulation or with fistulae, it might be desirable to have films taken at shorter intervals. In certain circumstances it might be advisable to prolong the interval between films. The venous phase is usually obtained about six seconds after the start of the injection.

Contrast Media

Most medical centers use 60 per cent methylglucamine diatrizoate (Renografin) or 50 per cent sodium diatrizoate (Hypaque). The amount and concentration will depend upon the site of introduction and the timing of the radiographic exposures. With a catheter or needle in the common carotid artery, 6 to 8 ml of contrast medium is usually sufficient. When the catheter is in the internal carotid artery, 6 ml is sufficient. Six milliliters is usually sufficient for the vertebral artery, and when a catheter in the subclavian artery is near the origin of the vertebral artery, 10 to 15 ml is sufficient. When the arch of the aorta is opacified to outline the major vessels in the neck, 40 ml of a more concentrated solution is used with a pressure apparatus so that the bolus of contrast medium is introduced within about 1.3 seconds.

Catheter Preparation

For simple percutaneous carotid catheterization, a PE 160 catheter is usually used. Either a 30-cm length of sterile catheter is obtained in a separate packet or a 30-cm length is cut from a reel of tubing. One end of the catheter is tapered by stretching it over a flexible guide wire (Fig. 9–9*A*), and the other end is attached to a connector (Fig. 9–10), which is then attached to a syringe. When thicker catheters are used, such as the radiopaque catheters for segmental opacification via the axillary or femoral route, the stretching of the catheter and ta-

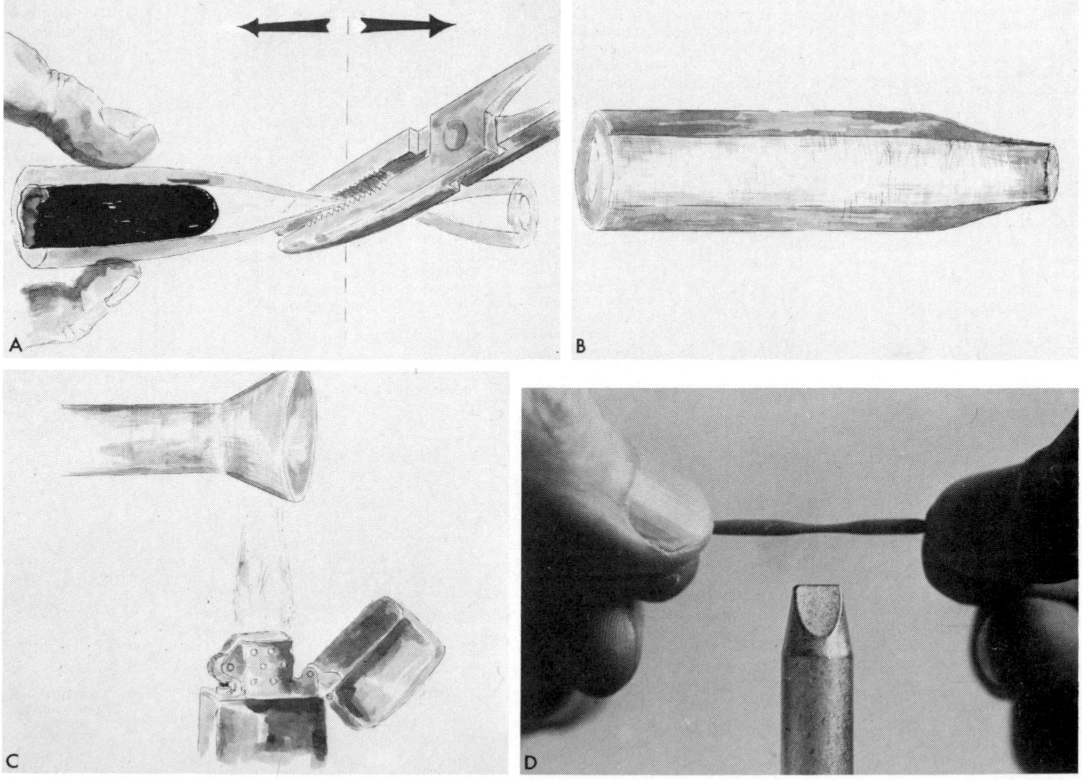

Figure 9–9 *A*. Preparation of catheter for angiography. *B*. Tip of catheter. *C*. Heat applied to end of catheter for flaring aperture. *D*. Note heating element in the center. Guide wire is in lumen of catheter.

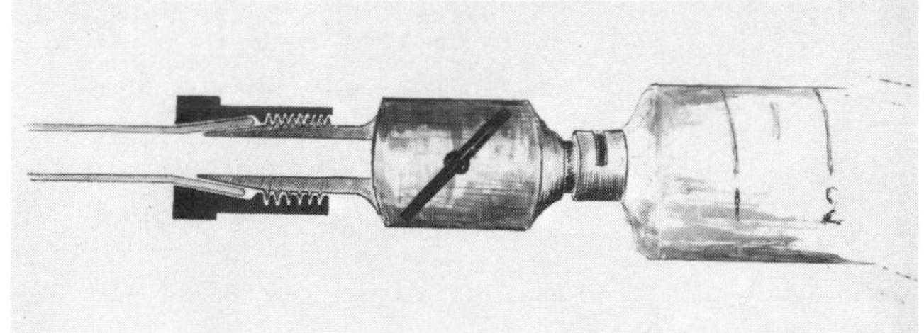

Figure 9–10 Connector between syringe and catheter.

pering of its end are facilitated by heating it over an open flame or radiant heat (Fig. 9–9*C* and *D*).

Every detail in the preparation of the catheters must be carefully followed, since omitting an apparently trivial step may result not only in an unsuccessful examination but also in most undesirable complications.

The vinyl and polyethylene catheters are prepared as follows. A suitable thickness and length of catheter having been selected, the rigid end of the guide is introduced into the catheter to within 1 cm of the end of the catheter. The tip of the catheter is now held in a pair of forceps and, while the catheter and guide are held in the other hand, this is stretched (Fig. 9–9*A*). The guide is now removed, and the catheter tip is cut with a sharp scalpel or pair of scissors just distal to its narrowing (Fig. 9–9*B*). In this way a tapered leading tip of catheter is obtained that will fit snugly over the guide and will pass easily through the skin and arterial wall. The more rigid catheters are prepared in a similar fashion by applying heat (from an open flame or a source of dry heat) over the region to be tapered (Fig. 9–9*C* and *D*). A few rapid passages through a spirit flame is usually all that is required. Should side openings be desired (with the larger bores), these may be drilled in the sides with either an ordinary sawed-off No. 18 (standard wire gauge) needle or a special instrument. The holes should be drilled with the channel directed backward so that the jets will leave the catheter retrogradely. These retrojets will counteract the recoil effect of the forward stream at the tip of the catheter. Three or four holes are usually sufficient and should be drilled in a spiral fashion around the catheter so as not to weaken it (Fig. 9–11). The opposite end of the catheter may be flared by holding it over a flame or a heating element, or using a flanged instrument, to accept the special connector (Fig. 9–10). When pressure injections are not used, the introduction of a closely fitting needle into this end will be quite satisfactory. Other radiopaque polyethylene and vinyl tubings are prepared in a similar manner. Some catheters are commercially available, preshaped and with a syringe adaptor attached.

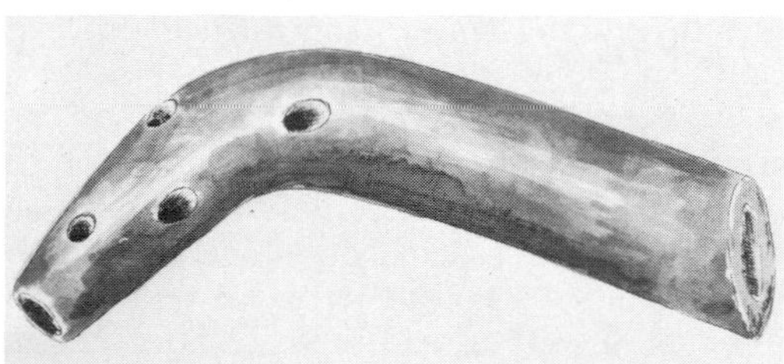

Figure 9–11 Note that the side openings in the catheter are directed backward so that the jet stream is directed backward.

Special connectors may, however, be used at this end. Figure 9–10 demonstrates their application. These are manufactured in various sizes and may be provided with a tap or a nonreturn valve. When the end of the catheter is too short to reach the pressure injector, a length of connector tubing must be used. This may be made of heavy duty tubing that will withstand high pressures. This tubing should have an internal diameter at least three times that of the catheter used. High-pressure connecting tubing sets are available in lengths of 25 cm (10 inches), 50 cm (20 inches), and 75 cm (30 inches) and will withstand pressures up to 100 lb per square inch or 7 kg per square centimeter. Luer-Lok connectors should be used when high pressures are anticipated.

To preshape the ends of the catheters, a thin rigid wire about 10 inches long may be inserted into the tapered end. The catheter end accommodating the wire may now be shaped (the stiff wire will retain the shape), and the end placed in boiling water for about five seconds. Next, the catheter is plunged into cold water, and the wire is removed. The "elastic memory" of the catheter insures that it will spring back into its shape after being straightened during the manipulations during passage of the spring guide and passage along the femoral or axillary artery. A variety of thicknesses and shapes should be available for use in each particular situation.

Carotid Angiography

Direct Puncture Techniques

Direct carotid artery puncture may be made into the common carotid artery, the internal carotid artery, or the external carotid artery. The site of puncture depends on the suspected pathological process and the information required. Denser opacification with greater intracranial definition will result from an internal carotid puncture. The external carotid circulation may be useful in demonstrating the collateral supply between the extracranial and intracranial circulation and also for the tumor circulation in meningiomas and other tumors and pathological processes supplied by the external carotid artery. If the internal carotid artery is selected for direct puncture, this should be attacked as high up in the neck as possible to avoid the carotid sinus, which is situated at the bifurcation. Furthermore, the internal carotid artery becomes progressively less mobile as it approaches the base of the skull and is therefore easier to puncture. The common carotid should be punctured as low down in the neck as possible to avoid the carotid sinus. Since most pathological conditions in the cervical carotid artery occur at the bifurcation, the injection should be made as low as possible to avoid puncturing the area and to visualize it radiographically.

About 3 ml of 2 per cent procaine hydrochloride is infiltrated into the skin and around the carotid artery. Larger amounts of local anesthetic will obscure the local anatomy and make palpation of the artery difficult. The procaine is introduced around the carotid artery, there being no necessity to infiltrate the wall of the vessel. An attempt is made to introduce the No. 18 (standard wire gauge) needle through the same opening made by the local anesthetic needle. No attempt is made to puncture the artery at this stage, but the needle is advanced with the right hand until its tip impinges on the wall of the vessel. The vessel is now anchored by placing the separated index and middle fingers of the left hand on either side of the needle, considering the operator on the right side (Fig. 9–12). The left carotid artery may be pulled over toward the vertebral bodies and trachea, and anchored, while the right carotid artery may be pushed toward the midline. With the right hand, the needle is briskly pushed into the lumen of the vessel. For beginners, it is perhaps easier to penetrate both walls of the vessel with the needle vertical to the long axis of the vessel; it is, of course, preferable to puncture only one wall. The needle is then tilted parallel with the vessel and is withdrawn slowly, using a rotary motion. Usually a characteristic flick is felt as the needle point leaves the distal wall of the vessel and pops into the lumen. This part of the puncture is performed with the bare needle, i.e., without a stylet or a connecting tube. The advantage of omitting the stylet lies in the recognition of the puncture of only one wall when blood under systolic pressure will spurt from the needle. This would be missed with a stylet in position. In young patients an extremely mobile vessel in the neck may resist puncture because of its elasticity and movements. A useful trick here is to embed a 2-inch 22-bore needle alongside the carotid artery and to anchor the vessel against this with the index and middle fingers.

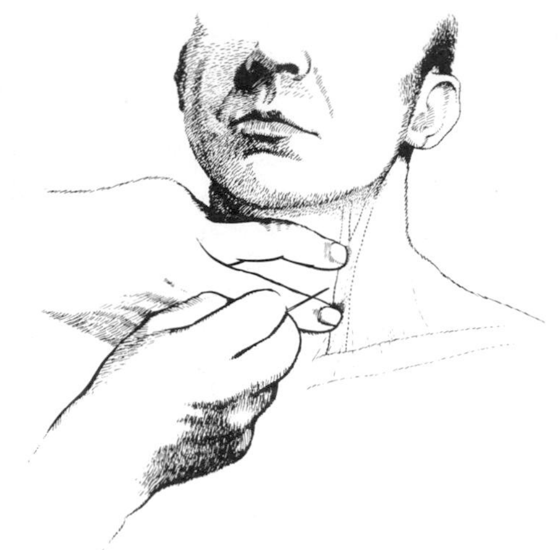

Figure 9–12 Technique of percutaneous carotid angiography.

The connecting tube, which has already been attached to a stopcock and a 20-ml syringe containing saline (stopcock is between tubing and syringe) is now attached to the needle, and saline infusion is continued until the examination is terminated; the saline may be heparinized. A continuous drip will release a pair of hands during the examination. It is not as satisfactory, however, as hand injection by a trained operator, who will immediately recognize displacement of the needle and immediately institute appropriate corrective measures. Cardiac patients should not be overloaded with saline.

To puncture the external carotid artery, the patient's neck is turned away from the side of injection. In this way the external and internal carotid arteries are separated. If a needle is introduced into the wrong vessel, it should be left in position and a puncture of the other vessel attempted. Leaving the first needle in position will aid in identifying the correct vessel.[169]

Saline is used only in 20-ml syringes and contrast medium in 10-ml syringes. This will prevent confusion. Ten milliliters of contrast medium—50 per cent sodium diatrizoate (Hypaque) or 60 per cent methylglucamine diatrizoate (Renografin)—is drawn up into the syringe and injected into the connecting tube. The plunger of the syringe containing the contrast medium should be well lubricated with saline to obviate jamming from crystallization of the contrast medium on its surface. At a given command, about 2 ml before the end of the injection, the technician starts exposing the films. Since the connecting tubing with catheter accommodates about 3 ml, only 7 ml of contrast medium is introduced.

The number of films and the time intervals between them will depend upon such factors as the vascular circulation rate, the disease present, and the information required. When an aneurysm is suspected, the arterial phase will perhaps supply the vital information, and a film in the intermediate or venous phase may demonstrate the pooling of contrast medium in the aneurysm. In occlusive disease, delayed films may show the collateral circulation. Arteriovenous malformations will require a very short interval between films because of the rapid shunt of arterial blood through the anastomotic vessels to the venous system. The circulation time in infants and children is faster than in adults.

Automatic injectors may be used and coupled to the exposure mechanism. In this way the exposure is started atuomatically after a predetermined amount of contrast medium has been introduced. When a rapid circulation is expected (in children and in patients with arteriovenous fistulae), the exposure should be started after about 3 ml of contrast substance has been introduced. The contrast material in the connecting tube and needle may act as an anticoagulant, to prevent clotting in the tube, which may allow the stopcock to be turned off at this stage in preparation for the next injection. The author, however, prefers to allow this amount of medium to drain away by opening the top; continuous saline perfusion should be resumed.

There are valid arguments for starting the examination with the anterosposterior projection, but equally convincing reasons for beginning with the lateral projection. Where biplane angiography is used, both views are obtained simultaneously.

If the contrast medium passes into the internal carotid artery, the patient may experience a burning sensation behind the eyes, whereas this sensation may be felt in the cheek, gums, and teeth if the medium enters the external carotid. Fifteen milliliters of saline injected rapidly usually produces blanching of the conjunctiva and skin over the face if the flow has entered the external carotid artery. It must be remembered, however, that with puncture of a common carotid or even of an internal carotid artery, this subjective sensation may be an unreliable indicator, and a scout film using 2 ml of contrast medium and the Polaroid cassette will show precisely which vessel has been entered.

With the needle (or catheter, as described later) in position, the 2 ml of contrast medium is injected and an exposure of the neck is made in the lateral projection, proximal to the intracranial course of the carotid artery. By using a cassette with a Polaroid film, the position of the needle and its relation to the vessels can be obtained within 10 seconds of film exposure. Similarly, the position of the catheter tip relative to the vessels in the neck may be appreciated. If the situation is not satisfactory, the needle or catheter may be adjusted.

The anteroposterior (modified) and lateral projections (Figs. 9–1 and 9–3) are usually all that are necessary. Under cer-

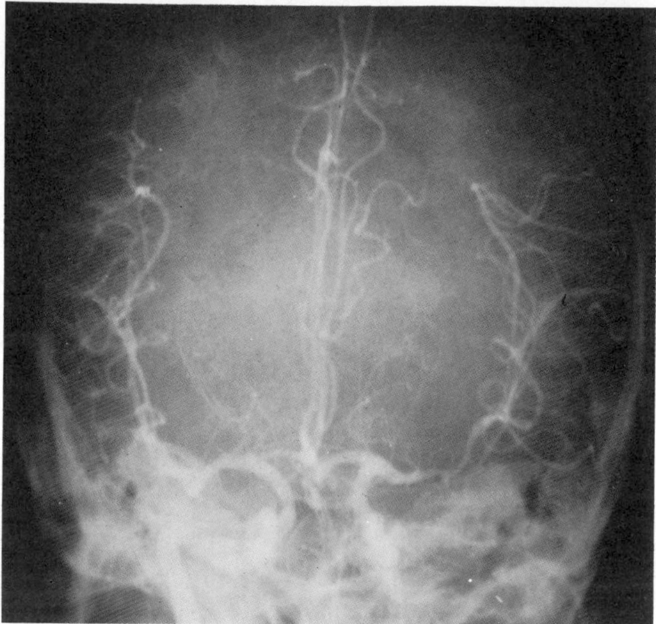

Figure 9–13 Right carotid angiogram with compression of the left carotid artery in the neck. Note that the contrast medium has passed from the right side to the left anterior, middle, and internal carotid arteries.

tain circumstances other views may be indicated. Compression of the contralateral carotid artery will usually result in filling of the vessels of the opposite hemisphere. In the anteroposterior projection, the two sides may now be compared and asymmetry will become obvious (Fig. 9–13).

Anterior communicating aneurysms may not fill unless the contralateral carotid artery is compressed. The presence or absence of contralateral flow is an important factor in determining the operative approach to aneurysms. Contralateral compression does not give a valid assessment of the flow from the uninjected to the injected side, but only evaluates the patency of the anastomosis from the injected to the uninjected side. Saltzman claims that compression of the ipsilateral vertebral artery during carotid artery injection will fill the posterior communicating and posterior cerebral arteries.[172,174]

If the ipsilateral anterior cerebral artery does not fill with the carotid injection, technical causes should be looked for before considering an anatomical basis. Poor filling of the carotid artery in the neck owing to spasm, hematoma, and extravascular passage of contrast medium is not infrequently associated with nonfilling of the anterior cerebral artery (Figs. 9–14 and 9–15). Partial withdrawal of the catheter may eliminate vascular spasm and permit demonstration of a normal vessel.

After removal of the needle, compression over the puncture site should be maintained for at least five minutes by "riding the carotid pulsations." The neck should then be carefully watched for an additional 15 minutes before the patient leaves the radiology department. Inspection at frequent intervals for the next 12 hours should be made.

Catheterization Techniques

The Seldinger apparatus with slight modifications can be used for carotid, brachial, and femoral catheterizations.[190] The author has dispensed with the large-size guide and uses only the small size for all angiography. The author has also found that the examination is facilitated by simply replacing the three-part special needle with the regular No. 18 (standard wire gauge) thin-walled needle. The technique for introducing the catheter into the carotid artery is the same as for the brachial and the femoral arteries.

With catheters larger than the PE 160, it is advisable to make a small nick in the skin and subcutaneous tissues with a tapered scalpel blade. This will facilitate the entry of the tip of the catheter through skin and soft tissues. A dilator may also facilitate vascular entry. Most punctures are performed percutaneously, but under certain circumstances, such as in infants, the brachial artery may have to be exposed operatively before puncture.

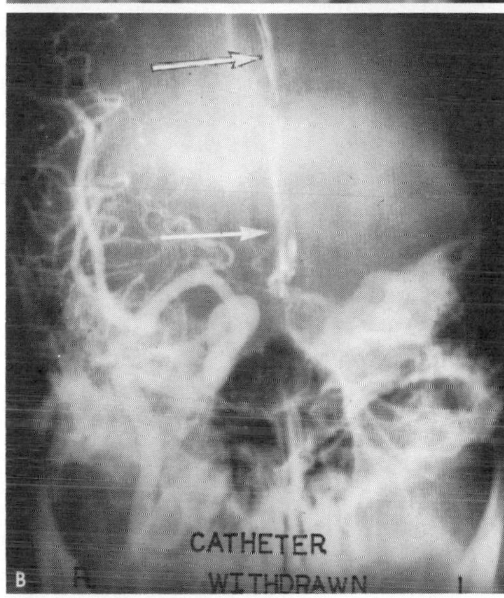

Figure 9–14 *A*. Note area of spasm in internal carotid artery from high placement of catheter tip. There is no filling of anterior cerebral artery. *B*. When catheter was withdrawn, a little contrast medium filled the anterior cerebral artery.

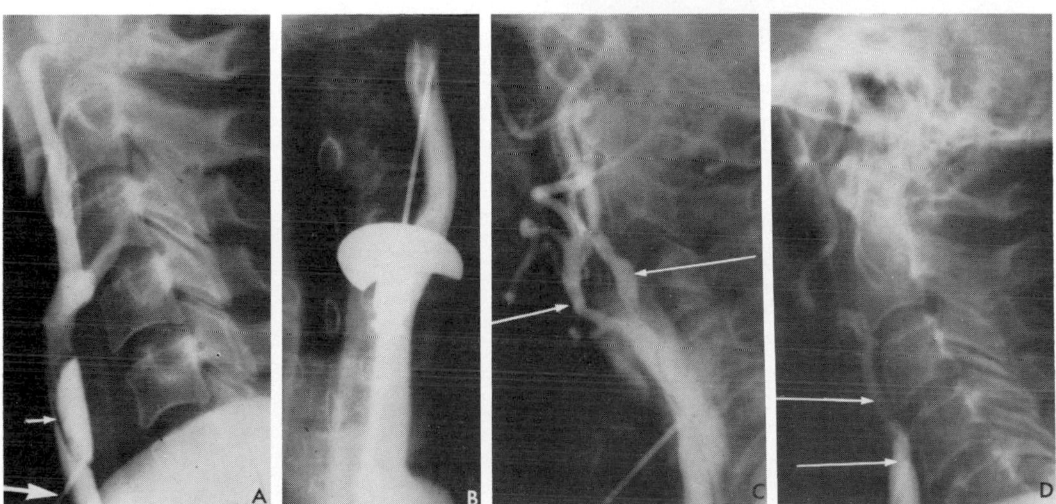

Figure 9–15 *A*. Subintimal injection of contrast medium. Note needle point and negative shadow (*smaller arrow*) representing an intimal flap. *B*. Injection into the carotid sheath simulating occlusive disease. *C*. Contrast medium injected partially into tissues of the neck and into the common carotid artery. There is partial filling of the internal and external carotid arteries. *D*. Second carotid injection into the same vessel. Note now no filling of internal carotid artery.

The Seldinger Technique

The common carotid artery is punctured as low in the neck as possible, using an 18-gauge thin-walled needle and the previously described technique. A Seldinger guide, 50 cm long, is introduced (flexible end first) into the needle and advanced about 3 cm beyond the tip of the needle (Fig. 9–16). If there is any resistance at all to the passage of the guide, the needle, without being removed, should be rotated through 180 degrees, and a second attempt made. Absolutely no effort should be used to overcome any resistance to the passage of the guide. If resistance is encountered, the introduction of a few milliliters of saline into the needle may result in better placement, and another attempt may be made to introduce the guide. If an attempt is made to overcome resistance during the introduction of the guide, a thrombus or atheromatous plaque may be dislodged. Furthermore, the end of the guide may be kinked and may catch on the end of the catheter, preventing withdrawal of the guide, or may catch on the artery wall, causing considerable difficulty during withdrawal of the guide. If resistance is still encountered, the guide should be removed, and with the needle still in the artery, an ordinary conventional angiogram should be performed.

If no resistance is encountered, the guide is advanced 3 cm beyond the tip of the needle, and the needle is removed over the guide. A 30-cm catheter (PE 160) that has been specially prepared is then threaded over the free end of the guide to approximate the skin surface. The catheter tip should fit snugly over the guide. Catheter and guide are now advanced, using a slight rotatory movement of the catheter and guide together, for about 4 cm. The guide is then withdrawn, leaving the catheter in position. Free flow of blood now issues from the end of the catheter, which is connected to an adapter and this to a syringe with saline.

If the special adapter is to be used, the catheter must be threaded through it before being threaded over the guide. Saline perfusion prevents clotting of blood in the cath-

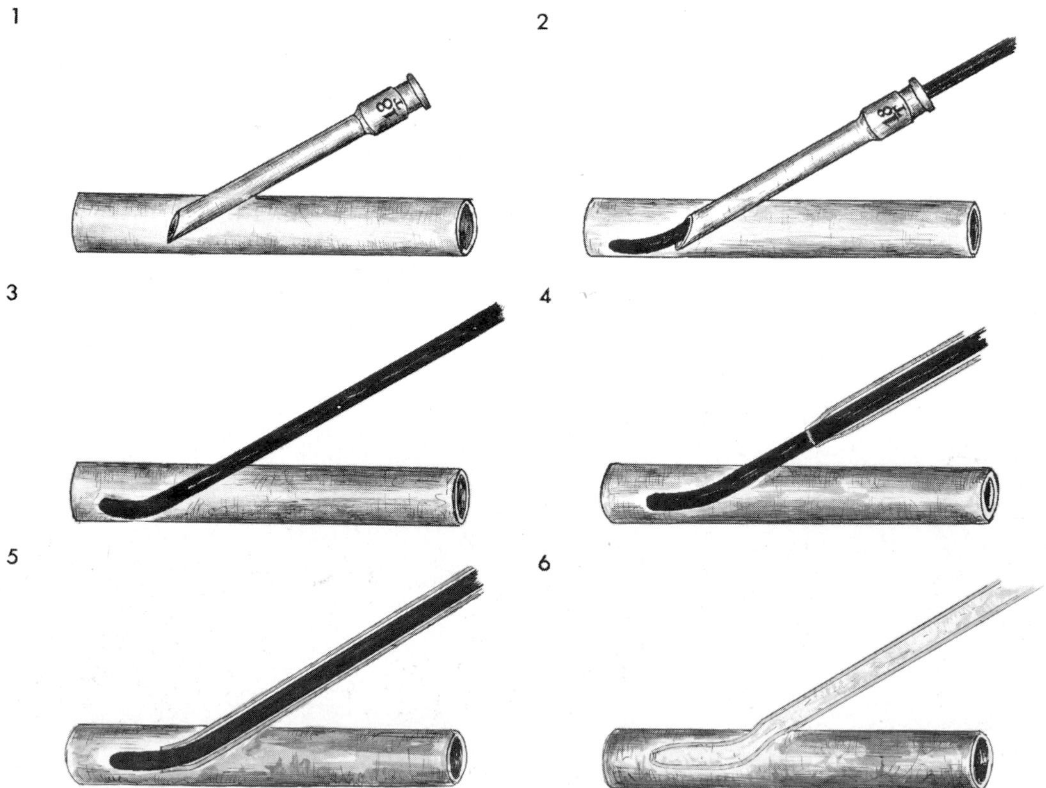

Figure 9–16 Schematic drawings illustrating the various steps of arterial catheterization.

eter, although the tube may be heparinized before use. Saline may be introduced into the catheter and the tap closed. A little blood, however, creeps into the tip of the catheter, and it is therefore necessary to perfuse with saline every minute or two. Before introducing saline, always open the stopcock and allow the blood to reflux through the tube. This is particularly important should the catheter remain unflushed for a few minutes. In this way embolization will be prevented if a clot does form.

The advancing catheter will enter the internal carotid artery from the common carotid artery 9 times out of 10 if the neck is flexed. In this position the internal carotid artery forms a direct line with the common carotid artery.[115,178] There is a far greater chance for external carotid cannulation if the neck is markedly extended during the passage from the common carotid artery.

The length of catheter inside the vessel lumen may be determined by measuring the length of catheter outside the vessel and subtracting this amount from 30 cm (allow 2 cm for passage through tissues in the neck). Should the catheter enter the external carotid artery, it may be withdrawn until its tip is in the common carotid artery; advancing it once again with the neck flexed will result in its entry into the internal carotid artery in most cases. Should the catheter again enter the external carotid artery, it may be withdrawn until the tip is present in the common carotid artery; the introduction of contrast medium here results in a simultaneous internal and external carotid angiogram.

With the catheter in position, 2 to 3 ml of saline rapidly injected will usually indicate whether the catheter is in the external or internal carotid artery. With the catheter in the external carotid artery, the patient usually has a slight burning or cold sensation along the distribution of the branches of the external carotid (i.e., the nose, mouth, tongue, and teeth). Slight blanching of the skin may also be observed on that side of the head. With the catheter in the internal carotid artery, there is usually no sensation or perhaps a slight burning sensation behind the eye on the side of the injection. There might be blanching of the skin over the distribution of the anastomosis of the ophthalmic artery.[91] These symptoms are markedly exaggerated when contrast medium is used.

Six to eight milliliters of medium (methylglucamine diatrizoate [Renografin] 60 per cent or sodium diatrizoate [Hypaque] 50 per cent) is now introduced, and the radiographic exposure is made 2 ml before the end of the injection. Exposures made with only 3 ml of contrast substance have resulted in perfectly adequate films. Accurate timing of exposure is necessary for success with these small amounts of contrast medium. Should subtraction techniques be contemplated, then radiographic exposure should be started a little before the injection is made so that the first film shows no contrast medium in the vasculature.

The common carotid artery may be punctured and the catheter introduced retrograde, down the carotid artery to outline the origin of this vessel. On the right, compression above the tip of the catheter will result in passage of contrast medium down the right common carotid to the innominate artery and to the subclavian artery and may outline the vertebral artery.[10,214] Ecker described opacification of the vertebral artery by compressing the right carotid artery just distal to the needle in its lumen.[42] The advantages and disadvantages of carotid catheterization are covered in greater detail elsewhere.[178] A catheter tip lying free in the lumen of the vessel is less likely to result in subintimal extravasation than a needle. Multiple projections may be obtained without fear of dislodging a rigid needle. Should a combined right carotid and vertebral angiogram be required, a catheter (PE 205 or 240) may be advanced retrograde down the common carotid artery. An injection at this stage will opacify the carotid tree. The catheter tip may then be advanced until it enters the innominate artery. Opacification will now be obtained of the vertebral artery and its branches.[10,178,214] A compression cuff on the right arm with distal compression of the carotid artery may give better definition of the vertebral tree. By using this technique with larger-lumen catheters, opacification of the aortic arch and its major branches has been obtained.[203]

At the completion of the examination the catheter is removed, and compression is applied to the puncture site for at least five minutes. Care must be taken to apply firm pressure and by "riding with the pulsations" not to occlude the circulation completely. Patients with atherosclerosis may require compression for longer periods, up to 20 minutes.

Weiner and associates described a technique of carotid catheterization via the exposed superficial temporal artery.[221] The superficial temporal artery is exposed under local anesthesia, and after a nick is made into the vessel, a catheter (PE 160) is inserted and advanced until its tip enters the common carotid artery. Introduction of saline into the catheter during its passage along the vessel facilitates negotiating bends in the vessel by straightening the short segment of the artery immediately ahead of the advancing catheter. This technique is more time consuming, but is useful when a puncture of the carotid in the neck or a catheter study via the axillary or femoral artery is difficult or contraindicated.

Segmental Selective Catheterization

The PE 205, 240, or the more rigid catheters will give the best results. A stab wound should be made in the skin after the preliminary steps already described for carotid catheterization. The catheter may be advanced under fluoroscopic control (an image intensifier will facilitate this part of the examination); the polyvinyl or polyethylene tube may be rendered opaque with contrast medium. The right radial, brachial, or subclavian artery may be punctured and the catheter advanced until its tip lies in the innominate artery (Fig. 9–17). The brachial artery may be punctured percutaneously in the antecubital fossa. After operative preparation of the area, as described previously, about 3 ml of 2 per cent procaine hydrochloride is infiltrated around the brachial artery at a point where it can be readily palpated. This is usually in line with the medial and lateral epicondyles. The index and middle fingers of the left hand anchor the vessel and immobilize it. The right hand is then used to introduce the No. 18 thin-walled needle into the brachial artery, using the same technique employed for the carotid artery puncture. Care must be taken to avoid damage to the median nerve. The brachial artery may be punctured in the bicipital groove, midway along the humerus,

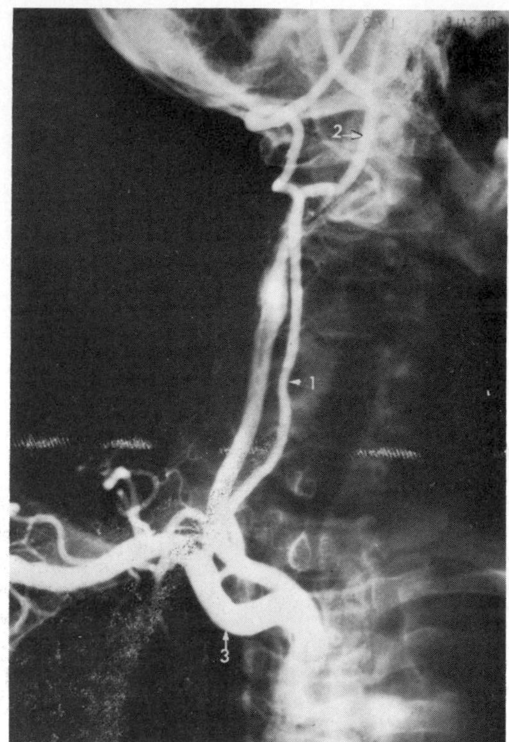

Figure 9–17 Brachial artery catheterization. Tip of catheter is in innominate artery. Note filling of vertebral artery (1) (origin stenosed), of common carotid and internal carotid arteries (2), and of subclavian artery (3).

as it passes from the posterior to the medial surface of this bone. Twelve to fifteen milliliters of 50 per cent Hypaque or 60 per cent Renografin introduced manually will result in adequate contrast of the carotid and vertebral arteries. Many workers have obtained contrast with the catheter tip in the brachial artery with or without a pressure injector. Thirty milliliters of 75 per cent Renografin introduced by pressure injector through a large cannula (No. 12) into the exposed right brachial artery may outline the carotid and vertebral arteries and their intracranial branches. Kuhn cuts down on the brachial artery and introduces a No. 8 cannula and 30 ml of 50 per cent Hypaque as rapidly as possible by hand.[103] A constricting bandage (Baumanometer cuff) around the arm, occluding the distal brachial artery during injection, may enhance the definition of the carotid and the vertebral arteries. A pilot injection of 2 ml of contrast medium is desirable to determine the precise position of the catheter in relation to the openings of the major vessels before the final bolus of medium is introduced.

In infants, Castellanos and Pereiras obtained excellent opacification of the aorta and its branches with the cannula or needle tip in the brachial artery.[23] This they have named "countercurrent aortography." Good intracranial opacification is obtained in infants with this technique, but results in adults are not as satisfactory. A recent revival of interest in it, however, has shown some promising results.[96]

Although not a catheterization technique, percutaneous injection of the right brachial artery has been used to outline the right subclavian, right vertebral, and right common carotid arteries and their branches. Percutaneous injection of the left brachial has been used to opacify the left subclavian and left vertebral arteries. The patient is premedicated as described earlier, and after the antecubital fossa is prepared, the course of the brachial artery is palpated. After infiltration with local anesthetic a No. 16 or No. 17 thin-walled short-beveled needle is introduced into the brachial artery. The needle is gently and carefully advanced up the lumen of the vessel. If difficulty is encountered in palpating the brachial artery in the antecubital fossa, it may be felt higher in the arm as it courses around the humerus (bicipital groove). A pilot dose of a few milliliters of contrast medium and an exposure with Polaroid film will quickly show the position of the needle in the vessel. One milliliter of Hypaque 50 per cent per kilogram of body weight is introduced with a pressure injector so that the bolus is injected in less than 1.5 seconds. Exposures are made 2 seconds later, at the rate of two or three exposures a second. The number and rate of exposures will depend on the suspected pathological condition. By using this technique, excellent definition of the major vessels in the neck is obtained, but opacification of intracranial vessels is not consistently good with simultaneous filling of the carotid and vertebral trees. The superimposed shadows often present a confusing picture.

Odman uses preshaped catheters and has successfully catheterized the various major vessels in the neck.[140] This author has selectively catheterized the carotid vessels via the femoral artery, using catheters with preshaped ends (Figs. 9–18 and 9–19).

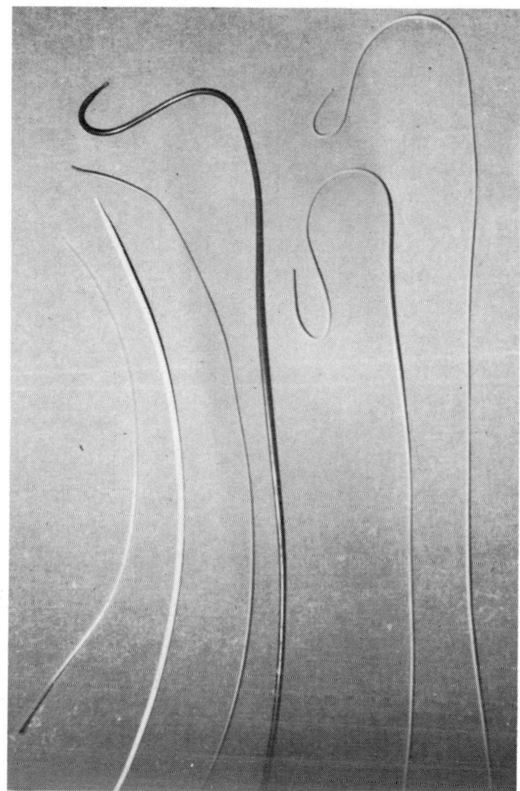

Figure 9–18 Catheters preshaped for selective introduction into the major vessels of the arch of the aorta.

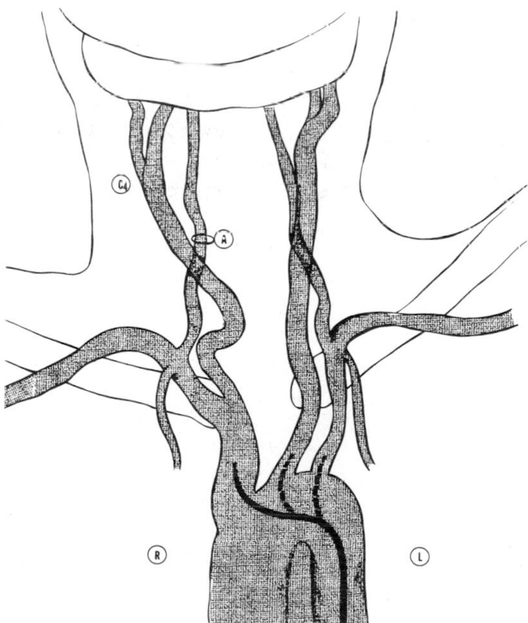

Figure 9–19 Drawing showing selective catheterization of major vessels in neck by a specially shaped catheter. C_4, level of fourth cervical vertebra; A, foramen transversarium.

This, at times, may be a tedious procedure; if any difficulty is encountered, a nonselective catheterization technique of the aortic arch will supply the information desired.

Rossi prefers the axillary route for selective catheterization of the major vessels of the neck.[166] When tortuous vessels resist the passage of the guide, he has used the "floppy guide" technique in which a variably adjusted length of the flexible end of the guide facilitates passage around curves.

Nonselective Catheterization or Aortic Arch Studies

The four avenues of approach here are the femoral, brachial, axillary, and common carotid arteries. Since the brachial artery is so notoriously liable to spasm and there is danger of compromising its circulation with a wide-bore catheter, the femoral or the axillary artery is the vessel of choice.[224] A radiopaque catheter with side openings or the PE 240 polyethylene catheter is introduced over the Seldinger guide. The tip of the catheter is premolded so that its bend will negotiate the arch of the aorta. (Image intensification will facilitate placement of the catheter.)

The right or left thigh (the author prefers the right) is prepared for the operative procedure as described earlier, and about 4 ml of 2 per cent procaine hydrochloride is infiltrated around the femoral artery 2 to 3 cm below the inguinal ligament. Puncture of the femoral artery above the inguinal ligament will make postpuncture compression difficult or impossible. After the skin is pierced at this level with a tapered scalpel blade, the No. 18 thin-walled short-beveled needle is introduced through the opening, the femoral artery is anchored with the index and middle fingers of the left hand placed on either side of the vessel, and the needle is introduced into the lumen of the vessel as in carotid arteriography. The metal spring guide is then introduced through the needle. Either of the following two methods may be followed:

1. The guide (of suitable length) is introduced until its tip is at the level that the catheter tip will assume. The catheter with side openings is now threaded over the guide and, with a rotary movement, is advanced through the skin and artery wall along the guide until its tip approximates the desired level. The guide is now removed.

2. The guide is introduced a few centimeters, and after the catheter has been threaded over it, the two are advanced together to the desired level, when the guide is removed. The tip should be placed in the ascending aorta about 2 to 3 cm proximal to the origin of the innominate artery. This location of its tip reduces the danger of its springing into a major branch during the pressure injection. Retrojets will maintain the position during the injection.

A pilot injection of 2 ml of contrast medium and an exposure of the neck in the anteroposterior projection will demonstrate the position of the tip of the catheter relative to the major branches and will also check the radiographic technique. Forty milliliters of 60 per cent Renografin or 50 per cent Hypaque is introduced by means of a mechanical pressure injector that introduces the bolus of contrast medium in less than 1.3 seconds. An oblique projection (right posterior oblique) will outline the aorta and its major branches. An anteroposterior projection of the head may be useful to demonstrate the cerebral circulation (Fig. 9–19). The lateral projection is not as helpful, since the vessels of the two sides are superimposed. The submentovertical position is often helpful for visualization of the intracranial circulation, since it obviates the superimposition of vessels that occurs in the lateral projection. After removal of the catheter, manual pressure over the puncture site should be applied for at least 15 minutes.

A tortuous iliac vessel may render introduction of the Seldinger guide difficult. The Gensini guide may facilitate passage around these sharp bends.[38,39] The spring metal guide (BD) also has a removable metal core that renders it much more flexible to negotiate the tortuous vessels. Rossi popularized the "floppy wire" technique.[166]

Vertebral Angiography

Contrast filling of the vertebral artery has been attempted by many maneuvers and often ingenious devices. Schechter and DeGutierrez-Mahoney demonstrated the evolution of the techniques that have been rewarding in the hands of each particular investigator.[180]

Direct Puncture Technique

The direct puncture of the vertebral artery will result in a high degree of intracranial definition, but will not always outline the origin of the vertebral artery. With the side-opening needle, however, contrast medium may be directed up or down the vertebral artery (Fig. 9–20).[177] The high cervical approach (suboccipital puncture of Maslowsky and Zielke and Weidner) has few followers.[123,235]

The anterior cervical approach is perhaps the simplest and the most rewarding of the direct vertebral puncture techniques.[110,201,207] The preparation of the patient is the same as for carotid angiography. Any level from C1 to C6 may be selected, but one should remember that when osteoarthritis is present a lower cervical approach may be more difficult. Unless there is an indication to examine the right vertebral artery (the right posterior inferior cerebellar artery arises from the vertebral artery a centimeter or two proximal to its union with the opposite vessel to become the basilar artery), the left side is usually selected. Statistically this is the larger vessel.[101,200] A submentovertical view of the base of the skull rarely demonstrates a significant difference in the size of the foramina transversaria, but the larger opening, when found, transports the larger vessel. It would be wise to attempt puncture of the vertebral artery on this side.

After the skin and subcutaneous tissue

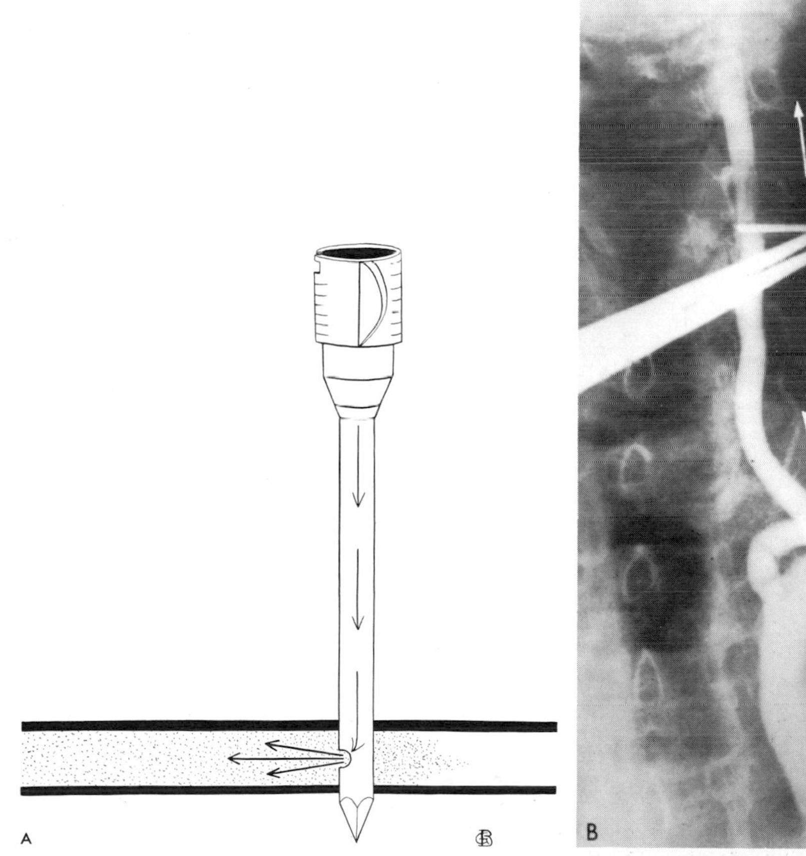

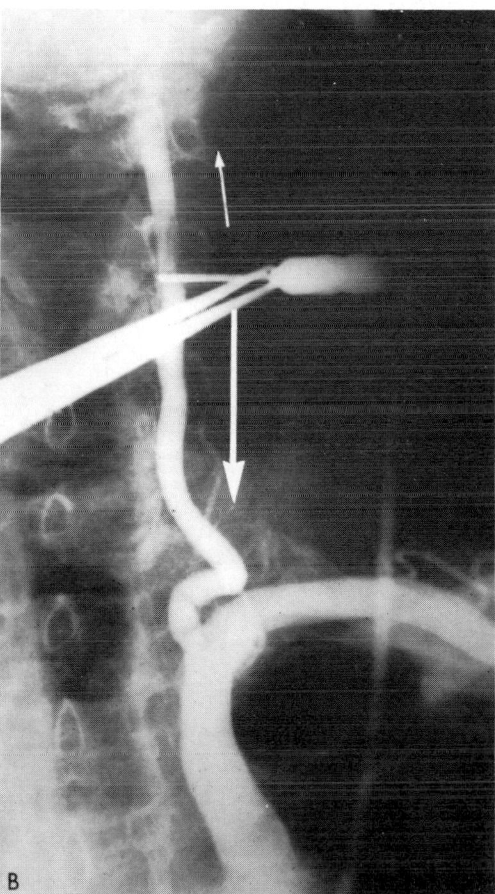

Figure 9–20 *A*. The vertebral artery is purposely transfixed by this needle, and the hub of the needle is rotated to direct the side opening at the end up or down the vessel. *B*. Vertebral angiogram produced by this technique using the anterior cervical approach and with the needle rotated so as to direct contrast medium from the side opening downward to outline the cervical course of the vertebral artery and its origin from the subclavian artery.

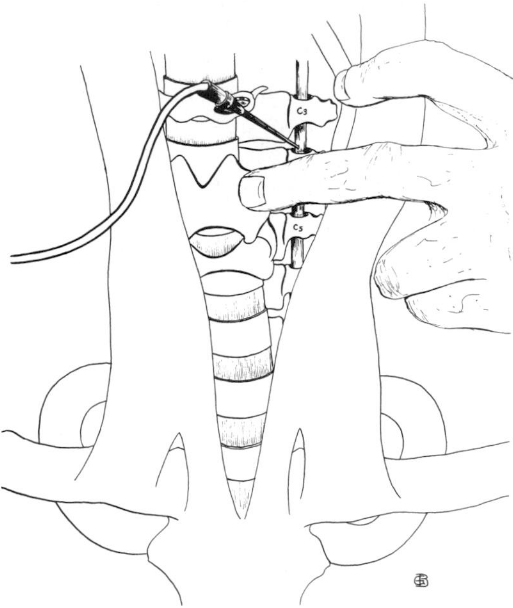

Figure 9–21 Technique of anterior cervical approach for vertebral angiography.

have been infiltrated with local anesthetic, the needle is advanced and local anesthetic is infiltrated around the intervertebral foramen. The vertebral arteriogram needle is attached to a plastic tube or other convenient connector; the system is filled with saline and connected to a syringe; the needle is introduced through the skin; and the syringe is disconnected from the connecting tube, rendering the system completely patent, so that any flow from the needle will spill freely from the end of the connecting tube. The right-handed operator displaces the trachea toward the opposite side; the carotid artery is displaced lateralward (Fig. 9–21). The right hand introducing the needle directs it between the anterior tubercles of the spine; an opening in the bony resistance will become apparent. Once the intervertebral foramen is entered, the tip of the needle is directed lateralward, and a few rapid short stabs are made inside the intervertebral foramen. The withdrawal movements of the needle should be very slowly and carefully executed, since the positioning of the hole in the needle relative to the vessel is critical.

It is unusual to actually feel the passage of the needle through the vertebral artery. Once flow is established, the connecting tube is attached to the syringe for perfusion with saline. There is no need to introduce contrast substance with great force. Approximately 6 ml of 60 per cent Renografin or 50 per cent Hypaque is used. Firm pressure on the plunger of the syringe is all that is required.

The connecting tube should be transparent, so that air bubbles may be recognized; should a faulty puncture produce blood mixed with cerebrospinal fluid, this will also be recognized. If the returned blood appears very dilute, this situation must always be suspected. Introduction of contrast medium under such circumstances has been reported and may have very undesirable effects.[17,205] To reduce this complication of the anterior approach, the vertebral needle is directed outward, i.e., away from the midline. If the needle with the side opening is used, the introduction of the needle may be vertical to the long axis of the neck. If an end-opening needle is used, the approach will differ in the sense that the hub of the needle is inclined caudally. Because of the anatomy of the parts, the side-opening needle is recommended. A notch on the hub of the needle indicates which way the opening faces (Fig. 9–20*A*).

To outline the cervical course of the vertebral artery and its origin from the subclavian artery, the side-opening needle may be rotated through 180 degrees without repuncturing the vessel, directing the orifice downward. The origin of the vertebral artery will be outlined by using this technique

(Fig. 9–20*B*).[177] The injection for opacification of the lower end of the vertebral artery should be made using a little more force than is used for the intracranial definition. It should be mentioned that even with the opening directed downward, contrast medium will eventually pass up the vessel to outline the basilar tree. Thus total vertebrobasilar opacification may be achieved with a single injection. Approximately 8 ml of 60 per cent Renografin or 50 per cent Hypaque is used with this retrograde technique.

With the end-opening needle, the vertebral artery may be catheterized. This has been attempted successfully but is not recommended. The lumen of the vertebral artery may be very small, and the removal of the guide may be difficult.

Catheterization Techniques

Catheterization of the vertebral artery from the brachial, radial, and femoral arteries employs the catheterization techniques already described.[27,76,112,154,156,157,204] In the hands of the experienced, a high success rate is claimed, and the examination is quite simple.

For partial segmental opacification of the vertebral artery, the brachial artery is punctured under local anesthesia, and the small-size Seldinger guide is introduced.[154] The brachial artery may be punctured where it is easily felt in front of the elbow or at a higher level where it runs in the bicipital groove. Cannulation is accomplished with a PE 205 catheter, although a PE 160 will often suffice. An appropriate length of catheter (usually 50 cm) should be introduced so that the tip lies opposite the vertebral artery. Side openings in the catheter are a distinct advantage. If a radiopaque catheter is used, fluoroscopic control for placement can be utilized. When a polyethylene tube is used, the introduction of a milliliter or two of contrast medium will show the position of the catheter. For the definitive study 12 to 15 ml of 60 per cent Renografin or 50 per cent Hypaque introduced as rapidly as possible by hand is usually sufficient. The cervical course of the vessel is well outlined, but the intracranial definition is usually not as good as that resulting from direct vertebral artery punctures (Fig. 9–22).

For partial segmental opacification of the vertebral artery without catheterization via a brachial artery injection, the technique must be modified slightly. A No. 12 or No. 14 needle is introduced into the brachial artery in the antecubital fossa. This may be the Robb-Steinberg needle or a thin-walled short-beveled needle. Thirty milliliters of 60 per cent Renografin is introduced as rapidly as possible by hand. Serial exposures should be made. A needle of smaller caliber (No. 17 thin-walled) may also be used with a pressure injector to introduce the contrast medium.

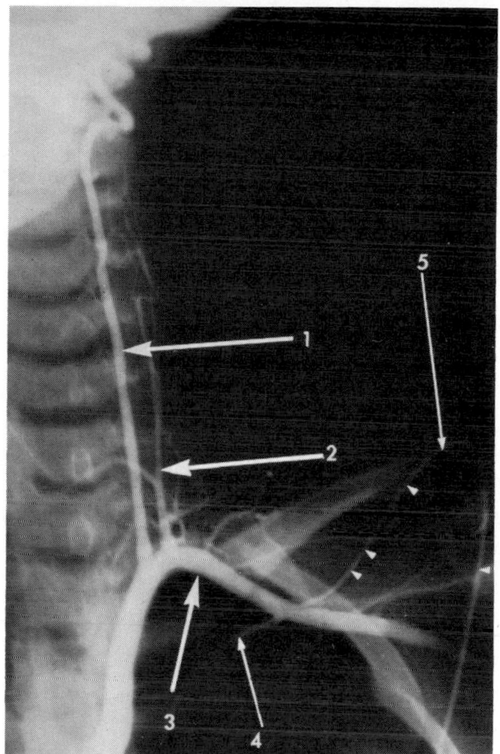

Figure 9–22 Catheter introduced percutaneously through a puncture of the left subclavian artery infraclavicularly. 1, Vertebral artery; 2, thyrocervical trunk; 3, subclavian artery; 4, internal mammary artery; 5, catheter (polyethylene PE 160).

With the femoral approach, the artery is punctured below the inguinal ligament under local anesthesia, and the catheter is advanced by using the usual technique. The femoral artery should be punctured at least 2 cm below the ligament to facilitate postinjection compression, and the artery should be compressed for at least 15 minutes after the catheter or needle is withdrawn.

Roy has described another approach in which he punctures the axillary artery and introduces a catheter, using the catheterization techniques previously described.[168] The axillary artery is palpated with either arm abducted. The author claims few complications and no spasm or thrombosis. Hanafee has used the axillary approach for selective catheterization of the vertebral artery.[69] Rossi has also used this technique with very good results.[165]

Since many variables are involved in catheterization techniques, including the length of catheter, the number and size of side openings, and the viscosity of the contrast medium, the pressure recording registered on the injector in no way resembles the pressure at the tip of the catheter. For this reason individual calibrations will have to be made by workers using these pressure injectors.

THE NORMAL ANGIOGRAM

Radiological Anatomy of the Arterial System

The three major vessels arising from the arch of the aorta are the innominate artery, the left carotid artery, and the left subclavian artery. The innominate artery divides into the right subclavian and right common carotid arteries, and the two vertebral arteries arise from the two subclavian arteries respectively (Fig. 9–23). Variations sometimes occur. A common trunk for the origin of the innominate and the left common carotid artery is a not uncommon variation in the Negro, and this

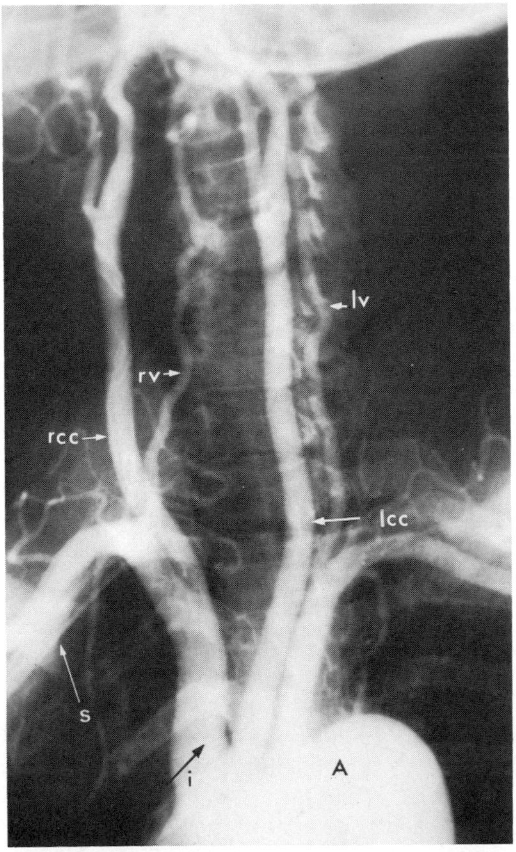

Figure 9–23 Aortic arch study with catheter introduced from the femoral artery with its tip in the ascending aorta. i, innominate artery; rcc, right common carotid artery; s, subclavian artery; lcc, left common carotid artery; rv, right vertebral artery; lv, left vertebral artery; A, aorta.

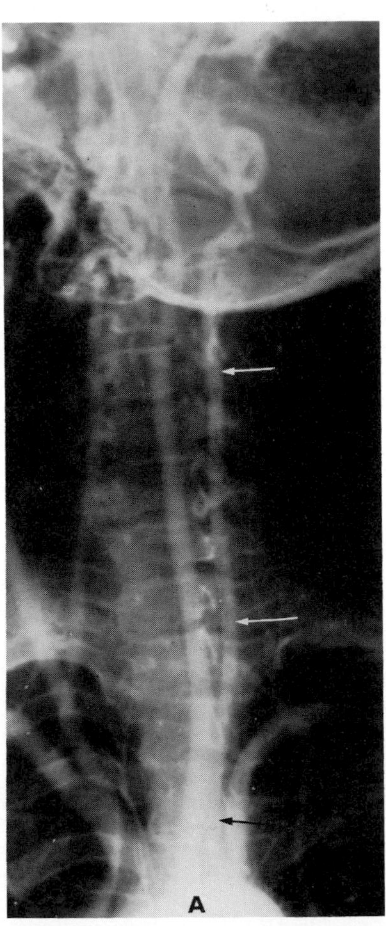

Figure 9–24 Aortic arch study. Note that the right vertebral artery arises from the subclavian artery, whereas the left vertebral artery indicated by three arrows arises directly from the arch of the aorta. A, aorta.

possibility should be kept in mind and suspected when the carotid arteries on both sides fill from an injection into the right subclavian or innominate artery. The vertebral arteries may arise directly from the arch of the aorta, a situation that should be considered when a subclavian injection does not opacify the vertebral artery (Fig. 9–24).

Carotid Arteries

The common carotid artery usually divides into the internal and external carotid arteries at the level of the superior margin of the thyroid cartilage.

The external carotid artery is anterior and medial to the internal carotid artery at its origin and, progressing cephalad, it assumes a lateral position. Branches of the external carotid artery enter the cranial cavity and assume an important role in the establishment of collateral pathways and supply to tumors.

Anatomists divide the internal carotid artery into four parts: cervical, petrous, cavernous, and cerebral (Figs. 9–25 and 9–26). The cervical internal carotid artery begins at about the level of the upper border of the thyroid cartilage and progresses vertically in the long axis of the common carotid artery to enter the skull through the carotid canal. It is here that the petrous portion of the carotid artery begins. The petrous portion is divided anatomically into the ascending portion, the knee, and the horizontal part. This horizontal or third part is the longest and runs anteriorly, upward, and medially. The petrous portion of the artery terminates as it passes between the lingula and the petrosal process of the sphenoid bone. It is here that the cavernous portion begins. The artery is situated between layers of the dura mater forming the cavernous sinus, where it is bathed in venous blood—the only site in the body where such a situation exists. The artery ascends and then runs along the carotid sulcus, and again curves upward on the medial side of the anterior clinoid process and perforates the dura mater to enter the subarachnoid space and assume its course as the cerebral portion. The meningohypophyseal trunk arises from the intracavernous portion of the carotid artery. The significance of hypertrophy of these vessels is discussed later.

The first branch of the cerebral carotid artery is the ophthalmic artery. Tiny vessels usually arise from the intracavernous portion of the artery to supply the wall of the cavernous sinus and its contents, but are not usually recognizable because of their tiny caliber unless they enlarge, when pathological change may be suspected. The normal radiological anatomy of the intracavernous artery has been well documented.[20] Its variations and their significance are discussed later. Having perforated the dura mater on the medial side of the anterior clinoid process, the internal carotid artery passes between the optic and oculomotor nerves and then gives off its anterior and middle cerebral artery branches. The course of the internal carotid artery including the intracavernous portion and the supraclinoid portion has been referred to as the "carotid siphon" by Moniz.[129]

The ophthalmic artery is the first intradural branch of the internal carotid artery. (Ruptured aneurysms at the site of origin of the ophthalmic artery will result in subarachnoid hemorrhage.) It passes laterally and inferiorly to enter the orbit through the optic foramen. The radiological anatomy of this vessel has been well covered by Lombardi.[119] The vessel is the major supply to the eyeball through the central retinal artery and also supplies the structures of the orbit and surrounding tissues. Occasionally the anterior meningeal artery takes origin from the ophthalmic artery (Fig. 9–27).[57] The ophthalmic artery forms the major collateral supply to the carotid siphon in occlusion of the carotid artery. In a large proportion of cases, the choroidal blush is recognized and outlines the back of the orbit. This is a useful landmark in expanding lesions of the orbit.

The posterior communicating artery is the next major branch of the internal carotid artery and arises from the dorsal aspect of the carotid siphon and courses posteriorly and medially to unite with the posterior cerebral artery; they both consitute part of the circle of Willis. This vessel, because of its tiny lumen, may not be opacified in the cerebral angiogram. When opacified, however, it may be seen as a fine shadow; occasionally it is well developed. Occasionally the posterior cerebral artery appears to arise directly from the internal carotid artery. The posterior communicating artery or posterior cerebral artery fills in a large proportion of cases. Saltzman found that

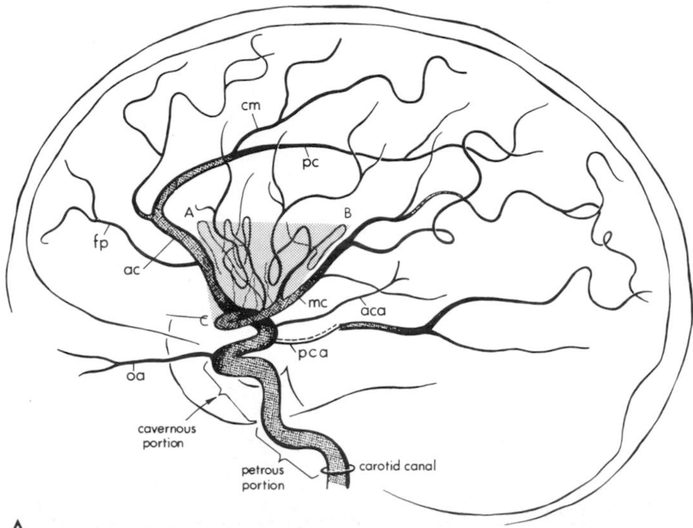

A

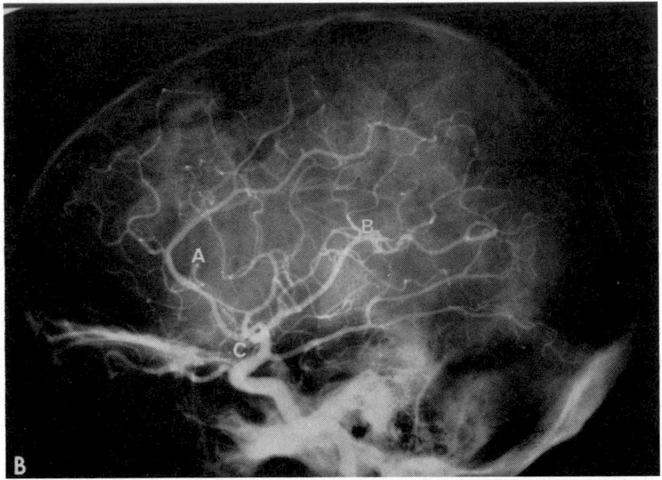

B

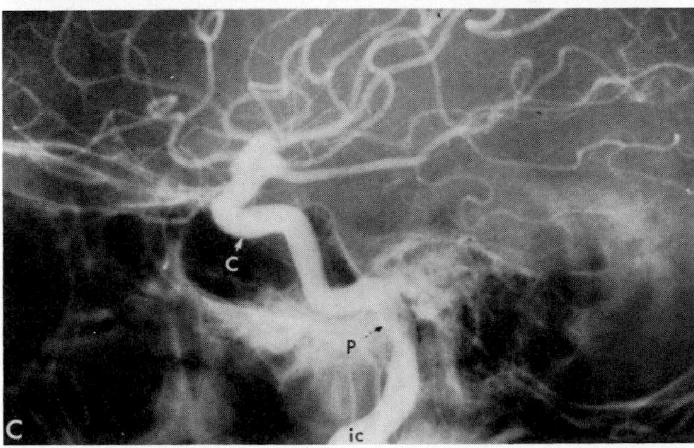

C

Figure 9–25 *A*. The triangle of Reil is constituted by selecting the most anterior branch of the opercular complex to leave the island. This is point A. Point B is the last branch to leave the island (angiographic sylvian point). The most anterior portion of the main stem of the middle cerebral artery is point C. mc, middle cerebral artery; ac, anterior cerebral artery; pc, pericallosal artery; cm, callosomarginal artery; fp, frontopolar artery; aca, anterior choroidal artery; pca, posterior communicating artery leading to the posterior cerebral artery; oa, ophthalmic artery. *B*. The triangle of Reil: points A, B, and C. *C*. Carotid angiogram. ic, internal carotid artery; p, petrous portion; c, cavernous portion.

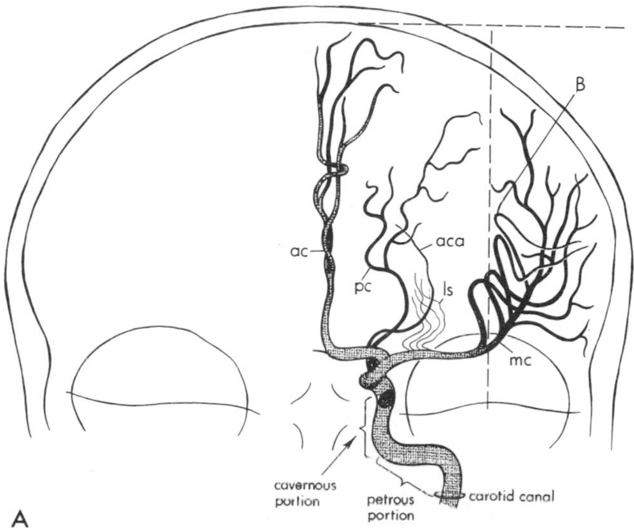

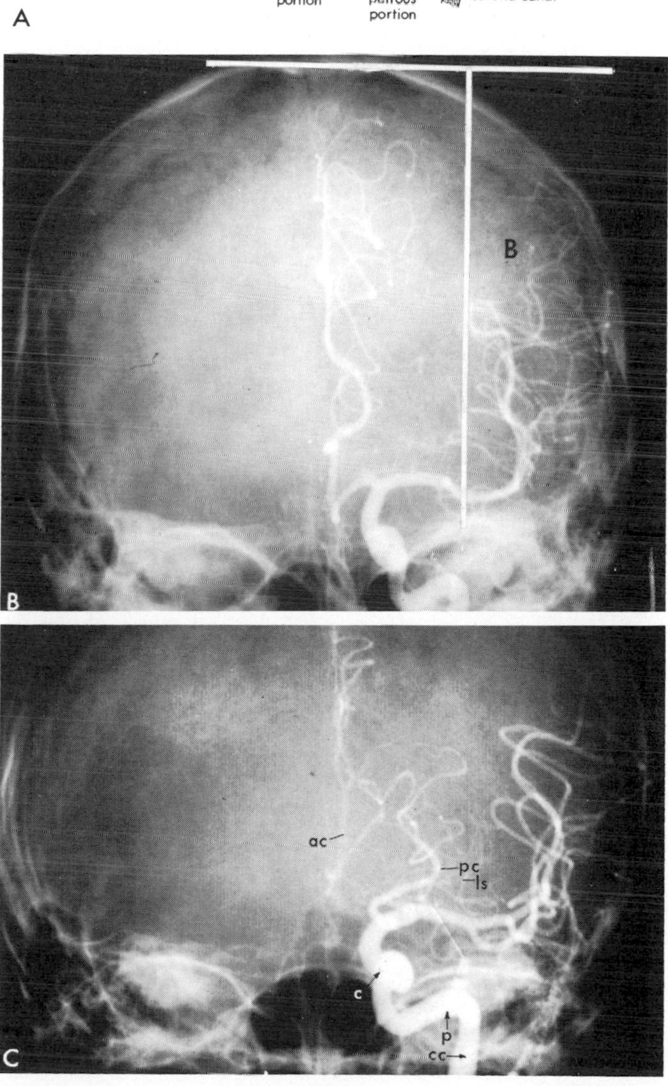

Figure 9–26 *A*. The angiographic sylvian point is the point at which the last branch of the middle cerebral artery leaves the island of Reil (B). In the frontal projection this should be halfway between a line drawn tangentially to the inner table of the skull and another line drawn parallel with and at the upper margin of the orbital roofs or the petrous crest, whichever is lower. ac, anterior cerebral artery; pc, posterior cerebral artery; aca, anterior choroidal artery; ls, lenticulostriate arteries; mc, middle cerebral artery. *B*. Construction of lines to evaluate the position of the angiographic sylvian point. *C*. Carotid angiogram. cc, carotid canal; p, petrous portion; c, cavernous portion; pc, posterior cerebral artery; ac, anterior cerebral artery; ls, lenticulostriate artery.

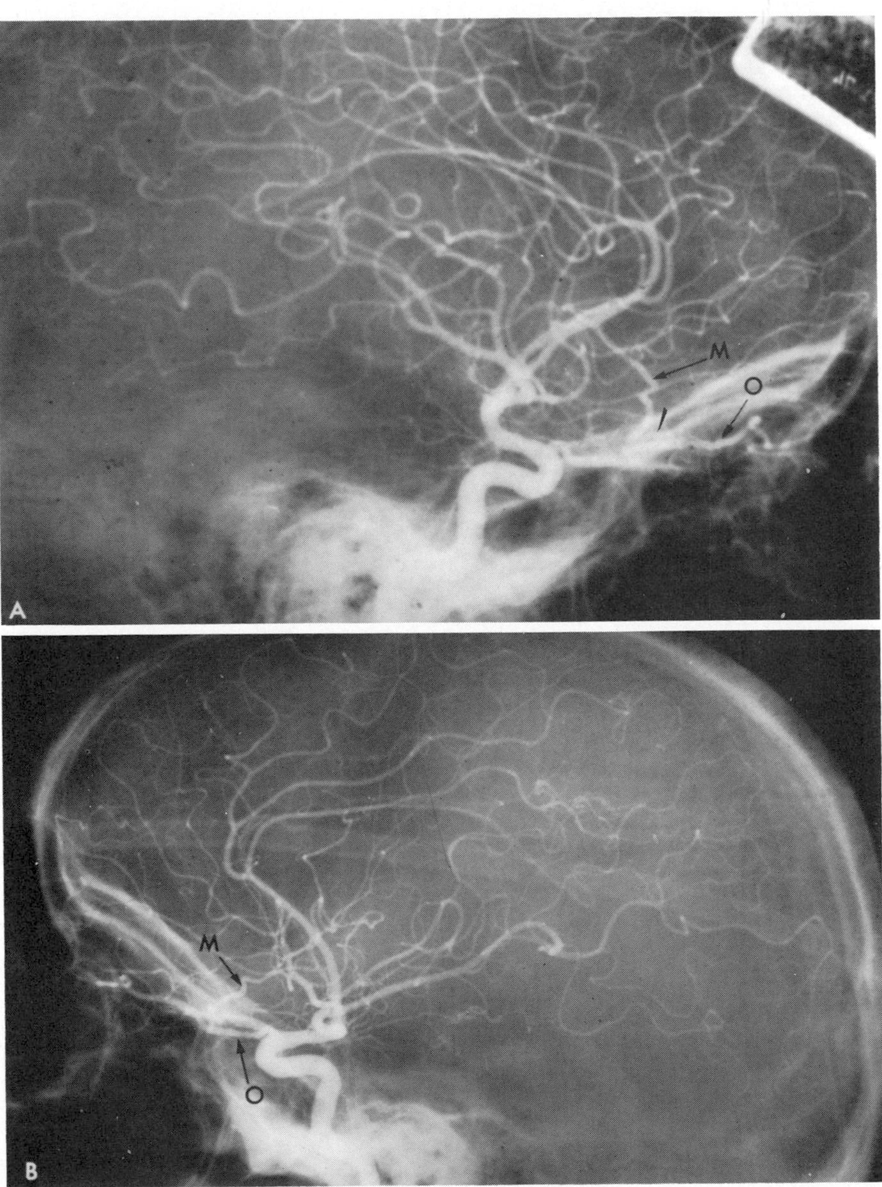

Figure 9–27 *A*. Right carotid angiogram showing the origin of the right meningeal artery (M) from the left ophthalmic artery (O). *B*. Left carotid angiogram in the same patient. Note origin of the left meningeal artery (M) from the left ophthalmic artery (O).

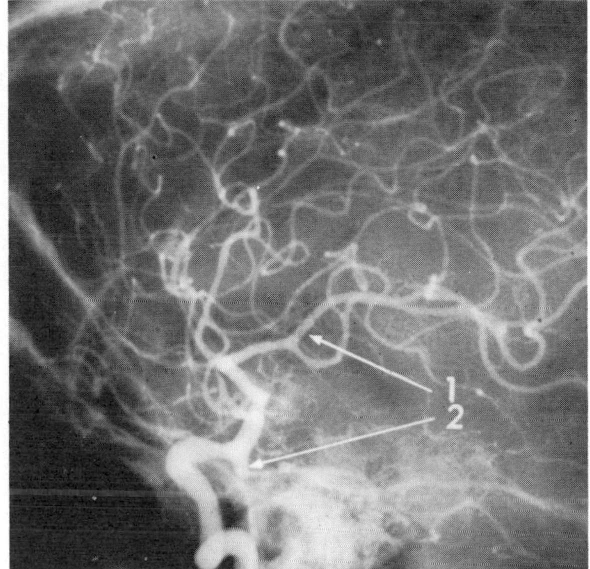

Figure 9–28 Carotid angiogram. The head has been purposely rotated into an oblique position to throw the branches of the middle cerebral artery (1) clear of the posterior cerebral artery. There is infundibular widening at the origin of the posterior cerebral artery from the internal carotid artery (2).

it did so in almost 50 per cent of internal carotid angiograms and in 30 per cent of common carotid angiograms.[172] Filling of this vessel depends upon various factors that alter hemodynamic flow. Vertebral artery compression during carotid angiography is one. At the origin of the posterior communicating artery, one sometimes sees infundibular widening of the carotid artery (Fig. 9–28).[273] It has not been conclusively established whether this represents an aneurysm or a preaneurysmal state. Hassler and Saltzman found anatomical defects in the wall of this widening in a few cases.[74,75] The significance of this finding becomes important when one is looking for a cause of subarachnoid hemorrhage.

Anterior Choroidal Artery

This is the next branch of the internal carotid artery, arising just distal to the posterior communicating artery, and can be identified in over 90 per cent of cases (Fig. 9–29). From its origin, which may show infundibular widening similar to that seen in the posterior cerebral artery, the anterior choroidal artery passes posteriorly and laterally and usually has a convex upward course. It finally enters the temporal horn and supplies the internal capsule and the choroid plexus of the inferior horn of the lateral ventricle. Occasionally a blush can be recognized angiographically that represents the choroid plexus. Sjögren refers to the cisternal and plexal course of the anterior choroidal artery, representing the length of artery from its origin through the cisternal space of the parasellar region and the length from its entry into the temporal horn to its supply to the choroid plexus.[196]

Anterior Cerebral Artery

This arises at the division of the internal carotid artery into its two major branches. It passes forward and medialward across the anterior perforated substance, above the optic nerve, to the commencement of the longitudinal fissure. The anterior communicating artery usually connects the anterior cerebral artery to the anterior cerebral artery of the opposite side. From this point the two vessels run alongside each other in the longitudinal fissure, curving over the genu of the corpus callosum as the pericallosal artery, and finally anastamosing with the branches of the posterior cerebral artery. The frontopolar branch of the anterior cerebral artery usually arises from the anterior cerebral artery just before the parent vessel takes a turn over the corpus callosum and passes toward the frontal lobe. The callosomarginal branch of the anterior cerebral artery distal to the frontopolar branch usually runs in the callosomarginal sulcus, but may emerge and return to the sulcus. This undulating course may be recognized in the frontal projection; the vessel wanders away from the midline and

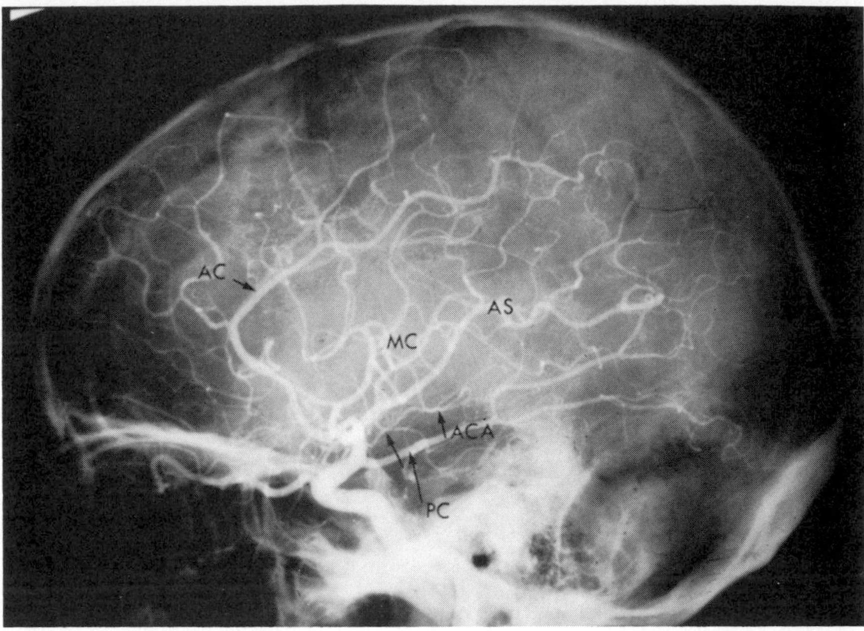

Figure 9–29 Normal carotid angiogram. AC, anterior cerebral artery; MC, middle cerebral group; PC, posterior cerebral artery; AS, angiographic sylvian point; ACA, anterior choroidal artery. (Also see Figure 9–66*A* for anterior choroidal artery.)

its fellow of the opposite side returns to the midline. In the lateral projection the vessel often runs a course roughly parallel to that of the pericallosal artery.

Middle Cerebral Artery

This is the largest branch of the internal carotid artery and often appears to be a continuation of this vessel. It at first passes lateralward in the sylvian fissure and then passes upward and backward over the island of Reil to distribute over the surface of the brain. The proximal portion of the middle cerebral artery is directed forward and lateralward and, if not horizontal, then usually a little downward; in the lateral projection it is therefore normally foreshortened. When the course of this portion of the middle cerebral artery is displayed in a well-centered lateral rádiograph, then abnormal displacement of the vessel should be suspected. The middle cerebral artery then trifurcates and continues between the island of Reil and the temporal lobe, and passing backward, divides into numerous branches before leaving the sylvian fissure (Fig. 9–30). Two groups of small branches arise from the horizontal segment of the middle cerebral artery, the medial and lateral lenticulostriate arteries. About two to six in number, these vessels pass directly upward to enter the anterior perforating substance (Fig. 9–31). The medial group supplies the medial ganglia (thalamus, caudate and lentiform nuclei) and the internal capsule, while the lateral group supplies the more laterally situated structures such as the putamen. In the anterior projection, the lenticulostriate arteries describe an S-shaped curve (Fig. 9–32). They are not always easy to recognize in the lateral projection, being superimposed on the other branches of the middle cerebral artery. The anterior temporal branch of the middle cerebral artery passes downward near the tip of the temporal lobe, and the orbitofrontal artery along the under surface of the frontal lobe. The ascending branches or the candelabra group (so called because it sometimes resembles a candelabra) is probably the most conspicuous group of the middle cerebral artery branches. The island of Reil is roughly triangular in shape and is covered in part by the operculum of the frontal, parietal, and temporal lobes.

The insular branches of the middle cerebral artery course over the island of Reil.

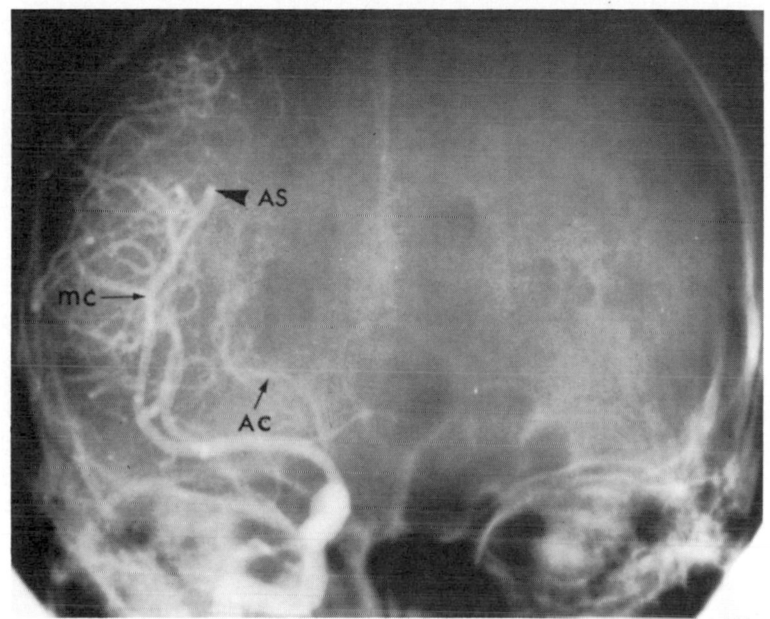

Figure 9–30 Carotid angiogram showing anterior choroidal artery (AC), middle cerebral artery (MC), and angiographic sylvian point (AS).

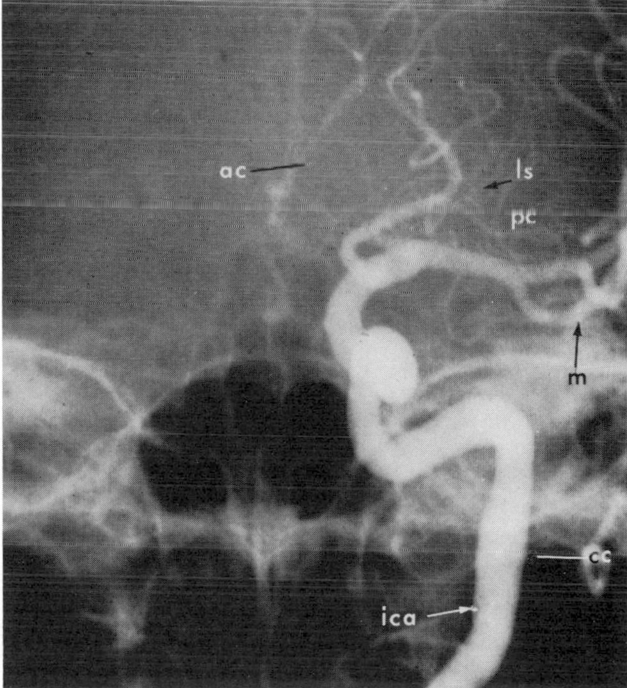

Figure 9–31 Carotid angiogram showing the fine lenticulostriate arteries (ls). m, middle cerebral arteries; ica, internal carotid artery; pc, posterior carotid artery; cc, carotid canal; ac, anterior cerebral artery.

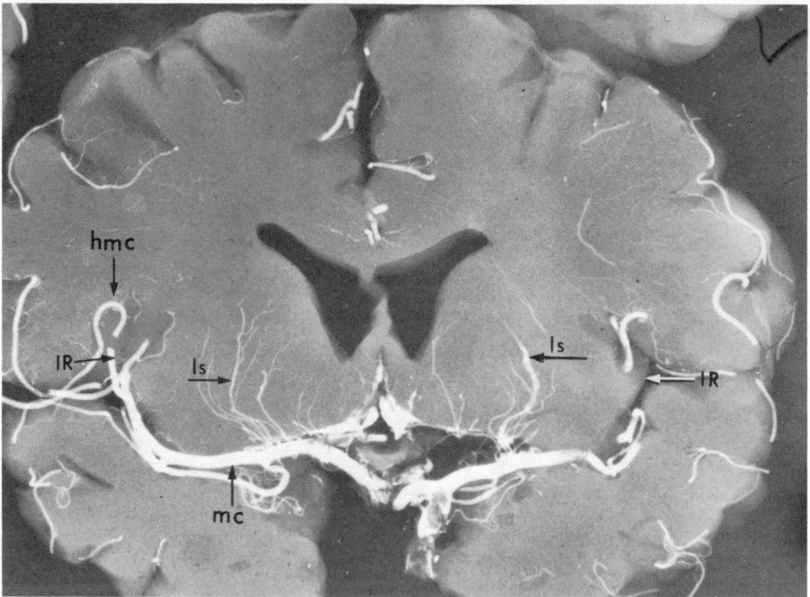

Figure 9–32 Postmortem angiogram using a barium and gelatin mixture. Note the course of the middle cerebral artery (mc) and the lenticulostriate arteries (ls) on both sides. The island of Reil (IR) is shown on both sides. Note the "hairpin bend" (hmc) of the middle cerebral artery.

As the branches that are directed upward meet the upper border of the island they enter a cul-de-sac and turn on themselves to run downward and then leave the sylvian fissure and are directed upward over the surface of the brain. Most of the branches pass upward and outward. Where the vessels turn on themselves or reverse direction, one may recognize a dense dot, the contrast-filled artery foreshortened. If these dots are joined by an imaginary line, we have the upper margin of the island of Reil. This is usually horizontal and constitutes the hypotenuse of the triangle of Reil (Figs. 9–25 and 9–33).

The course of the artery as it emerges from the sylvian fissure is usually recognizable, and one can predict the course of the sylvian fissure from this. The point of exit of the last of the insular branches to leave from the sylvian fissure is usually recognizable and has been termed the angiographic sylvian point (Figs. 9–25 and 9–26). In the anterior projection, the loops of the middle cerebral artery as they leave the sylvian fissure are readily recognizable. The lower loops are the anterior vessels, and the superior loops the posterior branches. The height of the angiographic sylvian point in the frontal projection is midway between the highest point of the skull and the upper margin of the orbit.[212] The distance between the angiographic sylvian point and the inner table of the skull varies from 30 to 43 mm.[212] The terminal branches of the middle cerebral artery pass backward and have been called, after Moniz, the posterior parietal, the angular, and the posterior temporal arteries. In infants and children the middle cerebral artery runs a more vertical course than in adults; this should not be misinterpreted as abnormal (Fig. 9–34).[211]

Vertebral Artery

For purposes of description, the normal roentgenological anatomy of the vertebral artery is divided into four segments: the origin of the vertebral artery from the subclavian artery to C6 (its usual site of entering the foramen transversarium); the course from C6 to C1; from C1 to its entry into the skull; and from its entry into the skull to its union with the opposite vertebral artery to become the basilar artery (Fig. 9–35).

Many variations of the origin of the vertebral artery have been described.[32,76,101,110] Of practical importance is absence of the vertebral artery in caroticobasilar anastomosis. Here the vertebral artery may arise from the carotid artery.[131] This situation

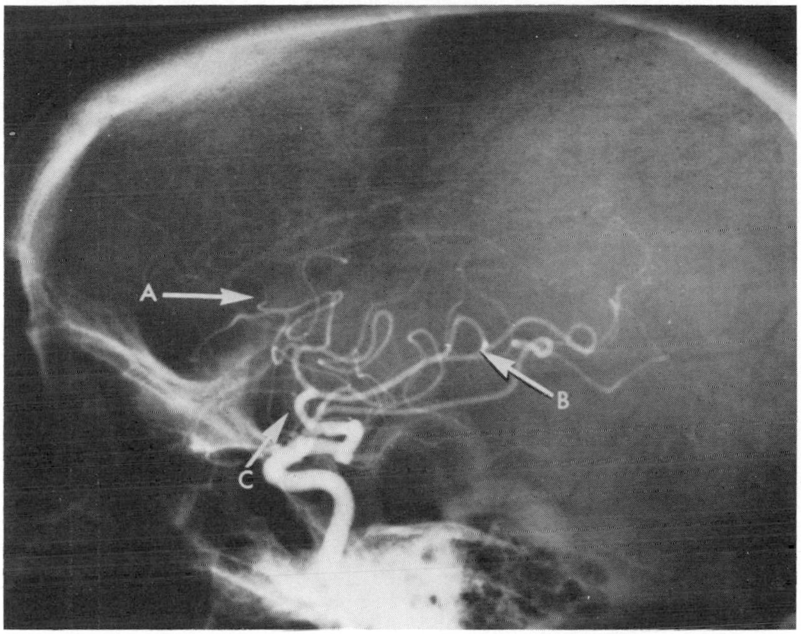

Figure 9–33 Carotid angiogram with only faint opacification of the anterior cerebral artery but with excellent filling of the middle cerebral artery group. Points A, B, and C constitute the triangle of Reil (see also Figure 9–25*A* and *B*).

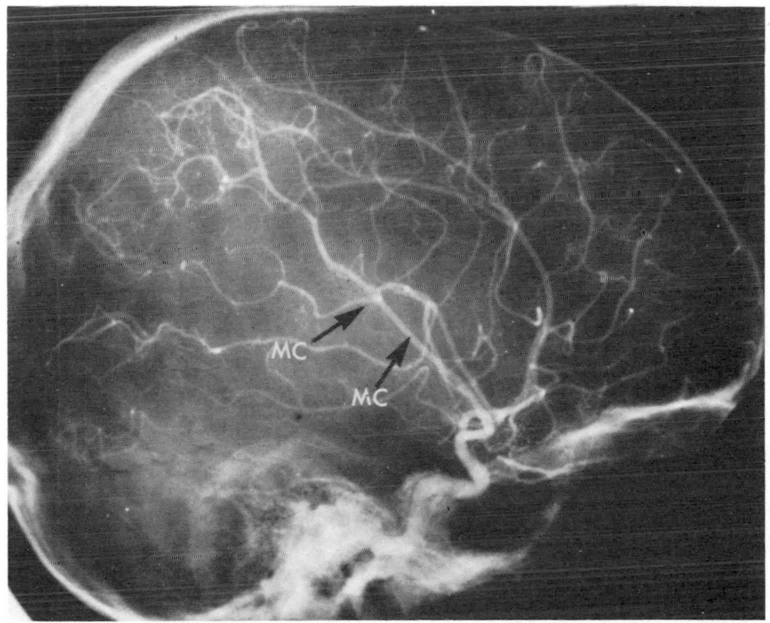

Figure 9–34 Carotid angiogram showing the middle cerebral artery running a more vertical course than usual. mc, middle cerebral artery.

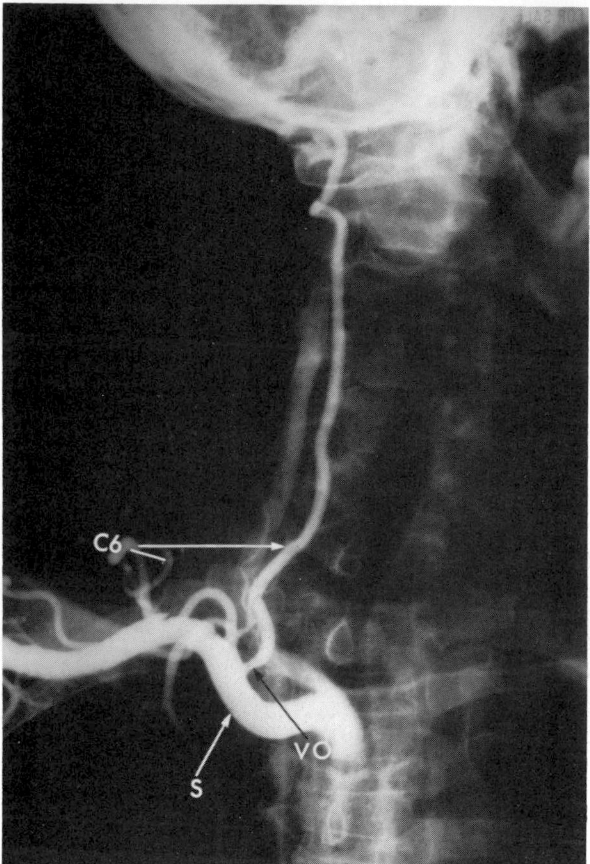

Figure 9–35 Subclavian opacification. The origin of the vertebral artery (VO) from the subclavian artery (S) is outlined. C6 is the level at which the vertebral artery usually enters the foramen transversarium. The origin of the vertebral artery to C6 is the first part. C6 to C1 is the second part.

may be misinterpreted as occlusive disease. The origin of the vertebral artery from the arch is of practical importance when vertebral angiography from the subclavian artery is attempted.

Variations of the second part are rare. Only a few anomalies have been described. Rivaglia, quoted by Krayenbühl and Yaşargil, described the vertebral artery leaving the canal between C2 and C3.[161] An incidental finding during angiography has been noted in which the vertebral artery entered the foramen transversarium at C3 (Fig. 9–36).

Multiple variations are seen in the third part. In some persons there may be differences between the two sides. In one case described by Krayenbühl and Yaşargil, there was no foramen in C1, so the artery went below C1.[101]

In the intracranial segment, or the fourth part, there are variations in the course of the vessels as they enter the basilar artery. Anatomical anomalies are rare. In Krayenbühl and Yaşargil's series, the vertebral artery in the lateral projection appeared to be parallel to the clivus in 47 per cent of cases (Fig. 9–37; see also Fig. 9–47) and slightly bent posteriorly in 39 per cent of cases or markedly bent posteriorly in 14 per cent of cases (Fig. 9–38).[101]

The displacement may be as much as 1 cm according to Lindgren.[110] Sergent and co-workers reported displacements in normal subjects of 0.8 to 1.2 cm, and Krayenbühl and Yaşargil noted a displacement of 1.6 cm in a normal vertebral angiogram.[101,191] The junction of the vertebral arteries may be projected approximately in the midline of the foramen magnum or definitely lateral to this (Figs. 9–39 and 9–40). The point of juncture of the two vertebral arteries varies considerably in the normal angiogram and may be quite laterally placed (compare with the tip of the basilar artery, which is usually midline). It is im-

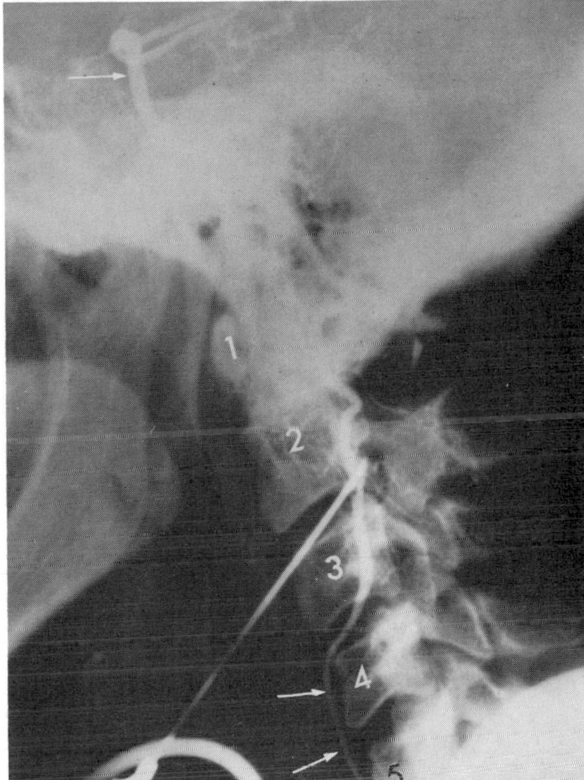

Figure 9–36 Vertebral angiogram. Note course of vertebral artery (*arrows*) in the lower cervical region where it enters foramen transversarium between C3 and C4.

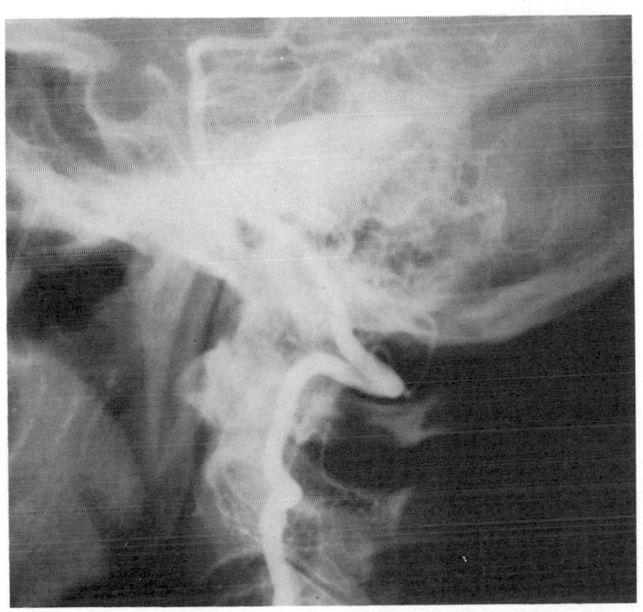

Figure 9–37 Note that the basilar artery is parallel to the clivus.

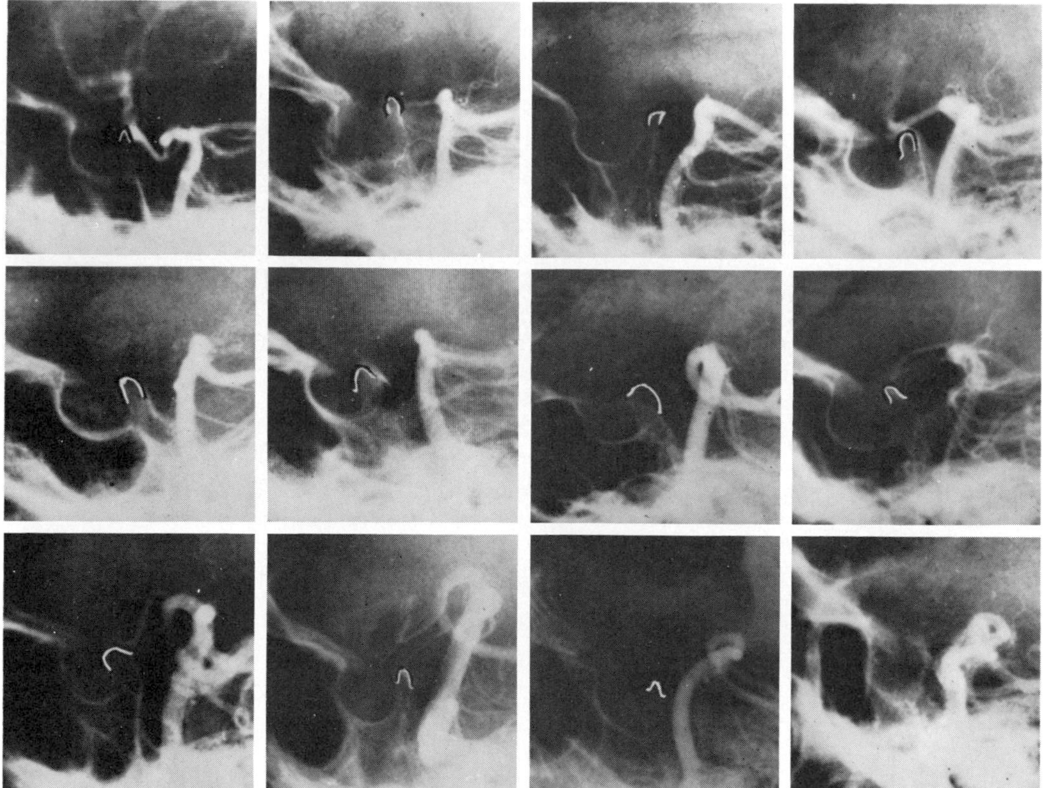

Figure 9–38 Twelve normal vertebral angiograms. The posterior clinoid has been retouched for identification. Note the variations in the height of the basilar artery and its distance (horizontal) from the tip of the posterior clinoid.

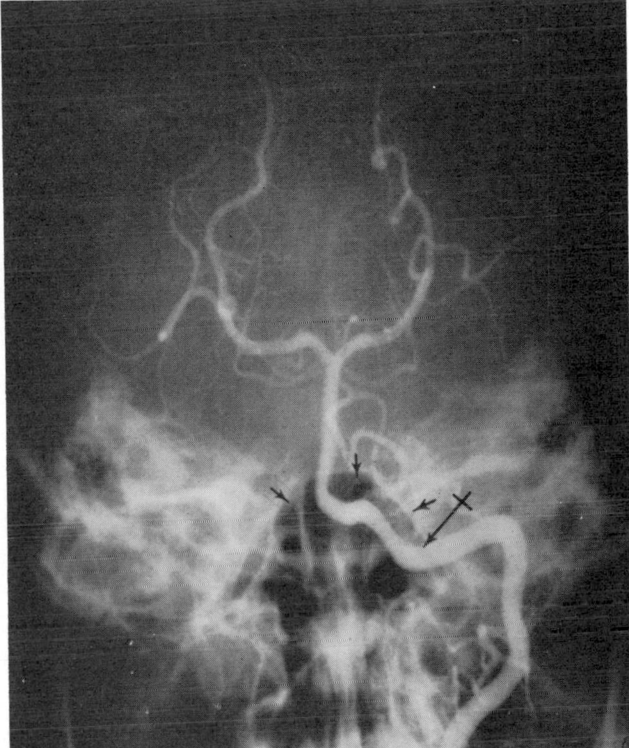

Figure 9–39 The junction of the two vertebral arteries is projected in the midline of the foramen magnum (*foramen magnum identified by arrows*); +→ represents the point of entry of the vertebral artery into the subarachnoid space.

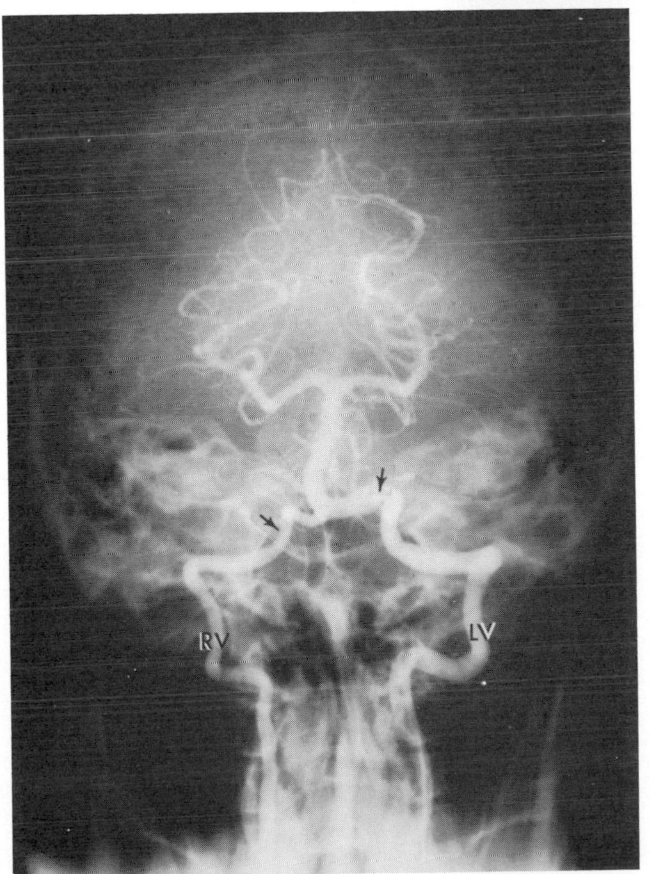

Figure 9–40 Vertebral angiogram. Note that the caliber of the vertebral artery on the left side (LV) is larger than that on the right side (RV). The junction of the two vertebral arteries is projected to the right of the midline. Note that the basilar artery is concave toward the vertebral artery of the larger caliber.

portant to recognize a laterally placed origin of the basilar artery and not interpret these findings as abnormal.[67]

Caliber of the Vertebral Artery

Stopford, examining these vessels in 150 cadavers, found a wider vertebral artery on the left in 51 per cent of cases, a wider vertebral artery on the right in 41 per cent of cases, and vertebral arteries of equal width in 8 per cent of cases.[200] Thus, in 92 per cent of cases, the vertebral arteries were of unequal width. Stopford also found an abnormally small vertebral artery on the right side in 9 per cent of cases (Fig. 9–41), abnormally small vertebral arteries on the left side in 5 per cent of cases, and abnormally small vertebral arteries on both sides in 1 per cent of cases.[200]

In a series of postmortem studies by Krayenbühl and Yaşargil, 42 per cent had wider vertebral arteries on the left side, 32 per cent had wider vertebral arteries on the right side, and 26 per cent had vertebral arteries of equal width. In 72 per cent the difference in caliber was clearly visible; in 20 per cent the caliber was minimal. They also found abnormally small vertebral arteries on the right side in 6.2 per cent, abnormally small vertebral arteries on the left side in 4.5 per cent, and abnormally small vertebral arteries on both sides in 0.75 per cent; in two cases, one vertebral artery was as thin as a string.[101] Of interest here is that when the foramina transversaria are of unequal size (this can be recognized in the basal view) the larger foramen transmits the larger vertebral artery.

The most dorsal point of the artery seen in the lateral angiogram corresponds with its entry into the subarachnoid space, and this is roughly the middle of the foramen magnum. In the fronto-occipital projection, the entrance into the subarachnoid space corresponds with the lateral margin of the foramen magnum (Fig. 9–39).

Height at Which Vertebral Arteries Join

In the Stopford series, 72 per cent joined below the inferior margin of the pons, 8 per cent joined above the inferior margin of the pons, and 19 per cent joined at the level of the olivary nucleus of the medulla. In the Krayenbühl and Yaşargil series, 66 per cent

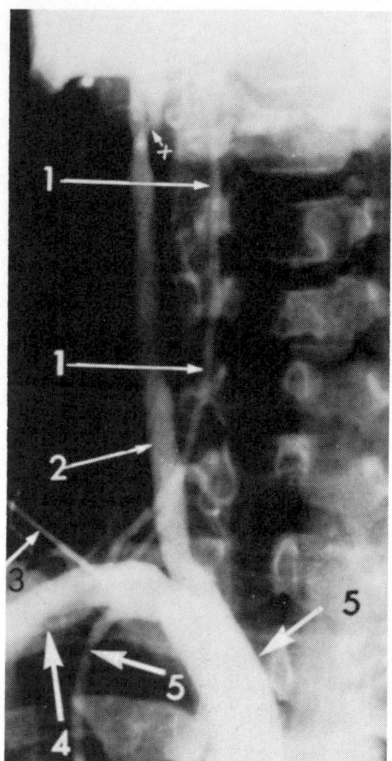

Figure 9–41 Supraclavicular puncture of the subclavian artery. Note needle (3), subclavian artery (4), innominate artery (5), common carotid artery (2), with marked narrowing at origin of internal carotid artery (x). Vertebral artery has a narrow and hypoplastic lumen (1).

joined at the inferior margin of the pons, 12 per cent above this point, and 22 per cent below this point; in one case they joined at the middle of the pons.[101]

Reflux Down Contralateral Side

Visualization of the contralateral vertebral artery depends on many factors. One important factor is the rate of injection. Compression of the ipsilateral vertebral artery over the supraclavicular region might promote reflux. Twenty to thirty per cent of cases show filling of the contralateral vertebral artery during percutaneous vertebral angiography.[157,206] Since there is no reflux in over 70 per cent of cases, the opposite vertebral artery must be opacified if pathological change such as an aneurysm at the origin of the posterior inferior cerebellar artery is suspected. Scatliff and associates investigated the factors involved in vertebral artery reflux.[175] Hypotension, turning of the head, and variations in the caliber of the vertebral artery were considered.

Posterior Inferior Cerebellar Artery

The first large artery arising from the vertebral is the posterior inferior cerebellar artery. The vessel usually arises from the vertebral artery 1 to 2 cm proximal to the origin of the basilar. The medial extension of the cerebellar hemisphere, which presents at or just above the foramen magnum, is called the cerebellar tonsil. A portion of the posterior inferior cerebellar artery is intimately associated with this part. The posterior inferior cerebellar artery arises from the vertebral artery and passes dorsolaterally with a caudal loop around the medulla, and then divides into a medial and a lateral branch. The lateral branch passes over the inferior surface of the cerebellum, while the medial branch runs along the medial aspect of the tonsil. The medial branch has a caudal loop and a cranial loop. The caudal loop passes under the cerebellar tonsil, and the cranial loop passes close to the caudal and lateral limits of the fourth ventricle. The vessel then distributes to the medial part of the cerebellar hemisphere. Thus, viewed at right angles to the median plane, a caudal loop is formed that defines the approximate outline of the caudal part of the tonsil, and a cranial arterial loop that indicates the cranial border of the tonsil.

By outlining this vessel with contrast medium it is possible to judge the position of the cerebellar tonsil and the caudolateral part of the fourth ventricle. Herniations of the tonsils may therefore be demonstrated by showing the hairpin bend of the posterior inferior cerebellar artery below the foramen magnum (Figs. 9–42 and 9–43).

Cases have been reported in which the origin of the posterior inferior cerebellar artery was from the basilar artery and in which one vertebral artery became the posterior inferior cerebellar artery, while the one on the other side continued to become the basilar artery; that is, there was nonfusion of the vertebral arteries.[101,157]

The posterior inferior cerebellar artery is unfortunately sometimes absent or too small to be clearly visualized during vertebral angiography. Krayenbühl and Yaşargil state that it is identified in the lateral projection in 88 per cent of cases, and not visualized in 12 per cent of cases.[101] In four cases, the loop of the posterior inferior cerebellar extended markedly below the foramen magnum. In 9 per cent of demonstrable posterior inferior cerebellar arteries, the loop was just below the foramen magnum in a narrow coil, while in 8 per cent the coil entered the foramen magnum in a broad sweep. Lindgren identified this vessel in the lateral projection in 90 per cent of cases.[111,112]

The posterior meningeal branches arising from the vertebral artery are sometimes recognized during angiography. These course along the inner table of the occipital bone. The anterior spinal artery can be identified in 50 per cent of vertebral angiograms. It may outline the anterior margin of the spinal cord, may act as a collateral pathway in occlusive disease, and may feed pathological processes, e.g., angiomas.[183,184]

Basilar Artery

The first part of the basilar artery, as seen in the lateral angiogram, is overlapped by the dense petrous bones. The artery then shows a curve with a ventral convexity. The variations in distance from the tip of the basilar to the dorsum sellae, according to Krayenbühl and Yaşargil, are as follows: in 39 per cent of cases 0.1 to 0.5 cm; in 48 per cent of cases 0.5 to 0.9 cm; in 13 per cent of cases 1.0 cm or more. The average is 0.6 cm; the minimum is 0.1 cm; the maximum is 1.4 cm.[101]

The point of basilar bifurcation also varies longitudinally. As a landmark, a line was projected backward from the anterior clinoids parallel to the baseline of the skull. In 51 per cent of cases the tip of the basilar was the same height; in 19 per cent of cases the tip of the basilar was less than half the height of the dorsum sellae; and in 30 per cent of cases the tip of the basilar was more than half the height of the dorsum sellae above. The maximum height above this line was 1.3 cm (Fig. 9–38). When the tip is projected above the posterior clinoids, the usual appearance in the lateral and anteroposterior projection is a W, like the handlebar mustache, but when projected below the posterior clinoids, the appearance in the lateral and anteroposterior projection is like a V or Y (Fig. 9–44). The W and V forms were described by Lindgren.[113]

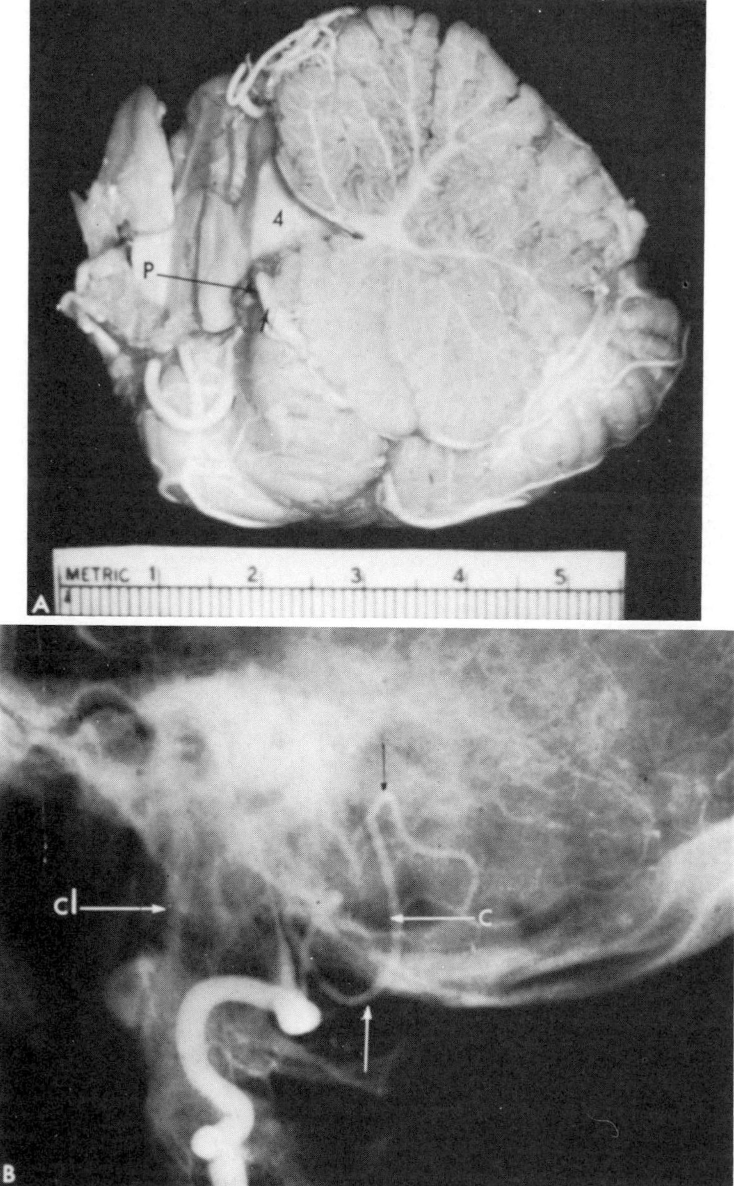

Figure 9–42 *A*. Postmortem injected specimen. Note the cranial loop of the posterior inferior cerebellar artery and its proximity to the fourth ventricle (↑). (Specimen by courtesy of Dr. Wollschlaeger.) *B*. Vertebral angiogram outlining the posterior inferior cerebellar artery. The caudal loop of the posterior inferior cerebellar artery outlines the inferior pole of the cerebellar tonsil (c), and the cranial loop (cl) is related to the caudolateral portion of the fourth ventricle.

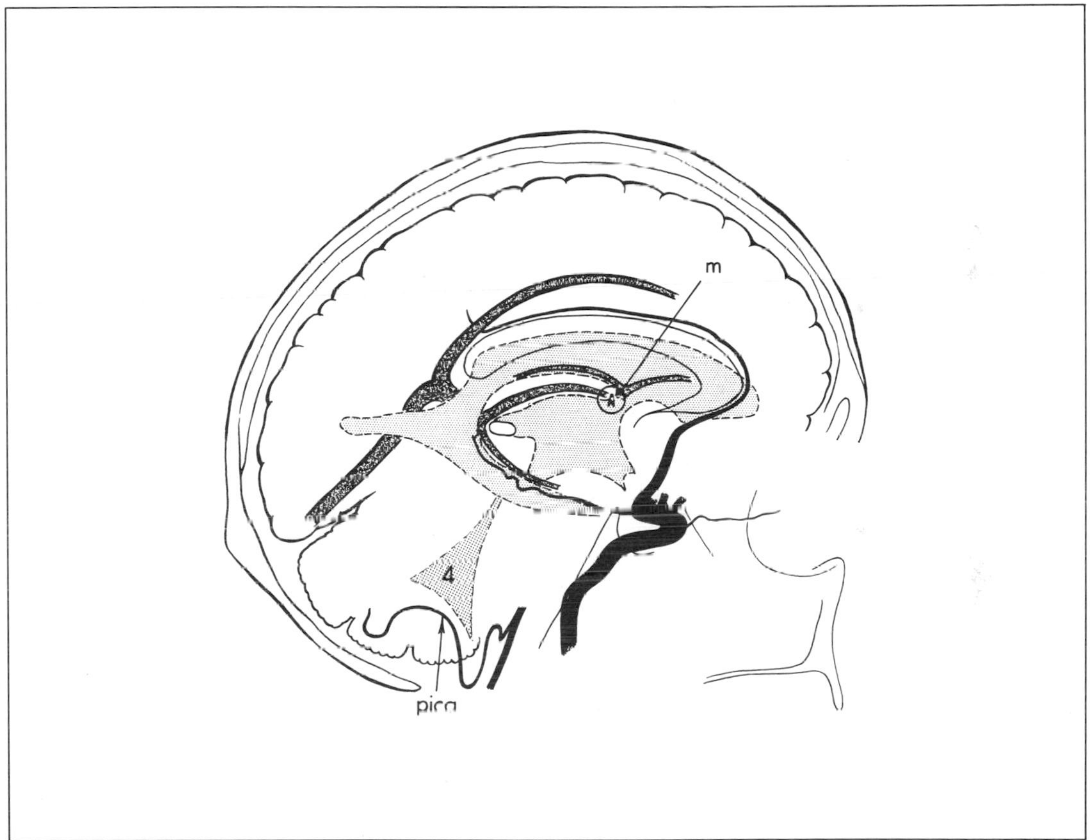

Figure 9–43 Diagram of relationship of ventricular system, arteries and veins. M, foramen of Monro; A, junction of thalamostriate vein, septal vein, and internal cerebral vein; 4, fourth ventricle; pica, posterior inferior cerebellar artery.

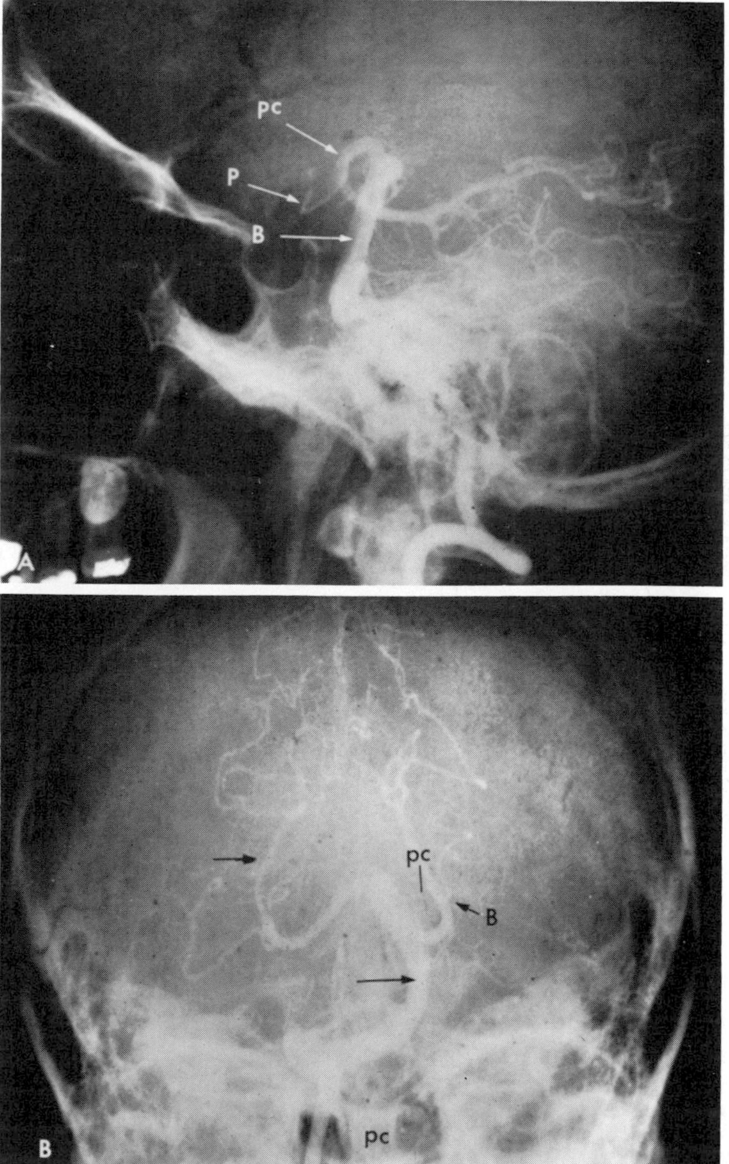

Figure 9–44 *A*. Lateral projection of a vertebral angiogram showing an elongated basilar artery extending for a considerable distance above the posterior clinoids. B, basilar artery; pc, posterior cerebral artery; p, posterior communicating artery. *B*. Anterior projection of the same vertebral angiogram. With the vertical extension of the basilar artery the configuration in the anterior projection is the W type.

Anterior Inferior Cerebellar Arteries

These are not seen in the lateral projections, as they are covered by the dense petrous bone. These vessels run laterally toward the auditory meatus. Some authors have described changes in the course of the vessel produced by acoustic neuromas.

Pontine Perforating Branches

These are sometimes seen in the lateral projection. They are five vessels running parallel to one another and posteriorly from the basilar artery to the pons.

Superior Cerebellar Arteries

These, in their most ventral part, follow the course of the posterior cerebral arteries and curve around the midbrain. This part of the artery may arch caudally in a single curve or show irregular loops. The majority of the branches of this artery are projected in a region that corresponds with the lateral projection of the tentorium. The superior cerebellar arteries divide into medial and lateral branches, which pass over the superior aspect of the cerebellum. Congenital anomalies are not common. The superior cerebellar arteries may arise from the posterior cerebrals, and two superior cerebellar arteries have been seen on the left and one on the right. Wollschlaeger and Wollschlaeger have shown numerous variations of the vessels arising from the basilar artery.[227]

Posterior Cerebral Arteries

The two posterior cerebral arteries course over the tentorium and, proximal to their bifurcation, pass straight back, or may even show a marked curve with a caudal convexity.[222] Usually, in most of their course, the two arteries run approximately the same course. The occipital branch of the posterior cerebral artery arches superiorly, and the branches are distributed in a wedge-shaped area in the occipital fossa. The calcarine branch of the posterior cerebral artery is more or less a straight continuation of the artery. The temporal branch of the posterior cerebral artery crosses the first part of the posterior cerebral artery and passes caudally. The lateral branches are projected in a triangular region, which in the lateral projection corresponds with the tentorium. In the anteroposterior projection there is no constant bilateral symmetry of the branches of the posterior

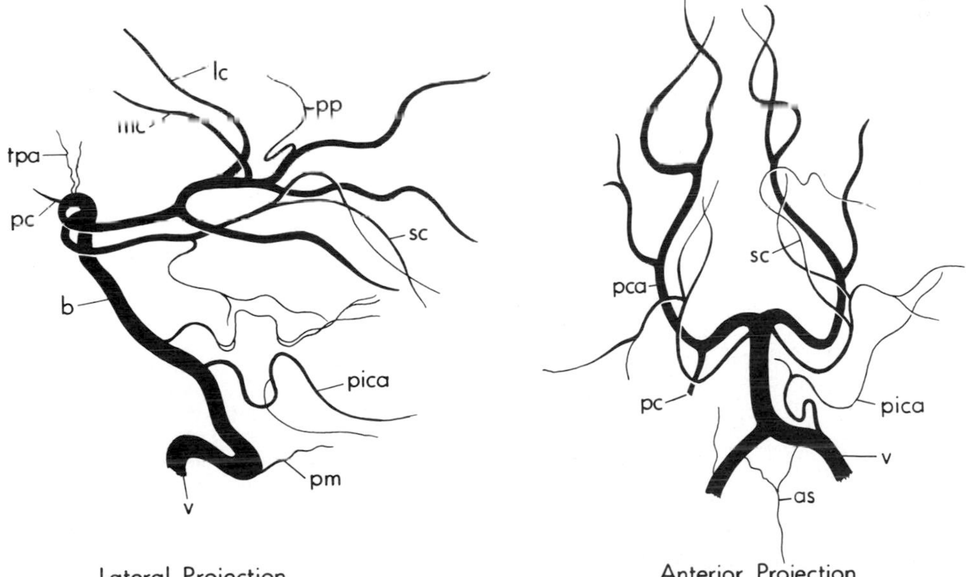

Figure 9–45 Vertebral arteriogram. v, vertebral artery; pm, posterior meningeal artery; pica, posterior inferior cerebellar artery; b, basilar artery; pc, posterior communicating artery; tpa, thalamoperforating arteries; sc, superior cerebellar artery; pp, posterior pericallosal artery; mc, medial posterior choroidal artery; lc, lateral posterior choroidal artery; as, anterior spinal artery; pca, posterior cerebral artery.

cerebral artery. The vessel gives off its temporal branch and then continues, forming a "Grecian vase" when viewed in the anterior projection, to divide into the occipital and calcarine branches (Fig. 9–45). Fetterman and Moran drew attention to the fact that with advancing age the posterior communicating arteries become reduced to filamentous strands, and this may explain the flow dynamics in which there may be filling of the posterior cerebral artery from both the carotid artery and the basilar artery or only from one of them.[50]

When one posterior cerebral artery fills from the carotid and one from the basilar artery, the resulting asymmetry may simulate a disease process (Fig. 9–46). Both posterior cerebral arteries may arise from the carotid artery while both superior cerebellar arteries arise from the basilar artery (Fig. 9–47). Saltzman reported an increased incidence of filling of the posterior cerebral artery and posterior communicating artery when the ipsilateral vertebral artery was compressed low in the neck.[172,174]

Posterior Choroidal Arteries

Lateral to the cerebral peduncle, the posterior cerebral artery gives off two posterior choroidal arteries—the medial branch, which supplies the choroid plexus in the third ventricle, and the lateral branch, which supplies the choroid plexus in the lateral ventricle. Branches also pass to the neighboring structures. The arteries first run parallel to the posterior cerebral and then, in the choroid fissure, swing around the medial posterior part of the thalamus to proceed upward in a concave curve forward. They extend at the same time in a medial direction and run laterally to and over the pineal body up into the tela choroidea of the third ventricle. Here, near the midline, they meet the internal cerebral vein, which they follow anteriorly in the roof of the third ventricle. The lateral posterior choroidal artery passes through the intraventricular foramen and supplies the choroid plexus in the upper part of the lateral ventricles. Only rarely can these vessels be identified in the anteroposterior

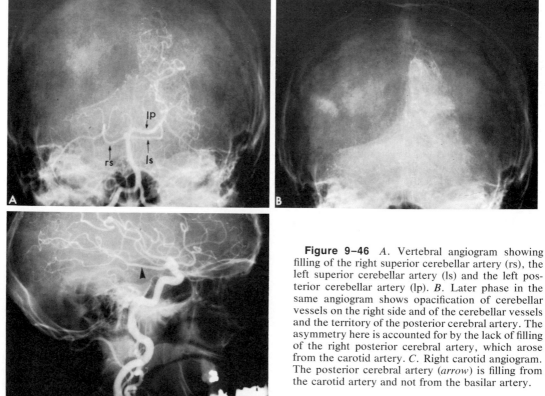

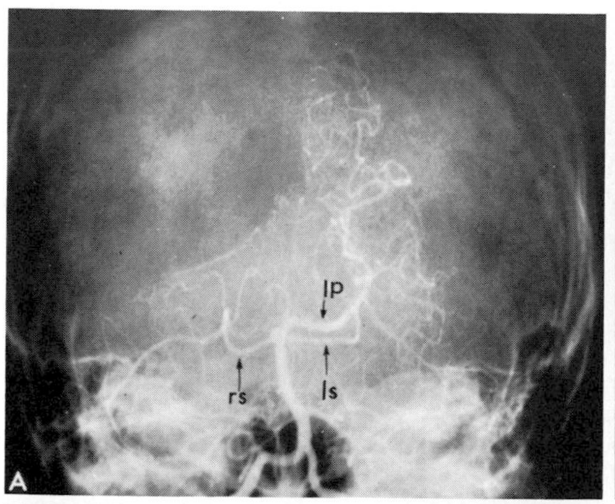

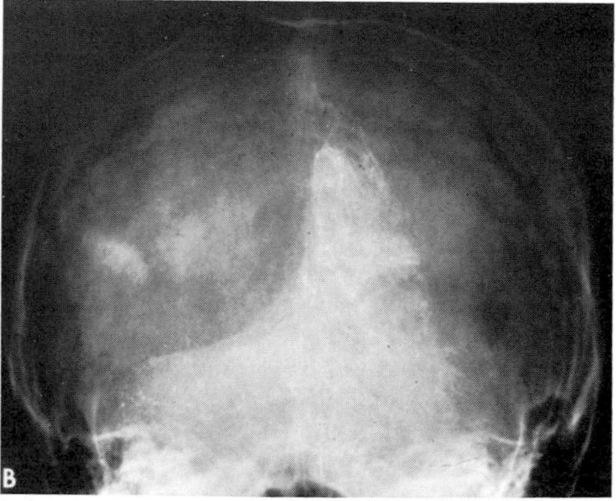

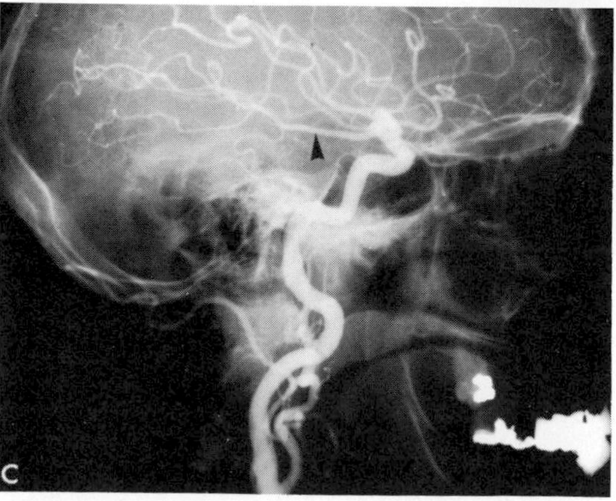

Figure 9–46 *A*. Vertebral angiogram showing filling of the right superior cerebellar artery (rs), the left superior cerebellar artery (ls) and the left posterior cerebellar artery (lp). *B*. Later phase in the same angiogram shows opacification of cerebellar vessels on the right side and of the cerebellar vessels and the territory of the posterior cerebral artery. The asymmetry here is accounted for by the lack of filling of the right posterior cerebral artery, which arose from the carotid artery. *C*. Right carotid angiogram. The posterior cerebral artery (*arrow*) is filling from the carotid artery and not from the basilar artery.

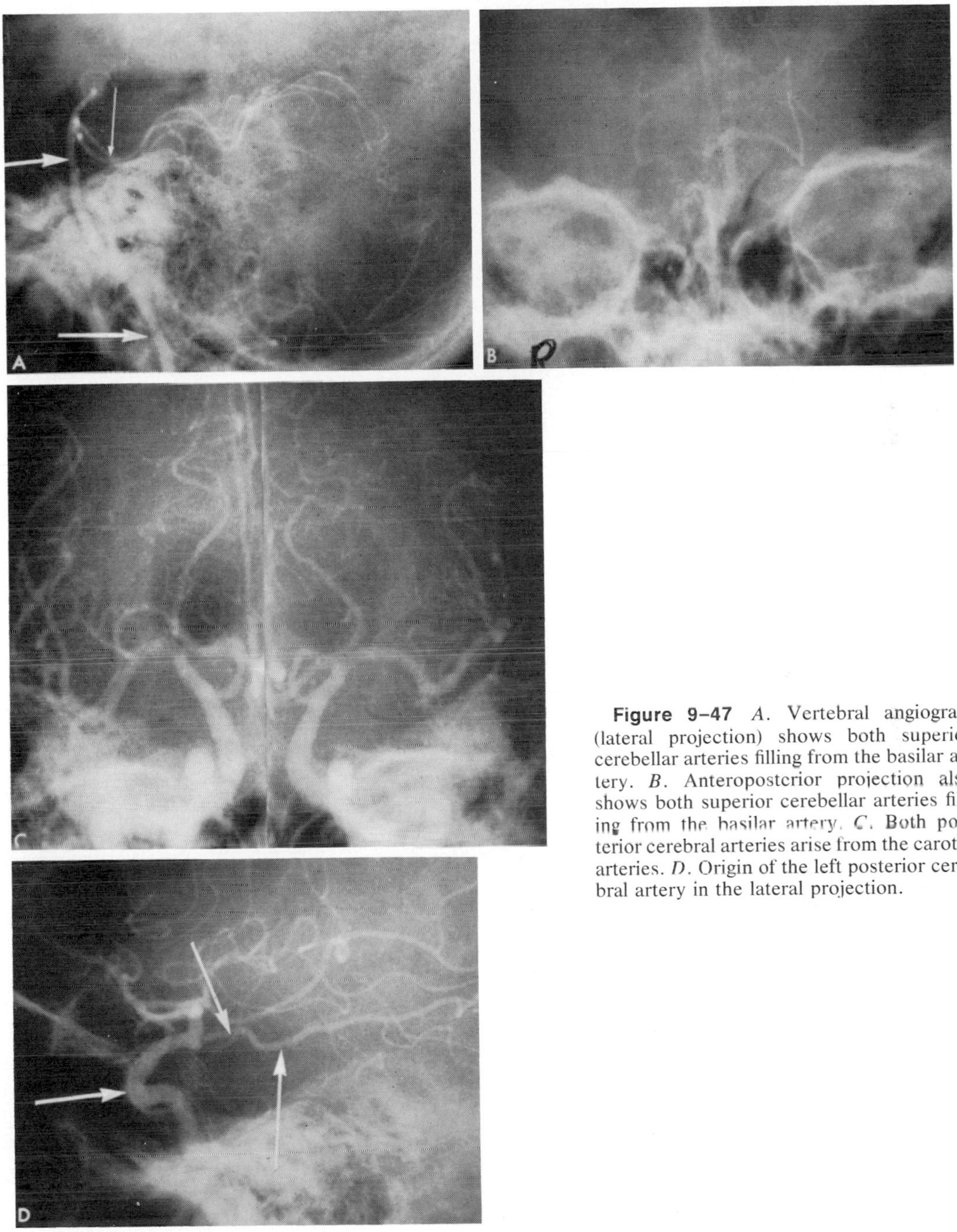

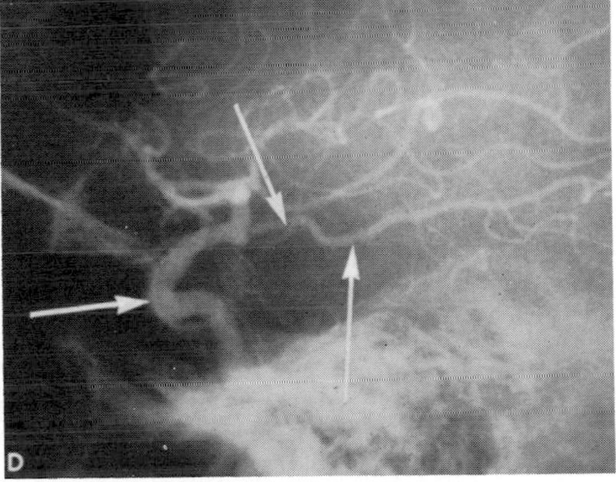

Figure 9–47 *A*. Vertebral angiogram (lateral projection) shows both superior cerebellar arteries filling from the basilar artery. *B*. Anteroposterior projection also shows both superior cerebellar arteries filling from the basilar artery. *C*. Both posterior cerebral arteries arise from the carotid arteries. *D*. Origin of the left posterior cerebral artery in the lateral projection.

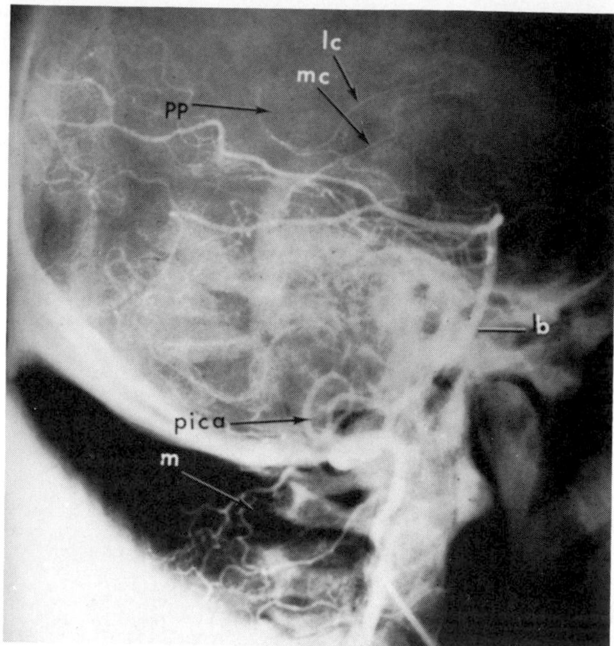

Figure 9–48 Vertebral angiogram. The lateral posterior choroidal arteries (lc) and the medial posterior choroidal arteries (mc) are outlined arising from the posterior cerebral artery. Note the course of the posterior pericallosal artery (pp) passing around the splenium of the corpus callosum. The posterior inferior cerebellar artery (pica) and the muscular branches (m) of the vertebral artery are identified. Note the basilar artery (b) parallel to the clivus.

projection. In the lateral view, two main arteries are usually distinguished, one on either side, each running a convex curve backward and upward from the posterior cerebral artery toward the interventricular foramen (Figs. 9–45 and 9–48). Except for deviations of a few millimeters, the pathways of these two main vessels usually coincide. A number of finer vessels are also seen along their course, but sometimes the branches are more distinct. The lateral posterior choroidal arteries form the largest curve, and situated anterior to them are the medial posterior choroidal arteries forming more narrow curves.

The main branch of the posterior choroidal artery arises from the posterior cerebral artery 1 to 2 mm posterior to the basilar artery. It usually runs backward together with the posterior cerebral artery, but in 15 per cent of cases, it courses 2 to 5 mm above and parallel to the posterior cerebral artery, which it then leaves in an upward curve. As a rule, the posterior choroidal arteries on either side differ from one another by only a few millimeters. There is no difference in the adult and in the child.[116]

Posterior Communicating Arteries

The posterior communicating and the anterior portion of the posterior cerebral artery give off some small branches—the thalamoperforating arteries—extending backward and upward. In 71 per cent of cases, according to Krayenbühl and Yaşargil, one or both posterior communicating arteries filled.[101] The posterior communicating arteries were not seen in 29 per cent of cases (Figs. 9–38 and 9–49). The posterior pericallosal artery (artery of the splenium of the corpus callosum) is sometimes seen arising from the posterior cerebral artery. It passes forward beneath the splenium to double back on itself and pass over the splenium of the corpus callosum (Fig. 9–48). The significance of this vessel is discussed in the section on the abnormal angiogram.[58]

Anastomoses of Vertebral-Basilar Tree with Carotid Tree

The vertebral and basilar tree anastomoses with the carotid tree in the following sites: (1) the posterior communicating artery and (2) the occipital branch of the external carotid artery and the vertebral artery in the neck (Fig. 9–49), (3) the anterior and posterior choroidal arteries, (4) the parieto-occiptal and callosomarginal branches, and (5) the posterior pericallosal artery and the pericallosal artery (Fig. 9–48), and (6) the persistent trigeminal artery (Fig. 9–50).

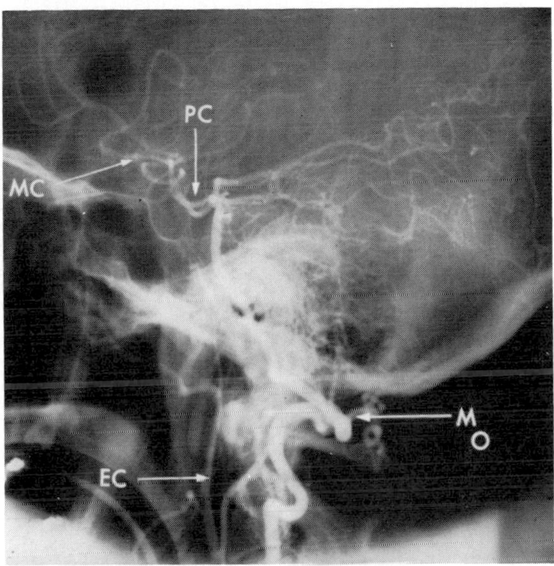

Figure 9–49 Vertebral angiogram. Both posterior communicating arteries (PC) have filled, and the anterior and middle cerebral arteries (MC) are outlined. The muscular branches of the vertebral artery are anastomosing with the occipital branch (M and O) of the external carotid artery, and other branches of the external carotid artery (EC) have filled.

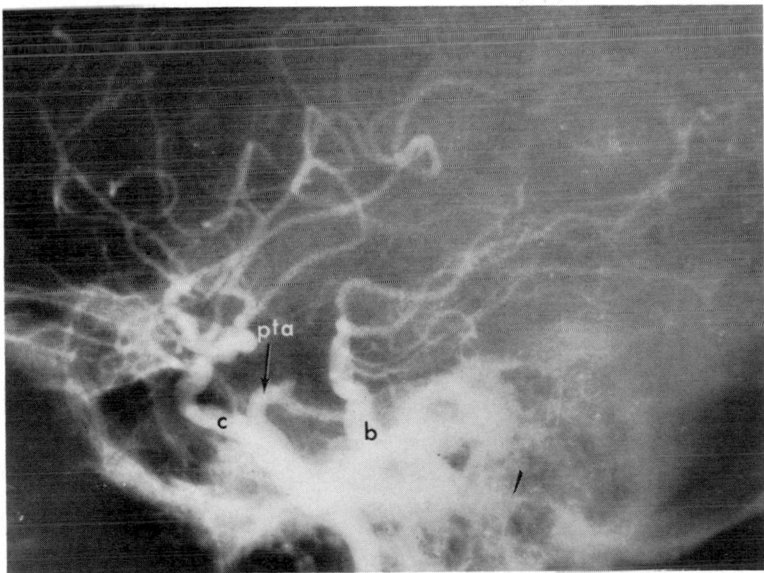

Figure 9–50 Carotid angiogram. The internal carotid artery (c) has filled, and the contrast medium has passed via a persistent trigeminal artery (pta) to the basilar artery (b). The vertebral artery on the same side of the trigeminal artery is usually absent.

Radiological Anatomy of the Venous System

The venous system may be conveniently described under the dural sinuses and superficial cortical veins, and the deep cerebral veins.

Dural Sinuses and Superficial Cortical Veins

The superficial sagittal or longitudinal sinus usually originates just above the nasion, and as it extends backward it increases in caliber to pass to the torcular

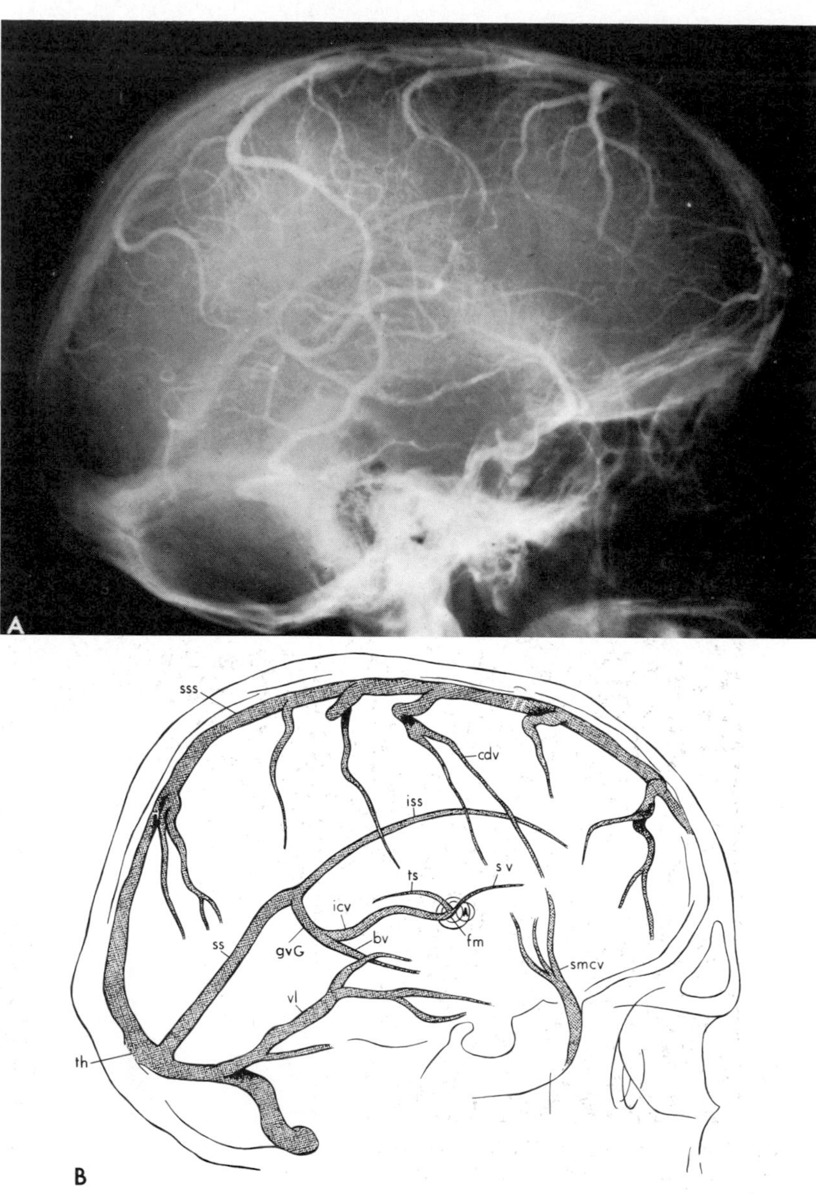

Figure 9–51 *A*. Venous phase of a carotid angiogram. *B*. Identification of structures shown in *A*. sss, superior sagittal sinus; ss, straight sinus; th, torcular Herophili; gvG, great vein of Galen; bv, basilar vein; icv, internal cerebral vein; ts, thalamostriate vein; fm, region of foramen magnum (i.e., junction of thalamostriate and septal and internal cerebral vein); sv, septal vein; smcv, superficial middle cerebral vein; cdv, cortical draining vein; iss, inferior sagittal sinus.

Illustration continued on opposite page.

Herophili and thence to the transverse or lateral sinuses to the jugular vein. The right lateral sinus is larger than the left, and not infrequently the superior sagittal sinus drains directly into the right transverse sinus. The cortical veins usually pass upward and enter the sagittal sinus against the stream (except the most anterior two or three tributaries). Streaming is often present where opacified and unopacified blood

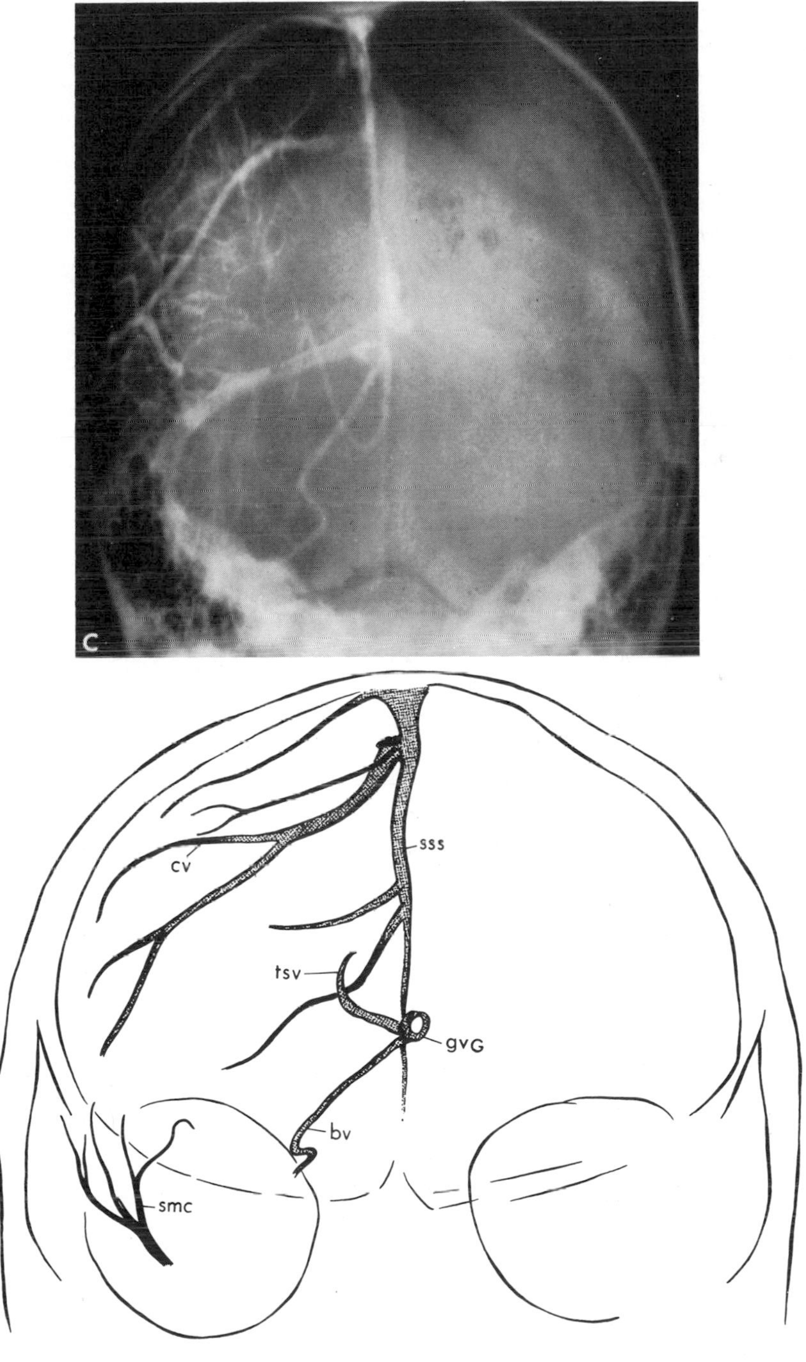

Figure 9–51 (*continued*) *C*. Venous phase of a carotid angiogram. There is some slight ventricular dilatation present. *D*. Identification of structures shown in *C*. sss, superior sagittal sinus; gvG, great vein of Galen; bv, basilar vein; tsv, thalamostriate vein; cv, cortical vein; smc, superficial middle cerebral vein.

mix. This accounts for thinning of the stream of contrast medium, which should not be mistaken for an organic defect (Fig. 9–51).

The inferior sagittal sinus courses in the free margin of the falx. The great vein of Galen passes into the straight sinus at the level of the junction of the free margin of the falx and the tentorial opening, and is directed backward and downward to enter the torcular. The petrosal sinuses are frequently identified and may provide a clue to the presence of angle tumors. The vein of Trolard is the largest superficial draining vein that enters the sinus. The vein of Labbé anastomoses with the vein of Trolard and usually enters the transverse sinus. The superficial middle cerebral vein runs in the sylvian fissure downward, outlining the temporal lobe, to enter the cavernous sinus. The dural sinuses are usually undisplaced by acquired cerebral disease. The deep cerebral veins may be displaced and are much more constant in position in the normal phlebogram.

Deep Cerebral Veins

The internal cerebral vein begins at the foramen of Monro by the union of the thalamostriate vein and the septal vein. The vessel is paired and runs in the roof of the third ventricle in the midline. The veins are arched upward and unite at the level of the quadrigeminal cistern to become the great vein of Galen. The thalamostriate vein is formed by veins from the walls of the lateral ventricle and the choroid plexus (Fig. 9–51*A* and *B*). The ependymal veins, if well opacified, will outline the lateral ventricles (Fig. 9–52). The thalamostriate vein, traced backward from the internal cerebral vein, extends backward and slightly upward in the groove between the caudate nucleus and the thalamus. In this portion it outlines the inferolateral aspect of the lateral ventricle. In the lateral projection the thalamostriate vein runs parallel to the internal cerebral vein. In the frontal projection, the vein has the shape of the horns of an African cow (Fig. 9–53). With ventricular dilatation, the arc becomes much wider, resembling a pair of short horns.[189] This is a much more reliable sign of ventricular dilatation than the shape of the anterior cerebral artery. The point where the thalamostriate vein enters the internal cerebral vein usually relates to the foramen of Monro. This has, therefore, been called the "venous angle" by Krayenbühl and Richter (Fig. 9–43).[100] Occasionally the thalamostriate vein enters the internal cerebral vein posterior to the foramen of Monro; here it forms a false venous angle and apparent shortening of the internal cerebral vein (Fig. 9–54).

The basilar vein, or the vein of Rosenthal, originates at the level of the temporal horn and anterior perforating substance in a group of small veins resembling a fine web. The vein passes backward around the brain stem to join the internal cerebral immediately before the origin of the great cerebral vein. The course of the basilar vein is similar to that of the posterior cerebral artery.

The veins of the posterior fossa may be divided into three groups: a superior group draining superiorly or deeply into the galenic system; an anterior group draining anteriorly into the petrosal sinuses; and a posterior group draining posteriorly or laterally into the torcular and neighboring straight and lateral sinuses.[81]

The anterior pontomesencephalic vein lies in front of the pons and extends into the depth of the interpeduncular fossa. The precentral cerebellar vein lies in the depth of the precentral cerebellar fissure. A detailed account of this venous drainage system is outside the scope of this text. The reader, if interested in more detail, is referred to the excellent work of Wolf, Huang, and Newman.[226]

THE ABNORMAL ANGIOGRAM

Extracranial Lesions

Vascular Occlusive Disease

Ischemic lesions of the brain may result from occlusive disease anywhere along the arterial tree leading to the brain. The common occurrence of infarction of the brain without demonstrable vascular occlusion confirms the observations of many previous workers. A number of authors have stressed the high incidence of extracranial vascular disease as a localized entity.[55] Fields and co-workers claim that over 25 per cent of strokes have their causative lesions situated extracranially.[51] In some cen-

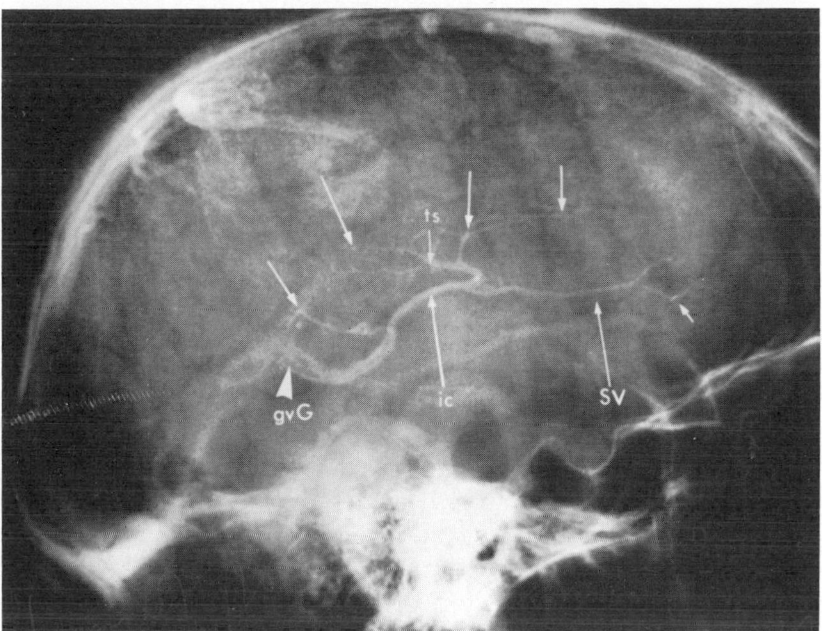

Figure 9–52 Venous phase of carotid angiogram to show the subependymal veins. Note the dense shadows created by the veins as they reverse direction. The shape and size of the ventricle can be determined from these shadows. ic, internal cerebral vein; ts, thalamostriate veins; gvG, great vein of Galen. Arrows point to subependymal veins (SV).

ters the operative correction of these lesions has been emphasized.[33,41,162]

The clinical picture produced by carotid occlusion is variable and may mimic other conditions such as neoplasms and space-occupying lesions. Even the most astute neurologists will, in some cases, admit to difficulty in distinguishing clinically between an internal carotid occlusion in the neck and one in the branches of the vessel in the head. Silverstein and associates examined 30 patients with proved occlusion

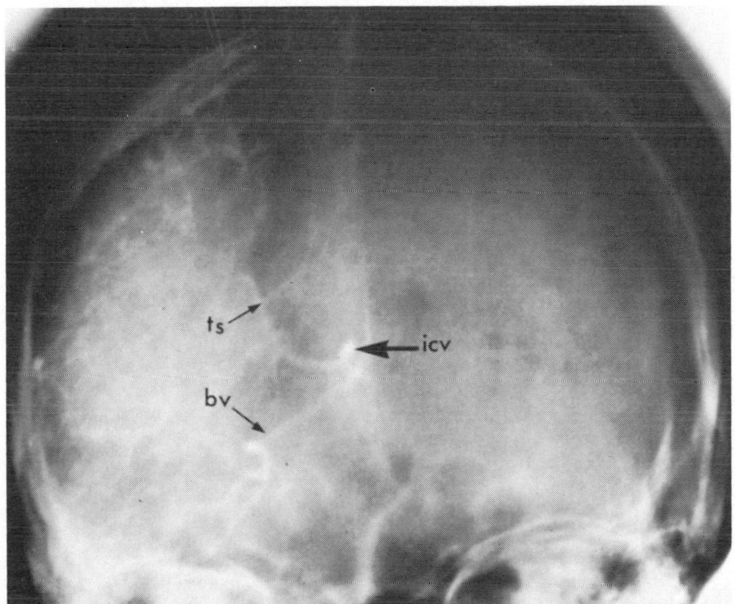

Figure 9–53 Venous phase of a carotid angiogram. ts, thalamostriate vein; bv, basilar vein; icv, internal cerebral vein. Note that there is some ventricular dilatation present.

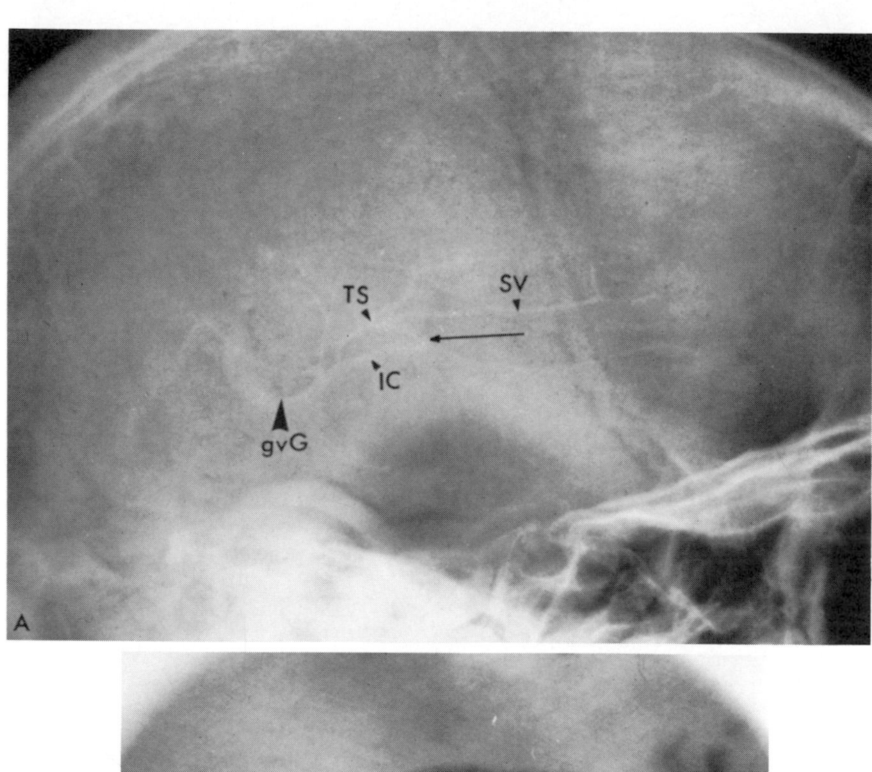

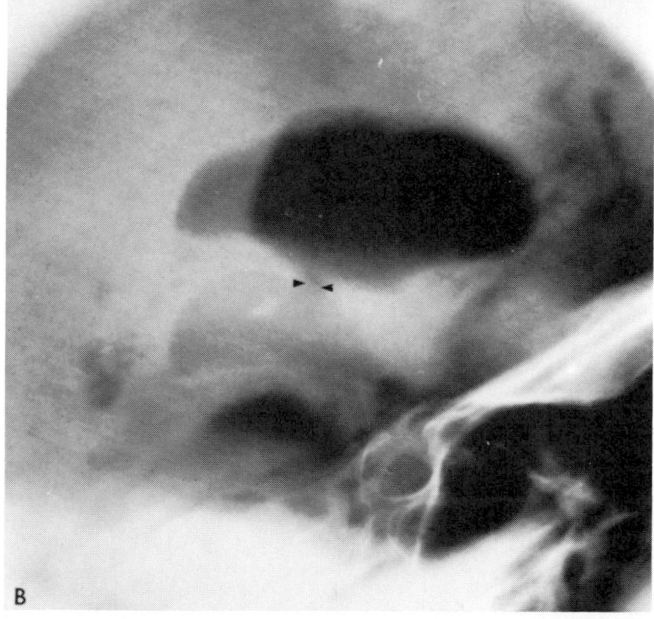

Figure 9–54 *A*. Venous phase of a carotid angiogram. The white dot indicated by the arrow is a false venous angle and does not represent the position of the foramen of Monro, which is identified in *B*. SV, septal vein; TS, thalamostriate vein; gvG, great vein of Galen; IC, internal cerebral vein. *B*. Air study showing the dilated ventricular system. The two arrows are directed to the foramen of Monro. Note that this does not correspond with the false angle.

of the common and internal carotid arteries in an attempt to evaluate certain procedures considered diagnostic for carotid occlusion.[195] Diminished carotid pulsations were present in only 17 per cent of these patients. An increase in carotid pulsations was reported, in two cases, on the occluded side. Carotid or intracranial bruits were not very helpful. Response to manual compression of the carotid artery was positive in 70 per cent of these cases, but many false positives do occur. Ophthalmodynamometric differences in retinal artery pressure were a fairly good diagnostic test. These clinical diagnostic modalities would sometimes, therefore, appear to be misleading, but a positive reaction would justify further investigation with angiography. Angiography plays a major role in the investigation and evaluation of patients with strokes. Many centers still limit their radiological examinations to the intracranial vasculature despite publications that emphasize the frequency with which an extracranial lesion is responsible for the patient's condition.[51]

Recent investigations have shown occlusive arterial disease in the cervical vessels in up to 80 per cent of patients with "stroke." Stenosis of the internal carotid artery at the bifurcation and stenosis of the vertebral artery at its origin are the most frequent findings. In 16 patients, all with severe neurological deficits, examined with aortocervical angiography as well as with selective angiography of the carotid and vertebral arteries, occlusive disease was found in 88 per cent. In 35 patients, many with intermittent strokes, examination with aortocervical angiography alone revealed disease in only 63 per cent. Aortocervical angiography alone revealed changes in the clinically relevant vessel in only 39 per cent, but selective angiography of the relevant vessel disclosed occlusive disease in 68 per cent of cases. These figures would indicate the value of a very careful investigation of the vascular tree, including selective vessel opacification. The validity of published reports of the incidence of disease may indeed be questioned when such a work-up is not undertaken. The incidence of carotid narrowing or occlusion in routine unselected autopsies is as high as 9.5 per cent.[55] By far the most common cause is atherosclerosis. The most common site of involvement is the carotid bifurcation.[8]

Hutchinson and Yates reviewed 100 patients who came to necropsy as the result of a cerebrovascular lesion or whose clinical history suggested such an event in the past.[85,86] In these 100 cases, the complete lengths of the vertebral and the carotid arteries were examined both radiologically and by dissection. Their findings indicate that unless the arch of the aorta is opacified with contrast medium during angiography, the origin of the major vessels leading from it will not be seen. Thus, occlusive disease of the origin of the common carotid and vertebral arteries will be missed. Significant stenosis or occlusion of the carotid artery was more common than that of the vertebral artery. In 5 per cent of cases a carotid and a vertebral artery were involved, the same incidence as for bilateral carotid involvement. The pathological

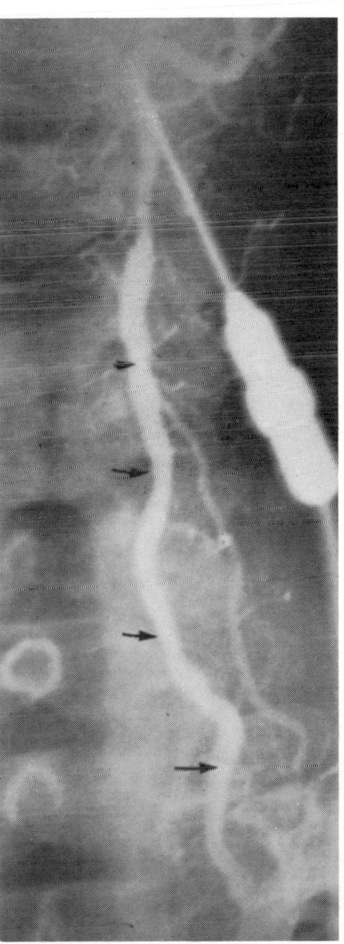

FIGURE 9–55 Vertebral angiogram. Note that at each level of cervical spondylosis there is narrowing of the caliber of the vertebral artery.

basis was always atheroma with an occasional addition of either old or recent thrombosis. A not uncommon finding was hemorrhage into the base of the plaques of atheroma. Recently the ulcerated atheroma appearing in the extracranial carotid circulation has been incriminated as a source of intracranial emboli. The most common sites of involvement were the internal carotid artery just beyond its origin near the bifurcation of the common carotid artery and the origin of the vertebral artery. Yates stressed the importance of cervical spondylosis and its effects on the cervical portion of the vertebral arteries (Fig. 9–55).[233] Bony outgrowths may displace the vessel, which, if already narrowed by atheroma, may undergo complete occlusion with movements of the neck. DeKleyn, Sheehan and co-workers, and Maslowski have shown the effect of extension and rotation of the neck on the vertebral artery.[35,124,192]

Of 646 patients examined angiographically by Fields and co-workers for symptoms suggesting cerebral insufficiency, 16 were found to have complete occlusions bilaterally.[52] The lesion usually involves the internal carotid artery just at and beyond its origin from the common carotid artery, but may extend to involve the external and common carotid arteries (Fig. 9–56). Little or no neurological deficit may occur even with complete occlusion, provided that adequate collateral channels are functioning. These channels may be via the circle of Willis or via the collaterals of the external carotid circulation.

Sites of anastomosis between the internal cerebral circulation and the extracranial circulation occur between the middle meningeal artery and the ophthalmic artery and between the superficial temporal artery, the external maxillary artery, and the ophthalmic artery (Fig. 9–57). The occipital branch of the external carotid artery frequently anastomoses with the muscular branches of the vertebral artery in the upper cervical region (Fig. 9–58). Intracranial anastomoses between the major vessels and their branches occur at the circle of Willis between the two anterior cerebral arteries through the anterior communicating artery and the two posterior communicating arteries. The cortical branches of the anterior, middle, and posterior cerebral arteries anastomose over the surface of the cortex (Fig. 9–59), and there is an anastomosis between the anterior and posterior choroidal arteries. The collateral circulation has been most adequately covered in the literature.[3,48,132,182,210,213,218]

Occlusive disease of the subclavian artery proximal to the origin of the vertebral artery may result in a reversal of blood flow in the ipsilateral vertebral artery from the basilar artery and thence to the subclavian

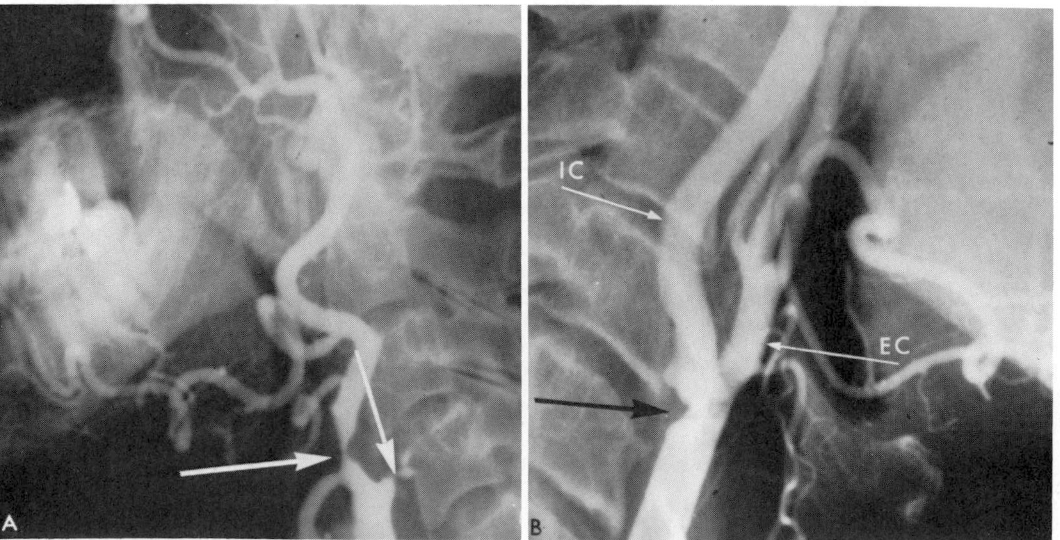

Figure 9–56 *A*. A carotid angiogram demonstrating complete occlusion of the internal carotid artery at its origin and a severe degree of narrowing of the external carotid artery. *B*. A defect in the lumen of the internal carotid artery at its origin (*black arrow*). IC, internal carotid artery; EC, external carotid artery.

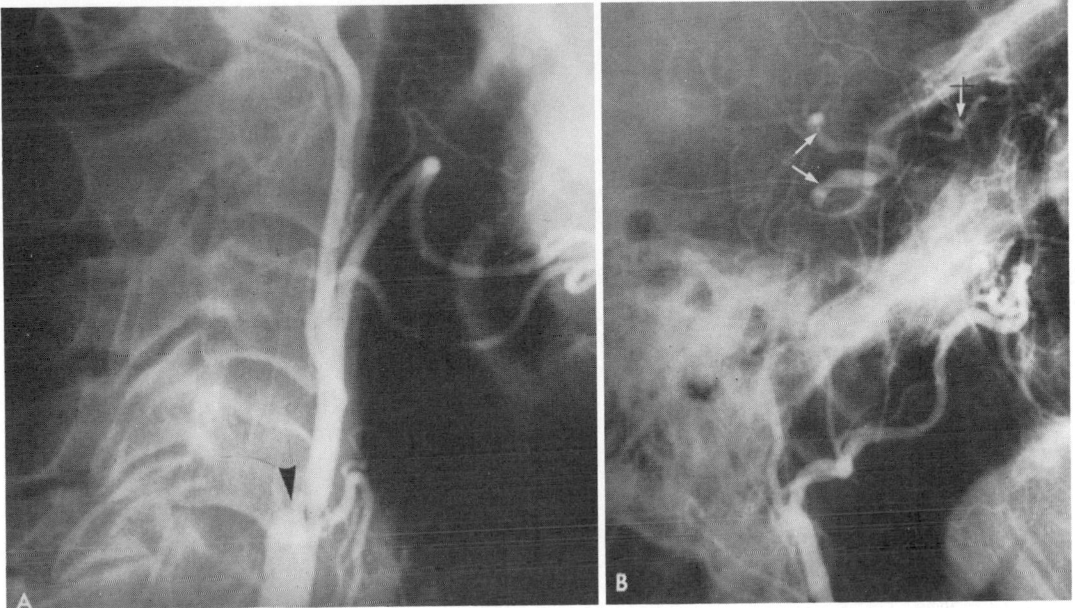

Figure 9–57 *A*. Carotid occlusion just beyond the origin of the internal carotid artery. There is also some narrowing of the lumen of the external carotid artery. *B*. Filling of the carotid siphon (→) via extracranial anastomoses such as the ophthalmic artery (+→).

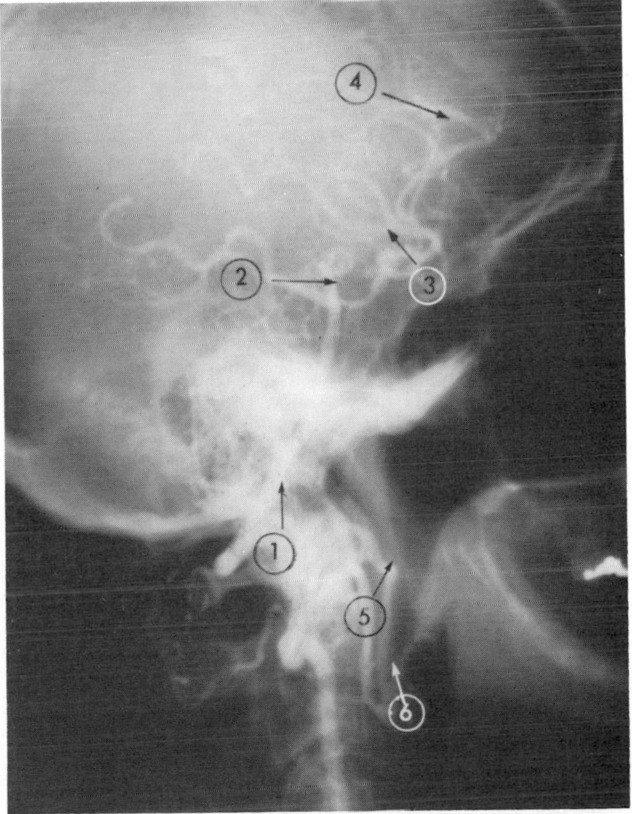

Figure 9–58 A vertebral angiogram in a patient with occlusion of the common carotid artery. Note filling of the vertebral artery (1), the basilar artery (2), the posterior communicating artery (3), the anterior and middle cerebral arteries (4), and filling of the occipital branch of the external carotid (5) and other branches (6) of the external carotid artery via the anastomosis in the neck between the muscular branches of the vertebral artery and the occipital artery. Note that the flow in the external carotid artery has reversed itself. On occasions the reverse flow continues from the external carotid artery to the bifurcation and then becomes anterograde up the internal carotid artery.

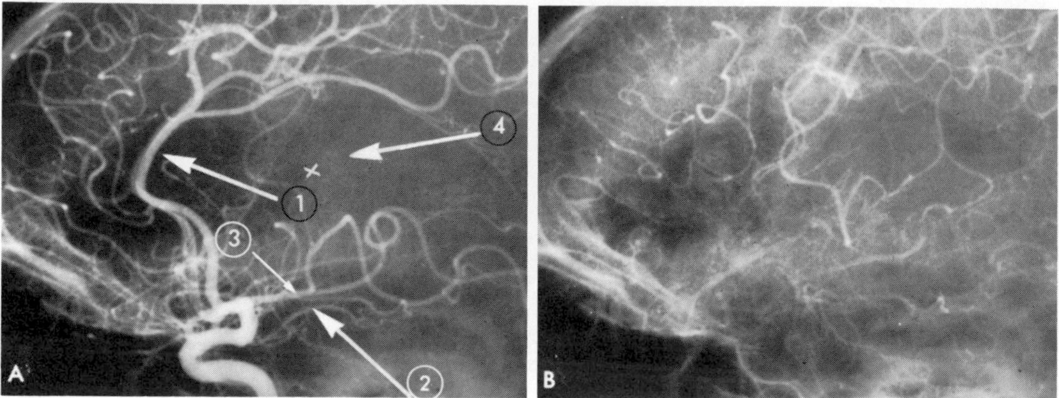

Figure 9–59 *A.* A carotid angiogram with filling of both anterior cerebral arteries (1), the anterior choroidal (2), and the posterior branches of the middle cerebral artery (3). The major branches of the island of Reil are missing; their absence results in a bare area (x and 4). *B.* Branches of the island of Reil filling retrogradely via the anterior cerebral artery branches.

artery beyond its point of occlusion. Contorni first described this interesting phenomenon, later named the "subclavian steal" by Reivich and associates.[25,158] This reverse flow in the vertebral artery may deprive the brain of blood and result in cerebral ischemia. It may occur also in occlusion of the innominate artery, when blood will reach the right vertebral, right subclavian, and right common carotid arteries via the basilar artery and the opposite vertebral artery. Other neck vessels may take part in

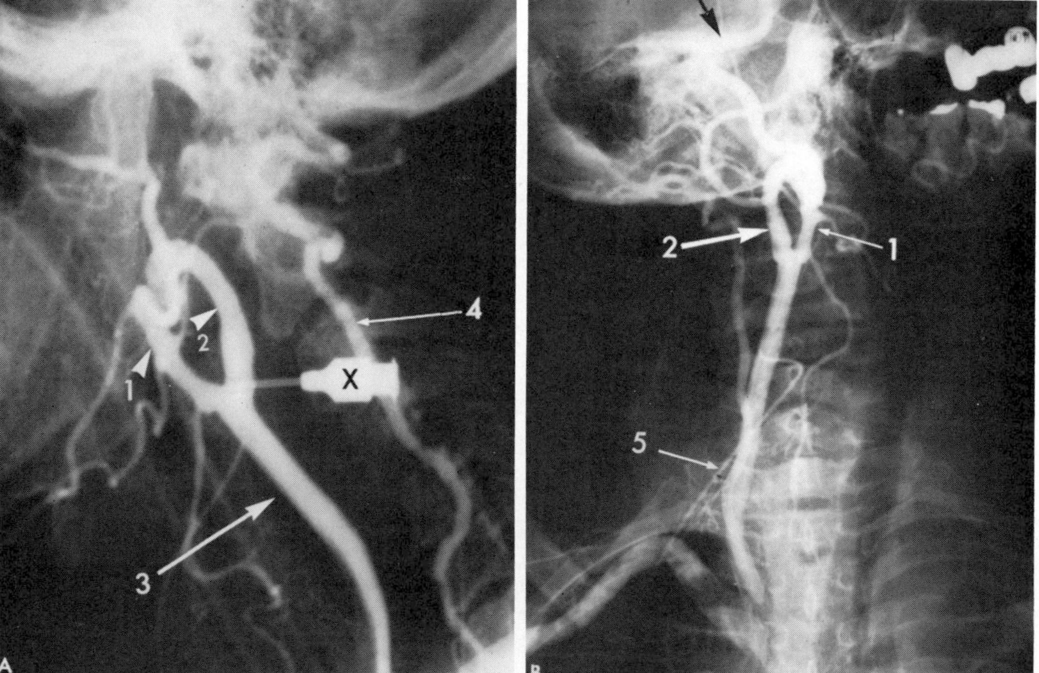

Figure 9–60 Right common carotid angiogram. *A.* Note that there is a kink in the internal carotid artery (2) without the passage of contrast medium beyond this point. The external carotid artery and its branches (1) have filled, and contrast has passed retrogradely down the common carotid artery (3) to the subclavian artery and anterogradely up the vertebral artery (4). Note the irregularities in the lumen of the vertebral artery. The needle (X) is artifactitious and is not related to the angiographic study. *B.* With the neck rotated, the kink no longer obstructs the flow of contrast into the internal carotid artery (*black arrow*). The polyethylene catheter (5) is in the common carotid artery.

establishing the flow to the occluded vessel.

Reports have appeared of kinks in the carotid and vertebral arteries that have resulted in ischemic attacks.[9,62,71,84,155,160] Hurwitt and co-workers state that kinked and buckled internal carotid arteries may be obstructed just as effectively as those with internal blocking lesions (Fig. 9–60).[84] Rarely do kinking and tortuosity of cerebral arteries alone give rise to symptoms of cerebral ischemia.[9] This is usually an incidental finding. In cases of diffuse atherosclerotic disease, stenosis, and vertebral artery compression by osteophytes, however, loops or kinks in a vessel may further embarrass the cerebral circulation and result in ischemic attacks (Fig. 9–55). In 241 patients with cerebrovascular disease, Harrison and Davalos operatively corrected buckling or tortuosity of carotid arteries in 39 of 46 cases demonstrating this phenomenon.[71] The curves in the vessel varied from S or V shapes to complete loops.

Aneurysms and Arterial Buckling

Dissecting aneurysms of the carotid artery are usually caused by trauma, the result of a subintimal injection of contrast medium or blunt injury to the neck. A rare spontaneous dissecting aneurysm of the internal carotid artery was reported by Anderson and Schechter.[4]

Aneurysms in the neck are rare. A pulsatile swelling in the neck is not infrequently misdiagnosed as an aneurysm. Tortuous and kinked vessels may be mistaken for aneurysms. Buckling or kinking of the major vessels in the neck occurs when the atherosclerotic aorta elongates and unfolds, and shadows of the tortuous vessels in the neck may be mistaken for aneurysms (Fig. 9–61).[187] In a case recently investigated by the author, the patient had received antimalarial, arsenical, and penicillin medications over a period of 20 years for a swelling in the neck diagnosed 20 years earlier as an aneurysm of the carotid artery. A bruit and thrill in the neck were elicited. An angiogram demonstrated a large carotid body tumor (see Fig. 9–66). Sutton reported a pulsatile mass in the tonsillar fossa that at angiography proved to be a large carotid aneurysm in the cavernous sinus that had eroded through the base of the skull and had presented in the tonsillar fossa.[205] One pulsatile mass in the tonsillar fossa examined angiographically by the author was a kink in the internal carotid artery; a second

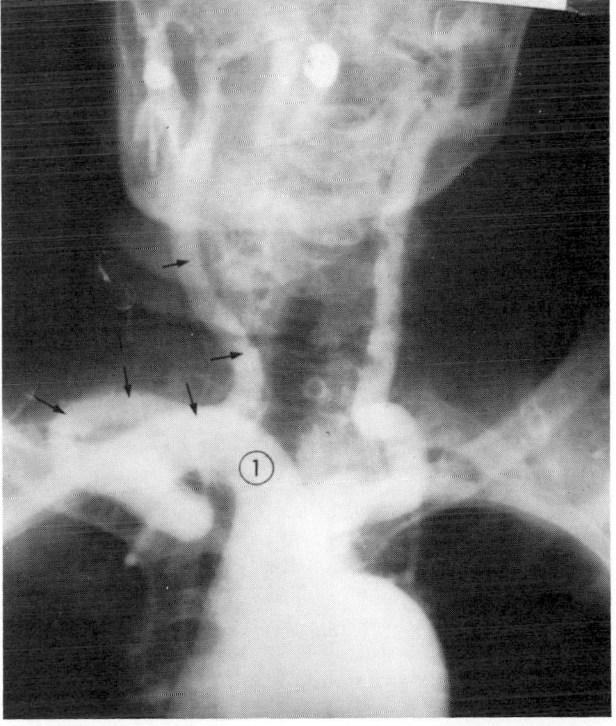

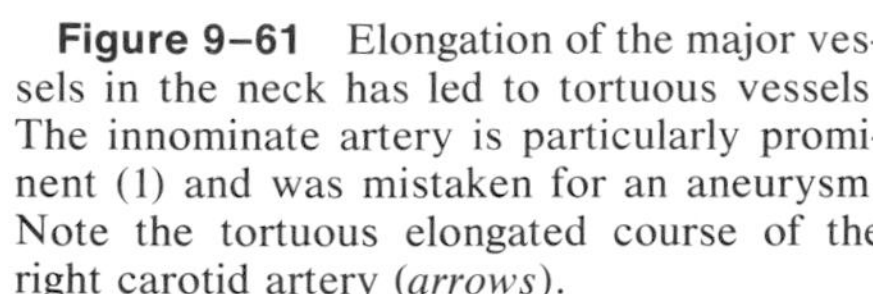

Figure 9–61 Elongation of the major vessels in the neck has led to tortuous vessels. The innominate artery is particularly prominent (1) and was mistaken for an aneurysm. Note the tortuous elongated course of the right carotid artery (*arrows*).

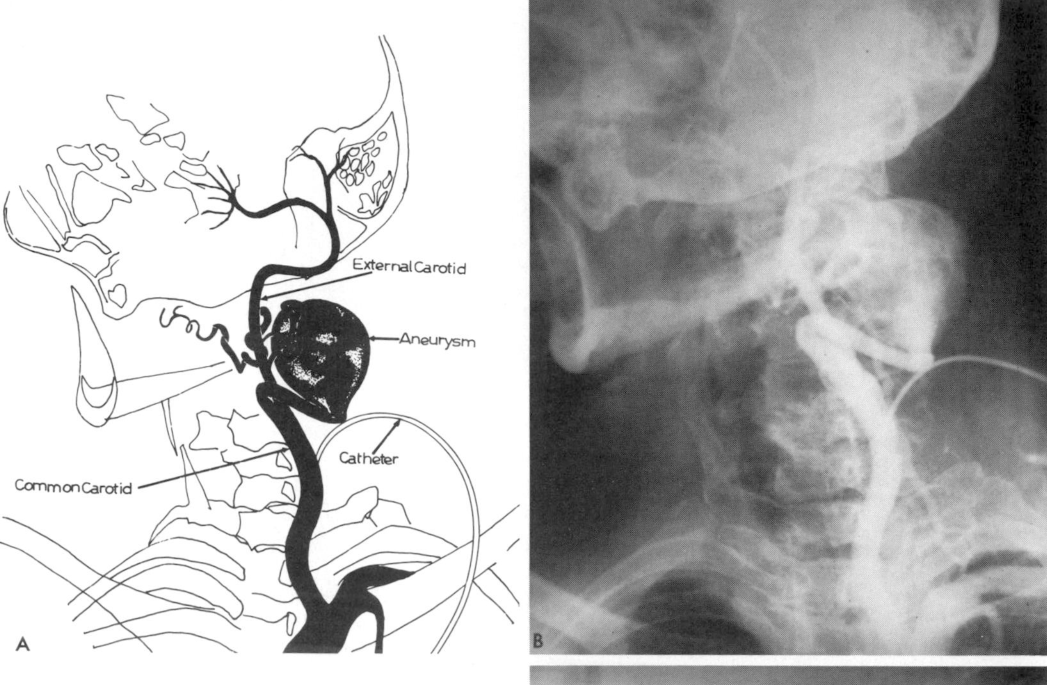

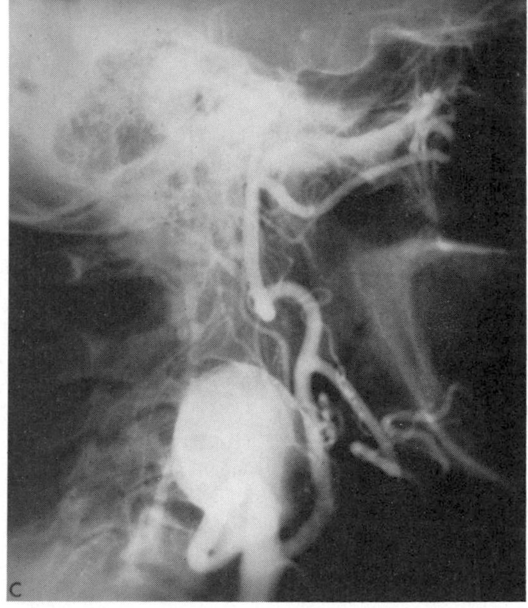

Figure 9–62 Aneurysm of the internal carotid artery. *A* and *B*. Note that the external carotid artery is unaffected. The tortuous internal carotid artery enters directly into the aneurysm. *C*. The lateral projection of the angiogram shows this to best advantage.

patient with a similar clinical presentation had an aneurysm of the internal carotid artery, which was resected with an end-to-end anastomosis of the carotid artery stumps.[24] Ullrich and Sugar reported a case of a carotid aneurysm in the neck with four other aneurysms in the head of the same patient.[217] Alexander and associates reported a case of bilateral extracranial aneurysms of the carotid arteries.[1] Other reports of extracranial aneurysms have appeared in the literature.[102,171] The internal carotid artery is almost invariably the vessel involved (Fig. 9–62).

Arteriovenous Fistulae

Most arteriovenous fistulae in the neck result from trauma, although there have been reports in the literature of their spontaneous occurrence. In a case reported elsewhere, this appeared to develop spontaneously in a patient at rest while listening to the radio.[65] Four weeks before hospitalization, the patient noted the sudden onset of occipital pain followed two hours later by a swishing noise in the head. On examination a to-and-fro murmur was heard over the posterior triangle of the neck. A vertebral angiogram demonstrated the fistula. Aronson reported a case of an arteriovenous fistula of the vertebral artery that followed trauma in a 23-year-old patient who, falling from a truck, struck his neck on the sharp corner of a box.[5] Arteriovenous fistulae of the vertebral artery have been described following percutaneous vertebral arteriography. Stab wounds (Fig. 9–63) and missile injuries are the most common causes.[236] Arteriovenous fistulae of the common carotid artery and jugular vein are rare and are usually associated with trauma. The author has demonstrated a fistula between the occipital artery and an adjacent vein that was caused by a gunshot wound. Tori and Garusi reported a case of a carotid-jugular fistula in which preoperative and postoperative angiography were performed in a 5-year-old child.[216] When the communication is large, the rapid shunting of blood from the arterial to the venous side may result in poor filling of the intracranial vessels. The carotid artery will also hypertrophy, and the arterialized large dilated jugular vein will be outlined almost immediately after the carotid opacification. Cardiomegaly follows large fistulae of some dura-

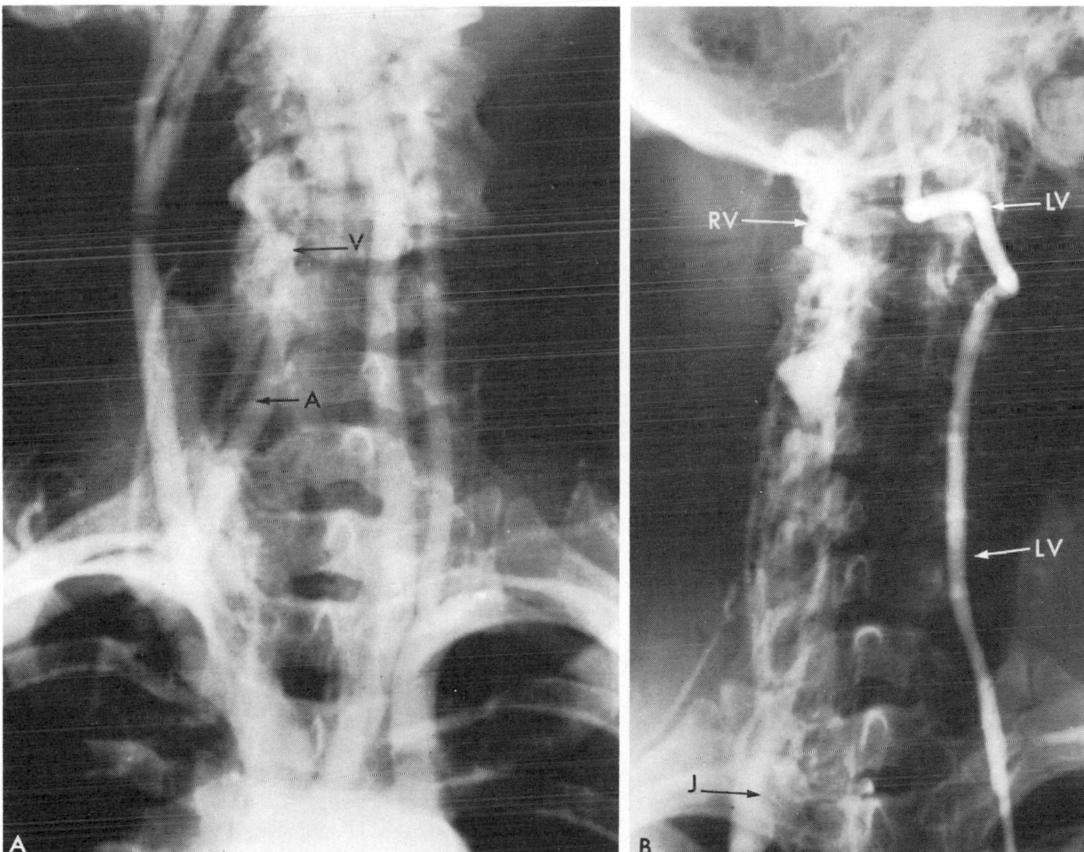

Figure 9–63 This patient was stabbed in the neck and developed a marked "whooshing" sound in the head. The weapon penetrated the vertebral artery and the surrounding venous plexus. *A*. An aortic arch study shows the fistula between the right vertebral artery (A) and the dilated veins (V). *B*. A left vertebral angiogram via the femoral artery shows the catheter in the left vertebral artery with opacification of the left (LV) and right (RV) vertebral arteries. Large veins can be seen transporting the contrast medium to the jugular veins (J).

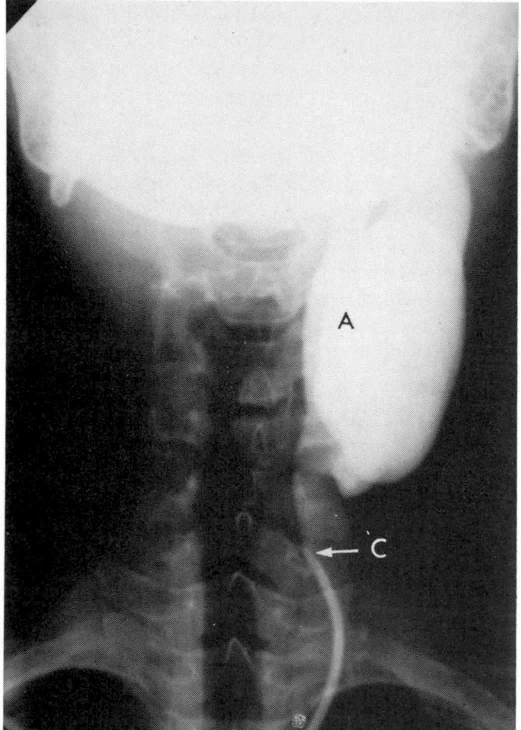

Figure 9–64 Left carotid angiogram via femoral catheterization with the catheter in the carotid artery (C). The large arterialized aneurysm of the jugular vein is well outlined (A).

tion, as may heart failure. We recently had the opportunity to investigate a 23-year-old man, retarded since birth, who was admitted for revision of an operatively induced right carotid-jugular fistula. This had been performed in 1949 to enhance cerebral blood flow and improve the patient's mental condition. The patient now presented with incipient cardiac failure. The large arterialized aneurysm of the jugular vein was resected (Fig. 9–64).

Congenital Lesions

The common carotid artery usually bifurcates opposite the third and fourth cervical vertebral bodies. It may, however, bifurcate at a much lower level. Anomalous origins of the carotid and vertebral arteries have been described. The incidence of these congenital anomalies has been placed as high as 52.3 per cent in the Negro adult male and 22.6 per cent in the Caucasian adult male. DeGaris and associates in postmortem examinations of 203 adult Negro males found 16 different patterns of branches of the aortic arch.[34] Some variation of the origin of the major vessels from the aorta was found in 75 per cent of stillborn fetuses studied by barium injection and dissection of the aortic arch.[238] Fisher reported a case of complete absence of both carotid arteries.[54] Many such congenital anomalies may be missed in a carotid angiogram unless the origin of these vessels is examined with particular attention.

Congenital anomalies of the origin of the vertebral artery appear to be more common than those of the carotid artery. The one vertebral artery may be absent in caroticobasilar anastomoses, and the vertebral artery may arise from the carotid artery.[131,202] Lindgren cited four cases in which the vertebral artery arose from the carotid artery in the neck, and Hauge also reported two cases in which the vertebral artery arose from sites other than the subclavian artery.[76,110] Krayenbühl and Yaşargil have noted quite a few variations of origin of the vertebral arteries in their postmortem studies.[101] Figure 9–65 shows the origin of the left vertebral artery from the arch of the aorta.

Variations in the second part of the course of the vertebral artery are rare. The vertebral artery may enter the foramen transversarium at a level above C6, but entry at C3 has been described by Silvan.[194] The present author has encountered a similar case (Fig. 9–36). Rivaglia has seen a vertebral artery leave the canal between C2 and C3 to enter the foramen magnum.[161]

Carotid Body Tumors

These are usually benign tumors that may invade locally. They are usually single, although Engstrom and Hamberger reported a case of bilateral carotid body tumors studied angiographically.[45] The present author has recently examined such a case. These tumors have a very characteristic appearance and, as previously stated, are often mistaken clinically for carotid aneurysms. Their extreme vascularity renders them pulsatile. The radiological appearances reported in 13 cases examined by the author were quite characteristic. Because of the extreme vascularity of the lesion, contrast medium introduced into the common carotid artery is soaked up like a sponge by the tumor that arises over the carotid body at the bifurcation of the common

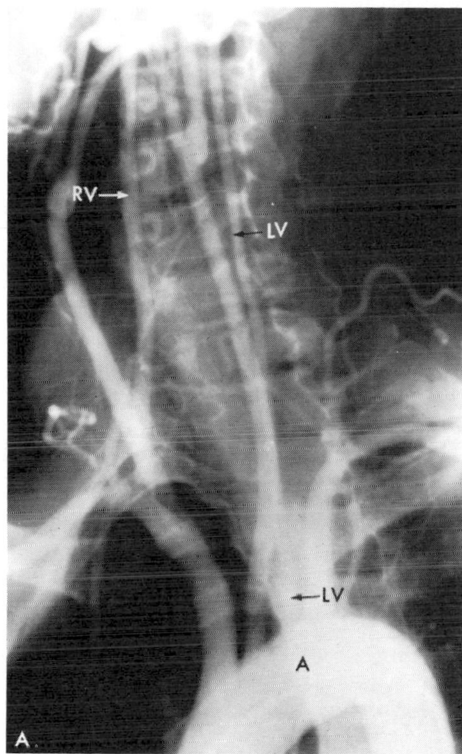

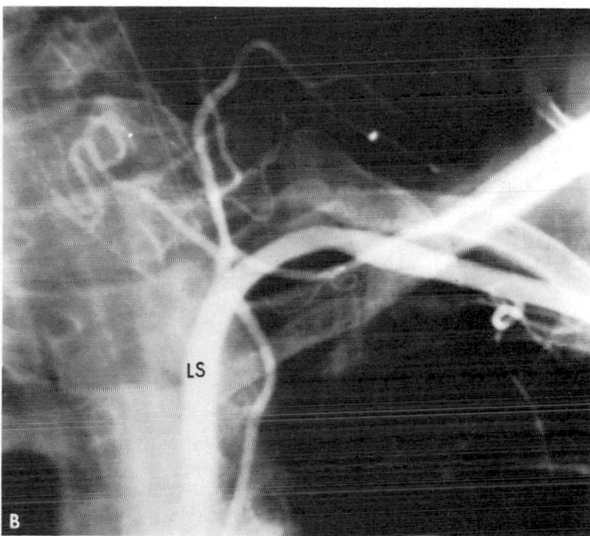

Figure 9–65 *A*. Arch study with tip of the catheter in ascending aorta. Note that the left vertebral artery (LV) arises directly from the arch of the aorta (A). RV, right vertebral artery. *B*. Left subclavian artery (LS) shows no origin of the left vertebral artery. (Courtesy of Dr. P. Rossi.)

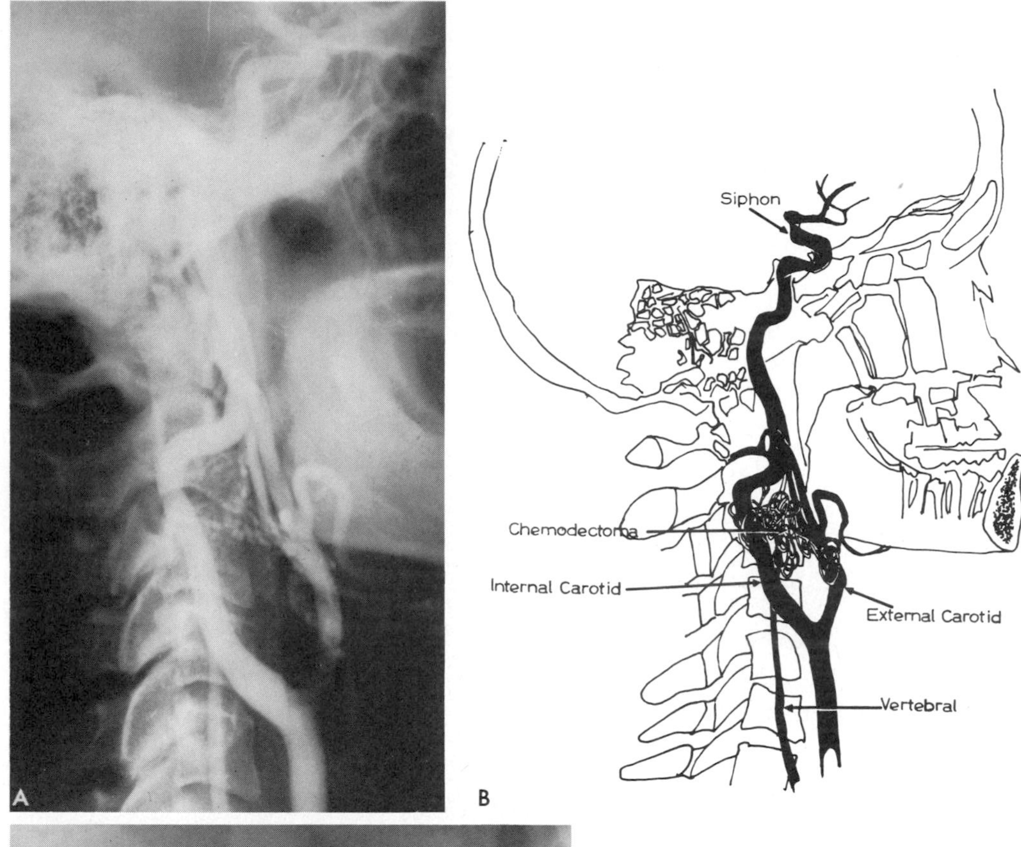

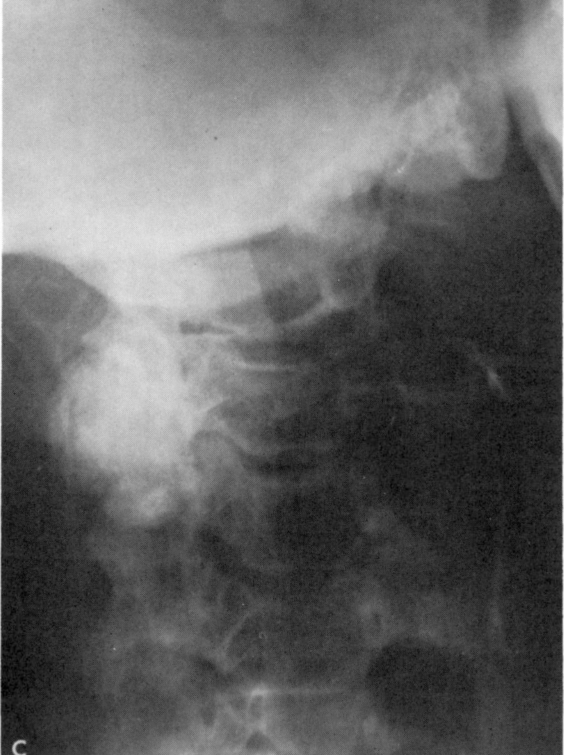

Figure 9–66 Carotid body tumor, mistaken clinically for an aneurysm of the carotid artery. *A* and *B*. Note the characteristic separation of the internal and external carotid arteries and the highly vascular tumor supplied by the external carotid artery and the vertebral artery. *C*. The marked vascularity of the tumor with an irregular margin is demonstrated.

carotid artery and usually engulfs the vessel, narrowing its lumen.[179] One of the most characteristic changes observed was the separation of the internal and external carotid arteries by the tumor mass (Fig. 9–66).[24]

False Occlusive Patterns of the Vessels in the Neck

The false passage of the needle with the introduction of contrast medium subintimally sometimes mimics the radiological appearances of occlusive and stenotic disease.[59,133,136,181] An injection beneath the intima of the artery may occlude the vessel temporarily and produce a pattern not unlike that of organic disease (Fig. 9–15). The flow distal to this point may be very slow and may simulate a narrowed lumen of the vessel, and sometimes the flow may be slowed to such an extent that streaming and layering of the heavier contrast medium may take place (Fig. 9–67). A needle or catheter in the external carotid artery may result in filling of only the external carotid artery and suggest internal carotid occlusion. This may not be recognized by the novice, but a film of the neck including the tip of the needle and the bifurcation of the carotid artery would clarify the position.

Spasm

It is sometimes difficult to distinguish radiologically between spasm and occlusive disease. Vessels in spasm usually show gradual tapering. Factors exciting spasm are, for example, contrast in the vessel wall or in the tissues outside the vessel, or a catheter threaded high up the carotid artery. A frequent site of spasm in vertebral angiography is the point where the vertebral artery crosses over the arch of C1. The change in the caliber of vessels during angiography has been demonstrated and supports the diagnosis of spasm.

The significance of internal carotid artery

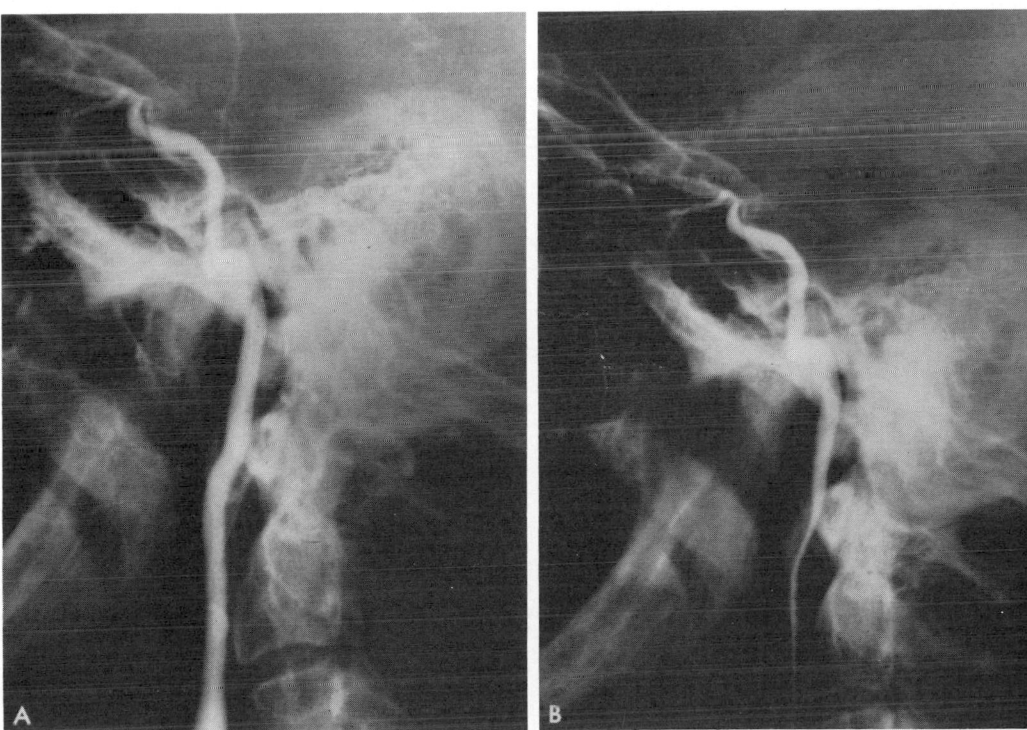

Figure 9–67 Internal carotid artery occlusion just distal to the origin of the ophthalmic artery. Because of slow flow, there is poor mixing of blood and contrast medium. The contrast medium with a higher specific gravity hugs the most dependent parts, in this case the posterior wall of the cervical internal carotid artery (the patient was in the supine position during this angiogram). The "streaming phenomenon" must be kept in mind when evaluating occlusive disease. *A*. The ophthalmic artery allows a runoff of the blood–contrast agent mixture, but it is slow enough to prevent through and through mixing. *B*. Further runoff through the ophthalmic artery has occurred, and unopacified blood is now passing along the carotid artery, above the attenuated layer of contrast medium.

occlusion at its origin has already been discussed. Rarely is the disease process situated further along the course of the vessel in the neck, although propagation of the thrombus distally from this point usually occurs. The region of the carotid siphon is not uncommonly involved, and linear streaks of calcification in this region seen on the plain film may direct one's attention to this area.

Intracranial Lesions

Occlusive Disease

Although angiography has proved to be a most valuable diagnostic test in revealing vascular occlusive disease in the neck, it has perhaps been less rewarding in the evaluation of patients who have suffered an occlusion of a vessel in the head. Various authors have indicated how erroneous the clinical diagnosis of stroke may be. The clinical diagnosis is often upset by the angiographic findings, and even the most astute physicians often find themselves unable to distinguish between middle cerebral occlusion and internal carotid artery occlusion before angiography. Various factors may be responsible for the so-called negative angiogram in the presence of a stroke. Autopsy casts of the cerebral arterial tree reveal an abundance of vessels. Even after the cast of the arterial tree is pruned, it is obvious and not surprising that only the larger branches of the part that remains will be represented and recognized in an angiogram during life. It is not surprising, therefore, that occlusion of a branch might remain unrecognized. Occlusion of a vessel may not be recognized when collateral vessels take over to irrigate the area deprived of its blood supply. Retrograde flow with a delay in local filling would confirm the presence of an occluded vessel, an observation that may only be made if serial films are taken.

Angiography may occasionally reveal a contrast stain in the presence of an infarct. Although most authors deny that there is anatomical evidence for the existence of direct connections between arteries and veins in the human brain, Hasegawa claims their presence.[72] Feindel and Perot have observed at operation cerebral veins partly or wholly filled with a stream of arterial blood.[49] These authors have outlined two major groups of cases showing this phenomenon: those in which there are structural changes, such as arteriovenous malformations, and those in which a local region of brain such as an infarct, uses oxygen inadequately. Cronqvist demonstrated a very specific angiographic pattern, which is characterized by regional rapid passage of the contrast medium.[28] Hence, early filling of veins may, on occasion, occur with a contrast blush. The regional hyperemia is due to the vasodilatory effects of the hypoxic tissue. Lassen refers to this as a state of "luxury perfusion," an unfortunate term since the tissue has an impaired oxygen consumption.[107] "Poverty perfusion" might perhaps be a more appropriate term. The presence of early-filling veins is not restricted to infarcts. When an early-draining vein is questioned in an angiogram, it is often helpful to examine the venous phase and trace the vessels backward to the arterial phase. The author has found this useful in distinguishing between an early-draining vein and artery.

Middle cerebral artery occlusion is more readily recognized in the lateral projection than in the anteroposterior, since the branches of the middle cerebral artery are superimposed in the latter, and occlusion of a single branch of the middle cerebral artery may not be so obvious. When the main stem of the middle cerebral artery is occluded, the stump of the vessel may be seen (Fig. 9–68*A*). Occlusion of the ascending frontoparietal artery is readily recognized, but nonfilling of the other branches is not as easily appreciated. With serial films, vessels irrigating the middle cerebral territory may be seen to fill in the late arterial stage from collateral supply from the anterior and posterior cerebral arteries (Fig. 9–68*B* and *C*).

The diagnosis of occlusion of the anterior cerebral artery on the basis of angiographic appearances must be made with caution, since anatomical variations of the circle of Willis are so frequent. Filling of an anterior cerebral artery after contralateral compression or injection of the other side may occur.

The radiological diagnosis of posterior cerebral artery occlusion must also be made with caution. In about one third of cases the posterior cerebral artery is of the fetal type and arises from the carotid ar-

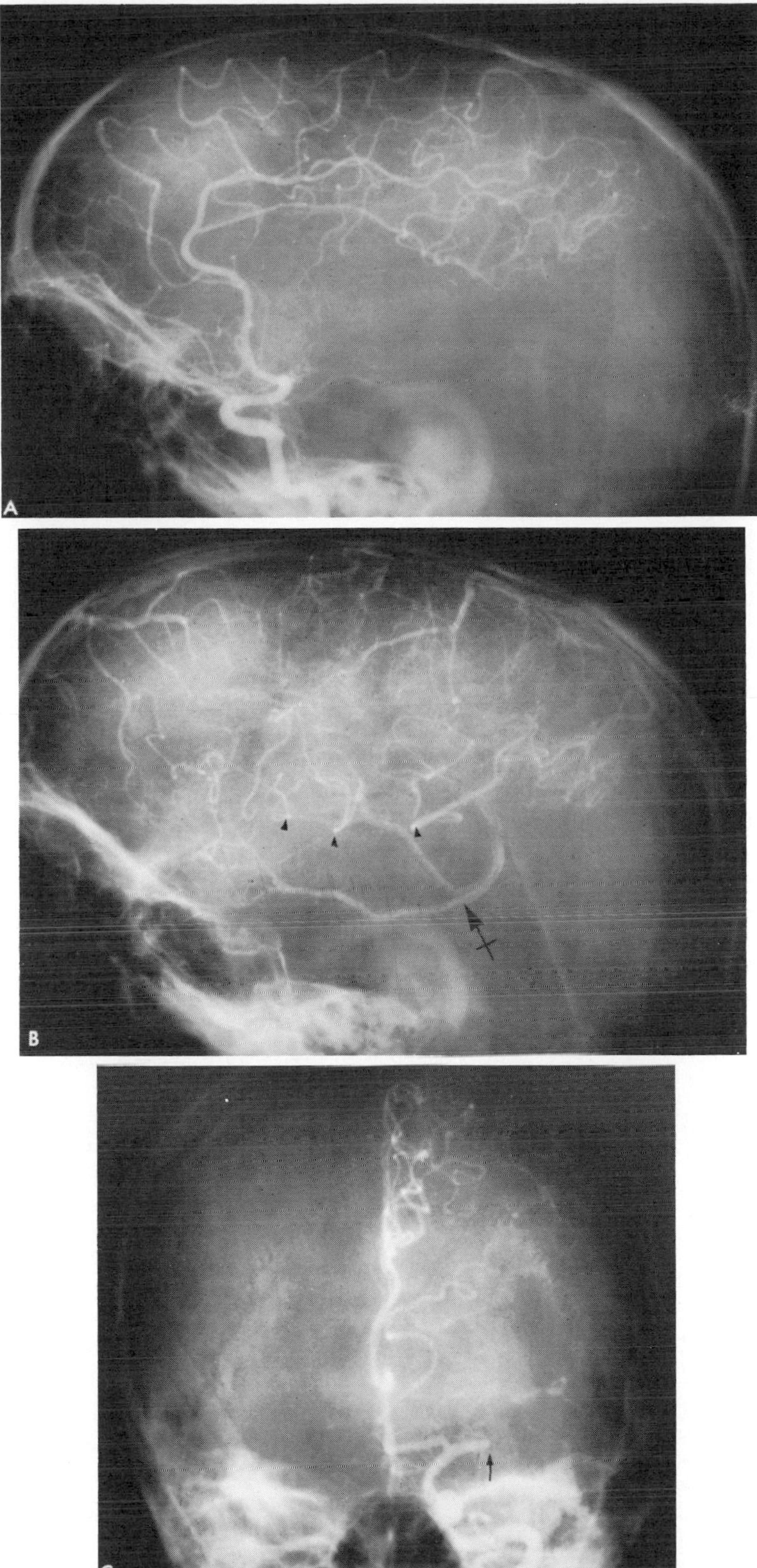

Figure 9–68 *A*. Lateral carotid angiogram showing nonfilling of branches of the middle cerebral artery. Only a stump (a few millimeters) has filled (cf. *C*). *B*. A later phase of the carotid angiogram. This now shows retrograde filling of branches of the middle cerebral artery (→). Note that these have eventually filled at a stage when the cortical veins and deep veins and dural sinus are filling (+→).

tery. On occasion, vertebral angiography will show filling of only the superior cerebellar arteries, because both posterior cerebral arteries fill from the carotid artery (Fig. 9–47). Anatomical studies of the circle of Willis explain the frequency of variation in the posterior circulation.[3,102,144,227] In all cases of nonfilling of a posterior cerebral artery, ipsilateral injection of the carotid artery must be done before the significance of this lack of opacification can be fully appreciated.

Factors apart from the anatomy may also be involved in the nonfilling of vessels. The differential in heads of pressure of the two vertebral arteries, spasm in the vessels, and the rate of injection may all influence the filling of individual branches of the circle of Willis. Saltzman has shown that by compressing the ipsilateral vertebral artery during carotid artery injection, filling of the posterior cerebral was frequently achieved when a previous injection had been unsuccessful.[172] Mones reported nonfilling of the posterior cerebral artery from either the basilar or ipsilateral carotid artery in four patients.[128] All these patients had homonymous field defects contralateral to the nonfilled artery. No postmortem confirmation was obtained.

The neuroradiologist is not frequently asked to undertake angiography on a patient who presents with the "classic" symptoms and signs of basilar thrombosis. This is a disease that usually does not respond to treatment currently available. It is more common for basilar thrombosis to be demonstrated radiologically in a situation of clinical uncertainty. Various angiographic factors must be seriously considered and their effects evaluated before the diagnosis may be made. Factors such as streaming, spasm washout from the opposite vertebral artery, temporary occlusion of the vertebral artery by the tip of the catheter or the needle end must be excluded, and strict angiographic criteria must be adhered to. There should be reflux down the

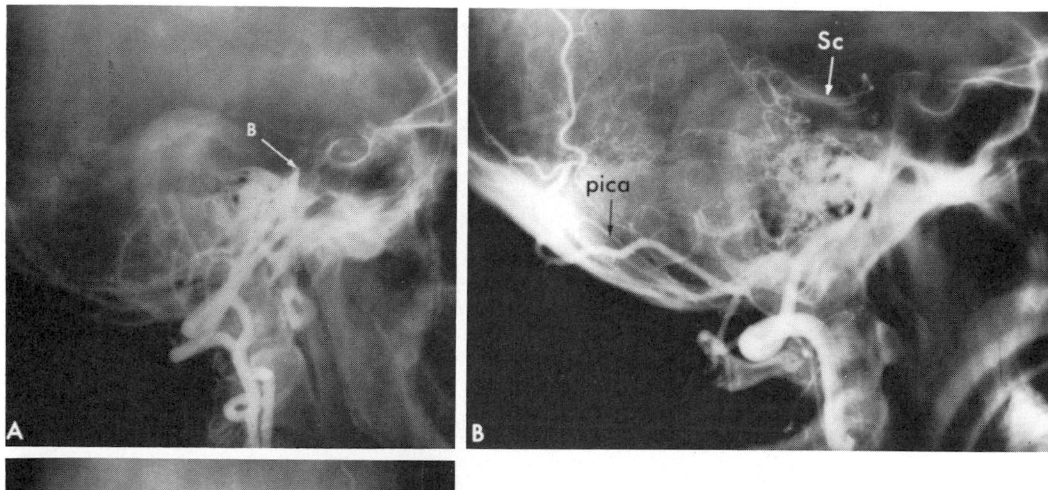

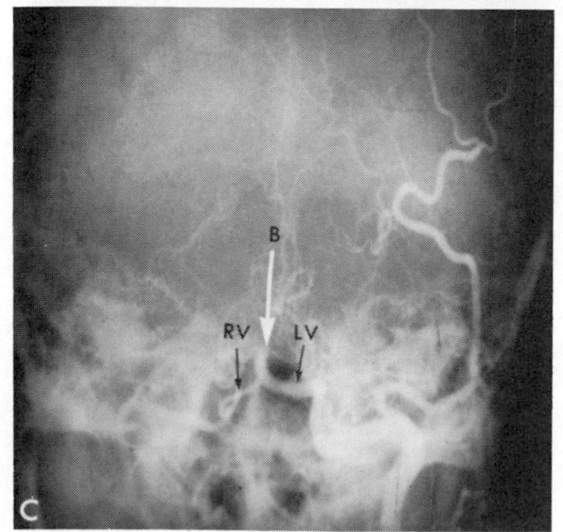

Figure 9–69 Vertebral angiography in two patients with basilar thrombosis. *A*. Note contrast medium has entered the basilar artery, which terminates abruptly. There is reflux down the opposite vertebral artery. *B*. Another patient, again with a sharp block of the basilar artery. *C*. There is reflux into the right hypoplastic vertebral artery (RV). Note that the posterior inferior cerebellar artery (pica) acts as a collateral pathway resulting in filling of the superior cerebellar arteries (Sc) and faint opacification of segments of the basilar artery. B, basilar artery block.

opposite vertebral artery. Rapid washout would suggest mechanical effects rather than organic disease. Collateral flow would also support the diagnosis (Fig. 9–69). A carotid angiogram might show filling of the tip of the basilar artery via the posterior communicating arteries.

It is usually not possible to distinguish radiologically between thrombosis and embolism purely on angiographic evidence. The shape of the defect in the vessel may, however, be suggestive; embolism appears as a defect concave toward the column of contrast medium. Migration of the point of obstruction also suggests embolism rather than thrombosis, although emboli may arise from an area of thrombus (Fig. 9–70).

Thrombosis of the longitudinal and transverse sinuses is rarely diagnosed in life and, even when suspected clinically, is rarely confirmed in the postmortem room. Krayenbühl has shown the characteristic changes in the venous phase of the cerebral angiogram.[98] Askenasy and associates illustrated the characteristic changes in three cases of venous sinus thrombosis.[6] All three cases had postmortem verification. In two cases cerebral angiography showed absence of filling of the superior sagittal sinus during the venous phase, with prominent deep veins draining the contrast medium.

Aneurysms

Intracranial aneurysms are not infrequently encountered at postmortem (0.5 to 3.7 per cent, according to various pathologists) and are the most common cause of spontaneous subarachnoid hemorrhage.[199] They are usually situated on the circle of Willis. Figure 9–71 shows the incidence of their location according to Bull.[19] Norlen and Paly claim that 15 per cent of intracranial aneurysms are situated in the posterior fossa and that 5 per cent of intracranial aneurysms arise from the vertebral artery.[137]

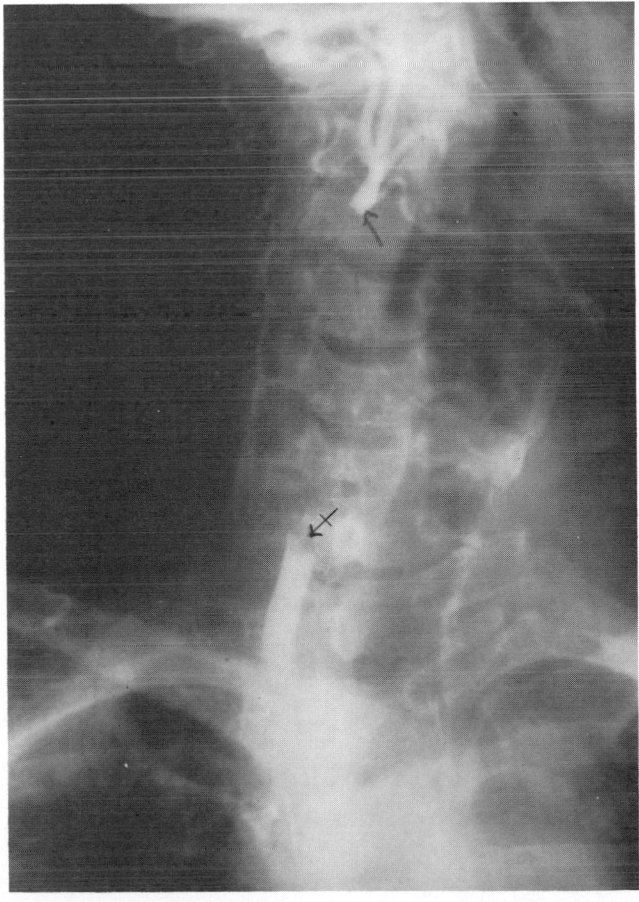

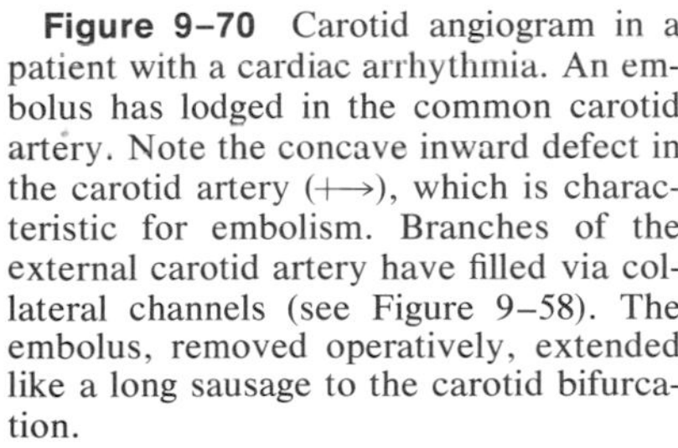

Figure 9–70 Carotid angiogram in a patient with a cardiac arrhythmia. An embolus has lodged in the common carotid artery. Note the concave inward defect in the carotid artery (⟶), which is characteristic for embolism. Branches of the external carotid artery have filled via collateral channels (see Figure 9–58). The embolus, removed operatively, extended like a long sausage to the carotid bifurcation.

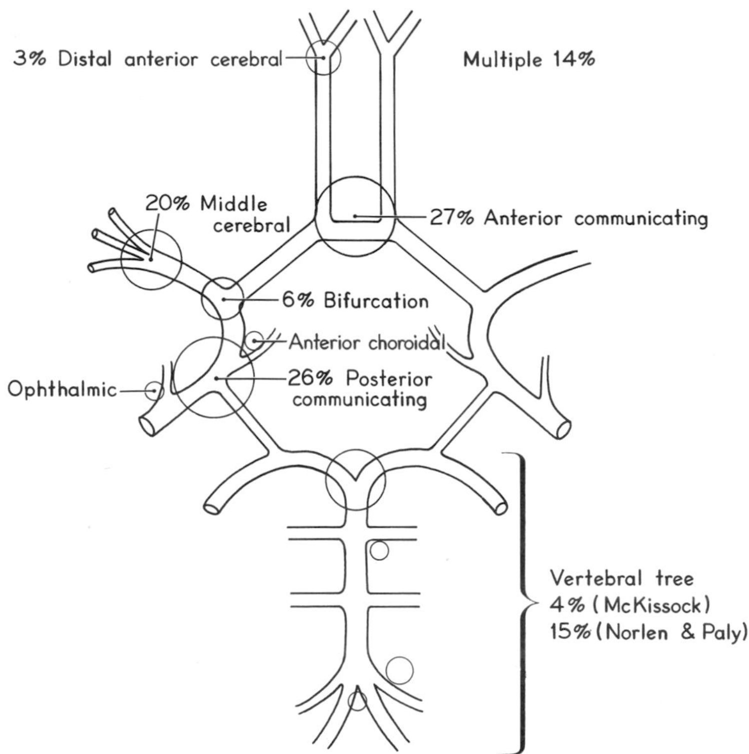

Figure 9–71 Analysis of the 1769 intracranial aneurysms collected by McKissock (from 1950 to 1960) by Bull. (From Schobinger, R. A., and Ruzicka, F. F., eds.: Vascular Roentgenology. New York, Macmillan Co., 1964. Reprinted by permission.)

Aneurysms may produce their effect by gradual expansion, acting as a mass lesion, and may compress adjacent structures. The great majority of aneurysms present clinically when they rupture into the subarachnoid space, into the cerebral tissue, or into the ventricles. Contrast medium may fill the lumen of the aneurysm depending upon the position of the sac during angiography, the presence of spasm around its neck, the presence of clot within its lumen and the phase of the angiographic series. An anterior communicating artery aneurysm may be clearly demonstrated in one film of the series and may no longer be seen in a film taken one second later. Multiple views may be required to establish the presence of an aneurysm and the anatomy of its attachment, i.e., whether a neck is present (Figs. 9–1 to 9–8 and 9–72).

In an analysis of McKissock's series of 1769 aneurysms, Bull found 14 per cent to be multiple.[18] Although Crawford claims that 12 per cent of aneurysms are multiple, a more recent large series claims that over 25 per cent are multiple.[26,147]

Although most aneurysms appear to be of congenital origin, at the point of bifurcation of the branches of the circle of Willis where the muscular layer of the wall is deficient, other factors involved in the production of these aneurysms are high blood pressure and atheromatous lesions in these vessels.[64] The congenital aneurysms are usually saccular; atherosclerotic aneurysms are fusiform and may be dissecting.[229]

Radiological evidence of rupture of an aneurysm may be displacement of other vessels by the presence of a hematoma, and spasm of vessels associated with the aneurysm. A few case reports have appeared of rupture during angiography.[89]

When multiple aneurysms are present and subarachnoid hemorrhage has occurred without localizing signs, it may be difficult to designate the offending aneurysm. Wood has offered criteria to determine the site of rupture when multiple aneurysms are present.[231] In order of decreasing dependability he lists the following angiographic signs: evidence of a mass (denoting hematoma or

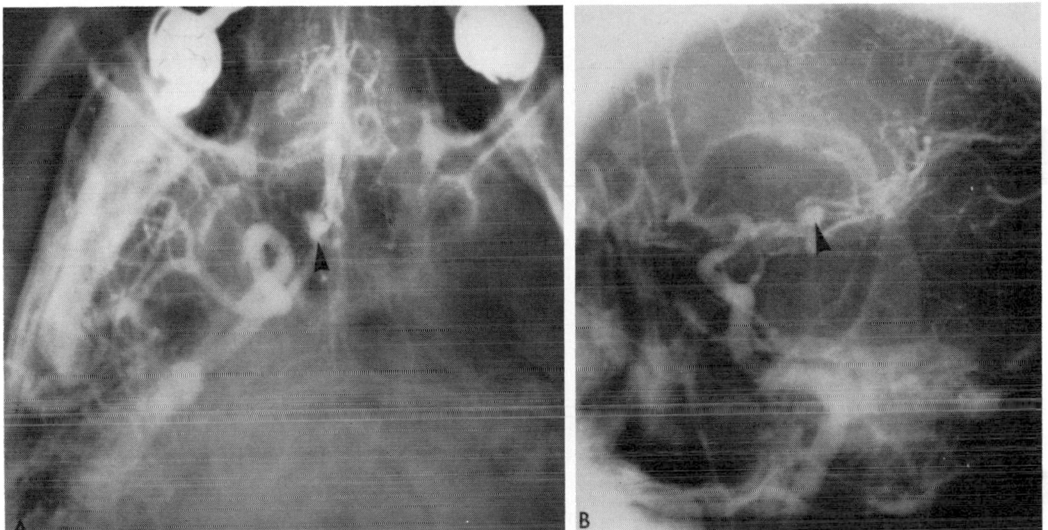

Figure 9–72 *A*. Multiple views may be required to demonstrate the presence of an aneurysm and its precise site of attachment. Submentovertical projection shows an aneurysm of the anterior communicating region. This was difficult to recognize in other projections. The submentovertical projection is also useful for aneurysms of the trifurcation of the middle cerebral artery. *B*. Perorbital view for an aneurysm arising at the trifurcation of the middle cerebral artery. The posterior inferior cerebellar artery is readily recognized in oblique views with the aneurysm projected through the open mouth. For other useful projections see Figures 9–1 to 9–8.

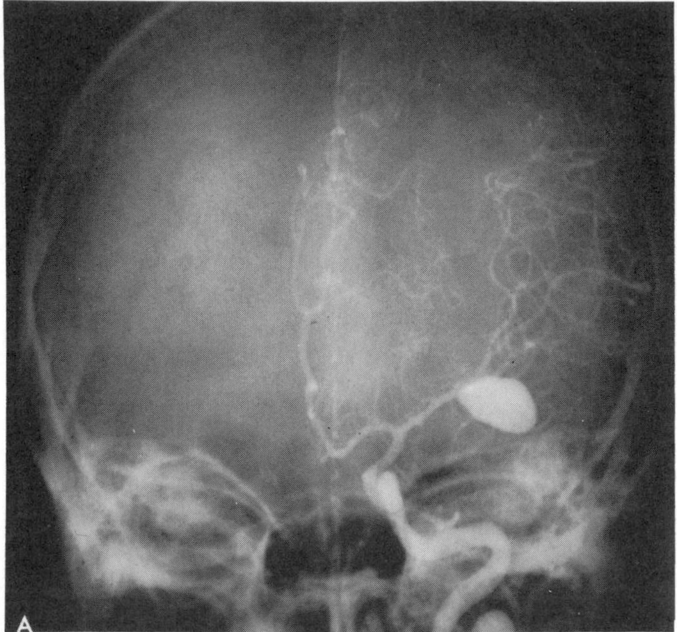

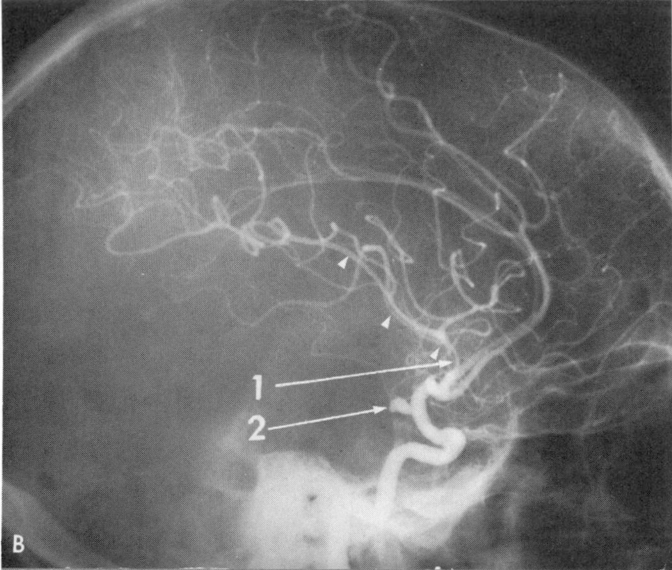

Figure 9–73 *A*. A large middle cerebral artery aneurysm. Note that there is a considerable displacement of the anterior cerebral artery across the midline and the middle cerebral artery has been displaced inward and upward. The aneurysm has bled and there is a surrounding hematoma. *B*. Posterior communicating aneurysm (2). The upward displacement of the middle cerebral artery and its branches (*white arrow heads*) and the narrowing of the main stem of the middle cerebral artery (1) suggest recent hemorrhage. Operation confirmed the presence of a temporal lobe hematoma.

edematous infarct) (Fig. 9–73); the size of the aneurysm (the greater it is, the more likely it was responsible for the subarachnoid hemorrhage); and the presence of spasm (not very valuable) (Fig. 9–74). By applying these criteria, he states, it should be possible to identify the ruptured aneurysm among multiple lesions in more than 95 per cent of cases. DuBoulay has reported on the natural history of intracranial aneurysms, and his contribution is well worth referring to in this respect.[40]

Of 403 consecutive cases of subarachnoid hemorrhage reported by Sutton, 77 per cent had lesions demonstrated by bilateral carotid angiography; the findings were negative in 23 per cent. Fifty-one of the ninety-one negative cases were further investigated by vertebral angiography. Unilateral vertebral angiography showed a lesion in 40 per cent of them. In 17 cases in which the findings of bilateral carotid and unilateral vertebral angiography were negative, a second vertebral angiogram on the contralat-

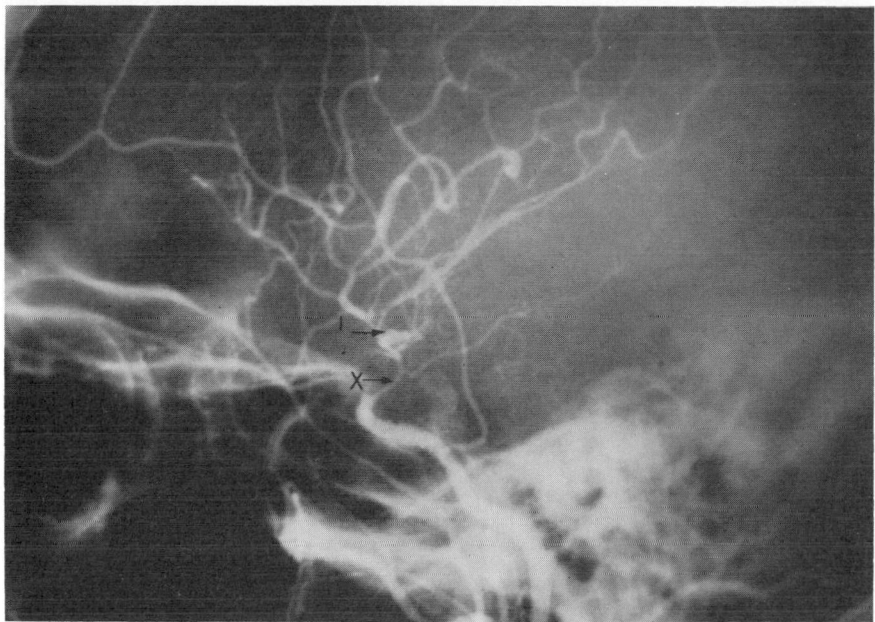

Figure 9–74 Anterior communicating aneurysm in a patient with subarachnoid hemorrhage. Aneurysm (1), which appears lobulated; spasm of carotid siphon (X).

eral side showed a lesion in 7 cases (Fig. 9–75).[205]

The importance of the posterior inferior cerebellar artery origin as a site for aneurysm formation is stressed here; it is the second most common site by far on the posterior circulation, the most common being the tip of the basilar artery (Fig. 9–76). Sixty per cent of aneurysms on the posterior circulation arise from the tip of the basilar artery and 20 per cent arise from the origin of the posterior inferior cerebellar artery.

Spatz and Bull reviewed 60 cases of spontaneous subarachnoid hemorrhage in which bilateral carotid angiography failed to reveal a source of bleeding.[198] In 16 cases, vertebral arteriography demon-

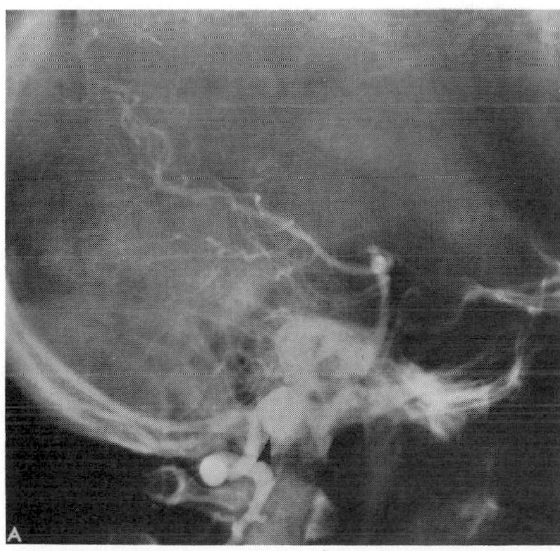

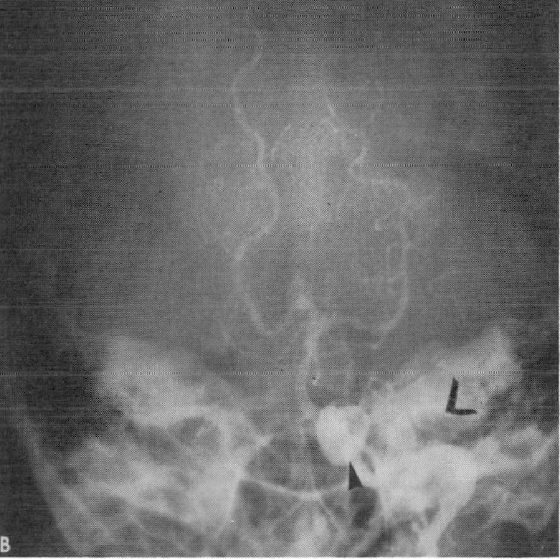

Figure 9–75 Left vertebral angiogram. Frontal (*A*) and lateral (*B*) projections demonstrate a left posterior inferior cerebellar artery aneurysm. Note that there is no reflux down the opposite vertebral artery; only when the contralateral side fills with contrast medium can the presence of an aneurysm be excluded.

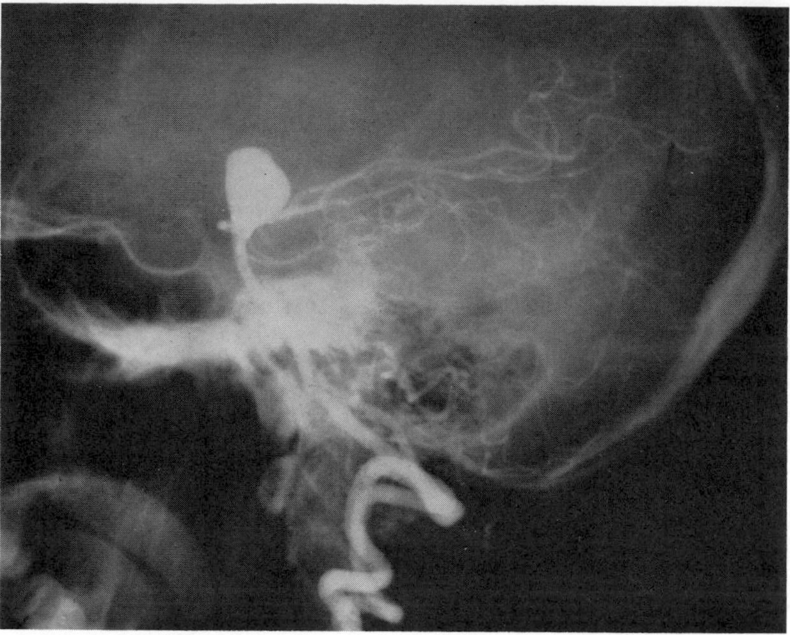

Figure 9–76 Aneurysm of the tip of the basilar artery. This is by far the most common site on the posterior circulation. This patient was admitted to hospital with spontaneous subarachnoid hemorrhage without localizing signs. Carotid angiography revealed an aneurysm arising from the right middle cerebral artery. During hospital stay bilateral third nerve palsy developed. A vertebral angiogram revealed a large terminal basilar aneurysm.

strated the lesion responsible for the bleeding. Eight of these were aneurysms and eight were angiomas. The diagnostic accuracy is considerably enhanced by a meticulous examination of the arterial tree in cases of subarachnoid hemorrhage.

Angiomas

Cushing and Bailey divided these into three groups: telangiectases, venous angiomas, and arterial (arteriovenous) angiomas.[29] Most angiomas appear to have arterial and venous components, and the terms "angioma" and "arteriovenous malformation" are here used synonymously.

These malformations vary in size and shape and may be superficially or deeply seated. They may be found supratentorially and in the posterior fossa and occasionally are situated both above and below the tentorium. Unless bleeding has occurred, these lesions are usually not space-occupying, but on occasions may be, and may even result in atrophy of surrounding cerebral structures.

Angiomas are not infrequently the cause of subarachnoid hemorrhage. The arteries supplying the angiomas are usually hypertrophied, but less so than the draining veins (Fig. 9–77). The venous return from these lesions to the deep or superficial system of veins depends on their size and situation. They are frequently supplied by the carotid and vertebral circulation, and an assessment of their extent and supply usually requires both vertebral and carotid angiography (Fig. 9–78).[6]

A large vascular glioblastoma may on occasion resemble an angioma radiographically, but the large tangle of vessels of more uniform size with an arterial supply and venous return typical for angioma will usually distinguish them. These large angiomas act like sponges and attract all the contrast medium, which passes rapidly from the arterial to the venous system. Definition and detail may be enhanced by the introduction of a larger bolus of contrast medium within a shorter time interval than usual; by using an automatic serialograph, both the maximum arterial and venous phases of the circulation will be obtained.

Aneurysms of the great vein of Galen are really arteriovenous malformations with secondary enlargement of the vein of Galen (Fig. 9–79). Reports of these have been published by Boldrey and Miller, Hirano

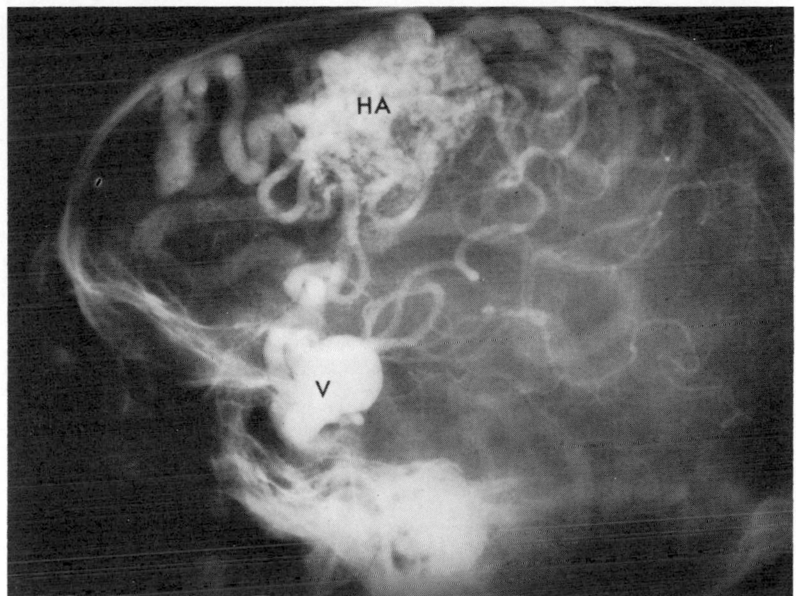

Figure 9–77 Carotid angiogram demonstrating a large arteriovenous malformation supplied by a tangle of hypertrophied arteries (HA). Large veins drain the malformation (V). There is also an aneurysm arising from the region of the anterior communicating artery.

and Terry, Poppen and Avman, and Litvak and associates.[13,79,114,150] The basic embryological defect is a fistula between primitive choroidal arteries and veins, with the resulting malformation related to the shifting of the vascular system with brain growth. This is discussed by O'Brien and Schechter.[139]

Although the combination of aneurysm and angioma is rare, they are associated more frequently than is accounted for by mere chance (Fig. 9–77).[15,147] Many sugges-

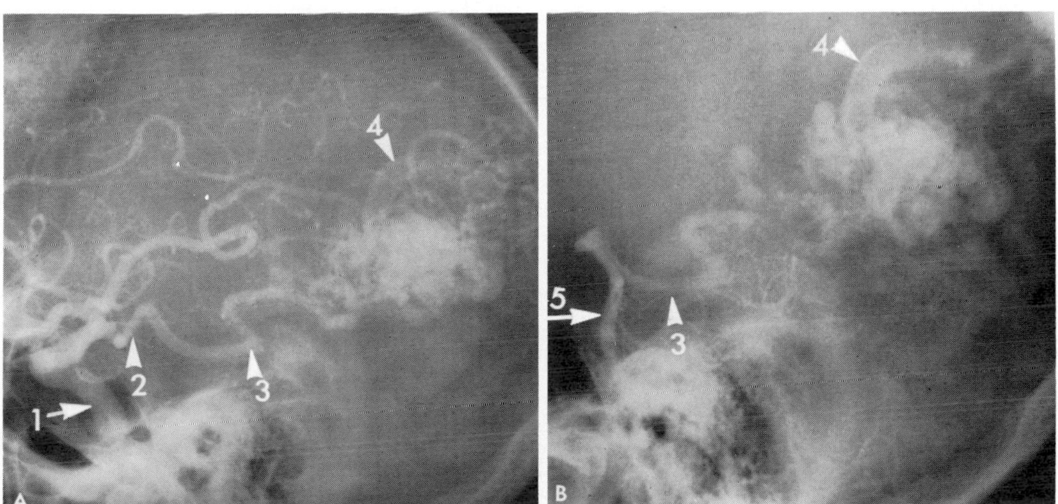

Figure 9–78 *A*. Carotid angiogram demonstrating a large angioma (1) supplied by a large hypertrophied posterior cerebral artery (2, 3). Note draining vein (4) during arterial phase. *B*. Vertebral angiogram in same patient showing angioma filled from basilar artery (5) via the posterior cerebral artery.

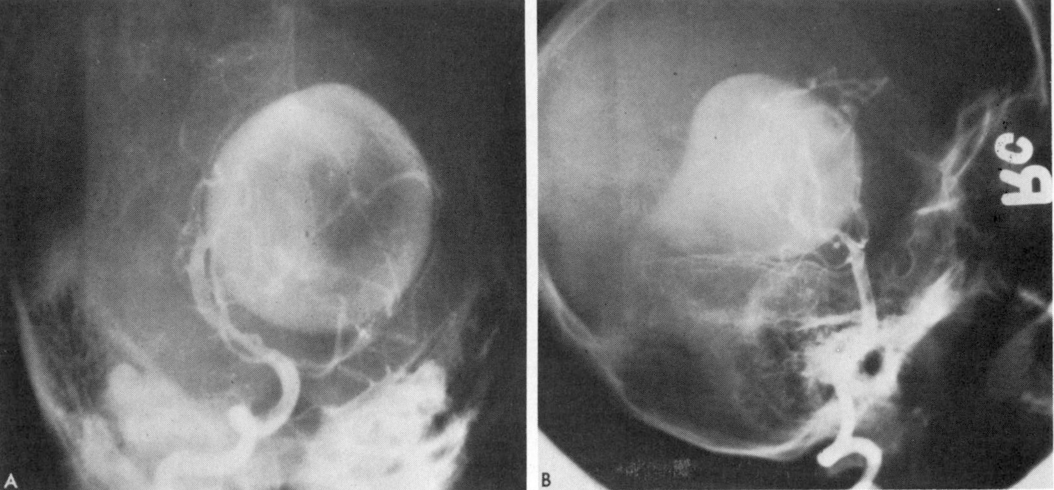

Figure 9–79 *A*. Right vertebral angiogram, anteroposterior Towne view. Here the aneurysm of the vein of Galen is filling from the right posterior cerebral artery. *B*. Lateral vertebral angiogram of same patient. Not only are the main stems of the posterior cerebral arteries filling the aneurysm of the vein of Galen, but enlarged choroidal arterial branches participate as well.

tions have been made as to the nature of the association. Its significance becomes obvious when the point of bleeding in intracranial hemorrhage must be determined. Spasm of vessels and the other radiological signs of a bleeding aneurysm may be helpful in this regard, as described earlier.

Tumors

Angiography may help not only in determining the presence and site of an expanding neoplasm but also in elucidating the nature of the mass. This information depends on two factors: the displacement of arteries and veins from their normal course, and the angioarchitecture of the tumor. The displacement of vessels depends on the size and situation of the tumor and on whether the growth is displacing or infiltrating. Displacements may also reflect such secondary changes as edema or swelling around the tumor and obstruction of cerebrospinal pathways with ventricular dilatation.

Some tumors are highly vascular, much more than normal brain, while others may have a poor blood supply. Tumor vessels differ from normal vessels in that they have irregular lumina and shapes. They are more tortuous than normal vessels, and connections may be present between arteries and veins. Malignant tumors may have numerous arteriovenous shunts within their substance. The latter may undergo necrosis, cystic changes, and even hemorrhage, causing areas of avascularity that may be recognized in the angiogram.

The circulation rate through a tumor may suggest the pathological condition present. Glioblastomas containing numerous arteriovenous shunts may show filling of the tumor vessels during the arterial phase only and early disappearance of the contrast medium, so that very little of the tumor may retain medium during the venous phase (Fig. 9–80). Meningiomas with a more homogeneous angioarchitecture consisting of numerous capillaries usually retain the contrast medium for a longer period, and the tumor opacification will still be present during the venous phase (Fig. 9–81). Metastatic deposits have a circulation rate that usually lies between those of glioblastomas and meningiomas (Fig. 9–82). Swelling of brain tissue may delay circulation time, and this will become manifest when the opacification of the tumor occurs later than that of the normal brain tissue.

Large avascular space-occupying masses such as cysts and abscesses may displace and crowd vascular channels on the periphery of a mass. These crowded normal cerebral vessels must be distinguished from the tumor vessels that form a halo or ring shadow on the surface of a glioblastoma (Fig. 9–83).

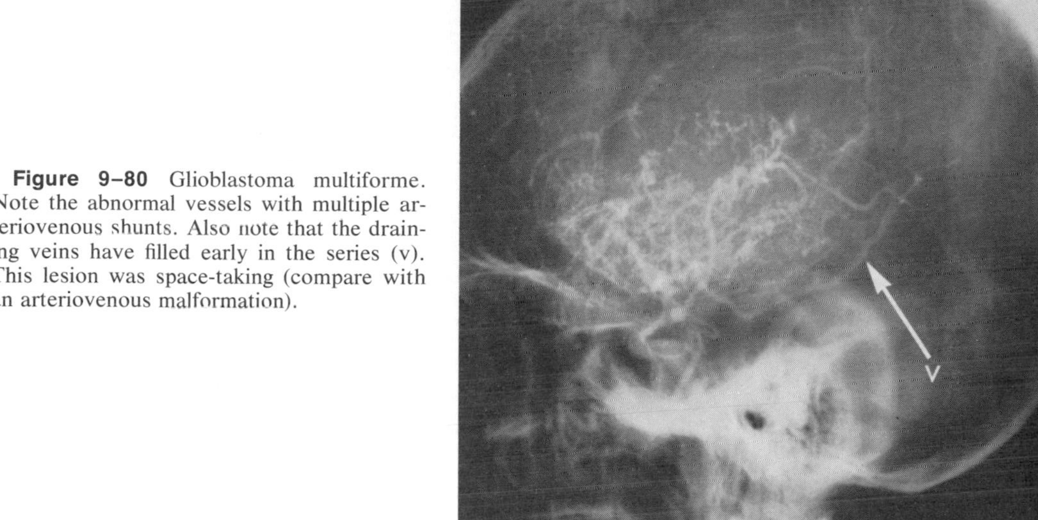

Figure 9–80 Glioblastoma multiforme. Note the abnormal vessels with multiple arteriovenous shunts. Also note that the draining veins have filled early in the series (v). This lesion was space-taking (compare with an arteriovenous malformation).

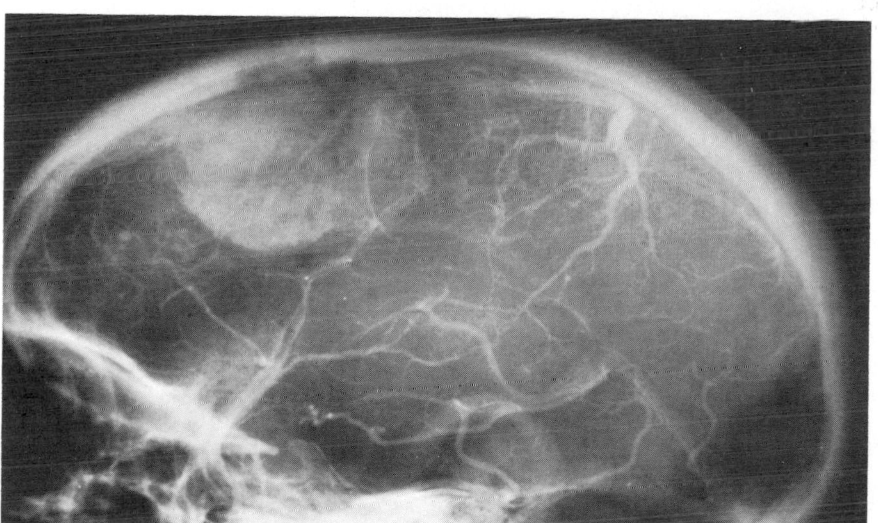

Figure 9–81 Venous phase of a carotid angiogram showing the tumor blush of a meningioma.

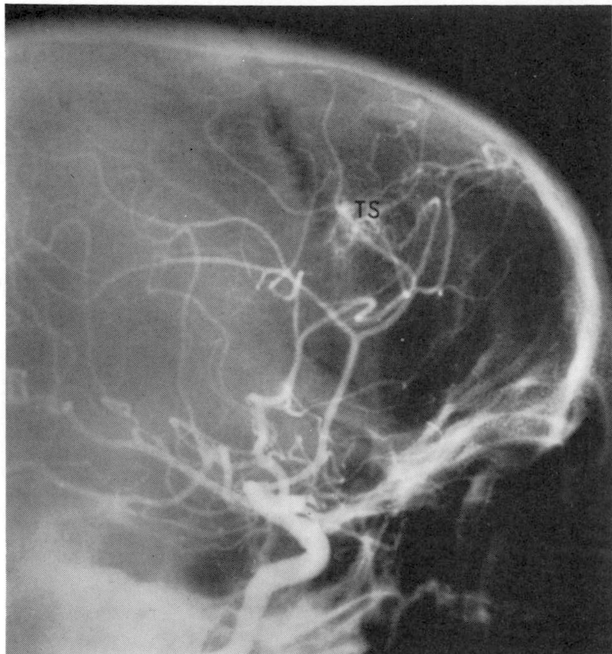

Figure 9–82 Carotid angiogram. Note the early filling of tumor vessels associated with a metastatic deposit. Although the tumor stain (TS) was seen in the venous phase, it disappeared quite rapidly, unlike that of a meningioma.

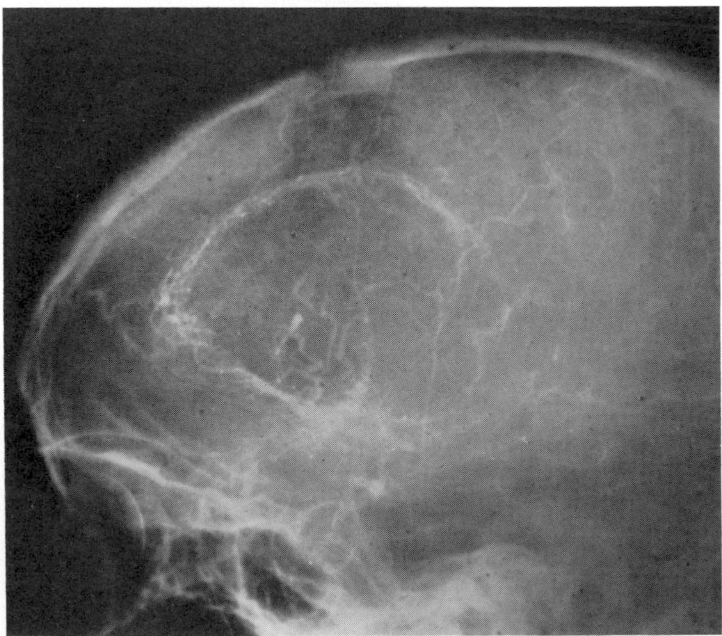

Figure 9–83 Carotid angiogram showing a halo of abnormal vessels surrounding a relatively avascular mass (this was a malignant glioma, astrocytoma grade III).

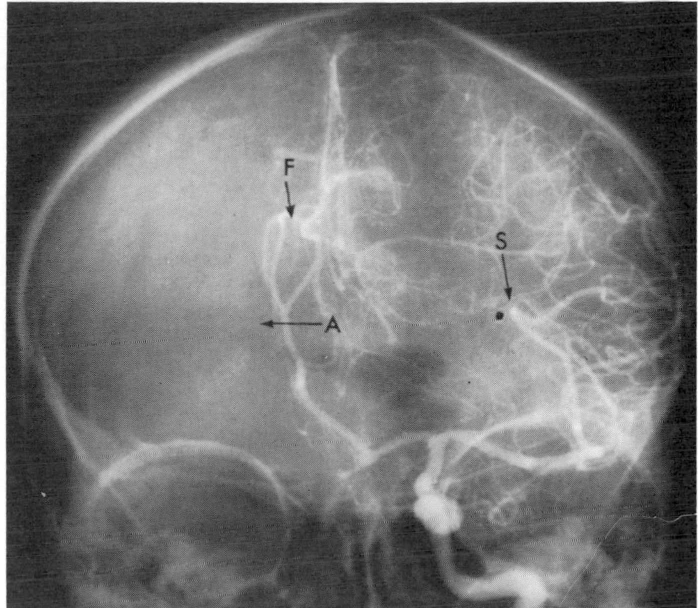

Figure 9–84 Displacement of the anterior cerebral artery (A) with falcine herniation (F) and downward displacement of the angiographic sylvian point (S) by a posterior frontal meningioma.

Displacement of Vessels

SUPRATENTORIAL LESIONS. The anterior cerebral artery will be displaced to the contralateral side by an expanding mass (Fig. 9–84). Masses deep in the temporal fossa, however, may not displace the artery (Fig. 9–85). The type of displacement varies with the situation of the mass. Anterior frontal masses cause maximum bowing of the vessel with minor displacements of the internal cerebral vein. With lesions situated further back, there will be more displacement of the internal cerebral vein than of the anterior cerebral artery (Fig. 9–86).

Displacement of vessels in certain situa-

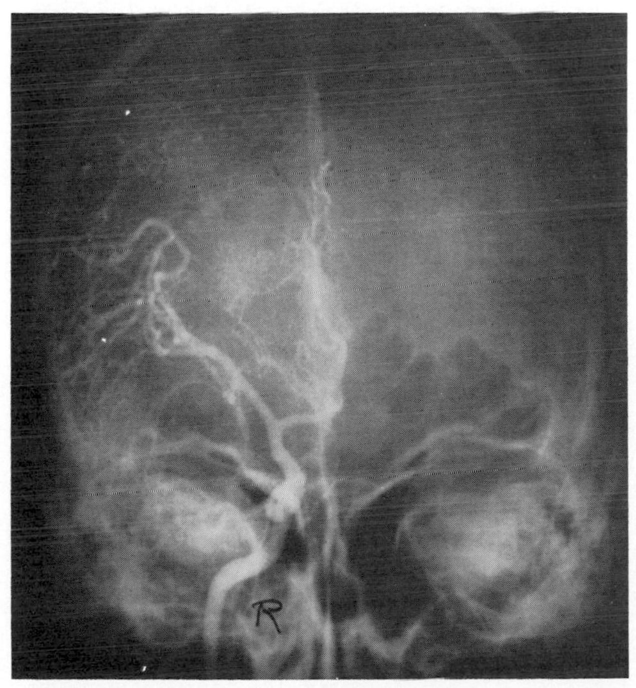

Figure 9–85 Upward and inward displacement of the middle cerebral artery by a temporal fossa meningioma. Note the stretched branches of the middle cerebral artery. There is little displacement across the midline of the anterior cerebral artery.

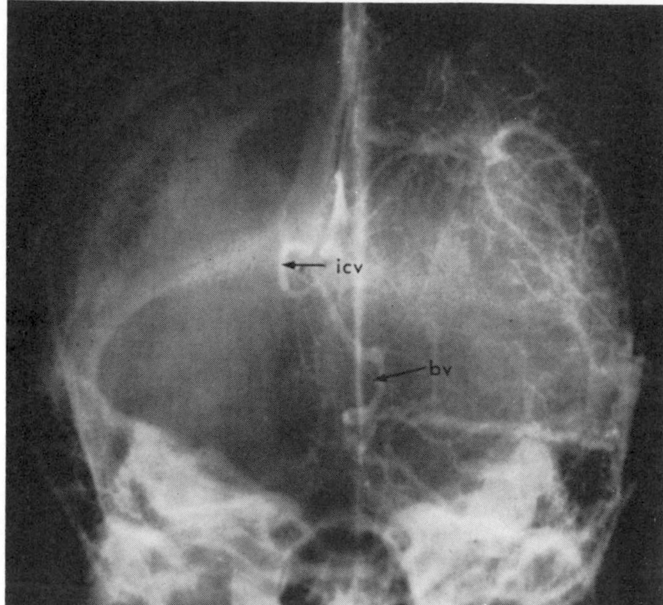

Figure 9–86 The internal cerebral vein (icv) is displaced more than the anterior cerebral artery when lesions are close to the midline. bv, basilar vein.

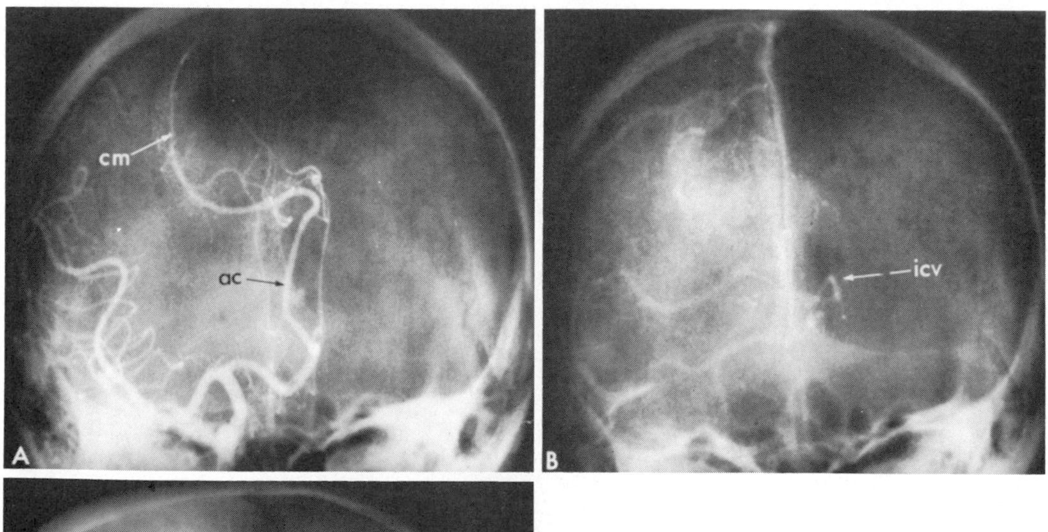

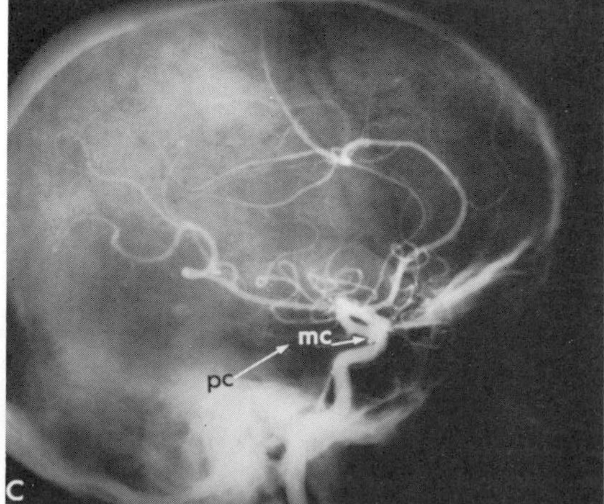

Figure 9–87 *A*. Falx meningioma. The displacement of vessels here is highly suggestive, almost pathognomonic for a falx meningioma. This shows the right anterior cerebral artery (ac) displaced toward the left, but the course of the callosomarginal artery (cm) is such that it cannot negotiate the falx. Since the tumor arises from the falx, this portion of the artery is displaced toward the right, i.e., the ipsilateral side. *B*. This shows the tumor stain and the displaced internal cerebral vein (icv). *C*. The callosomarginal artery is displaced laterally, the pericallosal artery (pc) depressed, and the roof of the triangle of Reil depressed (mc).

tions may provide evidence not only of a tumor mass, but of the specific nature of the tumor. Falx meningiomas may displace the pericallosal artery to the contralateral side and the callosomarginal artery to the ipsilateral side (Fig. 9–87). This sign is fairly specific, but may be mimicked by interhemispheric falx hematomas and interhemispheric empyemas.[22] A recently encountered exhibition of this sign was caused by a glioblastoma that had grown out of the hemisphere and had insinuated itself between the anterior cerebral artery and the falx. Tentorial meningiomas may displace the posterior end of the lateral ventrical or the posterior cerebral artery upward, while at the same time displacing the superior cerebellar artery downward (cf. Fig. 9–104). This is a fairly specific sign for tentorial meningiomas.[185]

Venous displacements and changes in the relative rate of filling of the superficial draining veins may be present with a comparatively normal arterial phase of the cerebral angiogram. The internal cerebral vein shows its maximum displacements with mass lesions approaching the midline (Fig. 9–86). The disproportionate displacement between the internal cerebral vein and the arterial tree may supply valuable diagnostic information. For instance, disproportionate displacement of the internal cerebral vein relative to the anterior cerebral artery would suggest a deep-seated lesion near the midline or a lesion situated more posteriorly.

The striothalamic vein and the septal vein are usually recognized in a lateral projection of the venous phase of a carotid angiogram (Fig. 9–88). The point of juncture usually represents the location of the foramen of Monro. Ring and Laine and coworkers have devised topograms of this point of juncture.[106,159] Although displacements of the "venous angle" may be appreciated by applying these topograms, caution must be exercised, since a false venous angle may be produced by a perforating vein entering behind the foramen of Monro (Fig. 9–54). Johansson has illustrated the normal and the displaced internal cerebral veins in a comprehensive monograph.[93]

When the major displacement of the anterior cerebral artery occurs along its distal course, falcine herniation will be more pronounced (Fig. 9–84). Subfrontal masses will displace the anterior cerebral artery upward and backward and will depress the carotid siphon (Fig. 9–89). The internal cerebral vein may be displaced backward, upward, and across the midline. Suprasellar masses may depress the carotid siphon

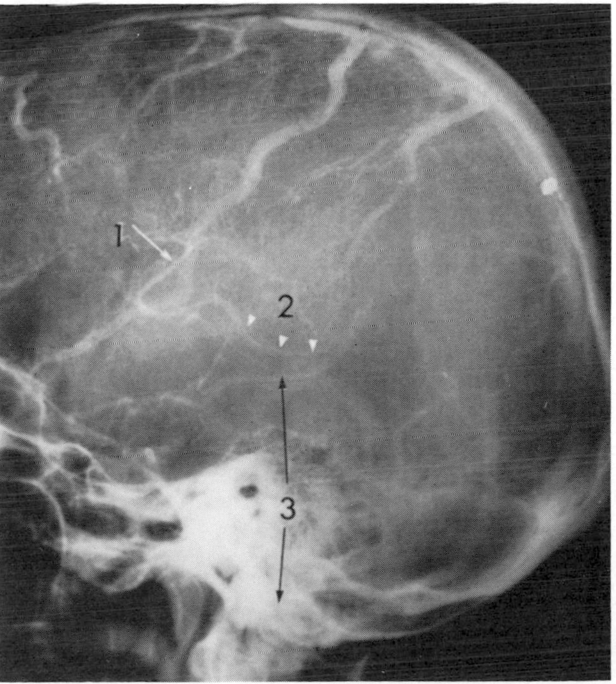

Figure 9–88 Venous phase of carotid angiogram. A large posterior parietal glioblastoma resulted in depression of the internal cerebral vein (2) and unfolding of the venous angle, manifested by a displaced thalamostriate vein (1). Note basal vein (3).

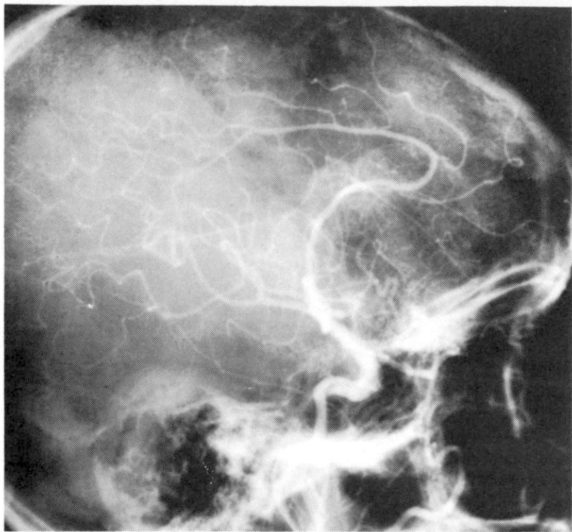

Figure 9–89 The typical upward and backward displacement of the anterior cerebral artery by an olfactory groove meningioma.

but elevate the anterior cerebral artery and the internal cerebral vein (Fig. 9–90).

Parasagittal tumors may simply depress the pericallosal and callosomarginal branches of the anterior cerebral arteries. The internal cerebral vein may also be depressed (Fig. 9–87*C*). When the tumor grows more to one side, the anterior cerebral branches will be displaced across the midline (Fig. 9–87).

The branches of the middle cerebral artery in the sylvian fissure are displaced upward in expanding lesions in the temporal lobe (Fig. 9–91). Usually some displacement of the anterior cerebral artery accompanies these middle cerebral artery displacements. (Although deep temporal lesions may not displace the anterior cerebral artery, they will usually displace the internal cerebral vein.) A parietal mass will dis-

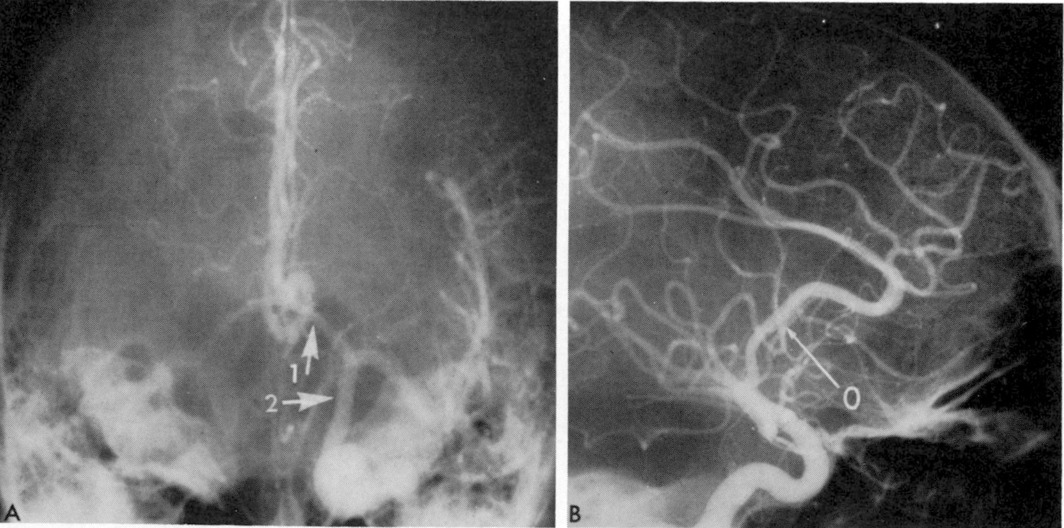

Figure 9–90 Carotid angiogram demonstrating the typical appearance of a suprasellar mass arising in the sella (chromophobe adenoma). Note that the carotid siphon (the intracavernous carotid artery and the supraclinoid internal carotid artery, 2) is displaced away from the midline, the anterior cerebral artery is arched upward (1 and 0), and the carotid siphon is depressed.

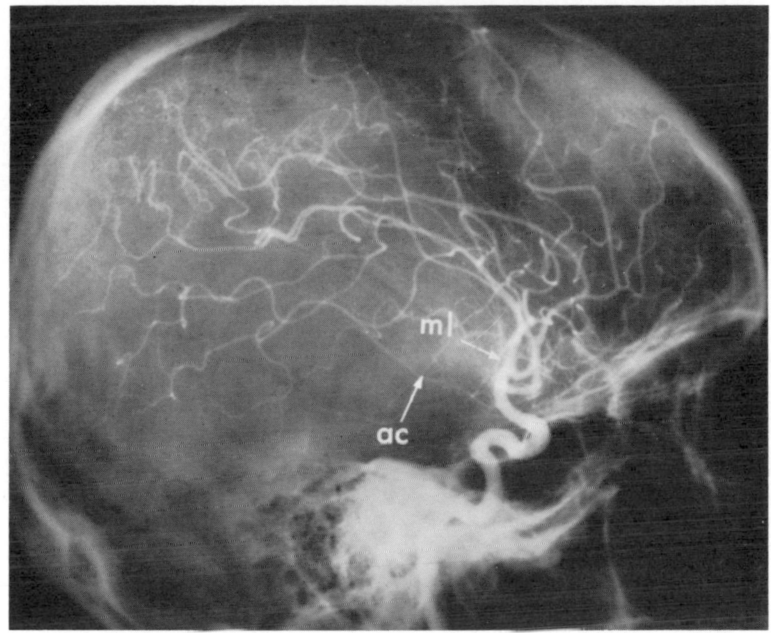

Figure 9–91 An avascular temporal lobe mass. The middle cerebral artery group is displaced upward, and the first portion of the middle cerebral artery (ml) is no longer foreshortened. The anterior choroidal artery (ac) is elevated and stretched.

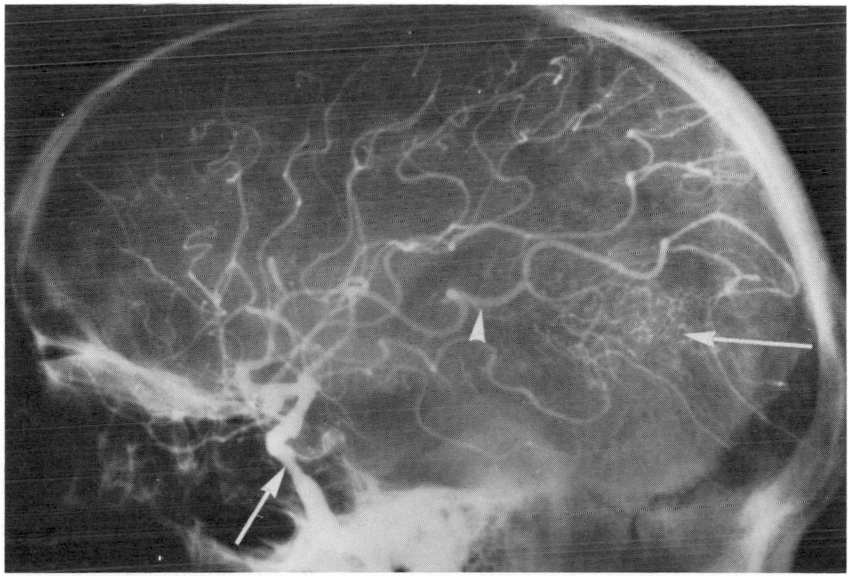

Figure 9–92 Carotid angiogram in a posterior parieto-occipital glioblastoma. Note the tumor vessels (*arrows*) and the apparent elevation of branches of the middle cerebral artery with ruching of the vessels (*white arrowhead*). Note atherosclerotic narrowing of the carotid siphon.

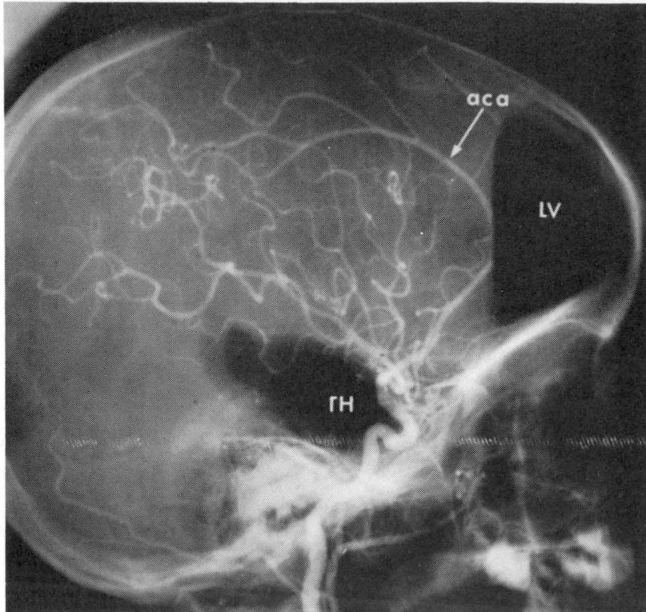

Figure 9–93 Carotid angiogram in a patient who had had a pneumoencephalogram a few days previously. Marked symmetrical dilatation of the entire ventricular system was present. Note the dilatation of both temporal horns (TH) and both frontal horns in the air study. Although the anterior cerebral artery (aca) is stretched and bowed, this is not an index of the degree of ventricular dilatation, since it lies in a trough between the two dilated lateral ventricles (LV).

place the sylvian group downward (Figs. 9–84 and 9–90). Lesions in the occipital lobe, if large enough, may displace the sylvian group upward and cause ruching of the vessel. This may actually appear to be a displacement of the middle cerebral artery (Fig. 9–92).

The anterior choroidal artery, which enters the temporal horn, may also show displacements. Temporal lobe lesions stretch this artery and may displace it upward (Fig. 9–91).

Dilatation of the lateral ventricles may be reflected in the stretched course of the anterior cerebral artery. A marked degree of ventricular dilatation, however, must be

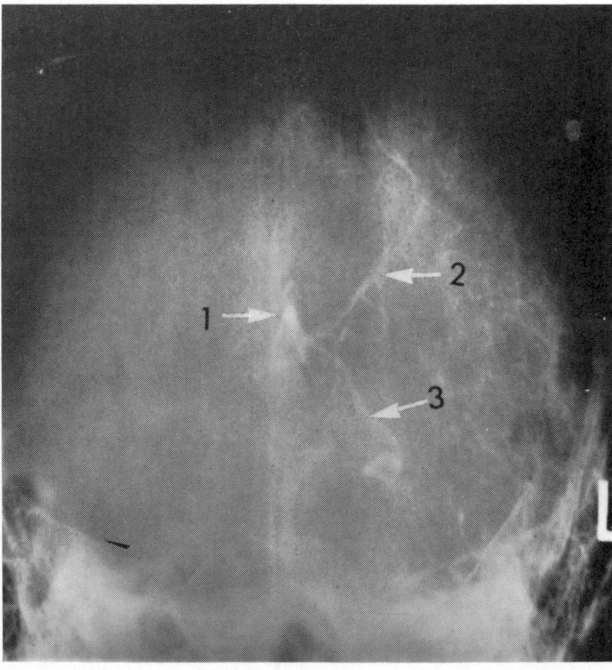

Figure 9–94 Venous phase of carotid angiogram. Note internal cerebral vein (1) is in midline. Thalamostriate vein (2) is separated abnormally from midline owing to ventricular dilatation. Basilar vein (3).

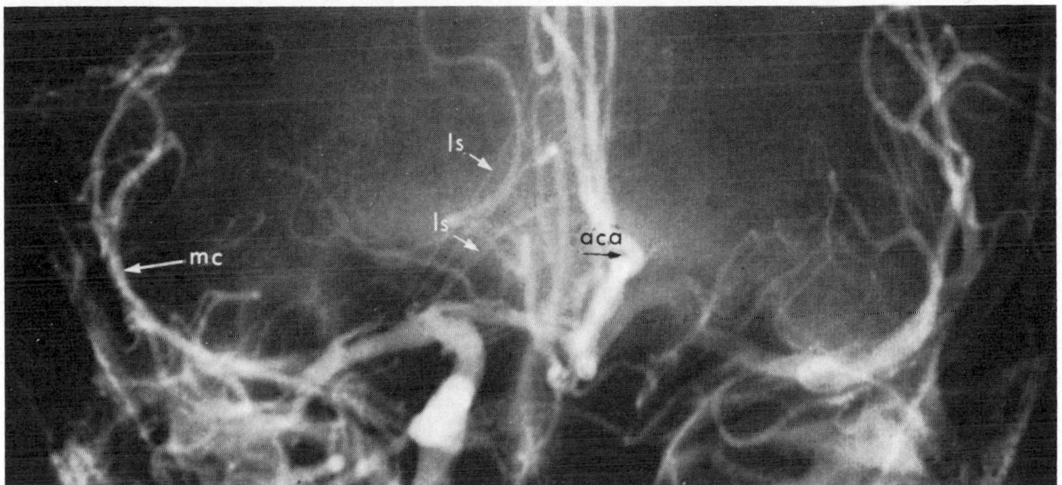

Figure 9–95 Carotid angiogram. Note the increased separation between the right middle cerebral artery (mc) and the anterior cerebral artery (aca). The right middle cerebral artery is stretched and displaced outward, and the lenticulostriate vessels (ls) are markedly displaced toward the midline. Compare with the left side.

present before these changes occur (Fig. 9–93). The thalamostriate vein, which runs along the lateral wall of the ventricle, will supply a much more sensitive indication of ventricular dilatation. Sears and associates have compared the appearance of these veins seen in the anteroposterior projection of the carotid phlebogram to a pair of bull's horns.[189] With dilatation of the ventricular system, they resemble a set of short horns, whereas normally they are convex inward (Fig. 9–94).

Although central expanding lesions display their maximum effect on the deep veins rather than on the larger arteries, angiographic magnification techniques that offer great detail and definition will allow displacement of the lenticulostriate arteries to be readily recognized (Fig. 9–95).[66]

Posterior Fossa Lesions. Carotid angiography may supply indirect signs of a posterior fossa expanding lesion. A midline anterior cerebral artery stretched and wide-swept because of dilatation of the lateral ventricles would suggest disease in the posterior fossa obstructing the cerebrospinal fluid pathway through the aqueduct of Sylvius. Air studies of the posterior fossa supply a more sensitive test of minor displacements of structures than does vertebral angiography, since minor changes and normal variations in the position of vessels in the posterior fossa may overlap. Vertebral angiography, however, may be more helpful in assessing the nature of the lesion rather than its precise localization.

Upward herniation through the tentorial opening may result in superior displacement of the superior cerebellar arteries and even the posterior cerebral arteries (Fig. 9–96). The cerebellar tonsillar herniations may displace the posterior inferior cerebellar artery below the foramen magnum (Fig. 9–97). (This may be seen, however, without herniation.)

Pontine and "angle" tumors may displace the superior cerebellar artery and the posterior cerebral artery (Fig. 9–98). Angle tumors may also displace or obliterate the petrosal sinus.[208] Smaltino claims to recognize angiographic changes in the course of the auditory artery.[197]

Extra-axial tumors can be distinguished from tumors of the pons and midbrain by vertebral angiography. In pontine lesions, the basilar artery may be in its normal position or displaced against the clivus, whereas in lesions originating in the clivus, such as meningioma, chordoma, or cholesteatoma, the basilar artery will be displaced backward (Fig. 9–99). Backward displacement of the basilar artery may also occur in infantile hydrocephalus.[108]

Thalamic tumors and tumors in the region of the pineal body may displace the posterior choroidal arteries upward, widening their curve. The great vein of Galen may be compressed and depressed by

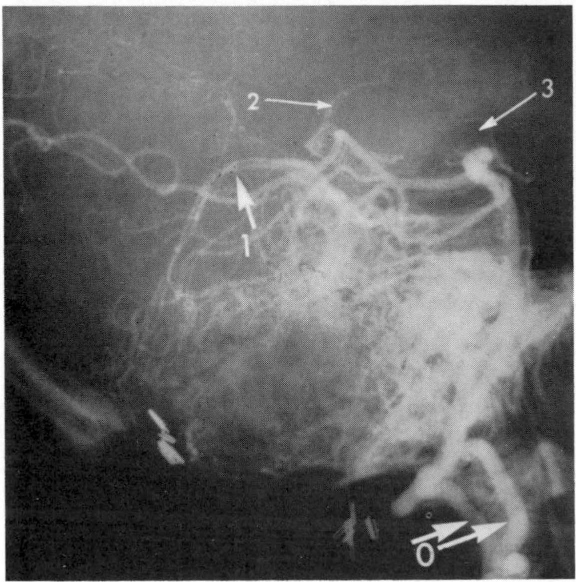

Figure 9–96 Posterior fossa metastatic deposit. A postoperative vertebral angiogram shows up herniation of the superior cerebellar arteries through the tentorial opening (1). The basilar artery is flat against the clivus. This latter sign has a little more significance in the infant. It is not a reliable sign of a mass lesion in the posterior fossa. 2, posterior choroidal arteries; 3, thalamoperforating arteries; 0, both vertebral arteries.

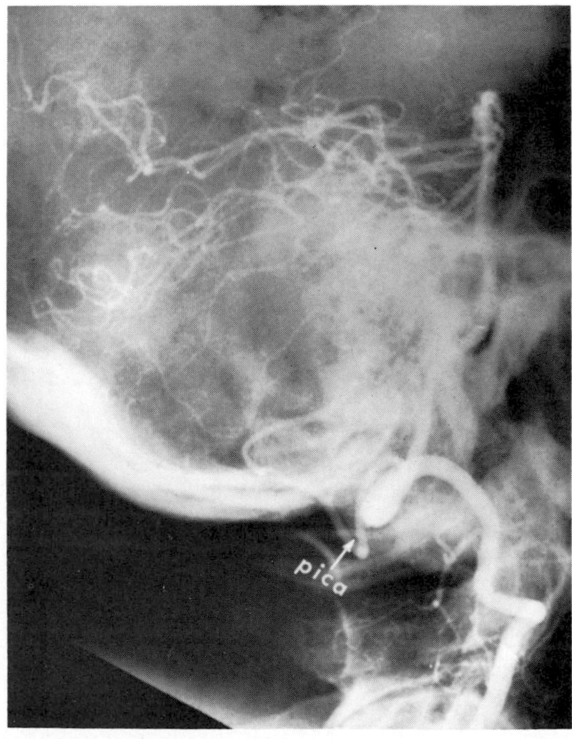

Figure 9–97 A vertebral angiogram in a patient with a posterior fossa metastatic deposit. The posterior inferior cerebellar artery (pica) has been displaced below the foramen magnum. This is evidence of tonsillar herniation but is not a very reliable sign since so many variations of the anatomy occur.

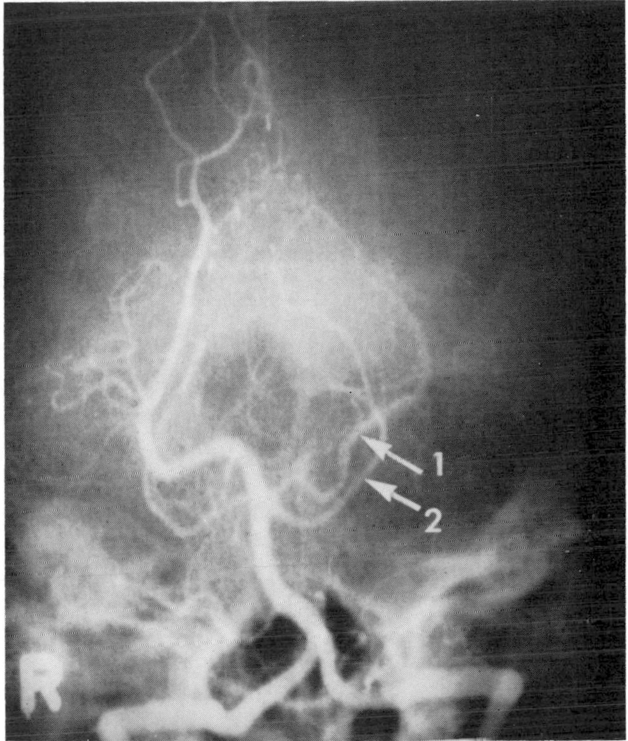

Figure 9–98 Vertebral angiogram in left acoustic neuroma. Note displacement of posterior cerebral artery (1) and superior cerebellar artery (2). A film taken three seconds later demonstrated tumor vessels.

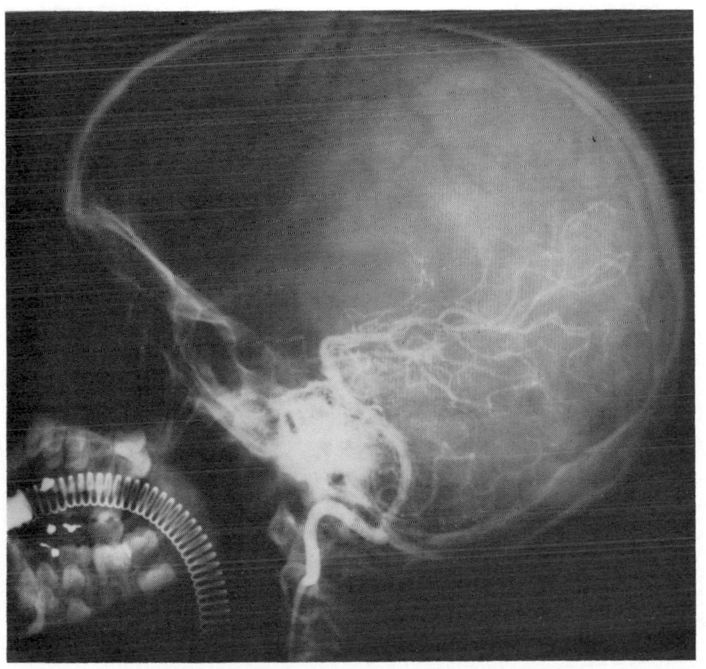

Figure 9–99 Typical displacement of the basilar artery by an extra-axial lesion. Note the displacement of the basilar artery away from the clivus produced by a clivus chordoma. Other extra-axial masses may produce similar changes. (Courtesy of J. W. D. Bull, National Hospital, Queen Square, London.)

tumors in this area (Fig. 9–88). Severe compression of this vessel may result in poor visualization during angiography.

The basilar artery also may be depressed and become accordion-like. This displacement may represent a large midline mass lying directly above the tip of the basilar artery.[176] The anterior choroidal artery, which usually has a curvilinear course with its convexity medially, will have to take a more oblique course around an uncal herniation and will appear stretched in the lateral projection.

Angioarchitecture of Tumor

The vascular architecture of and the rate of blood flow through a tumor will influence the angiographic appearance and often supply a histological diagnosis. Astrocytomas are usually less vascular than normal brain tissue, whereas glioblastomas, meningiomas, secondary deposits, and hemangioblastomas usually have an enriched blood supply.

GLIOMAS. These form the bulk of primary intracerebral tumors. Those of the glioblastoma multiforme group are highly vascular tumors consisting of tumor vessels arranged haphazardly. These vessels are of different sizes and shapes, and many arteriovenous shunts are present within the tumor mass (Fig. 9–80 and 9–92). The tumor fills during the arterial phase of the angiogram. Due to the vascularity of the mass and the arteriovenous shunts, the tumor may have emptied completely during the venous phase. It may sometimes be difficult to distinguish between a very vascular glioma and an arteriovenous malformation. The large feeding arteries and draining veins are usually more evident in malformations, which are usually not space-occupying unless they have hemorrhaged and a hematoma has formed.

Malignant gliomas frequently undergo degenerative changes and may contain necrotic areas, cysts, and hemorrhage. This may manifest itself radiologically in a hypervascularized area surrounding an avascular zone. This "ring sign" is seen most frequently in glioblastoma, but may also be present in metastatic deposits; it results from tumor vessels surrounding an area of necrosis (Fig. 9–83). In cysts and abscesses, a false ring sign may be present, but here the hypervascularized halo consists of compressed normal cerebral vessels, and no abnormal tumor vessels can be identified.

Some malignant gliomas have tumor vessels not unlike those just described, but with no visible communications between the arteries and veins. In these cases contrast filling of veins does not occur during the arterial phase. Greitz and Lindgren state that in this group, with the use of rapid serial angiography, the pathological drainage veins will be seen filled before the normal cerebral veins.[67] Some glioblastomas have a vascular supply poorer in vessels than normal adjacent brain, and others may have no difference in their vascular architecture.

The astrocytomas have a poorer blood supply than other gliomas. The angiographic demonstration of tumor vessels is rare, and, in fact, the brain may be less vascularized over this area. Arteriovenous fistulae are absent, and the diagnosis must be made on vessel displacements and areas of avascularity.

MENINGIOMAS. These tumors have angiographic characteristics that are recognizable in over half the cases.[113] Meningiomas are usually attached to the dura and show sites of predilection along the sagittal sinus, sphenoid ridge, and olfactory groove (Figs. 9–81, 9–84, 9–87, and 9–89). Rarely, these tumors are situated within the ventricles, where their characteristic appearances may be present (Fig. 9–100). In a review of 250 confirmed cases of meningioma by Gassel and Davies, 11 were situated in the lateral ventricles, and carotid angiography (performed in 2 cases) revealed displacement of vessels indicative of a deep mass.[63]

A hypertrophied anterior choroidal artery has been shown to supply the tumor.[7,47,82,220] Rogers reported a case of an intraventicular meningioma diagnosed by vertebral angiography.[163] A right carotid angiogram showed a doubtful displacement of the anterior cerebral artery. In an attempted left carotid arteriogram the needle inadvertently passed into the vertebral artery; the resultant angiogram revealed an intraventricular meningioma supplied by a large elongated posterior choroidal artery. An extensive tumor blush was seen in the venous phase. Intraventricular meningiomas may result in hypertrophy of the anterior choroidal artery (Fig. 9–101). Although other vascular intraventricular

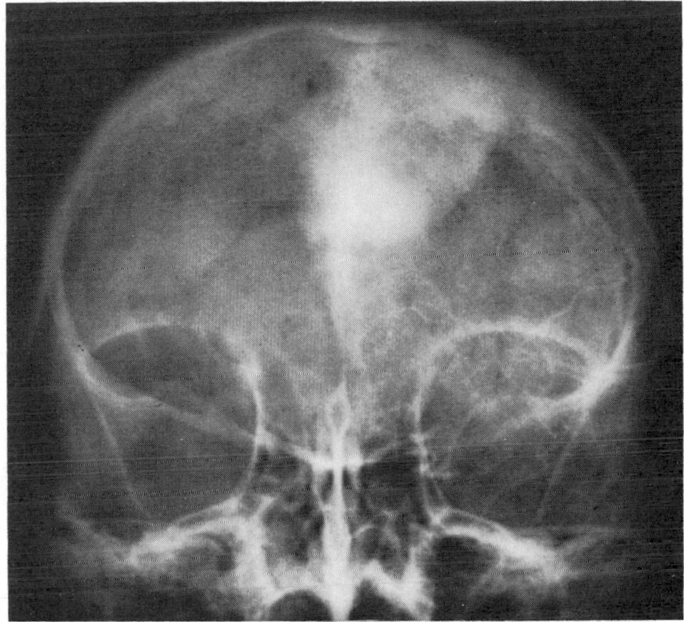

Figure 9–100 Venous phase of a carotid angiogram showing the typical "ground glass" opacification of a parasagittal meningioma.

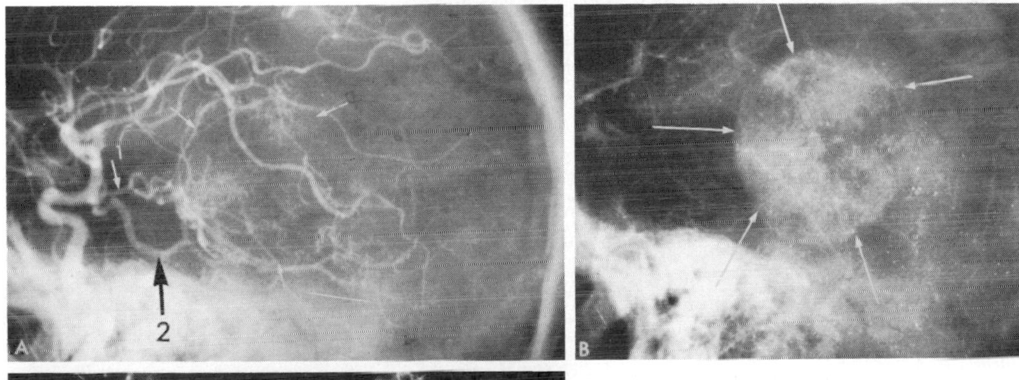

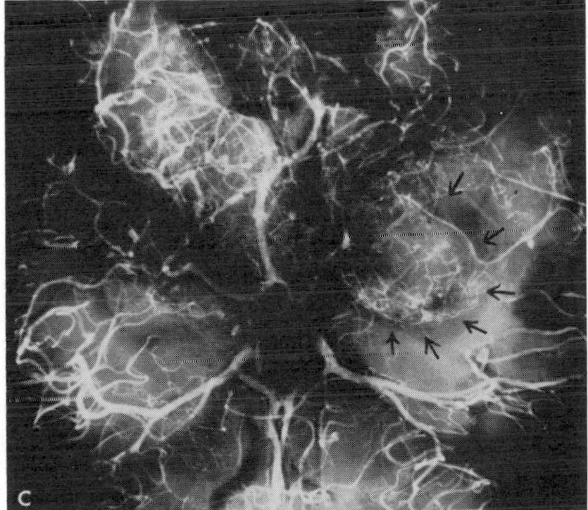

Figure 9–101 *A*. Intraventricular meningioma supplied by branches of the internal carotid artery. Note the hypertrophied anterior choroidal artery (1) and hypertrophied posterior cerebral artery (2) supplying the tumor. *B*. Film six seconds later shows homogeneous round smooth-edged area of opacification. Confirmed intraventricular meningioma. *C*. Postmortem angiogram of the intraventricular meningioma. Note the marked vascularity, position, shape, and attachment of the tumor.

tumors may hypertrophy these vessels, the margins of the tumor may not be smooth, and the other characteristics (persistence of tumor stain, location of tumor at the trigone of ventricle) may not be present. In two cases of intraventricular meningiomas seen by the present author both showed hypertrophy of the anterior choroidal arteries and one showed the characteristic tumor stain. Both were confirmed at postmortem. The tumor vessels of meningiomas usually have regular lumina and are characterized by many capillaries. The vessels may become filled during the arterial phase, and the capillaries usually remain filled until late in the venous phase. The stain is sometimes homogeneous like ground glass. Meningiomas are usually single, although multiple tumors have been reported.

Meningiomas often receive their blood supply from both external and internal carotid arteries (Fig. 9–102). The blood supply from the external carotid artery is usually mediated via the middle meningeal artery, but if the tumor has infiltrated the bone, it may receive blood via the other branches of the external carotid artery supplying the region (Fig. 9–103). When the tumor receives a supply from these vessels, they hypertrophy, and the segment of the vessel adjacent to the tumor may be larger than the stem vessel.

The tumor stain usually has a regular margin and is well outlined. With differential contrast filling of both the internal and the external carotid arteries, these changes may be more obvious. The appearance of a meningioma that receives this dual supply

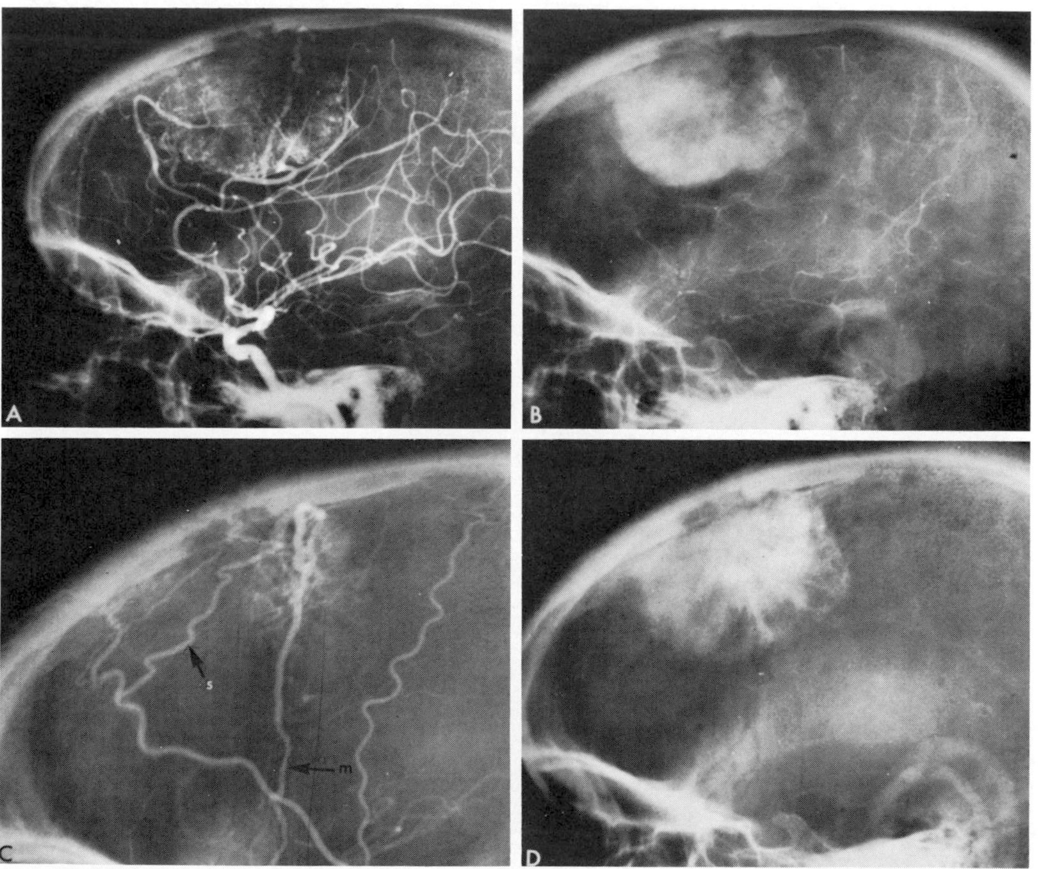

Figure 9–102 *A*. Internal carotid angiogram. Note the displacement of branches of the anterior cerebral artery by a large tumor stain. *B*. Later phase of the internal carotid angiogram showing more opacification of the tumor, principally distributed around the outside of the tumor. *C*. External carotid angiogram shows the middle meningeal artery (m) increasing in caliber as it approaches the tumor and involvement also of the superficial temporal artery (s). *D*. A later phase of the external carotid angiogram shows maximum opacification of the tumor in its center. There is less opacification of the periphery of the tumor, which is supplied by the internal carotid artery as is seen in *B*.

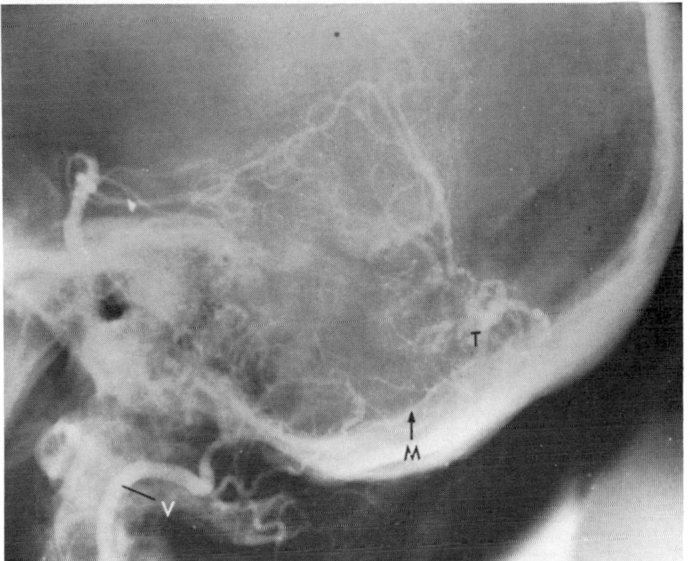

Figure 9–103 Posterior meningeal branch (M) of the vertebral artery (V) supplying a tentorial meningioma (T).

may be quite characteristic: the external meningeal vessels will follow the attachment of the tumor and will appear to supply the core of the tumor, while the surface of the tumor appears to derive its blood supply from the branches of the internal carotid artery. The "spoke wheel" angiographic appearance of meningioma referred to by Lindgren results because narrow, regular, tangled vessels are arranged in a radial fashion.[113] This vascular pattern appears to be most common in intraventricular and cerebellopontine angle meningiomas.

Even in the absence of tumor stain there are two situations in which the displacement of vessels is such that the diagnosis of a meningioma is almost certain. Falx meningiomas displace the main stem of the anterior cerebral artery to the contralateral side while the callosomarginal branches may be displaced ipsilaterally (Fig. 9–87). Similarly, tentorial meningiomas may displace the posterior cerebral arteries upward and the superior cerebellar arteries downward in the same patient (Fig. 9–104).[185]

Metastases. These tumors are usually round and well circumscribed. Hypernephromas are sometimes extremely vascular and may resemble glioblastomas (Fig. 9–82). When multiple separate accumulations of vessels are seen, the diagnosis of secondary deposits is most likely (Fig. 9–105).

Hemangioblastomas. These are usually situated in the cerebellum and are frequently multiple. Vascular displacement by these tumors is extremely slight, even in the presence of large cysts. In most cases these are, from the pathological standpoint, cystic lesions with a cherry-red mural nodule. The mural nodule consists of a conglomerate of vessels with regular lumina. A vertebral angiogram may demonstrate a hypertrophied vessel leading to the tumor with no obvious draining veins, which distinguishes it from an angioma. The tangle of vessels usually shows up as a dense, small, round, opacified nodule that may be surrounded by an avascular area resembling a cyst (Fig. 9–106). The appearance of these tumors is usually characteristic.[143]

Papillomas. These may show fine regular vessels not unlike those of a meningioma. The surface may be circumscribed but umbilicated. The lobulated surface of the papilloma may be seen during pneumoencephalography with air lying within the ventricle. The vessel supplying the tumor may be hypertrophied, as seen in Figure 9–107. Matson and Crofton state that the pneumographic demonstration of an intraventricular mass, in the presence of communicating hydrocephalus, is pathognomonic of this tumor.[125]

Acoustic neuromas. Displacement of vessels is more common than the demonstration of tumor vessels (Fig. 9–98). Olsson reviewed his vertebral angiographic findings in 14 acoustic nerve tumors.[142] In all cases the superior cerebellar artery ran

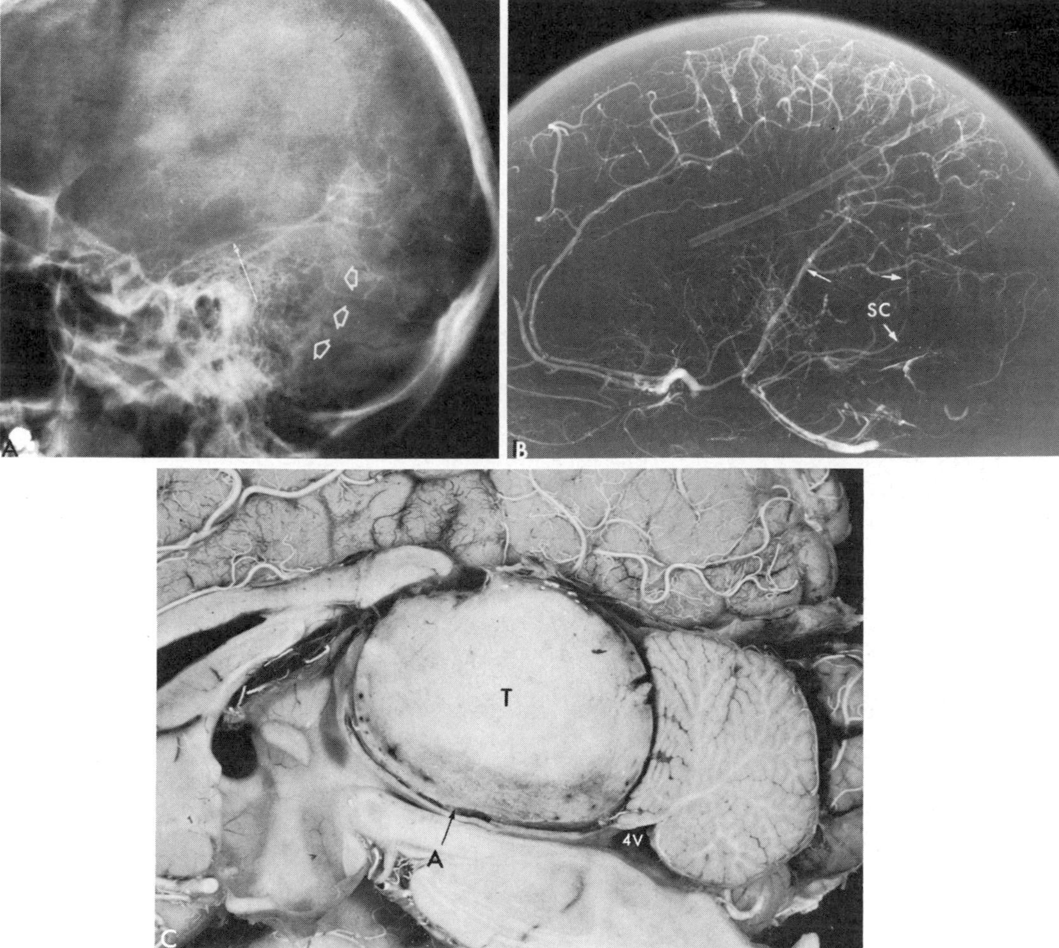

Figure 9–104 *A*. Tentorial meningioma with characteristic displacement of vessels. This shows the posterior cerebral artery displaced superiorly (*arrow*), while the superior cerebellar artery is displaced down and back (*arrowheads*). *B*. Postmortem angiogram showing in more detail the characteristic displacement of the posterior cerebral artery and the superior cerebellar artery (SC). *C*. The brain sliced in the sagittal plane through the midline shows the tumor (T), the aqueduct (A), and the fourth ventricle (4V).

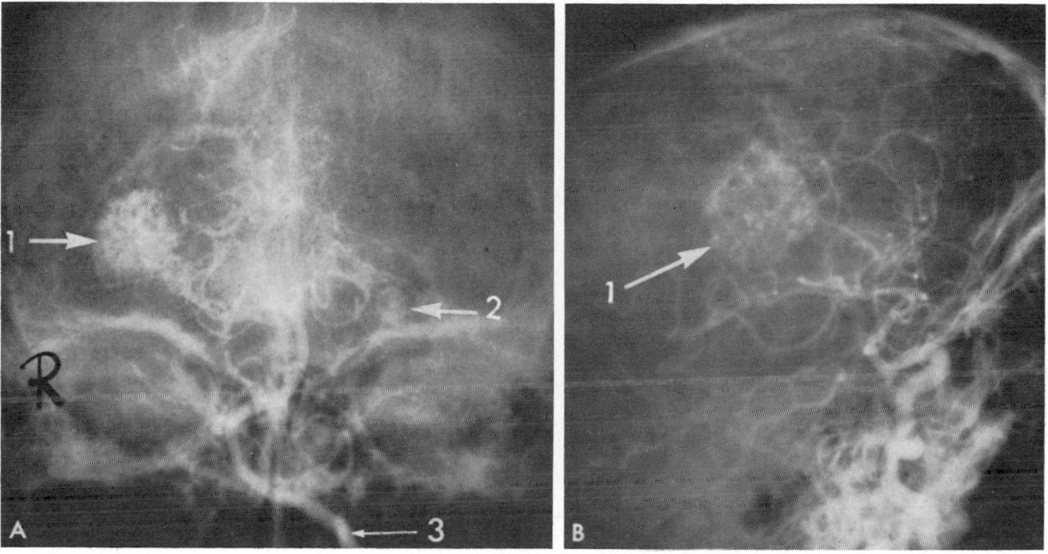

Figure 9–105 *A*. Vertebral angiogram showing two discrete areas of tumor vessels (1, 2). The vertebral artery (3) is filled with contrast medium. *B*. Carotid angiogram in the same patient showing a third discrete area of tumor opacification, hypernephroma of kidney with metastatic deposits outlined.

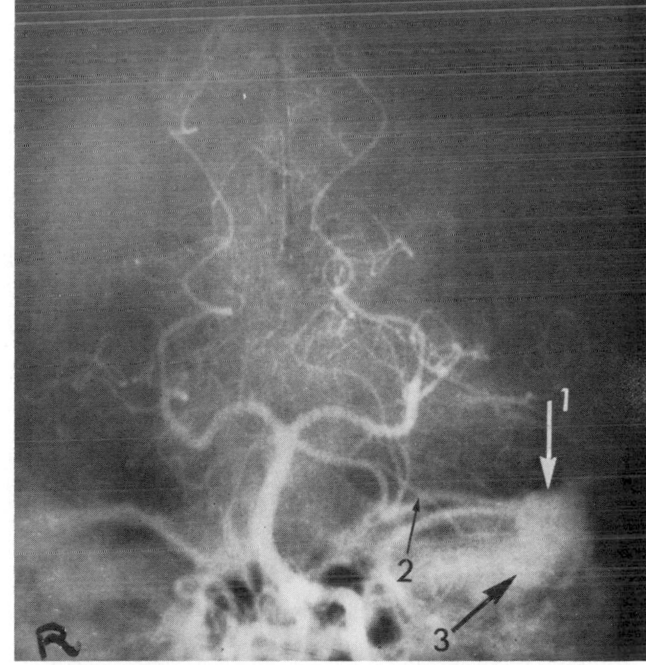

Figure 9–106 Vertebral angiogram demonstrating a hemangioblastoma. Note blood supply from branches of superior cerebellar artery (1, 2) and the posterior inferior cerebellar artery. 3, the opacified tumor. (Courtesy of Dr. Bernard Wolf.)

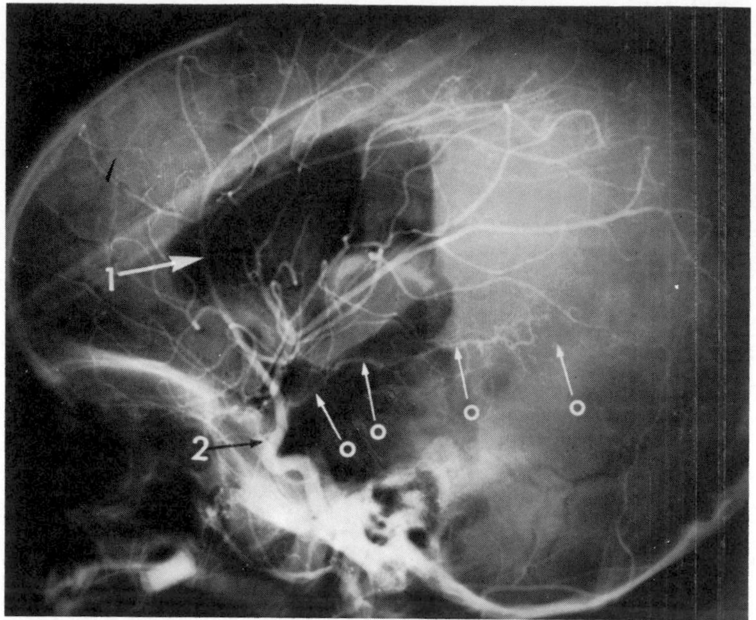

Figure 9–107 Carotid angiogram in a child with a papilloma of the choroid plexus of the lateral ventricle. Note the hypertrophy of the anterior choroidal artery (O, O, O, O), which supplies the plexus. The stretched wide-swept anterior cerebral artery (1) is an expression of the ventricular dilatation. 2, internal carotid artery.

an abnormal course. Nine cases showed abnormal tumor vessels related to the mass. Displacement or nonfilling of the petrosal vein is a significant finding in angle tumors.[208]

TUMORS IN THE REGION OF THE PINEAL GLAND. If these tumors are large enough, they will displace the great vein of Galen downward and the posterior choroidal arteries upward and backward.[116] Tumors in this region include pinealoma or teratoma, thalamic glioma, aneurysm of the great vein of Galen, meningioma of the free margins of the tentorium, and tumors of the quadrigeminal plate and splenium of the corpus callosum.

ORBITAL TUMORS. Krayenbühl has emphasized the value of carotid angiography in orbital lesions.[99] Displacements of the ophthalmic artery may be recognized, and vascular intraorbital tumors may fill from the ophthalmic artery. The ophthalmic artery may hypertrophy to supply tumors involving the roof and confines of the orbit.[36] Orbital phlebography and orbitography may be very helpful here, and may enhance the diagnostic potential considerably.

CEREBRAL ABSCESS. This lesion has no characteristic appearances. Vessels may be displaced, revealing an avascular mass.

PARASITES. Hydatid cysts will show displacement and marked stretching displacement and marked stretching of vessels around completely avascular areas.

Raised Intracranial Pressure

In marked elevation of intracranial pressure the circulation of contrast medium through the head is slowed. In a series of 17 cases reported by Pribram, in which narrowing of the carotid artery was seen in the neck and very little contrast medium entered the cerebral circulation, no organic disease was seen in the cervical vessels (Fig. 9–104*A* and *B*).[152] All were patients who had experienced an acute rise in intracranial pressure. The similarity of the angiographic appearances to those of carotid occlusion is stressed. The narrowing of the column of contrast medium in the neck is probably accounted for by layering in a slow circulation (Fig. 9–67), and not due to a narrowed lumen of the vessel.[188]

Herniation

Tentorial "Up" Herniation

These may occur with any posterior fossa expanding lesion. The superior cerebellar arteries may be displaced up through the tentorial opening. The posterior cerebral arteries, normally located above the tentorium, may be displaced further upward in severe herniations (Fig. 9–96).

Tonsillar Herniation

These may occur with supratentorial or infratentorial lesions that have resulted in increased intracranial pressure.

The caudal loop of the posterior inferior cerebellar artery passes under the cerebellar tonsil and may be displaced through the foramen magnum with tonsillar herniations (Fig. 9–97). This is not a very reliable sign, since a loop of the posterior inferior cerebellar artery is not infrequently seen below the foramen magnum unassociated with tonsillar herniations.

Tentorial "Down" Herniation

Tentorial herniations may be either up or down. Herniations of the temporal lobe down through the tentorial opening may occur with cerebral hemisphere swelling or supratentorial space-occupying lesions. In down herniations, the posterior communicating artery and the posterior cerebral artery may be displaced through the tentorial opening. The vessel, in order to negotiate the opening in the tentorium, must also be displaced medially. The artery may be displaced down in a bold curve or may show a stop-wedge deformity (Fig. 9–108). Filling of the posterior cerebral artery occurs in only one third of carotid angiograms, but the basal vein of Rosenthal is usually opacified. Since this vein follows the same course as the posterior cerebral artery, similar displacement of this vessel will occur. Since the veins are more easily compressed than the artery, opacification may be absent or difficult to recognize.

Trauma

The death toll in the United States in 1962 from motor accidents was 40,800. In 1964 in the United States, 10,000,000 disabling injuries occurred, killing almost 1,000,000 people. During 1967, an estimated 3,096,000 persons sustained injuries in moving motor vehicle accidents for which they required medical attention. With high-speed travel a routine of daily living, the major source of injuries in adults has moved to the highway and away from military accidents, industrial accidents, and sporting accidents. In 70 per cent of fatal highway accidents, brain damage was the cause of death.

Blunt trauma to the neck may result in thrombosis of the carotid arteries. This is due to subintimal tears of the intima with thrombus formation.[105,135] Penetrating injuries to the neck are usually the result of stab wounds and missile injuries. False aneurysms of the carotid artery may occur, but these are usually simple to manage.[184] When a major vessel such as the vertebral artery or the carotid artery is torn with the

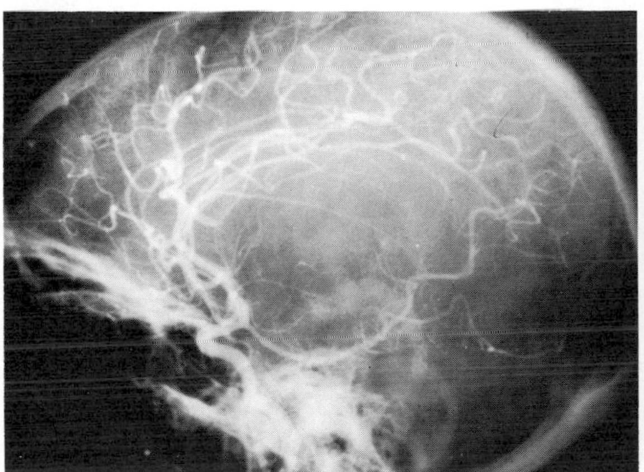

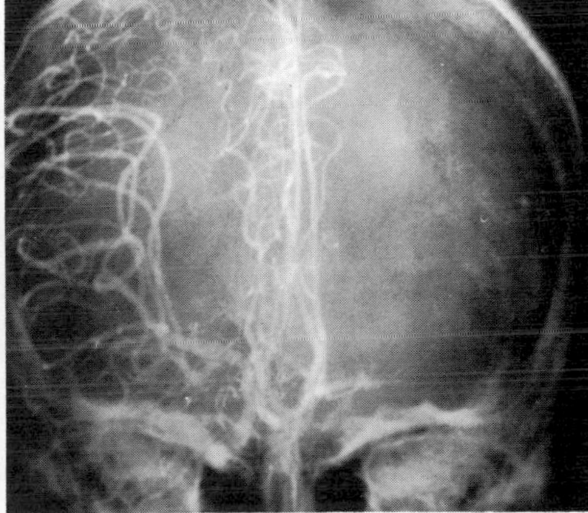

Figure 9–108 Temporal lobe tumor. Note the marked elevation of the middle cerebral artery complex, with stretching of these vessels and displacement toward the midline. There is marked transtentorial herniation of the temporal lobe revealed by the very marked displacement downward and to the midline of the posterior cerebral artery.

adjacent accompanying veins, an arteriovenous fistula may result. These are major surgical problems and may be very difficult to treat. Unless all the contributing arteries and draining veins are outlined, the operative management becomes complicated, often necessitating repeated operative attacks.[236]

Head injuries, open or closed, may result in raised intracranial pressure and may cause a situation in which blood flow in the cervical internal carotid artery is very slow. This may be due to thrombus formation in the internal carotid artery. Other mechanisms, however, are usually present to account for this pseudothrombosis. The raised intracranial pressure offers resistance to the passage of blood (and blood–contrast medium mixture) through the intracranial circulation. The passage of the column of contrast medium progresses to the base of the skull and then tapers to a very thin stream; little, if any, passes intracranially. The passage through the external carotid artery will, however, appear normal. In the experience of the author, such slow circulation has invariably been a sign of impending death. This phenomenon must be present bilaterally to invoke the agonal flow phenomena. Before making this diagnosis, therefore, it is incumbent to perform bilateral carotid angiography. That organic changes are not present in the neck vessels in these patients has been proved by the author in postmortem studies on patients at autopsy. These studies included postmortem angiography using barium gelatin injections and dissection of these vessels (Fig. 9–109).[141] However, when the intracranial vessels are not demonstrated sufficiently well in such patients to exclude an extracerebral hematoma (a remediable condition), a bilateral exploration is indicated. Traumatic aneurysms of the superficial

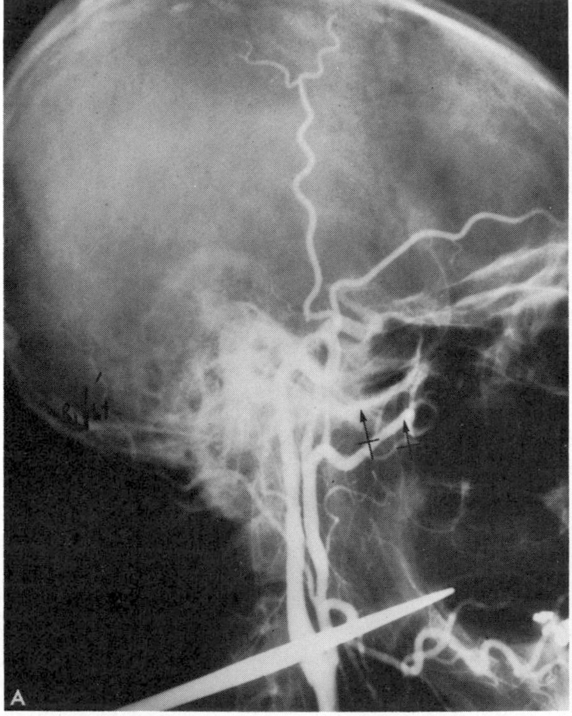

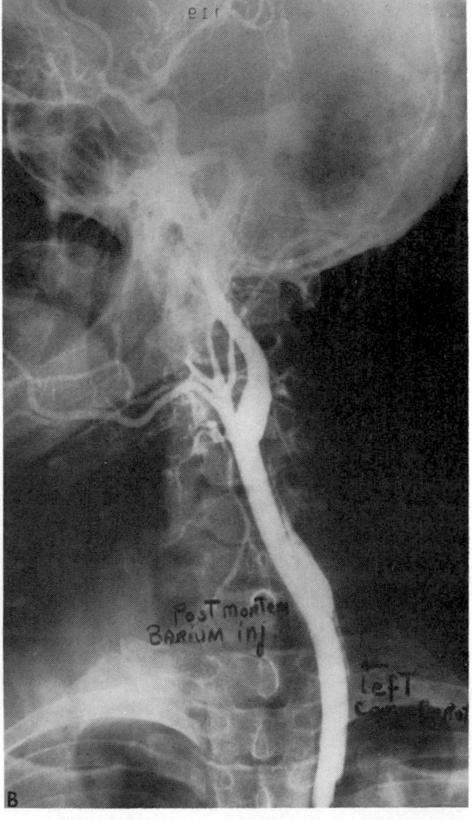

Figure 9–109 *A*. Common carotid angiogram in patient who has sustained severe head trauma. Agonal flow due to intracranial hypertension shows filling of external carotid artery and its peripheral branches (*arrows*), whereas the internal carotid artery is not opacified beyond the point of its passage beyond the anterior clinoid process. This phenomenon was present bilaterally. *B*. Postmortem angiogram reveals no organic obstruction in the vessels of the neck or head.

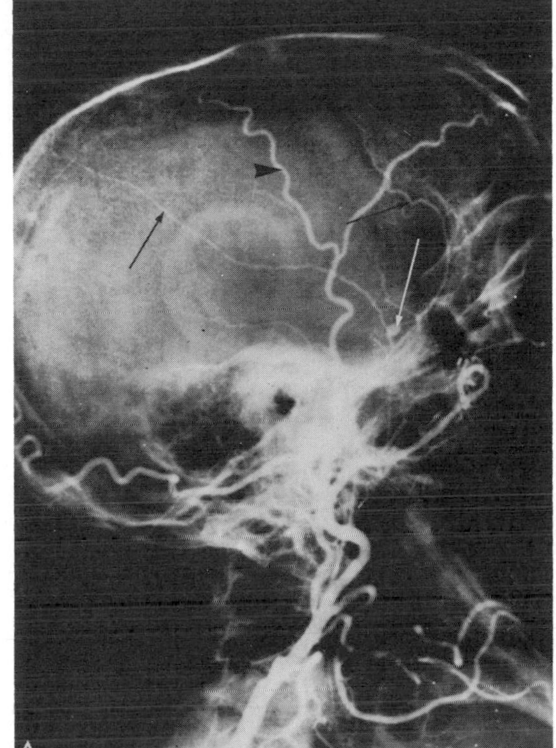

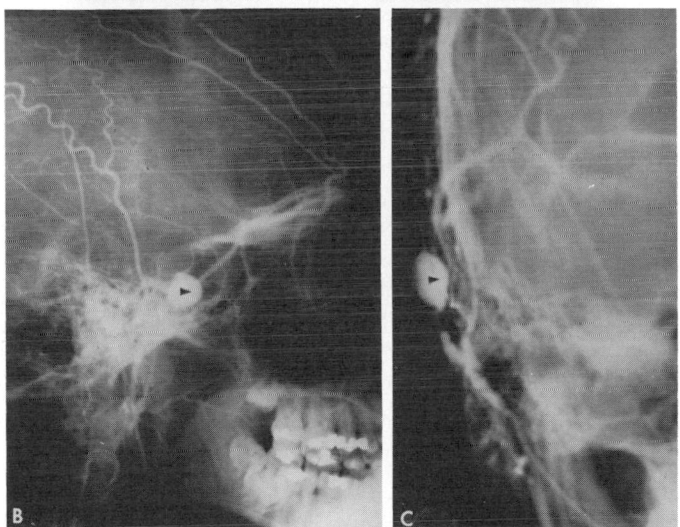

Figure 9–110 *A*. Right common carotid angiogram, lateral view. This patient has an occlusion of the internal carotid artery at its origin. The white arrow points to an aneurysm of the middle meningeal artery (*black arrows*), thought to be of congenital origin. The black arrowhead points to a branch of the superficial temporal artery. *B*. Right external carotid angiogram, lateral view. The small black arrowhead overlies a pseudoaneurysm of the superficial temporal artery. Note that this pseudoaneurysm is superimposed on the middle meningeal artery, which is intact. *C*. Right external carotid angiogram, anteroposterior view. The pseudoaneurysm is indicated by the small black arrowhead. This projection clearly shows the pseudoaneurysm arising from the superficial temporal artery and not from the middle meningeal artery.

temporal artery were more common in the days of "blood letting" and fencing.[46,78] Selective angiography of the external carotid artery will demonstrate the lesion (Fig. 9–110). This should not be confused with an aneurysm of the middle meningeal artery.[68] Nontraumatic aneurysms of the middle meningeal artery usually arise at points where the vessel branches.

The value of angiography in the management of head trauma is well established. Post-traumatic lesions that may be demonstrated by this technique are:

1. Subdural hematomas.
2. Epidural hematomas (middle meningeal) with significant accumulation of hematoma, with fistula formation between artery and accompanying dural venous or

diploic channels, or with formation of false aneurysm.

3. Intracerebral mass lesions, including cerebral contusion and edema and intracerebral hematoma.

4. Caroticocavernous fistula.

5. Aneurysm of carotid artery in its extracranial course and carotid-jugular fistula.

Additional information may be obtained about alterations in blood flow due to thrombosis of carotid or vertebral artery, pseudothrombosis (poor arterial filling due to raised intracranial or low systemic pressure or both), temporary occlusion of vessels (complete and incomplete, by spasm, herniation, and hematoma), and superior sagittal sinus thrombosis. Also, the presence of a lesion unrelated to the trauma may be disclosed.

Most authorities have accepted the value of angiography and have relegated the multiple blind burr hole exploration to the past. Even the most astute clinicians and skillful surgeons agree that, on occasion, even well-placed burr holes may miss a collection of blood that will be recognized on angiograms. Angiography may also reveal unsuspected lesions.

In cases of post-traumatic intracranial mass lesions, angiograms may occasionally be unrevealing to those unfamiliar with the radiographic principles involved. An understanding of these principles and recognition of some of the misconceptions of angiographic interpretation enhance the diagnostic value of the examination.

Trauma to the vessels outside the head has already been dealt with and we now direct our attention to lesions within the head.

Subdural Hematoma

The acute subdural hematoma is usually caused by tearing of the cortical veins as they enter the superior sagittal sinus. A fracture of the skull is usually not present. The fluid collection of blood spreads diffusely over the surface of the brain, displacing it in a more or less uniform fashion away from the inner table of the skull. In a short time, about a week, a membrane begins to form. Theories of the pathogenesis of the chronic subdural hematoma have been proposed, but these are not universally accepted. Putnam and Cushing believed that recurrent fresh hemorrhages into the hematoma account for its progressive enlargement.[153] Gardner suggested that osmotic attraction of cerebrospinal fluid through the semipermeable membrane is responsible for its growth.[61] Chronic subdural hematomas may present without a history of trauma, and the expanding mass may produce signs and symptoms indistinguishable from those produced by any expanding tumor in the head. The pathological distinction between an acute and chronic subdural hematoma is the presence of a membrane. As the diffuse subdural accumulation of blood becomes limited by this membrane and begins to expand in size, its shape changes from a thin blood clot with a concave medial surface to a lentiform shape (Fig. 9–111). The basis for Norman's angiographic differentiation between acute and chronic subdural hematoma depends on the shape of the bare area recognized angiographically.[138] A criticism of Norman's system of differentiation is offered later. Care must be exercised in the interpretation of these findings. The bare area may be missed completely if the central beam of the x-ray does not strike part of the fluid collection tangentially. Parietal lesions may be best examined with the head in a true anteroposterior position and the central x-ray beam displaced to the appropriate side. Lesions in the frontal region are best seen with the head turned toward the side of the lesion, and posterior lesions with the head turned away from the side suspected (Figs. 9–1 to 9–8 and 9–112).

The intermediate phase of the angiographic series shows opacification of the smaller vessels of the brain and is perhaps the most useful in recognizing these bare areas. Caution in the interpretation of the films is mandatory since three shadows may be projected onto the x-ray film: the anterior margin of the trough, the bottom of the trough, and the distal margin. Occasionally a chronic subdural hematoma may be mistaken for an acute one if a tangential view is not obtained. The venous phase, however, may be more revealing and show the characteristic biconvex shape (Fig. 9–113).[43,234] Frontal hematomas in the anteroposterior projection may only demonstrate a lateral displacement of the anterior cerebral artery without evidence of the classic bare area. On the lateral film, however, one sees a displacement posteriorly of the segment of the anterior cerebral artery distal to

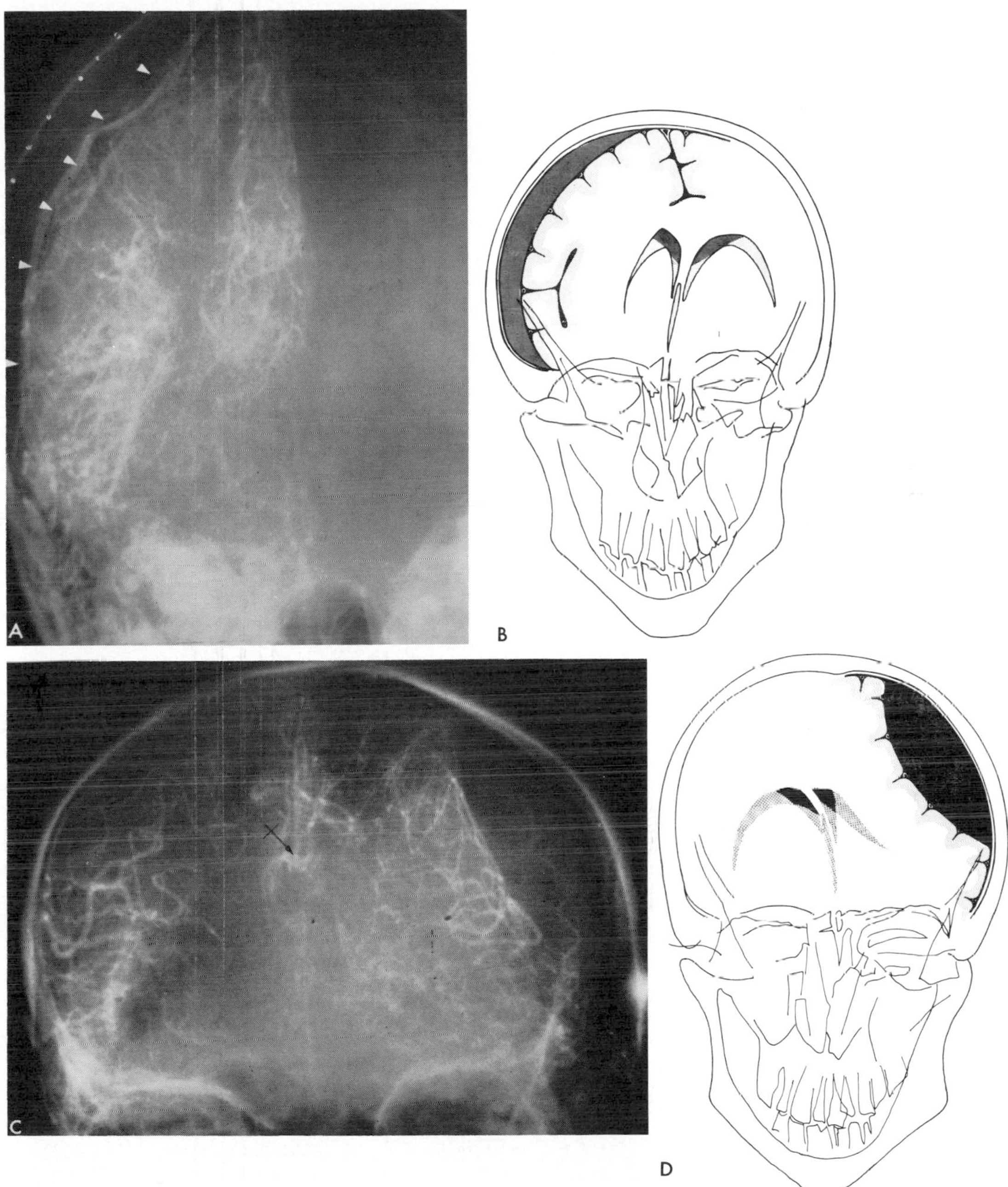

Figure 9–111 *A.* Acute subdural hematoma. Note that in the intermediate phase of the carotid angiogram a cortical vein outlines the surface of the brain and that vessels are prevented from reaching the inner table of the skull by the collection of blood. The "bare" area is crescentic in shape. *B.* Schematic representation of an acute subdural hematoma. *C.* Chronic subdural hematoma. The "bare" area is lentiform. Note crowding of branches of the middle cerebral artery and the shift across the midline of the anterior cerebral artery with "falcine" herniation (*arrow*). *D.* Schematic representation of a chronic subdural hematoma. Note the lentiform bare area.

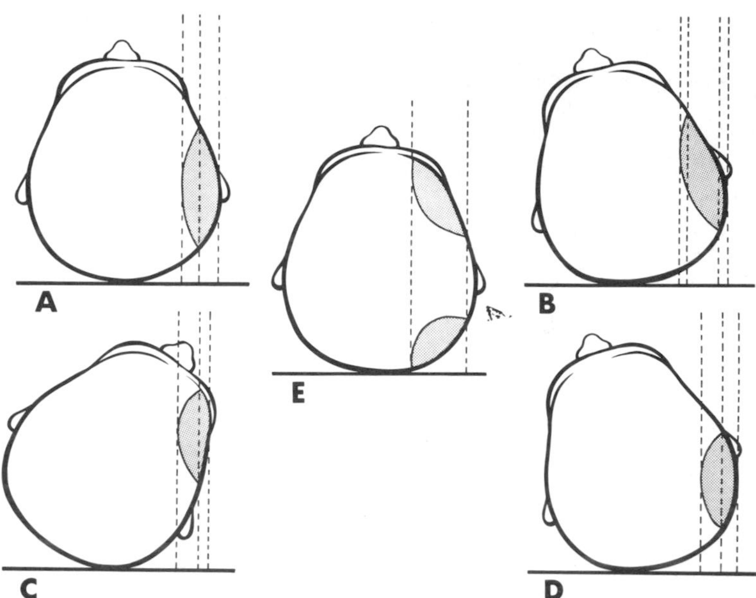

Figure 9–112 The shaded area represents the subdural collection of fluid or blood clot. In the anteroposterior projection *A*, a temporoparietal lesion will be recognized since the anterior and posterior margins of the depressed brain are projected within the margin of the vault of the skull. *B*. Note that the bare area in the same position will appear shallower since the head is inappropriately rotated and the beam is no longer projected tangentially to the bare area. *E*. One hematoma situated anteriorly and one situated posteriorly. Note that both of these may be missed in the anteroposterior projection. *C*. The optimal position of the head for an anteriorly located lesion. *D*. The optimal position of the head for a posteriorly located lesion.

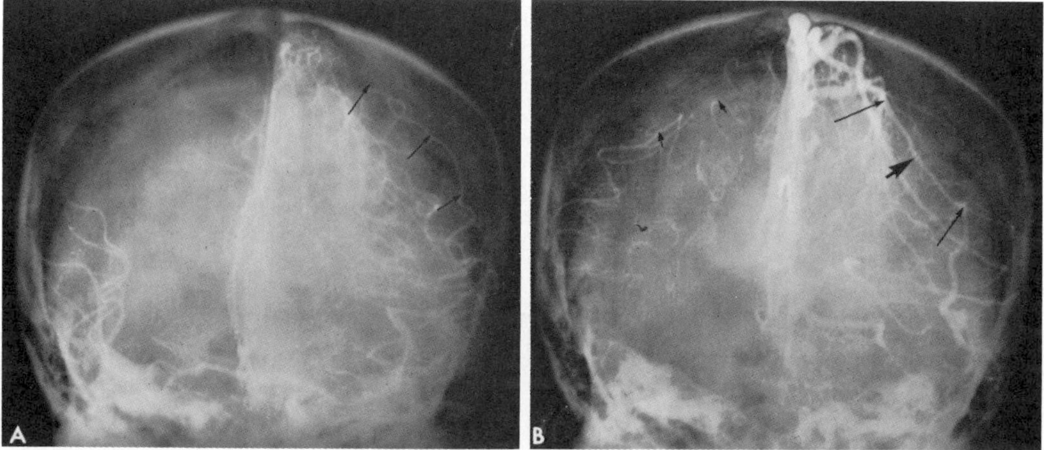

Figure 9–113 *A*. The arterial phase of a subdural hematoma. Since the most peripheral branches of the middle cerebral artery, representing the anterior margin of the trough, have an outward convex shape, the erroneous diagnosis of an acute subdural hematoma may be made. *B*. The venous phase shows cortical veins outlining the margin of a chronic subdural hematoma with a characteristic shape (*large arrows*). Note the disproportionate shift of the anterior cerebral artery and the presence of a chronic subdural hematoma on the opposite side (*small arrows*).

the anterior communicating artery, and one may occasionally be led to suspect a subdural hematoma because of the demonstration of a bare area between well-developed frontopolar branches and the inner table of the skull.

Since oblique films were discussed in the evaluation of the presence and shape of a subdural hematoma, it must be said that the "acute" shape of Norman's scheme may represent a chronic subdural hematoma. The author has no quarrel with the specificity of the "chronic" shape for chronic subdural hematoma, except that this may also represent an epidural hematoma (Fig. 9–114). The following observations support this contention: (1) not infrequently the "acute" shape is present in a patient with a history of trauma over four weeks previously, and with well-formed membranes as seen at operation; (2) postmortem observations have revealed the presence of membranes unassociated with a significant collection of fluid; and (3) Gannon has angiographically documented the resolution of a chronic subdural hematoma with a change in the shape from "chronic" to "acute."[60]

Hematomas at sites other than over the frontal, temporal, or parietal regions may be recognized angiographically. An interhemispheric hematoma may separate the two anterior cerebral arteries or the pericallosal and callosomarginal branches of the same anterior cerebral artery, displacing the pericallosal artery to the contralateral side and the callosomarginal artery to the ipsilateral side. This will produce the angiographic appearance of a bare area lying adjacent to the falx (Figs. 9–85 and 9–115). Jacobsen first described this angiographic sign.[90] Campbell and Campbell have angiograms that, taken after evacuation of an interhemispheric hematoma, show return of the anterior cerebral artery to its normal position and disappearance of the bare area.[21]

Infratemporal subdural hematomas elevate the branches of the middle cerebral artery and the basal vein of Rosenthal but are difficult to distinguish from intratemporal hematomas. When vessels appear stretched rather than displaced, an intracerebral situation is favored. There may be a minimal shift of the anterior cerebral artery in these lesions.

Vertebral angiography has been less helpful in the recognition of the rare posterior fossa subdural and epidural hematoma. In a recent publication, however, the suspected presence of a posterior fossa epidural hemorrhage was confirmed by vertebral angiography.[148] The posterior meningeal artery was displaced away from the table of the skull and was torn in several places, leaking contrast medium. The

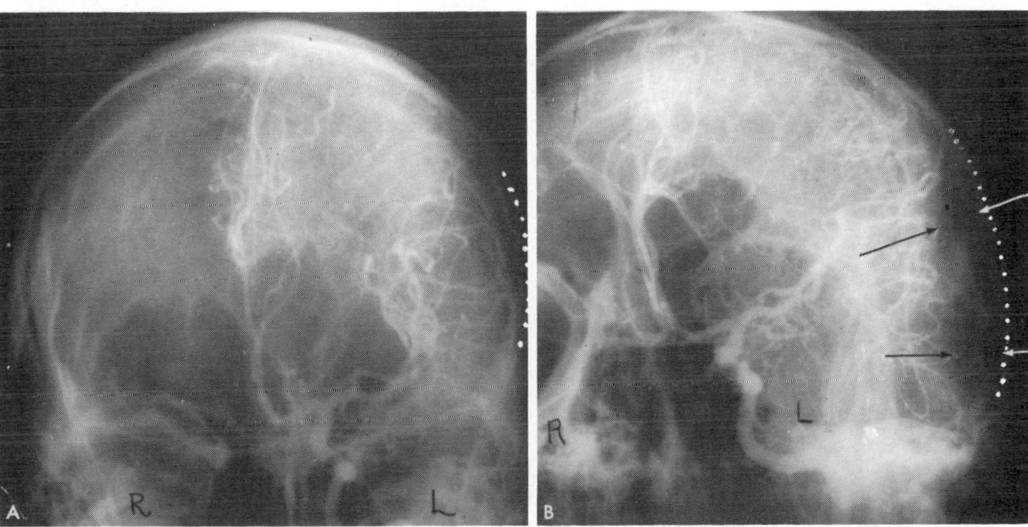

Figure 9–114 *A*. Left carotid angiography. Anteroposterior Towne view. There is a slight shift of the midline. No avascular space is demonstrated laterally. *B*. Left carotid angiography with the patient's head turned toward the opposite side. The posteriorly situated epidural hematoma is now demonstrated as an avascular space (*between white and black arrows*).

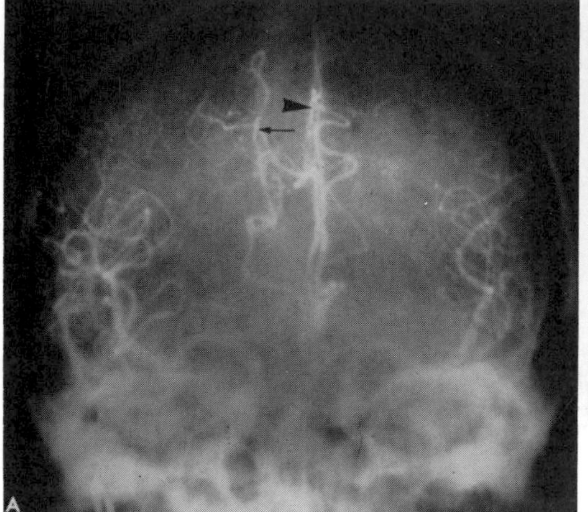

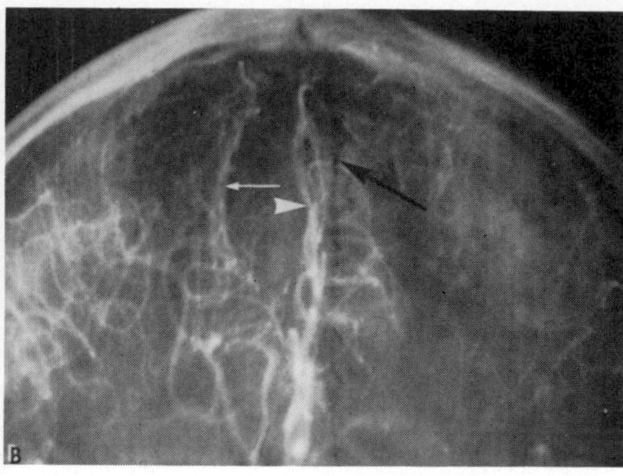

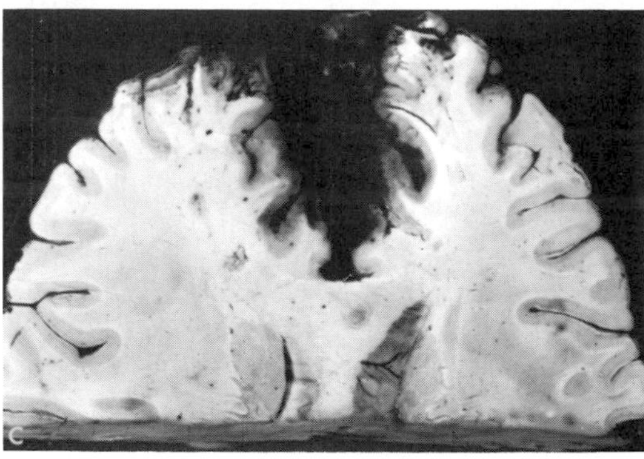

Figure 9–115 *A*. Right carotid angiography with compression of the left carotid artery, anteroposterior Towne view. Note the separation of the pericallosal artery (*black arrowhead*) and the callosal-marginal artery (*small black arrow*) by an interhemispheric subdural hematoma. *B*. Right carotid angiography with compression of the left carotid artery. The black arrow points to a linear fracture. This is another patient with an interhemispheric subdural hematoma separating the pericallosal artery on the right (*white arrowhead*) from the callosal-marginal artery (*small white arrow*). *C*. Note the large interhemispheric subdural hematoma. (Specimen by courtesy of Dr. LeMay.)

branches of the posterior inferior cerebellar artery were displaced away from the inner table of the skull. An epidural hematoma in the posterior fossa was successfully removed.

One usually examines the other side angiographically in head trauma, particularly when there is a disproportionate shift of the anterior cerebral artery across the midline relative to the depth of the bare area representing the extracerebral hematoma. Contralateral compression is useful to compare the two sides simultaneously, but should not be used as an excuse to neglect examining the opposite side in two projections.

Factors to be considered with a disproportionate shift of the anterior cerebral artery include: (1) a subdural or epidural collection of fluid on the opposite side (Fig. 9–116); (2) contusion, with swelling of the opposite cerebral hemisphere; (3) a low-placed middle fossa hematoma; (4) atrophy of the underlying brain allowing for accumulation of fluid without shift of the midline; and (5) resolution of the subdural collection.

Epidural Hematoma

These usually result from a tear of the meningeal arteries or veins, but may also originate from the dural sinuses and diploic channels. Although the initial tear may result in slow venous bleeding (the so-called chronic epidural hematoma), small arteries may be torn as the dura is stripped from the skull, and the bleeding becomes both venous and arterial.

Although early investigators doubted the feasibility of distinguishing angiographically between an epidural hematoma and a subdural hematoma, recognizable angiographic criteria exist that make such a distinction possible. They are:

1. Displacement inward of a meningeal artery.
2. Displacement of the sagittal sinus, torcular, or transverse sinus.

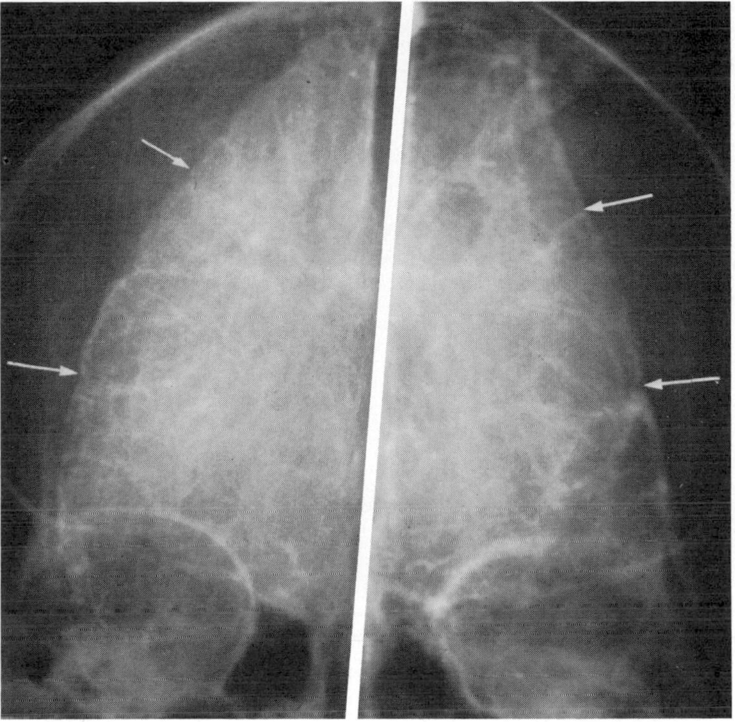

Figure 9–116 Bilateral chronic subdural hematomas. Note that the midline is relatively undisplaced, being balanced between the collections of fluid on either side.

3. Lentiform bare area with a history compatible with acute hematoma.
4. Irregular margin of the surface of the epidural hematoma.
5. Disproportionate shift of the anterior cerebral artery.
6. Leaking of contrast material from the torn vessel.
7. Fracture line crossing a vascular groove that accommodates a meningeal vessel.

Displacement of the meningeal arteries from the inner table of the skull is pathognomonic of an epidural hematoma, and the diagnosis depends upon the certainty with which the meningeal branches can be identified. A selective internal and external carotid angiogram is desirable and will facilitate this recognition, while a common carotid injection, although of less value, may also allow this distinction to be made (Fig. 9–117). Occlusion of the middle cerebral artery may produce an avascular area, and if common carotid angiography has been performed, the normal meningeal arteries superimposed over the bare area may produce a picture that could be mistaken for an epidural hematoma (Fig. 9–118).

Epidural hematomas are rare in infants and children because of the marked adherence of the dura to the inner table of the skull.[22] In the posterior fossa the dura may normally strip very easily from the inner table of the skull. The dura is less adherent in adults, but limits the spread of an accumulation of blood so that the collection assumes a lentiform shape. The angiographically bare area resembles the "chronic" subdural shape, and in the presence of a recent history is suggestive of an epidural hematoma, especially if a skull fracture transversing a meningeal channel is demonstrated (Fig. 9–114).

Irregularity of the medial surface of the lentiform bare area has been reported with epidural hematomas. This is presumably due to strands of dural tissue that limit its complete separation from the surface of the vault.

Since epidural hematomas have a limited surface area, being confined by the adherence of the dura to the skull, a small-volume hematoma that is lentiform in shape may be much thicker than an acute subdural hematoma of a much larger volume. Subdural hematomas tend to spread and oc-

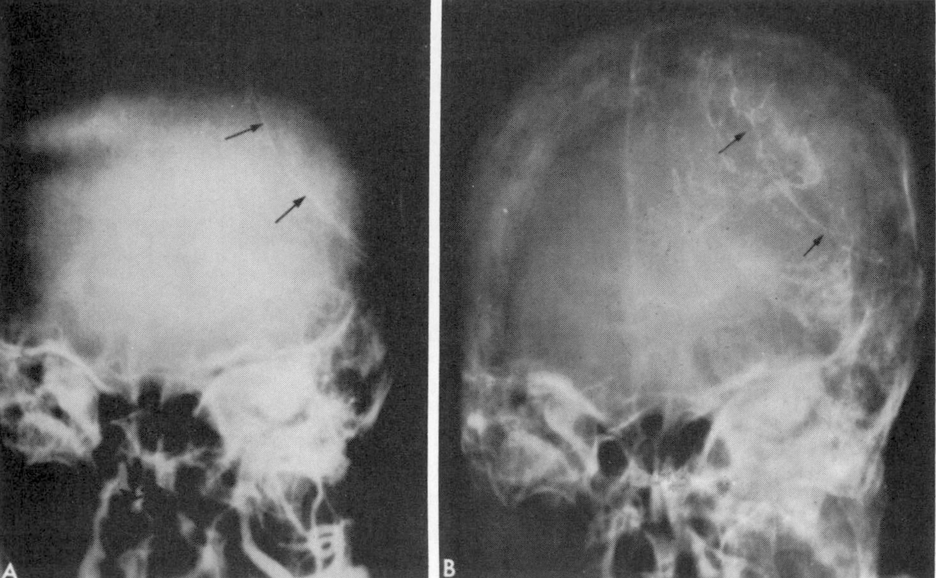

Figure 9–117 *A*. An epidural hematoma. Note filling of branches of the external carotid artery with inward displacement of the middle meningeal artery (*arrows*). *B*. This shows disproportionate shift of the anterior cerebral artery with pronounced inward displacement of the middle meningeal artery (*arrows*).

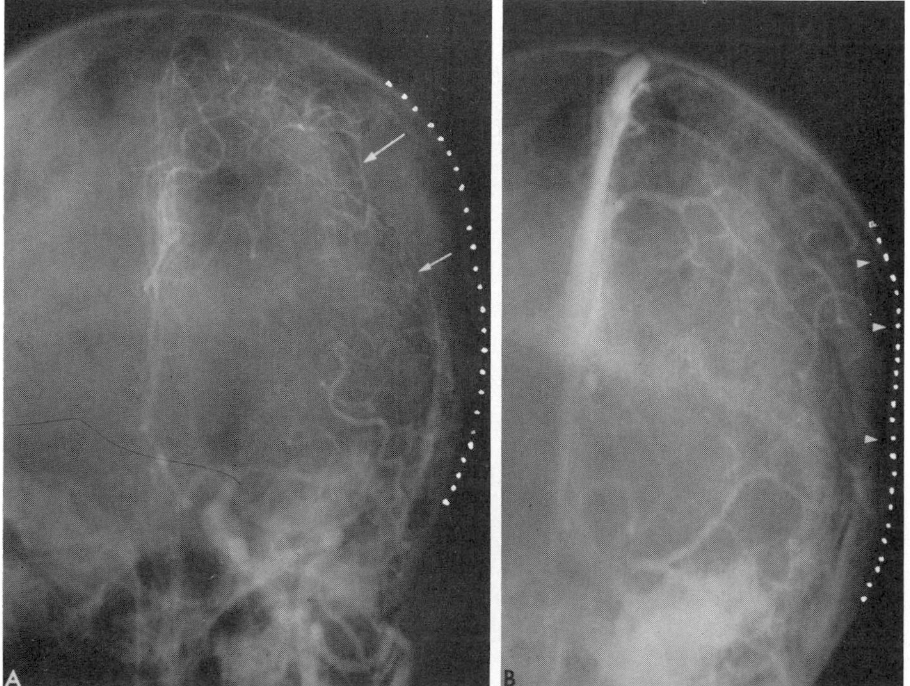

Figure 9–118 *A*. Left carotid angiogram, anteroposterior Towne view. There is an avascular space between the vascularized brain (*upper white arrow*) and the inner table of the skull (*white dots*). The middle meningeal artery (*lower white arrow*) is fortuitously superimposed on the inner border of this avascular space. Thus superficially there appears to be an epidural hematoma present, but in fact, the diagnosis here is occlusion of a branch of the middle cerebral artery. No extracerebral hematoma is present. *B*. Venous phase of angiographic series. The proximity of cortical veins (*white arrowheads*) to the inner table of the skull (*white dots*) rules out diagnosis of an extracerebral hematoma.

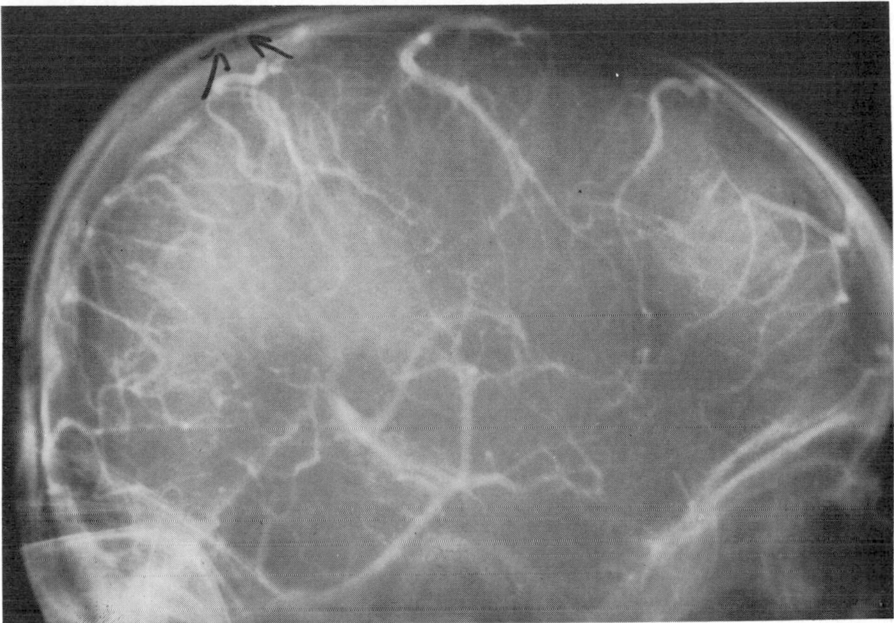

Figure 9–119 The two black arrows indicate a fracture extending across the midline to either side. Note that the superior sagittal sinus is displaced away from the inner table of the skull by an acute epidural hemorrhage.

cupy a larger surface area. There is, therefore, less shift of the midline structures in epidural hematomas than in subdural hematomas of comparable thickness. This accounts for the disproportionate shift of the middle structures in epidural hematomas (Fig. 9–114).

Separation of the superior sagittal sinus from the inner table of the skull is another pathognomonic angiographic sign of epidural hematoma and was first demonstrated by Wickbom (Fig. 9–119).[223] Bonnal described displacement of the torcular Herophili by a posterior fossa epidural hematoma, and Petit-Dutaillis and associates published a radiograph illustrating displacement of the torcular Herophili and sagittal sinus by a posterior fossa epidural hematoma (Fig. 9–120).[14,149] Other reports of separation of the sagittal sinus from the

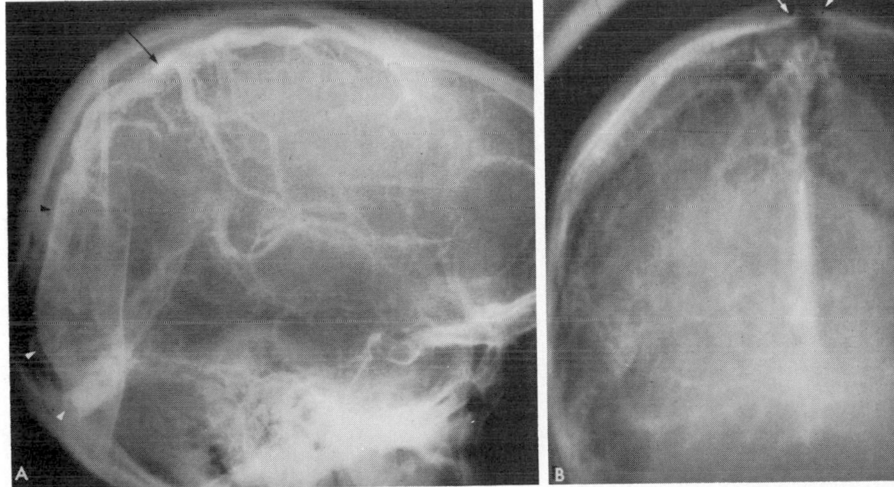

Figure 9–120 An epidural hematoma extending into the posterior fossa. Note the fracture extending into the sagittal suture (*white arrows*). Also note the separation of the superior sagittal sinus from the inner table of the skull. The transverse sinuses and the torcular Herophili have also been displaced from the inner margin of the skull (*black and white arrowheads*). Note separation of the superior sagittal sinus in the anteroposterior projection. This is an unequivocal sign of an epidural hematoma.

skull have appeared by Pecker and co-workers, Tiwisina and Stecker, McKissock and co-workers, and Alexander.[2,126,146,215] Caution must be exercised in the interpretation of this sign, since slight rotation of the skull in the lateral projection may cause misinterpretation of displacement of the sagittal sinus, or a superior sagittal sinus that is situated a little to the side may be mistakenly interpreted as a displaced sinus. Separation of the superior sagittal sinus from the skull in the anteroposterior projection is unequivocal (Fig. 9–120*B*).

Lohr recommended common carotid angiography to outline the middle meningeal artery.[118] Although he did not demonstrate leaking of contrast material from a torn meningeal vessel, he did demonstrate leaking from a branch of the middle cerebral artery. Since the majority of rapidly evolving epidural collections are recognized clinically and subjected to operation without angiography, and those of a more benign nature have angiograms made quite a few hours after the initial trauma, angiographic recognition of the bleeding site is unusual. Huber states that leaking contrast medium is not usually recognized when angiography is performed more than six hours after the initial trauma.[83] This, however, has not been true in the author's experience.

The extradural bleeding may originate from torn meningeal arteries, veins, dural sinuses, or diploic channels. The bleeding site usually identified at operation is the middle meningeal artery or one of its branches.

The rapidity with which the leaking contrast material appears and disappears during angiography usually precludes its entering only the epidural space, since a tremendous hematoma beyond all reasonable proportions would build up. Other workers, the author among them, have indicated that the leaking contrast material and blood is not a simple affair. As reports of this entity have accumulated in the literature, an analysis of the cases has led to the formulation and promulgation of rather rigid clinical diagnostic criteria.

Today it is generally accepted that the clinical spectrum seen with epidural hematomas is wide. Thus, although classic descriptions of the symptoms include the "lucid interval," such a history is obtained less than 50 per cent of the time—and although the classic description includes progression to a fatal outcome within hours, exceptions are fairly common.[88,127,167]

The explanation for this variability is complex. Certain anatomical factors may be responsible in part. One such is the strength of attachment of the dura to the skull. The dura is more adherent in children, especially along suture lines, and in females and in elderly people. Bradley, commenting on this fact in 1952, observed that certain subjects seem to be "immune" to epidural hemorrhage.[16] Another anatomical factor is the strength of the walls of the middle meningeal vessels. Hassler described congenital defects in the wall of the middle meningeal artery.[73] In addition to these anatomical factors, certain pathological features related to the injury influence the clinical picture. Two key ones are the site of the epidural hemorrhage (temporal location has the most rapidly progressive course) and the severity of injury to the underlying brain.

The use of angiography in epidural hemorrhage has revealed certain other factors that influence the clinical course. Observations of contrast material that has extravasated from a torn meningeal artery led to the following classification:

1. The extravasated contrast material may pass into the epidural space to form an epidural hematoma that progressively enlarges (Figs. 9–121*A* and 9–122).
2. The extravasated medium may pass out of the epidural space through the adjacent fracture line into the subgaleal area (Figs. 9–121*A* and 9–122).
3. The extravasated contrast material may be walled off by the formation of a pseudoaneurysm (Figs. 9–121*C* and 9–123).
4. The extravasated contrast material may pass into adjacent venous channels, thereby indicating the presence of an arteriovenous fistula. These venous channels may be within the diploë of the skull (Figs. 9–121*D* and 9–124) or they may be the veins that accompany the meningeal artery (Figs. 9–121*B* and 9–125).

Many reports of the extravasation of contrast material from the middle meningeal artery have been published.[83,111,117,215,219] Arteriovenous fistulae involving the middle meningeal vessels as a result of trauma or "spontaneous" fistulae shown angiographically have been reported.[12,53,87,109,121,170,225,238]

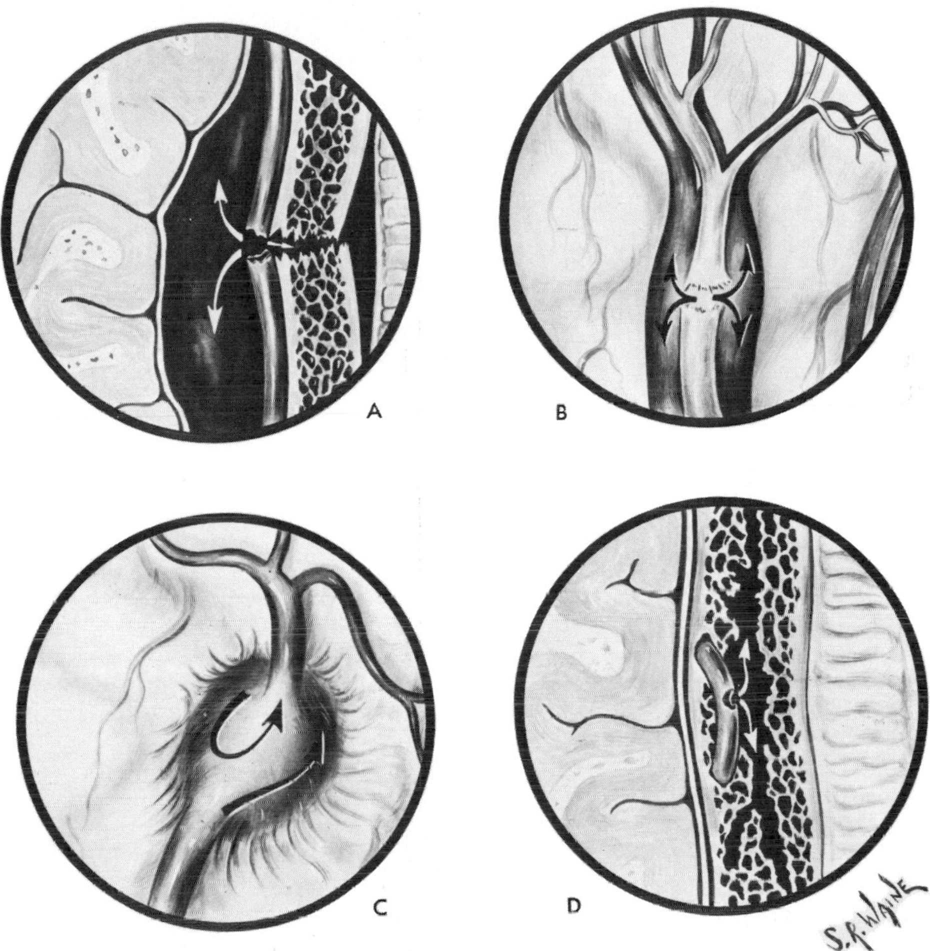

Figure 9–121 *A.* In this drawing the middle meningeal artery is not accompanied by a venous channel. A tear in the middle meningeal artery allows the extravasation of blood and contrast material into the epidural space or through the fracture line into the subgaleal space. (See also Fig. 9–122.) *B.* Where the middle meningeal artery is accompanied by a venous channel, blood and contrast material pass out of the torn meningeal artery into the venous channel. This fistula is a type of "protective mechanism." (See also Fig. 9–125.) *C.* A blood clot has sealed off a tear in the middle meningeal artery, forming a "pseudoaneurysm." This is another type of "protective mechanism." (See also Fig. 9–123.) *D.* A tear in the middle meningeal artery as it traverses the diploic space in the temporal area allows passage of blood and contrast material into the venous diploic channels. (See also Fig. 9–124.)

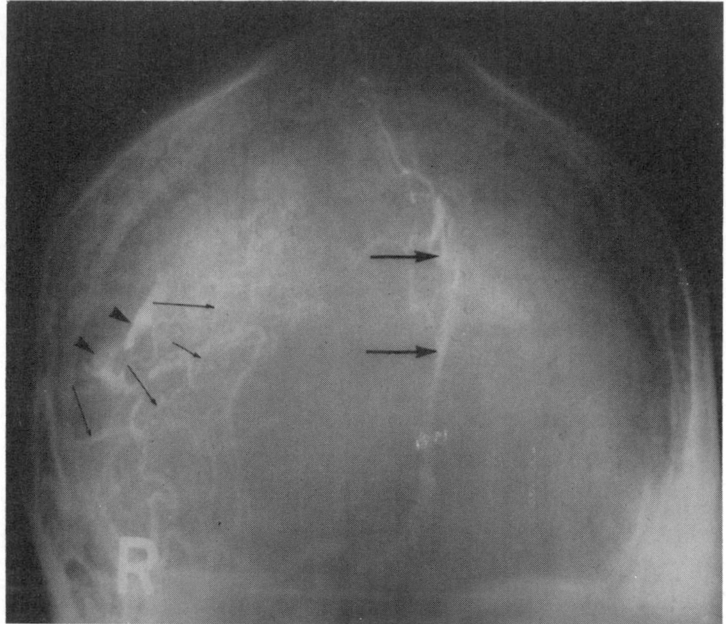

Figure 9–122 Right carotid angiogram, anteroposterior Towne view of arterial phase. An epidural hematoma is demonstrated here displacing the middle meningeal artery (*small black arrows*). The black arrowheads indicate collections of contrast material within the epidural space. On the lateral films these collections had a globular appearance. The large black arrows point to the right anterior cerebral artery, which is displaced to the left. The amount of displacement, however, is not commensurate with the thickness of the epidural hematoma (this is one of the radiological signs of the presence of an epidural hematoma).

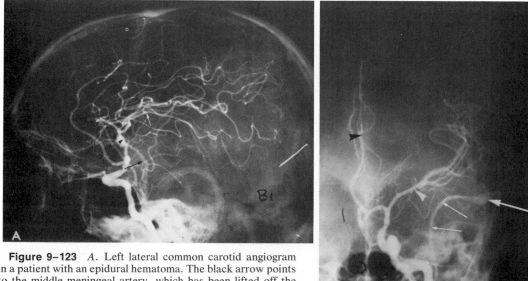

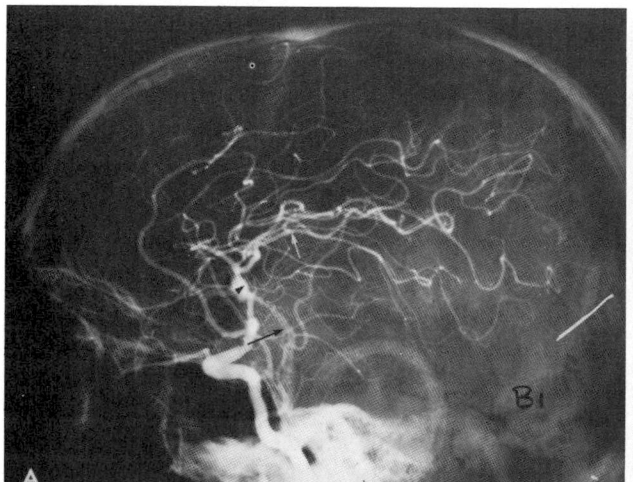

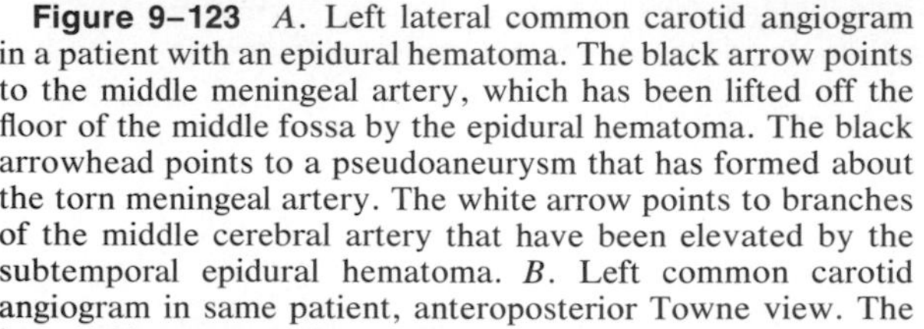

Figure 9–123 *A*. Left lateral common carotid angiogram in a patient with an epidural hematoma. The black arrow points to the middle meningeal artery, which has been lifted off the floor of the middle fossa by the epidural hematoma. The black arrowhead points to a pseudoaneurysm that has formed about the torn meningeal artery. The white arrow points to branches of the middle cerebral artery that have been elevated by the subtemporal epidural hematoma. *B*. Left common carotid angiogram in same patient, anteroposterior Towne view. The large white arrow points to the pseudoaneurysm. The small white arrows point to the displaced middle meningeal artery. The white arrowhead points to the displaced middle cerebral trunk. The black arrowhead indicates the left anterior cerebral artery, which is displaced only slightly. Angiography in this patient was performed 168 hours after the episode of trauma.

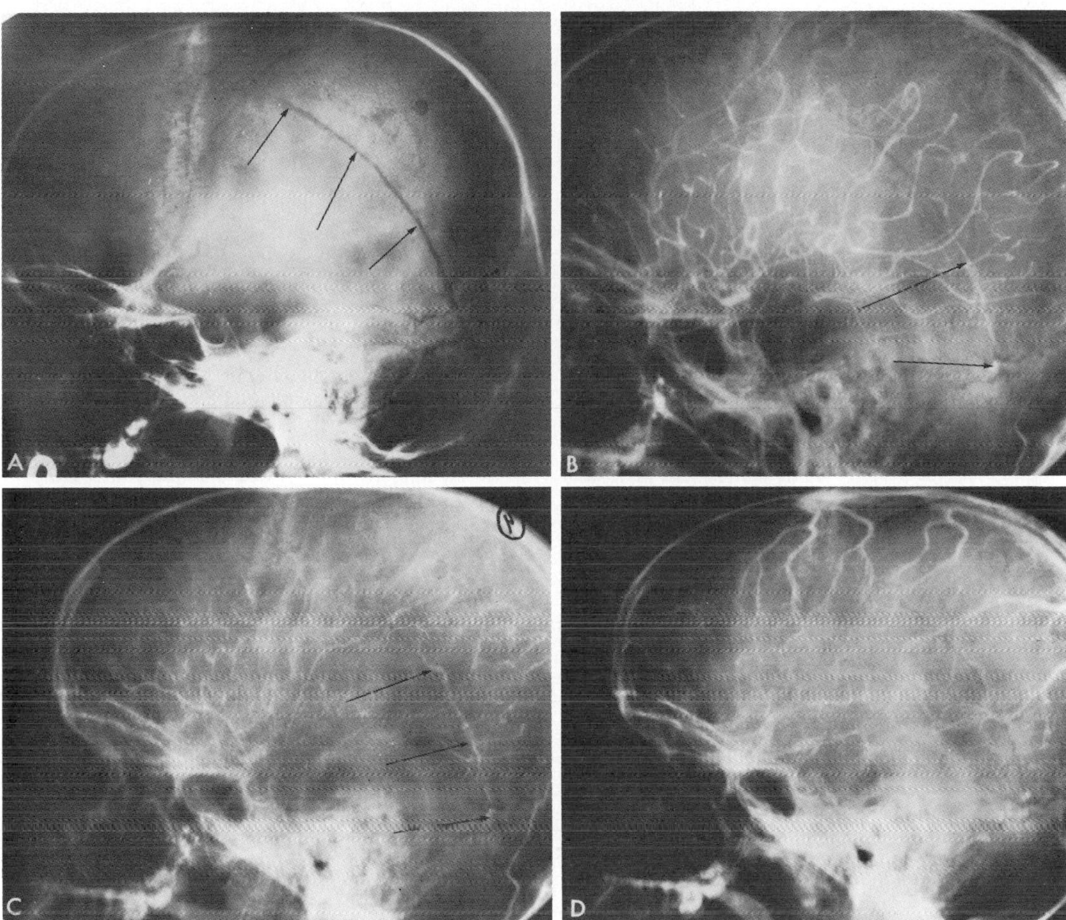

Figure 9–124 *A*. Lateral skull film of a 12-year-old boy who was struck by a baseball bat. The black arrows point to a linear fracture. *B*. Left common carotid angiogram in same patient. The black arrows point to extravasated contrast material along the fracture line. The extravasated contrast material has come from a torn meningeal vessel. *C*. Later film of the lateral angiographic series in same patient. The black arrows point to the accumulation of more extravasated contrast material along the fracture line. *D*. Later film of the angiographic series in same patient. Very little extravasated contrast material is still visible. Carotid angiography in this patient was performed 24 hours after the episode of trauma. The anteroposterior angiographic series showed no significant displacement of cerebral vessels and so no operation was performed for removal of extracerebral hematoma. The patient made a complete recovery without any form of operative intervention. The extravasated contrast material (and blood) is presumed to have run out of the middle meningeal artery, through the fracture, and into the subgaleal space, where a large hematoma was present.

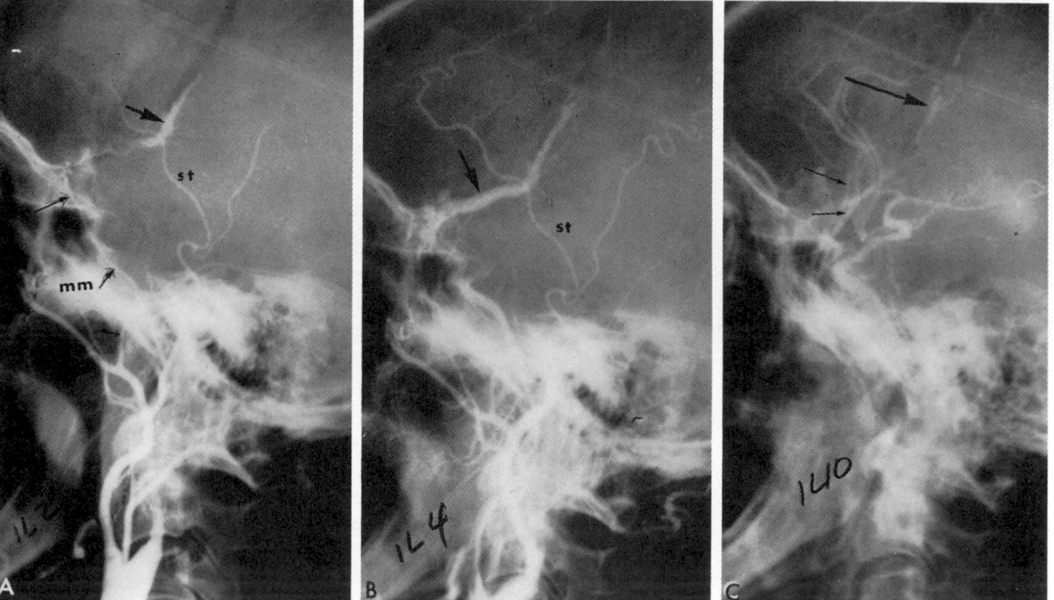

Figure 9–125 *A*. Left carotid angiogram, lateral view. The small black arrows point to the middle meningeal artery (mm). The large black arrow points to extravasated contrast material coming from this artery. The superficial artery is labeled st. *B*. Same patient as in *A*. More contrast material (*large black arrow*) has leaked out of the middle meningeal artery. *C*. Later phase of angiographic series in same patient. The large black arrow points to extravasated contrast material. The small black arrows point to contrast material that has found its way into the meningeal venous channels accompanying the meningeal artery. During this series contrast material in the internal carotid artery has slowly passed into the middle and anterior cerebral arteries. At the time of operation no significant collection of blood was noted in the epidural space.

Also, pseudoaneurysm formation of the middle meningeal artery has been reported.*

Of particular importance is the time interval between the injury and the angiographic studies. It is of special importance also that, in most of these cases, large amounts of contrast material were seen to leave the torn meningeal artery. Cases in which a tremendous outpouring of contrast material was seen many hours after the episode of trauma, without an epidural hematoma of a size commensurate with the production of the equation—flow times hours after injury—must clearly have had a "protective mechanism in operation." These findings with regard to the presence of extravasation many hours after the episode of trauma are not in accord with those of Huber.[83]

At this point, consideration is given to anatomical factors that the author believes to be responsible for the pattern emerging in any given case in which torn meningeal vessels initiate an episode of hemorrhage. The determining factor is the situation of the meningeal artery at the site of leakage. It may be encased by bone at this point, so that the extravasated material may find its way into diploic channels; the artery may be accompanied by venous channels at the site of the tear, resulting in fistula formation of the arteriovenous variety; finally, there may be no venous channel present adjacent to the torn meningeal artery, in which instance the extravasated material can accumulate only in the epidural space—unless the fracture site itself allows decompression. The anatomical relationships mentioned here are all presented in Figures 9–121 through 9–125.

The basis for an understanding of what is involved in fistula formation lies in the work of Jones.[94,95] This anatomist was intrigued by the anatomical explanation for the grooves on the inner table of the skull and found that the major channels accounting for these grooves were the accompanying meningeal veins rather than the meningeal artery itself (Fig. 9–126). According to Jones, this fact was discovered at an earlier date, but lost sight of for a time. Figures 9–

* See references 37, 80, 97, 104, 122, 145, 151, 169, 188, and 237.

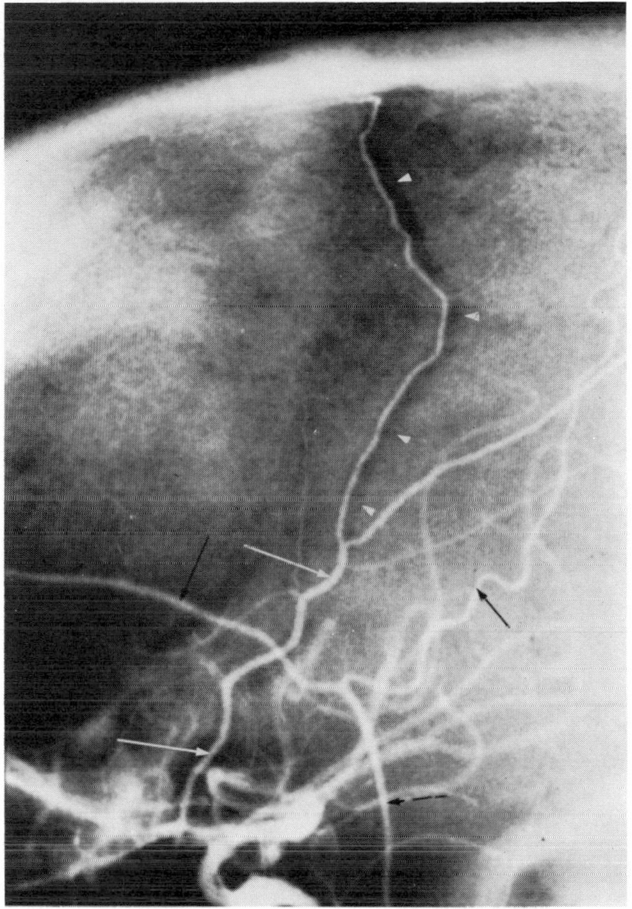

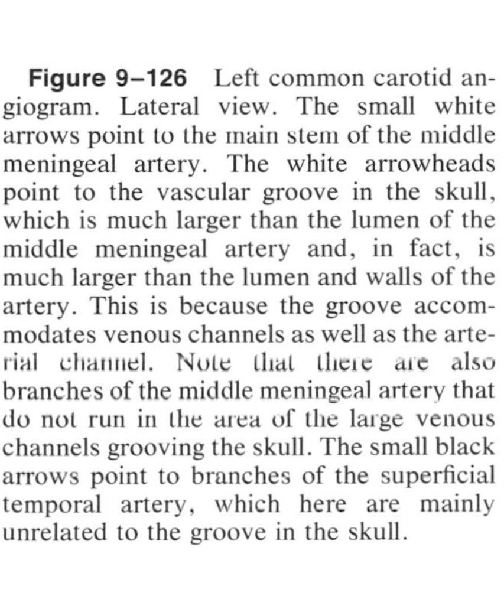

Figure 9–126 Left common carotid angiogram. Lateral view. The small white arrows point to the main stem of the middle meningeal artery. The white arrowheads point to the vascular groove in the skull, which is much larger than the lumen of the middle meningeal artery and, in fact, is much larger than the lumen and walls of the artery. This is because the groove accommodates venous channels as well as the arterial channel. Note that there are also branches of the middle meningeal artery that do not run in the area of the large venous channels grooving the skull. The small black arrows point to branches of the superficial temporal artery, which here are mainly unrelated to the groove in the skull.

121 through 9–125 illustrate passage of contrast material from a meningeal artery to an accompanying meningeal vein.

In pseudoaneurysm formation, extravasated blood from a torn vessel becomes walled off by a covering made up of fibrinous clot. Thus, the wall of the vessel does not form the wall of the aneurysm.

The lesions that must be considered in the differential diagnosis of a torn meningeal vessel with its resultant fistula formation or pseudoaneurysm formation are: (1) congenital aneurysms of the middle meningeal artery, (2) traumatic pseudoaneurysms of a branch of the external carotid artery in the scalp, and (3) extravasation of contrast medium from a lacerated cerebral vessel such as the middle cerebral artery.

"Congenital aneurysm" of the middle meningeal artery is a rare phenomenon.[11,143,237] Figure 9–110*A* illustrates such an aneurysm thought to be of congenital origin.

Angiograms demonstrating a pseudoaneurysm of a branch of the external carotid artery in the scalp have been presented by Wortzman.[232] Such pseudoaneurysms usually result from open injury, but may result from closed injury. Clinically, there is generally no difficulty in determining whether such a pseudoaneurysm is present, but angiographically they may overlie a meningeal artery and simulate a pseudoaneurysm of the middle meningeal artery (Fig. 9–110*B*).

Case reports of extravasation of contrast medium from torn cerebral vessels are extremely rare.[100,118,186] Another reported case is illustrated in Figure 9–127.

Intracerebral Mass Lesions

Cerebral Contusion and Edema. The temporal, frontal, and occipital lobes are the areas most frequently affected in cerebral trauma. The contrecoup phenomenon may

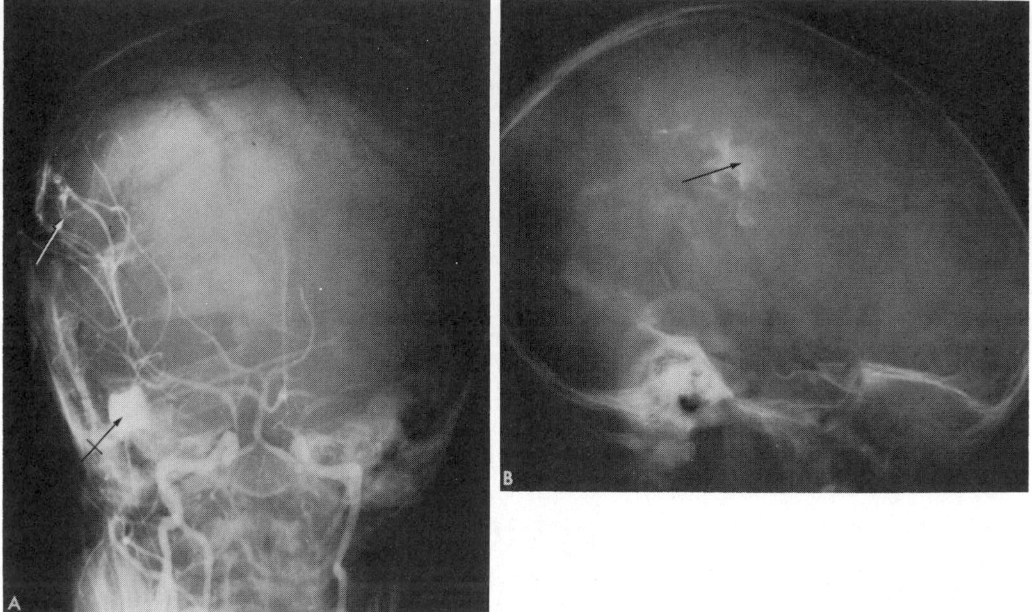

Figure 9–127 A young boy suffered severe head trauma with comminuted fractures of the skull. Angiography revealed displacement of intracranial vessels and a tear of a cortical branch of the middle cerebral artery with extravasation of contrast medium (*arrows*) over the cerebral cortex, pooling in cerebral sulci (*B*). +→, artifact.

result in greater damage on the side opposite the site of direct injury. An associated subdural or epidural hematoma may accompany the brain contusion and will produce the angiographic appearance of a mass lesion with appropriate displacement of vessels. Poor filling of cerebral vessels has been attributed by some to spasm. Swollen brain may account for failure of the midline angiographic structures to return to the midline after evacuation of epidural and subdural hematomas.

A localized segment of vascular narrowing or generalized spasm may result from trauma.[56] Angiograms will show the caliber of the vessels to be considerably narrowed, and the rate of flow of contrast through the cerebral circulation will be delayed. Repeat angiograms at a later date may reveal a return to normal of the caliber of the involved vessels.

INTRACEREBRAL HEMATOMA. These hematomas act as space-taking lesions that are angiographically avascular. Although some regression of vascular displacement may occur when contusion subsides, some displacement persists for a much longer period. These lesions may not be recognized without the benefit of angiography.[70]

Traumatic Occlusion of the Middle Cerebral Artery

This has been infrequently reported. Wolpert and Schechter reported four cases of traumatic middle cerebral artery occlusion demonstrated angiographically.[230] Collateral circulation from other vessels was established in three of these cases. The possible pathological factors to explain the occlusions include thrombosis of the middle cerebral artery, embolism of the middle cerebral artery, intracerebral hemorrhage causing direct arterial compression, arterial compression, arterial spasm, and a dissecting aneurysm of the middle cerebral artery.

Caroticocavernous Fistula

These usually result from a fracture involving the base of the skull, which may tear either the wall of the carotid artery as it passes through the cavernous sinus, or more frequently the branches of the inter-

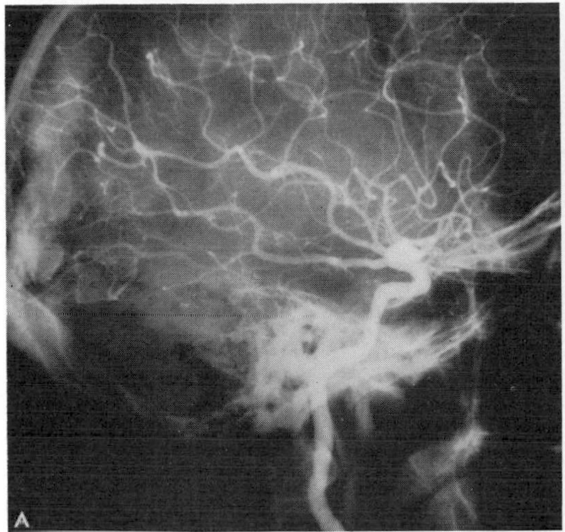

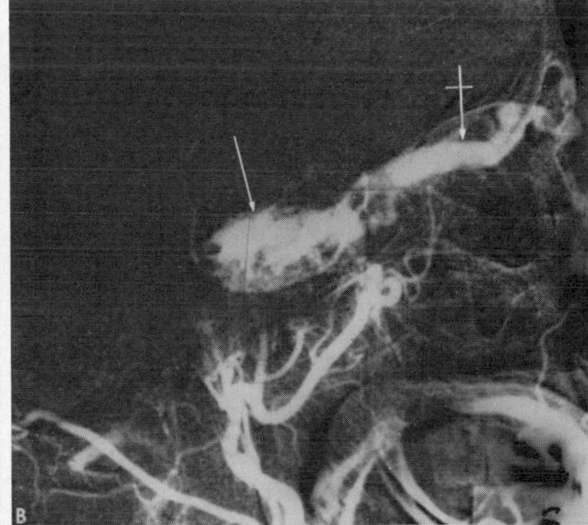

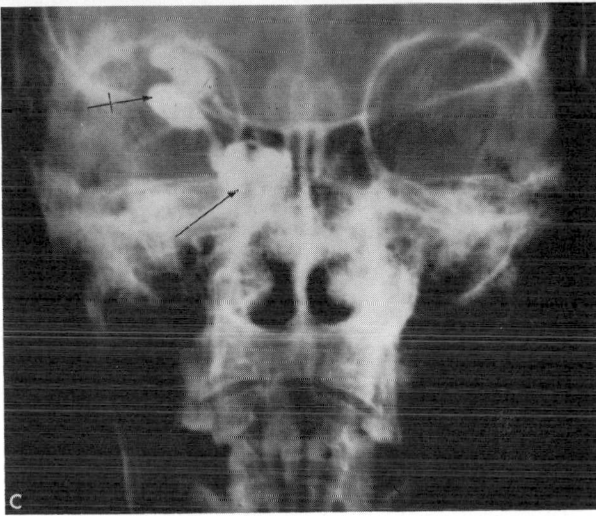

Figure 9–128 *A.* Right internal carotid angiogram in a patient with a carotid-cavernous fistula. Note that there is no opacification of the cavernous shunt. *B* and *C.* An external carotid angiogram shows filling of the branches of the external carotid artery and filling of the cavernous sinus (*arrow*) via numerous branches of an external carotid artery. The engorged orbital veins (+→) are well opacified.

nal or external carotid arteries as they enter the cavernous sinus. Penetrating wounds may also be responsible. Carotid and vertebral angiography should be performed to facilitate planning the proposed therapy. Unsuspected collateral channels have been responsible for some of the poor results of operation. In a recent series of cases reported by Rosenbaum and Schechter a fistula involving only branches of the external carotid artery was seen in one case.[164] Selective internal and external carotid angiography showed filling from the external carotid artery alone with no contribution from the internal carotid artery. The conventional trap procedure, as could be anticipated from the angiogram, did little to the fistulous communications (Fig. 9–128).

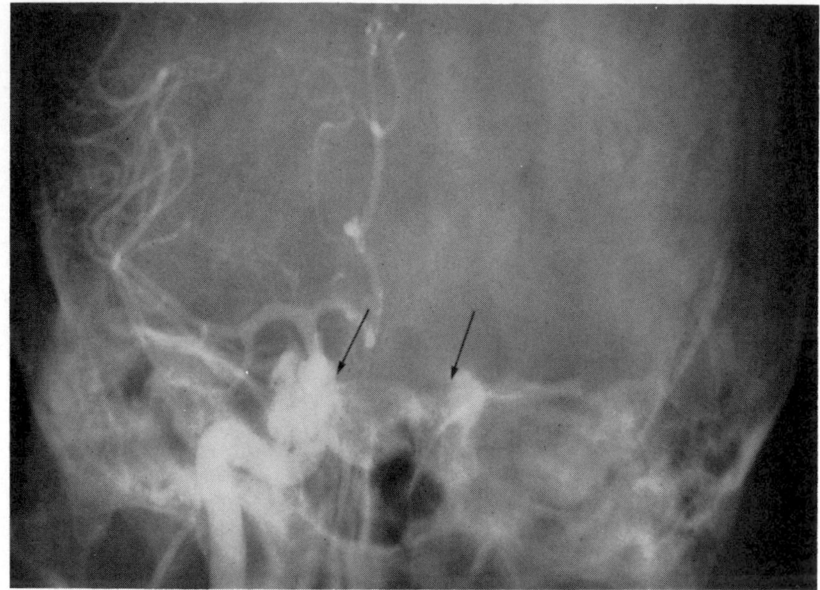

Figure 9–129 Left internal carotid angiogram in a patient with a left pulsating exophthalmos. Note filling of the left cavernous sinus with contrast medium and filling also of the right cavernous sinus (*arrows*).

The dramatic sudden onset of a pulsating exophthalmos is due to a communication between the branches of the carotid artery and the cavernous sinus. Contrast medium introduced into the carotid artery passes into the cavernous sinus and outlines the engorged ophthalmic veins (Fig. 9–128*B* and *C*). The cavernous sinus on both sides usually fills via the venous communications that are normally present between the cavernous sinuses of both sides (Fig. 9–129).[77,209]

REFERENCES

1. Alexander, E., Jr., Wigser, S. M., and Davis, C. H.: Bilateral extracranial aneurysms of the internal carotid artery. J. Neurosurg., *25*:437–442, 1966.
2. Alexander, G. L.: Extradural hematoma of the vertex. J. Neurol. Psychiat., *24*:381–384, 1961.
3. Alpers, B. J., Berry, R. G., and Paddison, R. M.: Anatomical studies of the circle of Willis in normal brain. Arch. Neurol. Psychiat., *81*:409–418, 1959.
4. Anderson, McD., and Schechter, M. M.: A case of spontaneous dissecting aneurysm of the internal carotid artery. J. Neurol. Neurosurg. Psychiat., *22*:195–201, 1959.
5. Aronson, N. I.: Traumatic arteriovenous fistula of the vertebral vessels. Neurology, *11*:817–823, 1961.
6. Askenasy, H. M., Kosary, I. Z., and Braham, J.: Thrombosis of the longitudinal sinus. Diagnosis by carotid angiography. Neurology, *12*:288–292.
7. Bagchi, A. K.: Lateral ventricle tumors. J. Indian Med. Ass., *29*:425–432, 1957.
8. Baker, H. L.: Angiographic investigation of cerebrovascular insufficiency. Radiology, *77*:399–405, 1961.
9. Bauer, R., Sheehan, S., and Meyer, J. S.: Arteriographic study of cerebral vascular disease. Arch. Neruol., *4*:119–131, 1961.
10. Berk, M. E.: Combined carotid-vertebral angiography. A selective procedure—preliminary report. Brit. J. Radiol., *33*:780–783, 1960.
11. Berk, M. E.: Aneurysm of the middle meningeal artery. Brit. J. Radiol., *34*:667–668, 1961.
12. Berkay, F.: A rare and interesting case of arteriovenous fistula between the middle meningeal artery and the greater petrosal sinus and surgical treatment. (In Turkish) Tip Fak. Mec., *26*:64–71, 1963.
13. Boldrey, E., and Miller, E. R.: Arteriovenous fistula (aneurysm) of the great cerebral vein (of Galen) and the circle of Willis. Report on two patients treated by ligation. Arch. Neurol. Psychiat., *62*:778–783. 1949.
14. Bonnal, J.: Hématome extradural de la fosse cérébelleuse. Rev. Neurol., *85*:439–443, 1951.
15. Boyd-Wilson, J. S.: The association of cerebral angiomas with intracranial aneurysms. J. Neurol. Neurosurg. Psychiat., *22*:218–223, 1958.
16. Bradley, K. C.: Extra-dural hemorrhage. Aust. New Zeal. J. Surg., *21*:241–260, 1952.
17. Bull, J. W. D.: Personal communication, 1960.
18. Bull, J. W. D.: Contributions of radiology to the study of intracranial aneurysms. Brit. Med. J., *2*:1701–1708, 1962.
19. Bull, J. W. D.: Short history of intracranial aneurysms. London Clin. Med. J., *3*:47–61, 1962.
20. Bull, J. W. D., and Schunk, H.: The significance

of displacement of the cavernous portion of the internal carotid artery. Brit. J. Radiol. *35*:801–814, 1962.
21. Campbell, J. A., and Campbell, R. L.: Angiographic diagnosis of traumatic head and neck lesions. J.A.M.A., *175*:761–768, 1961.
22. Campbell, J. B., and Cohen, J.: Epidural hemorrhage and the skull of children. Surg. Gynec. Obstet., *92*:257–280, 1951.
23. Castellanos, A., and Pereiras, R.: Retrograde or counter current aortography. Amer. J. Roentgen. *63*:559–565, 1950.
24. Conley, J. J., Chusid, J. G., and Schechter, M.M.: Angiography in head and neck surgery. Arch. Surg., *89*:609–619, 1964.
25. Contorni, L: Il Circulo collaterale vertebrovertebrale nella obliterazione dell'arteria subclavia alle sua origine. Minerva Chir., *15*:268–271, 1960.
26. Crawford, T.: Some observations on the pathogenesis and natural history of intracranial aneurysms. J. Neurol. Neurosurg. Psychiat., *22*:259–266, 1959.
27. Cronqvist, S.: Vertebral catheterization via the femoral artery. Acta Radiol., *55*:113–118, 1961.
28. Cronqvist, S.: *In* Third International Symposium on Cerebral Circulation. Thule. Salzburg, 1966.
29. Cushing, H., and Bailey, P.: Tumors Arising from Blood Vessels of the Brain. Angiomatous Malformations and Haemangioblastomas. Springfield, Ill., Charles C Thomas, 1928.
30. Dandy, E. W.: Ventriculography following the injection of air into the cerebral ventricles. Ann. Surg., *68*:5–11, 1918.
31. Dandy, E. W.: Roentgenography of the brain after the injection of air into the spinal canal. Ann. Surg., *70*:397–403, 1919.
32. Daseler, E. H., and Anson, B. J.: Surgical anatomy of the subclavian artery and its branches. Surg. Gynec. Obstet., *108*:149–174, 1959.
33. DeBakey, M. E., Crawford, E. S., and Fields, W. S.: Surgical treatment of patients with cerebral arterial insufficiency associated with extracranial arterial occlusive lesions. Neurology, *11*:145–149, 1961.
34. DeGaris, C. F., Black, I. H., and Riemenschneider, E. A.: Patterns of the aortic arch in American white and Negro stocks with comparative notes on certain other mammals. J.Anat., *67*:599–619, 1933.
35. DeKleyn, A.: Some remarks on vestibular nystagmus, Confin. Neurol., *2*:257, 1939.
36. Di Chiro, G.: Ophthalmic arteriography. Radiology, *77*:948–957, 1961.
37. Dilenge, D., and Wuthrich, R.: Traumatic aneurysm of the middle meningeal artery. (In French). Neurochirurgia, *4*:202–206, 1962.
38. Dotter, C. T.: Left ventricular and systemic arterial catheterization. A simple percutaneous method using a spring guide. Amer. J. Roentgen., *83*:969–984, 1960.
39. Dotter, C. T., and Gensini, C. G.: Percutaneous retrograde catheterization of the left ventricle and systemic arteries of man. Radiology, *75*:171–184, 1960.
40. du Boulay, G.: Some observations on the natural history of intracranial aneurysms. Brit. J. Radiol., *38*:721–757, 1965.
41. Eastcott, H. H. G., Pickering, G. W., and Rob, C. G.: Reconstruction of internal carotid artery in a patient with intermittent attacks of hemiplegia. Lancet, *2*:994–996, 1954.
42. Ecker, A.: The Normal Cerebral Angiogram. Springfield, Ill., Charles C Thomas, 1951.
43. Ecker, A., and Riemenschneider, P. A.: Angiographic Localization of Intracranial Masses. Springfield, Ill., Charles C Thomas, 1955.
44. Engestet, A.: Cerebral angiography with Per-Abrodil. Acta Radiol., Suppl. 56, 1944.
45. Engstrom, H., and Hamberger, C. A.: Bilateral tumor of the carotid body. Acta Otolaryng., *48*:390–396, 1957.
46. Erb, K. H., and Hahn, E.: Aneurysmen des Arteria temporalis als Folge von Mensurverletzungen. Zbl. Chir., *58*:2610–2613, 1931.
47. Falk, B.: Radiologic diagnosis of intra-ventricular meningiomas. Acta Radiol., *46*:171–177, 1956.
48. Fawcett, E., and Blackford, J. V.: The circle of Willis: an examination of 700 specimens. J. Anat. Physiol., *40*:63–70, 1906.
49. Feindel, W., and Perot, P.: Red cerebral veins. A report on arteriovenous shunts in tumors and cerebral scars. J. Neurosurg., *22*:315–325, 1965.
50. Fetterman, G. H., and Moran, T. J.: Anomalies of the circle of Willis in relation to cerebral softening. Arch Path., *32*:251–257, 1941.
51. Fields, W. S., Crawford, E. S., and DeBakey, M.E.: Surgical considerations in cerebral arterial insufficiency. Neurology, *8*:801–808, 1958.
52. Fields, W. S., Edwards, W. H., and Crawford, E. S.: Bilateral carotid artery thrombosis. Arch. Neurol., *4*:369–383, 1961.
53. Fincher, E. G.: Arteriovenous fistula between the middle meningeal artery and the greater petrosal sinus. Case report. Ann. Surg., *133*:886–888, 1951.
54. Fisher, A. G. T.: A case of complete absence of both internal carotid arteries. J. Anat. Physiol., *48*:37–46, 1913.
55. Fisher, M.: Occlusion of carotid arteries. Arch. Neurol. Psychiat., *72*:187–204, 1954.
56. Freidenfelt, H., and Sundstrom, R.: Local and general spasm in the internal carotid system following trauma. Acta Radiol. (Diagn.), *1*: 278–283, 1963.
57. Gabriele, O. F., and Bell, D.: Ophthalmic origin of the middle meningeal artery. Radiology, *89*:841–844, 1967.
58. Galloway, J. R., Greitz, T., and Sjogren, S. E.: Vertebral angiography in the diagnosis of ventricular dilatation. Acta Radiol. (Diagn.), *2*: 321–333, 1964.
59. Gannon, W. E.: Valves of the common carotid artery during angiography. Amer. J. Roentgen., *86*:1050–1057, 1961.
60. Gannon, W. E.: Interhemispheric subdural hematoma. J. Neurosurg., *18*:829–830, 1961.
61. Gardner, W. J.: Traumatic subdural hematoma with particular reference to the latent interval. Arch. Neurol. Psychiat., *27*:847–858, 1932.
62. Gass, H. H.: Kinks and coils of the cervical carotid artery. Surg. Forum, *9*:721–724, 1959.

63. Gassel, M. M., and Davies, H.: Meningiomas in the lateral ventricles. Brain, *84*:605–626, 1961.
64. Glynn, L. E.: Medial defects in circle of Willis and their relation to aneurysm formation. J.Path. Bact., *51*:213–222, 1940.
65. Gooddy, W., and Schechter, M. M.: Spontaneous arteriovenous fistula of the vertebral artery. Brit. J. Radiol., *33*:709–711, 1960.
66. Greenspan, R. H., Simon, A. L., Rickells, H. J., Rojas, R. H., and Watson, J. C.: In vivo magnification angiography. Invest. Radiol., *2*:419–431, 1967.
67. Greitz, T., and Lindgren, E.: Angiographic determination of brain tumor pathology. *In* Abrams, H. L., ed.: Angiography I. Boston, Little Brown and Co., 1961.
68. Gutstein, R. A., and Schechter, M. M.: Aneurysms and arteriovenous fistulas of the superficial temporal vessels. Radiology, *97*:549–557, 1970.
69. Hanafee, W. N.: Personal communication, 1963.
70. Hancock. D. O.: Angiography in acute head injuries. Lancet, *2*:745–747, 1961.
71. Harrison, J. H., and Davalos, P. A.: Cerebral ischemia. Surgical procedure in cases due to tortuosity and buckling of the cervical vessels. Arch. Surg., *84*:85–94, 1962.
72. Hasegawa, T., Ravens, J. R., and Toole, J. F.: Precapillary arteriovenous anastamosed "thoroughfare channels" in the brain. Arch. Neurol., *16*:217–224, 1967.
73. Hassler, O.: Medial defects in the meningeal arteries. J. Neurosurg., *19*:337–340, 1962.
74. Hassler, O., and Saltzman, G. F.: Histologic changes in infundibular widening of the posterior communicating artery. Acta Path. Microbiol. Scand., *46*:305–312, 1959.
75. Hassler, O., and Saltzman, G. F.: Angiographic and histologic changes in infundibular widening of the posterior communicating artery. Acta Radiol. (Diagn.), *1*:321–327, 1963.
76. Hauge, T.: Catheter vertebral angiography. Acta Radiol., suppl. 109, 1954.
77. Hayes, G. J.: External carotid-cavernous sinus fistulas. J. Neurosurg., *20*:692–700, 1963.
78. Heister, L.: General System of Surgery. London, 1750.
79. Hirano, A., and Terry, R. D.: Aneurysm of the vein of Galen. J. Neuropath. Exp. Neurol., *17*:424–429, 1958.
80. Hirsch, J. F., David, M., and Sachs, M.: Les anévrysmes artériels traumatiques intracrâniens. Neurochirurgie, *8*:189–201, 1962.
81. Huang, Y. P., and Wolf, B. S.: The veins of the posterior fossa—superior or galenic draining group. Amer. J. Roentgen., *95*:808–821, 1965.
82. Huang, Y. S., and Araki, C.: Angiographic confirmation of lateral ventricle meningiomas. A report of 5 cases. J. Neurosurg., *11*:337–352, 1954.
83. Huber, P.: Die Verletzungen der Meningealfasse bein Epiduralhamatöm im Angiogramm. Fortschr. Röntgenstr., *96*:207–220, 1962.
84. Hurwitt, E. S., Carton, C. A., Fell, S. C., Kessler, L. A., Seidenberg, B., and Shapiro, J.H.: Critical evaluation and surgical corrections of obstructions in the branches of the aortic arch. Ann. Surg., *152*:472–484, 1960.
85. Hutchinson, E. C., and Yates, P. O.: The cervical portion of the vertebral artery. A clinicopathological study. Brain. *79*:319–331, 1956.
86. Hutchinson, E. C., and Yates, P. O.: Caroticovertebral stenosis. Lancet, *1*:2–8, 1957.
87. Jackson, D. C., and du Boulay, G. H.: Traumatic arterio-venous aneurysm of the middle meningeal artery. Brit. J. Radiol., *37*:788–789, 1964.
88. Jackson, I. J., and Speakman, T. J.: Chronic extradural hematoma. J. Neurosurg., *7*:444–447, 1950.
89. Jackson, J. R., Tindall, G. T., and Nashold, B.S.: Rupture of an intracranial aneurysm during carotid arteriography. A case report. J.Neurosurg., *17*:333–336, 1960.
90. Jacobsen, H. H.: An interhemispherically situated hematoma. Case report. Acta Radiol., *43*:235–236, 1955.
91. Jaeger, R., and Whiteley, W. H.: Cerebral angiography by an intravascular intubation technique. Amer. J. Roentgen., *73*:735–747, 1955.
92. Jamieson, K. G.: Unusual case of extra-dural haematoma. Aust. New Zeal. J. Surg., *21*:304–307, 1952.
93. Johansson, C.: The central veins and deep dural sinuses of the brain. Acta Radiol., suppl. 107, 1954.
94. Jones, F. W.: Grooves upon ossa parietalia commonly said to be caused by arteria meningea media. J. Anat. Physiol., *46*:228–238, 1912.
95. Jones, F. W.: Vascular lesion in some cases of middle meningeal haemorrhage. Lancet, *2*:7–12, 1912.
96. Karras, B. G., Cannon, A. H., and Ashby, R. N.: Percutaneous left brachial aortography. Personal communication, 1960.
97. Kia-Noury, M.: Traumatisches intrakranielles Aneurysma der Arteria meningica media nach Schadelbasis-fraktur. Zbl. Neurochir., *21*:351–357, 1961.
98. Krayenbühl, H.: Cerebral venous thrombosis: diagnostic value of cerebral angiography. Schweiz. Arch. Neurol. Psychiat., *74*:261–287, 1954.
99. Krayenbühl, H.: The diagnostic value of orbital angiography. Brit. J. Ophthal., *42*:180–190, 1958.
100. Krayenbühl, H., and Richter, H. R.: Die Zerebrale Angiographie. Stuttgart, Georg Thieme, 1952.
101. Krayenbühl, H., and Yasargil, M. G.: Die Vaskularen Erkrankungen in Gebiet der Arteria Vertebralis und Arteria Basialis. Stuttgart, Georg Thieme, 1957.
102. Krayenbühl, H., and Yasargil, M. G.: Das Hirnaneurysma. Basel, J. R. Geigy, 1958.
103. Kuhn, R. A.: The normal brachial cerebral angiogram. Amer. J. Roentgen., *84*:78–87, 1960.
104. Kuhn, R. A., and Kugler, H.: False aneurysms of the middle meningeal artery. J. Neurosurg., *21*:92–96, 1964.
105. Lai, M. D., Hoffman, H. B., and Adamkiewicz, J. J.: Dissecting aneurysm of the cervical portion of the internal carotid artery secondary to non-penetrating neck injury. Acta Radiol. (Diagn.) *5*:290–295, 1966.
106. Laine, E., Delandtsheer, J. M., Galibert, P., and

Delandtsheer-Arnot, G.: Phlebography in tumours of the hemispheres and central grey matter. Acta Radiol., *46*:203–214, 1956.

107. Lassen, N. A.: The luxury perfusion syndrome and its possible relation to acute metabolic acidosis localized within the brain. Lancet, *2*:1113–1115, 1966.

108. La Torre, E., Occhipinti, E., and Pollicita, A., Backward displacement of the upper part of the basilar artery in infantile hydrocephalus. Acta Radiol. (Diagn.), *8*:385–399, 1969.

109. Leslie, E. V., Smith, B. H., and Zoll, J. G.: Value of angiography in head trauma. Radiology, *78*:930–939, 1962.

110. Lindgren, E.: Percutaneous angiography of the vertebral artery. Acta Radiol., *33*:389–405, 1950.

111. Lindgren, E.: Röntgenologie. Band II. *In* Olivecrona, H., and Tonnis, W., eds.: Handbuch der Neurochirurgie. Berlin, Springer-Verlag, 1954.

112. Lindgren, E.: Another method of vertebral angiography. Acta Radiol., *46*:257–262, 1956.

113. Lindgren, E.: Radiologic examination of the brain and spinal cord. Acta Radiol., suppl. 151, 1957.

114. Litvak, J., Yahr, M. D., and Ransohoff, J.: Aneurysms of the great vein of Galen and midline cerebral arteriovenous anomalies. J. Neurosurg., *17*:945–954, 1960.

115. Liverud. K.: Technique in percutaneous carotid and vertebral angiography with polyethylene catheters. J. Oslo City Hosp., *8*:220–242, 1958.

116. Lotgren, O. F.: Vertebral angiography in the diagnosis of tumors in the pineal region. Acta Radiol., *50*:108–124, 1958.

117. Lofstrom, J. E., Webster, J. E., and Gurdjian, E.S.: Angiography in the evaluation of intracranial trauma. Radiology, *65*:847–855, 1955.

118. Lohr, W.: Hirngefassverletzungen in arteriographischer Darstellung. Zbl. Chir., *63*:2466–2482, 1936.

119. Lombardi, G.: Radiology in Neuro-Ophthalmology. Baltimore, Md., Williams & Wilkins Co., 1967.

120. Luckett, W. H.: Air in the ventricles of the brain following a fracture of the skull. J. Nerv. Ment. Dis., *40*:326–328, 1913.

121. Markham, J. W.: Arteriovenous fistula of the middle meningeal artery and the greater petrosal sinus. J. Neurosurg., *18*;847–848, 1961.

122. Markwalder, H., and Huber, P.: Aneurysmen der Meningealarterien. Schweiz. Med. Wschr., *91*:1344–1347, 1961.

123. Maslowski, H. A.: Vertebral angiography. Percutaneous lateral atlanto-occipital method. Brit. J. Surg., *43*:1–8, 1955.

124. Maslowski, H. A.: International Meeting Society of British Neurological Surgeons and La Société de Neurochirurgiens de Langue Française, 1960.

125. Matson, D. D., and Crofton, F. D. L.: Papilloma of the choroid plexus in childhood. J. Neurosurg., *17*:1002–1027, 1960.

126. McKissock, W., Taylor, J. C., Bloom, W. H., and Till, K.: Extradural hematoma. Observations on 125 cases. Lancet, *2*:167–172, 1960.

127. McLaurin, R. L., and Ford, L. E.: Extradural hematoma. Statistical study of 47 cases. J.Neurosurg., *21*:364–371, 1964.

128. Mones, R.: Vertebral angiography. An analysis of 106 cases. Radiology, *76*:230–236, 1961.

129. Moniz, E.: L'encephalographie artérielle, son importance dans la localization des tumeurs cérébrales. Rev. Neurol., *342*:72–90, 1927.

130. Moniz, E., and Alves, A.: L'importance diagnostique de l'arteriographie de la fosse posterieure. Rev. Neurol., *40*:91–96, 1933.

131. Morris, L.: Arteriographic demonstration of the vertebral artery with special reference to percutaneous subclavian puncture. Brit. J. Radiol., *32*:673–679, 1960.

132. Mount, L. A., and Taveras, J. M.: Arteriographic demonstration of the collateral circulation of the cerebral hemispheres. Arch. Neurol. Psychiat., *78*:235–253, 1957.

133. Murphy, F., and Shillito, J., Jr.: Avoidance of false angiographic localization of the site of internal carotid occlusion. J. Neurosurg., *16*:24–31, 1959.

134. New, P. F. J.: True aneurysm of the middle meningeal artery. Clin. Radiol., *16*:236–240, 1965.

135. New, P. F. J., and Momose, K. J.: Traumatic dissection of the internal carotid artery on the atlantoaxial level secondary to non-penetrating injury. Radiology, *93*:41–46, 1969.

136. Newton, T. H., and Couch, R. S. C.: Possible errors in the arteriographic diagnosis of internal cartoid artery occlusion. Radiology, *75*: 766–773. 1960.

137. Norlen, G., and Paly, N.: Aneurysms of the vertebral artery. J. Neurosurg., *17*:830–835, 1960.

138. Norman, O.; Angiographic differentiation between acute and chronic subdural and extradural hematomas. Acta Radiol., *46*:371–378, 1956.

139. O'Brien, M. S., and Schechter, M. M.: Arteriovenous malformations involving the galenic system. Amer. J. Roentgen., *110*:50–55, 1970.

140. Odman, P.: Percutaneous selective angiography of the main branches of the aorta. Preliminary report. Acta Radiol., *45*:1–14, 1956.

141. Okay, N. H.: Angiographic studies of the factors causing cervical and intracranial flow. Brit. J. Radiol., *42*:676–681, 1969.

142. Olsson, O.: Vertebral angiography in the diagnosis of acoustic nerve tumors. Acta Radiol., *39*:265–272, 1953.

143. Olsson, O.: Vertebral angiography in cerebellar hemangioma. Acta Radiol., *40*:9–16, 1953.

144. Padget, D. H.: The circle of Willis: its embryology and anatomy. *In* Dandy, W.E., ed.: Intracranial Arterial Aneurysm. Ithaca, N.Y., Comstock Publishing Co., 1944.

145. Paillas, J. E., Bonnal, J., and Lavielle, J.: Angiographic images of false aneurysmal sac caused by rupture of median meningeal artery in the course of traumatic extradural hematomata. Report of three cases. J. Neurosurg., *21*:667–671, 1964.

146. Pecker, J., Javalet, A., and Stabert, C.: L'angiographie dans les traumatismes crâniens. J. Radiol. Electr., *40*:623–628, 1959.

147. Perret, G., and Nishioka, H.: Cerebral angiography. An analysis of the diagnostic value and complications of carotid and vertebral an-

giography in 5,484 patients. J. Neurosurg., *25*:98–114, 1966.

148. Perrot, P., Ethier, R., and Wong, A.: An arterial posterior fossa extradural hematoma demonstrated by vertebral angiography. Case report. J. Neurosurg., *26*:255–260, 1967.
149. Petit-Dutaillis, D., Guiot, G., Pertuiset, B., and LeBesnerais, Y.: Les hématomes extraduraux de la fosse cérébelleuse. Presse Méd., *64*:521–524, 1956.
150. Poppen, J. L., and Avman, N.: Aneurysms of the great vein of Galen. J. Neurosurg., *17*:238–244, 1960.
151. Pouyanne, H., Leman, P., Got, M., and Gouaze, A.: Traumatic arterial aneurysm of the left middle meningeal artery: Rupture one month after the accident; Temporal intracerebral hematoma; intervention. (In French). Neurochirurgie, *5*:311–315, 1959.
152. Pribram, H. F. W.: Angiographic appearances in acute intracranial hypertenison. Neurology, *11*:10–21, 1961.
153. Putnam, T., and Cushing, H.: Chronic subdural hematoma. Arch. Surg., *11*:329–393, 1925.
154. Pygott, F., and Hutton, C. F.: Vertebral angiography by percutaneous brachial artery catheterization. Brit. J. Radiol., *32*:114–119, 1959.
155. Quattlebaum, J. K., Upson, E. T., and Neville, R. L.: Stroke associated with elongation and kinking of the internal carotid artery: report of three cases treated by segmental resection of the common carotid artery. Ann. Surg., *150*:824–832, 1959.
156. Radner, S.: Intracranial angiography via the femoral artery. Preliminary report of a new technique. Acta Radiol., *28*:838–842, 1947.
157. Radner, S.: Vertebral angiography by catheterization. A new method employed in 221 cases. Acta Radiol., suppl. 87, 1951.
158. Reivich, M., Holling, H. E., Roberts, B., and Toole, J. F.: Reversal of blood flow through the vertebral artery and its effects on cerebral circulation. New Eng. J. Med., *265*:878–885, 1961.
159. Ring, B. A.: Variations in the striate and other cerebral veins affecting measurement of the "venous angle." Acta Radiol., *52*:433–447, 1959.
160. Riser, M., Geraud, J., Ducoudray, J., and Ribaut, L.: Dolichocarotide interne avec syndrome vertigineux. Rev. Neurol., *85*:145–147, 1951.
161. Rivaglia, cited by Perrig, H.: Zur Anatomie, Klinik und Therapie der Verletzungen und Aneurysmen der Arteria vertebralis. Beitr. Klin. Chir., *154*:272–307, 1931.
162. Rob, C. G., and Wheeler, E. B.: Thrombosis of internal carotid artery treated by arterial surgery. Brit. Med. J., *2*:264–266, 1957.
163. Rogers, V.: Vertebral angiography in the diagnosis of meningioma within the lateral ventricle. Brit. J. Radiol., *33*:326–328, 1960.
164. Rosenbaum, A. E., and Schechter, M. M.: External Carotid-cavernous fistulae. Acta Radiol. (Diagn.), *9*:440–444, 1969.
165. Rossi, P.: Personal communication, 1967.
166. Rossi, P.: Transaxillary selective catheterization of the carotid and vertebral arteries. Acta Radiol. (Diagn.), *5*:458–464, 1966.
167. Rowbotham, G. F., and Whalley, N.: Prolonged compression of the brain resulting from an extradural hemorrhage, J. Neurol. Neurosurg. Psychiat., *15*:64–65, 1952.
168. Roy, P.: Percutaneous catheterization of the axillary artery. Tenth International Congress of Radiology, 1962.
169. Ruggiero, G., and Jay, M.: Une technique pour l'arteriographie de l'artere carotide externe. Acta. Radiol., *50*:453–459, 1958.
170. Ruggiero, G., Calabro, A., Metzger, J., and Simon, J.: Arteriography of the external carotid artery. Acta Radiol. (Diagn.), *1*:395–403, 1963.
171. Rydell, J. R., and Jennings, W. K.: The surgical treatment of carotid aneurysm in the neck. West. J. Surg., Obstet. Gynec., *64*:385–390, 1956.
172. Saltzman, G. F.: Circulation through the posterior communicating artery in different compression tests. Acta Radiol., *51*:10–16, 1959.
173. Saltzman, G. F.: Infundibular widening of the posterior communicating artery studied by carotid angiography. Acta Radiol., *51*:415–421, 1959.
174. Saltzman, G. F.: Angiographic demonstration of the posterior communicating and posterior cerebral arteries. I: Normal angiography. Acta Radiol., *52*:1–20, 1959.
175. Scatliff, J. H., Hyde, I., and Gantot, H. J.: Vertebral artery reflux: a laboratory investigation of the non-obstructive causes of retrograde flow of contrast material in the contralateral vertebral artery. Radiology, *88*:63–74, 1967.
176. Scatliff, J. H., Kier, E. L., Zingesser, L. H., and Schechter, M. M.: Terminal basilar artery deformity secondary to suprasellar masses and third ventricular dilatation. Amer. J. Roentgen., *101*:61–67, 1967.
177. Schechter, M. M.: Total vertebrobasilar arteriography using a single vertebral puncture technique. J. Neurosurg., *18*:74–78, 1961.
178. Schechter, M. M.: Percutaneous carotid catheterization. Acta Radiol. (Diagn.), *1*:417–426, 1963.
179. Schechter, M. M., and Chusid, J. G.: Chemodectomas of the carotid bifurcation. Acta Radiol. (Diagn.), *5*:488–508, 1966.
180. Schechter, M. M., and De Gutierrez-Mahoney, C. G.: Vertebral angiography. Exhibited at International Congress of Neurosurgery, 1961.
181. Schechter, M. M., and Elkin, M.: The layering effect in cerebral angiography. Acta Radiol, *1*:427–435, 1963.
182. Schechter, M. M., and Zingesser, L. H.: The radiology of basilar thrombosis. Radiology, *85*:23–32, 1965.
183. Schechter, M. M., and Zingesser, L. H.: The anterior spinal artery. Acta Radiol. (Diagn.), *3*:489–495, 1965.
184. Schechter, M. M., and Zingesser, L. H.: The spinal arteries. Acta Radiol. (Diagn.), *5*:1124–1131, 1966.
185. Schechter, M. M., Zingesser, L. H., and Rosenbaum, A.E.: Tentorial meningiomas. Amer. J. Roentgen., *104*:123–131, 1968.
186. Schmidt, H., and Rossi, U.: Intracerebrale extravasation nach Hirnkortusion im Karotisangiogramm. Fortschr. Röntgenstr., *94*:505–508, 1961.
187. Schneider, H. J., and Felson, B.: Buckling of the

innominate artery simulating aneurysm and tumor. Amer. J. Roentgen., *85*:1106–1110, 1961.

188. Schulze, A.: Seltene verlaufsformen epiduraler Hematome. Zbl. Neurochir., *17*:40–47, 1957.
189. Sears, A. D., Miller, J. E., and Kilgore, B. B.: Diagnosis of cerebral atrophy from the anteroposterior carotid phlebogram. Amer. J. Roentgen., *85*:1128–1133, 1961.
190. Seldinger, S. I.: Catheter replacement of the needle in the percutaneous arteriography. A new technique. Acta Radiol., *39*:368–376, 1953.
191. Sergent, P., Rougerie, J., Pertuiset, B., and Petit-Dutailis, D.: L'angiographie vertebrale percutanée cervicale anterieure d'après 130 cas. Technique et bases de l'interpretation des cliches. Presse Méd., *60*:1415–1418, 1952.
192. Sheehan, S., Bauer, R. B., and Meyer, J. S.: Vertebral artery compression in cervical spondylosis, arteriographic demonstration during life of vertebral artery insufficiency due to rotation and extension of the neck. Neurology, *10*:968–986, 1960.
193. Shimidzu, K.: Beitrage zur Arteriographie des Gehirns einfache percutane Methode. Arch. Klin. Chir., *188*:295–316, 1937.
194. Silvan (1913): Quoted by Krayenbühl and Yasargil, see ref. 101.
195. Silverstein, A., Lehrer, G. M., and Mones, R.: Relation of certain diagnostic features of carotid occlusion to collateral circulation. Neurology, *10*:409–417, 1960.
196. Sjögren, S. E.: Anterior choroidal artery. Acta Radiol., *46*:143–157, 1956.
197. Smaltino, F.: Personal comments.
198. Spatz, E. L., and Bull, J. W. D.: Vertebral arteriography in the study of subarachnoid hemorrhage. J. Neurosurg., *14*:543–547, 1957.
199. Stehbens, W. E.: Intracranial arterial aneurysms. Aust. Ann. Med., *3*:214–218, 1954.
200. Stopford, J. S. B.: The arteries of the pons and medulla oblongata. J. Anat., *50*:131–164, 1916.
201. Sugar, O., Holden, L. B., and Powell, C. B.: Vertebral angiography. Amer. J. Roentgen., *61*:166–182, 1949.
202. Sutton, D.: Anomalous carotid basilar anastomosis. Brit. J. Radiol., *23*:617–619, 1950.
203. Sutton, D.: Discussion on the clinical and radiological aspects of diseases of the major arteries. Proc. Roy. Soc. Med., *49*:559–571, 1956.
204. Sutton, D.: Vertebral arteriography by percutaneous brachial artery catheterization. Note to the Editor. Brit. J. Radiol., *32*:283, 1959.
205. Sutton, D.: Arteriography, London, E. & S. Livingstone, Ltd., 1962.
206. Swann, G. F.: Vertebral arteriography using the Sheldon needle and modifications of it. Brit. J. Radiol., *31*:23–27, 1958.
207. Takahashi, K.: Die percutane Arteriographie der Arteria vertebralis und ihrer Versorgungsgebiete. Arch. Psychiat., *111*:373–379, 1940.
208. Takahashi, M., Wilson, G., and Hanafee, W.: Significance of petrosal vein in diagnosis of cerebellopontine angle tumors. Radiology, *89*:834–840, 1967.
209. Taptas, N. N.: Les anévrismes arterio-veineux carotido-caverneux. Neurochirurgie, *8*:385–394, 1963.
210. Tatelman, M.: Pathways of cerebral collateral circulation. Radiology, *75*:349–362, 1960.
211. Taveras, J. M., and Poser, C. M.: Roentgenologic aspects of cerebral angiography in children. Amer. J. Roentgen., *82*:371–391, 1959.
212. Taveras, J. M., and Wood, E. H.: Diagnostic Neuroradiology. Baltimore, Md., Williams & Wilkins Co., 1964.
213. Taveras, J. M., Mount, L. A., and Friedenberg, R. M.: Arteriographic demonstration of external-internal carotid anastomosis through the ophthalmic arteries. Radiology, *63*:525–530, 1954.
214. Tindall, G. T., and Culp, H. B., Jr.: Vertebral arteriography by retrograde injection of the right common carotid artery. Radiology, *76*:742–747, 1961.
215. Tiwisina, T., and Stecker, A. D.: The fresh cranio-cerebral injuries in vascular picture. (In German). Chirurg, *30*:344–349, 1959.
216. Tori, G., and Garusi, G. F.: Left carotid-jugular arteriovenous fistula. Radiol. Clin., *30*:76–85, 1961.
217. Ullrich, D. P., and Sugar, O.: Familial cerebral aneurysms including one extracranial internal carotid aneurysm. Neurology, *10*:288–294, 1960.
218. vander Eecken, H. M., and Adams, R. D.: The anatomy and functional significance of the meningeal arterial anastomosis of the human brain. J. Neuropath. Exp. Neurol., *12*:132–157, 1953.
219. Vaughan, B. F.: Middle meningeal haemorrhage demonstrated angiographically. Brit. J. Radiol., *32*:493–494, 1959.
220. Wall, A. E.: Meningiomas within the lateral ventricle. J. Neurol. Neurosurg. Psychiat., *17*:91–103, 1954.
221. Weiner, I. H., Azzato, N. M., and Mendelsohn, R. A.: Cerebral angiography. J. Neurosurg., *15*:618–626, 1958.
222. Wickbom, I.: Angiography of the carotid artery. Acta Radiol., suppl. 72, 1948.
223. Wickbom, I.: Angiography by post-traumatic intracranial hemorrhages. Acta Radiol., *32*:249–258, 1949.
224. Wickbom, I., and Bartley, O.: Arterial spasm in peripheral arteriography using the catheter method. Acta Radiol., *47*:433–448, 1957.
225. Wilson, C. B., and Cronic, F.: Traumatic arteriovenous fistulas involving the middle meningeal vessels. J.A.M.A., *188*:953–957, 1964.
226. Wolf, B. S., Huang, Y. P., and Newman, C. M.: Superficial sylvian venous drainage system. Amer. J. Roentgen., *89*:398–410, 1963.
227. Wollschlaeger, P. B., and Wollschlaeger, G.: Personal communication, 1968.
228. Wollschlaeger, P. B., and Wollschlaeger, G.: The interhemispheric subdural or falx hematoma. Amer. J. Roentgen., *92*:1252–1254, 1964.
229. Wolman, L.: Cerebral dissecting aneurysms. Brain, *82*:276–291, 1959.
230. Wolpert, S. M., and Schechter, M. M.: Traumatic middle cerebral artery occlusion. Radiology, *87*:671–677, 1966.
231. Wood, E. H.: Angiographic identification of the ruptured lesion in patients with multiple cerebral aneurysms. J. Neurosurg., *21*:182–198, 1964.

232. Wortzman, G.: Traumatic pseudo-aneurysm of the superficial temporal artery. A case report. Radiology, *80*:444–446, 1963.
233. Yates, P. O.: Pathological changes following proximal vertebral arterial stenosis. Proc. Roy. Soc. Med., *50*:663–665, 1957.
234. Zaclis, J., and Tenuto, R. A.: Diagnóstico angiográfico dos hematomas subdurais. Valor de fase venuso em incidência sagital. Arq. Neuropsiquiat., *13*:273–295, 1955.
235. Zielke, K., and Weidner, H.: Eine einfache und ungefährliche Punktionsmethode zue Kontrastmittelfüllung der Arteria vertebralis. Acta Neurochir., *9*:87–101, 1960.
236. Zilkha, A.: Les fistules arterioveineuses traumatiques du carr. Presented at the Eighth Neuroradiological Symposium. Paris, 1967.
237. Zingesser, L. H., Schechter, M. M., and Rayport, M.: Truths and untruths concerning the angiographic findings in extracerebral haematomas, Brit. J. Radiol., *38*:835–847, 1965.
238. Zingesser, L. H., Bernstein, J., Schechter, M.M., and Wollschlaeger, G.: The neuroradiologic significance of anomalies of the aortic arch. Presented at the meeting of the Association of University Radiologists, New Haven, Conn., 1963.

10

ENCEPHALOGRAPHY

PNEUMOENCEPHALOGRAPHY

Radiographic demonstration of the ventricular system was first obtained in 1912.[6] The patient was a man who had been injured in a streetcar accident. As a consequence of a fracture in the posterior wall of the frontal sinus, air had entered the ventricular system. Radiographs demonstrated the air-filled ventricles. It was not until 1918–1919, however, that Walter Dandy deliberately introduced air into the ventricles and into the subarachnoid space of the spinal canal for the purpose of demonstrating the intracranial cerebrospinal fluid-containing spaces.[2,3]

Pneumoencephalography and ventriculography are thus the oldest neuroradiological diagnostic modalities save for the application of the method of Röntgen to the examination of the bones and soft tissues of the head itself. These procedures remained the mainstay of neuroradiological diagnosis, even after the introduction of angiography, until relatively safe contrast media were discovered. Today, computed tomography and cerebral angiography have largely supplanted pneumography in the investigation of intracranial disease. There are, however, lesions of various sorts that are best diagnosed by means of air studies. Advances in our knowledge of the arteriographic and venographic anatomy relating to the ventricular and cisternal anatomy have enabled the expert who is well versed in the interpretation of angiographic studies to make well-informed statements about the exact situation and state of most parts of the ventricular system and cisterns, but the complete demonstration of all parts of the ventricular system and cisterns is possible only with the replacement of spinal fluid with contrast material, which may be either opaque or nonopaque. Thus, certain tumors that are large enough only to protrude into the subarachnoid cisterns, intraventricular lesions, juxtaventricular lesions, certain congenital anomalies, and conditions associated with atrophy of the brain are best studied in this manner (Figs. 10–1 and 10–2).

On the other hand, the angiographic techniques allow the investigation of space-occupying lesions to proceed without alteration of the pressures that have resulted from the intracranial mass lesion. The replacement of cerebrospinal fluid with air or even the addition of air to the cerebrospinal fluid spaces without removal of spinal fluid is the first in a series of events that may lead to shifts in the position of the brain and the mass lesion that will further jeopardize the patient's condition. At times, such shifts in the ventricular system may also give a false impression as to the location of a mass lesion.[12] This is true particularly when cerebral atrophy is present. Situations in which these considerations are vital and ways to minimize these effects are discussed in greater detail later in this chapter.

Preparation of the Patient

A wide variety of medications has been used to prepare the patient for pneumoencephalography. These are given to allay apprehension and to minimize the effects of the study on the vegetative nervous system. Intake of food and fluid should be restricted for several hours before the study is begun. A combination of barbiturates and atropine has, in the authors' experience, been the simplest and most effective way of

L. H. ZINGESSER AND M. M. SCHECHTER

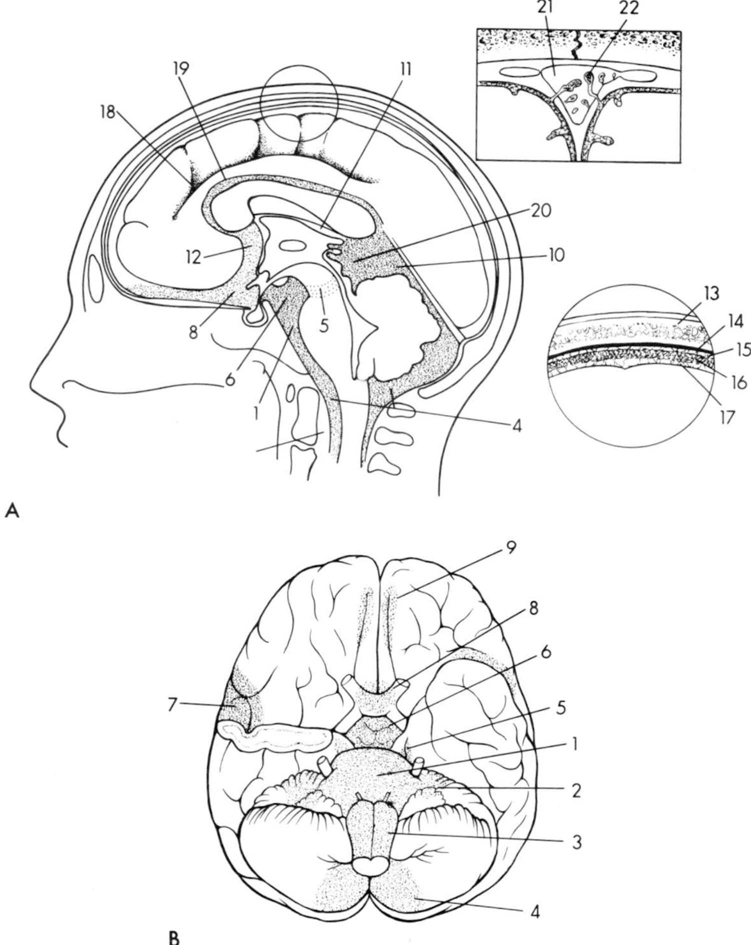

Figure 10–1 *A*. Sagittal view of subarachnoid cisterns. *B*. Basal view of subarachnoid cisterns. 1, Pontine cistern; 2, pontocerebellar cistern; 3, medullary cistern; 4, cisterna magna (vallecular portion communicates with outlet foramina of fourth ventricle); 5, ambient cistern; 6, interpeduncular cistern; 7, cistern of the sylvian fissure; 8, chiasmatic cistern; 9, cistern of the olfactory tract; 10, superior cerebellar cistern; 11, velum interpositum (when filled with air is called the cavum veli interpositi); 12, cistern of the lamina terminalis; 13, calvarium; 14, dura mater; 15, subdural space; 16, arachnoid; 17, subarachnoid space; 18, cistern of the cingulate sulcus; 19, cistern of the corpus callosum; 20, cistern of the quadrigeminal plate or cistern of the great vein of Galen; 21, superior sagittal sinus; 22, arachnoid villus.

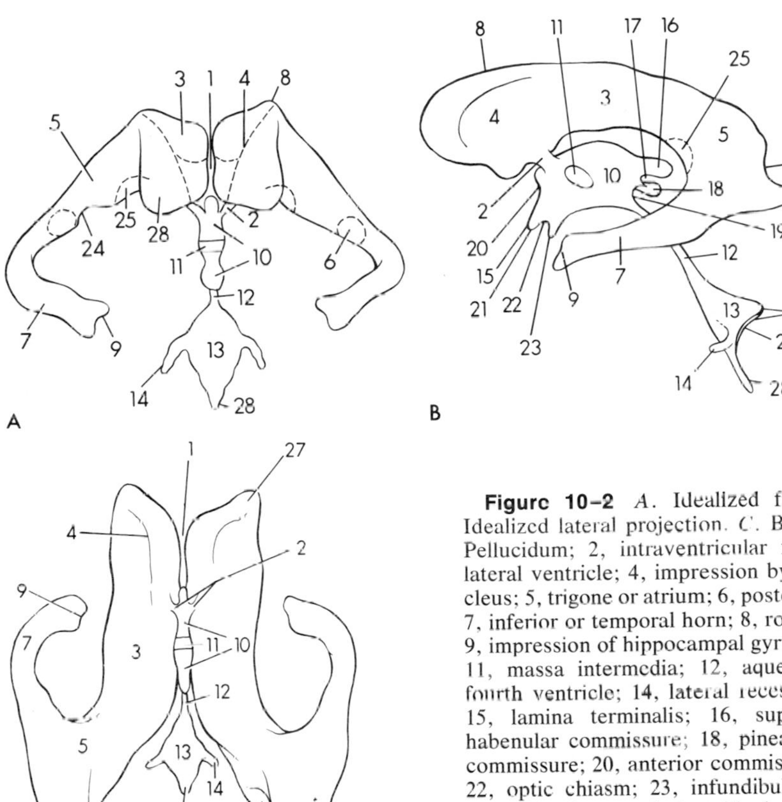

Figure 10–2 *A*. Idealized frontal projection. *B*. Idealized lateral projection. *C*. Basal view. 1, Septum Pellucidum; 2, intraventricular foramen; 3, body of lateral ventricle; 4, impression by head of caudate nucleus; 5, trigone or atrium; 6, posterior or occipital horn; 7, inferior or temporal horn; 8, roof of lateral ventricle; 9, impression of hippocampal gyrus; 10, third ventricle; 11, massa intermedia; 12, aqueduct of Sylvius; 13, fourth ventricle; 14, lateral recess of fourth ventricle; 15, lamina terminalis; 16, suprapineal recess; 17, habenular commissure; 18, pineal body; 19, posterior commissure; 20, anterior commissure; 21, optic recess; 22, optic chiasm; 23, infundibular recess; 24, calcar avis; 25, glomus of choroid plexus; 26, posterior superior recesses of fourth ventricle; 27, frontal horn; 28, foramen of Magendie; 29, impression of nodulus of cerebellum and choroid plexus.

TABLE 10–1 PEDIATRIC NEURORADIOLOGICAL PREMEDICATION

AGE (yr)	SECOBARBITAL (mg/kg)	CHLORPROMAZINE (mg/kg)	ATROPINE (mg/kg)
PNEUMOENCEPHALOGRAMS AND VENTRICULOGRAMS			
Newborn—2 yr	10–8	1.0	0.01
2–4	7–6	1.0	0.01
5–8	6–5	1.0	0.01
9–15	4–3	0.75–0.5	0.01 (up to 0.4 mg per patient)
ANGIOGRAMS AND MYELOGRAMS			
Newborn—2yr	8–7	1.0	0.01
2–4	6–5	1.0	0.01
5–8	5–4	1.0	0.01
9–15	4–3	0.75–0.5	0.01 (up to 0.4 mg per patient)

preparing patients for the study. Problems may arise in elderly individuals in whom the effect of barbiturates may be excitatory rather than sedative and in young persons in whom more medication may have to be used than seems appropriate for the weight of the patient. A dosage schedule of medication for pediatric patients is included here (Table 10–1).[4,9] It must be emphasized that there is a variability in response from patient to patient. In general, the younger the patient, the higher the per kilogram dose requirements.

General anesthesia is seldom used by the authors, for the morbidity of the procedure is probably increased in this way, but this may not be so in certain uncontrollable patients and where the general anesthetic is administered by experienced personnel.

Technique of Pneumoencephalography

The examination can be carried out via the lumbar or the cisternal route. There is usually no advantage to the cisternal route except when the lumbar route is blocked. The spinal puncture should be performed several days after any previous spinal puncture. Otherwise the spinal fluid that issues from the needle may be coming from a pool in the subdural space rather than from the subarachnoid space.

Selection of the proper needle is of great importance. The smaller the needle, the smaller the hole remaining when the needle is removed, and the less leakage of spinal fluid. This is an important consideration in patients with increased intracranial pressure. A 20-gauge needle in adults and a 22-gauge needle in children are recommended. The bevel of the needle should be short. This is very important, for the risk of injection of air into the subdural space is minimized with the short-beveled needle.

If it is necessary to collect spinal fluid for laboratory assay, this fluid should be collected immediately. A cellular response occurs very rapidly after the introduction of air, and the protein value may be altered also. Generally it is best to remove as little fluid as possible, especially in the early stages of the examination, and it is best to remove no fluid if intracranial pressure is raised.

The needle is introduced in the conventional way in the lumbar area and the usual sensations are felt as the needle penetrates the theca. When the stylet is removed, the spinal fluid should flow freely. If it does not, gentle manipulation of the needle may be required, for a fold of arachnoid or a nerve root may be blocking the needle even though it is centrally placed within the spinal canal. When a long-beveled needle is used, free flow of spinal fluid does not guarantee that the air introduced is going to pass into the subarachnoid space. Some workers believe that the needle should be introduced so that the bevel is longitudinally oriented. It is claimed that in this way the fibers of the dura are separated and not interrupted.

The patient should be comfortably seated. A "military" position of the head and neck is usually effective in directing the first air into the vallecular portion of the cisterna magna and thence into the foramen of Magendie. If the patient's neck and head are overflexed, the bulk of the air will pass over the surface of the cerebellum, which is desirable only if the pathological condition to be studied is located in that area. With overextension of the head and neck, the bulk of the air will pass into the pontine cistern and then go through the interpeduncular cistern to pass through a membrane usually located in that area to enter the cisterns at the base of the brain. From that location the air will pass around the lateral and anterior portions of the brain as it ascends to the high convexity.

The first films are critical in that they will indicate whether the needle is correctly placed, whether tonsillar herniation exists, and whether the posterior fossa is free of disease. Also, on later films cisternal air may obscure the aqueduct. The radiographic equipment that is employed should therefore provide for the necessity of obtaining horizontal and half-axial films of good quality with the patient erect. Apparatus that includes an upright Bucky grid for the half-axial films is a necessity. The lateral films obtained with a high-quality stationary grid, however, will be satisfactory. Some workers find the use of Polaroid films or image-intensification equipment to be advantageous in following the early passage of the air.

On these early films, careful attention is paid to the craniocervical junction. The cervical cord itself is evaluated, and one looks for evidence of tonsillar herniation. At times, the lobe of the ear overlies this area and simulates tonsillar herniation; it is advantageous to tape the ears forward in order to obviate this difficulty.

According to the path followed by the air on these early films, an adjustment in the position of the head and neck may have to be made to direct the air to the foramen of Magendie. If a large cisterna magna is present, considerable air may have to be introduced before the air-fluid level drops below the foramen of Magendie and air enters the fourth ventricle.

There are occasions when, in spite of proper positioning of the patient and correct placement of the needle (so that there is no evidence of subdural injection of air), the air does not enter the fourth ventricle. As long as there is no evidence of tonsillar herniation the study should be continued, introducing a total of at least about 30 cc of air. Oftentimes, the changes in the subarachnoid cisterns will afford valuable information. A tumor may be demonstrated in the cistern, and the size of the ventricles can be estimated if the air passes into the cistern of the corpus callosum. Disease in the fourth ventricle may account for the absence of filling of the ventricular system in some cases, but there are a significant number of cases in which nonfilling of the system occurs when the lesion is not in the posterior fossa. When the reason for nonfilling of the ventricles is thought to be increased intracranial pressure, an infusion of a hypertonic solution such as urea or mannitol may be helpful in getting the ventricles to fill.[11] Brow-up and brow-down films should be obtained even though the ventricles do not fill when the patient is erect because some air may enter the ventricles when the patient is repositioned for these views.

The patient with nonfilling of the ven-

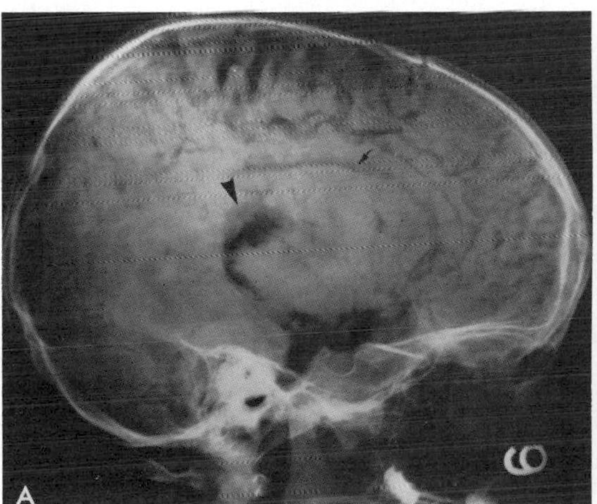

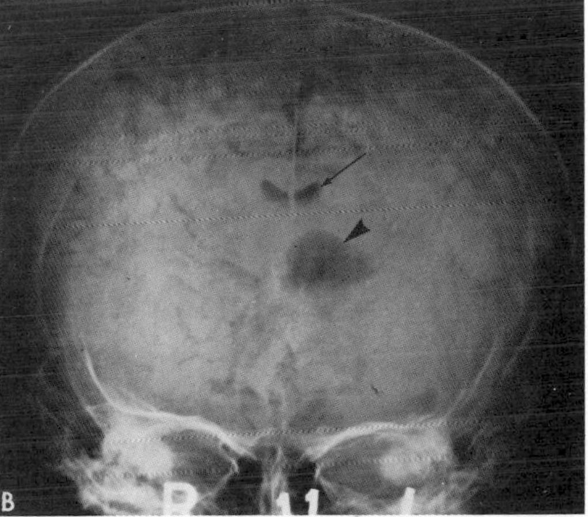

Figure 10–3 Lateral, *A*, and anteroposterior Towne, *B*, projections of patient with nonfilling of the ventricular system following the introduction of air via the lumbar route. The large arrowhead points to air in a portion of the wing of the ambient cistern. This cistern is dilated. The small arrow points to a dilated cistern of the corpus callosum. Note also the sulci of the convexity. The changes indicated here are *not* the result of atrophy, but usually indicate the presence of a tumor in the midline of the posterior fossa. Further studies—angiography or ventriculography—are needed to demonstrate the lesion in this case, but cisternal air may at times outline a portion of the tumor.

tricular system should be regarded with a high index of suspicion. A significant percentage of these patients will be shown, on other studies, to have an intracranial mass lesion. Dilatation of certain subarachnoid cisterns, particularly the wings of the ambient cisterns and the pericallosal cistern, is especially significant (in conjunction with nonfilling of the ventricular system) as an indication of pressure hydrocephalus (Fig. 10–3).

The air should be fractionally introduced in increments of about 10 cc. The first film should be taken after the introduction of the first 10cc. It should be a lateral film that is coned to show the posterior fossa and craniocervical junction.

The second film should be a tomogram or autotomogram of the posterior fossa. Equipment for doing midline tomography with the patient in the erect position is not generally available. Since autotomography is a most valuable and yet simple technique for the clear demonstration of the fourth ventricle and aqueduct free of confusing bone shadows caused by the overlying mastoid air cells, its technique is described. The patient rests his forehead against a sponge taped to the headstand, and the head is rocked from side to side either by the patient himself or with the assistance of the examiner. An exposure time of two or three seconds is used. The film so obtained will show in sharp focus those midline structures along the axis of rotation passing through the odontoid. Structures that are lateral to the axis of rotation will be blurred. It is desirable to obtain delineation of these structures before the cisterns have been flooded with air, for the air in the cisterns adjacent to the aqueduct will otherwise obscure the aqueduct (Fig. 10–4).

The fourth ventricle contains a number of recesses, the two lateral recesses, and the posterior superior recess. These compartments may be appreciated only in a general way on the initial films of the air study, which include a lateral film showing the passage of the first air into the fourth ventricle, an autotomogram, and a reverse Towne (half-axial) view (Fig. 10–5). Appreciation of these various compartments is enhanced when tomography in the coronal plane is employed, but since it is laborious and time-consuming, this procedure is not warranted unless disease is suspected in this area of the fourth ventricle. Information obtained from the routine films is sufficient in most cases. The rostral portion of the fourth ventricle (anterior medullary velum) generally is flat or convex inferiorly. The posterior portion of the fourth ventricle (posterior medullary velum) has a distinct convexity inward. The "indentation" should be recognized as normal, being due to the nodulus of the cerebellum and to the choroid plexus in the area. There are various measurements that relate the position of the fourth ventricle to bony landmarks. One of the most useful of these is based on

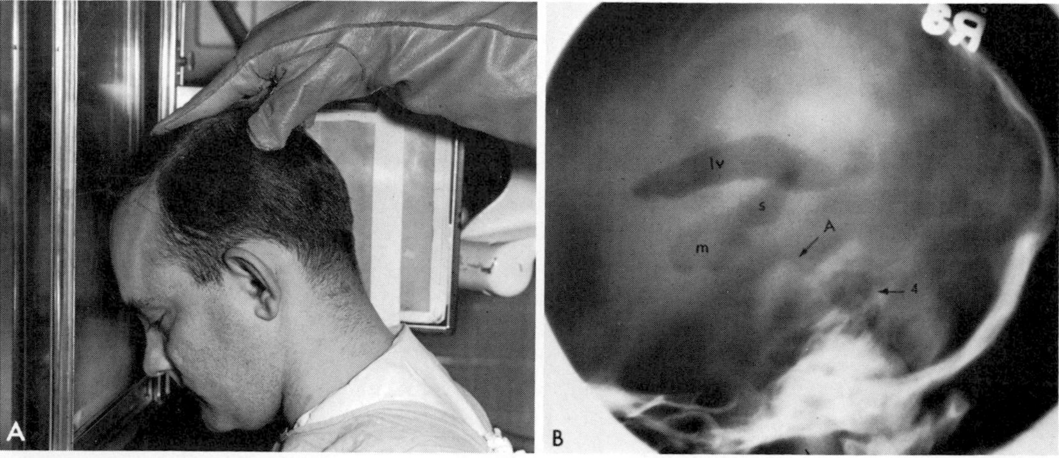

Figure 10–4 *A*. Patient positioned for autotomography. The patient's head will be rocked back and fourth while his forehead is pressed against the head unit. *B*. Autotomogram taken after the introduction of 10 cc of air. Structures outlined are the fourth ventricle (4), aqueduct (A), third ventricle (containing m, the massa intermedia, and s, the suprapineal recess), and a lateral ventricle (lv).

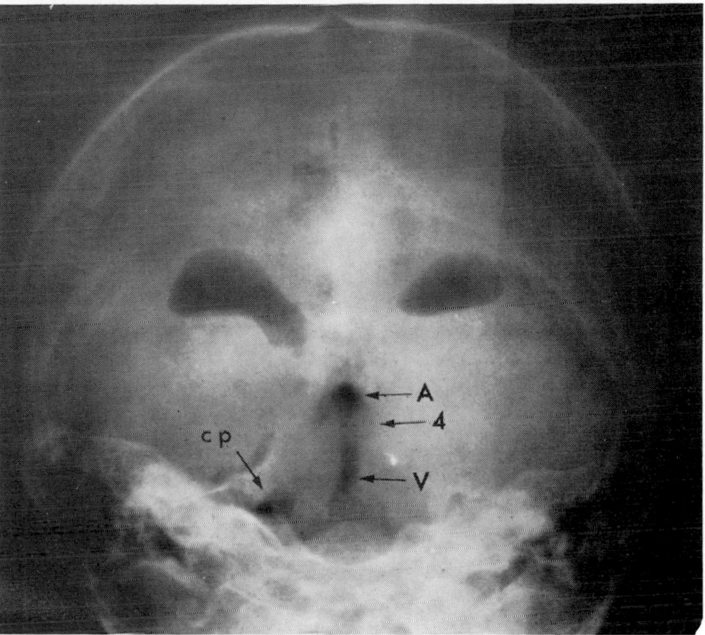

Figure 10–5 Reverse Towne projection. The vallecula (V), the fourth ventricle (4), and the point of entry of the aqueduct (A) into the fourth ventricle are demonstrated. In addition there is air in the right cerebellopontine angle (cp).

Twining's line: A line is drawn connecting the tuberculum sella and the torcular Herophili. The line is bisected. The midpoint should fall within and lie close to the floor of the fourth ventricle.[13]

The aqueduct should describe a gentle curve paralleling the curve of the inner table of the skull. Occasionally one sees a slight normal "kink" in the region of the quadrigeminal plate. A useful method of locating the position of the normal aqueduct is the Lysholm or Sahlstedt system. A line is drawn from the dorsum sellae to a point on the inner table of the skull. (The point may be selected anywhere along the inner table; the line that is thereby determined will pass through the aqueduct.) This line is then divided into thirds. The aqueduct should lie at the junction of the proximal and middle thirds.[7] In the postero-anterior half-axial projection, the fourth ventricle (including the lateral recesses), the aqueduct, and the posterior part of the third ventricle can be identified in the midline as the air passes through them.

In addition to the positions of the parts of the ventricular system just mentioned, the following cisterns should be demonstrated on these early films with the patient erect: the cisterna magna and the medullary, pontine, interpeduncular, ambient, crural, and chiasmatic cisterns. Extension of the head at the time the air is introduced may be necessary to direct the air into them. Reversing this maneuver (flexing the head) may be helpful when it is desired to direct air into cisterns above the cerebellum.

After all these structures have been demonstrated, an additional lateral film is obtained to demonstrate the roof of the lateral ventricles, and to ascertain whether there is enough ventricular air to carry out the remainder of the study. To expand on these two points, midline lesions such as parasagittal or falx meningiomas in the posterior frontal area may be demonstrated better on this than on subsequent lateral films mainly because the portion of the lateral ventricle affected most by such lesions is best displayed on this erect lateral film (Fig. 10–6). The second reason for taking this film is to ascertain whether enough air is present for the remainder of the examination. As a rough guide, enough air should be present within the lateral ventricles so that when the patient is turned brow-up the air-fluid level extends several centimeters posterior to the foramen of Monro. More air will be required in some patients than in others. Although the normal adult ventricular system contains only about 21 cc, most studies will require that twice this amount be introduced in order to obtain sufficient ventricular filling, and sometimes substantially more is required. This is so mainly because of the not inconsiderable fraction of air that

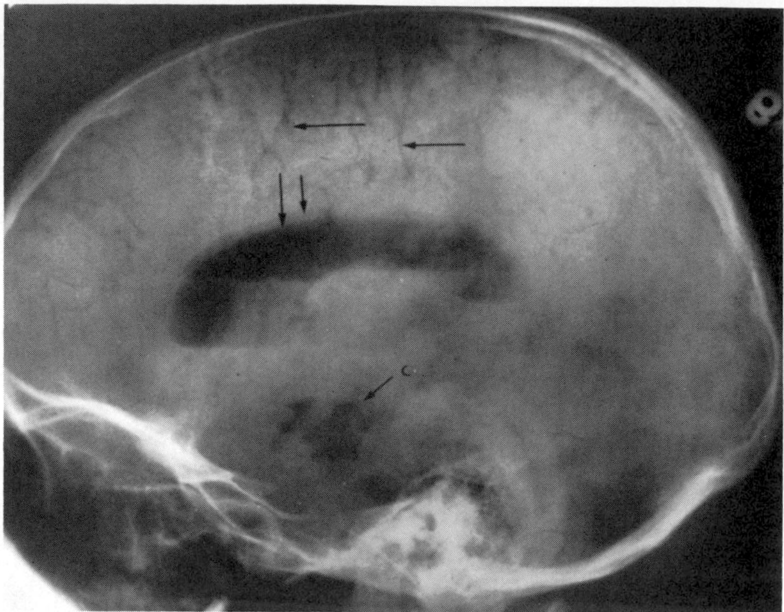

Figure 10–6 Lateral projection with the patient erect. The roofs of the two lateral ventricles are well demonstrated (*two vertical arrows*). The two horizontal arrows indicate a few of the sulci that are outlined by air. The arrow labeled c indicates the region of the interpeduncular cistern, which merges with the chiasmatic cistern anteriorly and the pontine cistern inferiorly.

passes into the cisterns rather than into the ventricular system.

It is important that the examination of the posterior fossa should be accomplished as rapidly as possible to minimize the amount of time the patient spends in the sitting position. This is especially true when the systemic blood pressure is low and when the intracranial pressure is elevated.

The next part of the examination is carried out with the patient in the brow-up position. Several films are obtained at this point, including two frontal views, an anteroposterior view, a Towne projection, and a lateral view (Fig. 10–7). On these films the anterior horns and a portion of the bodies of the lateral ventricles are demonstrated. Structures adjacent to these portions of the ventricular system, i.e., the genu and rostrum of the corpus callosum, the heads of the caudate nuclei, anterior portions of the thalamus making up the floor of the lateral ventricles, and the lateral wall of the body of the lateral ventricles should be identified. The septum pellucidum can be identified here and should be inspected because its displacement may indicate the presence of a mass lesion and also because it may be the primary site of a pathological process.

The type of displacement of the septum pellucidum may do more than indicate the presence of a mass lesion—it may indicate in a fairly precise way whether the lesion is high or low and whether it is anterior or posterior. Anterior or posterior placement of the lesion is, however, usually best indicated on the Towne projection, as this film displays the anterior portion of the septum pellucidum inferiorly and the more posterior portion of the septum pellucidum superiorly. An assessment of whether a lesion is high or low in location is best carried out by utilizing the configuration of the lateral angle of the lateral ventricle as well as the septum pellucidum and the anterior portion of the third ventricle.

Primary pathological conditions involving the septum pellucidum include a wide range of diseases. The septum may be congenitally absent (Fig. 10–8). It may be extremely thin as, for example, in patients with marked hydrocephalus, or it may be perforated as, for example, in boxers or because of the thinning resulting from extreme hydrocephalus. The septum may appear abnormally thick, and if this is so, a differentiation must be made between a cavum septi pellucidi, a primary tumor of the septum pellucidum, and a hemispheric

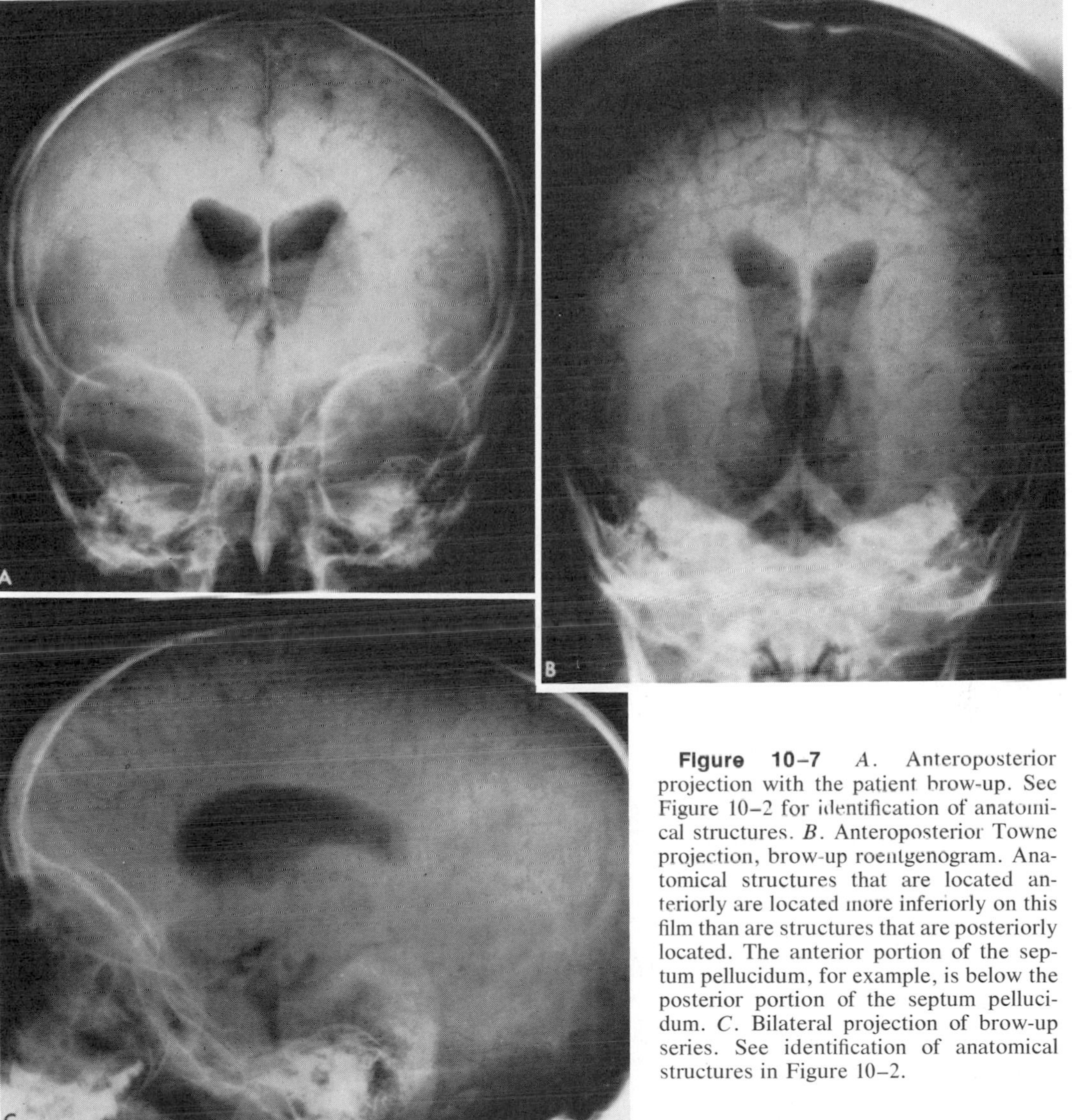

Figure 10–7 *A*. Anteroposterior projection with the patient brow-up. See Figure 10–2 for identification of anatomical structures. *B*. Anteroposterior Towne projection, brow-up roentgenogram. Anatomical structures that are located anteriorly are located more inferiorly on this film than are structures that are posteriorly located. The anterior portion of the septum pellucidum, for example, is below the posterior portion of the septum pellucidum. *C*. Bilateral projection of brow-up series. See identification of anatomical structures in Figure 10–2.

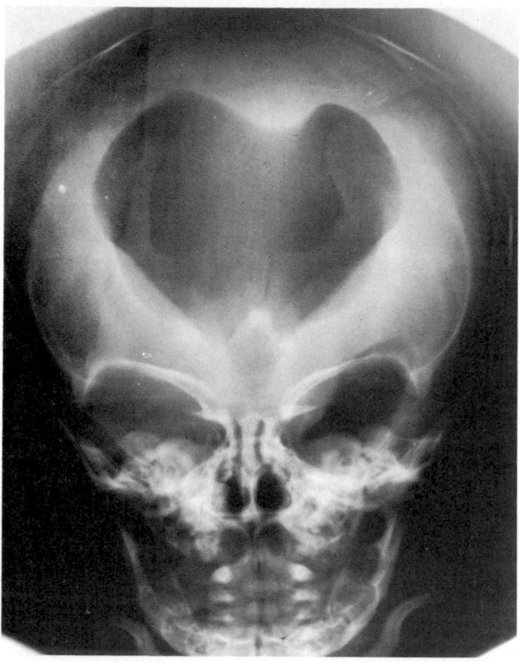

Figure 10–8 Brow-up anteroposterior film of patient with the Arnold-Chiari malformation. Absence of the septum pellucidum is demonstrated. The lateral ventricles are dilated and have a more pointed configuration anteriorly and inferiorly than is normal. Both these features are frequently seen in the Arnold-Chiari malformation.

lesion extending into the septum pellucidum, perhaps by way of the corpus callosum.

A cavum of the septum pellucidum may or may not fill with air at the time of the initial study. If it does not, it is not uncommonly filled on films taken a number of hours or a day later. Such a lesion, when fluid filled, does not usually bulge asymmetrically into the medial portions of the anterior horns. A primary tumor of the septum will usually, but not always, demonstrate some asymmetry. Features that would lead one to suspect that a thickening of the septum pellucidum is caused by a tumor extending into the septum pellucidum from the corpus callosum are abnormalities such as indentations along the roof of the lateral ventricle and perhaps the demonstration of an abnormally thick corpus callosum, as indicated by the air in the cistern of the corpus callosum and its distance from the air within the ventricles. Irregularity of the roof of the lateral ventricles may be a normal finding. In the interpretation of their meaning, degree and configuration of the irregular areas must be taken into account.

After the three brow-up films have been obtained, additional maneuvers should be carried out to demonstrate anterior portions of the ventricular system that may not have been clearly visualized. The first of these is designed to demonstrate the anterior portion of the third ventricle to advantage. With the patient brow-up (sometimes with his head hanging back in order to direct air from the lateral ventricles into the

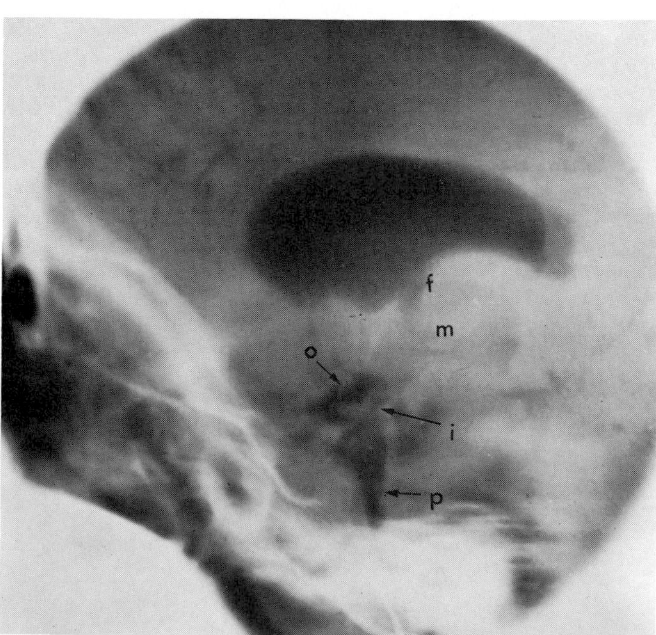

Figure 10–9 Brow-up autotomogram. The optic (o) and infundibular (i) recesses of the anterior portion of the third ventricle are visualized through the air in the chiasmatic cistern. The foramen of Monro is labeled f, the pontine cistern, p, and the massa intermedia, m.

anterior portion of the third ventricle), the patient's head is rocked from side to side while a two- or three-second exposure is carried out in the lateral projection. This film usually demonstrates well the two recesses of the anterior third ventricle—the optic and the infundibular recesses (Fig. 10–9). There are times, however, when these recesses are obscured by air in the cisterns adjacent. If the maneuver just described is repeated 24 hours following the introduction of the air, most or all of the cisternal air will have been absorbed so that the anterior third ventricle will no longer be obscured. Identification of these recesses within the third ventricle, the lamina terminalis, and the anterior commissure, and more posteriorly, the massa intermedia can then be made. The massa intermedia is quite variable in size. Confusion with a colloid cyst of the third ventricle (occurring just behind the foramen of Monro) is sometimes possible. A large massa intermedia and diverticulum of the anterior portion of the third ventricle as well as an absence of the septum pellucidum may be seen in patients with the Arnold-Chiari malformation. An accessory bundle of fibers (Meynert's commissure) may be seen in the anterior third ventricle in the Arnold-Chiari malformation (cf. Fig. 10–13).[5]

The other portion of the ventricular anatomy to be demonstrated with the patient in the brow-up position is the top of the temporal horn. Both temporal tips may be demonstrated if the patient's head is extended as far posteriorly as possible (off the edge of the table) and a film is taken with the beam directed through the orbits. Frequently, the lateral and supracornual clefts of the temporal horns can be identified if there is enough air in the temporal horns (Fig. 10–10). If this maneuver is unsuccessful because not enough air leaves the body of the lateral ventricle, then the horns can be filled one at a time. This is accomplished by turning the head to one side, then dropping the head below the edge of the table, and then turning the head brow-up into a neutral position. The perorbital view is again obtained in order to demonstrate each temporal horn.

After the anterior portions of the ventricular system have been demonstrated, the patient is turned into the brow-down position and three more films are obtained. These should include a posteroanterior view, a reverse Towne view (half-axial), and a lateral view (Fig. 10–11). Here the posterior portion of the bodies of the lateral ventricles, the occipital horns (when they are present), and the posterior portions of the temporal horns will be displayed. The term specifying the juncture of these portions of the ventricles is the "trigone"; sometimes the term "atrium" is used to de-

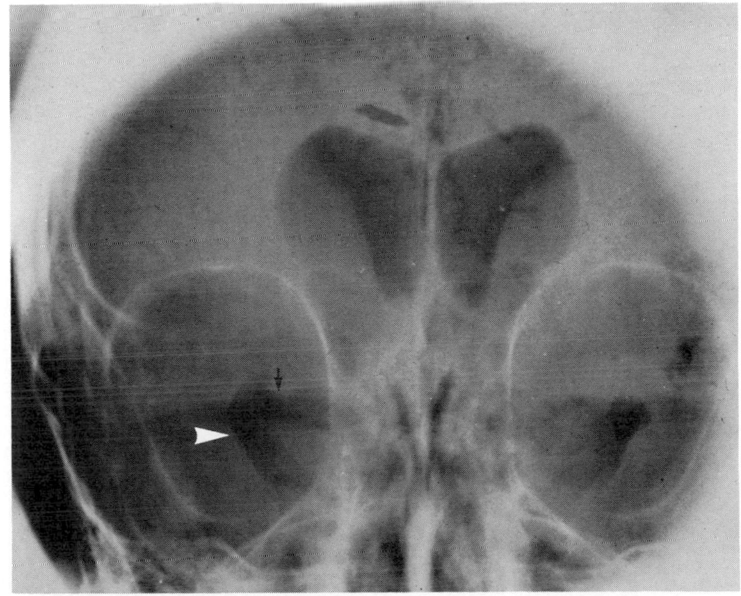

Figure 10–10 Anteroposterior projection of the temporal horns through the orbits. The large arrowhead indicates the lateral cleft and the small arrow indicates the supracornual cleft.

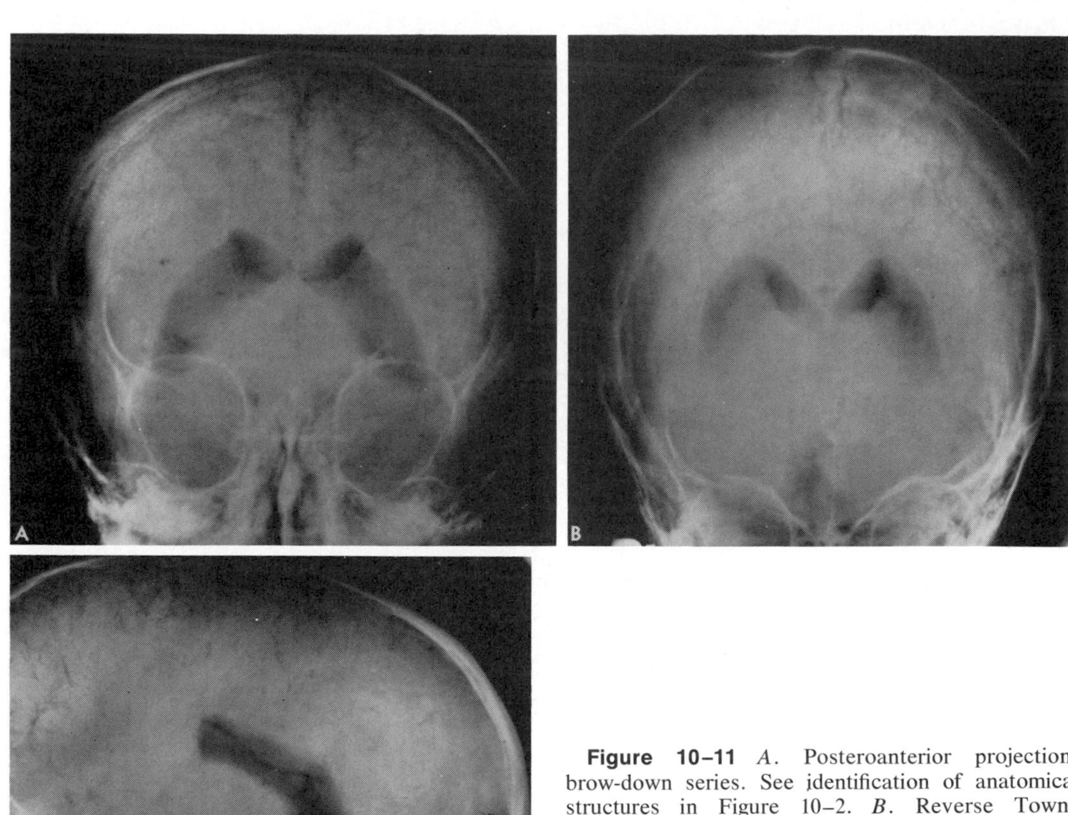

Figure 10–11 *A*. Posteroanterior projection, brow-down series. See identification of anatomical structures in Figure 10–2. *B*. Reverse Towne projection of brow-down series. *C*. Lateral projection of brow-down series.

note this area. Two features of the normal anatomy seen best on these views include the glomus of the choroid plexus of the lateral ventricle and the calcar avis.

The examination is usually complete at this point, but at times other views may be required. If the middle segment of the temporal horn has not deen demonstrated, it may be necessary to turn the patient into the decubitus position in order to obtain views of the temporal horn with a horizontal and a vertical x-ray beam. It may even be necessary to obtain films with the patient suspended upside down in order to trap considerable air in the temporal horns.

Films obtained 24 hours after injection of the air may be of aid in specific circumstances. As has been mentioned, cisternal air has largely disappeared by this time, and a better view of portions of the ventricular anatomy may be possible. Another reason for obtaining late films is that a porencephalic cyst may be demonstrated even when it did not fill previously. Also, a cyst of the septum pellucidum may require some time to fill with air. The ventricles usually appear larger at this time (Fig. 10–12).

Space allotted precludes all but an abbreviated presentation of lesions that may be demonstrated pneumoencephalographically. The illustrations selected show mainly those lesions that require an air study for optimal demonstration; most of them are closely related to the ventricular system (Figs. 10–13, 10–14, 10–15, 10–16, and 10–17).

Air in the cisterns or the absence of air in the cisterns may be of primary importance in neuroradiological diagnosis, as is indicated by the next set of illustrations. Atrophy of gray matter is indicated by dilation of sulci and by separation of cerebellar folia. Tumors may be large enough to be recognized in the cisterns, and yet they may have not reached a size sufficient to displace a portion of the ventricular system. Finally, the passage of air through the tentorial notch and up over the cerebral convexities is to be expected if the examination is properly conducted, and absence of these events may indicate a block in the subarachnoid pathways.

At times, it may be thought desirable to employ a gas other than air for the demonstration of the ventricular anatomy. A variety of gases has been employed, including carbon dioxide and nitrous oxide. Claims have been made for lesser morbidity with these gases than with air. Their absorption is more rapid, and in any event the gas that is found in the lateral ventricles after a period of time is a result of the partial pressures of these gases in the blood. In the authors' institution, carbon dioxide is used only to study a child with a ventricular-vascular shunt, and it must be stated that even in this circumstance, there is no report of an air embolus resulting from a pneumoencephalographic examination performed with air.

A discussion of the morbidity and mortality that may result from pneumoencephalography should include the following considerations: tonsillar herniation, air embolism, extracerebral hematoma formation, and meningitis, as well as the common events such as headache, nausea, and vomiting.

Tonsillar herniation is most apt to occur as a result of increased intracranial pressure. Further, it is more apt to occur in patients who have increased intracranial pressure as a result of a supratentorial mass lesion than in those who have increased intracranial pressure as a result of a mass lesion in the posterior fossa. It may be desirable to perform an air study by a spinal puncture in a patient who has increased intracranial pressure because the information obtained from cisternal air contrast is required or because it is considered unwise to go through the steps of ventriculographic procedure. In this situation, certain precautions should be observed. These include having the equipment and the personnel available for tapping the ventricles if evidence of tonsillar herniation develops. As always, the air should be introduced fractionally and in small increments. An inspection of early lateral films should be made for evidence of tonsillar herniation. No more air should be introduced than is necessary to demonstrate the lesion (and sometimes to exclude other lesions). After the diagnosis has been made, in patients with a high degree of intracranial pressure, it is advisable to follow the diagnostic procedure with the appropriate operative therapy or to institute ventricular drainage if the operation is to be delayed. The bad reputation that pneumoencephalography acquired in the investigation of patients with increased intracranial pressure is due, in part, to the

Text continued on page 368.

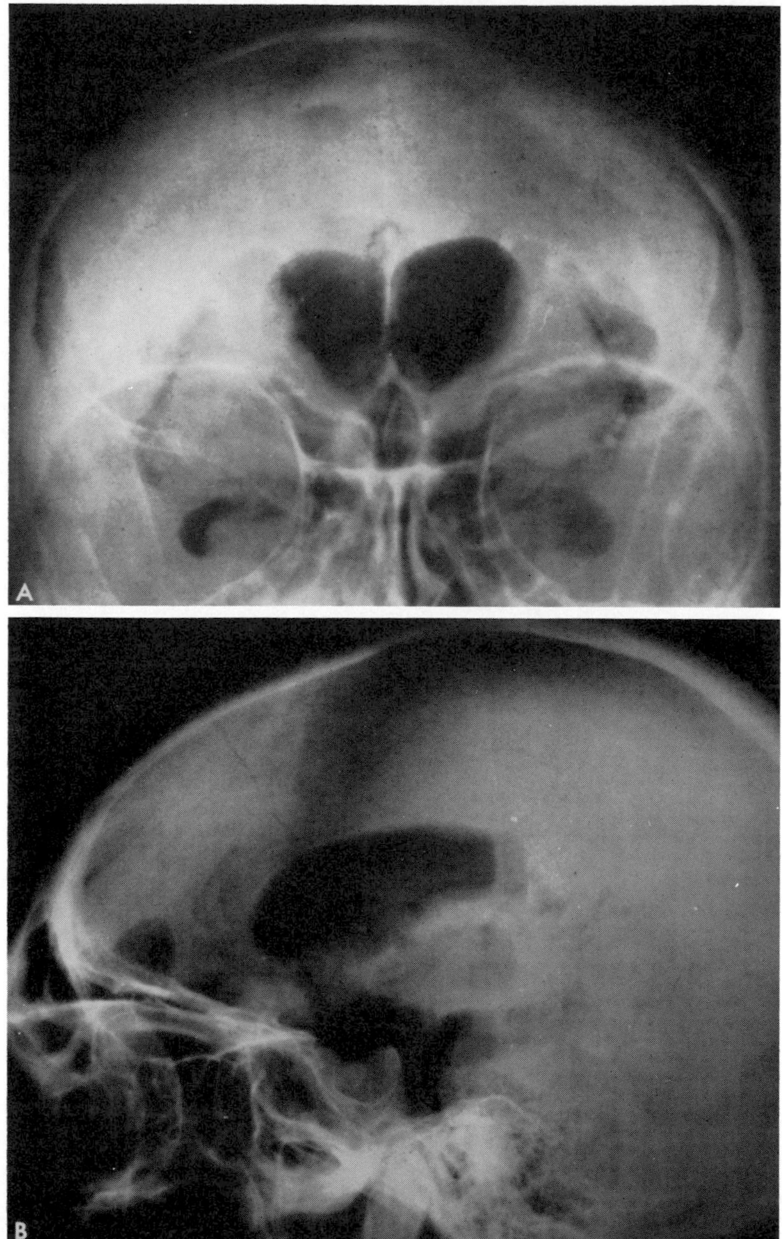

Figure 10–12 *A* and *B*. Anteroposterior and lateral films of patient with large porencephalic cyst in the left temporal lobe.

Illustration continued on opposite page.

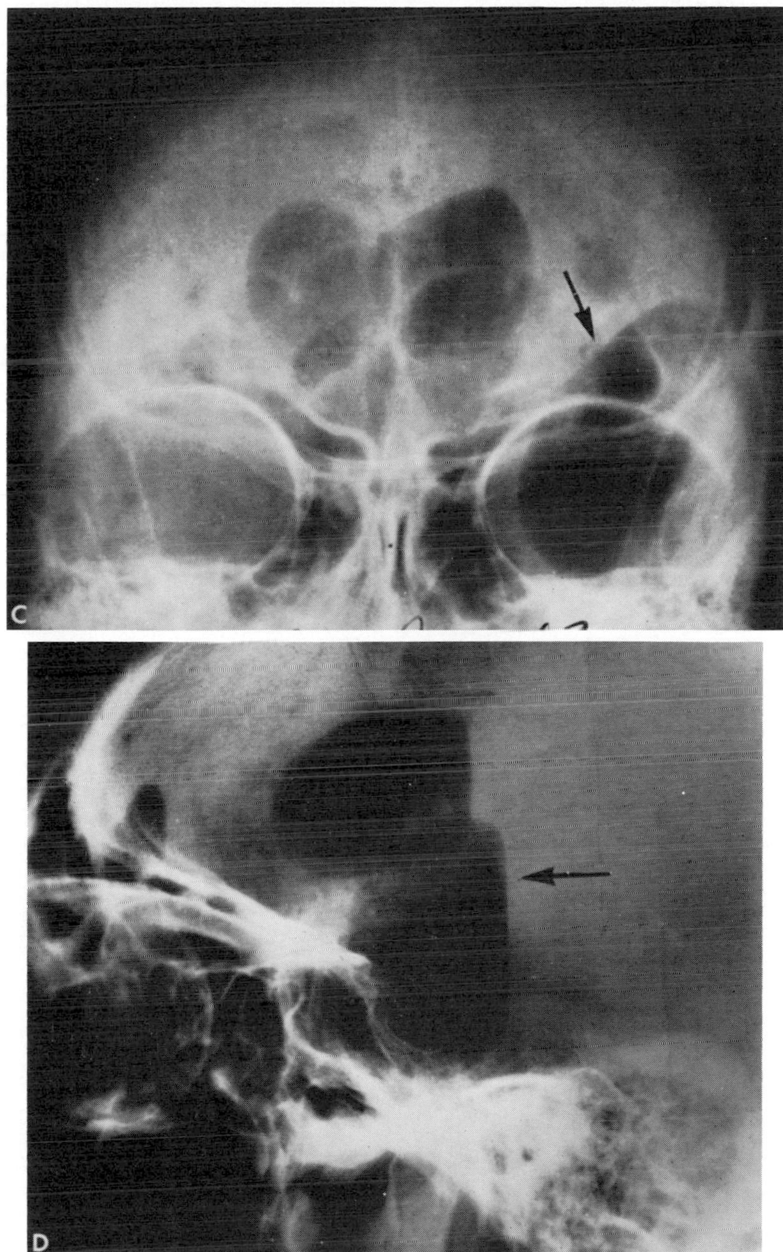

Figure 10–12 (*continued*) *C* and *D*. Same patient 24 hours later. The porencephalic cyst has filled with air.

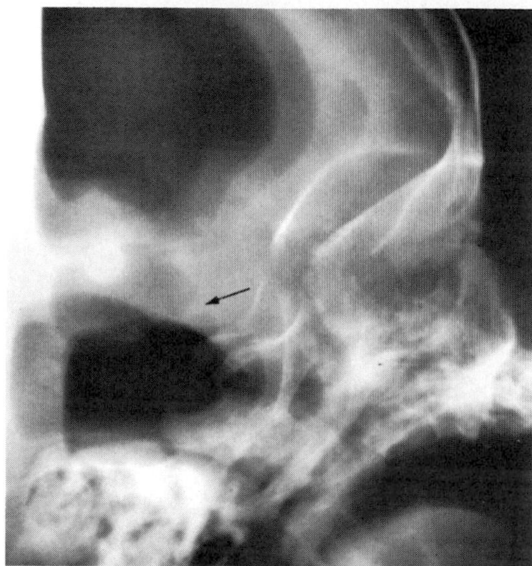

Figure 10–13 Same patient as in Figure 10–8. The arrow points to an accessory bundle of fibers (Meynert's commissure). This also is a common finding in the Arnold-Chiari malformation.

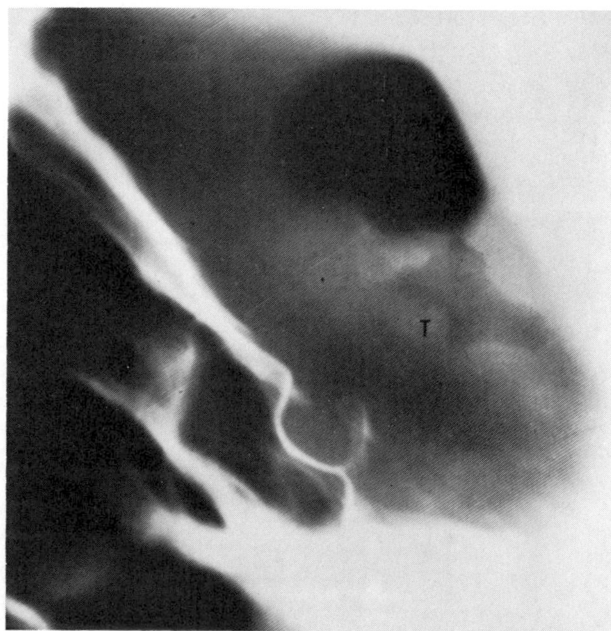

Figure 10–14 Autotomogram with the patient's head hanging back ("hanging-head autotomogram"). Air has spilled from the lateral ventricles into the anterior third ventricle. The recesses are splayed by a tumor (T) that was not demonstrated angiographically. The tumor, which was removed, proved to be a craniopharyngioma.

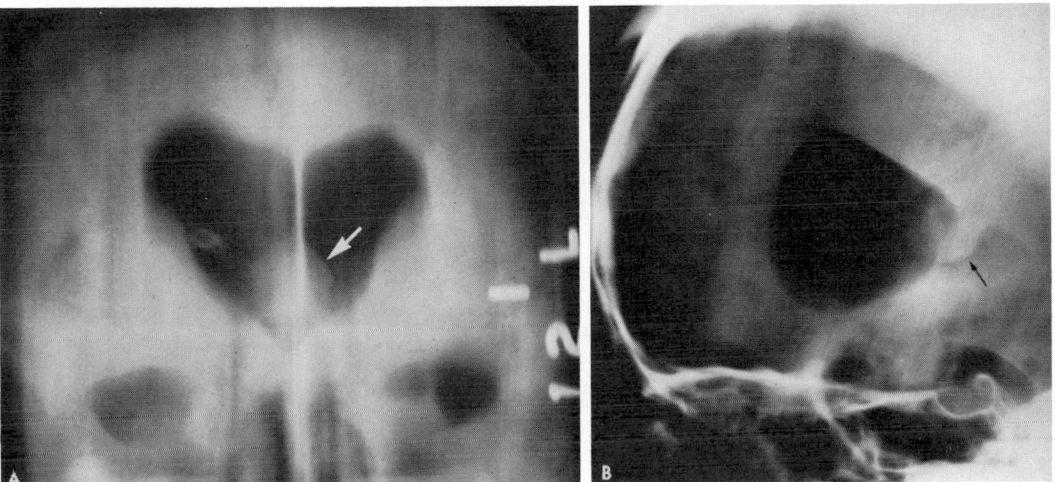

Figure 10–15 *A*. Brow-up anteroposterior tomogram demonstrating a colloid cyst of the third ventricle (*arrow*). These lesions may sometimes be diagnosed angiographically because of changes in the venographic phase that indicate a third-ventricular mass lesion. They are best delineated with air, however. Note also the shunt tube in the right lateral ventricle. *B*. Same patient as in Figure 10–15*A*, hanging-head lateral view. Air outlines the anterior aspect of the colloid cyst (*arrow*), which is located just behind the foramen of Monro.

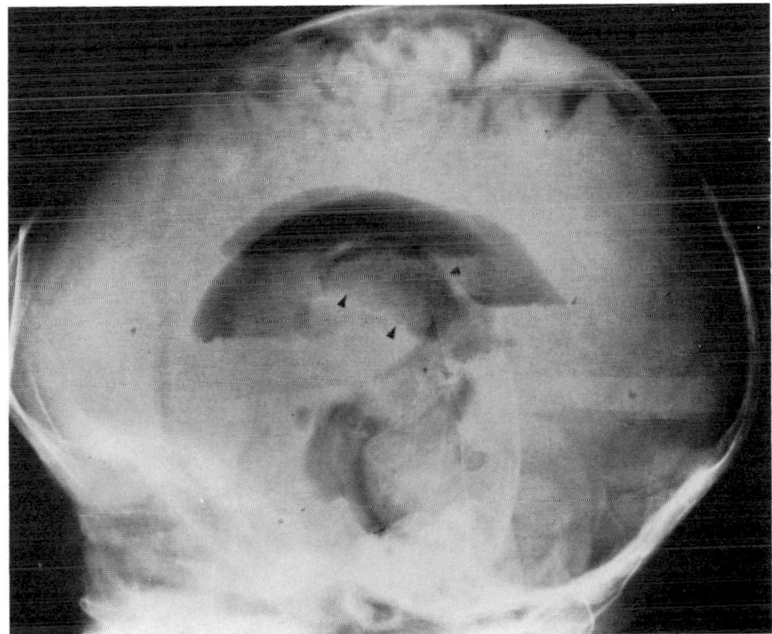

Figure 10–16 Lateral projection, patient erect. The arrowheads indicate a cavum veli interpositi above the third ventricle. This space communicates with the cisterns of the quadrigeminal plate posteriorly. This differentiates it from a cavum vergae, which fills after the ventricles fill and is always associated with a cavum septi pellucidi.

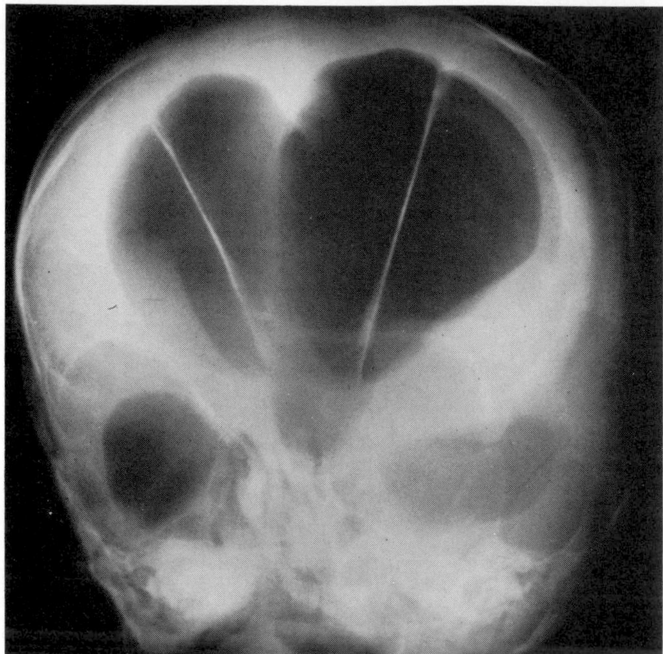

Figure 10–17 Ventricular bands in hydrocephaly resulting from ependymitis.

fact that large increments of air were introduced with no radiological control and that patients were put to bed for a considerable time after the completion of the procedure before operation was undertaken. The condition of a patient who has a ventriculographic study because of increased intracranial pressure may also deteriorate if the study is not followed with appropriate operative therapy.

Air embolization is an extremely serious complication of improperly conducted encephalographic examination. It occurs only when large amounts of air are introduced into the subdural space and will not occur if one adheres to correct technique. One should not be trapped into introducing large quantities of air into the subdural space in persistent attempts to "adjust" the needle so that the air may be introduced into the subarachnoid space. Frequently, the subarachnoid space is collapsed as more and more subdural air is introduced so that it becomes virtually impossible to achieve what is desired. It is best to terminate the study and to delay any further attempts to study the patient via this route for a period of several days.

Another serious complication that may occur is the production of an extracerebral (particularly a subdural) hematoma. This also is more apt to occur in a situation in which considerable subdural air has been introduced. It is even more likely if there is pre-existing cerebral atrophy. Bridging veins are more susceptible to injury if these factors are present. Another factor that may be important in this context is anticoagulation. Anticoagulation is a relative contraindication to pneumoencephalography.

A mild or moderate meningitis of the aseptic variety frequently follows pneumoencephalography, and this is indicated by a low-grade fever and by a cellular response in the spinal fluid. A more severe chemical meningitis may result if there are contaminating chemicals on the needle or tubing used in the performance of the procedure. Bacterial meningitis is infrequent. In an attempt to avoid this complication, some authorities have advocated using air that is filtered. There is no adequate proof that filtering the air will reduce the already low incidence of bacterial meningitis as a complication of pneumoencephalography.

The minor complications such as headache and vomiting are common and will subside after a relatively short period of time. These complications are often quite distressing to the patient and may preclude his cooperation in other neuroradiological studies. It is for this reason that pneumoencephalography is sometimes called a "sign-out procedure." It is interesting that headache seems to result mainly from air in the cisterns rather than in the ventricles. In fact, patients do not usually complain of headache until a quantity of air reaches the cisterns. It is also of interest, although not easy to explain, that patients with atrophy may experience no headache whatsoever. Some workers believe that introducing the air without removing spinal fluid reduces the incidence and severity of headache. Experience, however, does not confirm this belief.

VENTRICULOGRAPHY

Dandy, in 1918, succeeded in demonstrating the ventricular system in hydrocephalic infants by inserting a needle through an area of sutural diastasis and then through the brain into the ventricular system.[2] In adults, the puncture is carried out through twist drill holes or through burr holes in the calvarium. The hole may be placed posteriorly so that the atrium of the ventricle is entered, but there is danger that the needle may enter the vascular glomus lying on the floor of the atrium and cause a hematoma.

Often, the hole is made anteriorly through the coronal suture and 2.5 cm from the midline on the side of the nondominant hemisphere. Ventriculography may be performed through twist drill holes, and the contrast material introduced via a Scott cannula. A drill bit of adequate size to introduce the Scott cannula should be selected, and the hole should be drilled at the same angle at which the cannula is to be introduced. The cannula is directed toward the nasion and is slowly introduced until a "give" is felt; then the obturator is removed. Free flow of ventricular fluid indicates correct placement. Several sutures are placed around the hub of the cannula to affix the device to the scalp. Next, air is introduced; this can be done with the patient either brow-up or brow-down. It is best to do the exchange in the brow-up position if it is desired to study all parts of the ventricular system rather than just the posterior portions of the lateral ventricles, third ventricle, aqueduct, and fourth ventricle. If the air is to be introduced with the patient supine, the head should be turned so that the ventricle containing the tip of the cannula is dependent. In that position, more air can be introduced. Fractional instillation of air and removal of fluid can then be carried out. Enough air is instilled to carry out the study, and at the end-point the pressure is allowed to equilibrate with the atmopshere.

The first films are obtained with the patient's head hanging somewhat so that the air is able to find its way through the foramen of Monro into the third ventricle. Brow-up, anteroposterior, and lateral films are obtained, and if better definition of the anterior portion of the third ventricle is desired than is obtained on the lateral film, then autotomography (mentioned earlier in the section on pneumoencephalography) or tomography is carried out.

If there is a block in the foramen of Monro but no associated perforation of the septum pellucidum, then a puncture of the opposite lateral ventricle may have to be performed in order to establish the diagnosis firmly.

If the lesion is caudad to the anterior portion of the third ventricle, the brow-down films will be of importance. The patient is rapidly turned from the supine into the prone position so that the air in the anterior third ventricle passes into the posterior third ventricle and not (as will often happen is he is turned slowly) back through the foramen of Monro into the uppermost lateral ventricle. Four films are obtained as soon as possible after the patient is brow-down. It is advantageous to have the tube and film positioned for the first of these—the lateral film—before the patient is turned. If the aqueduct is large the air will pass rapidly through this structure, making its demonstration difficult; if the aqueduct is partially or completely blocked, however, then the timing is not so critical. After the lateral film is obtained, autotomography or tomography is carried out in order to better display the midline portions of the ventricular system. When properly performed this has the further virtue of demonstrating a shift of normally midline structures, for these structures will then be out of focus on the autotomogram or midline tomogram. Finally, a reverse Towne view and a posteroanterior view are obtained. At times the reverse somersault maneuver may be required to demonstrate the aqueduct and fourth ventricle.

If there is no obstruction to the ventricular system and the air passes out of the fourth ventricle into the cisterna magna, then by bending the patient's head and neck far forward, one can bring it into the spinal canal and then up again so that the cisterns may be studied. As indicated in the section on pneumoencephalography, the study of the cisterns may yield information that is of importance in establishing the diagnosis.

In the discussion on pneumoencephalography, mention was made of the place of ventriculography, and some of the fallacies about "risks" of pneumoencephalography, especially in the presence of increased intracranial pressure, were discussed. In situations in which there is nonfilling of the ventricular system with air introduced from below by spinal puncture, ventriculography is indicated if the nonfilling is not due to such "technical reasons" as subdural placement of the air and if the cisternal air present does not allow exact localization of the lesion. Also, if tonsillar herniation is present on preliminary pneumoencephalographic films, it may be wise to tap the ventricular system to relieve the pressure and either to continue the examination from below or to carry out the remainder of the examination from above.

There will be occasional instances when the ventriculographic examination will be greatly facilitated if an opaque contrast agent is used instead of air. The opaque material may be nonsoluble (and heavier than spinal fluid), as for example, iophendylate (Pantopaque), or it may be soluble meglumine iothalamate (Conray) or metrizamide.[1] A modification of the technique using a nonsoluble contrast agent such as Pantopaque is to use an emulsion of Pantopaque in ventricular fluid, which is then introduced into the ventricular system to coat the walls of the ventricles.[10]

If one is fortunate in placing the ventricular cannula, the tip will lie adjacent to the foramen of Monro. Introduction of Pantopaque into the third ventricle is then easily accomplished. If the tip of the cannula is not in such a position, the patient must be positioned so that the Pantopaque passing through the cannula will gravitate into the anterior horn of the lateral ventricle.

Only a few milliliters of Pantopaque are required for the complete demonstration of the aqueduct and fourth ventricle. With the Pantopaque in the anterior horn of a lateral ventricle, the patient's head and neck, which are flexed, are gradually straightened, and the head is tilted slightly to the side so that the lateral ventricle containing the Pantopaque is uppermost. As the head is gradually extended, about the time a neutral position is reached, the Pantopaque will pass through the medially placed foramen of Monro into the third ventricle. Then the patient is placed in the supine position, and lateral, anteroposterior, and Towne (half-axial) films are obtained. If these maneuvers are correctly performed, the Pantopaque will be in position to demonstrate the posterior part of the third ventricle and distal structures. Serial films may be required over a period of hours if maximal information is desired about the aqueduct in special circumstances.

If for some reason the Pantopaque has not entered the foramen of Monro with this maneuver, it will come to lie in the trigone or occipital horn, and can then be moved back into the frontal horn either by turning the patient upside down or by hanging his head back and turning it to the side so that the Pantopaque-containing ventricle is dependent. The Pantopaque will move into the body of the lateral ventricle; rapidly turning the patient into the prone position will cause the Pantopaque to flow into the anterior horn once more. Gradually, with the patient sitting, the flexed head and neck are again extended.

If a water-soluble contrast agent such as metrizamide or Conray is introduced instead, serial films must be obtained fairly rapidly in order to demonstrate the passage of this material through the ventricular system. A biplane angiographic unit may easily be programmed for this kind of study. Water-soluble agents presently used seem to evoke little inflammatory response within the ventricular system, but passage of these substances into the cisterns may provoke a chemical meningitis.

Complications of ventriculography include epidural hematoma, cerebral hemorrhage, and formation of porencephalic diverticula along the needle tract (most apt to occur in hydrocephalics) (Fig. 10–18).

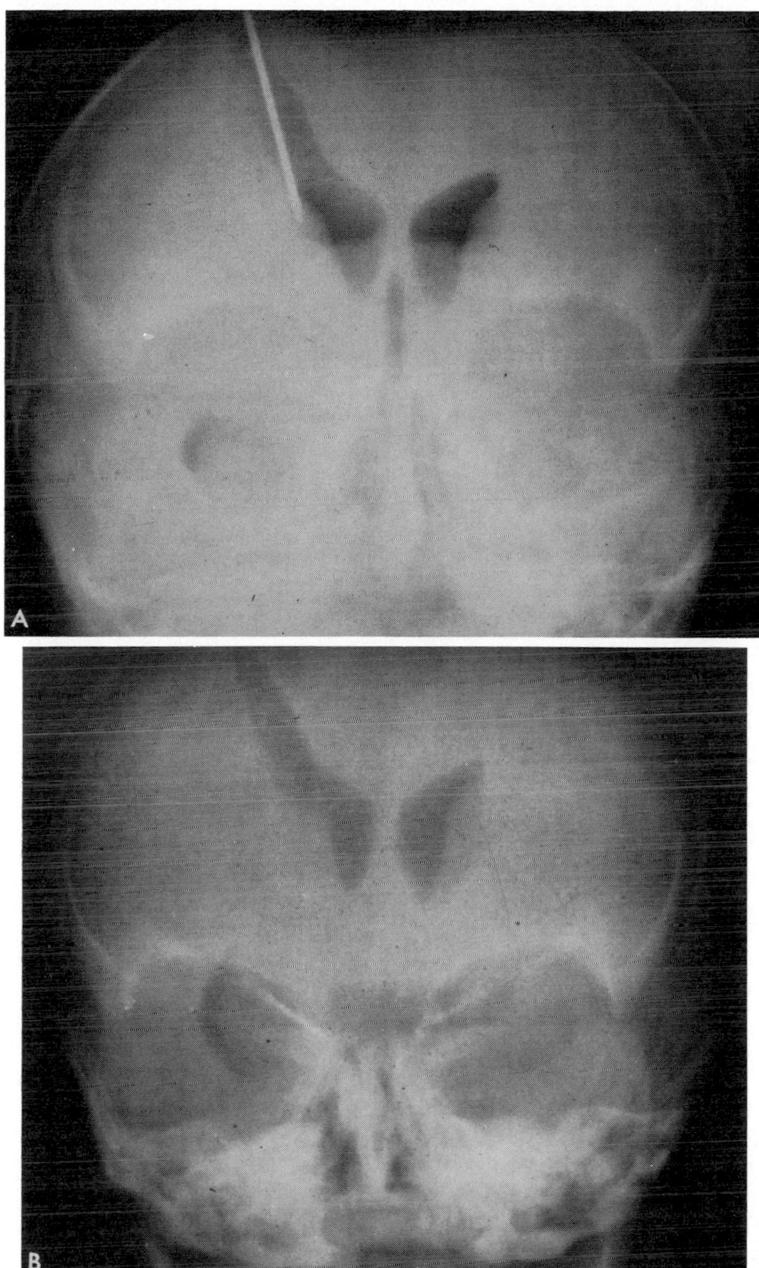

Figure 10–18 This set of anteroposterior roentgenograms taken during, *A*, and after, *B*, the introduction of air into the ventricular system illustrates the formation of an area of porencephaly along the needle tract.

EXAMINATION OF THE CEREBELLOPONTINE ANGLE WITH PANTOPAQUE

This procedure has its greatest usefulness in studying patients who are suspected of having a small lesion that is extra-axial in location and that is involving the eighth cranial nerve alone, or perhaps the eighth cranial nerve and other nearby nerves. Such a lesion may be confined entirely to the internal auditory meatus. The procedure should be undertaken after tomographic examination of the internal auditory meatuses in order to confirm or to supplement the results of this examination.

If the lesion is large and is suspected of lying primarily in the brain stem or cerebellum, then it is probably preferable to perform pneumoencephalography rather than an examination with Pantopaque, for more of the posterior fossa anatomy will be displayed with air than will be displayed with Pantopaque, especially if the examination with the opaque substance is conducted only with the patient in the prone position.

Examination of the cerebellopontine angle with Pantopaque carries with it a lesser morbidity than examination with air. There will probably be no discomfort or little discomfort, and for this reason the examination seems more appropriate in the patient who has only an impairment of hearing that might or might not be due to a small mass lesion. The examination procedure begins with the introduction of a few milliliters of Pantopaque into the lumbar subarachnoid space through a lumbar puncture.[14] The oily opaque material is then brought up into the cervical canal by tilting the patient head down while the head and neck are extended (patient's chin on sponge). In this way the opaque medium is brought over the hump in the thoracic area into the trough in the cervical area produced by the extension of the head and neck. No opaque medium will pass into the head as long as the tilt of the inclined table is not too steep. When sufficient opaque medium has been pooled in the cervical area, the examination may proceed. The inclined fluoroscopic table should at this time be in the neutral position. The sponge supporting the patient's chin is then removed, and the chin is tucked down toward the patient's chest. The Pantopaque will then begin to flow up onto the clivus. When the Pantopaque there begins to outline the area of juncture of the vertebral arteries, the patient's head is turned so that the side with the suspected lesion is lowermost. Pantopaque will run into the cerebellopontine angle. A slight tilt of the table may be required to bring the necessary amount of opaque medium into this location, but the tilt should be minimized so that the contrast agent does not escape the posterior fossa to pass into the middle fossa. The end-point of the examination is reached either when opaque medium has penetrated deeply into the internal auditory meatus or when it is clearly blocked by a lesion in this area. A bony ridge, the crista falciformis, is demonstrated at the depth of the meatus. Patients often experience a twinge of pain in the ear when the Pantopaque penetrates deeply into the meatus. Spot films are obtained with the patient's head in this oblique position and also with the patient's head turned back to neutral. If the chin remains tucked down, the meatus will be displayed through the orbit, and there will be no problem in interpreting the examination.

If the opposite meatus must be examined as well, then this side of the patient's head is placed against the table, and the opaque medium is pooled in this angle and meatus. Spot films are again obtained with the patient positioned obliquely, and then again with his head in neutral position.

For orientation it may be helpful to place a wax pellet containing an opaque substance, such as a piece of solder, within the patient's external auditory meatus at the beginning of the examination. This helps to identify the internal auditory meatus when the patient is in the oblique position.

Finally, the opaque medium should be recovered by tilting the head of the table upward. Small droplets may lodge against vascular structures or nerves; these can be dislodged by having the patient rock or shake his head from side to side.

The examination can be conducted without fluoroscopy if the patient is placed in the decubitus instead of the prone position. Tilting the patient so that the head is dependent and then neutralizing this angle directs the opaque medium into the appropriate meatus. In this technique, tomography may be used as a further refinement (Fig. 10–19).

When the examination of the cerebellopontine angle with Pantopaque is attempted

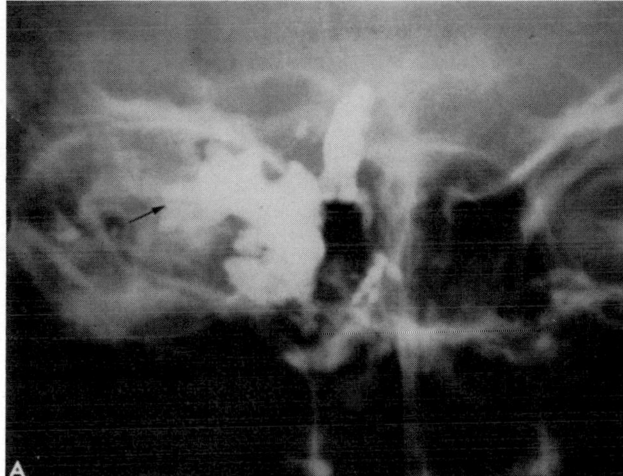

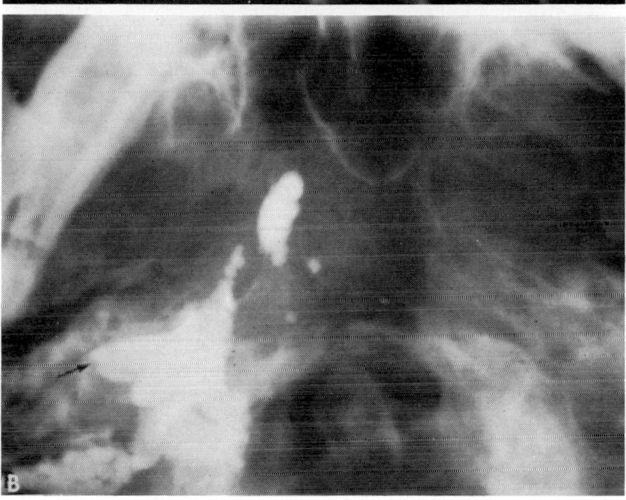

Figure 10–19 *A*. Perorbital view with the patient in right decubitus position. Pantopaque in the right internal auditory meatus is in contact with the crista falciformis (*arrow*), separating the vestibular and cochlear divisions of the eighth cranial nerve. *B*. Base view of patient in right lateral decubitus position. The crista falciformis (*arrow*) is again demonstrated. This study was performed to exclude a small eighth nerve tumor on the right as a cause for hearing loss.

in patients with large tumors, one commonly finds that the opposite meatus cannot be demonstrated. The brain stem is shifted in such a way as to block the access of the contrast medium to the contralateral cerebellopontine angle. This is one type of false positive result. Another source of false positive results is the variation in the depth of penetration of the subarachnoid space into the internal auditory meatus. Because of these problems, there may be a small percentage of false positives, even when the examination is conducted by an experienced person.

On the other hand, the low rate of morbidity associated with the procedure and the clarity of demonstration of the anatomy of the area recommend this technique, particularly in the diagnosis of small lesions.

RHOMBOENCEPHALOGRAPHY

This is a technique of examination of the posterior fossa with an oily opaque medium that was described by Mones and Werman in 1958.[8] In this procedure about 9 ml of Pantopaque is introduced into the lumbar subarachnoid space. The needle is then removed and the patient is placed in the supine position. He is tilted head downward about 80 degrees while his head is flexed. After about a minute in this position, he is brought back to about 70 degrees. Lateral and anteroposterior films are then obtained. The posterior foramen magnum, tonsils, fourth ventricle, and aqueduct may be clearly demonstrated in this fashion.

There are few instances in which the information obtainable with this procedure cannot be obtained in some other way, but it has the advantage at times of providing definition and clarity in difficult cases without resorting to Pantopaque ventriculography. The procedure has not gained widespread popularity, probably because of the fear of being unable to recover all of the Pantopaque from the head. Patients are likely to experience moderate to severe headache if the Pantopaque cannot be recovered.

REFERENCES

1. Campbell, R. L., Campbell, J. A., Heimburger, R. F., et al.: Ventriculography and myelography with absorbable radioopaque medium. Radiology, *82*:286, 1964.
2. Dandy, W.: Ventriculography following the injection of air into the cerebral ventricles. Ann. Surg., *68*:5. 1918.
3. Dandy, W.: Roentgenography of the brain after the injection of air into the spinal canal. Ann. Surg., *70*:397, 1919.
4. Erenberg, G.: Personal communication.
5. Goodling, C., et al.: New ventriculographic aspects of the Arnold-Chiari malformation. Radiology, *89*:626, 1967.
6. Luckett, W. H.: Air in the ventricles of the brain following a fracture of the skull. Surg. Gynec. Obstet., 213, 1913.
7. Lysholm, E., et al.: Das ventriculogramm. Acta Radiol. Suppl. 26, 1935.
8. Mones, R., and Werman, R.: Pantopaque fourth ventriculography via lumbar route (REG). J. Mount Sinai Hosp., N.Y., *25*:201, 1958.
9. Nellhaus, G., and Chutorian, A.: Narcosis for neuroradiologic procedures in children. Arch. Neurol., *10*:485, 1964.
10. Portera-Sanchez, A., Bravo, G., and Parera, C.: Emulsified Pantopaque ventriculography. J. Neurosurg., *21*:422, 1964.
11. Ruggiero, G.: Encephalography today. Acta Radiol., *5*:715, 1966.
12. Schechter, M. M., Zingesser, L. H., and Cuevas, C.: Dynamic displacements of intracranial structures simulating mass lesions. Amer. J. Roentgen., *98*:535, 1966.
13. Twining, E. W.: Radiology of the third and fourth ventricles. Parts I and II. Brit. J. Radiol., *12*:385 and 569, 1939.
14. Valvassori, G.: Abnormal internal auditory canal: the diagnosis of acoustic neuroma. Radiology, *92*:449, 1969.

11

SURGICAL CONSIDERATIONS OF VENTRICULOGRAPHY

HISTORICAL BACKGROUND

It is interesting that contrast ventriculography did not come into use earlier than it did. At the turn of the century, sites of election for benign ventricular puncture through silent areas of the brain had been determined. The external landmarks of Kocher and Keen provided, respectively, access to the frontal horn and the ventricular trigones. Cushing and others considered ventricular puncture useful for the sampling of cerebral spinal fluid under certain circumstances and for temporary relief of increased intracranial pressure.[6,27]

In 1913, W. J. Luckett demonstrated an air-filled ventricular system in a patient who had sustained a compound frontal fracture.[30] The diagnostic implication of air contrast within the ventricular system remained unrecognized, however, until 1918, when Walter Dandy reported his technique of "ventriculography."[7]

Dandy had long recognized the need for greater accuracy in tumor localization and had performed experimental ventriculography in dogs with the renal contrast materials of the day. These substances proved uniformly fatal. However, Halstead's reminder of "the remarkable power of intestinal gases to perforate bone on x-ray" prompted Dandy's choice of air as a suitable contrast medium.

The same clinical experience that led to the early reports of major morbidity and an up to 8 per cent mortality rate surrounding ventriculography also later provided guidelines for the prevention of these complications.[2,20,32] Thus, Dandy's original technique of air ventriculography has survived essentially without modification until today.[34,37,40]

Despite Dandy's disappointments with iodide contrast materials, the search continued for a positive contrast substance that would prove superior to air for demonstrating the midline ventricular system. Iodized oil (Lipiodol) and thorium dioxide (Thorotrast) were among the substances that were tried and abandoned. The need for precise landmarks for stereotaxic operations has been a renewed stimulus in the evolution of midline contrast ventriculography. Iophendylate (Pantopaque) and meglumine iothalamate (Conray 60) have proved acceptable agents but have some limitations. The physical properties of these materials have required advances in their technical placement, including direct transfrontal cannulation of the foramen of Monro.[41] Metrizamide (Amipaque) and Dimer-X are recent water-soluble positive contrast agents available for ventriculography.[5,17,19,28,39] Animal studies prove metrizamide is far less neurotoxic than other water soluble media.[5] Dimer-X is less likely to induce seizures than meglumine iothalamate.[28] The seizures induced by Dimer-X are controlled fully by intravenous diazepam (Valium).

INDICATIONS AND CONTRAINDICATIONS FOR VENTRICULOGRAPHY

Computer tomography has revolutionized the ease and reliability of diagnosis of almost every intracranial mass lesion. Be-

J. T. ROBERTSON AND I. C. DENTON, JR.

fore its development, except in infants and young children, arteriography and isotope brain scanning had replaced ventriculography as the procedures of choice in localizing supratentorial masses, and generally, there had been a marked decrease in the use of ventriculography on every major neurosurgical service. Ventriculography, however, is used for further elucidation when these more benign procedures yield equivocal results, and it is most useful in the demonstration of the third ventricle, aqueduct, and fourth ventricle. Ventriculography is used routinely in stereotaxic operations and may be used in patients having emergency operations for cerebral trauma.

Provided that the patient is a candidate for an operation, there are essentially no contraindications to ventriculography. The single most important guideline is that ventriculography should never be undertaken without preparation for subsequent operative intervention.

TECHNIQUES FOR VENTRICULOGRAPHY

Although the same basic principles of ventriculography apply to both children and adults, the technical approach to the ventricular system varies before and after closure of the cranial sutures.

In infants, ventriculography is usually performed by introducing an 18-gauge spinal needle through the scalp, which has been scrubbed and prepared for an operative procedure and injected with local anesthetic. The coronal suture is open and can be penetrated with ease. The needle is held in the sagittal plane on a line with the pupil while being advanced on a coronal plane in a line toward the inner canthus of the eye. It is advanced slowly, and the stylet is withdrawn at intervals. The appearance of cerebrospinal fluid should identify the ventricle at a depth not greater than 4 cm. Since repeated needle passes may increase the risk of hemorrhage and cortical damage, only in unusual circumstances should more than three attempts at ventricular puncture be made on either side without shifting to the opposite one. Occasionally the air will not pass into the opposite ventricle, and bilateral puncture may be necessary for a satisfactory exchange of air and ventricular fluid. In all cases, ventricular fluid pressure should be either estimated or measured and a small aliquot of fluid withdrawn for analysis.

If air ventriculography is performed in infants for purposes other than evaluation of hydrocephalus, complete fluid-air exchange will insure the best results. In order to maintain relatively normal pressure relationships, equivalent amounts of fluid and air should be exchanged in repeated aliquots of a few cubic centimeters. Adequate exchange is facilitated by positioning the head to create drainage of the fluid by gravity. In studying the patient with hydrocephalus, however, the smallest amount of air that will provide an adequate diagnosis should be used. The same principles of fluid-air exchange should be observed, but total exchange of air and fluid in the patient with hydrocephalus is seldom needed and can cause harm. In all cases, the exchanged room air should be filtered through several layers of sterile surgical sponge fitted around the stopcock.

In adults and in older children whose sutures are approaching closure, access to the ventricular system is provided by trephination (Fig. 11-1). Three standard points for the placement of trephines are recognized. Posterior parietal trephine openings, perhaps the most commonly used, are placed 8 cm above the inion at a point 2.5 to 3 cm lateral to the midline. The needle is directed along a line toward the inner aspect of the eye within the transverse plane of the supraorbital ridge. A Keen's point trephine opening 2.5 cm behind and 2.5 cm above the top of the ear provides access to the trigone of the lateral ventricle when the needle is directed at right angles to the cortex. The frontal horn of the ventricle may be approached by trephination at Kocher's point, 3 cm posterior to the normal hairline and 2.5 cm lateral to the midline. This position allows penetration of the anterior horn at its widest point. Twist drill holes made under local anesthesia can be used for rapid or elective access to the ventricular system.

Depending upon the trephination site that is selected, ventriculography may be performed in the sitting, semi-sitting, prone, or supine positions. If the patient is cooperative, an attempt should be made to use local anesthesia. Following placement of the trephine openings, usually bilaterally, the dura is incised in cruciate fashion and the brain

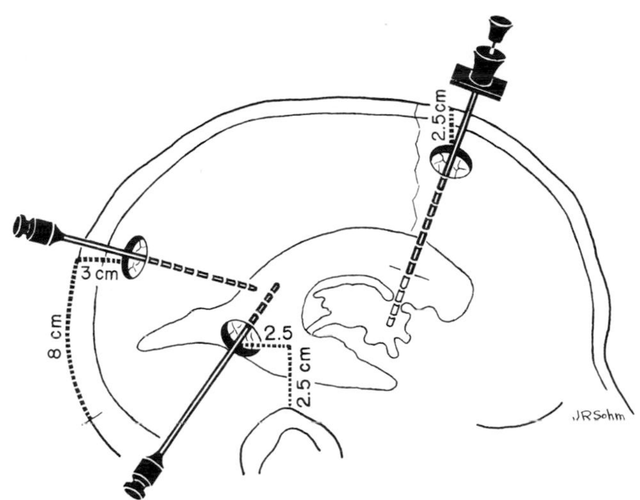

Figure 11–1 The three standard trephination sites used to gain access to the lateral ventricles. The anterior site, or Kocher's point, is 3 cm posterior to the normal hairline and 2.5 cm lateral to the midline. The Keen's point trephine opening permits tapping of the trigone of the lateral ventricle. It is 2.5 cm behind and 2.5 cm above the top of the ear. The posterior aspect of the lateral ventricle is approached through a posterior parietal trephine opening that is 8 cm above the inion and 2.5 to 3 cm lateral to the midline.

is punctured through a gyrus. Meticulous hemostasis should be obtained. The galea and skin may be closed prior to or after the ventricular puncture. Usually the initial attempt to place the needle in the ventricle is made on the side of the brain opposite to the one that is suspected of harboring the disease. The normal side of the brain is more likely to have the ventricle in a normal position and configuration. A blunt ventricular needle is considered safer than a sharp one and it affords a keen sensation of pressure as tissues of varying density are traversed. It transmits a distinct sensation of increased and then suddenly eased resistance as the ventricular wall is encountered.

When the needle is satisfactorily placed in the ventricle, a small amount of air should be instilled immediately in order to prevent possible ventricular collapse. The general principles already enumerated concerning repeated needle punctures, the estimation of cerebrospinal fluid, collection of fluid for analysis, and fluid exchange apply in the adult also.

In both children and adults, positive contrast ventriculography is used to best advantage in demonstrating alterations of midline ventricular configuration. The value of contrast ventriculography in stereotaxic operations is unquestioned. Several points concerning positive contrast ventriculography are noteworthy.

For positive contrast ventriculography, the technique of ventricular puncture should be modified so that a rubber catheter on a stylet may be directed into the third ventricle or placed near the foramen of Monro. Through frontal burr holes, the catheter is directed in the coronal plane toward the inner canthus of the eye and on a sagittal plane toward the opposite external auditory meatus. When the ventricle is encountered, a small bubble of air is introduced. The flexible catheter without its stylet, when introduced another 1 to 2 cm, will follow the floor of the frontal horn into the foramen of Monro. Prior to introduction of the contrast material, a lateral skull film should be taken to confirm the presence of the air bubble in the frontal horn.

Pantopaque and Conray 60 are the most frequently used contrast materials at present. As a general rule, the amount of contrast material used should be restricted to the amount necessary to achieve a satisfactory study. Three to four milliliters of undiluted Pantopaque will suffice. For an adequate Pantopaque study, head manipulation may be required to direct the transit of this nondispersible substance into the third ventricle, through the aqueduct, and into the fourth ventricle. Air-Pantopaque studies may be useful in evaluation of patients with hydrocephalus.[33] Myodil appears equally useful. Conray 60 may be injected after 4 to 6 ml of this substance have been diluted with an equal amount of spinal fluid. This highly dispersible material readily circulates throughout the ventricular system. It is widely accepted among neurosurgeons that no more than 10 to 12 ml of Conray 60 should be used at any one time. Greater quantities have, however, been used in the study of patients with hydrocephalus.[3] Shaw and co-workers have reported a marked increase in intracranial pressure when Conray 60 entered the posterior third ventricle, aqueduct, and fourth ventricle.[38] This pressure change may have resulted from induced vasodilatation resulting from brain stem stimulation.

Metrizamide is receiving considerable use in ventriculography in doses ranging from 2 to 15 ml.[39] Dimer-X is useful but more likely to induce seizures. These substances, like Conray 60, are usually injected into the nondominant frontal horn of the lateral ventricle.

Certain technical advances such as the chain guide technique for selective ventriculography may be quite useful, and seriography with a biplane serial changer shortens the procedure and allows minimal use of contrast media.[4,26]

COMPLICATIONS OF VENTRICULOGRAPHY

It is convenient to divide the complications of ventriculography into those of major and those of minor consequence. Subjective disturbances and seizure activity constitute the bulk of the minor complications. Pain, nausea, vomiting, and prostration are far less common with ventriculography than with pneumoencephalography. Nevertheless, minor degrees of discomfort do occur and may be associated with some alteration in vital signs such as mild temperature elevation and signs of meningeal irritation. These complaints are minimized if the contrast material does not get over the surface of the brain. Although transient electrocardiographic abnormalities may accompany fluid-air exchange, subjective complaints of palpitations or chest discomfort and objective electrocardiographic changes occurring some hours subsequent to ventriculography usually are related to cardiac disease rather than to the procedure.[10] Seizures occasionally occur with air ventriculography and are easily controlled in most cases. They occur far more frequently after the use of Conray 60 than after the use of air as the contrast medium.[36] These seizures are of two types. The most common is the generalized seizure occurring if the substance comes in contact with the cortex of the brain; these usually are easily controlled and self-limited. The second type of seizure is thought to be due to the irritation of the spinal cord or brain stem, resulting from excessive contrast material around these structures. These seizures, fortunately rare, require careful management. Respiratory support following pharmacological paralysis may be required to prevent the patient from becoming exhausted. This "spinal seizure" is likewise self-limited, usually disappearing within 24 hours. Metrizamide rarely causes seizure activity, and Dimer-X is less likely to produce a seizure than Conray 60.

The major complications of ventriculography fall into four general groups: infection, complications resulting from alterations in fluid dynamics, visual complications, and hemorrhage. As with any intracranial procedure, contamination of the operative field may lead to meningitis or brain abscess. The problem of infection very likely exceeds its reported incidence.[23] Nevertheless, with careful sterile techniques, significant complications from infections as a result of ventriculography are most unusual. If air is used, filtration of the air through multiple layers of an operative sponge before its introduction into the ventricular system effectively reduces the bacterial count of the ambient room air.[24] The use of oxygen for ventriculography would probably further reduce this likelihood of contamination. Theoretically, certain rare complications of ventriculography, such as cerebritis or ventriculitis, might occur in patients with septicemia or meningitis.[35] Such complications, however, appear to be quite rare. Ventricular tapping in the presence of an infected myelomeningocele may alter cerebral fluid dynamics, promoting an ascending infection.

The complications resulting from alterations of fluid dynamics are directly related to increased intracranial pressure and ventricular size.[25,31] In children with increased pressure, the development of a traumatic porencephalic diverticulum following ventricular puncture may occur with an incidence of approximately 9 per cent.[29] Multiple needle punctures at the same site also predispose to this complication. The porencephalic diverticulum assumes the form of a truncated cone with its base confluent with the ventricles and the apex beneath the gray matter. These diverticula may not be entirely innocuous; some authors have considered them responsible for seizure disorders and occult hemiparesis.[11]

Despite careful attention to air-fluid

exchange, alterations of fluid dynamics may allow compartmental shifts. For example, an upward herniation of the posterior fossa contents may occur in the presence of a posterior fossa mass. Likewise the supratentorial compartments are subject to such shifts.[13] Clinical deterioration may herald these disturbing events; they demand immediate craniotomy.

Visual complications are usually due to repeated attempts at ventricular puncture through the occipital cortex when posterior trephine openings are used. Typically, such complications may occur in cases with pseudotumor cerebri, in which small ventricles make it difficult to perform successful ventricular puncture without multiple needle passes. Although small permanent visual field defects may persist, most visual difficulties clear within a few days. In some cases with increased intracranial pressure, however, ventriculography may be followed by sudden blindness. One cause of blindness under such circumstances is compression of the posterior artery by cerebral herniation. Another cause of this sudden visual loss is presumed to be sudden pressure alterations resulting in blood flow shifts that promote optic nerve ischemia.

Intracerebral, intraventricular, subdural, and epidural hemorrhages have all been observed after ventriculography. Intracerebral hemorrhage is unusual when a blunt ventricular needle is used. Occult hemorrhage may not be manifested by bright bleeding through the needle at the time of ventricular puncture. At the time of x-ray studies of the ventricle, however, hemorrhage may be perceived as a mass in the region of cortical puncture. Intraventricular hemorrhage resulting from needle puncture may be due to injury of the glomus of the choroid plexus.[14] The radiographic demonstration of an intraventricular mass in the region of the choroid plexus signifies this complication. Most of these hemorrhages resolve spontaneously and do not require operative intervention. At a later date, benign calcification of the needle tract may attest to a previous hemorrhagic lesion incurred at the time of ventriculography.[15]

Although subdural hemorrhage may complicate pneumoencephalography, the development of a subdural hematoma following ventriculography is rare. Epidural hemorrhage, although unusual, may follow ventriculography.[12,21,22] Epidural hemorrhage in young people 16 years old or less has been reported at sites distant from the site of trephination, usually frontotemporal. At this age, the dura is usually quite elastic and less firmly applied to the inner table of the calvarium than it is in adults. It is presumed that epidural bleeding distant from the site of trephination results from traction on the dura by bridging cortical vessels following partial ventricular collapse. Subsequent hemorrhage occurs from the stripped calvarium. Experimental evidence from dog studies suggests that only 90 gm of nonpulsatile force is required to strip the dura from the calvarium, and once a collection is formed, the force required to expand the mass is further reduced.[18] The seriousness of this complication in young people undergoing ventriculography cannot be overemphasized, for only two survivors have been reported.[1] Since the dura of adults is more adherent than that of children, they rarely, if ever, manifest this complication.

In adults, epidural hemorrhage is more likely to occur at the trephination site where dural dissection may result from procedural factors. Benign epidural hemorrhage occurring at the site of trephination is frequently attested by button-like calcifications noted on x-rays taken at a later date.[42] Fortunately significant epidural hemorrhage at the site of trephination is a rare entity.

In both groups, the complication of epidural hemorrhage bears a direct relationship to ventricular size. In the patient with markedly enlarged ventricles, massive accumulations may occur before their presence is suggested by clinical deterioration. Unexplained anemia in a patient with hydrocephalus may offer a diagnostic clue to occult hemorrhage prior to clinical deterioration[43] Epidural hemorrhage can best be avoided by proper fluid-air exchange. Its presence may be detected radiographically at a late date, if the air has not been fully absorbed.

The overall number of deaths due to ventriculography is difficult to assess. The greatest factor compromising the accuracy of mortality rate figures after ventriculography is that the seriously ill patient frequently requires a subsequent craniotomy. For the same reason the incidence of seizures following ventriculography is difficult to define. The single most important principle concerning ventriculography is that immediate operative intervention must follow the demonstration of a mass lesion. Adherence to this and other principles has reduced the earlier mortality rate of 8 per cent to near zero.

REFERENCES

1. Arias, B. A., and Voris, H. C.: Extradural hemorrhage after ventriculography. Amer. J. Surg., *116*:109–112, 1968.
2. Cairns, H.: Observations on the localization of intracranial tumors: The disclosure of localizing signs following ventriculography. Arch. Surg., *18*:1936–1944, 1929.
3. Cornejo, S. G.: Positive contrast ventriculography using water soluble media (Conray). Presented at the meeting of the American Academy of Neurological Surgery. Mexico City, November 18–21, 1970.
4. Corrales, M.: The chain guide technique for selective ventriculography. Neuroradiology *9*(5):243–246, 1975.
5. Cronqvist, S.: Ventriculography with Amipaque. Neuroradiology, *12*(1):25–32, 1976.
6. Cushing, H.: Keen Surgery. W. W. Keen, ed. Philadelphia and London, W. B. Saunders Co., 1908, Vol. III, p. 172.
7. Dandy, W. E.: Ventriculography following the injection of air into the cerebral ventricles. Ann. Surg., *68*:5–11, 1918.
8. Davidoff, L. M., and Dyke, C. G.: The Normal Pneumoencephalogram. Philadelphia, Lea & Febiger, 1937.
9. Davidoff, L. M., and Epstein B. S.: The Abnormal Pneumoencephalogram. 2nd Ed. Philadelphia, Lea & Febiger, 1955.
10. Davie, J. C.: EKG alterations observed during fraction pneumoencephalography. J. Neurosurg., *20*:321–328, 1963.
11. Dekabon, A. S.: Is needle puncture of the brain entirely harmless? Neurology (Minneap.), *8*: 556–557, 1958.
12. Del Viron, R. E., and Armenesse, B.: Ematoma epidurale acutospontaneo depo decompress ventriculari in corso di idrocephalo, Minerva Neurochir., *5*:43–48, 1961.
13. Dyke, C. G.: Acquired subtentorial pressure diverticulum of a cerebral lateral ventricle. Radiology, *39*:167–174, 1942.
14. Dyke, C. G., Elsberg, C. A., and Davidoff, L. M.: Enlargement in the defect in the air shadow following ventriculography. Amer. J. Roentgen., *33*:736–743, 1935.
15. Falk, B.: Calcification in the track of the needle following ventricular puncture. Acta Radiol., *35*:304–308, 1951.
16. Ferguson, L.: Filling patterns in contrast ventriculography, J. Neurol. Neurosurg. Psychiat., *37*(4):449–454, 1974.
17. Finck, M., and Vogelsang, H.: Experience with Dimer-X 1-ventriculography. Neuropaediatrie, *6*(4):339–346, 1975.
18. Ford, L. E., McLaurin, R. L.: Mechanism of extradural hematoma. J. Neurosurg., *20*:760–769, 1963.
19. Gonsette, R. E.: Metrizamide as contrast medium for myelography and ventriculography. Preliminary clinical experiences. Acta Radiol. (Stockh.), (Suppl.) *335*:346–358, 1973.
20. Grant, F. C.: Ventriculography: A review based on the analysis of 392 cases. Arch. Neurol. Psychiat., *14*:513–533, 1925.
21. Haft, H., Liss, H., and Mount, L. A.: Massive epidural hemorrhage as a complication of ventricular drainage. J. Neurosurg., *17*:49–54, 1960.
22. Higazi, I.: Epidural hematoma as a complication of ventricular drainage. Report of a case and review of literature. J. Neurosurg., *20*:527–528, 1963.
23. Hook, E. B.: Central nervous system infection in hydrocephalic children following ventriculography. Clin. Pediat., 481–483, 1965.
24. Hook, E. B., and Vesley, D.: The efficacy of sterile gauze as a filter of air ventriculography in pneumoencephalography. Neurology (Minneap.), *15*:1078–1080, 1965.
25. Jefferson, G.: The balance of life and death in cerebral lesions. Surg. Gynec. Obstet., *93*:444–458, 1951.
26. Karle, L., and Gjerris, F.: Conray ventriculography carried out as seriography on a biplane serial changer. Neuroradiology, *5*(3):145–149, 1973.
27. Keen, W. W.: Exploratory trephining and puncture of the brain. Med. News, *53*:603–609, 1888.
28. Kunze, S., Klinger, M., and Schiefer, W.: Central ventriculography with Dimer-X. Acta Neurochir. (Wien), *28*:41–63, 1973.
29. Lorber, J., and Emery, J. L.: Intracerebral cyst complicating ventricular needling in hydrocephalic infants: A clinical pathologic study. Develop. Med. Child Neurol., *6*:125–139, 1964.
30. Luckett, W. J.: Air in the ventricles of the brain following a fracture of the skull. Surg. Gynec. Obstet. *17*:237–240, 1913.
31. Marini, G., and Taveras, J. M.: Influence of ventricular size on mortality and morbidity following ventriculography. Acta Radiol., *1*:602–608, 1963.
32. Masson, C. B.: The disturbances in vision and in visual fields after ventriculography. Bull. Neurol. Inst. N.Y., *3*:190–209, 1934.
33. Papatheodorou, C. A., and Teng., P.: Air-Pantopaque ventriculography in congenital hydrocephalus and myelomeningocele. Acta Radiol. (Diag.) (Stockholm), *91*:647–655, 1964.
34. Pendergrass, E. P.: Indications and contra-indications of encephalography and ventriculography. J.A.M.A., *94*:408–411, 1931.
35. Petersdorf, R. G., Swarner, P. R., and Garcia, M.: Studies on the pathogenesis of meningitis. II. J. Clin. Invest., *41*:320–327, 1962.
36. Picaza, J. A., Hunter, S. E., and Cannon, B. W.: Axial ventriculography. J. Neurosurg., *33*:297–303, 1970.
37. Riggs, H. W.: The dangers and mortality of ventriculography. Bull. Neurol. Inst. N.Y., *3*:210–231, 1934.
38. Shaw, M. M., Miller, J. D., and Steven, J. L.: Effect of intracranial pressure of meglumine iothalamate ventriculography. J. Neurol. Neurosurg. Psychiat., *38*:(10):1022–1026, 1975.
39. Suzuki, S., Ito, K., and Iwabuchi, T.: Ventriculography with non-ionic water soluble contrast

medium—Amipaque (metrigamide). J. Neurosurg., *47*:79–85, 1977.
40. Walker, E. A.: A History of of Neurological Surgery. New York, Hafner Publishing Co., 1967, pp. 27–29.
41. Vinas, F. J.: Iodoventriculography by direct catheterization of third ventricle in posterior fossa lesions of childhood. J. Neurosurg., *21*:492–496, 1964.
42. Whisler, W. W., and Voris, H. C.: Ossified epidural hematoma following posterior fossa exploration. J. Neurosurg., *23*:214–216, 1965.
43. Youmans, J. R., and Schneider, R. C.: Post-traumatic intracranial hematomas in patients with arrested hydrocephalus. J. Neurosurg., *17*:590–597, 1960.

12

DIAGNOSTIC BIOPSY FOR NEUROLOGICAL DISEASE

This chapter is designed to assist the neurological surgeon in deciding when to perform a biopsy, the choice of tissue, technical aspects of the biopsy, and the method of preserving the tissue to provide maximal information. Rarely will the surgeon personally fix and process the tissue. He should, however, be prepared to be a responsible partner with the pathologist in insuring the overall success of the procedure. Even in a large institution, the neurological surgeon should be more than a technician who removes the biopsy specimen. In smaller hosptials, the surgeon may have to organize the entire procedure. Few general pathologists have developed standard procedures for handling brain, muscle, or peripheral nerve biopsies, and they may look to the neurological surgeon for direction.

The text, tables, and references on fixation, stains, and special studies may be used to help the pathologist to organize processing procedures, to determine whether the biopsy should be forwarded to a research center, to preserve the specimen in a way that makes such referral feasible, and to provide a quick reference on fixatives and storage procedures at hours when the pathologist is not available for consultation.

Table 12–1 lists the tissues that have been examined for diagnosis of neurological disorders. They include brain, tumor tissue, peripheral nerve, muscle, bone, temporal artery, rectal mucosa, appendix, skin, and even organs such as liver, kidney, tonsils, gingiva, and tooth pulp. Needle biopsy of bone has been advocated for rapid, relatively atraumatic diagnosis of many neurological disorders.* Neurological complications of the procedure have been few but have been recorded occasionally, however.[151,182] Many biopsies, in particular those of skeletal muscles, contain arteries that may reveal a systemic arteritis such as polyarteritis nodosa. Indeed, temporal artery biopsy is the procedure of choice for diagnosis of cranial giant cell arteritis.[22,30,205,219]

In recent years, biopsies of many nonneural tissues have been used to identify metabolic and degenerative disorders formerly diagnosed by brain biopsy.[53,54,167,242] Rectal biopsy has been used extensively to identify intraneuronal storage material in myenteric plexus neurons, although several authors have questioned the specificity of findings without use of electron microscopy.† Appendectomy also has been used effectively to identify storage material in myenteric ganglion cells.[75,144,184,228]

Skin biopsies may be used both as a source of fibroblasts for cell cultures and enzyme assays and for direct light or elec-

* See references 5, 15, 115, 166, 197, 233, 243.

† See references 25, 31, 32, 61, 66, 80, 117, 124, 125, 145, 160, 163, 208, 237, 238.

W. G. ELLIS, J. R. YOUMANS, AND P. M. DREYFUS

TABLE 12–1 DIAGNOSTIC BIOPSY FOR NEUROLOGICAL DISEASE: SUITABLE TISSUES

Brain: cerebral cortex–white matter, subcortical nuclei, meninges, cerebellum
Tumor tissue
Peripheral nerve
Skeletal muscle
Bone: skull, vertebra, intervertebral disc
Temporal artery
Rectal mucosa, appendix
Skin
Viscera: liver, kidney
Oral cavity: tonsils, gingiva, tooth pulp

tron microscopic detection of inclusion material characteristic of certain metabolic disorders.*

Visceral biopsies—especially of liver, kidney, or adrenals—are valuable for diagnosis of metabolic diseases that produce a diffuse storage of substances such as lipid or glycogen.† In other conditions, such as Reye syndrome or Wilson disease, a primary liver disease may be associated with cerebral dysfunction, and the neurological disorder may be diagnosed indirectly by liver biopsy.[196,241] Gingival biopsy is a source of fibroblasts for cell culture and may be used for identification of amyloid in generalized amyloidosis. Prior to development of enzymatic assays, several metabolic disorders were diagnosed histologically and histochemically by identification of storage material in tonsillar lymphoid tissue or nerves in the tooth pulp.[28,29,68]

During the past two decades, biopsy has been replaced by other techniques for diagnosis of many neurological diseases.[54,167,242] This is particularly true in demyelinative or infectious diseases and inborn metabolic errors.‡ Also in the past two decades, techniques applied to biopsy tissues have changed. Electron microscopy and immunohistochemical procedures have become extremely important in the study of some neurological disorders, including the identification of many neoplasms.§ Biochemical analysis of biopsy specimens has become far more important in the diagnosis of many disorders than slide histochemistry.‖ Enzyme histochemistry and brain tissue culture, have few, if any, applications as diagnostic procedures for neurological disease.

* See references 39, 42, 54, 142, 150, 169, 170.

† See references 28, 29, 68, 81, 106, 150, 169, 195, 198.

‡ See references 28, 29, 47, 68, 112, 138, 150, 169, 215.

BRAIN BIOPSY

Indications

When confronted with what appears to be a progressively crippling and incurable neurological disease, patients and their families are anxious to have an accurate diagnosis and prognosis. Brain biopsy may be indicated when there is no alternative diagnostic procedure and the biopsy can be obtained safely. Table 12–2 outlines the general indications for brain biopsy in adults and children.¶

In earlier decades, brain biopsy was used to diagnose many diseases that now may be confirmed by enzymatic and serological techniques. Table 12–3 outlines diseases that have been diagnosed by brain biopsy in the past. Today, these diseases may be divided into those for which there are reliable laboratory tests other than biopsy, those in which biopsy of organs other than brain is useful for diagnosis, and finally those diseases in which no reliable antemortem alternative to brain biopsy is available (Tables 12–4, 12–5, and 12–6).

§ See references 23, 41, 59, 91, 93, 96, 120, 122, 126, 127, 143, 144, 162, 170, 173, 188, 200, 218, 223.

‖ See references 28, 29, 68, 106, 108, 150, 169, 215.

¶ See references 19, 20, 21, 26, 53, 54, 118, 121, 146, 154, 156, 159, 167, 242.

TABLE 12–2 BRAIN BIOPSY: SYMPTOM INDICATIONS

ADULT
Dementia
Central nervous system infection—unknown cause
CHILD
Dementia
Progressive loss of motor function
Increasing dyskinesia or cerebellar dysfunction
Developmental arrest
Intractible seizures—with or without myoclonus
Central nervous system infection—unknown cause

TABLE 12–3 DISEASES PREVIOUSLY DIAGNOSED BY BRAIN BIOPSY

DEGENERATIVE DISORDERS
- Presenile and senile dementias
  - Alzheimer disease (including senile brain disease)
  - Pick disease
- Neuroaxonal dystrophy
  - Infantile neuroaxonal dystrophy†
  - Hallervorden-Spatz disease
- Progressive poliodystrophy of childhood (Alpers disease)

INBORN METABOLIC DISORDERS: PROVED OR SUSPECTED
- Sphingolipid disorders
  - Neuronal storage diseases: Tay-Sachs disease and related disorders*
  - Neurovisceral storage diseases: Niemann-Pick and Gaucher diseases*
  - Myelination diseases: metachromatic leukodystrophy,* Krabbe disease*
- Mucopolysaccharide and mucolipid disorders: Examples, Hurler disease,* generalized gangliosidosis*
- Glycogen storage diseases: Example, Pompe disease*
- Ceroid-lipofuscinosis (Batten disease)*
- Leukodystrophies of unknown cause
  - Sudanophilic leukodystrophies: adrenoleukodystrophy,* Pelizaeus-Merzbacher and Seitelberger variants
  - Spongy degeneration of white matter (Canavan disease)
  - Alexander disease (leukodystrophy with Rosenthal fibers)
- Lafora disease (progressive myoclonic epilepsy)†

DEMYELINATIVE DISEASES
- Multiple sclerosis*
- Schilder disease and transitional cases*

INFECTIONS OF THE NERVOUS SYSTEM
- Viral encephalitis; example, *Herpesvirus hominis**
- Subacute sclerosing panencephalitis*
- Creutzfeldt-Jakob disease
- Leptomeningitis of unknown cause

* Alternative to brain biopsy available.
† Possible alternative to brain biopsy available.

TABLE 12–4 ALTERNATIVES TO BRAIN BIOPSY: DISEASES DIAGNOSED BY BIOPSY OF OTHER TISSUES

DISEASE	TISSUE	FINDINGS	REFERENCES
Ceroid-lipofuscinosis (Batten disease)	White blood cells, appendix, rectum, liver, skin, muscle, nerve, conjunctiva	Cytoplasmic inclusions: dense, pleomorphic, fingerprint, and curvilinear bodies	7, 31, 32, 39, 42, 54 66, 75, 90, 114, 124, 142, 144, 184, 228
Infantile neuroaxonal dystrophy	Peripheral nerve, muscle	Swollen terminal axons and motor end-plates	7, 143
Lafora familial myoclonic epilepsy	Liver, muscle	PAS-positive bodies	40, 164, 195
Adrenoleukodystrophy	Adrenal cortex, testes	Cells distended with lamellated lipid	198

TABLE 12–5 ALTERNATIVES TO BRAIN BIOPSY: DISEASES DIAGNOSED BY LABORATORY TESTS

DISEASE	LABORATORY TEST	SPECIMEN	ALTERNATE PROCEDURE	REFERENCES
Tay-Sachs disease, related gangliosidoses	Enzyme assay	Serum; cultured skin fibroblasts, leukocytes, amniotic fluid cells	Rectal biopsy, chemical analysis of urinary sediment (Sandhoff disease)	32, 54, 60, 117, 124, 138, 167, 169
Niemann-Pick disease	Enzyme assay	Serum; cultured skin fibroblasts, leukocytes, amniotic fluid cells	Biopsy of liver, skin, lymph node, bone marrow, rectal mucosa	28, 54, 117, 138, 167, 170
Gaucher disease	Enzyme assay	Serum; cultured skin fibroblasts, leukocytes, amniotic fluid cells	Biopsy of liver, lymph node, bone marrow; urinary sediment chemical analysis	29, 54, 60, 138, 167
Globoid cell leukodystrophy (Krabbe disease)	Enzyme assay	Serum; cultured skin fibroblasts, leukocytes, amniotic fluid cells	Peripheral nerve biopsy (electron microscopic examination); urinary sediment chemical analysis	7, 54, 60, 138, 167, 215
Metachromatic leukodystrophy	Enzyme assay	Urine; serum; cultured skin fibroblasts, leukocytes, amniotic fluid cells	Urinary sediment microscopic examination or chemical analysis, peripheral nerve or renal biopsy	7, 54, 60, 68, 138, 167
Ceramidase deficiency (Farber lipogranulomatosis)	Enzyme assay	Cultured skin fibroblasts	Biopsy of skin nodule	158
Cerebrotendinous xanthomatosis	Cholestanol assay	Plasma, bile, skin	Skin biopsy	18
Acid cholesteryl ester hydrolase deficiency (Wolman disease)	Enzyme assay	Cultured skin fibroblasts or leukocytes	Rectal biopsy, liver biopsy	81, 117
Mucopolysaccharidoses (types I, II, III, VI, VII)	Enzyme assay	Cultured skin fibroblasts, leukocytes, or amniotic fluid cells	Urinary excretion of mucopolysaccharide; cultured skin fibroblast and amniotic fluid cell microscopic examination; biopsy of liver, skin, rectum	54, 117, 150, 170
Mucolipidoses (e.g., GM_1 or generalized gangliosidosis)	Enzyme assay	Urine, cultured skin fibroblasts, leukocytes, amniotic fluid cells	Biopsy of liver, skin, bone marrow, lymph node, rectum	54, 117, 125, 169, 170
Glycogenoses (e.g., type II with central nervous system involvement)	Enzyme assay	Tissue biopsy	Liver, skin, or muscle biopsy (microscopic or biochemical examination)	54, 106, 170
Multiple sclerosis and related disorders	Myelin basic protein or immunoglobulin identification (oligoclonal IgG)	Cerebrospinal fluid	None	47, 112
Viral encephalitis	Virus isolation	Cerebrospinal fluid	Rising serum and cerebrospinal fluid antibody titers	239
Subacute sclerosing panencephalitis	Elevated measles virus antibodies	Serum, cerebrospinal fluid	Electroencephalogram, elevated cerebrospinal fluid immunoglobulins, virus isolation from lymph nodes	112, 242

TABLE 12-6 DISEASES DIAGNOSED ONLY BY BRAIN BIOPSY

DISEASE	BIOPSY FINDINGS
Alzheimer disease	Senile (neuritic) plaques and intraneuronal neurofibrillary tangles
Pick disease	Neuronal loss and intraneuronal Pick bodies
Creutzfeldt-Jakob disease (subacute spongiform encephalopathy)	Neuronal loss, astrogliosis, vacuolated neuropil (status spongiosus)
Progressive poliodystrophy of childhood (Alpers disease)	Neuronal loss, astrogliosis, lipid-filled phagocytes, vacuolated neuropil (status spongiosus)
Hallervorden-Spatz syndrome	Swollen dystrophic axons and iron deposits in basal ganglia
Spongy degeneration of white matter (Canavan disease)	Vacuolar degeneration of white matter, relative axonal preservation, Alzheimer II astrocytes in gray matter
Leukodystrophy with Rosenthal fibers (Alexander disease)	White matter demyelination with perivascular Rosenthal fibers
Sudanophilic leukodystrophies (including congenital and Pelizaeus-Merzbacher types)	Sudanophilic myelin degenerative products, relative axonal preservation, patchy islands of myelin preservation

In adult dementia, biopsy may be performed for prognosis, genetic counseling, and family reassurance. It is important to identify possible familial disorders with vague clinical presentations that are characterized by mental deterioration. Concern of other family members is allayed if the biopsy reveals a nonfamilial condition. In addition, genetic counseling can be given to parents in the childbearing age groups.

Since dementia usually is associated with cerebral cortical atrophy and ventricular dilation, it is important to distinguish primary hydrocephalus from enlargement of the ventricles secondary to Alzheimer disease or another type of presenile dementia. A cerebral cortical biopsy may be performed at the time of ventricular shunting.[43] It will provide information regarding the likelihood of recovery of mental function. Also, the identification of a progressive dementing disease will lessen concern about shunt dysfunction in the patient whose cerebral function deteriorates further after insertion of the shunt.

In many progressive neurological disorders of childhood, the basic pathophysiological mechanism is poorly understood and it may not be possible to establish the diagnosis without biopsy of the brain. In such cases, the clinician and the patient's parents must choose between the biopsy and postmortem examination as a means of establishing the correct diagnosis. If waiting for the autopsy is chosen, it should be arranged in advance and done within 30 minutes of death.[87,116,223,224] Longer delay between death and tissue processing may lead to ultrastructural artifacts and may alter the activity of some enzymes.

Besides progressive mental deterioration, other indications for brain biopsy in infants and children are: general developmental arrest, progressive dysfunction of cerebellum or basal ganglia, and severe untreatable seizures, particularly those associated with myoclonus. Certain inborn errors of metabolism that ultimately lead to progressive neurological deterioration may appear relatively stable at the onset. Thus, developmental arrest should trigger the same intense diagnostic efforts as are made for rapidly progressive mental deterioration. With progressive cerebellar dysfunction, biopsy of the cerebellum may be performed, although this procedure is somewhat more hazardous than cerebral cortical biopsy.

Intractable seizures accompanied by generalized myoclonus occur in infancy and childhood. Many cases are sporadic, and the biopsy is of little value. In familial cases, the diagnosis of Lafora disease, or Unverricht myoclonus epilepsy, may be made by the detection of specific inclusion bodies in the cytoplasm of cerebral or cerebellar neurons.[82]

For unusual cases, central nervous system infection of undetermined cause may be an indication for brain biopsy. In some patients acute onset of unilateral cerebral dysfunction may be associated with signs of meningoencephalitis. In other patients systemic and cerebrospinal fluid signs of chronic infection persist, yet no cause can be indentified by either serological tests or cultures of blood and cerebrospinal fluid. Biopsy of the brain and leptomeninges may be performed to obtain tissue for cultures and histological identification of the cause. The prime example would be herpes simplex encephalitis, which is amenable to treatment with adenine arabinoside.[2,239] Tissue handling for the identification of central nervous system infections differs from that used for the diagnosis of neoplasia or metabolic disorders. A skilled microbiologist must provide the necessary expertise.

Diseases with Alternative Laboratory Tests

Inborn Metabolic Errors

Inherited enzymatic deficiencies have been discovered in four major groups of metabolic disorders that, in the past, were diagnosed by brain or visceral biopsy. These groups are disorders of sphingolipids (e.g., Tay-Sachs disease), mucopolysaccharides (e.g., Hurler disease), mucolipids (e.g., generalized gangliosidosis), and glycogen (e.g., Pompe disease).* In the many diseases within each category, one or more chemical compounds, which usually are the substrates for the deficient enzymes, gradually accumulate in the brain or other tissues. At present, these diseases are most accurately diagnosed by documenting lack of specific enzyme activity in cultured leukocytes or skin fibroblasts, cultured amniotic fluid cells, excised tissue, and in some diseases, the serum or urine.

Study of tissue morphology is useful if enzymatic studies are not diagnostic or an unsuspected disorder is encountered. Table 12–5 indicates the tissues from which biopsies may be taken to diagnose excessive substrate storage if noninvasive techniques should fail. The choice of tissue or fluid for diagnosis depends upon the disease and the degree of certainty required in the individual case. Proof of an abnormal storage substance in an organ requires less tissue than biochemical identification of the particular substance.

If the disease has already been identified within a family, the simple histological demonstration of neuronal or visceral storage abnormalities may be sufficient evidence of disease in a family member who develops symptoms. In this case, the type of storage material need not be identified again. Small biopsy specimens from peripheral nerve, rectal mucosa, or bone marrow are suitable to prove the presence of storage material histologically or by electron microscopy, even though the specimens are too small for complete biochemical analysis. Needle biopsy of liver often provides enough tissue for microassay of common storage materials, and should be the first step in biochemical analysis of an unknown neurovisceral storage disease. If enzyme assays and liver needle biopsy both fail, then lymph node, muscle, splenic, or open liver biopsy should produce sufficient tissue mass for nonenzymatic biochemical analysis. If the abnormal storage of the substance occurs only in the central nervous system, then brain biopsy will be required to provide tissue for the analysis.

Biochemical analysis of the urine will provide the diagnosis in many patients with inborn errors of metabolism. Mucopolysaccharidoses may be subclassified partially on the basis of urinary excretion compounds, although in several subtypes enzyme assays are required for precise diagnosis.[150] Excessive substrate has been measured biochemically in the urinary sediment of patients with globoid cell leukodystrophy, metachromatic leukodystrophy, Gaucher disease, and Sandhoff variant of gangliosidosis.[60] In metachromatic leukodystrophy, urinary sediment may be stained metachromatically by cresyl violet or toluidine blue, but interpretation of test results may be difficult.[68]

Many inborn errors of metabolism produce inclusions of variable specificity in the leukocytes. Certain mucopolysaccharide and mucolipid disorders may be diagnosed by the presence of metachromatic lymphocyte inclusions.[54] Leukocyte inclusions found in other disorders provide useful collateral information but generally lack specificity to qualify as confirmatory tests in undiagnosed cases.

Skin biopsy is a relatively minor procedure that may be performed alone or as part of other biopsies such as those of nerve and muscle. Cultured skin fibroblasts are used for enzymatic analysis in lipid, mucopolysaccharide, and mucolipid disorders; however, skin cells may contain sufficient abnormal storage material to permit diagnosis by metachromatic or other stains and by electron microscopy.[54,150,169,170]

Not every inborn metabolic error produces diagnostic morphological changes in the brain or other organs, and hence biopsy diagnosis is not feasible. The aminoaci-

* See references 28, 29, 54, 68, 106, 118, 150, 167, 169, 215, 242.

durias, lipoprotein abnormalities, galactosemia, Lesch-Nyhan syndrome, and the porphyrias produce no characteristic histological changes in the brain. Systemic amyloidosis may produce cerebral amyloid deposits, and Wilson disease produces characteristic abnormalities in subcortical nuclei, but brain biopsy rarely has been used for diagnosis of either disease. Leigh's subacute necrotizing encephalomyelopathy involves chiefly brain stem and spinal nuclei from which biopsies cannot be taken safely.[53,82]

Demyelinative and Infectious Diseases

Multiple sclerosis and certain cases of the related Schilder disease often may be diagnosed by detection of myelin basic protein or oligoclonal bands of IgG in cerebrospinal fluid by using a variety of techniques.[47,112] In the past subacute sclerosing panencephalitis was diagnosed only by brain biopsy. Now the disease is easily detected by elevated serum measles antibody titers and confirmed by cerebrospinal fluid immunoglobulin findings similar to those in multiple sclerosis.[82,112,242]

Occasionally, *Herpesvirus hominis* infections of the central nervous system may be diagnosed by histological examination of brain tissue prior to completion of cerebrospinal fluid virus cultures. In these cases tissue usually is excised as part of operative decompression for increased intracranial pressure. Recently, the promising results of adenine arabinoside in treatment of herpes simplex encephalitis has renewed interest in brain biopsy for rapid diagnosis of cerebral infections.[2,239] Brain biopsy is recommended to exclude encephalitis that does not respond to this drug. Virus in the excised tissue may be identified quite rapidly by immunofluorescence techniques, tissue smear, or rapid electron microscopic procedures long before routine viral cultures or even histological sections are available.[2,41,130,188] Speed of diagnosis is important because early treatment carries the best prognosis.

Brain Diseases Diagnosed by Biopsy of Other Tissues

Four brain diseases may be diagnosed by biopsy of tissues other than brain. They are Batten ceroid-lipofuscinosis, infantile neuroaxonal dystrophy, Lafora myoclonic epilepsy, and adrenoleukodystrophy. Each of these disorders is familial and produces dementia, blindness, seizures, and ataxia or paralysis in infancy or early childhood. Each causes great parental concern. None has an enzymatic deficiency or other biochemical abnormality that permits consistent diagnosis without biopsy of tissue.[177] In the past, brain biopsy was the only method available for antemortem diagnosis.[53,82,103,198] In recent years other tissues, as outlined in Table 12–4 have been found to contain specific histological or ultrastructural changes.* If future studies prove that these changes are consistent in all cases, then the need for brain biopsy will be eliminated.

Diseases Diagnosed by Brain Biopsy Only

Diseases in which diagnosis can be confirmed only by brain biopsy may be put into two categories: presenile-senile dementias and childhood leukodystrophies (see Table 12–6). Each causes characteristic histological or ultrastructural changes in the brain that permit biopsy diagnosis. None produces changes in peripheral nervous system or viscera that are specific enough to support biopsy diagnosis.

Alzheimer disease and senile brain disease are identical histologically and are separated only by age of onset. Senile brain disease is a specific illness. Indeed, dementia is a specific illness and not an invariable result of aging. Dementia occurring after 65 years of age deserves the same careful evaluation as does dementia in the patient under that age.[43]

Creutzfeldt-Jakob disease, or subacute spongiform encephalopathy, is a dementing disease caused by an infectious agent of an unknown type.[8] Its infectious origin has been proved by transmission of disease to subhuman primates and nonprimates by inoculation with human brain tissue. The manner by which humans become infected is unknown. No systemic manifestations of infection or immunological response have been detected, and the infectious agent has not been identified by electron microscopy.

---

* See references 7, 31, 32, 39, 40, 42, 54, 66, 75, 90, 114, 124, 142–144, 164, 184, 195, 198, 228.

Except for characteristic electroencephalographic changes in some forms of the disease, diagnosis depends upon demonstration of spongiform encephalopathy by biopsy or autopsy.

A histologically similar condition in children is called progressive poliodystrophy of childhood, or Alpers disease. This syndrome encompasses cases of many kinds, including postanoxic or postepileptic cerebral degeneration and several familial conditions. Transmission to subhuman primates has not been accomplished. Occasional cases of childhood dementia without other obvious causes may be diagnosed by brain biopsy on the basis of a peculiar spongiform encephalopathy.[53,82,226]

Another childhood neurodegenerative disorder with characteristic histological changes is Hallervorden-Spatz syndrome.[62,82] This condition, probably related to infantile neuroaxonal dystrophy, generally presents as a dystonic movement disorder with dementia. Dystrophic axons and iron deposits may be identified by needle biopsies of globus pallidus, but cerebral cortex rarely shows diagnostic changes.

Two childhood leukodystrophies that have no proved enzyme defect but that show characteristic histological changes in cerebral white matter are spongy degeneration of white matter, or Canavan disease, and leukodystrophy with Rosenthal fibers, or Alexander disease.[53,54,82] Cerebral biopsy must be sufficiently deep in each case to include adequate amounts of white matter.

A third type of leukodystrophy, classed under the general heading of sudanophilic leukodystrophy, probably comprises several diseases with entirely different causes.[54] The terms "Schilder disease" and "sudanophilic leukodystrophy" have been used interchangeably in the past to cover any generalized white matter disorder with sudanophilic end products of myelin breakdown and no other identifying criteria. Some cases are related to multiple sclerosis, others to adrenoleukodystrophy, and still others to Pelizaeus-Merzbacher disease, in which islands of preserved myelin remain in the midst of sudanophilic white matter degeneration. Brain biopsy findings in these cases may be quite nonspecific or may reveal the typical myelin islands. All these leukodystrophies except Alexander disease produce minor but unfortunately nonspecific changes in peripheral nerves.[7]

Operative Techniques

The area of the skull to be exposed will be decided by the portion of the brain from which the biopsy is to be taken. The skull opening should be large enough to permit an adequate biopsy. Usually a free bone flap made with the air drill is suitable. After opening the dura, cautery should not be used on the cortex until the biopsy specimen has been obtained. Sharp dissection with the scalpel is used to outline the biopsy specimen, which should include one gyrus and one half of the gyrus on either side, as shown in Figure 12–1. The specimen should be approximately as deep and as long as it is wide. The cautery should not be used until the pathologist confirms that an adequate amount of tissue has been removed.

Biopsy Site

The biopsy usually is taken from the nondominant middle frontal gyrus unless the disease is localized to another specific area (Table 12–7). Another common site is preoccipital cortex in approximately Brodmann's area 19.[230]

The majority of conditions diagnosed by brain biopsy either are generalized in the brain or, as in Alzheimer disease, preferentially involve frontal cortex. Biopsy sites in patients suspected of having Pick or Creutzfeldt-Jakob disease should be determined by areas of maximal atrophy as seen by computed tomography or pneumoen-

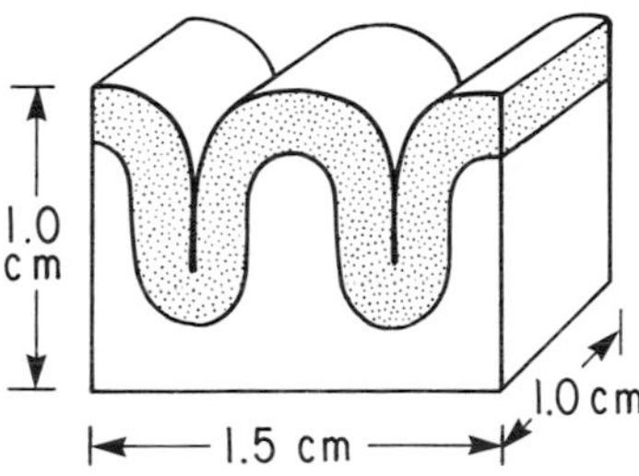

Figure 12–1 Drawing of minimum-sized biopsy of brain for adequate sampling of gray and white matter. Care must be taken to insure that one whole untraumatized gyrus is included and that sufficient white matter is obtained.

TABLE 12–7 PREFERRED BRAIN BIOPSY SITES

DISEASE	PREFERRED BRAIN SITE	ALTERNATIVES
Alzheimer disease	Frontal cortex	Preoccipital cortex
Pick disease	Temporal cortex	Frontal cortex
Creutzfeldt-Jakob disease	Preoccipital cortex	Frontal cortex
Herpes encephalitis	Temporal cortex	Frontal cortex (inferior)
Lafora myoclonic epilepsy	Cerebellar cortex	Frontal cortex
Hallervorden-Spatz syndrome	Globus pallidus	—

cephalography. Pick disease often preferentially involves the anterior two-thirds of the superior temporal gyrus, although it may be predominantly bifrontal. Creutzfeldt-Jakob disease may involve occipital cortex initially. Usually this disease is rapidly progressive, and by the time biopsy is considered, there will be diagnostic changes in the frontal cortex. Occasionally, however, biopsy is performed too early or in the wrong area, and the histological changes are nonspecific.[118]

Anterior temporal and inferior frontal lobes are the usual sites of maximal involvement of herpes simplex encephalitis. Biopsy localization is important in establishing a correct diagnosis, and all available clinical and radiographic techniques should be used to identify the site of maximal involvement.[239] The preferred site for biopsy in subacute sclerosing panencephalitis is the temporal lobe. Fortunately biopsy rarely is required to confirm this diagnosis.

The cerebellum is the preferred biopsy site to identify Lafora bodies in familial myoclonic epilepsy. Frontal cerebral cortex is an alternate site, but the cerebrum may not contain the bodies. Needle biopsy of the globus pallidus is required to obtain diagnostic tissue in Hallervorden-Spatz syndrome.[62] Stereotaxic needle biopsy of the head of the caudate nucleus has been performed for research in Huntingdon chorea and porphyria, and needle biopsies of other subcortical nuclei have been obtained at the time of stereotaxic operation for various movement disorders.[98]

In patients with *long-standing* slowly progressive diseases, biopsies *should not* be obtained from areas of *maximal* involvement. These areas may show only gliosis, necrosis, or calcification. Neurons with pathognomonic inclusions or white matter with characteristic myelin changes may have been replaced by nonspecific repair changes.

Tissue Requirements

A block of cerebral cortex and white matter measuring 1.5 by 1 to 1.5 cm is the ideal cerebral biopsy specimen, as shown in Figure 12–1. The specimen generally will include an entire gyrus and half of the gyri on each side. The pathologist should be present in the operating room at the time of the biopsy and should inspect the specimen to insure that the size is adequate and specifically that sufficient white matter is obtained.

Until adequate tissue has been obtained, hemorrhage can be controlled with Gelfoam soaked in a thrombin solution. After adequate tissue has been obtained, hemostasis can be accomplished with the cautery. A watertight closure of the dura should be made. The bone should be wired into place and the scalp closed in the usual manner.

Complications of Brain Biopsy

Although Kaufman and Catalano reported morbidity at a rate of 13 per cent, the overall incidence of complications with brain biopsy is low in most series and is barely mentioned in others.[118] The possible complications of brain biopsy are numerous (Table 12–8). Epilepsy, intracerebral hemorrhage, subdural hematoma or fluid accumulation, mild and usually transient hemiparesis, porencephaly, postoperative fever of unknown cause, cerebrospinal fluid leak, and wound infection have been reported

TABLE 12–8 POSSIBLE COMPLICATIONS OF BRAIN BIOPSY

Epilepsy and electroencephalographic abnormalities
Subdural hematoma or fluid accumulation
Intracerebral hemorrhage
Hemiparesis, mild, usually transient
Porencephaly
Cerebrospinal fluid leak
Secondary wound infection
Unexplained postoperative fever
Spread of primary infection to other sites
Contagion of slow virus infections

one or more times.* Death has been rare and generally has been attributed to the underlying brain disease.[118] Epilepsy may occur immediately after biopsy or may be a long-term complication. Elian reported a 20 per cent incidence of focal seizures and a 75 per cent incidence of focal electroencephalographic abnormalities as delayed effects of brain biopsy.[71]

Theoretically, spread of a primary nervous system infection is possible, especially with virus or fungi, but has not been reported. Anesthetic complications, such as pneumonia and pulmonary embolism, may be problems, since many candidates for brain biopsy, especially children, have poor respiratory control and are bedridden.

There has been a special interest in the potential for transmission of slow virus disease by contact with infected tissues. Several factors contributed to these concerns. First, kuru, the New Guinea slow virus disease, was identified and its transmission by contact with infected human tissues was confirmed.[8] Next, Creutzfeldt-Jakob disease was transmitted to subhuman primates, and human tissues were found to be infective even after prolonged formalin fixation or routine sterilization.[8] With the stage set, three events happened in rapid succession. Human-to-human transmission of Creutzfeldt-Jakob disease was reported by corneal transplantation; two patients were accidentally inoculated with the virus via inadequately sterilized depth electrodes in the brain; and the virus was identified in the brain tissue of a well-known neurological surgeon who died after a long dementing illness.[17,67,85] Thereafter, the Creutzfeldt-Jakob disease agent was feared to be highly contagious and to survive most sterilizing techniques. After brain tissue from patients with familial Alzheimer disease produced spongiform encephalopathy in subhuman primates, blood and tissues from such patients also were considered potentially infectious.[49]

Some neurosurgeons have refused to perform brain biopsies on patients who were suspected of having Creutzfeldt-Jakob disease. This reluctance to handle tissue infected with slow virus probably is not justified. Although the tissue must be handled carefully, no accidental human transmission has been documented among laboratory workers, surgeons, or pathologists during the more than 20 years that they have been investigated by the National Institutes of Health.[86] This experience includes many autopsies performed in New Guinea under primitive unsterile conditions and numerous laboratory accidents that have been thoroughly investigated. A detailed analysis of the operative procedures performed by the neurological surgeon who died with Creutzfeldt-Jakob disease reveals that none of his patients, either child or adult, were identified as having the disease or a possible childhood equivalent.[201]

There probably is a correlation between previous brain or eye operations and contracting Creutzfeldt-Jakob disease.[8,86]

Against this background, the report by Gajdusek and co-workers should offer both caution and reassurance. The most positive aspect of their report is that the Creutzfeldt-Jakob agent is inactivated by autoclaving for one hour at 250°F under 15 pounds per square inch pressure or by immersion for two hours in 5 per cent sodium hypochlorite (household bleach), iodophore, or phenolic disinfectants.[81,86,220,221] These procedures protect operating room personnel from accidental inoculation by soiled instruments prior to washing and resterilization. Excessively strong bleach solutions may destroy the finish on delicate instruments, however. The same techniques protect laboratory workers, cleaners, and morticians from contaminated cerebrospinal fluid, blood, biopsy, and autopsy tissues. Disposable materials and wound dressings should be decontaminated before disposal to protect maintenance personnel. No specific isolation procedures are indicated. The concern for the safety of subsequent patients using anesthetic equipment is unfounded, since Creutzfeldt-Jakob disease is not spread via the respiratory tract.

All physicians, whether they be neurosurgeons, anesthesiologists, or pathologists, share the responsibility of establishing the diagnosis and prognosis for patients with presenile dementia. In view of the 10 per cent familial incidence of Creutzfeldt-Jakob disease, the diagnosis should be established if the indications for brain biopsy are met.[8] Fear of being infected is not a valid reason for physicians or other medical personnel to shirk the responsibility.

* See references 20, 71, 118, 154, 156.

TABLE 12–9 BRAIN BIOPSY: TISSUE STUDIES INDICATED

SUSPECTED DISEASE	LIGHT MICROSCOPY*			ELECTRON MICROSCOPY†	MICRO-BIOLOGY	BIOCHEMISTRY	ANIMAL INOCULATION	IMMUNOFLUORESCENCE MICROSCOPY	ENZYME HISTOCHEMISTRY	TISSUE CULTURE
	Routine	*Silver*	*Lipid*							
Alzheimer and Pick diseases	X	X		X			R		R	R
Creutzfeldt-Jakob disease	X	X		X			R		R	R
Neuronal storage disorders	X		X	X		X			R	
Leukodystrophy or demyelination	X	X	X	X		X			R	
Encephalitis	X	X		X	X			X		R
Axonal dystrophy	X	X	X	X		R			R	
Poliodystrophy	X	X	X	X		X	R		R	
Totally unknown disorder	X	X	X	X	X	X	R	R	R	R

Key: X, study essential or very useful for diagnosis; R, study often performed for research purposes.

* Routine, routine stains on paraffin-embedded tissue; silver, Von Braunmühl's silver impregnation on frozen sections of formalin-fixed tissue; lipid, lipid stains on frozen sections of formalin-fixed or unfixed tissue.

† Light microscopy of 1-μ sections and electron microscopy on epoxy-embedded tissue.

Tissue Handling

The amount of tissue removed and how it is handled is determined by the studies to be performed (Table 12–9). The pathologist should be in the operating room to receive the tissue and subdivide it under sterile conditions that are not available in the pathology laboratory.

The specimen should be delivered from the operating table on a smooth, firm, slightly moistened surface, such as a Teflon-coated sheet, a wooden tongue blade, or an inverted metal pan. The soft tenacious white matter may cling to the sides of the deep medicine glass and may be partially absorbed into a moistened sponge. Usually the biopsy tissue is subdivided into three portions for light microscopy, electron microscopy, and either microbiological or chemical studies. Sterile handling of the tissue is needed for the isolation of infectious organisms, animal inoculation, or tissue culture. A number of solutions and containers should be available in the operating room for use in handling and fixing the tissue. They include 10 per cent neutral buffered formalin or formol-calcium; electron microscopy fixative (Karnovsky's 2 per cent paraformaldehyde–2.5 per cent glutaraldehyde solution or 2 to 4 per cent phosphate-buffered glutaraldehyde); sterile wide-mouth screw-top bottles for virological or animal inoculation studies; nonsterile wide-mouth screw-top bottles and aluminum foil for biochemical studies; and tissue culture medium in sterile containers, if indicated. Fuming containers of isopentane and liquid nitrogen need not be brought into the operating room. If tissue must be frozen rapidly for immunofluorescence or enzyme histochemical studies, this may be done in the laboratory after the initial operating room dissection.

Initial Dissection

Table 12–10 summarizes the initial subdivision of the specimen and the steps in its preservation. This dissection of the specimen is performed most conveniently on a sterile table in a corner of the operating room. The cube of cortex should be oriented with the pial surface up. First, trim away the irregular outer 2 mm on each side. This slightly traumatized peripheral tissue is suitable for microbiological, animal inoculation, tissue culture, or biochemical studies if gross blood is removed. Tissue obtained by a second biopsy at the depth of the wound also will be traumatized and should be used for similar nonmorphological studies. Cut down the depths of the sulci on either side of the major gyrus in the middle of the specimen. Set aside tissue from the half gyri on each side. Then, a 2-

TABLE 12–10 BRAIN BIOPSY: INITIAL PROCESSING

STUDY	TISSUE AMOUNT	TISSUE PRESERVATION	REFERENCES
Light microscopy			
Routine	3-mm slab	10% neutral buffered formalin	12, 55, 83, 135, 181, 207
Silver	3-mm slab	10% neutral buffered formalin	12, 55, 83, 135, 181, 207
Lipid	3-mm slab	10% formalin (neutral buffered or formol-calcium)	12, 55, 83, 135, 181, 207
Electron microscopy	½ of 3 mm slab	Karnovsky's or glutaraldehyde	99, 100, 113, 123, 130, 136, 137, 148, 149, 223, 224, 240
Viral culture	0.5 cc	Sterile container; transportation on wet ice or freeze at −70°C	
Biochemistry	0.5–1 cc	Freeze at −70°C	21
Immunofluorescence microscopy	3-mm slab	Freeze rapidly (isopentane–liquid nitrogen); store at −70°C	9, 212
Animal inoculation	0.5 cc	Sterile container; store at −70°C	8, 76
Tissue culture	0.5 cc	Mince sterilely; transport in Eagle's medium at room temperature or 37°C	76, 88, 206
Enzyme histochemistry			
Hydrolases	½ of 3-mm slab	1–2 hours in 1–4% buffered formalin, then store in buffered sucrose solution	12, 83, 135, 137, 181
Oxidative and other enzymes	½ of 3-mm slab	Freeze rapidly (isopentane–liquid nitrogen); store at −70°C	12, 83, 135, 137, 181

to 3-mm-thick slice should be cut from two opposite sides of the major gyrus and set aside. A central slab of cortex and white matter at least 3 mm thick will remain. This remaining central slab is bisected lengthwise, and one half is placed in fixative for electron microscopy. The second half of this central optimally preserved slab is available for other special morphological studies; e.g., silver impregnations, immunofluorescence or enzyme histochemical analysis.

From the tissue removed from the ends of the specimen, several subdivisions are made. (1) The two best-oriented 2- to 3-mm-thick slices of cortex and white matter are fixed in either 10 per cent neutral buffered formalin or formol-calcium. (2) At least 0.5 cc of tissue (gray and white matter) is put in a sterile closed container, which is kept on wet ice and transferred to a microbiology laboratory where it will be inoculated directly into bacteriological or fungal or viral culture media, or frozen for later viral culture. (3) If biochemical rather than microbiological studies are indicated, the 0.5 cc of tissue just mentioned may be stored frozen in an unsterile container. (4) Tissue cultures may be performed with any of the tissue fragments that may be distorted or slightly traumatized as long as the tissue is neither ischemic nor cauterized.

Material for viral culture may remain in the sterile contaner at 4° C for six to eight hours without harm. If the tissue cannot be delivered to the virology laboratory during that interval, it should be frozen and kept at −70° C. Material for anaerobic culture should be transported to the laboratory either in a syringe or in a closed anaerobic specimen collector.

Material for biochemical analysis should be placed in a wide-mouthed container to facilitate retrieval of the frozen material without breaking the container. Many biochemists prefer to wrap the tissue in aluminum foil before placing it in the container. This maneuver prevents the soft brain tissue from adhering to the container wall and permits its easy removal. The majority of biochemical studies may be performed on tissue stored for long periods of time at −70° C.

Tissue to be used for such morphological studies as enzyme histochemical analysis or immunofluorescence microscopy should be frozen rapidly by immersion in either isopentane or Freon that has been cooled by liquid nitrogen. After freezing, the tissue may be stored in a laboratory deep freezer or transported on dry ice at −70° C. Ice crystals form and distort the architecture of the tissue if it is frozen slowly by placing it directly in a deep freezer or if it is repeatedly frozen and thawed. The tissue should not be plunged directly into liquid nitrogen, since a layer of gas will develop around the specimen and slow its freezing. A new transport medium, polyvinylpyrrolidone, is now available commercially and permits tissue storage and transportation for up to 24 hours without significant alteration of ultrastructure or enzyme activty.[137]

To obtain tissue cultures of brain biopsies, sterile cortex or white matter or both should be moistened with small amounts of culture medium, minced into 1-mm cubes, and immersed in one of several sterile media. Eagle's basal medium with 10 to 20 per cent fetal calf serum and antibiotics or Leibovitz L-15 medium with 20 per cent fetal calf serum is suitable.[76,89,206] The tissue then may be stored briefly at 37° C until transported at room temperature to the tissue culture laboratory.

Subsequent Studies

Light Microscopy

One slice of formalin-fixed gray and white matter is embedded in paraffin, and sections are stained with hematoxylin-eosin, phosphotungstic acid–hematoxylin, periodic acid–Schiff, Luxol fast blue–cresyl violet, or equivalent myelin and Nissl stains. Silver techniques for axons, such as Bodian's method, and lipid stains, such as Sudan black or Nile blue sulfate, may be attempted on paraffin sections but generally are unsatisfactory.

One slice of formalin-fixed tissue should be retained unembedded for such silver and lipid techniques. Von Braunmühl's silver method is the preferred technique to demonstrate the neuritic (senile) plaques and neurofibrillary tangles of Alzheimer disease and the Pick bodies in Pick disease. If only paraffin sections are available, the periodic acid–Schiff stain often demonstrates neuritic plaques better than the silver methods for paraffin. Under no circumstances is a hematoxylin and eosin–stained section sufficient to exclude Alzheimer disease, because both plaques and tangles may remain virtually invisible unless differentially stained.

If a sphingolipidosis, a related storage disorder, or leukodystrophy is suspected, a preliminary battery of lipid stains should include oil red-O, Sudan black, and acidified cresyl violet for sulfatide metachromasia. Toluidine blue is an additional confirmatory stain for metachromasia, and Nile blue sulfate is a relative simple stain for both phospholipids and neutral lipids. These stains in addition to the periodic acid–Schiff stain for glycogen and the alcian blue stain for mucopolysaccharides also may be applied to sections of frozen unfixed tissue. Other semispecific lipid stains are available but cannot replace biochemical analysis.

Electron Microscopy

The material embedded in epoxy resin for electron microscopy is valuable not only for its ultrastructural features but also for the light microscopic changes visible in 1-μ-thick sections.[136] In these sections many early lesions may be identified owing to the increased microscopic resolution in thin sections, and paraffin artifacts such as vacuolization and cell shrinkage are avoided. This tissue has been fixed and embedded by procedures that differ radically from those used for paraffin and frozen sections; therefore changes, no matter how slight, that are present in both paraffin and epoxy sections probably are not artifacts. The neuropil vacuolization characteristic of Creutzfeldt-Jakob spongiform encephalopathy closely resembles paraffin artifacts and should be identified in both paraffin and epoxy sections before a diagnosis is made.

BIOPSY OF TUMOR

Tumor biopsy and diagnosis of tissue type is an essential guide for making decisions regarding treatment and prognosis. The procedure represents an exchange of information between neurosurgeon and pathologist. The neurosurgeon should supply information on the location of a tumor, which may be helpful to the pathologist if it occurs in a characteristic site. Table 12–11 lists nervous system neoplasms according to their usual locations. Table 12–12 lists the types of mass lesions that most often occur in typical sites. Other information that is useful in interpretating the pathological changes includes general tissue texture, tumor vascularity, tumor necrosis, discreteness of tumor-brain interface, peritumoral edema, cysts and their contents, and xanthomatous degeneration.[36–38]

TABLE 12–11 COMMON LOCATIONS OF NERVOUS SYSTEM NEOPLASMS

NEOPLASM	LOCATIONS
Astrocytoma, well differentiated	Cerebral white matter, optic nerve, optic chiasm, third ventricle wall (thalamus-hypothalamus), brain stem (pons), cerebellum, upper spinal cord
Astrocytoma, anaplastic; glioblastoma multiforme	Cerebral white matter (chiefly frontal) including corpus callosum; much less often brain stem and spinal cord
Oligodendroglioma	Cerebral white matter, corpus callosum, subcortical nuclei
Ependymoma	Fourth ventricle, lower spinal cord and filum terminale, less often deep in cerebrum
Microglioma	Cerebrum, including basal ganglia
Hemangioblastoma	Cerebellum, less often medulla and spinal cord
Meningioma	Cerebral convexity: attached to inner dural surface: parasagittal (middle third), Sylvian fissure, mid- and inferior parietal area Brain base: parasellar area, tuberculum sellae, olfactory groove, sphenoid wing, cerebellopontine angle, foramen magnum Spinal cord; commonly thoracic, intradural Intraventricular
Schwannoma	Attached to sensory nerve roots in cerebellopontine angle, spinal intradural space; less often extradural or extending through intervertebral foramen
Neurofibroma	Peripheral and autonomic nerves, usually in multiple neurofibromatosis
Germinoma	Pineal, suprasellar
Chordoma	Sacrum, clivus
Dermoid cyst	Midline posterior fossa, lumbosacral spinal canal
Epidermoid cyst	Cerebellopontine angle, parapituitary area and middle cranial fossa, within frontal or parietal bone, fourth ventricle, spinal canal
Metastatic neoplasms	Superficial cerebral white matter, cerebellum, vertebral body, spinal epidural space

The Pathology Report

The pathology report should contain a series of descriptive phrases that lead to a clinically useful diagnosis. The diagnosis should contain the basic cell type, an estimation of malignancy, and clinically important secondary changes that either aid in planning therapy or correlate with clinical, operative, and laboratory findings. Table 12–13 lists the usual components of a microscopic description of a tumor. Except for purely research procedures, all the pathological techniques applied to neural neoplasms are designed to provide information about the 13 items listed in Table 12–13. Table 12–14 outlines the use of these components in making the three-part diagnosis.

TABLE 12–12 MASS LESIONS EXPECTED IN TYPICAL SITES

SITE	LESION
Cranial convexity (extradural space, cranium, or both)	Abscess, metastatic neoplasm, epidermoid cyst, less often meningioma
Cerebral convexity (subdural space)	Meningioma, hematoma, abscess, metastatic neoplasm, epidermoid cyst
Cerebral cortex, white matter	Astrocytoma–glioblastoma multiforme, metastatic neoplasm, oligodendroglioma, abscess or granuloma, acute infarct, organizing hematoma, focal encephalitis (Herpesvirus, papova virus), traumatic edema and contusion, rarely ependymoma or microglioma
Corpus callosum	Glioblastoma multiforme, lipoma, oligodendroglioma
Subcortical nuclei (basal ganglia, diencephalon)	Astrocytoma, oligodendroglioma, metastatic neoplasm, hematoma, abscess
Parasellar region	Pituitary adenoma, meningioma, craniopharyngioma, germinoma, epidermoid or dermoid cyst, aneurysm; hypothalamic, medial temporal lobe or optic chiasm astrocytoma; sarcoidosis or other granuloma
Optic nerve	Astrocytoma, meningioma, sarcoidosis
Subfrontal area	Meningioma, nasopharyngeal carcinoma, olfactory neuroblastoma, focal encephalitis (Herpesvirus)
Clivus	Chordoma, meningioma
Cerebellopontine angle	Schwannoma, meningioma, epidermoid cyst, ependymoma, glomus jugulare tumor, metastatic neoplasm
Brain stem	Astrocytoma, metastatic neoplasm, abscess
Pineal region	Germinoma, true pineal tumor, glioma, tentorial meningioma
Cerebellum, fourth ventricle	Astrocytoma, medulloblastoma, hemangioblastoma, metastatic neoplasm, ependymoma, abscess, hematoma, infarct
Ventricles (lateral, third)	Choroid plexus papilloma, meningioma, colloid cyst, extension of other neoplasms (astrocytoma, subependymoma, ependymoma)
Spinal cord	Astrocytoma (upper), ependymoma (lower and filum terminale), hemangioblastoma
Spinal subdural space	Meningioma, schwannoma, neurofibroma, lipoma, dermoid and epidermoid cysts, less often metastatic neoplasms
Spinal epidural space, spine	Metastatic neoplasms (carcinoma, lymphoma, myeloma), abscess or granuloma, chordoma, lipoma, herniated disc

TABLE 12–13 SURGICAL PATHOLOGY REPORT: TUMOR DESCRIPTION

Reports of microscopic examination of tumors include descriptions of the following components:

1. Basic tumor cell nucleus and cytoplasm: size, shape, staining properties
2. Fiber production by tumor cells
3. Other specialized cytoplasmic structures
4. Specialized cellular interrelationships
5. Degree of tumor cell pleomorphism: nucleus, cytoplasm
6. Mitosis population
7. Blood vessels: number, morphology, evidence of proliferation
8. Necrosis: degree, pattern
9. Fibrous stroma: pattern, cell content, relationship to neoplastic cells
10. Peritumoral edema
11. External relationships of tumor cells to brain, ependyma, meninges, bone, operative margins
12. Hemorrhage
13. Calcification

Tumor Cell Identification

The four major means of tumor cell identification are outlined in Table 12–15. Each has its value and its pitfalls. The first criterion, resemblances between normal and neoplastic cells, is used universally and successfully in examination of well-differentiated neoplasms. Errors occur when poorly differentiated cells are confused

TABLE 12–14 SURGICAL PATHOLOGY REPORT: TUMOR DIAGNOSIS

The diagnostic portion of a tumor pathology report contains three parts. Each part is based chiefly on data described under the 13 items listed in Table 12–13.

DIAGNOSIS COMPONENT	MAJOR DESCRIPTIVE DATA ITEM USED
Basic tumor cell type	1–4
Degree of malignancy	5–11
Useful clinical correlates	7–13

TABLE 12–15 TUMOR CELL IDENTIFICATION CRITERIA

RESEMBLANCE TO CELLS OF EMBRYO, NORMAL ADULT, OR ANOTHER TUMOR
- Nuclear size, shape, staining properties
- Cytoplasmic outline, stain affinity: may require metallic impregnations*

SPECIFIC TUMOR CELL PRODUCTS
- Cytoplasmic glial fibrils: displayed by special stains, electron microscopy*
- Nissl bodies and argyrophilic neurofibrils in neurons*
- Intracellular filaments: meningiomas*
- Extracellular material: collagen, reticulin, basement membrane, amyloid*
- Secretory granules: biogenic amines, pituitary hormones, melanin, mucin*

SPECIALIZED CELLULAR INTERRELATIONSHIPS
- Glial cells: ependymal rosettes, ependymoma and astroblastoma gliovascular structures
- Neurons: rosettes of neuroblastoma, retinoblastoma, medulloblastoma
- Mesenchymal cells: meningioma whorls and desmosomes*, schwannoma palisades
- Carcinoma: acinus, zonula adherens, desmosomes*

TYPICAL TUMOR LOCATION
- Helpful in small tumors (e.g., subependymoma, choroid plexus papilloma)

* Special techniques may be required for some characteristics in this group.

with embryonic cells or when minor cell features are compared. For example, not every triangular cell with a prominent nucleolus is a neuron.

The second set of cell identification criteria requires demonstration of specific tumor cell products. The demonstration usually is based on specialized techniques such as histochemical analysis, metallic impregnation, electron microscopy, and immunohistochemical or biochemical analysis of tumor tissue. When the specific tumor cell products can be identified, these techniques are quite useful. Unfortunately, they are most likely to fail when they are most needed to diagnose the poorly differentiated neoplasm.

The highly specialized interrelationships among tumor cells make up the third set of cell identification criteria. These interrelationships are easily seen with routine stains in well-differentiated neoplasms. Special stains or impregnations may be required for poorly differentiated tumors, while in highly anaplastic examples, only electron microscopy may reveal abortive attempts to maintain characteristic cell-to-cell contacts.

If a tumor is in a typical location, its cell type may be inferred from the site of origin. Two examples of this fourth identification criterion are subependymoma and choroid plexus papilloma. Another tumor that arises in a typical location, "pinealoma," illustrates a pitfall in this method of tumor identification. Multiple tumor types arise in the pineal region, each with a different cell of origin, biological activity, or mode of treatment. Other criteria, therefore, must be used to identify the cell type of pineal tumors.

Tumor Malignancy

The histological factors important in estimating tumor malignancy are given in Table 12–16. Increased cell population in a particular area, for instance cerebral white matter, may be the major indication of a well-differentiated neoplasm. Cell nuclei in such a slowly growing tumor are slightly larger and darker than nonneoplastic nuclei and usually occur in irregular clusters, often in pairs or quartets. Their resemblance to normal or reactive astrocytes indicates a low degree of malignancy, and the only diagnostic problem is identifying the presence of a neoplasm. Nuclear pleomorphism is a more accurate indication of growth rate in a glioma than is the number of mitoses, which are relatively rare.[105] Estimating the degree of cellular dedifferentiation or cellular immaturity is a second means of measuring malignancy. Cells look less and less mature as they become more malignant. Many ma-

TABLE 12–16 INDICES OF TUMOR MALIGNANCY

DIRECT EVIDENCE OF CELL PROLIFERATION
- Hypercellularity
- Mitoses
- Hyperchromatic nuclei
- Nuclear pleomorphism
- Increased cell labeling index*

EVIDENCE OF DEDIFFERENTIATION—CELLULAR IMMATURITY
- Variations in cellular size and shape
- Loss of specialized cytoplasmic function*

INDIRECT EVIDENCE OF MALIGNANCY
- Tumor angiogenesis
- Stromal proliferation
- Tumor necrosis
- Relationship to adjacent structures
  - Peritumoral edema
  - Narrow glioma-brain transition
  - Satellitosis of tumor cells around normal structures
  - Invasion of adjacent tissues

* Special techniques required.

lignant cells are so poorly differentiated that their basic cell line is unidentifiable. In a few cases, special procedures may be used to determine cell turnover in a neoplasm. These procedures include determination of cell labeling indices by autoradiography and identification of cells in the S phase of the mitotic cycle by immunoenzymatic techniques.[105,132]

Biopsy Procedure

The tissue should be obtained from viable portions of the tumor. Necrotic foci, which are common in central portions of malignant glial tumors and metastatic lesions, should be avoided. Cautery should be used sparingly near the tissue that is slated for biopsy. The specimen should be dissected free with sharp instruments and with as little trauma as possible to the specimen. For frozen sections, the tissue should be transferred to a firm smooth-surface container, such as a shallow plastic cup. It may be covered with a slightly moistened sponge, but should not be placed on the sponge or immersed in saline or fixative.[187] Immersion of the tissue in a fluid adds to ice crystal artifacts in subsequent frozen sections, while extrication of soft glial tumor fragments from the meshes of a sponge is tedious and time consuming.

Complications

Several factors tend to lessen the postoperative neurological deficits that follow an excisional tumor biopsy. The excision generally is limited to removal of tumor and includes only minimal amounts of normal tissue. Also, the internal decompression accomplished by removing the inner portions of the tumor reduces intracranial pressure. Postoperative hemorrhage may complicate either tumor excision or needle biopsy.[52] A rare complication of tumor biopsy is spread of neoplastic cells either within the operative field, through the cerebrospinal fluid pathways, or outside the central nervous at the incision site and via venous and lymphatic channels to lymph nodes, lung, or other viscera.[189] Since the successful tumor cell implantation is so rare, it is not a contraindication to tumor biopsy and excision.

Needle Biopsy

Needle biopsy is an alternative to tumor excision and may be indicated with deep-seated neoplasms such as thalamic or pontine astrocytomas whose excision would be hazardous and with lesions in highly characteristic locations, e.g., medulloblastoma, that are quite radiosensitive.[48,70,98,234] Computed tomography may be used to assist needle placement.[131,139] The major drawback to needle biopsy is the difficulty of establishing a histological diagnosis with small tissue samples. Often, the biopsy is not truly representative of the tumor. The narrow tissue core often is vacuolated or distorted owing to trauma, and only a few central cells are well preserved and in proper alignment. Unless the needle is extremely sharp, it is difficult to sample firm fibrous neoplasms without tearing artifacts. Well-differentiated astrocytomas, unfortunately the most common tumors in thalamus and brain stem, are composed of widely separated mature astrocytes. Such tumors are difficult to distinguish from normal white matter or reactive gliosis if only a small tissue sample is available for examination. If the pathologist is familiar with squash or touch preparations, and can identify normal brain tissue in these preparations, they may be preferable to frozen sections for intraoperative diagnosis of small needle biopsy specimens.

The principal risk of needle biopsy is the induction of serious intracranial hemorrhage. In one large survey of complications from stereotaxic operations of all kinds, an 8 per cent incidence of intracranial hematomas was noted and there was a mortality rate of 5 per cent.[52] The majority of the serious hematomas were intracerebral, chiefly thalamic. Fourteen per cent of patients suffered a motor deficit, presumably from vascular occlusion. Seizures have not been reported as a complication of needle biopsy.

Cytological Techniques

A second alternative to excisional biopsy for tumor diagnosis is cytological examination of cerebrospinal fluid combined with precise radiographic localization of the lesion. Such techniques may be used with suprachiasmatic lesions such as craniopharyngioma and dysgerminoma and posterior fossa tumors of childhood such as ependymoma or medulloblastoma.[189]

Intraoperative Diagnosis

Indications

Indications for intraoperative diagnosis include confirmation that the lesion has been located, differentiation of neoplastic from nonneoplastic lesions, differentiation of metastatic from primary intracranial neoplasms, subclassification of primary intracranial neoplasms, and estimation of malignancy. These latter two findings are important to the neurological surgeon in planning the extent of the resection of a tumor.[37,38]

Touch, Squash, and Smear Techniques

Slides for these techniques should be made prior to freezing the tissue. Many pathologists prefer cytological techniques to examination of frozen sections, and others use both. Specimens that are unusually small or soft in consistency may provide more information when examined as touch preparations than as frozen sections.

The techniques are relatively simple and rapid. For touch imprints, the glass slide is pressed briefly to the unfixed tissue surface, air dried, then fixed for two minutes in 95 per cent alcohol and stained by the Giemsa method. Hematoxylin-eosin stain may be applied after only one minute in alcohol. A more rapid technique involves simple flooding or immersion of the slide in a polychrome stain followed by a wash and water mount.[38]

The smear or squash method involves the smearing of a tiny tissue fragment between two glass slides in the same manner used in making peripheral blood smears. The slide then is dried on a hot plate for 30 to 60 seconds, or fixed as for the touch imprints. The slide then may be flooded with polychrome stain or stained with either hematoxylin-eosin, eosin–methylene blue, toluidine blue, or phosphotungsic acid–hematoxylin.*

* See references 24, 110, 111, 140, 141, 153, 157, 192.

Frozen Sections

After touch preparations have been made, the unfixed specimen is mounted on a chuck and arranged to keep multiple tissue fragments in the same plane of section. This permits simultaneous sampling of the entire specimen without tedious sectioning deeply into the block. The block may be flooded with coolant spray and frozen in the cryostat chamber or rapidly frozen by immersion in super-cooled isopentane or Freon.

Sections may either be stained by immersion in hematoxylin and eosin stain or may be flooded with or immersed in a commercially available polychrome stain.[37,38] Polychrome stains shorten the procedure but may stain capriciously. A reticulin stain is useful in differentiating a pituitary adenoma from a normal pituitary gland in frozen sections.[229]

Most of the time required for producing a frozen section diagnosis is consumed in freezing and sectioning the tissue. A certain amount of trial and error is required to determine the optimal temperature and section thickness for each specimen. Sections should be ready for staining within five minutes.

Frozen sections alone have an accuracy of approximately 90 per cent in grouping material into general diagnostic categories, but are less accurate for subclassifying gliomas and determining their degree of malignancy. Accuracy may be improved by also using touch or smear preparations. Probably the most treacherous task in neuropathology is differentiating between normal white matter, early infarction, reactive gliosis, and well-differentiated astrocytoma by frozen sections.

Several problems are common in frozen section diagnosis. Often, the initial specimens come from cerebral cortex and do not contain obvious neoplasm. Often, just beyond the edge of a glioma, widely separated neoplastic cells cluster around neurons and blood vessels or line up beneath the pia mater. These cell configurations should signal a need for additional deeper specimens.[199] The degree of malignant change in a glial neoplasm frequently is underestimated in frozen sections. Mitoses are rare in gliomas, and indices of malignancy such as nuclear hyperchromia and pleomorphism often are mimicked by freezing artifacts. Furthermore, the frozen section specimens usually come from tumor periphery, which often is better differentiated and lacks the secondary degenerative features so helpful in estimating malignant change. Malignant changes in nerve sheath or meningeal tumors also may be overlooked in frozen sections because of nuclear distortion and irregular nuclear staining. A final problem in frozen section diagnosis is failure to differentiate astrocytoma from the less common glial tumors such as oligodendroglioma and ependymoma. The most useful histological clue to the presence of a nonastrocytic glial tumor is the cellular monotony of oligodendroglioma and ependymoma. In these tumors, cells are tightly packed together but fail to show the nuclear and cytoplasmic pleomorphism that results from the high-density living conditions of neoplastic astrocytes.

Tissue Techniques

Light Microscopy

Fixation

Although the majority of neural tumors can be diagnosed by examining tissue fixed in 10 per cent neutral formalin buffered with sodium phosphate, many of the new pathological techniques require special initial fixation and cannot be applied to formalin-fixed tissue. The pathologist should become involved early in the handling of the tissue in order to select the special techniques that may add to the diagnostic accuracy. For this reason, many pathologists prefer to examine frozen sections of all neural tumors and, on the basis of frozen section findings, choose fixatives best suited to the diagnostic problem. Under no circumstances is saline a suitable environment for the specimen, since it causes distortion of the cells and increases the number of artifacts.

Special fixatives are preferred for certain histological techniques (Table 12–17). Formalin–ammonium bromide (FAB) is the best fixative for metallic impregnations of glial cells; Cajal's gold chloride for astrocytes; and Hortega's silver carbonate methods for immature astrocytes, oligodendroglia, and microglia. Zenker's mercuric chloride–potassium dichromate solution may be used as the initial fixative to enhance glial fiber staining with the phosphotungstic acid–hematoxylin (PTAH) stain, but tissue must be removed from Zenker's solution within 24 hours to avoid excessive brittleness. Zenker-formalin (Helly's solution) and Heidenhain's "susa" solution are useful variations to improve glial fiber demonstrations in paraffin-embedded material and yet avoid the tissue brittleness caused by regular Zenker's solution. Fixatives in which picric acid is added to formalin or other solutions (e.g., Bouin's and Halmi's solution) preserve secretory granules well in pituitary tumors.*

Nuclear detail is enhanced, particularly in highly cellular neoplasms such as lymphomas, by a mercuric chloride–sodium acetate–formalin solution known as B-5, which is similar to the Heidenhain's "susa" solution.[133] This fixative is also excellent for light microscopic immunoenzymatic techniques.

If no decision upon proper fixation can be made at the time of operation, or if such fixatives are not available, a holding-transport

* See references 12, 55, 83, 113, 135, 181, 189, 207.

TABLE 12–17 COMMON TUMOR TISSUE PROCEDURES: SUMMARY

TUMOR	FIXATIVE	LIGHT MICROSCOPY STAINS	ELECTRON MICROSCOPY FINDINGS	OTHER PROCEDURES
Glial	Zenker FAB	PTAH Hortega (frozen sections)	Glial filaments	Glial fiber immunohistochemical studies
Neuronal	Formalin	Bielschowsky (frozen sections)	Neurofilaments and tubules	
Neuronal and paraganglionic	Orth (dichromate)	Chromaffin reactions	Biogenic amine granules	Autofluorescence techniques
Pituitary	Bouin	PAS–orange G and variations	Hormonal secretory granules	Hormonal immunohistochemical studies

medium containing polyvinylpyrrolidone may be used. This will permit storage for 24 hours without injury to ultrastructure, enzymes, or many other chemical constituents.[137]

Fixation of most biopsy specimens is complete within 24 hours. Tiny fragments (1 to 2 mm) may be fixed for two hours and then embedded, but at least overnight fixation is preferable for larger neural tissue blocks. Not all fixed tissue should be embedded in paraffin if diagnostic problems are anticipated. Formalin- or formalin–ammonium bromide–fixed tissue must be retained for frozen sections when it will be necessary to use oil-red O or another Sudan lipid stain for lipid-filled stromal cells in hemangioblastomas; Bielschowsky or other silver impregnations for neurofibrils in neurons and neuroblasts; or Cajal gold chloride and Hortega silver carbonate impregnations for glial cells. Regardless of the initial fixative, formalin is the best solution for long-term tissue storage.

Stains

Hematoxylin and eosin staining of paraffin sections solves the majority of diagnostic problems in neuropathology as well as in general pathology. Such diagnoses are made on purely morphological criteria for tumors with a single clearly identifiable cell type. Special stains or other procedures are needed, however, for some complex tumors made up either of multiple tumor cell lines or cells of uncertain origin. These special stains help to identify glial and neuronal elements of the tumor, collagen and reticulin fibers in either the tumor or its stroma, and diagnostically important cytoplasmic inclusions or secretory material within tumor cells. Mallory's phosphotungstic acid–hematoxylin technique is the most useful method for staining glial fibers for paraffin sections because glial and collagen fibers usually stain in contrasting colors.[135] This stain is also useful in examination of peripheral nerves and nerve sheath tumors because myelin and collagen also stain contrasting colors. Unfortunately, fibrin and many immature collagen fibers stain the same deep blue color as do glial fibers, and confirmatory reticulin stains are recommended.[94] Pituitary adenomas fixed in Bouin's solution should be stained chiefly by variations on the periodic acid–Schiff–orange G method.*

Demonstration of biogenic amines in neuronal tumors and paragangliomas is important diagnostically, but the difficulties of staining these substances consistently are betrayed by the large number of techniques recommended in the histochemical literature.† In general, dichromate fixative (Orth's solution) is used for chromaffin reactions to display biogenic amines in neuronal tumors and paragangliomas.[12,83,203] Frozen tissue, either unfixed or fixed briefly in paraformaldehyde–glyoxylic acid, is required for autofluorescent demonstration of biogenic amines in these neuronal tumors.[11,14,78,168] Direct biochemical measurements of biogenic amines in excised tumor tissue may be the best diagnostic method at times.[35,161]

Electron Microscopy

The major use of electron microscopy in tumor diagnosis is cell identification of poorly differentiated neoplasms. Table 12–18 lists ultrastructural features that are useful in the identification of primary brain tumors. None of the characteristics is absolutely diagnostic of a specific cell type. Table 12–19 lists the ultrastructural features of malignant neoplasms that commonly metastasize to the central nervous system. These characteristics often help to identify the cell of origin and aid in the search for an occult primary tumor.[41,93] Because electron microscopy requires prompt tissue fixation, both the neurosurgeon and the pathologist must understand the initial steps in tissue preservation.‡

The most workable approach to specimen selection is to fix at least a small portion of every tumor specimen for electron microscopy. This material may be discarded later if initial light microscopic examination eliminates the need for electron microscopy. Soon, perhaps, all pathologists will accept the use of a "universal" fixative that will preserve ultrastructure and at the same time permit a wide variety

---

* See references 33, 77, 83, 95, 96, 101, 102, 133, 135, 147, 174–176.

† See references 1, 11, 14, 23, 50, 51, 57, 74, 78, 83, 97, 109, 168, 173, 202, 203, 236.

‡ See references 99, 100, 113, 130, 148, 188, 240,

TABLE 12–18 DIAGNOSTIC ULTRASTRUCTURE: PRIMARY INTRACRANIAL AND NEURAL TISSUE NEOPLASMS

NEOPLASM	ULTRASTRUCTURAL FEATURES	REFERENCES
Astrocytoma, glioblastoma multiforme	Compact 6-nm intracytoplasmic filaments	189
Ependymoma	Microvilli, basal bodies, cilia, zonula adherens formation, 6-nm cytoplasmic filaments	185, 189, 232
Oligodendroglioma	Concentrically laminated cell processes	186, 189
Meningioma		
Fibroblastic, meningothelial, transitional	Whorls of interlacing cell processes, desmosomes, compact or whorled 10-nm intracytoplasmic filaments	189
Angioblastic	10-nm intracytoplasmic filaments, basement membrane material	189
Schwannoma, neurofibroma	Basement membranes investing Schwann cells, long-spaced collagen	183
Medulloblastoma	Dense core vesicles, incomplete synapses (very rare)	189
Central ganglioglioma, neuroblastoma, pineocytoma	Dense core vesicles, synapses, axonal processes with neurofilaments and microtubules	165, 190
Retinoblastoma	Dense core vesicles, cilia, terminal bars, microvilli	180
Peripheral neuronal tumors: neuroblastoma, ganglioneuroma, ganglioneuroblastoma	Dense core vesicles, synapses, axonal processes with neurofilaments and microtubules	92, 155, 173
Pheochromocytoma, paraganglioma	Dense core vesicles	35, 92, 104, 155, 173
Pituitary adenoma	Secretory granules with characteristic size ranges	79, 126–128, 171

of special stains to be used on light microscopic sections.[148,149]

Problems

The most serious problem in surgical electron microscopy is an error in tissue sampling. The second problem is artifacts due to damage of the ultrastructure by the electrocautery. Another source of artifacts is incomplete tissue fixation due to immersion of thick tissue fragments. These problems are produced within the first five minutes after the tissue is removed. Several steps may be taken to decrease their frequency.

TABLE 12–19 DIAGNOSTIC ULTRASTRUCTURE: COMMON METASTATIC NEOPLASMS

NEOPLASM	ULTRASTRUCTURAL FEATURES
Adenocarcinoma	Mucin granules, microvilli Apical zonula occludens Lumen formation
Squamous carcinoma	Tonofibrils, desmosomes Glycogen
Melanoma	Melanosomes, promelanosomes
Lymphomas, leukemias	No specialized cellular attachments, few or no cellular inclusions

Tissue Selection

Representative portions of viable tumor should be excised cleanly without cauterization. In a large tumor, the most suitable tissue lies just inside the growing tumor rim where neovascularity and necrosis are minimal.

The tumor border often is indistinct, particularly in well-differentiated glial tumors, and alternative sampling techniques must be used. If multiple frozen sections are required to identify tumor tissue, the pathologist should set aside under a moist gauze approximately one fourth of each frozen section specimen. Fragments that are representative of tumor may then be fixed for electron microscopy.

Another method, particularly for large en bloc dissections, is to section immediately the unfixed tumor specimen into broad 2-mm-thick slabs. After overnight immersion in a fixative for electron microscopy, viable tumor will be more sharply demarcated from normal brain and necrosis or cautery artifact. If the slabs of tissue do not exceed 2 mm in thickness, all parts will be equally well fixed. One or more areas then may be selected for electron microscopy, and the remaining tissue can be stored in fixative for possible additional sampling. The broad thin slabs maintain specimen orientation in heterogeneous tumors from which multiple areas should be sampled and correlated with the tissue patterns seen on gross examination or light microscopy.

Fixation

Surgical pathology requires an immersion fixative that penetrates rapidly and deeply, preserves proteins and cytoplasmic organelles well, and will not overfix tissue stored for long periods of time. Most agents are composed of varied combinations of two basic fixatives, formaldehyde or glutaraldehyde, and two basic buffer systems, phosphate or cacodylate. Each ingredient has strong points and weak points. Glutaraldehyde, the research fixative preferred especially for perfusion studies, preserves secretory granules, microtubules, and other proteins, and also preserves many enzyme functions. Glutaraldehyde, however, penetrates tissue slowly for only short distances, and lengthy immersion produces unmanageable tissue brittleness. Formaldehyde, on the other hand, penetrates tissue rapidly and deeply, and will not produce brittle tough tissue with prolonged fixation. Formaldehyde, however, preserves secretory granules, microtubules, and other proteins poorly; and rapidly destroys most enzymes.

An excellent fixative for electron microscopic work is a phosphate-buffered glutaraldehyde-formaldehyde mixture called Karnovsky's solution. A final mixture of 2 per cent paraformaldehyde and 2.5 per cent glutaraldehyde in 0.1 M phosphate buffer (pH 7.3) maintains both the tissue preservation qualities of glutaraldehyde and the penetration and long-term storage qualities of formaldehyde.[99,100] Fixative penetrates faster at room temperature, but buffers maintain pH better over long periods of time at 4° C. Therefore, after initial fixation at room temperature, the specimen should be refrigerated until embedment.

A few laboratories have championed the use of a universal fixative, suitable for both light microscopy of paraffin-embedded material and electron microscopy of plastic-embedded material.[148,149,223,224] One recommended universal fixative contains 4 per cent commercial formaldehyde and 1 per cent glutaraldehyde in phosphate buffer.[149] Most electron microscopists have avoided commercial formaldehyde because of the harmful effects of additives and have mixed formaldehyde from the paraformaldehyde powder. Perhaps, as just suggested, currently available commercial formaldehyde solutions are not as harmful to ultrastructure as previously thought, if they are well buffered. The small amount of glutaraldehyde in the solution does not interfere with sectioning of paraffin-embedded blocks or any of the usual light microscopic stains.

The 10 per cent neutral buffered formalin ordinarily used in histopathology laboratories is harmful to tissue ultrastructure and is not an adequate substitute for the previously mentioned fixatives. All is not lost, however, if tissue lands in the wrong solution. Newer embedding and microscopy techniques help cover up many technical errors.

Several situations require fixation by glutaraldehyde alone. Immunologically active binding sites are better preserved by glutaraldehyde than by formaldehyde. One per cent phosphate-buffered glutaraldehyde is suggested for pituitary immunocytochemical study with peroxidase methods.[209] Other investigators prefer paraformaldehyde-fixed tissues. Noradrenalin is said to be demonstrated easily in formaldehyde-fixed material, but adrenalin is not.[51]

Semi-Thick Sections

The term "thick section" or "semi-thick section" indicates a 1-μ-thick section of plastic-embedded tissue cut with a freshly fractured glass knife on a special microtome. Such sections are mounted on glass slides, stained, and examined under a light microscope.

This technique bridges the gap in magnification and orientation between light and electron microscopy. One-micron sections add to the clarity of image and fine detail visible in thicker paraffin sections. Semi-thick sections also are used to sample blocks and select for electron microscopy those tissue areas that best represent the tumor seen in paraffin sections.[136]

Water-Soluble Embedding Media

Water-soluble embedding media such as glycol methacrylate have been introduced recently for two purposes: to permit light microscopic examination of 1-μ-thick tissue sections stained with a wide range of histological stains, and to facilitate electron microscopic immunocytochemical studies.[129,209] Many pathologists have abandoned paraffin embedment of small biopsies and place the entire specimen in methacrylate. Light microscopy of these thin sections reveals many fine fibrils, cell-to-cell contacts, and cellular inclusions that would go undetected in the thicker paraffin sections.

Immunohistochemistry

Value and Indications

Four applications of immunohistochemical methods appear to be feasible in neuropathology. The first is the identification by immunoperoxidase techniques of glial fibrillary acidic protein in neoplastic astrocytes.[88,185,232] Use of this immunological marker for astrocytes is rapidly becoming almost routine in some laboratories for diagnosis of gliomas, particularly because the techniques are suitable for paraffin-embedded material. Another protein marker for mature astrocytes has been identified biochemically.[235]

A second use is identification of hormones in normal and neoplastic anterior pituitary cells by means of both light and electron microscopic modifications of these techniques.*

The third application of immunohistochemistry is in the diagnosis of metastatic tumors. Many malignant neoplasms present initially as nervous system metastases, and search for the primary lesion is difficult or fruitless. Immunopathological techniques may identify the origin of such metastatic neoplasms by detecting organ-specific tumor cell antigens. Many tumor-related antigens, such as carcinoembryonic antigens, are only semi-specific, but even these are useful in excluding certain organs, for example, the nervous system, as the origin of tumors with large amounts of carcinoembryonic antigen.[91] A partial list of neoplasms with detectable specific or semi-specific antigens includes lymphoma, myeloma, smooth and striated muscle tumors, neuroblastoma, choriocarcinoma, colonic carcinoma, hepatoma, and breast carcinoma. As additional organ-specific antigens are identified on neoplastic cells, the value of the technique will increase.[235]

The fourth use is estimation of tumor labeling index and degree of malignancy by using antinucleoside antibodies.[132]

Immunohistochemical Techniques

Two basic methods are used to localize antigen-antibody complexes in tissue sections, cell cultures, cell suspensions, or touch preparations. Immunofluorescence methods use antibodies bound to a fluorescent substance, while immunoenzymatic methods use antibodies bound to an enzyme, usually horseradish peroxidase, which can be visualized with stains such as diaminobenzidine–hydrogen peroxide.†

For light microscopic immunofluorescence techniques, tissue must be frozen rapidly in either dry ice–acetone or liquid nitrogen–isopentane and stored in a freezer, and cryostat sections must be prepared. For light microscopic immunoenzymatic techniques, tissue should be fixed in B-5 for two to four hours, transferred to 80 per cent alcohol, and embedded in paraffin. Formalin-fixed tissue also may be used. For electron microscopy, a dilute fixative such as 1 per cent paraformaldehyde should be used and followed by Araldite or glycol methacrylate embedment.

Research Procedures

Occasionally, neurosurgeons affiliated with research institutions will be asked to obtain neoplastic tissue for highly specialized studies of limited clinical value. These studies include cell and organ cultures, enzyme histochemical analysis, scanning electron microscopy, and biochemical analysis. Generally each research laboratory specifies tissue handling techniques, but a few general guide lines for tissue processing and preservation are provided for reference. Table 12–20 summarizes tissue handling for these procedures.

---

* See references 95, 96, 101, 102, 120, 122, 162, 174–176.

† See references 9, 58, 59, 88, 123, 174–176, 212, 216, 231.

TABLE 12–20 BRAIN TUMOR SPECIAL TISSUE PROCEDURES: INITIAL HANDLING

PROCEDURE	TISSUE HANDLING	REFERENCES
Histochemical analysis		
Autofluorescence—of biogenic monoamines	Attach unfixed tissue to cryostat chuck and freeze rapidly in either dry ice powder or liquid nitrogen–isopentane OR	78
	Fix for several minutes in 0.5% paraformaldehyde* and 2% glyoxylic acid, then freeze	11, 14, 23, 168
Immunofluorescence	Rapidly freeze unfixed tissue as above	212
Immunoenzymatic	B-5† fixative for 2 to 4 hours followed by 80% alcohol and paraffin embedment	133, 178, 212, 216
Enzyme		
Hydrolytic enzymes	Fix overnight in 1 to 4% paraformaldehyde, store at 4°C in buffered sucrose	12, 55, 83, 135, 181
Oxidative enzymes	Freeze rapidly in isopentane–liquid nitrogen Store at −70°C	
Electron microscopy Immunoenzyme	Fix in dilute paraformaldehyde 24 hours, 1% glutaraldehyde $1\frac{1}{2}$ hours or 1% paraformaldehyde–1% glutaraldehyde for $1\frac{1}{2}$ hours and embed in Araldite or glycol methacrylate	123, 162, 209, 212
Transmission	Fix in Karnovsky's solution (2% paraformaldehyde–2.5% glutaraldehyde) and store indefinitely, fix in 2.5% glutaraldehyde for 1 to 2 hours, then store in buffer	99, 100, 222
Scanning	Same as for transmission electron microscopy	99, 100
Cell and organ culture	Mince sterilely, place in culture medium (e.g., Puck's, Eagle's, Hank's), and store briefly at room temperature or 37°C Ship in nutrient medium at 4°C on wet ice	13, 89, 134, 179, 191, 232
Biochemical analysis	Freeze and store at −70°C	161

* Mixed from a powder with phosphate or cacodylate buffer, pH 7.3.
† Mercuric-chloride sodium acetate-formalin.

PERIPHERAL NERVE BIOPSY

Diabetes and alcoholism are the principal causes of peripheral neuropathy; it has, however, many other causes.[7,27,227] Table 12–21 lists peripheral nerve disorders and the associated pathological changes. Unfortunately, owing to the small number of relatively nonspecific pathological changes, peripheral nerve biopsy has only a minor role in diagnosis. Biopsy may, nevertheless, be highly accurate for vasculitis, amyloidosis, leprosy, metachromatic and globoid leukodystrophy, neoplastic infiltration of peripheral nerve, and chronic relapsing polyneuritis.* Biopsy also is useful in diagnosis of such generalized or central nervous system disorders as ceroid-lipofuscinosis, even though no peripheral nerve dysfunction may occur.[39,114] It adds little, however, to the diagnosis of the acute or subacute toxic-metabolic distal polyneuropathies. Since vasculitis, leprosy, and chronic relapsing polyneuritis are treatable or reversible disorders, their accurate identification is important. Biopsy diagnosis also aids in genetic counseling of patients who have heredofamilial neuropathies such as Charcot-Marie-Tooth disease and primary amyloidosis, and in identifying the make-up of diffuse neurological or neuromuscular disorders of unknown type. Table 12–22 lists the clinical settings in which the biopsy is most valuable.

Selection of Nerve

The nerve from which the biopsy is to be taken should be accessible and easily located, expendable, involved by disease, and protected from incidental trauma or entrapment. The sural nerve meets these criteria and is the favorite biopsy site in cases of symmetrical distal sensory or sensorimotor polyneuropathy and lower extremity mononeuritis multiplex.†

An alternative to the sural nerve for biopsy is the superficial radial nerve. It innervates the skin of the lateral part of the dorsum of the hand. Sensory loss after

* See references 54, 68, 73, 204, 210, 215.

† See references 6, 7, 27, 69, 152, 214, 217.

TABLE 12–21 COMMON PERIPHERAL NERVE DISORDERS

CAUSE	USUAL PATHOLOGICAL CHANGES
Metabolic and deficiency disorders	
Vitamin deficiency, alcohol	Axonal degeneration
Diabetes mellitus, uremia	Axonal degeneration, secondary segmental demyelination
Toxins	
Organophosphorus compounds	Axonal degeneration
Arsenic, vincristine	Axonal degeneration
Lead	? Demyelination
Diphtheria toxin	Segmental demyelination
Ischemia	
Vasculitis: polyarteritis nodosa	Epineurial arterial inflammation, occlusion Nerve trunk necrosis, scar Distal wallerian degeneration
Diabetes mellitus (mononeuritis)	Epineurial arterial occlusion Nerve trunk necrosis, scar Distal wallerian degeneration ? Selective myelin ischemia
Infection	
Leprosy	Interstitial fibrosis Many organisms, little inflammation
Herpes zoster	Hemorrhagic necrotizing inflammation with inclusion bodies in ganglia and roots
Immune postinfectious reaction	
Guillain-Barré syndrome	Mononuclear infiltrates Demyelination: focal and acute
Chronic relapsing polyneuritis	Segmental demyelination Interstitial fibrosis, onion bulbs Mononuclear infiltrates (few)
Neoplastic infiltration	
Carcinoma, lymphoma	Infiltration of nerve by tumor cells
Genetic disorders of peripheral nerve	
Hypertrophic neuropathies (Charcot-Marie-Tooth, Dejerine-Sottas, Refsum diseases)	Nerve fiber loss, interstitial fibrosis, onion bulbs
Amyloidosis	Interstitial amyloid, ischemia
Fabry disease	Lamellated cytoplasmic inclusions
Genetic disorders of central and peripheral nervous systems	
Leukodystrophies: metachromatic, globoid cell	Myelin breakdown or absence Characteristic lipid storage
Motor neuron diseases: amyotrophic lateral sclerosis	Axonal degeneration (little seen in peripheral nerves)
Ceroid-lipofuscinosis	Specific cytoplasmic inclusions

TABLE 12–22 INDICATIONS FOR PERIPHERAL NERVE BIOPSY: SIGNS AND SYMPTOMS

CLINICAL PRESENTATION	POSSIBLE CAUSES
Mononeuritis multiplex	Vasculitis: polyarteritis nodosa, rheumatoid arthritis
Palpable peripheral nerves	Amyloidosis; leprosy; Refsum, Dejerine-Sottas, or other genetic neuropathies; plexiform neurofibroma, carcinomatous infiltration
Postinfectious or recurrent polyneuropathy	Chronic relapsing polyneuritis
Progressive polyneuropathy with central nervous system involvement; often heredofamilial	Leukodystrophy, ataxia telangiectasia
Progressive motor loss, particularly in infants	Infantile polyneuropathy, progressive spinal muscular atrophy, primary myopathy

excision of this nerve is more noticeable to the patient than the loss over the lateral surface of the ankle and foot after sural nerve biopsy. The anterior tibial nerve is a mixed sensorimotor nerve that is accessible just above the ankle; however, the approach to this deeply situated nerve may damage extensor tendon sheaths.[27,69,214,217]

Other nerves that have been used for biopsy include the greater auricular, superficial peroneal, deep peroneal, saphenous, and anterior tibial on the dorsum of the foot.[213,214] Each of these nerves either fails the criteria given earlier or has been studied so rarely that normal quantitative values are not available.

Operative Techniques—Sural Nerve Biopsy

The patient is most comfortable in a lateral decubitus position, partially rotated to prone, exposing the area between the Achilles tendon and the lateral malleolus of the uppermost leg. The ankle is supported by a sandbag, the knees separated by a pillow, and the under leg slightly flexed. An alternative position is prone with the ankle partially everted.*

One per cent lidocaine is injected into the skin along a line lateral to and parallel with the Achilles tendon. The incision extends 7 to 10 cm along this depression, beginning about 1 cm proximal to the lateral malleolus. Sural nerve and small saphenous vein run together on the deep fascia. Usually the nerve lies deep (medial) and anterior to the vein. The nerve usually measures slightly over 1 mm in diameter when first encountered but may be 2 to 3 mm at the proximal end of the incision. The sural nerve is composed of many fascicles that branch at a minimally acute angle. Multiple branches just proximal to the malleolus help to identify the nerve. The vein is larger

* See references 6, 7, 69, 152, 214, 217.

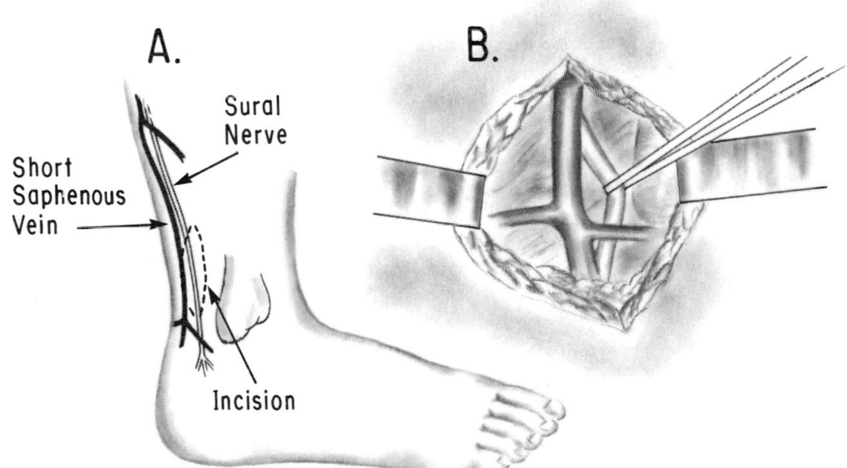

Figure 12–2 Dotted line shows incision site. The course of the small (short) saphenous vein may be identified by asking the patient to stand. The engorged vein will become visible and its course marked on the skin. *B.* Note position of nerve (retracted with ribbon tie) relative to overlying small saphenous vein and its branches. In a minority of patients, the sural nerve divides into two parallel branches at the incision site.

and branches at right angles, but may be extremely fibrotic and white with no grossly visible lumen. A nerve stimulator or immediate frozen section examination is useful to identify the nerve (Fig. 12–2).

After a 3- to 5-cm segment of nerve has been freed from adjacent tissues by gentle dissection, the proximal end should be transsected cleanly either with sharp scissors or, preferably, with a scalpel or razor blade against a wooden tongue blade. Prior to transsection, the nerve proximal to the site may be infiltrated with a small amount of anesthetic, and the patient should be warned of the impending sharp pain. Occurrence of this pain is added evidence that a nerve rather than a vein has been excised. The nerve need not be ligated, but the proximal stump should retract beyond the incision line and not become entrapped within the healing skin. The skin should be closed with 4-0 nylon suture in an interrupted mattress stitch and covered with an elastic pressure dressing. After biopsy, the patient may walk but should keep the leg elevated when seated. Sutures may be removed in 10 to 14 days.

The specimen should be placed in a moistened sponge for transport to the pathologist.

Some surgeons prefer a fascicular biopsy in which only approximately one third of the fascicles at a given level are excised in a strip 2 to 4 cm long.[214,217]

Complications

Transient sensory abnormalities are common after nerve biopsy, but serious complications are rare. They include wound infection, neuroma formation, and slow wound healing.[7,69,214,217] Asbury and Johnson believe that development of a painful neuroma may be avoided by allowing the proximal end of the nerve to retract beyond the skin incision.[7] Arterial occlusive disease, venous stasis, ulceration, or other trophic skin changes that complicate the neuropathy or underlying general illness may prohibit lower extremity biopsy.

Sensory loss after sural nerve transsection is expected over the lateral part of the ankle, heel, and foot, but rarely does this persist more than several weeks. In one series, 60 per cent of patients had no symptoms at the end of one year, 30 per cent had mild intermittent symptoms that eventually disappeared, and only 10 per cent had persistent paresthesias or dysesthesias.[69,214] Patients with severe sensory neuropathy rarely suffer additional symptoms from the biopsy.

Tissue Techniques

General Aims and Strategies

Light microscopy, lipid histochemical analysis, electron microscopy, teased single-fiber studies, morphometric analysis, biochemical assays, and in vitro electrophysiological or metabolic studies may be performed on the excised nerve segment. The first four techniques listed usually provide clinically important information. The clinical application of morphometric and biochemical studies varies with the disease and the skill of the investigator.

Before the widespread use of electrodiagnostic techniques, nerve biopsy often was performed to determine whether disease was present. Currently, the biopsy is used to characterize the disease process as fully as possible.

Electron microscopy is valuable in the analysis of axonal abnormalities; separation of wallerian degeneration from primary axonal disease; the examination of unmyelinated axons, which often escape light microscopic view; and the analysis of cytoplasmic inclusions in Schwann cells and perineurial fibroblasts.

Subdivision and Fixation

Table 12–23 summarizes tissue studies and required material. Tissue to be frozen unfixed and stored for lipid histochemical, biochemical, or immunofluorescence studies should be excised from each end of the specimen initially. A 1-cm segment is required for each of these studies. Lipid histochemistry is analyzed on frozen sections of either unfixed or formalin-fixed tissue. Lipid histochemical studies are indicated in almost all cases except obvious vasculitis or tumor infiltration. Biochemical studies, if available, are indicated in heredofamilial and combined peripheral and central nervous system disorders, particularly in suspected inborn errors of metabolism. Immunofluorescence studies are chiefly of research interest.

TABLE 12–23 PERIPHERAL NERVE BIOPSY: TISSUE STUDIES

PROCEDURE	SPECIMEN LENGTH (CM)	FIXATION	DURATION OF FIXATION, STORAGE
Light microscopy			
Paraffin sections	1	Heidenhain's "susa"	24 hr; switch to formalin
Frozen or paraffin sections	1	Formalin (neutral) or formol-calcium	Indefinitely
Frozen sections (optional)	1	Freeze rapidly	Store indefinitely in −70°C freezer
Electron microscopy	1	3.6% to 4% glutaraldehyde	1 to 2 hours; store in buffer
Teased single fiber preparations	1	3.6% to 4% glutaraldehyde	1 to 2 hours; store in buffer or 100% glycerine (see text)
Biochemical analysis (optional)	1	Freeze rapidly	Store indefinitely in −70°C freezer
Immunofluorescence studies (optional)	1	Freeze rapidly	Store indefinitely in −70°C freezer

A 3- to 4-cm nerve segment should be stretched slightly and allowed to dry for one minute on a small cardboard or note card. Two alternative techniques for maintaining a slight stretch on the nerve during fixation have been described. One is to insert fine sutures in each end of the specimen and tie them to a small self-retaining retractor, which is then immersed in a single all-purpose fixative.[7] The other is to place sutures or small hooks at each end of the specimen and attach weights to one end before suspending it in the fixative.[27,60,211]

If a universal fixative is used, the entire specimen, firmly attached to cardboard, may be fixed for one hour in 3.6 to 4 per cent phosphate-buffered glutaraldehyde solution, then subdivided for light microscopy, electron microscopy, and teasing.

Preferably, the specimen should be subdivided into 1- to 2-cm segments while still attached to the cardboard. The nerve is sectioned with a very sharp razor blade or scalpel, and the cardboard is then trimmed with fine scissors. These small cardboard rafts with nerve attached are immersed in at least three separate fixatives.

A 1-cm length of nerve is immersed in Heidenhain's susa fixative for no more than 24 hours, then embedded in paraffin, or if necessary, stored in neutral buffered formalin. An additional 1-cm length is immersed in either neutral buffered formalin or formol-calcium and stored for either frozen section lipid stains or later paraffin embedment.

A 2-cm segment is fixed for one hour in 3.6 or 4 per cent phosphate-buffered glutaraldehyde. Then the specimen is removed from the cardboard and halved. One half is divided into cross and longitudinal sections, returned to glutaraldehyde for one hour, then stored in buffer at 4° C until osmication and embedment in Epon or Araldite.[7,27,172]

The other half of the glutaraldehyde-fixed tissue is used for teased single-fiber preparations. Ideally, the specimen should be washed twice for 15 minutes each time in buffer, fixed for 4 to 6 hours in 0.1 M phosphate-buffered 2 per cent osmium tetroxide, washed again, immersed for 12 hours in a 66 per cent glycerin and water mixture, and stored in 100 per cent glycerin at 4° C until dissection.[7] Pragmatically, the one-hour limit in glutaraldehyde is important, but the initial wash may stretch to several hours or overnight with minimal distortion.

The formol-calcium–fixed segment is also suitable for teased preparations if not used in other ways.[27]

The remaining unfixed tissue may be frozen in either isopentane–liquid nitrogen or dry ice powder, or if histological features are not important, simply placed in a freezer and stored at −30° C to −70° C until used. Rapid freezing in Freon or isopentane cooled by liquid nitrogen is important, however, to avoid distortion by ice crystals in histological preparations. Many accurate biochemical studies may be performed on a 1-cm segment of peripheral nerve, particularly if epineurium and perineurium have been dissected away before freezing.[34]

Subsequent Studies

Carefully oriented cross and longitudinal paraffin sections should be stained with hematoxylin and eosin, Luxol fast blue–cresyl violet, and Weil-Weigert stains for myelin; a connective tissue stain such as hematoxylin–van Gieson or Masson's trichrome, which stains collagen and myelin contrasting colors; PTAH, which also stains myelin and collagen differentially; and Bodian's silver impregnation for axons. Luxol fast blue is compatible with the PAS stain and also with Bodian's axon stain.[27,135,181] Frozen sections of either unfixed or formol-calcium–fixed nerve should be stained with cresyl violet–acetic acid for sulfatide metachromasia, and oil red O and Sudan black for neutral lipid debris of degenerating myelin.

The majority of pathological changes are easily seen by light microscopy in 1-μ-thick sections of epoxy-embedded specimens. These sections, mounted on glass slides, may be stained with methylene blue–azure II, Paragon epoxy stain, toluidine blue, or para-phenylenediamine.[7] Segmental demyelination occasionally is identified in longitudinal sections of epoxy-embedded nerves, and cross sections are ideal for morphometric studies.

SKELETAL MUSCLE BIOPSY

Muscle biopsy may be indicated in primary diseases of skeletal muscle, central and peripheral nervous system disease, and certain generalized inflammatory, vascular, or metabolic disorders that are reflected in skeletal muscle.*

Signs and Symptoms

Five symptom complexes that may lead to muscle biopsy are: progressive muscular weakness or atrophy; congenital muscular weakness or atrophy with or without progression; multifocal or diffuse muscle pain, cramps, tenderness, and weakness; fever with disseminated visceral and cutaneous lesions of unknown type; and posttraumatic muscle weakness and atrophy that fail to respond to treatment.

Disease Entities

Neurogenic Muscular Atrophy

Muscle weakness due to denervation may be identified in muscle biopsies by patterns of fiber atrophy or by a characteristic distribution of muscle fiber types, as determined by enzyme histochemical analysis. Denervation may be due to peripheral nerve or spinal motor neuron disease. Muscle biopsy is useful in distinguishing at least four major subtypes of denervation: amyotrophic lateral sclerosis or motor neuron disease, the many forms of spinal muscular atrophy such as Werdnig-Hoffmann disease, chronic peripheral neuropathies of slowly progressive disorders such as Charcot-Marie-Tooth disease, and the more rapidly progressive toxic or metabolic polyneuropathies.[65] Biopsy may be used to differentiate neurogenic muscular atrophy from such nonspecific conditions as disuse atrophy, aging, and debility. The majority of muscle biopsies contain nerve twigs, which also may reveal evidence of disease if examined carefully. Disease of the motor end-plate usually is not diagnosed by muscle biopsy unless highly specialized techniques are used.[10,44–46]

Inflammatory Myopathy

Biopsy diagnosis prior to treatment is important in the diffuse muscle inflammation of such diseases as polymyositis, dermatomyositis, lupus erythematosus, scleroderma, and rheumatoid arthritis. Disseminated inflammatory foci may be identified in polyarteritis nodosa, trichinosis, toxoplasmosis, and sarcoidosis.[3]

Dystrophic Myopathy

Biopsy diagnosis of muscular dystrophy is important in order to exclude treatable myopathies such as polymyositis and to differentiate dystrophy from neurogenic disorders that carry different prognoses and genetic patterns.[4] Enzyme fiber typing may be used to identify subtypes of dystrophic myopathy—in particular, myotonic dystrophy, which produces few identifiable histological changes.[65]

Metabolic Myopathies

Muscle biopsy may be used to diagnose inherited disorders of glycogen metabolism, either generalized diseases such as acid maltase deficiency (Pompe disease) or myopathies such as myophosphorylase deficiency (McArdle disease).[106] Other conditions with biopsy-demonstrable muscle ab-

* See references 3, 4, 10, 63–65, 107.

normalities include primary amyloidosis, paroxysmal myoglobinuria, and carnitine or carnitine-palmitoyl transferase deficiency.[3,64] Periodic paralysis causes no diagnostic change in muscle, and steroid myopathy produces only nonspecific findings. Muscle biopsy is extremely useful, however, in screening patients for malignant hyperthermia, an autosomal dominant trait and a potentially lethal reaction to certain anesthetic agents.[72,108,193,194]

Selection of Biopsy Site

The site of the muscle biopsy is determined by the distribution of weakness or electrophysiological abnormalities, and by the tempo of the disease. The muscle should be only moderately abnormal to avoid areas of nondiagnostic end-state fibrosis and fatty replacement. Muscle that is only mildly involved by a long-standing progressive disease may show the most characteristic changes, while a severely weak muscle may be ideal in an acute disease. Tender or irritable muscle should be selected in cases of a suspected multifocal inflammatory disease. The usual proximal muscles from which specimens are taken are deltoid, biceps, and quadriceps (usually vastus lateralis). Intrinsic hand muscles should be avoided, if possible. Palmaris brevis is occasionally sampled as a distal muscle. Preferred distal lower extremity muscles are peroneal, anterior tibial, and gastrocnemius. Gastrocnemius should be avoided in adults, however, because of denervation changes that are common with nerve root compression or polyneuropathy unrelated to the muscle disorder. Use of standard biopsy sites is helpful when normal data for fiber diameter and fiber type distribution are to be applied. Gastrocnemius muscle is difficult to orient in a true transverse plane to measure fiber diameters.

External intercostal muscle biopsy has been advocated for generalized diseases, although normal histological variations in this muscle are not yet known.[211] Muscle biopsies should not be taken at the site of previous electromyography or medication injection in order to avoid tissue with needle-induced necrosis and inflammation.

Motor point biopsy is a specialized technique to identify abnormalities in terminal motor axons and motor end-plates.[10,44–46] This procedure involves intravital injection of methylene blue into the muscle near the site of innervation and excision of the muscle after a five-minute delay. Motor points are determined by electrical stimulation and usually lie in a zone midway between origin and insertion for longitudinally oriented fibers. This procedure, as well as the specialized histological preparations that follow it, generally are not indicated in a diagnostic biopsy. Routine biopsy of the area near motor nerve insertion, however, will increase both the number of nerve twigs found in the specimen and the likelihood of identifying both nerve and muscle abnormalities in the same specimen. An alternative method is simultaneous biopsy of a nerve and muscle through the same incision such as can be done with the anterior tibial nerve and peroneus brevis muscle at the ankle.[69,214] Biopsy of sural nerve and gastrocnemius muscle through a single very long incision rarely is indicated. Two relatively short, ideally located incisions are preferable—one for nerve and one for muscle.

Biopsy Technique

Open Biopsy

Muscle biopsy should be performed under local anesthesia unless part of a more serious operative procedure. One per cent lidocaine (Xylocaine) without adrenalin is infiltrated into skin and subcutaneous tissues, and a 3- to 4-cm incision is made over the muscle belly parallel to the muscle fibers. The anesthetic is injected into the exposed muscle sheath prior to incision. Additional anesthetic may be applied directly to the muscle surface if needed but should not be injected into the muscle.

A segment of muscle oriented in the long axis of the muscle bundles is gently isolated from adjacent tissue and either grasped at one end by fine forceps or sutured at each end.[65] The specimen is then excised cleanly with either a fresh scalpel or very sharp curved scissors. After excision, fascia is closed with absorbable suture to prevent herniation.

To maintain tension, the sutured muscle segment may be tied to a wooden tongue depressor. A preferable technique for obtaining multiple specimens for special studies is to excise the single specimen without sutures, subdivide the block into several longitudinally oriented segments, and attach each segment to a firm surface. The specimens may be stapled to cardboard or pinned to a sheet of soft dental wax. The bond achieved by simply letting the muscle dry onto a tongue blade or note card usually will not prevent contracture artifacts.

These specimens should be kept in a slightly moistened sponge for 15 to 20 minutes before submersion in fixative. Special muscle biopsy clamps are available but rarely are worthwhile, except for specialized research studies that require absolutely isometric fixation.

Needle Biopsy

Duchenne first used a needle or "harpoon" to obtain muscle biopsies in 1866.[56] Bergstrom designed a muscle biopsy needle to obtain specimens rapidly for biochemical studies.[16] Although the amount of tissue is quite small, the specimens are suitable for morphological studies. The method has become increasingly popular as histological, histochemical, and ultrastructural techniques and diagnostic criteria have become more refined.

Under local anesthesia, the biopsy instrument is inserted through a 5-mm skin incision and thrust 2 to 4 cm into the muscle, usually the vastus lateralis. Then the obturator is advanced and tissue is excised from deep within the muscle. The procedure is rapid and has few subjective or objective side effects. The major problem lies in performing adequate diagnostic studies on the small specimens, which are difficult to orient.

Needle biopsy is not recommended in disseminated focal disease such as polyarteritis, in which biopsy success depends upon finding randomly scattered lesions; in complex diagnostic problems that require numerous special studies; or in a hospital where the pathologist rarely examines such biopsies.

Complications

Relatively few complications occur from muscle biopsy.[65] Many patients report transient pain at the moment of muscle excision and a pressure sensation of tingling at the biopsy site for 24 hours. Rarely, hematomas and wound infections are seen, but biopsy does not limit mobility or cause permanent symptoms.

Initial Tissue Handling

The number of tissue subdivisions and specialized fixatives required for histological diagnosis depend upon the disease suspected and the techniques preferred by the pathologist (Table 12–24). Hematoxylin and eosin–stained paraffin sections are sufficient to identify vasculitis in patients with few signs of myopathy and in whom neither enzyme muscle fiber typing nor electron microscopy is needed. On the other hand, many neurologists and pathologists who specialize in muscle disease have abandoned paraffin embedment and make all diagnoses on unfixed frozen cross sections stained with a large battery of enzymatic and nonenzymatic stains.[65] For specimens

TABLE 12–24 MUSCLE BIOPSY: STUDIES INDICATED

	STUDIES				
DISEASE CATEGORY	*Light Microscopy**	*Thick Sections†*	*Electron Microscopy‡*	*Enzyme Histochemistry*	*Biochemistry*
Neurogenic atrophy	X	X		X	
Dystrophic myopathy	X	X		X	
Inflammatory myopathy	X	(X)		(X)	
Vasculitis	X				
Congenital myopathy	X	X	X	X	X
Metabolic myopathy					
Glycogen	X	X	X	X	X
Lipid	X	X	X	X	X
Hyperthermia	X			X	X

Key: X, essential; (X), preferred but not essential.

* Light microscopy of routinely stained paraffin or frozen sections.
† Light microscopy of stained 1-μ plastic sections.
‡ Electron microscopy of thin sections.

TABLE 12–25 MUSCLE BIOPSY: INITIAL HANDLING

PROCEDURE	SPECIMEN SIZE	FIXATIVE	DURATION OF FIXATION, STORAGE
Light microscopy	1.5 × 1 × 0.5 cm	10% formalin	48 hours or more
Electron microscopy	0.2 × 1 × 1 cm slab	Karnovsky	24 hours or more
		4% Glutaraldehyde	1 to 2 hours, then store in buffer
Enzyme histochemical analysis	0.5 cm cube	Transport at 4°C slightly damp	Up to 24 hours delay before freezing
		Freeze rapidly in Freon cooled by liquid nitrogen	Store in deep freezer or ship on dry ice
Biochemical analysis	0.5 to 1 cc	Freeze rapidly in Freon cooled by liquid nitrogen	Store in deep freezer or ship on dry ice

handled in the majority of pathology laboratories some compromise between these extremes is indicated. This compromise requires subdivision of tissue and use of multiple fixatives if sufficient tissue is available. Paraffin sections are useful for surveying a large volume of tissue for focal lesions. Epoxy-embedded tissue is useful for examining fine detail by light and electron microscopy.[65,200] Frozen sections are needed to subdivide muscle fibers into enzymatic types and identify type-related abnormalities (Table 12–25).[3,65,225]

Light Microscopy

For paraffin embedment, a specimen at least 1.5 by 1 by 0.5 cm (approximately half of the average specimen) should be fastened securely to a firm smooth surface, as indicated previously, and immersed in either 10 per cent neutral formalin, Bouin's, or Zenker's fixative. Fixation in formalin or Bouin's solution should continue at least 48 hours, but Zenker's solution will produce brittleness if tissue remains in it for more than 24 hours.

Electron Microscopy

For electron microscopy, a 2-mm-thick tissue slab, approximately 1.0 cm across, should be immersed in either Karnovsky's formaldehyde-glutaraldehyde solution or 3.6 to 4 per cent phosphate-buffered glutaraldehyde.[65,211] As for other tissues, Karnovsky's solution is preferred because it penetrates better and the tissue can be stored for long periods prior to embedment. If glutaraldehyde is used, the specimen should be changed to buffer after one or two hours.

Enzyme Histochemistry

For enzyme histochemical analysis, one or more tissue blocks each 0.5 cm in diameter should be frozen rapidly and stored until frozen sections can be cut. Biopsies performed at some distance from the enzyme histochemistry laboratory may be transported on wet ice (4° C) in a gauze sponge very slightly moistened with saline (wring out as much saline as possible) and sealed in a watertight container. A delay of 4 to 6 hours between biopsy and freezing is quite compatible with excellent enzyme localization, and delays even up to 24 hours are tolerable if the specimen is kept refrigerated and slightly moist. Delay is far better than tissue distortion by ice crystals that result from freezing in an improper manner.

If the specimen must be frozen prior to shipment, the muscle should be oriented in transverse section on a thin flat piece of cork and surrounded by gum tragacanth or other medium for embedding frozen sections.[65] The mounted specimen then is lowered into a wide-mouthed container of Freon or isopentane cooled in a liquid nitrogen bath. The instantly frozen muscle attached to the cork should be sealed in a very small airtight plastic bag. Storage in a larger container may permit desiccation. The specimen then may be shipped on dry ice and stored in a freezer until processing. Direct immersion of muscle in liquid nitrogen should be avoided because of the protective gas layer that forms around the specimen, which slows cooling and produces ice crystals.

Biochemical Analysis

If biochemical studies are indicated, an additional 1-cc specimen should also be frozen rapidly, sealed in a small airtight container, and transported on dry ice to the appropriate laboratory. When sending an entire biopsy preserved in more than one way, package the frozen material separately from specimens immersed in fixative to avoid accidental freezing of fixed material during shipment. Frozen tissue remaining after enzyme histochemical studies should be stored in small airtight containers and used as reserve tissue for biochemical analysis.

Studies Recommended

Light Microscopy

Hematoxylin and eosin–stained paraffin sections are sufficient for diagnosis of cases with the classic findings of neurogenic muscle atrophy, vasculitis, or inflammatory myopathy. Azure eosinate is a useful stain to highlight inflammatory cell infiltrates. Serial sections may be required to identify focal vasculitis or differentiate polymyositis from primary vasculitis with extension of inflammatory cells into adjacent muscle fibers.

Several other staining methods generally are indicated in more complex cases: phosphotungstic acid–hematoxylin for demonstration of muscle fiber striations (A bands), collagen, and rod bodies; Gomori's trichrome for demonstration of muscle fibers, myelin, axons, collagen, and "ragged red fibers"; Verhoeff–van Gieson technique for collagen and myelinated axons; undigested and digested PAS for glycogen. Many of these stains also may be used on frozen sections of unfixed tissues; in fact, frozen sections are preferable to paraffin embedment for the trichrome stain.

Studies of terminal axons and motor endplates generally are performed at specialized centers under the direct supervision of experienced research workers. Several approaches are used: silver impregnation by the Bielschowsky-Gros technique on frozen sections of formalin-fixed tissue, cholinesterase localization, and vital staining by methylene blue followed by biopsy and examination of squash preparation.[3,10,44–46]

Electron Microscopy

A portion of most muscle biopsies should be fixed initially for electron microscopy.[65,200] Generally this material is not embedded until preliminary light microscopic studies have indicated the diagnostic problems that are involved. Based on purely clinical criteria, electron microscopy rarely is indicated for diagnosis of inflammatory myopathy or neurogenic atrophy; however, many unusual ultrastructural changes of research interest have been described in these conditions (e.g., the discovery of intranuclear viruslike particles in muscle biopsies from patients with collagen-vascular disease.[200]

Electron microscopy is essential in all cases of infantile myopathy and in metabolic myopathy at any age.

Enzyme Histochemistry

Enzyme histochemical analysis of frozen sections is essential to muscle biopsy diagnosis in all but the most obvious cases. Two major muscle fiber types are identified by their enzyme content: type 1 fibers with high levels of oxidative enzymes, and type 2 fibers with high levels of routine adenosine triphosphatase (ATPase). Type 2 fibers may be further subdivided according to the relative amounts of these enzymes.[65,225] Highly diagnostic patterns of fiber type distribution characterize neurogenic muscular atrophy, disuse atrophy, and certain subtypes of dystrophic myopathy. These patterns cannot be detected in routine stains of paraffin-embedded sections, although type-related variations in lipid and glycogen content may be identified in frozen sections. Enzyme histochemistry provides the most useful information in the early stages of many disorders.

Biochemical Analysis

If a metabolic myopathy is suspected, a variety of biochemical studies may be performed on unfixed frozen tissue. The tissue remaining uncut after enzyme histochemical studies is suitable, but in most cases an additional 0.5 to 1.0 gm is preferred.

In the many subtypes of glycogen storage disease that affect muscle, biochemical studies may detect the specific enzyme defect in addition to the increased glycogen content.[106] Two abnormalities of lipid metabolism in muscle have been identified biochemically: carnitine deficiency and carnitine palmitoyl transferase deficiency.[64] In the former, increased muscle lipid may be identified histochemically, but in the latter, muscle biopsy may be normal. Precise diagnosis depends upon biochemical analysis of frozen muscle in both diseases.

Malignant hyperthermia is the third myopathy, presumably metabolic, that requires enzyme histochemical and biochemical diagnosis by specialized laboratories. Because the condition is an autosomal dominant trait, not only involved patients but family members must be screened for it.[72,108,193,194]

REFERENCES

1. Abell, M. R., Hart, W. R., and Olson, J. R.: Tumors of the peripheral nervous system, Hum. Path., *1*:503–51, 1970.
2. Adams, J. H., and Urquhart, G. E. D.: Early diagnosis of herpes encephalitis (letter). New Eng. J. Med., *297*:1288, 1977.
3. Adams, R. D.: Diseases of Muscles: A Study in Pathology. 3rd Ed. Hagerstown, Md., Harper & Row, 1975.
4. Appel, S. H., and Roses, A. D.: The muscular dystrophies. *In* Stanbury, J. B., Wyngaarden, J. B., and Fredrickson, D. S., eds.: The Metabolic Basis of Inherited Disease. 4th Ed. New York, McGraw-Hill Book Co., 1978, pp. 1260–1281.
5. Armstrong, P., Green, G., and Irving, J. D.: Needle aspiration/biopsy of the spine in suspected disc space infection. Brit. J. Radiol., *51*:333–337, 1978.
6. Asbury, A. K., and Connally, E. S.: Sural nerve biopsy: Technical note. J. Neurosurg., *38*:391–392, 1973.
7. Asbury, A. K., and Johnson, P. C.: Pathology of Peripheral Nerve. Philadelphia, W. B. Saunders Co., 1978.
8. Asher, D. M., Gibbs, C. J., Jr., and Gajdusek, D. C.: Pathogenesis of subacute spongiform encephalopathies. Ann. Clin. Lab. Sci., *6*:84–103, 1976.
9. Avrameas, S., Ternynck, T., and Guesdon, J. L.: Some general remarks about immunoenzymatic techniques. *In* Feldman, G., Druet, P., Bignon, J., and Avrameas, S., eds.: Immunoenzymatic Techniques. Proceedings of the First International Symposium on Immunoenzymatic Techniques, Paris, April 2–4, 1975. Amsterdam-Oxford, North-Holland Publishing Co., 1976, pp. 1–6.
10. Awad, E. A.: Motor-point biopsies in carcinomatous neuropathy. Arch. Phys. Med., *49*:643–649, 1968.
11. Axelsson, S., Bjorklund, A., Falck, B., Lindvall, O., and Svensson, L. A.: Glyoxylic acid condensation: A new fluorescence method for the histochemical demonstration of biogenic monoamines. Acta Physiol. Scand., *87*:57–62, 1973.
12. Bancroft, J. D.: Histochemical Techniques. 2nd Ed. London and Boston, Butterworth & Co., 1975.
13. Barker, M., Wilson, C. B., and Hoshino, T.: Tissue culture of human brain tumors. *In* Kirsh, W. F., Grossi-Paoletti, E., and Paoletti, P., eds.: The Experimental Biology of Brain Tumors. Springfield, Ill., Charles C Thomas, 1972, pp. 57–84.
14. Battenberg, E. L. F., and Bloom, F. E.: A rapid, simple and more sensitive method for the demonstration of central catecholamine-containing neurons and axons by glyoxylic acid induced fluorescence. I. Specificity. Psychopharmacol Comm., *1*:3–13, 1975.
15. Bergstrom, B., Drettner, B., and Stenkvist, B.: Transnasal aspiration biopsy of central skull base destructions. Acta Cytol., *17*:425–430, 1973.
16. Bergstrom, J.: Percutaneous needle biopsy of skeletal muscle in physiological and clinical research. Scand. J. Clin. Lab. Invest., *35*:609–616, 1975.
17. Bernoulli, C., Siegfield, J., Baumgartner, G., Regli, F., Rabinowicz, T., Gajdusek, D. C., and Gibbs, C. J., Jr.: Dangers of accidental person-to-person transmission of Creutzfeldt-Jakob disease by surgery. Lancet, *1*:478–479, 1977.
18. Bhattacharyga, A. K., and Connor, W. E.: Familial diseases with storage of sterols other than cholesterol (cerebrotendinous xanthomatosis, and β-sitosterolemia and xanthomatosis). *In* Stanbury, J. B., Wyngaarden, J. B., and Fredrickson, D. S., eds.: The Metabolic Basis of Inherited Disease. 4th Ed. New York, McGraw-Hill Book Co., 1978, pp. 656–669.
19. Biemond, A.: Indications, legal and moral aspects of cerebral biopsies. *In* Proceedings of the Fifth International Congress of Neuropathology, Zurich, Aug. 31 to Sept. 3, 1965. Amsterdam, Excerpta Medica Foundation, 1966, pp. 362–375.
20. Blackwood, W.: Cerebral biopsy. *In* Vinken, P. J., and Bruyn, G. W., eds.: Handbook of Clinical Neurology. Vol. 10, Leucodystrophies and Poliodystrophies. Amsterdam, Elsevier–North Holland Publishing Co., 1970, pp. 680–687.
21. Blackwood, W., and Cumings, J. N.: The combined histological and chemical aspects of cerebral biopsies. *In* Proceedings of the Fifth International Congress of Neuropathology, Zürich, Aug. 31 to Sept. 3, 1965. Amsterdam, Excerpta Medica Foundation, 1966, pp. 364–371.
22. Blodi, F. C.: The temporal artery biopsy as a diagnostic procedure in ophthalmology. Trans. Aust. Coll. Ophthal., *1*:26–33, 1969.
23. Bloom, F. E., and Battenberg, E. L. F.: A rapid, simple and sensitive method for the demonstration of central catecholamine-containing neurons and axons by glyoxylic acid–induced fluorescence. II. A detailed description of methodology, J. Histochem. Cytochem., *24*:561–571, 1976.
24. Bloustein, P. A., and Silverberg, S. G.: Rapid cytologic examination of surgical specimens. Path. Annu. 12:Part 2:251–278, 1977.
25. Bodian, M., and Lake, B. D.: The rectal approach to neuropathology. Brit. J. Surg., *50*:702–714, 1963.
26. Boltshauser, E., and Wilson, J.: Value of brain biopsy in neurodegenerative disease in childhood. Arch. Dis. Child., *51*:264–268, 1976.
27. Bradley, W. G.: Disorders of Peripheral Nerves.

Oxford, Blackwell Scientific Publications, 1974, pp. 105–215.

28. Brady, R. O.: Sphingomyelin lipidosis: Niemann-Pick disease. *In* Stanbury J. B., Wyngaarden, J. B., and Fredrickson, D. S., eds.: The Metabolic Basis of Inherited Disease, 4th Ed. New York, McGraw-Hill Book Co., 1978, pp. 718–730.
29. Brady, R. O.: Glycosyl ceramide lipidosis: Gaucher's disease. *In* Stanbury, J. B., Wyngaarden, J. B., and Fredrickson, D. S., eds.:The Metabolic Basis of Inherited Disease. 4th Ed. New York, McGraw-Hill Book Co., 1978, pp. 731–746.
30. Brennan, J., and McCrary, J. A., III.: Diagnosis of superficial temporal arteritis. Ann. Ophthal., *7*:1125–1129, 1975.
31. Brett, E. M., and Berry, C. L.: Value of rectal biopsy in paediatric neurology: Report of 165 biopsies. Brit. Med. J., *3*:400–403, 1967.
32. Brett, E. M., and Lake, B. D.: Reassessment of rectal approach to neuropathology in childhood. Review of 307 biopsies over 11 years. Arch. Dis. Child., *50*:753–762, 1975.
33. Brookes, L. D.: A stain for differentiating two types of acidophil cells in the rat pituitary. Stain Techn., *43*:41–42, 1968.
34. Brown, M. J., Pleasure, D. E., and Asbury, A. K.: Microdissection of peripheral nerve: Collagen and lipid distribution with morphological correlation. J. Neurol. Sci., *29*:361–369, 1976.
35. Brown, W. J., Barajas, L., Waisman, J., and Quattro, V. D.: Ultrastructural and biochemical correlates of adrenal and extra-adrenal pheochromocytomas. Cancer. *29*:744–759, 1972.
36. Burger, P., and Vogel, F. S.: Surgical Pathology of the Nervous System and its Coverings. New York, John Wiley & Sons, Inc., 1976.
37. Burger, P., and Vogel, F. S.: Frozen section interpretation in surgical neuropathology. I. Intracranial lesions. Amer. J. Surg. Path., *1*:323–347, 1977.
38. Burger, P., and Vogel, F. S.: Frozen section interpretation in surgical neuropathology. II. Intraspinal lesions. Amer. J. Surg. Path., *2*:81–95, 1978.
39. Carpenter, S., Karpati, G., and Andermann, F.: Specific involvement of muscle, nerve, and skin in late infantile and juvenile amaurotic idiocy. Neurology (Minneap.), *22*:170–186, 1972.
40. Carpenter, S., Karpati, G., Andermann, F., Jacob, J. C., and Andermann, E.: Lafora's disease: Peroxisomal storage in skeletal muscle. Neurology (Minneap.), *24*:531–538, 1974.
41. Carr, I., and Toner, P. G.: Rapid electron microscopy in oncology. J. Clin. Path., *30*:13–15, 1977.
42. Ceuterick, C., Martin, J. J., Casaer, D., and Edgar, G. W. F.: The diagnosis of infantile generalized ceroidlipofuscinosis (type Hagberg-Santavuori) using skin biopsy. Neuropädiatrie, 7:250–260, 1976.
43. Coblentz, J. M., Mattis, S., Zingesser, L. H., Kasoff, S. S., Wiśniewski, H. M., and Katzman, R.: Presenile dementia: Clinical aspects and evaluation of CSF dynamics. Arch. Neurol. (Chicago), *29*:299–308, 1973.
44. Coërs, C., and Telerman-Toppet, N.: Morphological and histochemical changes of motor units in myasthenia. Ann. N.Y. Acad. Sci., *274*:6–19, 1976.
45. Coërs, C., and Woolf, A. L.: The Innervation of Muscle: A Biopsy Study. Oxford, Blackwell Scientific Publications, 1959.
46. Coërs, C., Telerman-Toppet, N., and Gérard, J-M.: Terminal innervation ratio in neuromuscular disease: I. Methods and Controls, II. Disorders of lower motor neuron, peripheral nerve and muscle. Arch. Neurol. (Chicago), *29*:210–214 and 215–222, 1973.
47. Cohen, S. R., Brune, M. J., Herndon, R. M., and McKhann, G. M.: Cerebrospinal fluid myelin basic protein, and multiple sclerosis. Advances Exp. Med. Biol., *100*:513–519, 1978.
48. Conway, L. W.: Stereotaxic diagnosis and treatment of intracranial tumors including an initial experience with cryosurgery for pinealomas. J. Neurosurg., *38*:453–460, 1973.
49. Cook, R. H., and Austin, J. H.: Precautions in familial transmissible dementia: Including familial Alzheimer's disease. Arch. Neurol. (Chicago), *35*:697–698, 1978.
50. Corrodi, H., and Jonsson, G.: The formaldehyde fluorescence method for the histochemical demonstration of biogenic monoamines: A review of the methodology. J. Histochem. Cytochem., *15*:65–78, 1967.
51. Coupland, R. E., Kobayashi, S., and Crowe, J.: On the fixation of catecholamines including adrenaline in tissue sections. J. Anat., *122*:403–413, 1976.
52. Crevier, P. H.: Post-stereotaxic intracranial hematomas. Acta Neurochir. (Wien) suppl., *21*:71–73, 1974.
53. Crome, L., and Stern, J.: The Pathology of Mental Retardation. 2nd Ed. Edinburgh, Churchill Livingstone, 1972, pp. 483–485.
54. Crome, L., and Stern, J.: Inborn lysosomal enzyme deficiencies. *In* Blackwood, W., and Corsellis, J. A. N., eds.: Greenfield's Neuropathology. 3rd Ed. Chicago, Yearbook Medical Publishers, Inc., 1976, pp. 501–580.
55. Culling, C. F. A.: Handbook of Histopathological and Histochemical Techniques. 3rd Ed. London, Butterworth & Co., Ltd., 1974.
56. Curless, R. G., and Nelson, M. B.: Needle biopsies of muscle in infants for diagnosis and research. Develop. Med. Child. Neurol., *17*:592–601, 1975.
57. DeLellis, R. A., and Roth, J. A.: Norepinephrine in a glomus jugulare tumor: Histochemical demonstration. Arch. Path. (Chicago), *92*:73–75, 1971.
58. Denk, H., Radaszkiewicz, T., and Whitting, C.: Immunofluorescence studies on pathologic routine material: Application to malignant lymphomas. Beitr. Path. *159*:219–225, 1976.
59. Denk, H., Syré, G., and Weivich, E.: Immunomorphological methods in routine pathology. Application of immunofluorescence and the unlabeled antibody-enzyme (peroxidase-antiperoxidase) technique to formalin fixed paraffin embedded kidney biopsies. Beitr. Path., *160*:187–194, 1977.
60. Desnick, R. J., Dawson, G., Desnick, S. J., Sweeley, C. C., and Krivitt, W.: Diagnosis of

glycosphingolipidoses by urinary sediment analysis. New Eng. J. Med., *284*:739–744, 1971.

61. Dobbins, W. O., III.: Diagnostic usefulness of rectal biopsy. Med. Ann. D.C., *40*:223–226, 1971.
62. Dooling, E. C., Schoene, W. C., and Richardson, E. P., Jr.: Hallervorden-Spatz syndrome. Arch. Neurol. (Chicago), *30*:70–83, 1974.
63. Dubowitz, V.: Muscle biopsy: Technical and clinical aspects. Ann. Clin. Res., *6*:69–79, 1974.
64. Dubowitz, V.: Muscle Disorders in Childhood. Major Problems in Clinical Pediatrics, Vol. XVI. London, W. B. Saunders Co. Ltd., 1978.
65. Dubowitz, V., and Brooke, M. H.: Muscle Biopsy: A Modern Approach. Major Problems in Neurology, Vol. 2. London, W. B. Saunders Co. Ltd., 1973.
66. Duckett, S., Cracco, J., Lublin, F., and Scott, T.: Electron microscopical diagnosis of lipidosis with the use of rectal biopsy. Amer. J. Dis. Child., *127*:704–705, 1974.
67. Duffy, P., Wolf, J., Collins, G., DeVoe, A. G., Streeter, B., and Cowen, D.: Letter to Editor. Possible person-to-person transmission of Creutzfeldt-Jakob disease. New Eng. J. Med., *290*:692–693, 1974.
68. Dulaney, J. T., and Moser, H. W.: Sulfatide lipidosis: Metachromatic leukodystrophy. *In* Stanbury, J. B., Wyngaarden, J. B., and Fredrickson, D. S., The Metabolic Basis of Inherited Disease. 4th Ed. New York, McGraw-Hill Book Co., 1978, pp. 770–809.
69. Dyck, P. J., and Lofgren, E. P.: Nerve biopsy: choice of nerve, method, symptoms, and usefulness. Med. Clin. N. Amer., *52*:885–893, 1968.
70. Edner, G.: Stereotaxic brain tumor biopsy—5 years' experience. (Abstract) Acta Neurochir. (Wien), *31*:261, 1975.
71. Elian, M.: Late effects of brain biopsy. J. Neurol., *211*:95–104, 1975.
72. Eng, G. D., Epstein, B. S., Engel, W. K., McKay, O. W., and McKay, R.: Malignant hyperthermia and central core disease in a child with congenital dislocating hips: Case presentation and review. Arch. Neurol. (Chicago), *35*:189–197, 1978.
73. Enna, C. D., Jacobson, R. R., and Mansfield, R. E. An evaluation of sural nerve biopsy in leprosy. Int. J. Leprosy, *38*:278–281, 1970.
74. Eränkö, O., and Räisänen, L.: Demonstration of catecholamines in adrenergic nerve fibers by fixation in aqueous formaldehyde solution and fluorescence microscopy. J. Histochem. Cytochem., *14*:690–691, 1966.
75. Erdohazi, M., and Read, C. R.: A histological study of the appendix vermiformis—a possible alternative to rectal biopsy in neurological diagnosis. Develop. Med. Child. Neurol., *9*:98–101, 1967.
76. Espana, C., Gajdusek, D. C., Gibbs, C. J., Jr., and Lock, K.: Transmission of Creutzfeldt-Jakob disease to the Patas monkey (*Erythrocebus* patas) with cytopathological changes in *in vitro* cultivated brain cells. Intervirology, *6*:150–155, 1975–1976.
77. Ezrin, C., and Murray, S.: The cells of the human adenohypophysis in pregnancy, thyroid disease and adrenal cortical disorders. *In* Bernoit, J., and DaLage, C., eds.: Cytologie de l'Adenohypophyse. Paris, Editions du Centre National de la Recherche Scientifique, 1963, pp. 183–200.
78. Falck, B., and Owman, C.: A detailed methodological description of the fluorescence method for the cellular demonstration of biogenic monoamines. Acta Univ. Lund, Sec. II, *7*:1–23, 1975.
79. Farquhar, M. G., Skutelsky, E. H., and Hopkins, C. R.: Structure and function of the anterior pituitary and dispersed pituitary cells. In vitro studies. *In* Tixier-Vidal, A., and Farquhar, M. G., eds.: The Anterior Pituitary. New York, Academic Press, 1975, pp. 83–135.
80. Fenson, A. H.: Letter to editor: Rectal biopsy or biochemistry for the diagnosis of neurological disorders. Develop. Med. Child. Neurol., *17*:253–254, 1975.
81. Fredrickson, D. S., and Ferrans, V. J.: Acid cholesteryl ester hydrolase deficiency (Wolman's disease and cholesteryl ester storage disease). *In* Stanbury, J. B., Wyngaarden, J. B., and Fredrickson, D. S., eds.: The Metabolic Basis of Inherited Disease. 4th Ed. New York, McGraw-Hill Book Co., 1978, pp. 670–687.
82. Friede, R. L.: Developmental Neuropathology. New York, Springer-Verlag, 1975.
83. Gabe, M.: Histological Techniques. New York, Paris, Masson-Bier–Springer-Verlag, 1976.
84. Gajdusek, D. C., Gibbs, C. J., Jr., and Asher, D. M.: Letter to the editor New Eng. J. Med., *298*:976, 1978.
85. Gajdusek, D. C., Gibbs, C. J., Jr., Earle, K., Dammin, G. J., Schoene, W. C., and Tyler, H. R.: Transmission of subacute spongiform encephalopathy to the chimpanzee and squirrel monkey from a patient with papulosis atrophicans maligna of Köhlmeier-Degos. *In* Proceedings of the X International Congress of Neurology, Barcelona, Spain, Sept. 8–15, 1973. Amsterdam, Excerpta Medica Foundation, 1974, pp. 390–392.
86. Gajdusek, D. C., Gibbs, C. J., Jr., Asher, D. M., Brown, P., Diwan, A., Hoffman P., Nemo, G., Rohwer, R., and White, L.: Precautions in medical care of, and in handling materials from, patients with transmissible virus dementia (Creutzfeldt-Jakob disease). New Eng. J. Med. *297*:1253–1258, 1977.
87. Gilchrist, K. W., Gilbert, E. F., and Esterly, J. R.: Pediatric necropsies by general pathologists. Arch. Path. Lab. Med., *102*:223, 1978.
88. Gilden, D. H., Wroblewska, Z., Eng, L. F., and Rorke, L. B.: Human brain in tissue culture. Part 5. Identification of glial cells by immunofluorescence. J. Neurol. Sci., *29*:177–184, 1976.
89. Gilden, D. H., Devlin, M., Wroblewska, Z., Friedman, H., Rorke, L. B., Santoli, D., and Koprowski, H.: Human brain in tissue culture: I. Acquisition, initial processing, and establishment of brain cell cultures. J. Comp. Neurol., *161*:295–306, 1975.
90. Goebel, H. H., Zeman, W., and Pilz, H.: Significance of muscle biopsies in neuronal ceroid-

lipofuscinoses. J. Neurol. Neurosurg. Psychiat., *38*:985–993, 1975.

91. Goldenberg, D. M., Sharkey, R. M., and Primus, F. J.: Carcinoembryonic antigen in histopathology: Immunoperoxidase staining of conventional tissue sections. J. Nat. Cancer Inst., *57*:11–22, 1976.

92. Greenberg, R., Rosenthal, I., and Falk, G. S.: Electron microscopy of human tumors secreting catecholamines. Correlation with biochemical data. J. Neuropath. Exp. Neurol., *28*:475–500, 1969.

93. Gyorkey, F., Min, K-W, Krisko, I., and Gyorkey, P.: The usefulness of electron microscopy in the diagnosis of human tumors. Hum. Path., *6*:421–441, 1975.

94. Hahn, J. F., and Netsky, M. G.: Brain tumors of mixed tissue origin: Staining procedures to distinguish glial from connective tissue. Southern Med. J., *70*:539–542, 1977.

95. Halmi, N. S.: The current status of human pituitary cytophysiology. New Zeal. Med. J., *80*:551–556, 1974.

96. Halmi, N. S., and Duello, T.: "Acidophilic" pituitary tumors: A reappraisal with differential staining and immunocytochemical techniques. Arch. Path. Lab Med., *100*:346–351, 1976.

97. Hamberger, R., and Norberg, K. A.: Histochemical demonstration of catecholamines in fresh frozen sections. J. Histochem. Cytochem., *12*:48–49, 1964.

98. Hankinson, J., Hudgson, P., Pearce, G. W., and Morris, C. J.: A simple method for obtaining stereotaxic biopsies from the human basal ganglia: A case of cerebral porphyria. Acta Neurochir. (Wien), suppl. 21:227–233, 1974.

99. Hayat, M. A.: Principles and Techniques of Electron Microscopy: Biological Applications. New York and London, Van Nostrand Reinhold Co., Vol. 1, 1970, Vol. 2, 1972.

100. Hayat, M. A.: Basic Electron Microscopic Techniques. New York, Van Nostrand Reinhold Co.,1972.

101. Herlant, M.: The cells of the adenohypophysis and their functional significance. Int. Rev. Cytol., *17*:299–382, 1964.

102. Herlant, M., and Pasteels, J. L.: Histophysiology of human anterior pituitary. Meth. Achiev. Exp. Path., *3*:250–305, 1967.

103. Herman, M. M., Huttenlocher, P. R., and Bensch, K. G.: Infantile neuroaxonal dystrophy. Report of a cortical biopsy and review of the recent literature. Arch. Neurol. (Chicago), *20*:19–34, 1969.

104. Horoupian, D. S., Kerson, L. A., Saiontz, H., and Valsamis, M.: Paraganglioma of cauda equina: Clinicopathologic and ultrastructural studies of an unusual case. Cancer, *33*:1337–1348, 1974.

105. Hoshino, T., Wilson, C. B., and Ellis, W. G.: Gemistocytic astrocytes in gliomas. An autoradiographic study. J. Neuropath. Exp. Neurol., *34*:263–281, 1975.

106. Howell, R. R.: The glycogen storage diseases. *In* Stanbury, J. B., Wyngaarden, J. B., and Fredrickson, D. S., eds.: The Metabolic Basis of Inherited Disease, 4th Ed. New York, McGraw-Hill Book Co., 1978, pp. 137–159.

107. Hughes, J. T.: Pathology of Muscle. Major Problems in Pathology. Vol. 4. Philadelphia, W. B. Saunders Co., 1974.

108. Isaacs, H.: Comments on predictive tests for malignant hyperthermia. *In* Aldrete, J. A., and Britt, B. A., eds.: Second International Symposium on Malignant Hyperthermia. New York, Grune & Stratton, Inc., 1977, pp. 351–362.

109. Jacobowitz, D., and Koelle, G. B.: Histochemical correlations of acetylcholinesterase and catecholamines in postganglionic autonomic nerves of the cat, rabbit, and guinea pig. J. Pharmacol. Exp. Ther., *148*:225–237, 1965.

110. Jane, J. A., and Bertrand, G.: A cytological method for the diagnosis of tumor affecting the central nervous system. J. Neuropath. Exp. Neurol., *21*:400–409, 1962.

111. Jane, J. A., and Yashon, D.: Cytology of tumors affecting the nervous system. Springfield, Ill., Charles C Thomas, 1969.

112. Johnson, K. P., Arrigo, S. C., Nelson, B. J., and Ginsberg, A.: Agarose electrophoresis of cerebrospinal fluid in multiple sclerosis: A simplified method for demonstrating cerebrospinal fluid oligoclonal immunoglobulin bands. Neurology (Minneap.), *27*:273–277, 1977.

113. Jones, G., Gallant, P., and Butler, W. H.: Improved techniques in light and electron microscopy. J. Path., *121*:141–148, 1977.

114. Joosten, E., Gabreëls, F., Stadhouders, A., Bolmers, D., and Gabreels-Feston, A.: Involvement of sural nerve in neuronal ceroid-lipofuscinoses: Report of two cases. Neuropädiatrie, *4*:98–110, 1973.

115. Jowsey, J.: The Bone Biopsy. New York and London, Plenum Medical Book Co., 1977.

116. Kalimo, H., Garcia, J. H., Kamijyo, Y., Tanaka, J., Viloria, J. E., Valigorsky, J. M., Jones, R. T., Kim, K. M., Mergner, W. J., Pendergrass, R. E., and Trump, B. F.: Cellular and subcellular alterations of human CNS: Studies utilizing in situ perfusion fixation at immediate autopsy. Arch. Path. (Chicago), *97*:352–359, 1974.

117. Kamoshita, S., and Landing, B. H.: Distribution of lesions in myenteric plexus and gastrointestinal mucosa in lipidoses and other neurologic disorders of children. Amer. J. Clin. Path., *49*:312–318, 1968.

118. Kaufman, H. H., and Catalano, L. W., Jr.: Diagnostic brain biopsy: A series of 50 cases and a review. Neurosurgery, *4*:129–136, 1979.

119. Ketenjian, A. Y.: Muscular dystrophy: Diagnosis and treatment. Orthop. Clin. N. Amer., *9*:25–42, 1978.

120. Kovacs, K., Corenblum, B., Strek, A. M. T., Penz, G., and Ezrin, C.: Localization of prolactin in chromophobe pituitary adenomas: Study of human necropsy material by immunoperoxidase technique. J. Clin. Path., *29*:250–258, 1976.

121. Kovarsky, J., Schochet, S., and McCormick, W.: Modern use of the biopsy in the diagnosis of neurological disease. J. Iowa Med. Soc. *62*:424–428, 1972.

122. Kruseman, A., Bots, G., Lindeman, J., and Schaberg, A.: Use of immunohistochemical and morphologic methods for the identification

of human growth hormone-producing pituitary adenomas. Cancer, *38*:1163–1170, 1976.
123. Kuhlmann, W. D.: Ultrastructural immunoperoxidase cytochemistry. Progr. Histochem. Cytochem. *10*:1–57, 1977.
124. Lake, B. D.: Diagnosis of "Tay-Sachs" disease, Batten's disease and Wolman's disease. *In* Seakins, J. W. T., Saunders, R. A., and Toothill, C., eds.: Treatment of Inborn Errors of Metabolism. Edinburgh, Churchill Livingstone, 1973.
125. Landing, B. H., Silverman, F. N., Craig, J. M., Jacoby, M. D., Lahey, M. E., and Chadwick, D. L.: Familial neurovisceral lipidosis. Amer. J. Dis. Child., *108*:503–522, 1964.
126. Landolt, A. M.: Ultrastructure of human sella tumors. Correlation of clinical findings and morphology. Acta Neurochir. (Wien), suppl. 22:1–167, 1975.
127. Landolt, A. M., and Hosbach, H. U.: Biological aspects of pituitary tumors as revealed by electron microscopy. Pathologica, *66*:413–436, 1974.
128. Landolt, A. M., and Rothenbühler, V.: The size of growth hormone granules in pituitary adenomas producing acromegaly. Acta Endocr. (Kobenhavn), *84*:461–469, 1977.
129. Lee, R. L.: 2-hydroxyethyl methacrylate embedded tissues—a method complementary to paraffin embedding. Med. Lab. Sci., *34*:231–239, 1977.
130. Leet, N. G., and Chalcroft, J. P.: Rapid method for processing entire biopsy pieces for light and electron microscopy. Lab. Pract., *23*:59–60, 1974.
131. Lewander, R., Greitz, T., and Wilkins, J.: Stereotactic computer tomography for biopsy of gliomas. Acta Radiol. [Diagn.] (Stockholm), *19*:867–888, 1978.
132. Liebeskind, D., Hsu, K. C., Elequin, F., Mendez, L., Ghossein, N., Janis, M., and Bases, R.: Novel method of estimating the labeling index in clinical specimens with the use of immunoperoxidase-labeled antinucleoside antibodies. Cancer Res., *37*:323–326, 1977.
133. Lillie, R. D., and Fullmer, H. M.: Histopathological Technic and Practical Histochemistry. 4th Ed. New York, McGraw-Hill Book Co., 1976, pp. 52–53.
134. Lumsden, C. E.: The study by tissue culture of tumours of the nervous system. *In* Russell, D. S., and Rubinstein, L. J., eds.: Pathology of Tumors of the Nervous System. 3rd Ed. Baltimore, Williams & Wilkins Co., 1971, pp. 39–41.
135. Luna, L. G.: Manual of Histologic Staining Methods of the Armed Forces Institute of Pathology. 3rd Ed. New York, McGraw-Hill Book Co., 1968.
136. Lynn, J. A.: "Adjacent" sections—a bridge in the gap between light and electron microscopy. Hum. Path., *6*:400–402, 1975.
137. Magnusson, B. C., Heyden, G., and Arwill, T.: Histochemical tests on lipids in the oral and skin epithelia in the mouse. Histochemie, *34*:249–256, 1973.
138. Malone, M. J.: The cerebral lipidoses. Pediat. Clin. N. Amer., *23*:303–326, 1976.
139. Maroon, J. C., Bank, W. O., Drayer, B. P., and Rosenbaum, A. E.: Intracranial biopsy assisted by computerized tomography. J. Neurosurg., *46*:740–744, 1977.
140. Marshall, L. F. and Jennett, B.: Smear biopsy in neurosurgical diagnosis. Arch. Neurol. (Chicago), *29*:124–126, 1973.
141. Marshall, L. F., Adams, H., Doyle, D., and Graham, D. I.: The histological accuracy of the smear technique for neurosurgical biopsies. J. Neurosurg., *39*:82–88, 1973.
142. Martin, J. J., and Jacobs, K.: Skin biopsy as a contribution to diagnosis in late infantile amaurotic idiocy with curvilinear bodies. Europ. Neurol., *10*:281–291, 1973.
143. Martin, J. J., and Martin, L.: Infantile neuroaxonal dystrophy: Ultrastructural study of the peripheral nerves and of the motor end plates. Europ. Neurol., *8*:239–250, 1972.
144. Martin, J. J., and Martin, L.: Ultrastructural study of the appendix as a contribution to the diagnosis of juvenile amaurotic idiocy. Medikon, *2*:165–168, 1973.
145. Massey, E. M.: A review of rectal biopsy. Southern Med. J., *63*:315–317, 1970.
146. McCormick, W. F.: Biopsy as an adjunct to the study of the natural history of strokes. *In* Fields, W. F., and Moossy, J., eds.: Stroke: Diagnosis and Management—Current Procedures and Equipment. St. Louis, Mo., Warren H. Green, Inc., 1973, pp. 256–263.
147. McCormick, W. F., and Halmi, N. S.: Absence of chromophome adenomas from a large series of pituitary tumors. Arch. Path. (Chicago), *92*:231–238, 1971.
148. McDowell, E. M.: Fixation and processing. *In* Trump, B. F., and Jones, R. T., Eds.: Diagnostic Electron Microscopy. Vol. 1. New York, John Wiley & and Sons, 1978, pp. 113–139.
149. McDowell, E. M., and Trump, B. F.: Histologic fixation suitable for diagnostic light and electron microscopy. Arch. Path. Lab. Med., *100*:405–414, 1976.
150. McKusick, V. A., Neufeld, E. F., and Kelly, T. E.: The mucopolysaccharide storage diseases. *In* Stanbury, J. B., Wyngaarden, J. B., and Fredrickson, D. S., eds.: The Metabolic Basis of Inherited Disease. 4th Ed. New York, McGraw-Hill Book Co., 1978, pp. 1282–1307.
151. McLaughlin, R. F., Miller, W. R., and Miller, C. W.: Quadriparesis after needle aspiration of the cervical spine. J. Bone Joint Surg., *58-A*:1167–1168, 1976.
152. McLeod, J. G., Walsh, J. C., and Little J. M.: Sural nerve biopsy Med. J. Aust., *2*:1092–1096, 1969.
153. McMenemey, W. H.: An appraisal of smear-diagnosis in neurosurgery. Amer. J. Clin. Path., *33*:471–479, 1960.
154. McMenemey, W. H.: The cerebral biopsy. *In* Bailey, O. T., and Smith, D. E., eds.: The Central Nervous System: Some Experimental Models of Neurological Diseases. Baltimore, Md., Williams & Wilkins Co., 1968, pp. 291–299.
155. Misugi, K., Misugi, N., and Newton, W. A.: Fine structural study of neuroblastoma, ganglioneuroblastoma, and pheochromocytoma. Arch. Path. (Chicago), *86*:160–170, 1968.
156. Moossy, J.: Diagnostic cerebral biopsy. *In*

Toole, J. E., ed.: Special Techniques for Neurological Diagnosis. Contemporary Neurology Series No. 3. Philadelphia, F. A. Davis Co., 1969, pp. 184–194.

157. Morris, A. A.: The use of smear technique in the rapid histologic diagnosis of tumors of the central nervous system. Description of a new staining method. J. Neurosurg., *4*:497–504, 1947.

158. Moser, H.: Ceramidase deficiency: Farber's lipogranulomatosis. *In* Stanbury, J. B., Wyngaarden, J. B., and Fredrickson, D. S., eds.: The Metabolic Basis of Inherited Disease. 4th ed. New York, McGraw-Hill Book Co., 1978, pp. 707–717.

159. Müller, J. E.: The cerebral cortical biopsy. *In* Tedeschi, C. G., ed.: Neuropathology: Methods and Diagnosis. Boston, Little, Brown & Co., 1976, pp. 415–418.

160. Myers, G. J., Hedley-Whyte, E. T., and Fagan, M. E.: Re-evaluation of the role of rectal biopsy in diagnosis of pediatric neurological disorders. Neurology (Minneap.), *23*:27–34, 1973.

161. Nagatsu, T.: Biochemistry of Catecholamines: The Biochemical Method. Baltimore, Md., University Park Press, 1973.

162. Nakane, P. K.: Identification of anterior pituitary cells by immunoelectron microscopy. *In* Tixier-Vidal, A., and Farquhar, M. G., eds.: The Anterior Pituitary. New York, Academic Press Inc., 1975, pp. 45–61.

163. Nelson, J. S.: Rectal biopsy in the diagnosis of pediatric neurologic disorders. Develop. Med. Child Neurol., *16*:830–831, 1974.

164. Neville, H. E., Brooke, M. H., and Austin, J. H.: Studies in myoclonus epilepsy (Lafora body form). IV. Skeletal muscle abnormalities. Arch. Neurol. (Chicago), *30*:466–474, 1974.

165. Nielsen, S. L., and Wilson, C. B.: Ultrastructure of a "pineocytoma." J. Neuropath. Exp. Neurol., *34*:148–158, 1975.

166. Nordenstrom, B.: Percutaneous biopsy of vertebrae and ribs. Acta Radiol. [Diagn.] (Stockholm), *11*:113–121, 1971.

167. Noronha, M. J.: Cerebral degenerative disorders of infancy and childhood. Develop. Med. Child Neurol., *16*:228–241, 1974.

168. Nygren, L. G.: On the visualization of central dopamine and noradrenaline nerve terminals in cryostat sections. Med. Biol., *54*:278–285, 1976.

169. O'Brien, J. S.: The gangliosidoses. *In* Stanbury, J. B., Wyngaarden, J. B., and Fredrickson, D. S., eds.: The Metabolic Basis of Inherited Disease. 4th Ed. New York, McGraw-Hill Book Co., 1978, pp. 841–865.

170. O'Brien, J. S., Bernett, J., Veath, M. L., and Paa, D.: Lysosomal storage disorders: Diagnosis by ultrastructural examination of skin biopsy specimens. Arch. Neurol. (Chicago), *32*:592–599, 1975.

171. Olivier, L., Vila-Porcile, E., Racadot, O., Peillon, F., and Racadot, J.: Ultrastructure of pituitary tumor cells: A critical study. *In* Tixier-Vidal, A., and Farquhar, M. G., eds.: The Anterior Pituitary. New York, Academic Press Inc., 1975, pp. 231–276.

172. Onishi, A., Offord, K., and Dyck, P. J.: Studies to improve fixation of human nerves. Part 1. Effect of duration of glutaraldehyde fixation on peripheral nerve morphometry. J. Neurol. Sci., *23*:223–226, 1974.

173. Pearse, A. G. E.: The cytochemistry and ultrastructure of polypeptide hormone-producing cells of the APUD series and the embryologic, physiologic, and pathologic implications of the concept. J. Histochem. Cytochem., *17*:303–313, 1969.

174. Phifer, R. F.: Human adenohypophyseal stains. *In* Clark, G., ed.: Staining Procedures Used By The Biological Staining Commission. 3rd Ed. Baltimore, Md., Williams & Wilkins Co., 1973, pp. 166–170.

175. Phifer, R. F., Midgley, A. R., and Spicer, S. S.: Immunohistologic and histologic evidence that follicle-stimulating hormone and luteinizing hormone are present in the same cell type of the human pars distalis. J. Clin. Endocr., *36*:125–141, 1973.

176. Phifer, R. F., Spicer, S. S., and Hennigar, G. R.: Histochemical reactivity and staining properties of functionally defined cell types in the human adenohypophysis. Amer. J. Path., *73*:569–587, 1973.

177. Pilz, H., Goebel, H. H., and O'Brien, J. S.: Isoelectric enzyme patterns of leukocyte peroxidase in normal controls and patients with neuronal ceroid-lipofuscinoses. Neuropädiatrie, *7*:261–270, 1976.

178. Pinkus, G. S., and Said, J. W.: Specific identification of intracellular immunoglobulin in paraffin sections of multiple myeloma and macroglobulinemia using an immunoperoxidase technique. Amer. J. Path., *87*:47–55, 1977.

179. Ponten, J.: Neoplastic human glial cells in culture. *In* Fogh, J., ed.: Human Tumor Cells in vitro. New York, Plenum Press, 1975, pp. 178–179.

180. Popoff, N. A., and Ellsworth, R. M.: The fine structure of retinoblastoma. In vivo and in vitro observations. Lab. Invest., *25*:389–402, 1971.

181. Rális, H. M., Beesley, R. A., and Rális, Z. A.: Techniques in Neurohistology. London, Butterworth & Co., 1973.

182. Ramgopal, V., and Geller, M.: Iatrogenic Klebsiella meningitis following closed needle biopsy of the lumbar spine: Report of a case and review of literature. Wisconsin Med. J., *76*:41–42, 1977.

183. Ramsey, H. J.: Fibrous long-spacing collagen in tumors of the nervous system. J. Neuropath. Exp. Neurol., *24*:40–48, 1965.

184. Rapola, J., and Haltia, M.: Cytoplasmic inclusions in the vermiform appendix and skeletal muscle in two types of so-called neuronal ceroid-lipofuscinosis. Brain, *96*:833–840, 1973.

185. Rawlinson, D. G., Rubinstein, L. J., and Herman, M. M.: In vitro characteristics of myxopapillary ependymoma of the filum terminale maintained in tissue and organ culture systems. Light and electron microscopic observations. Acta Neuropath. (Berlin), *27*:185–200, 1974.

186. Robertson, D. M., and Vogel, F. S.: Concentric lamination of glial processes in oligodendrogliomas. J. Cell Biology, *15*:313–334, 1962.

187. Rosen, V., and Ahuja, S. C.: Ice crystal distor-

tion of formol-fixed tissues following freezing. Amer. J. Surg. Path., *1*:179–181, 1977.

188. Rowden, G., and Lewis, M. G.: Technical method. Experience with a three-hour microscopy biopsy service. J. Clin. Path., *27*:505–510, 1974.

189. Rubinstein, L. J.: Tumors of the central nervous system. *In* Atlas of Tumor Pathology, 2nd Series, Fascicle 6. Washington, D.C., Armed Forces Institute of Pathology, 1972.

190. Rubinstein, L. J., and Herman, M. M.: A light- and electron-microscopic study of a temporal-lobe ganglioglioma. J. Neurol. Sci., *16*:27–48, 1972.

191. Rubinstein, L. J., Herman, M. M., and Foley, V. L.: In vitro characteristics of human glioblastomas maintained in organ culture systems: Light microscopy observations. Amer. J. Path., *71*:61–80, 1973.

192. Russell, D. S.: The wet-film technique in neurosurgery. *In* Dyke, S. C., ed.: Recent Advances in Clinical Pathology. London, J. & A. Churchill Ltd., 1951, pp. 455–462.

193. Ryan, J. F.: The early treatment of malignant hyperthermia. *In* Gordon, R. H., Britt, B. A., and Kalow, W., eds.: International Symposium on Malignant Hyperthermia. Springfield, Ill., Charles C Thomas, 1973, pp. 430–440.

194. Ryan, J. F., and Kerr, W. S., Jr.: Malignant hyperthermia: A catastrophic complication. J. Urol., *109*.879–883, 1973.

195. Sakai, M., Austin, J., Witmer, F., and Trueb, L.: Studies in myoclonus epilepsy (Lafora body form). II. Polyglucosans in the systemic deposits of myoclonus epilepsy and in corpora amylacea. Neurology (Minneap.), *20*:160–176, 1970.

196. Sass-Kortsak, H., and Bearn, A. G.: Hereditary disorders of copper metabolism (Wilson's disease [hepatolenticular degeneration] and Menkes' disease [kinky-hair or steely-hair syndrome]). *In* Stanbury, J. B., Wyngaarden, J. B., and Fredrickson, D. S., eds.: The Metabolic Basis of Inherited Disease. 4th Ed. New York, McGraw-Hill Book Co., 1978, pp. 1098–1126.

197. Schajowicz, F., and Derqui, J. C.: Puncture biopsy in lesions of the locomotor system: Review of results in 4050 cases including 941 vertebral punctures. Cancer, *21*:531–548, 1968.

198. Schaumberg, H. H., Powers, J. M., Raine, C. S., Suzuki, K., and Richards, E. P., Jr.: Adrenoleukodystrophy A clinical and pathologic study of 17 cases. Arch. Neurol. (Chicago), *32*:577–591, 1975.

199. Scherer, H. J.: Structural development in gliomas. Amer. J. Cancer, *34*:333–351, 1938.

200. Schochet, S. S., Jr., and Lampert, P. W.: Diagnostic electron microscopy of skeletal muscle. *In* Trump, B. F., and Jones, R. T., eds.: Diagnostic Electron Microscopy. Vol. 1. New York, John Wiley & Sons, 1978, pp. 209–251.

201. Schoene, W.: Personal communication, 1979.

202. Sherwin, R. P.: Histopathology of pheochromocytoma. Cancer, *12*:861–877, 1959.

203. Sherwin, R. P., and Rosen, V. J.: New aspects of the chromoreactions for the diagnosis of pheochromocytoma. Amer. J. Clin. Path., *43*:200–206, 1965.

204. Sima, A. F., and Robertson, D. M.: Involvement of peripheral nerve and muscle in Fabry's disease. Histologic, ultrastructural and morphometric studies. Arch. Neurol. (Chicago), *35*:291–301, 1978.

205. Simkin, P. A., Sumner, D. S., and Ricketts, H.: Letter to editor: Diagnosing giant cell arteritis. Arthritis Rheum., *16*:702, 1973.

206. Slack, P. M., Dayan, A. D., Slavin, G., and Tyrrell, D. A. J.: Morphological and virological investigations of cell strains cultured from the brain in Jakob-Creutzfeldt disease and subacute sclerosing panencephalitis. Brit. J. Exp. Path., *56*:377–387, 1975.

207. Smith, A., and Bruton, J.: Color Atlas of Histologic Staining Techniques. Chicago, Yearbook Medical Publishers, Inc., 1977.

208. Smith, P., Dickson, J. A. S., and Lake, B. D.: Rectal biopsy in the diagnosis of neurological disease in childhood. Brit. J. Surg., *63*:313–316, 1976.

209. Spaur, R. C., and Moriarty, G. C.: Improvements of glycol methacrylate: I. Its use as an embedding medium for electron microscopic studies. J. Histochem. Cytochem., *25*:163–174, 1977.

210. Steinberg, D.: Phytanic acid storage disease: Refsum's syndrome. *In* Stanbury, J. B., Wyngaarden, J. B., and Fredrickson, D. S., eds.: The Metabolic Basis of Inherited Disease. 4th Ed. New York, McGraw-Hill Book Co., 1978, pp. 688–706.

211. Stern, L. Z., Gruener, R., and Anderson, R. M.: External intercostal muscle biopsy. Arch. Neurol. (Chicago), *32*:779–780, 1975.

212. Sternberger, L. A.: Immunocytochemistry. 2nd Ed. New York, John Wiley & Sons, 1979.

213. Stevens, J. C., Lofgren, E. P., and Dyck, P. J.: Histometric evaluation of branches of peroneal nerve: Technique for combined biopsy of muscle nerve and cutaneous nerve. Brain Res., *52*:37–59, 1973.

214. Stevens, J. C., Lofgren, E. P., and Dyck, P. J.: Biopsy of peripheral nerve. *In* Dyck, P. J., Thomas, P. K., and Lambert, E. H., eds.: Peripheral Neuropathy. Philadelphia, W. B. Saunders, Co., 1975, pp. 410–423.

215. Suzuki, K., and Suzuki, Y. Galactosylceramide lipidosis: Globoid cell leukodystrophy (Krabbe's disease). *In* Stanbury, J. B., Wyngaarden, J. B., and Fredrickson, D. S., eds.: The Metabolic Basis of Inherited Disease. 4th Ed. New York, McGraw-Hill Book Co., 1978, pp. 747–769.

216. Taylor, C. R., and Burns, J.: The demonstration of plasma cells and other immunoglobulin-containing cells in formalin-fixed, paraffin-embedded tissues using peroxidase-labeled antibodies. J. Clin. Path., *27*:14–20, 1974.

217. Thomas, P. K.: The quantitation of nerve biopsy findings. J. Neurol. Sci., *11*:285–295, 1970.

218. Thomas, P. K.: The value of electron microscopy in nerve biopsy. Proc. Roy. Soc. Med., *63*:468–470, 1970.

219. Townes, D. E., and Blodi, F. C.: The diagnostic value of temporal artery biopsy. Trans. Amer. Ophthal. Soc., *66*:33–44, 1968.

220. Traub, R. D., Gajdusek, D. C., and Gibbs, C. J., Jr.: Precautions in conducting biopsies and au-

topsies on patients with presenile dementia. J. Neurosurg., *41*:394–395, 1974.

221. Traub, R. D., Gajdusek, D. C., and Gibbs, C. J., Jr.: Letter to editor: Precautions in autopsies on Creutzfeldt-Jacob disease. Amer. J. Clin. Path., *64*:287, 1975.
222. Trump, B. F., and Jones, R. T.: Diagnostic Electron Microscopy. Vol. 1. New York, John Wiley & Sons, 1978.
223. Trump, B. F., Valigorsky, J. M., Jones, R. T., Mergner, W. J., Garcia, J. H., and Cowley, R. A.: The application of electron microscopy and cellular biochemistry to the autopsy: Observations on cellular changes in human shock. Hum. Path., *6*:499–520, 1975.
224. Trump, B. F., Valigorsky, J. M., Dees, J. H., Mergner, W. J., Kim, K. M., Jones, R. T., Pendergrass, R. E., Garbus, J., and Cowley, R. A.: Cellular change in human disease: A new method of pathological analysis. Hum. Path., *4*:89–109, 1973.
225. Tunell, G. L., and Hart, M. N.: Simultaneous determination of skeletal muscle fiber, Types I, IIA, and IIB, by histochemistry. Arch. Neurol. (Chicago), *34*:171–173, 1977.
226. Urich, H.: Malformation of the nervous system, perinatal damage, and related conditions early in life. *In* Blackwood, W., and Corsellis, J. A. N., eds.: Greenfield's Neuropathology. London, Edward Arnold, Ltd., 1976, pp. 445–447.
227. Urich, H.: Disease of peripheral nerve. *In* Blackwood, W., and Corsellis, J. A. N., eds.: Greenfield's Neuropathology. London, Edward Arnold, Ltd., 1976, pp. 688–770.
228. van Haelst, U. J., and Gabreëls, F. J. M. The electron microscopic study of the appendix as early diagnostic means in Batten-Spielmeyer-Vogt disease. Acta Neuropath. (Berlin), *21*:169–175, 1972.
229. Velasco, M. E., Sindely, S. O., and Roessmann, U.: Reticulum stain for frozen-section diagnosis of pituitary adenomas. J. Neurosurg., *46*:548–550, 1977.
230. Vigouroux, R. P., Toga, M., Choux, M., Baurand, Ch., Dubois, D., and Perrimond, H.: Intérêt de la biopsie cérébrale chez l'enfant dans les affections cérébrales chroniques. Neurochirurgie, *13*:385–398, 1967.
231. Vogt, A., Takamiya, H., and Kim, W. A.: Some problems involved in postembedding staining. *In* Feldmann, G., Druet, P., Bignon, J., and Avrameas, S., eds.: Immunoenzymatic Techniques. Proceedings of the First International Symposium on Immunoenzymatic Techniques, Paris, April 2–4 1975. Amsterdam-Oxford, North-Holland Publishing Co., 1976, pp. 109–115.
232. Vraa-Jensen, J., Herman, M. M., Rubinstein, L. J., and Bignami, A.: In vitro characteristics of a fourth ventricle ependymoma maintained in organ culture systems. Light and electron microscopic observations. Neuropath. Appl. Neurobiol., *2*:349–364, 1976.
233. Wallace, S.: Interventional radiology. Cancer, *37*:Conf. suppl.:517–531, 1976.
234. Waltregny, A., Petrov, A., and Brotchi, J.: Serial stereotaxic biopsies. Acta Neurochir. (Wien), suppl. 21:221–226, 1974.
235. Warecka, K.: Immunologic differential diagnosis of brain tissues. *In* Deutsch, A. S., Moses, K., Rainer, H., and Stacher, A., eds.: Molecular Base of Malignancy. Stuttgart, Georg Thieme Verlag, 1976, pp. 110–113.
236. Waris, T., Rechardt, L., and Partanen, S.: Simultaneous demonstration of cholinesterases and glyoxylic acid-induced fluorescence of catecholamines in stretch preparations. Acta Histochem. (Jena), *58*:194–198, 1977.
237. Weintraub, W. H., Heidelberger, K. P., and Coran, A. G.: A simplified approach to diagnostic rectal biopsy in infants and children. Amer. J. Surg., *134*:307–310, 1977.
238. Whitehead, R.: Mucosal Biopsy of the Gastrointestinal Tract. Major Problems in Pathology. Vol. 3. Philadelphia, W. B. Saunders Co., 1979.
239. Whitley, R. J., Soong, S-J., Dolin, R., Galasso, G. J., Ch'ien, L. T., Alford, C. A., and the Collaborative Study Group: Adenine arabinoside therapy of biopsy-proved herpes simplex encephalitis: National Institute of Allergy and Infectious Diseases Collaborative Antiviral Study. New Eng. J. Med., *297*:289–294, 1977.
240. Whittaker, D. K., and Williams-Jones, D. G.: Biopsy techniques for electron microscopy. J. Path., *103*:61–63, 1971.
241. Wigger, H. J.: Frozen section of liver in the diagnosis of Reye syndrome. Amer. J. Surg. Path., *1*:271–277, 1977.
242. Wilson, J.: Investigation of degenerative disease of the central nervous system. Arch. Dis. Child., *47*:163–170,1972.
243. Wright, M. G.: Vertebral trephine biopsy. Rheumatol. Rehab., *14*:208–211, 1975.

13

CEREBROSPINAL FLUID

The cerebrospinal fluid has been the subject of monographs, chapters, and innumerable general articles.* Davson and Fishman have published exhaustive reviews.[89,91,143] This chapter brings together for the clinician, especially the medical and surgical neurologist, a current concept of the fluid's biology and nature in relation to its dynamics and composition, and its reactions in health and various states of nervous system and systemic disease. Although impressive improvements in our radiological techniques seem to have decreased the total number of indications for sampling the fluid, this procedure continues to be of great value in clinical practice and is a useful source of information to researchers in most fields of neuroscience.

HISTORICAL BACKGROUND

A review of what is known about cerebrospinal fluid reflects the great discoveries of medicine, pathology, and biology in general, albeit with a moderate lag period. Before 1885, when Corning punctured the subarachnoid space to introduce cocaine in a living patient, the existence of the fluid was recognized, but only scant data about its anatomy and physiology were recorded.[72,299] An abrupt increase in knowledge about this fluid was initiated when Wynter and Morton removed the fluid through a cutdown in 1891.[305,475] At the same time, Quincke removed it through a percutaneous approach.[343,344] By the early 1920's, Dandy was directly puncturing the ventricles and Ayer had introduced the technique of cisternal puncture.[12,84]

This new-found easy accessibility of the cerebrospinal fluid was introduced to the medical world at the dawn of microbiology, and an intensive investigation of its bacteriological and cellular content rapidly began. Significant advances have kept pace with the march of microbiological science. For example, fluorescent antisera specific for many common microbial diseases can be applied to the fluid's sediment for fast and reliable recognition of intracellular or extracellular organisms.[30,131,198,329] Virological techniques, such as immunoelectronmi croscopy and cellular fusion, and quantitation of milligrams of antibody synthesized by cerebrospinal cells and the central nervous system await application.

Cytological techniques have advanced significantly since the paper of Widal and co-workers appeared in 1901.[116,191,265,457] Although differential cell counting had been moderately reliable for years, its utility increased when, in 1960, Marks and Marrack emphasized the importance of the addition of albumin to reduce drying artifacts.[276] More recently, the introduction of cytocentrifugation and Millipore filter collection of cells has further broadened interest in differentiating cells in the cerebrospinal fluid.† Immediate fixation of cerebrospinal fluid cells has been shown to increase appreciably the yield and quality of cellular material from the spinal fluid. Methods of examining exfoliated cells, as introduced by Papanicolaou in 1935, are now more often applied to spinal fluid sediment when

* See references 14, 20, 35, 66, 76, 82, 112, 138, 139, 142, 144, 154, 181, 211, 216, 221, 250, 264, 269, 287, 292–296, 298, 299, 312, 319, 334, 369, 370, 398, 402, 410, 449, 469, 474.

† See references 115, 308, 371, 392, 394, 404, 428.

W. W. TOURTELLOTTE AND R. J. SHORR

an intracranial neoplasm is suspected.[308,327] The use of tissue culture to establish the type of cell and its immunoglobulin synthetic ability has been introduced recently.[69,113,146,366] Furthermore, the immunological reactivity of lymphocytes in the cerebrospinal fluid appears to differ from that of those in the blood.[5,248,257]

Shortly after the turn of the century (1906), Wassermann described a serological test for syphilis.[448] The following year it was applied to the spinal fluid, and the importance of syphilis as a cause of mental illness was established. Advances in this area were few until Nielsen and Reyn described the delicate but highly sensitive *Treponema pallidum* immobilization test.[315] Further studies have since led to simple, valid, scientific tests utilizing fluorescent antibody reagents prepared from treponemal antigen.

Advances in the determination of the chemical constituents of the cerebrospinal fluid paralleled the advances in analytical chemistry at the turn of the century. Mestrezat's milestone monograph in 1912 reviewed the accumulated knowledge.[295,296] Little about the state of health or disease of the nervous system can be specified from the quantitative determinations of sodium, chloride, phosphate, urea, and other substances in the spinal fluid, since their concentration closely reflects the blood concentration; but studies employing radioactive isotopes of these components have increased knowledge about the formation, circulation, and absorption of the fluid. Additionally, quantitative chemical studies of the acid-base homeostasis of it and the blood during the course of treatment of the blood electrolyte abnormalities in diabetic acidosis and uremia (by dialysis) revealed that a moderately slow correction of the systemic abnormalities improved neurological function more definitively than did fast correction.[339] This was the result of the lag that existed between the electrolyte concentrations of the central nervous system and the blood.

Levels of glucose and its metabolic intermediates have been of value in following the course of infections and neoplasia of the nervous system. The fluid lipid profile could become important in reflecting nervous system disease, since it is not under the direct influence of the serum lipid concentrations.

Microtechniques for the determination of neurotransmitters, such as catecholamines and gamma-aminobutyric acid, and neuroregulators such as endorphins are now available. Active investigation in this area may prove to be of great value in diagnosis and in following the course of treatment.

Of great clinical importance is the determination of protein in the cerebrospinal fluid. The fluid is a dilute protein solution (about 40 mg per 100 ml), and its concentration was estimated only semi-quantitatively until the sulfosalicylic acid turbidity test was improved and spectrophotometric methods were introduced.* The introduction of a number of nonspecific tests (Lange colloidal gold curve, gum-mastic curve, zinc sulfate turbidity, Pándy phenol test, and Nonne-Apelt test) led to an understanding that the spinal fluid protein comprises several different types of proteins. For the most part these tests indicate an increase of gamma globulin.[186,406,407]

Advances in protein chemistry have led to more refined fractionation of this protein. In 1942 Kabat and co-workers applied the Tiselius free electrophoresis procedure to large quantities of cerebral spinal fluid.[214,399] They proved that spinal fluid was similar to serum in protein composition. Microelectrophoretic techniques such as paper, agar, and starch electrophoresis (other supporting media have also been used) soon followed.[458] Study of essentially all neurological diseases has yielded only a few unique pherograms. More recently, quantitative fluid chromatography, immunoelectrophoresis, radial immunodiffusion, electroimmunodiffusion, isoelectric focusing, isotachophoresis, and radioimmunoassay have been introduced; most protein fractions can now be determined by one of these methods.

Quantitative isotachophoresis will perhaps be of great importance, especially as applied to the gamma globulin region by the method of Delmotte.[100] Under active investigation are ways to measure the daily synthesis of cerebrospinal fluid oligoclonal IgG bands in those diseases in which they exist, which should assist the diagnosis of and evaluation of the treatment of those diseases.[407,409,417]

---

* See references 86, 106, 263, 355, 389, 426, 446.

The use of radioactively labeled proteins such as IgG and albumin has demonstrated important properties of the blood-brain barrier. It is now possible with an empirical formula to calculate the daily synthesis of IgG by the nervous system, a synthesis that does not occur under normal circumstances.[407,409,417]

Radioactive albumin studies and advances in immunochemistry have, additionally, established albumin as the marker of the efficiency of the tight junctions of the microcirculation of the brain.[407,417] Accordingly, measurement of albumin in many clinical laboratories has replaced the total protein determination, as described later in the section on proteins.

Intensive study of cerebrospinal fluid enzymes has mirrored research into those in serum, but only limited information has been forthcoming.[129]

Determination of peptides such as myelin basic protein, endorphins, and neurohormones can be made by means of chromatography and radioimmunoassay. The relationship of these constituents to nervous system and systemic disease is of great interest, and helpful information should be forthcoming in the near future

Spectrophotometric studies of xanthochromia have increased the understanding of hemorrhagic processes such as traumatic lumbar puncture, spontaneous subarachnoid hemorrhage, subdural hematoma, and other cerebrovascular accidents.*

The study of the cerebrospinal fluid pressure correlates was begun with the Queckenstedt procedure in 1916.[342] More recently, Lundberg and others, utilizing, among other methods of measurement, pressure transducers implanted in the cerebrospinal fluid space and the central nervous system, have demonstrated temporal variations in the pressures in these compartments that were not recognized earlier.[268] Their value lies in monitoring treatment of intracranial disease with agents to control cerebral edema or antineoplastic agents, and in postoperative states.[268,439]

Radiological examination of the subarachnoid space began in 1918 when Dandy removed spinal fluid from the subarachnoid space and replaced it with air to produce increased contrasts on x-rays.[85] He discovered that distortion of the normal shape of the spinal cord and brain could indicate disease. Significant advances in pneumoencephalography to localize lesions have been limited to injection of air under pressure and tomography. More recently, air myelography has been of great value in evaluation of spinal cord syrinx and cervical spondylosis by virtue of its ability to measure the size of the cord precisely and to serve as substitute for opaque media when a patient demonstrates a contrast medium allergy.

In 1922, iodized oil was injected into the spinal subarachnoid space by Sicard and Forestier.[377] Occasionally this contrast medium is passed into the posterior fossa and ventricles to enhance roentgenographic contrasts or introduced into the ventricles to evaluate the flow of cerebrospinal fluid.

Metrizamide (Amipaque), a water-soluble and nonionic contrast medium, has gained favor for myelography and cisternography.[173] Among other advantages, it is removed from the cerebrospinal fluid space by diffusion rather than by aspiration with a needle. Additionally, this method coupled with computed tomography should be useful in quantitating volume as well as flow rates of the cerebrospinal fluid.[114,173]

In therapy, the subarachnoid space has been used for injecting anesthetic agents, antibiotics, antineoplastic agents, and corticosteroids and other immunosuppressant medications; for drainage of fluid; and for lavage of the cerebrospinal fluid compartment. Techniques for measuring and predicting the concentration of drugs injected into the fluid either intrathecally or systemically are not ideal. Progress will depend on the development of micromethods for drug assays, as well as methods to assure uniform distribution of drugs in the cerebrospinal fluid space. The volume injected, the rate of injection, the specific gravity of the substance injected, the position of the patient, and the diffusion coefficients seem to be the most important variables. Additional knowledge is also needed concerning the formation, circulation, absorption, and total volume of the cerebrospinal fluid; the turnover of its various constituents; and the blood–cerebrospinal fluid–central nervous system barriers in both health and disease.

* See references 18, 233, 356, 425, 431.

BIOLOGY OF THE CEREBROSPINAL FLUID AND ITS SPACES

Cerebrospinal Fluid Spaces, Circulation, and Interfaces

Free circulation is necessary for the fluid to maintain its normal characteristics.[74,298] The path of circulation leads from the lateral ventricles into the third ventricle through the interventricular foramina (Monro) and through the cerebral aqueduct (Sylvius) into the fourth ventricle. From the fourth ventricle there is a potential continuation into the central canal of the spinal cord down to the terminal ventricle (fifth ventricle), which ends bluntly just above the filum terminale. In humans the central canal usually is obliterated by the twelfth year. From the fourth ventricle, the fluid communicates with the subarachnoid space by three routes—the two lateral foramina of Luschka and the medial aperture in the roof of the fourth ventricle called the foramen of Magendie. These foramina direct fluid into the cisterna magna, and from there it circulates through the subarachnoid space of the cerebellar hemispheres, through the basilar cisterns, and caudally to the spinal subarachnoid space. Fluid arriving in the basilar cisterns (premedullary, prepontine, and cerebellopontine) follows a course through the interpeduncular and prechiasmatic cisterns, the sylvian fissures and callosal cisterns, to the lateral and frontal hemispheric subarachnoid space. A dorsomedial flow from the basilar cisterns leads the fluid through the ambient cisterns and the cisterna venae magnae cerebri to the medial and posterior cerebral hemispheric subarachnoid space.[298] The fluid comes in contact with the arachnoid villi in its course cephalad, in proximity to the superior longitudinal and other dural venous sinuses, and in its course caudad, in proximity to the spinal nerve arachnoid villi.[372] In health, the arachnoid villi of the dural sinuses are responsible for absorption of the fluid. The arachnoid villi along spinal roots have not been shown to be involved in the physiological absorption of fluid.[193]

An average of 140 ml of fluid is present within the cerebrospinal fluid space. Of this, 23 ml is found within the ventricles, 30 ml within the spinal cord subarachnoid space, and the remainder in the cerebral cisterns and cerebral subarachnoid space.[91] The fluid's flow in the spinal cord subarachnoid space is complex. It predominantly flows caudad in the posterior portion of the space and cephalad anteriorly. Additionally, there is a gentle eddy in both directions.[108,109]

The question arises concerning an alternative pathway of flow of the fluid. In health, 500 ml per day flows from the choroid plexus, which is the fountainhead of its formation. It goes through the ventricular and subarachnoid spaces to the arachnoid villi, which constitute the major site of absorption. In experimental animals with stenosis of the aqueduct of Sylvius that obstructs the flow of fluid from the ventricles, however, an alternative flow has been seen.[277] It leaves the ventricles via the ependymal surface and traverses the substance of the brain, exiting through the pia mater into the cerebral subarachnoid space, to be absorbed in the arachnoid villi.

Understanding of the interfaces of the cerebrospinal fluid system is aided by the classic concept of the intracranial and intravertebral volume as consisting of three fluid compartments with interposed barriers of varying anatomical and functional characteristics. The spaces are the intravascular, the intracellular, and the extracellular. The extracellular space of the intracranial and vertebral volume includes the cerebrospinal fluid's space and the extracellular space of the central nervous system. The cerebrospinal fluid's space is considered an extension of the extracellular space of the nervous system, with which it freely communicates. Hence, the fluid's space is actually a lacuna of the extracellular space of the nervous system.[91,92,319–321,346]

The intracerebral volume of the cerebrospinal fluid's space consists essentially of the lateral ventricles, third ventricle, and fourth ventricle. The fluid in these spaces is separated from the extracellular space of the nervous system by the ependyma. The ependyma does not act as a barrier to solutes, in contrast to the intercellular bridges of the choroid plexus epithelium, which are a barrier to solutes.[345,346,348]

The fluid in the subarachnoid space is contained by the inner pia mater and the outer arachnoid. The arachnoid completely invests the brain and spinal cord. It is the outer limit of the blood-brain barrier, manifested structurally by tight intercellular bridges.[348] In contrast to the arachnoid membrane, the pia exactly follows the contour of the central nervous system. Passage of solutes from the fluid across the pia mater is unrestricted, as it is across the ependyma. Both pia and arachnoid themselves are avascular and depend on diffusion from the spinal fluid and underlying tissue for their nutrition.[469]

There are reservoirs for the cerebrospinal fluid outside the major ones of the ventricular system, the cerebral cisterns, and the spinal and subarachnoid spaces. These other reservoirs are the Virchow-Robin perivascular spaces, extensions around the cranial nerves, and extensions around the spinal nerve roots.

Blood vessels that supply the brain and spinal cord must pass through the arachnoid membrane to enter the nervous system. They are covered by the arachnoid membrane, a delicate network of collagenous fibers, which in turn is covered by a layer of flat mesothelial cells. These mesothelial cells join the pia mater within the nervous tissue, but do not fuse with it, hence forming a cul-de-sac. This space is referred to as the Virchow-Robin perivascular space and is continuous with the adjacent subarachnoid space. In health the fluid moves within these spaces as a gentle eddy in both directions. Terminal arterioles, capillaries, and smaller venules are not invested with the arachnoid-mesothelial covering; i.e., the Virchow-Robin perivascular spaces do not penetrate the brain very deeply.[250,348]

The possibility of yet another interface in the nervous system was recently suggested by the studies of Prineas that demonstrated what appear to be lymph vessels in it.[340] In white matter not involved with the disease process from patients with multiple sclerosis, motor neuron disease, and adrenoleukodystrophy, he was able to demonstrate thin-walled channels in the perivascular spaces identical to the lymphatic capillaries in other body tissues in both structure and contents. Although cerebral lymphatic drainage by way of the nasal mucosal lymphatics and lymphatics in the spinal nerve root area that interact with the systemic lymphatic system has been generally acknowledged in the past, prior to Prineas's work there was no anatomical evidence for a lymphatic compartment in the nervous system.[120,122,145]

Cerebrospinal Fluid Formation and the Choroid Plexus

The choroid plexus is a villous tuft enclosing a core of highly vascular connective tissue.[112,312] It has been estimated that there are 100 million choroid plexus cells, with an approximate surface area of 150 to 200 sq cm. The plexus lies within the ventricles. It is lined by a columnar epithelium that is continuous with and embryologically homologous with the ependymal epithelium. Its capillaries differ from those in most central nervous tissue by having fenestrations or pores similar to those seen in capillaries in the remainder of the body. The only other parts of the central nervous system with this type of capillary are the supraoptic nucleus, infundibulum, and area postrema. The basement membrane of the capillary endothelium separates it from the choroid epithelial cells. The epithelium has zonulae occludentes, which are rings of tight intercellular junctions just below the intraventricular surface. The choroidal surface is covered with microvilli and cilia. Extracellular fluid is present between the capillary endothelium and the choroid epithelium. It is postulated that the natural leak of albumin, IgG, and other serum proteins up to a molecular weight of about 200,000 daltons is due to their ability to traverse the capillary fenestrae, then diffuse through the extracellular space, cross the ependyma, and enter the cerebrospinal fluid space.[406,407]

The choroid plexus is capable of both absorption and secretion, and it has been compared to the proximal renal tubule.[142,309] It is functionally and morphologically suited to both secretory and absorptive activity.[91,348] It can produce a nonproteinaceous fluid at 0.35 ml per minute, its normal rate of secretion, against a pressure head of 700 mm of water. Its barrier function is demonstrated among many other ways by the fact that silver ions, for example, from the blood are deposited in the basement membrane of the capillaries without reaching the epithelial cell. Trypan blue, while crossing the endothelial cell and the basement membrane, does not pass the epithelial tight junctions. On the other hand, bromide and iodide are absorbed by the choroid plexus.[91,177] Other substances, such as ionized calcium, can be seen to move freely in both directions. There are many examples of simultaneous absorption and secretion of nonphysiological substances as well as of substances treated differentially according to the direction of transport across the plexus.

Recognition of the absorptive capacity of the choroid plexus has led to the application of Fishman's provocative test of this function.[142] Just as acetazolamide decreases cerebrospinal fluid production, probenecid blocks the disappearance of penicillin, para-aminohippurate, and phenol red from the fluid. This effect is similar to its action on the renal tubule. Additionally, some monoamine catabolites, which are decreased in the cerebrospinal fluid in patients with Parkinson's disease or phenothiazine-induced dyskinesias, are shown to increase in this fluid after probenecid administration. This type of evidence has led to the concept of the choroid plexus as the site of specific removal of organic anions from the cerebrospinal fluid.

The ventricular ependyma, site of the cerebrospinal fluid–central nervous system extracellular space interface, is continuous with the choroid epithelium. The ependyma has no pores, only sparse tight junctions, and does not have a basement membrane.[345] The ependymal epithelium covering the area postrema and the infundibulum, however, have zonulae occludentes.[44] Neuroglia are found between the ependyma and subjacent capillaries, with glial processes extending deep into the parenchyma. In health, the ependymal contribution to the cerebrospinal fluid probably is very small. The belief that it has secretory function is supported by the continuous production of fluid in animals whose choroid plexus has been removed.[91–93]

On the other hand, the interface between the cerebrospinal fluid and the central nervous system extracellular space at the pial-glial lining, particularly over the cerebral cortex and spinal cord, is characterized by a basement membrane and the absence of zonulae occludentes.[250] Functional characteristics remain less well characterized, but fluid exchange is found to be essentially unrestricted, although perhaps less so than over the ependyma–cerebrospinal fluid interface.[348]

Except for the cerebrospinal fluid, the extracellular volume and its constituents in the central nervous system have been difficult to determine. Early electron microscopic work that showed almost complete absence of extracellular space in the brain was probably incorrect. More recent studies indicate that the extracellular volume of the central nervous system is approximately 20 per cent of its total volume.[323,443] Also there is evidence of a circulation of the extracellular fluid to and from the cerebrospinal fluid.[345]

Cerebrospinal Fluid Absorption and the Arachnoid Villi

The arachnoid villi, along with the choroid plexus, are the major blood–cerebrospinal fluid interfaces.* They are an outcropping of arachnoid cells through the dural membrane into the endothelially lined venous sinuses. Doubt exists whether they are entirely lined within the sinus by the sinus endothelium. According to early descriptions, the villi contained essentially open channels in communication with the venous sinus that opened and closed in response to changes in cerebrospinal fluid pressure. These descriptions have been supplanted by the demonstrations that cells in the arachnoid villi are traversed by channels formed by the continous formation and destruction of giant vacuoles by the arachnoid cells.[436–438] This dynamic process probably leads to a limited number of large transcellular channels being present at any one time. Flow through the arachnoid vacuolar channels has been shown to be pressure dependent, with increases in the fluid's pressure leading to increased flow rates.[205]

Although the contributions of other fluid compartments must be kept in mind, the clinical approach to the dynamics of the cerebrospinal fluid must be based on the overwhelming contribution of the choroid plexus in its production and the preponderance of the arachnoid villi in its resorption.[396,454] Net flow of the fluid is a function of the rate of its formation and removal. Cutler and co-workers have shown that while the choroid plexus secretes at a constant rate of 0.35 ml per minute, the arachnoid villi have the capacity to absorb five times this much fluid. Additionally, a pressure of at least 60 mm of water is necessary in the fluid to operate the arachnoid villi absorptive mechanism.[82]

* See references 92, 96, 121, 167, 168, 454.

The active pumping of the fluid due to choroid plexus pulsations secondary to the cardiac pulse may be the most important factor in its intraventricular flow, but other mechanisms may also operate. Effects of respiratory variations, cerebral arterial pulsations, and the ciliary action of the ventricular ependyma may contribute to the process.[91] In addition, it has been suggested that the cerebral arachnoid villi act as a "suction pump," with a pressure gradient from subarachnoid space to dural venous sinus of approximately minus 60 mm of water.[298]

In the spinal subarachnoid space, the cardiac pulsation, Valsalva-like maneuvers, and postural effects probably all play a role in flow of the fluid, but removal of significant amounts by the spinal arachnoid villi does not occur.[109,193]

Clinical assessment of the healthiness of ventriculosubarachnoid flow is aided by an intraspinal dose of isotope that, failing to enter the ventricles, follows instead the course of fluid leaving the ventricles for the arachnoid villi of the cerebral convexities.[108]

Rates of formation and flow of the fluid can be measured directly with ventriculocisternal perfusion, whereby marker substances introduced into the ventricles and measured in the cisternal fluid give an indication of these values by their declining concentrations.[82,91,320,330,348] More recently, computed tomographic measurement of decreasing metrizamide concentration in the ventricles has produced similar results.[359] Absorptive capacity of the arachnoid villi may be assessed by infusion manometrics, discussed further in the section on lumbar puncture.[219]

Cerebrospinal Fluid Pressure

The authors studied 105 normal young adults who were 18 to 25 years of age. The spinal fluid pressures measured in the lateral recumbent position ranged from 94 to 216 mm of spinal fluid, with an average value of 150 mm and a standard deviation of ±33.[158–160] Similar values are found in older adults with a slight drift toward lower pressures with increasing age. In the sitting position, the average normal adult has a pressure, measured by lumbar puncture, of 400 mm of water. In the newborn, the normal range is 15 to 80, and from 6 to 8 years onward, the values are the same as those for adults.[91]

This average cerebrospinal fluid pressure of 150 mm of water with the effect of gravity removed has been attributed to the compliance of meningeal elements. The classic formula of the Monro-Kellie hypothesis remains generally relevant. The total volume of the rigid cranium and spinal column remains constant. Any increase in volume of one of the components (nervous tissue, blood, or cerebrospinal fluid) must be at the expense of others. Normal cerebrospinal fluid pressure will be maintained until the limits of the compensatory mechanisms are exceeded.[348]

Study of compensatory mechanisms for dealing with increasing intracranial pressure has led to the concept of compliance and resistance factors in the craniospinal axis.[4,38,237,278] Low-volume, rapid increases in intracranial pressure, such as the transmitted arterial and respiratory pulsations or the initial small volume of infused artificial cerebrospinal fluid during manometric studies, may cause little increase in cerebrospinal fluid pressure owing to the compliance component of the brain and spinal cord. The compliance component is thought to comprise the compressibility of intracerebral vessels (predominantly veins) and the distensibility of the spinal meninges. The ability of the compliance elements to compensate for increased pressures is greatly limited in practical terms by the effect on cerebral perfusion of decreasing vascular volume of the cerebral compartment.[282] This compliant compensatory device accounts for the early, relatively slow rise of the exponential curve of pressure and volume relationships within the skull and spinal column.[237,278]

When, in the short term, the compliance factor is exhausted, the rapid phase of the exponential pressure-volume curve is reached, reflecting the resistance component of the compensatory system. The resistance component is in essence equivalent to cerebrospinal fluid venting through the arachnoid villi. This resistance is pressure-dependent and may, morphologically, be related to the limited number of vacuolar transcellular channels through the villi, which have been shown not to increase in size in response to increased pressure of the fluid.[205]

The introduction of isovolumetric pressure transducers has made possible accurate measurements of variations in cerebrospinal fluid pressure, rather than of the mean pressure as shown by the clinically used displacement manometer.[159] With increased intracranial pressure, the arterial and respiratory pulses are seen to be altered. Unusual pressure responses of the fluid may also be measured.[123,268] Under all circumstances, the arterially transmitted pulsations are more marked in the ventricular compartment than in the spinal subarachnoid space, where they represent about 40 per cent of the amplitude of the ventricular pulse. With increases in intracranial pressure, the amplitude of the arterially transmitted pressure pulse, normally about 50 mm of water in the ventricles, 40 mm in the cisterna magna, and 30 mm in the lumbar sac, approaches the pulse pressure measured in the systemic arterial system. Variations of pressure caused by respirations or Valsalva maneuvers tend to be the same throughout the cerebrospinal fluid system, since both cranial and spinal veins drain into the superior vena cava.[462] In situations of increased intracranial pressure, in contradistinction to the magnification of the arterially transmitted pulse pressure, the respiratory and Valsalva-induced pressure changes become less and less evident.

Plateau waves, or A waves, of pathological variations in pressure have been described in association with increased intracranial pressure.[268] These are sudden elevations of pressure to a level higher than 50 mm of mercury. They usually last 5 to 20 minutes, but may be longer, and they decrease as rapidly as they appear. These waves usually are seen in the presence of moderate intracranial hypertension (20 to 40 mm of mercury) and are associated with the presence of papilledema and concurrent transient neurological dysfunction. They have also been seen during rapid eye movement sleep and in patients with normal-pressure hydrocephalus.[123] They occur at intervals of minutes or hours. Rhythmic variations of intracerebral pressure (B and C waves) occur at a frequency of 1 or 2 per minute in relation to underlying pathological respiratory patterns (e.g., Cheyne-Stokes) and at 4 to 8 per minute in relation to arterial pressure variations. The plateau waves appear to be of great clinical importance, and their appearance relates to the degree of intracranial pressure decompensation.

In general terms, intracranial hypertension may be conceived as resulting from increased production, inadequate circulation, or decreased absorption of the cerebrospinal fluid, or to intracranial volume increases in the tissue or intravascular components.[82,126,220] Expansion of brain tissue may result from cerebral edema, hemorrhage, neoplasm, or abscess.[99] Cerebral edema may be the result of increased capillary permeability in cases of hypertensive encephalopathy, carbon dioxide retention, infections, Reye syndrome, trauma, or rapidly expanding brain tumors.[439] Intravascular expansion may result from hypercapnia or profound hypoxia, from drugs such as halothane, or from decreased venous drainage in congestive heart failure or the superior vena cava syndrome.[250] Intracranial hypertension seen during convulsions may be considered here, since this phenomenon may be secondary to increased intracranial blood volume as a result of autonomic sympathetic discharge during a tonic seizure.[124] Conversely, increased intracranial pressure itself may cause convulsions, and the transient increases in intracranial pressure that occur normally at the onset of sleep and on waking may be magnified in the presence of an already existing increased intracranial pressure (as in hydrocephalus), which may account for the occurrence of childhood seizures at these times of the day, the so-called "pressure-fits."[124,361]

Mass lesions will not increase intracerebral pressure until they reach about 90 ml in volume, if acute, or much larger, if chronic.

Obstruction to the flow of the cerebrospinal fluid may be in the ventricles, at the junction of the ventricular system and subarachnoid space, or may represent a defect in absorption. In obstructive hydrocephalus, the output of the choroid plexus will continue to be 0.35 ml per minute until the secretory pressure of the plexus is exceeded by a hydrostatic pressure of about 700 mm of water.[82] Pulsations of the plexus may be necessary to produce ventricular enlargement; this, however, has not been proved.[27,35,91,92]

In noncommunicating hydrocephalus it is possible that cerebrospinal fluid can be shunted by a rupture of the anterior wall of the third ventricle, by rupture of the occipital horn of the lateral ventricle, or by its passage through the brain substance to the cerebral subarachnoid space.[99,277]

Overproduction of cerebrospinal fluid has not been documented as a cause of increased intracranial pressure. As would be expected as a corollary, choroid plexectomy does not benefit the hydrocephalus that is seen in some patients with choroid plexus papilloma.[285]

Defects of absorption may produce increased cerebrospinal fluid pressure, and this mechanism has been implicated in communicating hydrocephalus, pseudotumor cerebri, the Guillain-Barré syndrome, tumor of the spinal cord or cauda equina, poliomyelitis, following subarachnoid hemorrhage, and possibly in normal-pressure hydrocephalus.[17,143,261]

Increased spinal fluid pressures (over 200 mm of water on lumbar puncture) may be measured in conditions not associated with increased intracranial pressure. It may be seen in a tense patient in whom abdominal muscle contraction and breath holding may result in decreased venous return from the cranial and spinal vaults. Postural effects, including having the head above the horizontal, arm pressure on the jugular vein, and marked obesity, may produce it.[334]

Low spinal fluid pressures may have a number of causes.[23,143,235,424] They include spinal subarachnoid block, decrease in vascular volume, barbiturate intoxication, leakage of fluid through holes in the arachnoid, otorrhea, rhinorrhea, or lumborrhea; the last of which may be caused by lumbar puncture, tears in the lumbar nerve sheaths secondary to trauma, or operative trauma to the nerve sheaths.[247,251,252] Primary intracranial hypotension may also exist. A large decrease in pressure on removal of a small amount of fluid indicates a small (lumbosacral) reservoir, and one should suspect a spinal subarachnoid block. Conversely, a small decrease in pressure on removal of a large amount of fluid suggests a large reservoir. The Ayala quotient (closing lumbar pressure multiplied by 10 divided by opening pressure after removal of 10 ml of fluid) has been used to express this phenomenon; it is, however, of little clinical value.[11,91] On the other hand, study of normal individuals shows linear regression of pressure when 20 ml is withdrawn at a rate of 1 ml per minute. The normal closing pressure is 30 per cent less than the opening pressure. These findings should help to define whether a young adult patient does indeed have normal cerebrospinal fluid pressure.[160]

Blood-Brain-Cerebrospinal Fluid Barriers

All these barriers taken together are commonly referred to as the blood-brain barrier. The concept that one mechanism exists in both health and disease to control the passage of all substances through this blood-brain barrier, however, is an oversimplification.* No unitary theory suffices to explain the rate of entry, the steady-state concentration, the length of persistence, or the rate of disappearance of all substances found in the brain. A number of factors affect how each substance enters, equilibrates in, persists in, and disappears from the brain. They include rate of formation and flow of cerebrospinal fluid, energy-dependent active transport, carrier-facilitated diffusion, pinocytosis, and passive diffusion.[143,348] In addition, binding of blood constituents by plasma proteins, intracellular affinity for various compounds, physical barriers to molecular size, lipid solubility and state of ionization of charged compounds, metabolic barriers such as enzymatic degradation of some compounds by membranes themselves, and metabolic turnover rates all play a role.[321,322]

There are virtually no pinocytes in the arachnoid membrane that surrounds the cerebrospinal fluid space. Furthermore, except in the choroid plexus, area postrema, intercolumnar tubercle, supraoptic crest, neurohypophysis, median eminence, and pineal gland, there are tight junctions in the microcirculation of the central nervous system. These factors emphasize that the central nervous system and its fluid space are in a moderately isolated compartment.

Clinical estimation of the integrity of the barrier by radioisotope brain scanning techniques as well as computed tomography utilizing contrast media normally excluded by the blood-brain barrier is well known.[348] Biochemical estimation of the integrity of the endothelial tight junction barrier may be undertaken by analysis of the albumin in

* See references 42–46, 91, 147, 218, 250, 348, 375, 417.

the cerebrospinal fluid, as discussed further in the section on proteins. This molecule is produced only in the liver. It is found in increased amounts in the spinal fluid (in the presence of normal blood serum albumin concentrations) in association with barrier damage, i.e., damage to the microcirculation endothelial tight junctions.[78,407,417]

A unique type of circulation exists between the cerebrospinal fluid and the central nervous system. The fluid acts as a lacuna of the nervous system's extracellular space and operates as a sink to regulate, in part, the concentration of solutes in this space.[217,319,323,441] Such action is possible because the total volume of about 140 ml is replaced about three and a half times per day, primarily by secretions generated by the choroid plexus. The fluid exits by flow to the blood via the arachnoid villi.

The effect of "ordinary" stress on the efficiency of the barrier should be noted. For example, it has been shown that inhalation of elevated concentrations of carbon dioxide significantly increases the susceptibility of mice to intravenously inoculated type II poliovirus.[374] Furthermore, hypotonicity and hypertonicity of the blood can widen the tight junctions of the capillary endothelium of the nervous system and lead to breakdown of the barrier. Accordingly, the proposal is warranted that in disease the barrier could modulate a reaction of the cerebrospinal fluid.[347,348]

A function of the barrier that is frequently passed over because it is difficult to study in the human is the passage of circulating core immune network leukocytes into the nervous system. In diseases such as pneumonia without meningitis or leukemia without central nervous system infiltration, the patient may have a high blood leukocyte count and normal cerebrospinal fluid leukocyte and differential counts. From this observation, the conclusion that blood leukocytes do not pass freely across the barrier is warranted.[417] On the other hand, in certain neurological diseases, pleocytosis can consist of essentially polymorphonuclear cells (and mononuclear cells, or a combination). It is the authors' opinion that these different types of leukocytes are recruited to the central nervous system by chemotactic agents generated by lesions in the system. Identification of the chemotactic agents and their origin might supply another missing piece in the puzzle of the molecular immunopathogenesis of the inflammatory response in the nervous system.[417]

Composition of the Cerebrospinal Fluid

The cerebrospinal fluid is clear and colorless except in some neonates (see section on cerebrospinal fluid in infancy and prematurity). Continuous spectrophotometric analysis from 400 to 615 mμ indicates that it is different from water in that it has a slight absorption from 400 to 420 mμ.[18,403,410] Its total absorption over this wavelength range is 1.371 ($\pm$0.736 standard deviation) optical densities.[403] It normally contains 1.8 ($\pm$1.2) leukocytes per cubic millimeter and no erythrocytes. The differential count reveals 16 ($\pm$9.5) per cent monocytes, 17 ($\pm$15) per cent small and 63 ($\pm$ 17.7) per cent large lymphocytes, less than 4 per cent cells that cannot be easily classified, and no polymorphonuclear cells. The total protein content is 38.2 ($\pm$ 10.4) mg per 100 ml and the IgG is 9.9 ($\pm$2.5) per cent of the total protein.[406] The glucose content is 61 mg per 100 ml (65 per cent of blood plasma value in the fasting state). The chloride ion content is 124 mEq per liter (120 per cent of blood plasma value), and the total lipid concentration is 1.25 ($\pm$ 0.243) mg per 100 ml, which is composed of phospholipids, nonphosphorus sphingolipids, cholesterol, cholesterol esters, and neutral fats.[91,423,442] Many other constituents are present in small quantities (Table 13–1).* There is a definite relationship between most constituents in cerebrospinal fluid and those in blood plasma.[91,348] With the exception of trace proteins, all substances found in the fluid are found in the blood.[91,240,348] Not all substances found in the blood, however, are found in the fluid; for example, beta-lipoprotein and fibrinogen.[91,348] Because of this relationship with the blood, certain changes from the normal cerebrospinal fluid values are merely a reflection of the changes in blood plasma concentration and have nothing to do with nervous system disease. Hence, it is imperative to do simultaneous blood plasma studies when interpreting values for most constituents in the fluid, particularly glucose and chloride ion concentrations.

---

* See references 40, 91, 212, 332, 384, 406, 440, 445.

A gradient for many constituents of the fluid exists along the cerebrospinal axis. The best-known gradients are those of total protein and glucose.[91,348] In terms of the total protein gradient, the ventricular fluid contains approximately 10 mg, the cisternal fluid 20 mg, and the lumbar fluid 40 mg per 100 ml. Glucose concentration in the ventricles is about 60 mg per 100 ml, while it is 50 mg per 100 ml in the cisternal fluid and 40 mg per 100 ml in the lumbar sac. Accordingly, to standardize the lumbar sampling, the authors recommend the removal of lumbar fluid at a standard rate, viz., 1 ml per minute, to obtain a total of 20 ml when clinical judgment indicates it is safe. The collection tubes should be carefully marked and numbered.

Cerebrospinal Fluid Function

In early embryological stages, the fluid may play a nutritive role, but with the approach of maturity this function probably is lost except in the case of the avascular arachnoid, pia, and ependyma.[469] The mechanical functions of the fluid are the most widely accepted.[91,143] It may lubricate and serve as a buffer between the compressible brain and spinal cord and the more rigid fibro-osseous framework of the dura and skull and vertebral column. The brain may thus be protected against injury. The weight of the adult brain has been calculated to be only 50 gm when it is suspended in the fluid.[293] Changes in brain volume may be accommodated in part by decreases in the fluid volume, as in the case of expanding intracerebral lesions, or by increases in the fluid volume as in hydrocephalus ex vacuo.[91,143]

Cerebrospinal fluid is unique among body fluids. It not only fills the ventricles and surrounds the central nervous system but also probably penetrates it by way of the Virchow-Robin spaces. Moreover, it is in close contact with but separated by a barrier from the blood supply of the central nervous system as well as from the blood and lymphatic supply of its covering membranes. Tschirgi was one of the first investigators to present evidence to support the hypothesis that the fluid is a circulating pool in communication with the extracellular fluid. The pool surrounds the brain and is an expansion of its extracellular space. It is approximately 150 ml in volume, and is filled with a type of "diluted" extracellular fluid.[441]

The cerebrospinal fluid circulates through the ventricles and subarachnoid space at the rate of 500 ml per day. Oldendorf has reviewed the data that have been accumulated to advance the argument that it nonspecifically clears solutes from the extracellular space of the brain; i.e., it constitutes a low-concentration compartment (a "sink") in widespread close contact with the extracellular fluid, resulting in diffusion of solutes into it.[319,320,323,467] In turn, these solutes are returned to the blood by flow through the macropinocyte system of the arachnoid villi. It might be said that the sink action of the cerebrospinal fluid serves the function of a lymphatic system adapted to the nervous system. On the other hand, Davson and Segal perfused the ventricles of rabbits with silicone instead of artificial cerebrospinal fluid.[93] The escape of ^{14}C-sucrose, an extracellular space marker, from the central nervous system was largely prevented by replacement of fluid by silicone. The data suggested that the removal of ions by a flow mechanism from the extracellular space was relatively unimportant, since the silicone should have carried the extracellular fluid as efficiently as did artificial cerebrospinal fluid. They suggested that the mechanism for escape of solutes from extracellular space to the cerebrospinal fluid is simple diffusion through stationary extracellular fluid.

The cerebrospinal fluid is in contact with the extracellular space by the ependyma and possibly the Virchow-Robin spaces. The ependyma behaves like a loosely knit membrane presumably with large gaps between its cells; moreover, according to Brightman and co-workers, it is permeable to large molecules such as ferritin (500,000 daltons).[41]

The extent to which the Virchow-Robin perivascular spaces follow small vessels is still not settled; if they penetrate at least to the arteriolar level, they could offer a potential communication between extracellular fluid and cerebrospinal fluid in the subarachnoid space.

As already noted, controversy regarding the size of the nervous system extracellular space continues, but the critical point is that there is an adequate amount of space for the free diffusion of compounds,

TABLE 13-1 COMPOSITION OF NORMAL LUMBAR CEREBROSPINAL FLUID

CONSTITUENT	UNITS	AVERAGE VALUE
Xanthochromic index	optical density	1.371
Total protein	mg/100 ml	38.2
Prealbumin	%	4
Albumin	%	62
Globulins		
Alpha-1	%	5
Alpha-2	%	5
Beta	%	9
Tau (beta 2)	%	6
Gamma*		10
IgG	μg/ml ($\pm$2 SD) by EID†	18.8 (6.1–58.5)
IgG	μg/ml ($\pm$2 SD) by RIA†	14.6 (4.2–51.2)
IgM	ng/ml ($\pm$2 SD) by RIA†	51.3 (7.3–361)
IgA	μg/ml ($\pm$2 SD) by RIA†	1.32 (0.32–5.5)
Protein-bound carbohydrates	mg/100 ml	2
Myelin basic protein‡	ng/ml	$<$4
Betaendorphin††	pmol/L	72 (61–93)
Enzymes (see text and references)		
Complement		
C3	mg/100 ml	0.46–1.4
C4	mg/100 ml	0.09–0.4
Glucose§	mg/100 ml	61
Lactate	mg/100 ml	19
Pyruvate	mg/100 ml	0.9
Lactate/pyruvate ratio		11.0
Citric acid	mM/L	0.3
Inositol	mM/L	0.2
Total phospholipids	mg/100 ml	0.38
Cephalins	mg/100 ml	0.10
Lecithins	mg/100 ml	0.18
Plasmalogens		Qualitative
Lysolecithin	mg/100 ml	0.03
Diphosphoinositide		Qualitative
Sphingomyelin	mg/100 ml	0.10
Nonphosphorus sphingolipids	mg/100 ml	0.08
Total cholesterol	mg/100 ml	0.40
Free	mg/100 ml	0.12
Esterified	mg/100 ml	0.27
Free	%	33
Neutral fat	mg/100 ml	0.42
Total lipid	mg/100 ml	1.25
Fatty acids		
Free		Qualitative
Total		
Protein bound lipid		
Alpha-1 lipoprotein		Qualitative
Gamma lipoprotein		Qualitative
Total leukocytes	cells/cu mm	1.8
Lymphocytes	%	79
Large	%	63
Small	%	16
Monocytes	%	17
Leukocytes that cannot be further characterized	%	4
Polymorphonuclear		0
Sodium	mEq/L	141
Potassium	mEq/L	3.3
Calcium	mEq/L	2.5
Magnesium	mEq/L	2.4
Total base	mEq/L	155
Chloride	mEq/L	124
Bicarbonate	mEq/L	21
Inorganic phosphate	mgP/100 ml	1–1.5
Copper	μg/100 ml	6.2
Iron	μg/100 ml	38
Lead	μg/100 ml	14–38
Aluminum	μg/100 ml	12.5
Carbon dioxide	mm Hg	46
pH		7.31

TABLE 13–1 COMPOSITION OF NORMAL LUMBAR CEREBROSPINAL FLUID (*continued*)

CONSTITUENT	UNITS	AVERAGE VALUE
Nonprotein nitrogen	mg/100 ml	19
Ammonia	μg/100 ml	6.4
Urea	mg urea N/100 ml	11
Uric acid	mg uric acid N/100 ml	0.6
Creatinine	mg creatinine N/100 ml	4
Neuraminic acid	mg neuraminic acid N/100 ml	0.28
Glutamine	mg/100 ml	12.6
Gamma aminobutyric acid**	pmol/ml	273 ± 121
Glucosamine	mM/L	0.1
Free amino acids§	All expressed as micromoles/100 ml¶‖	
Glutamic acid		0.8
Taurine		0.6
N-acetylaspartic acid		
Aspartic acid		0.02
Glycine		0.7
Alanine		2.6
Serine		2.5
Threonine		2.5
Lysine		2.1
Arginine		1.8
Histidine		1.3
Valine		1.6
Leucine		1.1
Isoleucine		0.4
Phenylalanine		0.8
Tyrosine		0.8
Proline		
Methionine		0.3
Ornithine		0.6
Homocarnosine		0.3
Vitamin C	mg/100 ml	3.7
Folate	μg/ml	23.6
Total solids	gm/L	1.0
Specific gravity		1.008
Neurotransmitter catabolites		
Homovanillic acid (HVA)¶	ng/ml	48
5-HIAA	ng/ml	31.5

* IgG and IgA are expressed in micrograms (μg) per milliliter; IgM is expressed in nanograms (ng) per milliliter.

† See Mingioli, E., Storober, W., Tourtellotte, W., Whitaker, J., and McFarlin, D.: Quantitation of IgG, IgA, and IgM in the CSF by radioimmunoassay. Neurology (Minneap.), *28*:991, 1978.

‡ See Cohen, S. R., Herndon, R. M., and McKhann, G. M.: Radioimmunoassay of myelin basic protein in spinal fluid. An index of active demyelination. New Eng. J. Med., *295*:1455, 1976.

§ See Maker, S. M., Clarke, D. D., and Lajtha, A. L.: Intermediary metabolism of carbohydrates and amino acids. *In* Siegel, G. J., et al., eds.: Basic Neurochemistry. 2nd Ed. Boston, Little, Brown & Co., 1976.

‖ See Sourkes, T. L.: Parkinson's disease and other disorders of the basal ganglia. *In* Siegel, G. J., et al., eds.: Basic Neurochemistry. 2nd Ed. Boston, Little, Brown & Co., 1976.

¶ Various neurological diseases excluding parkinsonism. See Ouvrier, R. A.: Progressive dystonia with marked diurnal fluctuation. Ann. Neurol., *4*:412–417, 1978.

** Neethling, A. C., McCarthy, B., and Taljaard, J. J. F.: Gamma-aminobutyric acid in CSF. Lancet, *1*:211, 1980.

†† Domschke, W., Dickschas, A., and Mitzness, P.: C.S.F. beta-endorphin in schizophrenia. Lancet, *2*:425, 1979.

whether it accounts for 8, 13, or closer to 20 per cent of the total brain weight.

From an immunological standpoint, the cerebrospinal fluid may act as a disseminator of inflammatory exudate (white cells and gamma globulins) and gamma globulins synthesized within the central nervous system.[406,408]

The functional significance of hormones found within the cerebrospinal fluid remains unclear. The fluid may influence pituitary function by altering concentrations of hormones in the neurohypophyseal portal circulation.[348] The concentration of electrolytes in and the pressure of the cerebrospinal fluid may also have functional significance in terms of the medullary centers involved in respiratory and vasomotor control.[338,339]

NATURE OF THE CEREBROSPINAL FLUID IN HEALTH AND DISEASE

Turbidity

Turbidity of the fluid usually is due to the presence of cells and becomes evident in the presence of 400 or more leukocytes or

200 or more erythrocytes per cubic millimeter. A "fatty"-appearing spinal fluid can be seen after an iophendylate (Pantopaque) myelogram. It has been found in a patient presenting with an intracerebral hematoma with concurrent severe hyperlipoproteinemia (type V), in which case it appears turbid, pinkish, and milky.[478]

Coagulation

Normal cerebrospinal fluid does not contain fibrinogen and therefore does not clot.[47] If the total protein content of the fluid is greater than 100 mg per 100 ml, however, this macromolecule could be present in sufficient concentration for clot formation. Furthermore, the higher the protein concentration, the more rapid the formation of the fibrin clot. If a sample of fluid is suspected of having a sufficient fibrinogen concentration at the time of sampling, the following qualitative test may be performed. Store a tube of fluid at 4°C for about 12 hours. If fibrinogen is excessive, a thin thread will develop and may be seen floating after a gentle shake of the tube. Quantitation of fibrinogen is tedious and is probably less sensitive than this qualitative method.

Because of potential clotting of the cerebrospinal fluid, cell counting should always be done as soon as possible after withdrawing the sample. Leukocytes, especially polymorphonuclear cells, have a propensity to adhere to the clot, resulting in an artifactually low total leukocyte count and an erroneous differential cell count.

In most cases when total protein concentration is sufficiently elevated, a fibrin clot will develop. There are, however, notable exceptions to this rule. In the Guillain-Barré syndrome and in brain subarachnoid hemorrhage, conditions that are frequently accompanied by a very high total protein level, the fluid seldom clots. This failure to clot most likely occurs because, at least in subarachnoid hemorrhage, the serum entering the fluid is defibrinated at the site of the lesion. The remainder of the serum proteins diffuse into the fluid and result in a high total protein content without fibrinogen.

It is recommended that if a high protein content is suspected on clinical grounds or if a clot develops while the fluid is being obtained, the fluid should be collected in a tube containing an anticoagulant so that accurate cell and differential counts may be obtained. The authors' recommended procedure is detailed in the section of this chapter dealing with standardized laboratory procedures.

The most marked elevation of protein levels in fluid in the lumbar sac occurs with the blockage of the subarachnoid space around the spinal cord at a level above the lumbar puncture needle entry site. Such blockage may result in loculation of fluid below the block, and the fluid may be yellow, clot spontaneously, and have a protein content as high as 5 gm per 100 ml (Froin syndrome).[99,154]

Even though a clot develops, analysis for total protein and all proteins except fibrinogen in the supernatant fluid of a centrifuged specimen remains valid. The amount of fibrinogen necessary for fibrin formation is small, 0.01 to 0.02 mg per 100 ml, and a cerebrospinal fluid fibrinogen level above 1 mg per 100 ml has never been reported.[47]

Hemorrhagic Cerebrospinal Fluid

Normal cerebrospinal fluid never contains erythrocytes. If it has erythrocytes their presence is due either to faulty technique in entering the subarachnoid space or to a subarachnoid hemorrhage. A decision regarding the cause usually can be made at the time the sample of fluid is acquired.*

Even in a patient who has had a subarachnoid hemorrhage, it is possible to obtain clear fluid in the lumbar sac for several hours after the ictus. Accordingly, when a spontaneous cerebral subarachnoid hemorrhage is suspected on clinical grounds, it is advisable to wait at least two hours before doing a lumbar puncture so that the blood has time to traverse from the cerebrum to the lumbar subarachnoid space.[447]

At the time of lumbar puncture, if the first few drops show a bloody tinge, then fluid should be collected in five different tubes. In the first tube, 16 drops should be collected, and a waiting period of two minutes should then be allowed with the stylet remaining in place. The maneuver is repeated five times with 1-ml samples collected in separate numbered tubes. This technique of collection permits time for nat-

---

* See references 18, 233, 356, 403, 425, 431, 447.

ural clotting processes to ensue, for rinsing of the needle, and for mixing of clear fluid from the surrounding area and its entrance into the hemorrhagic puncture site. When the hemorrhagic fluid is due to faulty technique, the following can be observed: (1) The fluid appears to be the clearest in the fifth tube; this impression may be confirmed by cell counts of the first and fifth tubes. During the early phases of subarachnoid hemorrhage, the erythrocyte counts in serial tubes may remain the same or increase. In the resolution stage it is possible to see some decrease in the erythrocyte counts in serial tubes. (2) The fluid may clot if the red cell count is more than 250,000 per cubic millimeter in cases of traumatic puncture, but not in cases of spontaneous subarachnoid hemorrhage, since as noted earlier, the fluid has been defibrinated at the site of the hemorrhage. (3) The supernatant fluid will be clear spectrophotometrically, unless the hemorrhage exceeded 12,000 erythrocytes per cubic millimeter.[431] (4) In traumatic puncture, the leukocyte count and total protein concentrations are increased in proportion to the number of erythrocytes present, viz., about one white blood cell per 1000 erythrocytes and approximately 1.5 mg per 100 ml protein per 1000 erythrocytes, while in subarachnoid hemorrhage the fluid takes on additional inflammatory qualities ("hematogenous meningitis").[447] (5) The presence of crenated red cells is of no important differential utility, since erythrocytes have a tendency to become crenated rather quickly in the presence of cerebrospinal fluid. (6) If erythromacrophages are found on differential staining with Wright's stain, then spontaneous subarachnoid hemorrhage is confirmed.[371] (7) A repeat tap at the next higher interspace should give clear fluid if the hemorrhage was due to faulty technique. (8) More recently applied measurement of fibrinogen split products in the fluid may, in the future, aid in the differential diagnosis.[192]

The means by which erythrocytes disappear from the cerebrospinal fluid has been studied in dogs.[291] Radioactive tagged erythrocytes were noted in the arachnoid villi and in the systemic reticuloendothelial system. Presumably the nasal lymphatics are the important entry point into the systemic lymphatic system. In addition, erythrophagocytosis and autolysis of red cells is of importance.

If possible, entry into the subarachnoid space of a patient who is receiving anticoagulants or who has a severe clotting abnormality should be avoided. Subarachnoid, subdural, or epidural hemorrhages may result.[236,334]

Xanthochromia

Semantically, xanthochromia implies any yellow discoloration. The level of pigmentary changes within the cerebrospinal fluid may be described by use of a xanthochromic index by which the optical density of the fluid is measured over wavelengths from 400 to 615 mμ and the area subtended by the graph is summated. Normal values are 1.371 $\pm$ 0.736 optical densities with a 95 per cent range of 0 to 2.[403,425] This method measures all pigments present and remains accurate as long as total spinal fluid protein is less than 100 mg per 100 ml. Additionally, quantitation of specific blood pigments in supernatant fluid after centrifugation (i.e., oxyhemoglobin, methemoglobin, and bilirubin) can be simply, reliably, and validly determined by spectrophotometric analysis and the application of Kronholm's equations.[233] Other pigments that can be specifically characterized are carotene and melanin.[269]

In the course of a one-time subarachnoid hemorrhage, oxyhemoglobin is found within 2 hours of the ictus (owing to lysis of red cells), peaks at about 36 hours, and disappears within 7 to 10 days in the absence of further bleeding; it may be seen after up to 30 days with persistence of hemorrhage.[18,233,403,425,431]

Oxyhemoglobin in supernatant fluid appears pinkish on inspection with the naked eye when the concentration reaches about 1 mg per 100 ml. It is quantitated spectrophotometrically at a wavelength of 415 mμ.[18,233,403]

Bilirubin in the cerebrospinal fluid gives it a yellowish tinge.[18,233] It depends for its formation on the action of arachnoid cell heme oxygenase on hemoglobin and thus only appears in vivo and will not change in content with the specimen after the sample has been drawn.[356] In one-time subarachnoid hemorrhage, bilirubin appears about 10 hours after the hemorrhage, peaks at 48 hours, and persists for two to three weeks.[18,425] Bilirubin is also the cause of the xanthochromia noted in fluid with a high protein content (greater than 150 mg per 100 ml), and in jaundiced patients.[403] High serum levels of bilirubin (around 10 to 16 mg per 100 ml, or less if the blood-brain barrier is abnormal) must be reached for this effect, however. The cerebrospinal fluid concentration is about one tenth to one hundredth that of the serum.[28]

Methemoglobin can be detected any time after the appearance of oxyhemoglobin,[233,425] but is usually only seen in encapsulated or loculated hematomas.[18] Cerebrospinal fluid spectrophotometry has been reported to be even more sensitive than computed tomography in diagnosing cerebrovascular disease.[387]

The "pseudoxanthochromia" produced by hyperbilirubinemia, carotenemia, and high fluid protein content is also noted when rubber cork stoppers are used to close the collection tubes. In most centers, this practice has been replaced by the use of plastic caps.[351]

Quantitation of blood pigments and cell counts in cerebrospinal fluid following spontaneous subarachnoid hemorrhage permits some conclusions to be drawn. Leakage of an aneurysm can be confirmed, but of more practical importance is that a precise quantitation of blood pigments on serial samples can substantiate continued leakage if it should occur.[425]

Cells

Handling of the cerebrospinal fluid from the time of sampling is now fairly standard for cellular analysis; generally about 5 ml collected in a plastic-capped tube is sent to the laboratory. This procedure may be altered, for example, in suspected subarachnoid hemorrhage, in which case several samples are sent for serial cellular analysis. Additionally, if a clot develops or is suspected clinically, the fluid should be collected in a tube containing an anticoagulant as specified in the section on standardized laboratory procedures. Furthermore, when fluid is collected during pneumoencephalography, a progressive increase of mononuclear cells to over 100 per cubic millimeter after exchanging 50 to 100 ml of fluid with air is a regular finding. Thus it becomes important that the cellular examination of the fluid be done on the first few milliliters that are collected.[394]

Numerous methods have been developed for preparing the fluid for cytological examination. They include various sedimentation techniques, filtration methods, centrifugation, and special preparatory techniques for electron microscopy.* All have their relative merits and disadvantages. Clean equipment and proper mixing of specimens are essential for analyzing a fluid that contains a small number of cells. The total cell count can be performed on undiluted fluid unless the number of cells is too high, in which case Hayem's solution is recommended as the diluent. The leukocyte count should be done by employing a dye that contains acetic acid. It is convenient to make a constriction pipet so that the acid dye can be brought to the first constriction and the spinal fluid to the second constriction, resulting in a 1 to 9 dilution of the cerebrospinal fluid before mixing. A Fuchs-Rosenthal chamber (total volume 3.2 cmm) is recommended, because it is the largest commercially available chamber.[403]

For the purposes of differential cell counting, the authors' laboratory employs centrifugation (4° C, 900 rcf, 10 minutes). The supernatant is removed with a Lang-Levy pipet and 5 μl of 20 per cent albumin is added before smearing of 1 μl on clean glass cover slips. The albumin prevents drying artifacts and may make up for the low oncotic pressure of normal fluid, which under most circumstances leads to rapid lysis and morphological alterations in the cell.[276,404] The fluid should be processed as rapidly as possible after sampling, since cellular disintegration, especially of polymorphonuclear cells, may occur. If the total protein content is relatively high (more than 100 mg per 100 ml), a fibrous clot may form in several hours, leading to withdrawal of some or all of the cells from the fluid. Cell counts and differential analysis of cells may, however, be made with reliability for up to 48 hours if the fluid is stored at 4° C, no clot develops, and the cell composition does not include excessive polymorphonuclear cells.[403,404]

With the techniques just described and application of Wright's stain, the authors

* See references 169, 170, 190, 191, 229, 230, 276, 308, 371, 392, 394, 404, 472.

have found the following normal values in 135 normal university students (18 to 35 years of age).[406] 1.8 leukocytes per cubic millimeter with a standard deviation of 1.2. The upper limit of normal is 5. The mean percentage distribution of various cell types is as follows (with standard deviations in parentheses): large lymphocytes 65 per cent (±17.7), small lymphocytes 17 per cent (±15.1), monocytes 16 per cent (±9.5), with 4 per cent of the cells difficult to classify. Fewer lymphocytes may be seen in ventricular than in lumbar fluid.[269]

Many laboratories employ stains other than Wright's for routine cellular differentiation, probably most commonly the Giemsa technique. Methyl green pyronine is used for plasma cells; Papanicolaou's stain is used particularly for tumor cytology; Prussian blue may distinguish iron deposits from melanin; lipids within cells may be detected with Sudan stains; carbohydrates may be stained with periodic acid–Schiff techniques; and acridine orange staining makes fluorescence microscopy possible. The nitroblue tetrazolium reaction has been applied to cerebrospinal fluid cells; the presence of granulocytes active in bacterial phagocytosis results in a positive reaction. The nitroblue tetrazolium test is considered to be positive if more than 12 per cent of the granulocytes react. Positivity of this test is seen in the proliferative and chronic phases of bacterial and mycotic meningitides, but usually is negative in viral infections. Its clinical utility in this regard remains under investigation.[481]

Immunological techniques employing direct or indirect immunofluorescence may demonstrate bacterial and viral antigens in the cells of the cerebrospinal fluid in patients suspected of having encephalitides.* Investigation of the source of the cells has been aided by autoradiographic techniques.[317,318] The general concept has emerged that normally all cells in the fluid are derived from circulating blood and probably are passing through the nervous system, as is the case for other organs. On the other hand, cells of the leptomeningeal mesenchyme may differentiate into monocytes or lymphocytes, the only cells seen in the cerebrospinal fluid under normal circumstances. In pathological conditions, proliferation and further differentiation of the normally present leukocytes may take place, and more likely, the leukocytes may be recruited by an unknown chemotactic agent generated by injuries of the nervous system.[417] In circumstances involving dysfunction of the blood-brain barrier, nonnative cells such as erythrocytes can appear. Disappearance of the cells from the fluid most likely is due to autolysis and phagocytosis as well as to removal via the arachnoid villi.[18,291,371]

The authors' hypothesis that a barrier exists to keep lymphocytes from migrating from the blood to the central nervous system or the cerebrospinal fluid is described in the section on blood–central nervous system–cerebrospinal fluid barriers. Other immunological techniques (rosette formation, mitogen stimulation, and specific viral sensitization) have been applied to cerebrospinal fluid lymphocytes, and it has been shown that, as in the peripheral blood, the majority represent thymus-derived (T) cells, although the percentage of T cells in the fluid is even higher than that in peripheral blood (about 95 per cent of cerebrospinal fluid lymphocytes are T cells).[155] Further subfractionation of T cells in the fluid has shown that the great majority have Fc receptors and are thus considered to have a suppressor role.† Lymphocytes and monocytes are normally present in the fluid and increased numbers of them do not have a specific diagnostic value. The increase implies a subacute process and has been reported in encephalitis due to virus or mycobacterium and in mycosis. Additionally, resolving bacterial infections, tumor, response to foreign material, or injuries in general can result in mononuclear pleocytosis.‡

The presence of cerebrospinal fluid cells other than lymphocytes and monocytes, such as polymorphonuclear cells, eosinophils, basophils, plasma cells, macrophages, and tumor cells, is always abnormal, even when the total leukocyte count is normal. The presence of macrophages is never normal. Phagocytosis in the fluid is a function of both granulocytes and macrophages, the latter of which function primarily as phago-

* See references 30, 97, 98, 131, 198, 245, 302, 329, 404.

† See references 5, 10, 157, 228, 248, 257, 273, 306.

‡ See references 99, 143, 174, 269, 292–294.

cytes of microbes, erythrocytes, and lipids. Monocytes are generally not active in phagocytosis, but transformed monocytes may phagocytose essentially any foreign material. The term "macrophage" does not imply a particular cell line, although they are thought to be derived from monocytes, presumably originating in the circulating blood.[230,371] Lipid-laden macrophages ("foam cells") are common in Tay-Sachs disease.[418,430] Lipophages have been reported after Pantopaque myelography, and siderophages and erythrophages after subarachnoid hemorrhage.*

The presence of polymorphonuclear cells is never normal in the cerebrospinal fluid.[406] Polymorphonuclear granulocytes are predominant in the early, exudative phase of pyogenic infections and may also increase in the early period of viral infections, in tuberculous meningitis, in sterile hematogenous meningitis, or in meningeal irritation induced by the presence of other foreign material. The largest increase, up to several thousand, occurs in the pyogenic infections. It is possible that counts in the fluid can be higher than those in the blood. Deep-seated cerebral and extradural abscesses and subdural hemorrhage may also produce a neutrophilic response in the fluid ("sympathetic meningitis").[269,292–294]

The presence of eosinophils in the cerebrospinal fluid is never normal.[233a,406] They may be seen rarely in infectious processes, or even after subarachnoid hemorrhage, in which case they generally represent less than 1 per cent of the total cells, although they may be more numerous in viral meningitis. Eosinophilia in the fluid is seen most often in the pleocytosis that accompanies tuberculous meningitis. It may be seen in patients with urticaria or allergic bronchial asthma, or those with indwelling catheters, and has been noted after subarachnoid hemorrhage, Pantopaque myelography, and intrathecal injection of penicillin, radioactive iodine–labeled serum albumin, and other materials. Persistent cerebrospinal fluid eosinophilia is most commonly associated with parasitosis, particularly cerebral cysticercosis.[33]

Plasma cells are seen only in abnormal cerebrospinal fluid.[406] When present, they are thought to be of hematogenous origin, possibly from the immune reaction in the diseased brain, and derived from transformed lymphocytes; they are especially typical of viral diseases and chronic infections such as syphilis, tuberculosis, sarcoidosis, parasitosis, and subacute sclerosing panencephalitis.[274] They also occur with collagen diseases of the nervous system. They may be seen with a normal total cell count in the Guillain-Barré syndrome, occasionally after subarachnoid hemorrhage, and with malignant tumors of the nervous system.[371] It has been proposed that relative plasmacytosis is indicative of multiple sclerosis, but the authors' results do not support this postulate.[371,406] Plasma cells are considered tissue residents whose persistent presence depends on the presence of in situ antigenic stimulation. The authors conceive of the presence of plasma cells in the fluid as resulting from exfoliation from inflammatory lesions of the nervous system that extend into the cerebrospinal fluid space.[417]

In addition to blood elements not normally seen in cerebrospinal fluid, other abnormal cells may be identified by various techniques. Giant cells may be of tumorous origin (especially in glioblastoma multiforme and various carcinomas) or of leptomeningeal origin. The latter generally represent specialized macrophages, such as the "foreign body" giant cells seen after subarachnoid hemorrhage, cerebral contusion, intraspinal injection of contrast medium, or placement of ventricular drains. Basophilic giant cells resembling megakaryocytes may be seen in cerebral mycoses and occasionally in childhood encephalitides.[371] Malignant cells may be identified in less than half the cases, and benign neoplasms may be accompanied by free cells in the fluid in even fewer cases.[276,308,371,428] In meningeal leukemia or carcinomatosis, cellular recovery may be increased by repeated samplings, and these methods have had their greatest clinical value in pediatric leukemic patients.[115]

Microbes

Differentiation of bacterial from nonbacterial encephalomeningeal infections is important, and examination of the cerebrospinal fluid may be helpful.[404] Intact bacterial organisms often can be identified on gram-

* See references 115, 308, 371, 392, 394, 402–404, 428.

stained smears of the fluid. This identification usually is of timely import. The fluid should not be refrigerated, since some organisms, particularly *Neisseria meningitidis*, are extremely fragile and others may proliferate if it is kept at 37° C. Prior treatment of the patient with antibiotics may prevent growth of the bacteria in the culture medium.

In pyogenic infections, examination of the fluid usually will reveal gram-negative intracellular diplococci of *Neisseria meningitidis*, plump gram-negative bacilli of *Escherichia coli*, or chains of gram-positive *Diplococcus pneumonia*. Artifacts commonly are misinterpreted by inexperienced investigators.

Although tuberculous organisms may be revealed by acid-fast techniques, the number of organisms is quite small and negative results are common.

Fungal infections pose other difficulties. *Cryptococcus neoformans* is easily recognized with India ink stains of wet mounts of the fluid or by the authors' albumin method that utilizes fix-dried smears stained by Wright's method.[404] *Coccidioides immitus* rarely is seen on examination of the fluid, and identification of the organisms will depend on culture.

Many viral agents can be cultured. To do the culture, several milliliters of the fluid should be collected in a sterile, tightly sealed tube and immediately frozen at −70 degrees C.[393] Direct visualization is done best with electromicroscopy, although immunofluorescence techniques are occasionally helpful.[302]

Cerebrospinal Fluid Protein

The protein is the most frequently abnormal component of the cerebrospinal fluid in clinical practice.[104] In addition, the study of cerebrospinal fluid protein has shed much light on two important aspects of neurophysiology: the blood-brain barrier and neuroimmunology.

Regardless of at which point along the neuroaxis it is sampled, the cerebrospinal fluid is a dilute protein solution. It has about $^1/_{200}$ the concentration of protein in the systemic blood circulation. The protein concentration in the fluid may be measured and subfractionated by numerous methods. Detailed description of how the proteins are analyzed are given in the section of this chapter dealing with standardized laboratory techniques.

The total protein concentration in the fluid is influenced by the site of sampling and the age, sex, and degree of activity or recumbency of the patient.*

Total protein level is lowest in the ventricles, intermediate in the cisterna magna, and highest in the lumbar sac. The authors studied 105 normal university students age 18 to 35 years and found that the average lumbar cerebrospinal fluid protein value in this group was 38.2 mg per 100 ml with a standard deviation of 10.4. Levels change from 5 to 15 mg per 100 ml in the ventricles to 15 to 25 mg per 100 ml in the cistern and 15 to 52 mg per 100 ml in the lumbar sac.[91] According to others the protein content is highest at birth (approximately 100 mg per 100 ml), decreases to low levels by 3 months (about 25 mg per 100 ml), reaches adult levels by 1 year, remains relatively constant until 40 years of age, and then gradually increases to reach levels up to about 72 mg per 100 ml in the elderly.[91,269,293] There appears to be slightly more protein in the fluid of males than in that of females, but the statistical significance of this difference remains in doubt. Prolonged recumbency also increases the protein level.[269]

Increased cerebrospinal fluid protein may be iatrogenic. For example, slight increases are seen in patients receiving phenothiazines. Increased protein levels may also be a reflection of increased serum proteins in cirrhosis, myxedema, sarcoidosis, collagen-vascular diseases, lymphogranuloma venereum, and multiple myeloma.[99]

Froin's Syndrome

Froin's syndrome originally was described in a case of localized spinal meningitis with subarachnoid block. There was xanthochromia, pleocytosis, and coagulation of the fluid.[154] The designation was later limited to a state in which the fluid contained more than 500 mg protein per 100 ml without frank purulence.[99] This may be seen in chronic meningitis, especially syphilitic (rarely in acute or subacute) meningitis, in obstruction of the spinal subarachnoid space secondary to inflammation or

* See references 40, 64, 79, 102, 193, 452.

tumor, and in acute and subacute polyneuritis.

Albuminocytological Dissociation

While inflammatory processes tend to cause simultaneous increases in the cells and proteins in the fluid, several processes tend to produce an increase in the protein without concomitant cellular proliferation ("albuminocytological dissociation"). This dissociation may occur in acute polyradiculitis (Guillain-Barré syndrome), in diphtheritic polyneuritis, during the convalescent phase of acute anterior poliomyelitis, with cerebral infarctions, during and after convulsive seizures, in sarcoidosis, in myxedema, and with cerebral or spinal cord neoplasms, especially tumors of the cerebellopontine angle.[64,99] Acoustic neuroma is almost always associated with an increased protein level. Perhaps the increase in protein with this tumor results from its proximity to the foramen of Luschka, which is the exit of the fluid from the ventricle. Passage of the fluid over the tumor with an abnormal blood-brain barrier may permit passage of serum proteins into the cerebrospinal fluid.[319] Tumors close to the lateral ventricle seem to produce higher protein levels than tumors located farther from the ventricles. Increased protein in patients with tumors of the central nervous system may be due to obstruction of the flow of the fluid, to local venous obstruction, to heavy tumor vascularization that does not have capillary endothelium with tight junctions, and to tumor breakdown.[42,99]

Low Protein Levels

Low protein levels (less than about 15 mg per 100 ml) may be seen in children less than 3 to 6 months old; with benign intracranial hypertension (pseudotumor cerebri), acute water intoxication, and hyperthyroidism; and after pneumoencephalography or other procedures in which large amounts of fluid are removed.[99]

Protein Fractions

Application of electrophoretic and immunoelectrophoretic techniques to the total cerebrospinal fluid protein has demonstrated that with few exceptions, the proteins are a direct reflection of the serum proteins; that is, the same ones are found in the serum as in the fluid.* It appears that all serum proteins with molecular weights less than 200,000 daltons gain access to the fluid, and that alterations in serum proteins lead to alterations in the proteins in the fluid.[290,456] In the normal person, there are two "specific" cerebrospinal fluid proteins, i.e., proteins found in the fluid but not in normal serum. They are known as trace proteins (beta trace and gamma trace protein) and tau protein (also known as beta-2 globulin). Beta-2 globulin appears to be immunologically identical to serum transferrin, but with four neuraminic acid groups removed, most likely the result of the action of neuraminidase.[240] The origin of the trace proteins is controversial. They are found in extracts of nervous tissue and in the urine and are small molecules (less than 30,000 daltons).[253,325] Within the neuraxis, they probably diffuse into fluid from the nervous system itself. On the other hand, prealbumin, while normally found in the blood, is found in larger amounts in the fluid. The situation results from concentration of the prealbumin by the choroid plexus during secretion of the fluid.[240,253]

Under normal circumstances, two serum proteins, macroglobulin and fibrinogen, do not gain access to the cerebrospinal fluid.[105]

As noted, specific central nervous system proteins make a minor contribution to the fluid's proteins and the very large proteins are excluded from it. About 90 per cent of the protein is composed of albumin, beta globulin, and IgG.[266] These three proteins account for 58, 20, and 10 per cent respectively of normal fluid protein.

The cerebrospinal fluid albumin is derived exclusively from the blood.[407] It is synthesized only in the liver, enters the nervous system through natural leaks in the microcirculation of the choroid plexus, and sinks into the fluid space. It has not been shown to be synthesized within the nervous system or to undergo metabolism within it. This lack of catabolism of albumin by the nervous system becomes an important factor when one is attempting to use albumin as a measure of the integrity of the blood-brain barrier.[407,414] It is removed from the fluid via the arachnoid villi. The differential concentration of albumin along the cerebrospinal fluid space probably is related to dif-

* See references 53, 54, 61, 67, 103, 150, 240, 241, 255, 262, 266, 290.

ferences in flow of the fluid in the ventricular and cisternal compartments and around the spinal cord.[194]

Experiments with labeled albumin have shown that in the normal situation and in the pathological conditions in which there is breakdown of the blood-brain barrier, the serum albumin equilibrates with the albumin in the spinal fluid.[194,407,409,417] The normal blood-brain barrier tends to exclude albumin from the central nervous system at the microcirculation (capillary-venule) endothelium tight junction. At equilibrium the cerebrospinal fluid albumin will equal $^1/_{230}$ of the serum concentration.[46] Breakdown of the blood-brain barrier allows further entry of albumin, and equilibrium with the serum will be reached at higher levels of cerebrospinal fluid albumin, the exact amount depending upon the degree of barrier damage.

An increase in the cerebrospinal fluid albumin concentration may result from: (1) hemorrhage into the cerebrospinal fluid (with the hemorrhagic fluid containing about 230 times the concentration of albumin found in the pre-existing fluid), (2) persistent elevation of the serum value (since equilibration with the fluid will occur), (3) a lesion of the choroid plexus (since its secretion contains no albumin), (4) damage of the blood-brain barrier (with excess albumin in the nervous tissue sinking into the fluid), and (5) blockage of the flow of fluid, particularly in the spinal subarachnoid space.

In the absence of serum albumin abnormalities, choroid plexus lesions, hemorrhage, and spinal block, cerebrospinal fluid albumin may be used as a specific marker of the capillary endothelial tight junction of the blood-brain barrier. Indeed, most clinical situations in which it is generally accepted that breakdown of the barrier to proteins is involved will be associated with increased total cerebrospinal fluid protein concentrations, reflecting an increase in the albumin, a molecular marker of an abnormality of the capillary endothelial tight junctions.

In summary, a significantly elevated cerebrospinal fluid albumin concentration is often due to dysfunction of the blood-brain barrier. When the albumin concentration is abnormal, so is the total protein level. In all cases in which total protein content is greater than 65 mg per 100 ml, the albumin level will be found to be significantly elevated (i.e., 32 mg per 100 ml or more).[417] Because of the high degree of correlation between the total protein and albumin, a significantly elevated total protein concentration generally reflects a breakdown in the blood-brain barrier, and its measurement is a clinically convenient method of evaluating the barrier.

For historical reasons, the Lange colloidal gold reaction is mentioned briefly. In the past it was used in the diagnosis of neurosyphilis. Although gamma globulin causes coagulation of the gold suspension, the test must be considered nonspecific, since falsely negative results may be obtained because of interference by beta globulin, alpha globulin, and albumin. Instability of the gold suspension also may lead to erratic results. The colloidal gold reaction, as well as other nonspecific tests such as the gum-mastic reaction and the zinc sulfate turbidity test, has essentially been replaced by the newer more specific tests for specific protein fractions.[266,406,429]

Studies employing radioactively labeled immunoglobulin G (IgG) have shown that it, like albumin, reaches an equilibrium with serum IgG.[195] While it may be conclusively stated that albumin synthesis does not take place within the central nervous system, even in neurological diseases such as multiple sclerosis and subacute sclerosing panencephalitis, this cannot be stated for IgG.[77,83] In certain neurological diseases, most notably multiple sclerosis, subacute sclerosing panencephalitis, neurosyphilis, and toxoplasmosis, a pool of cerebrospinal fluid IgG and IgM not derived from serum is a constant finding.[461] For example, Frick and Scheid-Seydel were the first to show that in multiple sclerosis, from 16 to 92 per cent of the cerebrospinal fluid IgG is derived from a source other than serum.[137,151–153]

In multiple sclerosis, neither hemorrhage, which does not occur, nor blood-brain barrier dysfunction, which occurs in only about 20 per cent of patients, can explain the increased IgG found in the fluid.[406,417] The choroid plexus usually is functioning normally, and flow dynamics are seldom altered. The source of the extravascular IgG, presumably produced by the central nervous system, in these neurological diseases (particularly multiple sclerosis) is lymphoplasmacytes.[130,340,380]

There is overwhelming evidence that the central nervous system can perform as an immunological tissue, e.g., that it can synthesize in situ IgG that can be detected by the presence of cerebrospinal fluid IgG oligoclonal bands and measured by an empirical formula.*

Protein IgG Quotients

IgG to Total Protein Ratio

Regardless of disease, the IgG concentration varies with the amount of total protein in the cerebrospinal fluid.[2,213,407] This quotient will remain normal because of the increase in IgG in the fluid due to abnormal transudation from the serum, since other proteins included in the total protein (e.g., albumin) will be increased in a proportional amount, no matter how extensive the damage to the blood-brain barrier. An increase in the quotient for IgG to total protein signals an extravascular source of IgG, i.e., de novo synthesis within the central nervous system.[407]

Albumin to IgG Ratio

This is a ratio similar to that of IgG to total protein, and should be more discriminative, since total protein will include normally present IgG due to leakage as well as IgG produced de novo in the central nervous system. In fact, clinically, little difference is found between these two ratios. The authors have found that 73 per cent of patients with multiple sclerosis have an elevated albumin to IgG ratio, which is practically identical to the incidence (67 per cent) found when the IgG to total protein ratio is applied.[406,407,409]

Beta Globulin to Gamma Globulin Ratio

Bergmann and associates, and Cosgrove and Agius, utilizing paper electrophoresis, found that 90 per cent of patients with multiple sclerosis demonstrated a decreased beta globulin to gamma globulin ratio.[26,73] Since the average concentration of beta globulins is unchanged in multiple sclerosis, this is an artifactual ratio and merely measures an increase in IgG.[105] Even though the ratio is an artifact of calculation, it remains sensitive and is therefore included in this discussion.

Cerebrospinal Fluid Gamma Globulin to Serum Gamma Globulin Ratio

This ratio increases in multiple sclerosis.[26,368] The increase may be the result of either in situ IgG synthesis in the nervous system or of a change in the blood-brain barrier (with transudation of serum gamma globulin into the fluid). Since it does not separate out the serum gamma globulin transuded across a damaged blood-brain barrier, this quotient would be expected to be abnormally increased in any patient with a damaged barrier; hence its utility in supporting the diagnosis of multiple sclerosis is decreased when the blood-brain barrier is slightly damaged, as it is in about 20 per cent of these patients.[406] Moreover, a dysfunction of the blood-brain barrier almost always is associated with an increase in total protein in the fluid, and greater breakdown of the barrier will lead to the fluid's protein having a pattern more and more like that of the serum. As a result the quotient loses its value as a means of distinguishing between increased gamma globulin derived de novo from the central nervous system and that diffused across a damaged blood-brain barrier.

Link's IgG Index

The IgG index is equal to the ratio of cerebrospinal fluid IgG to serum IgG divided by the ratio of its albumin to the serum albumin, i.e., (IgG csf/IgG serum)/(Albumin csf/Albumin serum). Increased values were found in 86 per cent of patients with multiple sclerosis.[254]

Calculation of de novo IgG Synthesis in Central Nervous System

An empirical formula has been developed to calculate the de novo central nervous system IgG synthesis rate. It is based on physiological principles governing the passage of albumin and IgG across the blood-brain barrier.† To validate the formula, radiolabeled IgG and albumin obtained from

---

* See references 101, 240, 253, 405–417, 419–421, 427.

† See references 81–83, 151–153, 162, 256, 407, 408, 417.

pooled normal individual sera were followed from the blood to the cerebrospinal fluid over a 21-day period in patients with clinically definite multiple sclerosis.[409] IgG synthesis rates were calculated by using the isotope exchange method and compared with the values obtained with the authors' empirical formula. There was excellent concordance between the two methods, from a low rate of synthesis of 5 mg per day to a high rate of 120 mg per day. To further validate the formula and to determine whether the blood-brain barrier in multiple sclerosis processes normal serum IgG differently from IgG derived from autologous sera, an experiment with double-radiolabeled IgG was performed. Results show that in multiple sclerosis, the blood-brain barrier processes IgG from normal serum in the same way as IgG derived from autologous multiple sclerosis serum. Accordingly, the empirical formula, which requires only one sample of cerebrospinal fluid and matched serum, can reliably and validly estimate the rate of de novo IgG synthesis in the central nervous system in multiple sclerosis.[407,409,417] In 1970, Tourtellotte proposed an empirical formula to estimate the amount of IgG synthesized per day by the central nervous system in multiple sclerosis based on blood and cerebrospinal fluid values.[407] This formula, as recently revised and used in this study, is:

$$\text{de novo CNS IgG}_{SYN} = \left[\left(\text{IgG}_{CSF} - \frac{\text{IgG}_S}{369}\right) - \left(\text{Alb}_{CSF} - \frac{\text{Alb}_S}{230}\right)\left(\frac{\text{IgG}_S}{\text{Alb}_S}\right) 0.43\right] \times 5$$

where de novo CNS IgG_{SYN} represents the IgG in milligrams per day in the cerebrospinal fluid derived from extravascular sources, i.e., synthesized primarily within the blood-brain barrier by lymphoplasmacytes. IgG_{CSF} is the IgG concentration (in milligrams per 100 ml) found in the patient's cerebrospinal fluid, and IgG_S is the patient's serum IgG concentration (in milligrams per 100 ml). The number 369 is a ratio constant that quantitatively determines the proportion of IgG that normally passes by filtration from the serum into the cerebrospinal fluid across an intact blood-brain barrier.[409,417] It is the quotient of the average normal serum IgG concentration divided by the average normal cerebrospinal fluid IgG concentration. Thus, $\text{IgG}_S/369$ is the IgG that is expected to cross from the serum to the cerebrospinal fluid, on the basis of the patient's serum IgG concentration and the normal cerebrospinal fluid serum ratio.

Alb_{CSF} is the albumin concentration (in milligrams per 100 ml) found in the patient's cerebrospinal fluid, while Alb_S is the patient's serum albumin concentration (in milligrams per 100 ml). The number 230 represents a constant that determines the proportion of albumin that normally passes by filtration from the serum into the cerebrospinal fluid across an intact blood-brain barrier. It is the quotient of the average normal serum albumin concentration divided by the average normal cerebrospinal fluid albumin concentration. Thus, $\text{Alb}_{CSF} - (\text{Alb}_S/230)$ is a term that represents the excess albumin in the fluid that has crossed a damaged blood-brain barrier. This term is then multiplied by $(\text{IgG}_S/\text{Alb}_S) \times (0.43)$ to convert (on a molar basis) the excess albumin in the fluid to excess IgG that has crossed the damaged barrier with the albumin, assuming a one-to-one molecular equivalence.[206] To calculate the daily IgG synthesis, this entire equation is then multiplied by 5 to convert the concentration in milligrams per 100 ml to the amount present in the 500 ml that, on the average, is formed each day.

Other Cerebrospinal Fluid Proteins

In addition to normal protein components of cerebrospinal fluid and their alterations, myelin basic protein has undergone intensive measurement and investigation.[70,71,456b] Myelin basic protein accounts for approximately 40 per cent of the total protein of the myelin sheath, with a molecular weight of about 18,000 daltons.[88] Increased levels of this protein may be present in the fluid of patients with transverse myelitis and metachromatic leukodystrophy, and it may be a sensitive indicator of a process of active demyelination.[70,71]

Most of the constituents of the humoral arm of the immune response, for the most part proteins (e.g., specific antibodies, complement, and immune complexes), have all been investigated in the cerebrospinal fluid.*

Enzymes that have been measured include glutamic-oxalacetic transaminase, lactic dehydrogenase, creatine phosphokinase, esterase, peptidase, aldolase, beta-glucuronidase, leucine amino peptidase, isocitric dehydrogenase, 2′,3′-cyclic nucleotide 3′-phosphohydrolase (a myelin marker enzyme), and proteinases, among others.† Increased activity of particular enzymes may be seen with tumors or infarction, but the findings have not been specific enough for clinical application. Increased enzyme levels may also result when the total protein in the fluid is increased owing to dysfunction of the blood-brain barrier.

The discovery of endogenous opiate receptors in the brain has led to the recognition of enkephalins and endorphins as endogenous peptides with morphinelike qualities both in vivo and in vitro.[200] Beta-endorphin probably is synthesized within the brain. The endorphin levels are higher in brain and cerebrospinal fluid than in plasma.[207] They are decreased in the cerebrospinal fluid of patients with chronic schizophrenia and those receiving neuroleptic medication.[118]

Serology

Classic serological tests of the cerebrospinal fluid have been applied in suspected cases of neurosyphilis and in following the clinical course of these cases. In addition to *Treponema pallidum*, a wide variety of bacterial, viral, and parasitic pathogenic antigens in the cerebrospinal fluid have been identified by other complement-fixation tests and cellular immunofluorescence techniques.[329]

When *T. pallidum* or similar treponemas invade a human host, multiple antibodies are formed.[359a] They are of two basic types: antibodies directed against the treponema itself, and reaginic antibodies, or antibodies against antigens presumably released by interaction of the treponema with normal tissue constituents. The most widely used test for reaginic antibody is known as the Venereal Disease Research Laboratory (VDRL) test. Other tests include the Kline cardiolipin test, the Kahn standard test, the Kolmer test, and the Wassermann test. Examples of nonreaginic treponemal antibody tests include the *Treponema pallidum* immobilization test (TPI), the *Treponema pallidum* complement-fixation test, the fluorescent treponemal antibody (FTA) test, and the Reiter complement-fixation test. The *Treponema pallidum* immobilization test is the most specific, but is performed by the fewest laboratories. Additional nontreponemal (reaginic) tests include the rapid plasma reagin, which uses a modified Venereal Disease Research Laboratory antigen and agrees well with the latter.

Certain important points must be kept in mind when interpreting the reaginic tests. All of them are measurements of a reaction of the patient's serum or cerebrospinal fluid with an artificial antigen (lecithin and cardiolipin). Quantitative titers are the most important factor, and serial dilutions are of utmost importance. A "false negative" reaction may be noted in the prozone phenomenon, in which the specimen gives a negative reaction when undiluted but a positive one (i.e., shows flocculation) when diluted, indicating a great excess of reaginic antibody. This result will occur in approximately 1 per cent of tests. Serum reaginic titers are negative or low in early syphilis, but nearly all patients with secondary syphilis have higher titers (usually greater than 1:32). The titers will fall again in late untreated syphilis. A substantial change in titers is more important in assessing activity or response to treatment than a single titer value. In primary syphilis, the titers rapidly return to negative with treatment; this change requires 24 months in secondary syphilis. About 5 per cent of patients will remain serofast at low titers (less than 1:8) even with adequate treatment, and a larger proportion of patients treated during tertiary or latent syphilis will remain serofast. In these cases, reinfection may be indicated by a rise in titer.[21,107,270,435]

Twenty to forty per cent of all serum reaginic tests give biological false positive reactions, of which two thirds will convert to negative within six months. Of patients with false positive reaginic tests (that is, those with negative fluorescent treponemal

* See references 69, 175, 178, 179, 197, 224, 226, 227, 234, 260, 300, 316, 335, 354, 477.

† See references 15, 129, 208, 311, 313, 353, 357.

antibody absorption reactions) lasting more than six months, approximately half will eventually receive a diagnosis of syphilis.[288] The most common causes of biological false positive serum reaginic tests are autoimmune diseases, hyperglobulinemia, drug addiction, and aging (about 10 per cent of patients over the age of 70 have a false positive VDRL test).[435]

Treponemal tests, while specific for *Treponema,* are still not specific for *T. pallidum,* and positive tests may be seen in yaws, pinta, and bejel. The test becomes positive within two weeks of the primary infection, and stays *positive for life* in 90 per cent of patients, in both serum and cerebrospinal fluid. The fluorescent treponema antibody (FTA) test measures the presence of IgG directed against treponemas; the *Treponema pallidum* immobilization (TPI) test measures the ability of antibody complement complexes to immobilize a suspension of living treponemes extracted from rabbit testis. The fluorescent treponemal antibody absorption (FTA-ABS) test now in wide use employs dried *T. pallidum* on a glass slide as an antigen. The patient's serum is absorbed with nonpathogenic treponemal strains and is added, and then fluorescent anti–human gamma globulin antibodies are added. As noted earlier, the test becomes positive early in the disease and remains so despite antibiotic treatment, implying only previous infection and not necessarily active disease. It is currently the most sensitive and specific test available.[288,359a,435] In neonates, a similar test (FTA-ABS-IgM) is employed, replacing anti–human IgG with anti–human IgM, which cannot cross the placental barrier.[222,359a] For follow-up of the response to treatment, the VDRL remains the test of choice.[204,270,435,460]

Additional serological techniques applied to cerebrospinal fluid include the quellung reaction (capsular swelling of bacteria concentrated by centrifugation on exposure to specific antisera), which may lead to a rapid identification of organisms such as *Hemophilus influenzae, Neisseria meningitidis,* and *Diplococcus pneumoniae.*[329]

Bacterial antigens may also be detected rapidly by counterimmunoelectrophoresis (capsular polysaccharides of *H. influenzae, N. meningitidis,* and *D. pneumoniae,* and the teichoic antigen of *Staphylococcus aureus*). Cryptococcal antigen may be measured by a latex agglutination test (with a titer greater than 1:8 being essentially diagnostic), and this test is more specific than the more commonly applied tests for cryptococcal antibody, which may be falsely negative owing to the patient's inability to mount an adequate antibody response.[329]

Complement-fixing antibodies against most viruses causing encephalitis can be measured at specialized centers; usually, however, these are only helpful retrospectively.[57,245]

Serological tests in toxoplasmosis have been helpful. High titers in the fluid indicate active disease in the nervous system with local antibody production. A similar situation holds for trypanosomiasis as well as for parasitic infestations such as cysticercosis.[128,242,352]

In addition to the classic pathogens, amebae such as *Naegleria* and *Acanthamoeba-Hartmannella* (or free-living amebae), that were thought to be nonpathogenic, have more recently been identified as the cause of meningoencephalitis; examination of the fluid has been of little benefit in these cases, however. Diagnosis is dependent on serological studies of the serum and specialized brain tissue studies.[117]

Serological tests are now available for, among others, the viruses of choriomeningitis, poliomyelitis, mumps, lymphogranuloma inguinale, Eastern and Western equine encephalitis, and Coxsackie and echoviruses.[131,245,329,404]

Glucose and Intermediates

The normal cerebrospinal fluid glucose value ranges from 50 to 80 mg per 100 ml, i.e., 60 to 70 per cent of serum glucose concentration. Although it is higher in the ventricles, it never reaches the serum values.[370] Entry and exit of glucose from the fluid are by carrier-mediated transport (fast component) and by simple diffusion (slow component).[140] Removal of glucose from the fluid also may depend to some degree on absorption and on the metabolic activity of tissue close to the spinal fluid (the brain as a "glucose sink"). Increases and decreases in the cerebrospinal fluid glucose will reflect hyperglycemia and hypoglycemia respectively, although the lag period for plasma equilibration consists of about 90 minutes. Thus cerebrospinal fluid and serum samples must be taken simultaneously, ideally with the patient fasting. In order to suppress metabolism by concomitant cells in the specimen, the fluid should be collected in tubes containing fluoride.[404]

It is of practical interest that injury of the floor of the fourth ventricle can cause hyperglycemia and hence increased spinal fluid glucose concentration that is not responsive to insulin. There are other central lesions that are probably related to the floor of the fourth ventricle and also produce hyperglycemia.[90]

Acute bacterial infections and several viral infections produce marked reduction of cerebrospinal fluid glucose, as do certain other diffuse meningeal affections such as meningeal carcinomatosis, leukemic meningitis, and subarachnoid hemorrhage.[25,133,465]

Many carbohydrate intermediates may be measured in the cerebrospinal fluid.[246] The pyruvate to lactate ratio (normal 1 : 11) has been used as an indicator of normal metabolism of the central nervous system.[303] Lactate is known to increase in meningitis, reflecting the simultaneous decrease in cerebrospinal fluid glucose, and probably represents local anaerobic metabolism secondary to the effects of leukocytes and possibly bacterial endotoxin.[142,175a,243] Increased lactate has been thought to be pathognomonic of bacterial as opposed to viral meningitis, with levels above 35 mg per 100 ml indicative of bacterial infection.[231] The lactate level has also been used to evaluate response to treatment, with more rapid reductions tending to correlate with clinical improvement.[231,243] Lactic acid is also increased in perinatal posthemorrhagic encephalopathy, in uremia, and after a convulsion, and an increased level may be correlated with severity of head trauma.[444] Large increases in the levels of lactate in cerebrospinal fluid have been demonstrated in experimental subarachnoid hemorrhage, with halving of the abnormal level within 24 hours. Highly elevated lactate levels in the fluid have been suggested as presumptive evidence, in the presence of a normal lactate to pyruvate ratio (ca. 11:1), of a spontaneous subarachnoid hemorrhage.[376]

The level of citric acid is higher in the fluid than in plasma by a factor of about 2, and higher in the lumbar than in the ventricular fluid. It may accumulate to three times its normal value below a block of the spinal subarachnoid space.[175a,272]

Chlorides

The normal cerebrospinal fluid chloride concentration is 110 to 130 mEq per liter, which gives a ratio of 1.2 when divided by the blood plasma concentration (100 mEq per liter). This relative concentration is maintained under essentially all conditions, with increases directly reflecting changes in the plasma chloride concentration. A low chloride level is a bad prognostic sign in tuberculous meningitis because it reflects the severe concomitant systemic electrolyte imbalance. In practical terms, chloride levels in the fluid give the clinician little useful information.[91,99]

Acid-Base Balance

Acid-base characteristics of the cerebrospinal fluid have been studied in detail; specific central nervous system mechanisms of acid-base homeostasis, however, outside of well-understood renal and pulmonary mechanisms, remain poorly understood.* Lacking the protein and phosphate buffer systems of the blood, the cerebrospinal fluid acts essentially as a simple bicarbonate buffer system, following the well-known Henderson-Hasselbalch relationships. The fluid is slightly acidic compared with arterial blood, the cerebrospinal fluid pH being 7.31 compared with the 7.41 of arterial blood. Carbon dioxide tension in the fluid is higher (average 48 mm of mercury) than that of arterial blood (38). Bicarbonate concentrations are similar in both fluids (23 mEq per liter). pH may vary from the ventricles to the lumbar cerebrospinal fluid. With changes in systemic acid-base balance, the fluid remains most stable in subacute or chronic metabolic acidosis, and less stable in metabolic alkalosis and in respiratory acidosis or alkalosis. Clinical signs and symptoms of neurological dysfunction seem to be most closely related to spinal fluid pH rather than to alterations in the systemic arterial acid-base balance. Nu-

* See references 56, 232, 338, 339, 365, 379.

merous factors are involved in the homeostasis of the pH of the fluid. Of importance in this respect is the seemingly exquisite sensitivity of the medullary pH receptor and its effects on ventilation.[48] The entire spectrum from life-threatening hypoventilation to maximal hyperventilation (about 45 liters per minute) may be seen over a range of pH in fluid that may go as low as 0.05 unit.[379] Factors that may be involved in regulation of the fluid's pH include the normally positive electrical potential of the fluid (about 6 mv with respect to plasma), the secretion of bicarbonate by the choroid plexus, the contribution of acid metabolites by the brain tissue (e.g., in head trauma or meningitis), the effect of cerebral blood flow on the cerebral arteriovenous difference in carbon dioxide tension (and its effect on cerebrospinal fluid P_{CO_2}), and the possibility of an active hydrogen ion–bicarbonate ion pump between the fluid and the plasma.[32,171] In acute ventilatory changes, pH of the fluid reflects changes in plasma carbon dioxide tension reasonably well, but the slope of pH change is somewhat less than that seen in the arterial blood. Studies in neonates have shown essentially the same relationships.[232]

Lipids

Interest in lipids in the cerebrospinal fluid has increased as methods of determining minute amounts of lipids have become available.[149,307a,335a,423,442] The lipid concentration in serum is approximately 500 times as great as that in cerebrospinal fluid, and lipid concentrations in the fluid, unlike many other components, seem to be independent of the blood lipid concentrations.[349,423] Certain serum lipids, e.g., beta-lipoprotein, are absent from normal cerebrospinal fluid, and conversely, lipids such as cephalins are in much higher concentration in the fluid than in the serum.[423]

Analysis of the cerebrospinal fluid lipid profile has been done in diseases other than multiple sclerosis and primary dysmyelinating disease.* They include hyperlipemias, myxedema, retrobulbar neuritis, and others. In myxedema, the lipid levels are elevated in relation to the increase in total cerebrospinal fluid protein noted in this condition. Abnormal lipid profiles in retrobulbar neuritis and Tay-Sachs disease are probably due to alterations of in situ central nervous system lipids. Finally, any condition resulting in breakdown of the blood-brain barrier, particularly neoplasms and meningitis, results in increases of lipid in the form of beta- and other lipoprotein in the fluid.

Prostaglandins, 20-carbon cyclopentane carboxylic acids, might be discussed as neurotransmitters or hormones, but for simplicity and brevity, are included with other lipid moieties.[466] Prostaglandins have vasoactive, synaptic, and other effects. They may be measured directly in the fluid by radioimmunoassay. Of particular interest at this time is prostaglandin F_2 alpha. Prostaglandin F_2 alpha is considerably increased within five days after cerebral stroke and returns to normal levels within one month, the degree of decrease of its concentration in the fluid corresponding to regression of symptoms. It has been proposed as a prognostic and follow-up measurement in such patients.[125]

Neurotransmitters

The burgeoning field of neurochemistry has led to numerous investigations into levels of well-known neurotransmitters in brain tissue and in cerebrospinal fluid as well as attempts to relate levels of various constituents to disease states and degrees of disease activity. Even a somewhat lengthy summary would be difficult. It seems reasonable, however, to summarize by stating that measurement of various neurotransmitters in cerebrospinal fluid has met with difficulties relating to variability in their levels in brain and in the ventricular as compared with the cisternal fluid and lumbar fluid, as well as to difficulties in quantitation.†

There are several categories of neurotransmitters under current investigation: (1) the monoamines (the catecholamines, serotonin, histamine, and dopamine); (2) the amino acids (gamma-aminobutyric acid, glycine, glutamine, and aspartic acid); (3) the polypeptides (substance P—an un-

* See references 6, 155a, 307a, 335, 406, 409a, 418, 422, 430, 431a, 478.

† See references 34, 75, 87, 303, 328, 385, 451, 470, 473.

decapeptide—and the endorphins); (4) the cyclic nucleotides (cyclic AMP and cyclic GMP); and (5) the carboxylic acids (the prostaglandins—20-carbon cyclopentane carboxylic acids).* More detailed information and a historical perspective are to be found in several excellent reviews.[297,378,433]

Monoamine transmitters essentially comprise norepinephrine, serotonin, and histamine. Their respective catabolic products, which have been measured in cerebrospinal fluid, are 4-hydroxy,3-methoxyphenylethylene glycol. 5-hydroxy indoleacetic acid. and 5-hydroxytryptamine, respectively. Amino acid transmitters, polypeptide transmitters, cyclic nucleosides, and prostaglandins have been mentioned.

Homovanillic acid of the cerebrospinal fluid, the breakdown product of dopamine, has been found to be decreased in Parkinson's disease, Shy-Drager syndrome, Jakob-Creutzfeldt disease, parkinsonian dementia of Guam, epilepsy, Gilles de la Tourette syndrome, motor neuron disease, progressive supranuclear palsy, olivopontocerebellar degeneration, Huntington's disease, multiple sclerosis, dystonia musculorum deformans, senile and presenile dementia, and dominant striatonigral degeneration.[326] In addition, low levels have been seen in fasting states and after 12 hours of recumbency.

The alcohol metabolite of noradrenaline is 4-hydroxy,3-methoxyphenylethylene glycol (HMPG). The cerebrospinal fluid of patients with Korsakoff's psychosis has been found to have abnormally low levels of this constituent.[286] In addition, it as well as 5-hydroxyindoleacetic acid (5HIAA) is reduced in lumbar fluid after complete or partial spinal lesions in man.[11,51] Abnormal levels of 5-hydroxytryptamine (5HT) also may be found in patients with intracranial or spinal lesions, including trauma.[203,301]

Other Constituents

Physical characteristics of the cerebrospinal fluid include a total solid concentration of 1.0 gm per liter, resulting in a specific gravity of 1.008 (1.006 to 1.009). It is probable that normal fluid has a slightly greater total osmolarity than the blood plasma.[91,189,289]

Major cations in the fluid are sodium, potassium, calcium, and magnesium. The sodium concentration of the fluid is identical with that in plasma (133 to 145 mEq per liter). Alterations in the concentration of sodium reflect changes in plasma levels and not neurological disease.[17,363,364] The potassium content remains remarkably stable at 3.0 mEq per liter, less than the plasma concentrations of 4.5 mEq per liter, and its concentration is unaffected by changes in plasma potassium or by neurological disease.[36,91] The average spinal fluid calcium value is 2.5 mEq per liter (5 mg per 100 ml) or about half the blood plasma value, probably representing the free or diffusible serum fraction. The calcium concentration is well maintained even with marked changes in parathyroid activity, but does increase proportionately with increases in protein.[37,55,183,471] The spinal fluid magnesium concentration of 2.4 mEq per liter is 30 per cent higher than that in the normal blood serum. It does not rise with increases in serum magnesium. Decreases in magnesium are seen in meningitis, probably secondary to dysfunction of the blood-brain barrier, and are also noted in parallel to the decreased serum values in cirrhosis and other hypomagnesemias, but the 1.3:1 ratio is maintained. Hypomagnesorrhachia has also been noted in some patients with ischemic brain disease.[37,68,183,471]

Major cerebrospinal fluid anions comprise chloride, bicarbonate, and phosphate.[91,369] The inorganic phosphorus content of the fluid is 0.48 mg per liter compared with a serum value of 1.3. Its measurement remains of little clinical value.

The iron content of the cerebrospinal fluid varies between 23 and 50 μg per 100 ml; low values have been reported in tuberculous meningitis and high values have been seen in pernicious anemia, amyotrophic lateral sclerosis, and parkinsonism, and in conjunction with increased total protein.[225]

Plum found the copper content to be normal in multiple sclerosis, epilepsy, and various other neurological and psychiatric conditions.[336] Zinc concentration is extremely low in the fluid, the fluid to serum ratio is

---

* See references 1, 161, 200, 201, 238, 360, 434. 440, 445, 450.

low, and the concentration seems to be independent of changes in serum zinc.[471] Manganese, selenium, and cadmium have also been studied; the importance of manganese in its relationship to dopamine is emerging, but little can be said as yet about the clinical usefulness of measurement of these elements.[52]

Deoxyribonucleic acid (DNA) concentration in the fluid has been measured.[249,453] The value for control subjects is 0.42 ± 0.05 μg per 100 ml. Higher concentrations were found in patients with brain tumors, infectious diseases, and degenerative diseases.[453] There are no significant changes in concentration with aging.

Nonprotein nitrogen includes urea, creatinine, ammonia, uric acid, free amino acids, and neuraminic acid.[91] The cerebrospinal fluid concentrations are given in Table 13–1. Urea concentrations reflect and are identical to those in serum. Creatinine concentration is about two thirds of plasma value and reflects changes in plasma concentrations well. When the concentration of blood ammonia is about 50 μg per 100 ml, which is considered normal, the spinal fluid value will be approximately 6 μg per 100 ml. The spinal fluid reflects the elevated blood values to some extent in hepatic insufficiency.[199] Cerebrospinal fluid uric acid is 6 per cent of normal plasma value and is probably all diffusible; it has been noted to increase in meningitis.[59]

Essentially all free amino acids have been identified in the spinal fluid.[188,259,307,479] Overall total concentration is about one tenth that in plasma. Some (serine and phenylalanine) show relatively elevated levels, but few correlations with disease are possible except for hereditary ataxias, in which increased concentrations have been reported. Glutamine, the amide of glutamic acid, is found in high concentration—equal to the plasma concentration—in the spinal fluid. Furthermore, it is 10 to 30 times as concentrated as any other amino acids measured in the fluid.[91] Its level has been found to be elevated in chronic liver disease and markedly elevated in hepatic encephalopathy. Values in patients with chronic liver disease without encephalopathy of 21.0 ± 6.2 mg, in patients with encephalopathy of 40.3 ± 14 mg, and in normal subjects of 12.6 ± 5.1 mg per 100 ml (mean and one standard deviation) have been noted.[199]

Vitamin C accumulates in the cerebrospinal fluid. The normal serum concentration is 1.6 mg per 100 ml, and the corresponding cerebrospinal fluid value is 3.7 mg per 100 ml. The dietary content of vitamin C can influence both the serum and spinal fluid values. The levels of most other vitamins have been determined in the spinal fluid.[386] Cerebrospinal fluid folate concentration is normally three times that of serum, with low levels being associated with dementia and mental retardation.[211]

Many hormones have been measured in cerebrospinal fluid, usually by radioimmunoassay. The levels of melatonin, ACTH, somatostatin, thyrotonin, prolactin, luteinizing hormone, follicle stimulating hormone, and gonadotropin have been measured, among others.[187,212,332] Melatonin is secreted by the pineal gland in response to retinal stimuli. It has a diurnal secretion pattern and goes directly into the fluid rather than into the blood. The hypothalamus probably is the end-organ. Pituitary hormones in the fluid have been found to be decreased in patients with neurological diseases and those with pituitary tumor without suprasellar expansion. If there is suprasellar expansion of the tumors, the level of at least one of these hormones usually is elevated.[212] Cerebrospinal fluid somatostatin levels have been shown to be increased in patients with neurological disease, and it has been suggested that they indicate damage of brain or spinal tissue.[332]

Cerebrospinal Fluid in Infancy and Prematurity

In newborn premature infants the fluid is usually xanthochromic, the cell count is about 10 leukocytes per cubic millimeter, the protein concentration 100 mg per 100 ml, and the sugar content equal to that of plasma.

In normal infancy, the fluid usually is clear. The cell count is 10 and falls to the adult level by the second month. The protein concentration is 80 mg per 100 ml (predominantly albumin), and falls to 20 mg per 100 ml by six months, remaining there for two years, after which it begins to rise to approach the adult level later in childhood.[91,102,258,283]

Postmortem Findings

Fluid taken minutes after death reveals marked abnormalities in most constituents. Examination of postmortem cerebrospinal fluid generally is of benefit only for microbiological studies.[91,369,370] The pressure is zero, and the fluid must be aspirated. The cell count rises modestly, and the total protein rises to very high levels shortly after death; however, this is not always the case.[412] It has been reported that a spinal fluid glucose value greater than 200 mg per 100 ml suggests diabetes, excluding the parenteral administration of glucose ante mortem. The added findings of acetone and of carbon dioxide less than 10 volumes per cent in the fluid support the diagnosis of diabetic acidosis. On the other hand, cerebrospinal fluid glucose levels lower than 100 mg per 100 ml permit the exclusion of severe hyperglycemia. Urea content of more than 200 mg per 100 ml, and especially with confirmatory urinary findings, indicates renal failure. Urea concentration less than 100 mg per 100 ml with a creatinine level less than 2.5 mg per 100 ml tends to rule out renal failure. The bromide concentration rapidly approaches the serum value.

PUNCTURE OF THE CEREBROSPINAL SPACE

Contraindications

Lumbar puncture is contraindicated in acute trauma to the spinal column, especially in the lumbar area, in the presence of certain infectious processes, in increased intracranial pressure due to space-occupying lesions, and when the patient has a coagulation defect.[99,334] It should not be done if there are infections in skin or subcutaneous tissues, such as erysipelas, carbuncles, or decubitus ulcers, in the region of the puncture site. It may be dangerous in tuberculous osteitis of the vertebra and in cases in which there is infection near the cranial cavity as in osteomyelitis of the skull, lateral or cavernous sinus thrombosis, suppuration of the mastoid air cells or paranasal sinuses, or basilar skull fractures that have created an extracranial passage manifested by otorrhea or rhinorrhea. It has been suggested that a change in the pressure relationships of the spinal fluid may cause transmission or spread of the infection to the meninges and subarachnoid space. Similarly, in cases of brain abscess, changes in pressure may cause rupture of the abscess and dissemination of the infection. Increased intracranial pressure from brain tumors or other space-occupying lesions, e.g., (subdural or epidural hematoma), particularly when papilledema or signs of uncal herniation (third nerve palsy with altered state of consciousness) are present, should be a contraindication to lumbar puncture. Furthermore, lumbar puncture in the presence of tumors of the posterior fossa is more dangerous than with supratentorial tumors. The tonsils of the cerebellum may herniate into the foramen magnum, compressing the medulla oblongata. Lumbar punctures in patients with basilar impression or the Arnold-Chiari malformation may be relatively contraindicated because of the same potential tonsillar herniation. Cardiorespiratory arrest may occur when the pressure is released below. With supratentorial tumors, however, equally fatal herniation of the hippocampus through the incisura of the tentorium cerebelli may occur.

If the history and examination suggest that increased intracranial pressure is due to meningitis or subarachnoid hemorrhage, lumbar puncture is not contraindicated.[404]

Indications

Examination of the cerebrospinal fluid is necessary to establish the diagnosis of infectious meningitis.[400,404,464] It should be common practice to do the examination in order to rule out or confirm the possibility of meningitis in a patient with a fever of undetermined cause, even when meningeal signs are minimal. Naturally, any febrile patient with meningeal signs must have the examination.[404]

The initial examination of the fluid should be completed in less than one hour.[404] Since the reaction of the subarachnoid space to a specific class of microorganisms is reasonably consistent, the initial data usually fit a pattern. On the basis of several accepted profiles indicating infections, it is possible to choose for immediate administration an appropriate antimicrobial agent or agents that are most likely to be specific.

To justify this speedy approach to the administration of specific antimicrobial agents, which carries a modest risk of error, it should be remembered that in recent years the prompt administration of appropriate therapeutic agents has reduced the mortality rate and complications of meningoencephalitis more than any other factors such as development of new antimicrobial agents (with the distinct exception of adenine arabinoside in the treatment of herpetic meningoencephalitis), route of administration of the agent, or development of new general supportive measures.[132,258,456a]

If serological tests of the serum for syphilis are positive, it is mandatory to examine the cerebrospinal fluid to confirm or rule out a luetic syndrome of the nervous system.[243a]

Examination of the fluid is also useful to establish the diagnosis of spontaneous subarachnoid hemorrhage, especially if the CT scan is unrevealing.[425] If computed tomography positively shows intracerebral, intraventricular, or subarachnoid blood, the examination of the fluid may be bypassed in favor of an angiographic procedure. If the CT scan shows no intracranial bleeding, but the fluid findings are consistent with a spontaneous subarachnoid hemorrhage, an angiogram should be done. In 25 per cent of the patients reported in the Cooperative Study of Intracranial Aneurysms and Subarachnoid Hemorrhage angiographic studies appeared normal in the presence of subarachnoid hemorrhage proved by examination of the fluid.[362]

Lumbar puncture may be indicated to measure cerebrospinal fluid pressure in certain patients, regardless of whether further analysis of the fluid is desired. Lumbar puncture gives valuable information for evaluating patients who have not developed papilledema or in whom its presence is questionable (for example, in many cases of pseudotumor cerebri, papilledema does not develop). Also, low-pressure syndromes may be definitely diagnosed.[99]

The Queckenstedt test, which can detect partial or complete block of the subarachnoid space, is of some clinical value.[159,237]

Further indications for lumbar puncture of the subarachnoid space may arise in patients in whom abnormal cerebrospinal fluid dynamics are suspected.[468] An abnormality in the Katzman infusion test to evaluate the sufficiency of the arachnoid villi, for example, will lend support to a diagnosis of normal-pressure hydrocephalus.[31,219] Additionally, the rate of formation of the fluid may be gauged approximately by the Masserman withdrawal test.[91,280,281] Compliance of the nervous system may be measured by use of lumbar puncture, but has no important clinical correlate.[278] On the other hand, assessment of a patient's linear pressure decay curve may be of value clinically in establishing the condition of the cerebrospinal fluid space.[160]

The cytological examination of the fluid is useful to screen for neoplasia of the nervous system or leukemic meningitis.[371]

Indications for lumbar puncture also include instillation of foreign substances for diagnostic or therapeutic purposes. Iophendylate (Pantopaque) or metrizamide (Amipaque) is injected to evaluate spinal and cerebral contours as well as contours of the subarachnoid and intraventricular spaces. When performing these diagnostic instillations, the surgeon should routinely obtain pressure readings and collect samples of fluid prior to introducing the contrast medium.

Therapeutic applications of the lumbar puncture include the intrathecal instillation of antimicrobial, anti-inflammatory, and antineoplastic agents, as well as spinal anesthetic agents.[165,166] It is the authors' practice to inject these solutions through a Millipore filter (0.15μ). Therapeutic removal of fluid by lumbar puncture has been recommended for the treatment of pseudotumor cerebri, some forms of infantile hydrocephalus, intractable headache secondary to subarachnoid hemorrhage, and paraplegia following aortography.[164,304] Other indications for puncture of the cerebrospinal space are discussed elsewhere in this chapter.

Technique of Percutaneous Lumbar Puncture

When the lumbar puncture is used for diagnosis, the following minimum routine should be observed: measure the pressure and perform a Queckenstedt test if indicated. Collect the first few drops of fluid in a tube and inspect it for blood. If it is bloody, the routine described in the section on hemorrhagic cerebrospinal fluid should be followed. If the fluid is clear, approximately 3 ml should be collected in each of three tubes and in a fourth one if bacteriological analysis is indicated. The closing pressure should be obtained if there is interest in checking for a normal pressure decay curve.[160] The appearance of the fluid is recorded, and total cell, leukocyte, and differential counts are done on tubes 1 and 3. A smear should be made of the spinal fluid sediment obtained after centrifugation of tube 2. The supernatant fluid from the second tube should be used for quantitative determination of total protein, albumin, IgG, glucose, and a nontreponemal antigen test for syphilis (VDRL). Tube 4 is handled with sterile precautions and, without centrifugation, is sent to the microbiology laboratory.

Since the interpretation placed on the results of cerebrospinal fluid examination can be only as good as the methods used, comments on technique are appropriate. The pressure may be obtained through a 22-gauge needle with an Ayer's water manometer, but the best results are obtained with a pressure transducer.[159,160,275,287] The needle is in proper position if straining, coughing, and pressure on the abdomen will alter the pressure appreciably; in addition, the heart beat and wider respiratory excursions should be visible. If the pressure is elevated, it should be observed for three to five minutes before the fluid in the manometer is taken for analysis (microtechniques are available for cell counts and total protein determination) and the procedure is discontinued. Care should be taken to position the patient properly so that complete relaxation is assured, the jugular vein is not compressed by the underlying arm, and the head is at the same level as the needle. Furthermore, if increased intracranial pressure is anticipated, a small needle (25 or 26 gauge) should be used and every precaution taken to avoid fluid loss.

The authors have had extensive experience with small-bore needles of 25 or 26 gauge. These needles can be placed without a guide. With them the post–lumbar puncture syndrome is greatly reduced and, if it does occur, is mild.[176,424,432] Iophendylate (Pantopaque) can be injected through these needles only if it is warmed to body temperature, and it cannot be removed through them. Furthermore, the pressure has to be obtained by filling the manometer with spinal fluid via syringe, utilizing the third post on the stopcock. The manometer is filled to the 200 mark, and in about five minutes it either falls to the normal pressure or comes to a higher steady state. Utilizing a pressure transducer obviates filling the manometer. Also, when a small-bore needle is used, the fluid must be removed with a syringe. The authors recommend the removal of 1 ml per minute.

When a spinal subarachnoid space block exists, removal of a few milliliters of fluid will produce a marked decrease in the pressure; normally (i.e., in the absence of block) the pressure should fall, on the average, 30 per cent of the opening pressure if fluid is removed at the rate of 1 ml per minute for a total volume of 20 ml. The fluid may be yellowish and may clot (Froin syndrome). A Queckenstedt test should be done to confirm a spinal subarachnoid block and should be followed by instillation of iophendylate (Pantopaque) or metrizamide (Amipaque) for an immediate myelogram. A repeat puncture to inject contrast medium for myelography may be impossible because the subarachnoid space is difficult to impale. On the other hand, contrast media can be instilled via cisternal or lateral cervical puncture.[480]

If the fluid clots spontaneously during the procedure, it should be collected in a tube containing anticoagulant (dry sodium citrate or ethylenediaminetetraacetic acid [EDTA]). The additive will prevent clot formation and permit cytological studies such as total cell and differential counts.

The Queckenstedt Test

The Queckenstedt test may be used to demonstrate a block of the spinal subarachnoid space above the puncture site and thrombosis of the lateral sinus.[159,237] The test is indicated in patients with signs and symptoms of a spinal cord lesion, but is contraindicated in those with intracranial disease other than suspected lateral sinus thrombosis.

A 22-gauge needle may be used, but a 20- or 18-gauge spinal needle yields more precise data. Before the test, pressure on the abdomen and straining should cause a rise of lumbar pressure of 50 to 200 mm of water, even in the presence of a spinal subarachnoid block, and this is a good indication that the lumbar needle is properly placed.

The Queckenstedt test is performed by

observing the effect of compression of the jugular veins on the resting lumbar cerebrospinal fluid pressure. With the patient in the lateral recumbent position, jugular venous compression causes decreased venous return from the brain, producing a temporary increase in the volume of the cranial contents. The increased intracranial pressure so caused is transmitted to the spinal fluid throughout the system and is measured with the lumbar manometer. An assistant should compress and release the jugular veins quickly when requested, taking care not to cause pain by undue pressure. The pressure should be applied quickly and firmly but not so firmly as to obstruct the internal carotid arteries.

Normally, 10 seconds of bilateral jugular compression will cause the pressure in the lumbar manometer to rise at least 150 mm of water higher than the opening pressure. Upon release of jugular compression, the pressure returns almost to baseline within 10 to 20 seconds.

If cervical cord disease such as cervical spondylosis is suspected, it is recommended that the jugular compression be repeated with the neck in the neutral position, in hyperextension, and in flexion.

If the fluid pressure does not rise and fall promptly, the test is abnormal. In the case of spinal cord disease, it is recommended that a myelogram be done immediately. If lateral venous thrombosis is suspected, a carotid angiogram with late filming is necessary to prove the diagnosis.

Linear Pressure Regression

The linear pressure regression is obtained by first obtaining a steady-state opening pressure for five minutes. It may be measured by connecting a standard pressure manometer or a pressure transducer to a 26-gauge needle. Then fluid is withdrawn at a controlled rate of 1 ml per minute via syringe aspiration. After 20 ml has been removed, the pressure is recorded again. When this controlled technique is used, the average closing pressure should be 30 per cent lower than the opening pressure. Analysis of the pressure by this standardized method should give a more accurate indication of the opening and closing pressures than their mere randomized measurement.[160]

Masserman Cerebrospinal Fluid Formation Test

The rate of formation of the cerebrospinal fluid may be estimated by use of a modified Masserman test.[91,280,281] Fluid is removed by lumbar puncture at a rate of 1 ml per minute until the pressure falls to 60 mm of water, a pressure at which absorption of the cerebrospinal fluid by the arachnoid villi presumably stops.[82] The amount of spinal fluid removed to reach 60 mm of water is recorded. The pressure is then monitored without further removal of fluid until it returns to the pretest value (opening pressure). The amount of fluid removed divided by the time required for the restoration of the opening pressure is the formation rate of the fluid. The normal value is 0.35 ml per minute. No obvious clinical correlates of abnormal test results have been forthcoming.

Katzman Cerebrospinal Fluid Absorption Test (Infusion Manometrics)

That the infusion tests might be diagnostic of "normal-pressure hydrocephalus," as first described by Adams and co-workers, is controversial.[3,219,310] Infusion of fluid into the subarachnoid space by lumbar puncture remains a useful tool for evaluating defects of absorption of fluid in patients who do not have an obstructive form of hydrocephalus. Strict indications for performing infusion manometrics remain unsettled, although it is frequently used along with isotope cisternography, computed tomography of the brain, and pneumoencephalography in the evaluation of the presenile dementias.

In the original technique of Katzman and Hussy, normal saline or artificial cerebrospinal fluid was infused into the spinal subarachnoid space; and the change in hydrostatic pressure, the volume, and the rate of infusion were measured.[202,219] Assuming under normal circumstances that reabsorption of cerebrospinal fluid must at least equal formation (about 0.35 ml per minute), infusions were begun at this rate. It was then demonstrated that normal reabsorptive capacity is equal to at least twice the rate of normal formation of fluid, i.e., 0.76 ml per minute. With infusion at this rate, a steady-state pressure of 295 mm of water is reached within 30 minutes. Abnormal absorptive capacity is indicated by a rise in pressure to 300 to 600 mm of water, usually within 20 minutes. It was also shown that most normal patients have absorptive capacities of 3 to 4 times the normal formation rate, and that half of normal patients can absorb at a rate up to 8 to 10 times the normal formation rate. Essentially all patients with later pathologically proved Alzheimer's disease have normal reabsorption of fluid.[310]

Rather than using variable infusion rates, Ekstedt has performed infusion manometrics by infusing fluid under constant pressure and recording differences in flow rates.[127,388] This method reveals similar information and, in addition, that a "critical opening pressure" for cerebrospinal fluid reabsorption, a pressure of 10 to 50 mm of water, must be reached before reabsorption occurs.

In any infusion manometric study, the use of artificial cerebrospinal fluid (Elliot's B solution) in place of normal saline appears to minimize the poststudy syndrome consisting of pain, paresthesia or paralgesia of the legs and buttocks, vomiting and defecation, piloerection and sweating.[127] Occasionally, mental excitation may also occur during the examination. With artificial cerebrospinal fluid used in place of normal saline these complications may be eliminated, but occasional mild irritative meningitis of short duration may occur.

Complications of Lumbar Puncture

The post–lumbar puncture syndrome may occur several hours after the lumbar puncture. One of three individuals experiences mild, moderate, or severe frontal and occipital postural headache and occasionally nuchal pain. These symptoms are relieved by recumbency. In severe cases, nausea, vomiting, diaphoresis, and malaise may accompany the headache in the erect posture. These symptoms also are relieved by recumbency. The syndrome usually lasts four days, but may persist for two weeks or more. The symptoms are not related to removal of the usual amounts of fluid taken at the time of lumbar puncture, and adequate fluid collection should not be forgone in an attempt to avoid the occurrence of post–lumbar puncture headache. The syndrome is the result of a dural rent caused by the insertion of the spinal needle. The headache is caused by traction on and dilatation of intracranial vessels. It has been shown that use of a 26-gauge spinal needle, rather than a 22-gauge needle, will decrease the incidence of the syndrome to 10 per cent and result in its having a milder and shorter course.[424,432]

Chronic post–lumbar puncture syndrome (lumborrhea) secondary to chronic cerebrospinal fluid leakage has been treated with the injection of about 10 ml of autologous blood into the spinal epidural space, accelerating the sealing of the cerebrospinal leak.[110,247,251]

More serious complications are much less common than the headaches.[99,269,293] They include injury to the nerve roots and the intervertebral cartilage. The latter may result in a herniation of the disc. Injury of blood vessels may result in significant hemorrhage, particularly in patients who are receiving anticoagulants, are thrombocytopenic, or have liver disease. Septic meningitis may occur owing to faulty sterile technique. "Settling" of the spinal cord tumor can follow decompression of the sacculated fluid below. Rupture of a brain abscess or spread of infection from extradural foci such as Pott's disease or epidural abscesses or from the middle ear or nasal mucosa in patients suffering from basilar skull fracture complicated by otorrhea or rhinorrhea may result. Abortion may be induced in the first trimester of pregnancy.[99] More recently a late complication of lumbar puncture has been recognized, particularly in children. Intraspinal epidermoid tumors may result from displacement of skin elements into the spinal canal and present with progressive back and leg pain, lordosis, and difficulty in walking years after the lumbar puncture.[19] The process is thought to result from the use of spinal needles with ill-fitting stylets or without stylets.

Post–lumbar puncture cerebellar tonsillar or hippocampal gyral herniations have been attributed to lumbar puncture, particularly in patients with posterior fossa or other brain tumors. It has been suggested that the true incidence of this complication may approximate 1 to 2 per cent; others, however, report high incidences with mortality rates approaching 40 per cent.[99,269,293]

The introduction of foreign substances (anesthetics, air, contrast media, and the like) into the subarachnoid space is accompanied by mild or moderate meningeal reactions. The fluid removed within the first day may show a pleocytosis (usually less than 1000 cells), increased total protein, normal sugar, and sterile cultures. These reactions are quickly reversible and rarely result in significant arachnoiditis, radiculitis, or myelitis.[381] When they occur, they are found to be caused by contamination of the instruments with either sterilizing agents or detergents used for cleaning the equipment. It is claimed that the incidence of such complications is lower with metrizamide than with iophendylate.[182]

In addition to local effects, vasovagal reactions leading to respiratory or cardiac arrest resulting secondarily in anoxic damage to the brain have been reported.[99,269,293]

Alternative Procedures to Lumbar Puncture

Lumbar puncture may be difficult because of patient obesity, spinal arachnoiditis, or spinal column bony deformities; in this case cisternal puncture or lateral cervical puncture may be used.[480] Additional indications for these procedures include failure of lumbar puncture due to spinal subarachnoid block, injection of contrast medium for myelography to outline the rostral level of spinal subarachnoid block, and administration of amphotericin-B when arachnoiditis prevents lumbar injections. The same contraindications hold for lateral cervical and cisternal puncture as for lumbar puncture.

Because of the proximity to the medulla oblongata and major blood vessels, cisternal puncture carries more danger than lumbar puncture. Accordingly, a trained surgical neurologist should perform this procedure. Lateral cervical puncture is potentially capable of injuring the spinal cord and is best done under x-ray control by a neuroradiologist or a neurological surgeon.[480] As with lumbar puncture, a traumatic tap and nerve root injury may occur. Although a syndrome resembling post–lumbar puncture headache may develop, it is less common with lateral cervical and cisternal punctures than with the lumbar puncture.[99,269,293,294,480]

Indications for percutaneous ventricular puncture in infants include relief of increased intracranial pressure prior to intracranial operations, relief of pressure from inoperable tumors, and ventriculography. Dye may be injected to differentiate obstructive from nonobstructive hydrocephalus; failure of the dye to appear in the lumbar area after several minutes supports the diagnosis of obstructive hydrocephalus. The procedure should be performed by trained neuroradiologists or surgical neurologists.[99,269,293,294]

STANDARDIZED LABORATORY TESTS

Anticoagulation of Cerebrospinal Fluid

The procedure used to prevent coagulation of cerebrospinal fluid is as follows: Remove the top from a vacuum tube (Vacutainer) that contains dried EDTA-K_3 (0.05 ml of a 30 per cent solution) and dissolve the crystals in 1 ml of sterile 0.15 M sodium chloride solution. Let 1 ml (16 drops) of fluid drip directly from the needle into the tube and shake the Vacutainer as each drop of fluid falls in.

Even though the anticoagulant is hypertonic compared with the fluid, it appears to have no cytomorphological effect on the leukocytes. On the other hand, the use of heparin has resulted in many artifacts in leukocytes. It has also been found that adding cerebrospinal fluid directly to the dried crystals does not prevent coagulation.[404]

Cell Counts

Cell counts should be done with clean and dry equipment. To obtain valid results, the original specimens should be thoroughly mixed immediately before testing.[404] Mixing of the sample can be efficiently accomplished with a vortex-type mixer. The total cell count can be done on undiluted fluid unless it is too high, in which case Hayem's solution should be used to make the appropriate dilutions.

In making the leukocyte count, a dye containing acetic acid should be used (crystal violet, 0.2 gm; glacial acetic acid, 40 ml; phenol 5 per cent, 3 drops; to which is added 10 ml of water and the solution is then filtered). It is convenient to make a constriction pipet so that the acid dye can be brought to the first constriction and the spinal fluid to the second constriction, resulting in a 0.9 dilution of the fluid.[403] Thorough mixing of the dye and lysis of the erythrocytes can be accomplished in three minutes by using a Burton Pipette Shaker.

For both the total cell and the leukocyte counts a Fuchs-Rosenthal counting chamber, which has a total volume of 3.2 cmm, is recommended. It is the largest commercially available chamber. After the chambers have been charged, three to five minutes are required for adequate settling of the cells.

Differential Cell Count

The differential cell count is done on at least 3 ml of fluid after aliquots have been taken for the total cell and leukocyte counts. The fluid is concentrated by centrifugation at 4° C at 900 rcf for 15 minutes.[404] The supernatant fluid is decanted and saved for other tests. The tubes are recentrifuged for a few minutes, and the remaining supernatant fluid is removed with a micropipet. To the sediment is added 5 μl (or more if a large amount of sediment is present) of 20 per cent albumin in 0.15 M sodium chloride. The albumin solution prevents drying artifacts and can be stored frozen. The diluted sediment is mixed thoroughly with a vortex-type mixer, and approximately 1 μl of suspension is transferred to a glass cover slip. The drop is smeared by placing another cover slip on it and then quickly pulling the slips apart. The smear dries immediately. A number of smears, which keep well for days at room temperature under a dust cover and for years in a sealed bag at −90° C, should be made, since many stains can be used on these dried smears. Two hundred and fifty consecutive cells should be noted for the differentiated cell count.

Since polymorphonuclear cells may disintegrate and clump, it is important for the cell counts to be done immediately. Also, if the total protein content is moderately high (more than 100 mg per 100 ml), a stringy, delicate fibrin clot may develop and withdraw some or all of the cells from the fluid. On the other hand, accurate, reliable cell counts and differentials can be made for up to 48 hours if the fluid is kept at 4° C and no clot develops. Recovery of cells by this method has been studied in the authors' laboratory. Fifteen samples were studied before centrifugation, with total cell counts ranging from 2 to 717 cells per cubic millimeter and leukocyte counts from 1 to 692. The recoveries after centrifugation and resuspension of the sediment in albumin for the total cell count and leukocyte counts were 90 per cent ± 6.7 and 93 per cent ± 6.9, respectively.[403,404]

Staining of Cells in Cerebrospinal Fluid

Wright's stain of the dry smears permits identification of the various types of leukocytes as well as erythrocytes, bacteria, cryptococci, inclusion bodies within the leucocytes due to cytomegalic inclusion body disease, and neoplastic cells.[403,404] Gram stain, methylene blue, and Ziehl-Neelsen stains also work well.

With the Wright's stain, the cytoplasm of the cryptococci stains a distinct reddish purple in contrast to bluish staining of the nuclei of leukocytes. Occasionally the mucinous capsule stains reddish purple. Dry smears for the quellung reaction with specific antiserum, which contains methylene blue, have identified *Hemophilus influenzae*, pneumococci, meningococci, and *Diplococcus pneumoniae*. A positive test is manifested by a swollen capsule that is stained with methylene blue. This procedure requires only 30 minutes and can be helpful and timesaving in identifying the microbe that is causing the meningitis.[404]

Also helpful and timesaving is the application of fluorescent antibody reagents to dry smears to identify the more common bacterial and viral pathogens associated with meningoencephalitis.[30,131,302,404] It would appear that the indirect fluorescent antibody technique is preferable.

Cultures of Cerebrospinal Fluid

Immediate cultures are obtained by permitting two drops of fluid to fall directly from the needle into tubes containing each of the following: sheep blood broth, chocolate agar slant, tryptose broth, thioglycollate broth, and Sabouraud's agar. These tubes should be taken immediately to the microbiological laboratory for culturing. If a technician is not available, it is essential that the specimens be incubated by placing the tubes with sheep broth and Sabouraud's agar in the 37° C incubator, the chocolate slant in the candle can, and the tryptose broth in the refrigerator.

A large volume of fluid, up to 20 ml if possible, collected under the most sterile conditions should be stored at 4° C if the microbiologist is not available. It will be centrifuged to concentrate the sediment, which will then be studied more extensively and with more elaborate methods to attempt to identify the infectious organism and to determine the sensitivity of the identified organism to various antimicrobial agents.

Glucose Determination

The quantitative analysis for cerebrospinal fluid glucose is the same as it is for blood glucose. The same precautions should be taken in its collection. Pipette 0.5 ml of cerebrospinal fluid into a Vacutainer for blood glucose determination that contains sodium fluoride. Mix well and refrigerate at 4° C to inhibit further glycolysis. A simultaneous blood glucose test is indispensable for a meaningful interpretation of the glucose level of the fluid. The test is best done with the patient in the fasting state.

Qualitative Fibrinogen Determination

Tube 1 should be used for a qualitative fibrinogen test. It should be kept at 4° C. If fibrinogen is present, a fiberlike clot will be present after about 12 hours. After centrifugation, the supernatant fluid can be used for other noncellular tests such as electrophoresis and albumin and IgG determinations.

Electroimmunodiffusion Technique to Determine Albumin and IgG

For this procedure, a commercial kit* is available that is based on the authors' electroimmunodiffusion procedure.[429] Simultaneous determination of IgG and albumin in 5 μl of neat cerebrospinal fluid and serum diluted 1:200 is possible. With these data, the daily de novo central nervous system IgG synthesis can be calculated according to the empirical formula described earlier.[409,417]

* Antibodies, Inc., Davis, Calif.

Identification of Cerebrospinal Fluid IgG Oligoclones by Immunofixation

Panagel (Worthington Corp.) is utilized as the supporting medium, and 3 μl of fluid containing 1.0 μg of IgG is applied. Electrophoresis, followed by immunofixation by layering a monospecific IgG antiserum over the separated proteins, is followed by staining with Coomassie blue.[62,271] Preliminary concentration of the fluid is not required when the IgG concentration exceeds 10 mg per 100 ml. When the IgG concentration is less than this value, concentration by a pressure micro–collodion bag filtration system is necessary (average recovery of IgG is greater than 90 per cent).† In lieu of concentration of fluid, multiple applications of as many as five 3-μl samples of unconcentrated cerebrospinal fluid, totaling 1 μg of IgG, have been found to be equivalent to preliminary concentration. This procedure is 20 times as sensitive as conventional agarose electrophoresis. The addition of IgG immunofixation validates cathodic proteins as IgG.

REACTIONS OF THE CEREBROSPINAL FLUID IN DISEASE

The cerebrospinal fluid examination provides important information when high pressure readings, an abnormal Queckenstedt test, xanthochromic fluid, spontaneous clotting of fluid, high total cell counts and abnormal differential cell count, microorganisms, positive serological tests, increased total protein or albumin values, and increased de novo central nervous system IgG synthesis are discovered.

It is not always possible, however, to determine when a constituent of the fluid is abnormal. Mathematically ± 2 standard de-

† Sartorius-Membranfilter GMBH, Gottingen, Germany.

viations on each side of the mean should include 95 per cent of all normal observations if the distribution curve is normal. If the normal data are skewed either toward low values or high values, the 2.5 to 97.5 percentile range is an adequate mathematical way to describe a range that includes 95 per cent of all normal observations. The consequence of using the 95 per cent normal range is that any value that falls above or below this limit has one chance in 20 of being normal ($p \leq 0.05$). These are good odds in favor of the normal and if anything probably too lenient; i.e., disease may occur before it reaches these extremes.

There are situations in which it is easy to tell that the fluid is abnormal, and there may even be changes in it that can be considered pathognomonic of certain diseases, for example, extreme values or phenomena such as xanthochromia and clots or the appearance of new substances such as red blood cells, microorganisms, or malignant cells.

One may find obvious neurological disease in a patient whose cerebrospinal fluid proves to be normal. There must be many explanations for this phenomenon, but it would appear that the most important reason is that the disease is too far away from the cerebrospinal fluid space. On the other hand, there may be a reaction in the fluid but the abnormality may not have reached or could not reach the lumbar puncture needle because of a block, or the mildly reactive fluid may have been too much diluted by normal fluid.

The investigation of the cerebrospinal fluid has led to many related discoveries, such as the role in the central nervous system of neurotransmitters, cyclic nucleotides, hormones, enzymes, and other constituents referred to earlier. Much of this information cannot yet be applied to the clinical investigation of an individual patient. The following section therefore presents the disease entities and cerebrospinal fluid profile for which useful clinical correlates have been identified.

Infections

Acute Bacterial (Purulent) Meningoencephalitis

With meningoencephalitis or meningitis the fluid is usually under increased pressure (about 200 to 1000 mm of water) and pleocytosis is noted (generally 500 to 10,000 leukocytes and rarely as many as 50,000), predominantly polymorphonuclear cells in the early phases.[50,60,163,185,404] In certain cases a higher leukocyte count has been recorded in the fluid than in the peripheral blood. Also high erythrocyte counts may suggest that dural thrombophlebitis exists. The protein content is increased (from 50 to 1000 mg per 100 ml), and the fluid may clot; the glucose level is low (usually less than 50 mg and sometimes less than 10 mg per 100 ml) and must be expressed in relation to that of a simultaneously drawn blood sample. Cerebrospinal fluid and blood are best obtained with the patient in the fasting state, and to inhibit carbohydrate metabolism the collection should be made in a tube containing fluoride.

Identification of the infecting organism on stained smears of the sediment or clot has been the classic method of bacteriological diagnosis.[404] It has been recognized, however, that prior antibiotic treatment may make such determinations impossible, and diagnostic techniques to identify bacterial products in the fluid rather than viable organisms have aroused increased interest.[135] Both bacterial endotoxin and specific polysaccharide antigens have been identified in the fluid.[284] The *Limulus* lysate assay is a rapid and sensitive test for the presence of gram-negative endotoxin in the cerebrospinal fluid, plasma, and urine, although it cannot distinguish between different gram-negative organisms.[8,358] Its success rate approaches 100 per cent in *Hemophilus* and meningococcal infections. The latex agglutination test, employing latex particles coated with specific antibodies, has also been applied, with a 70 to 90 per cent rate of success, and may be performed in less than three minutes to identify the presence of specific cell wall polysaccharide antigens. Low antigen concentration in cerebrospinal fluid has also been found to be of good prognostic value in meningococcal, pneumococcal, *Hemophilus,* and *Escherichia coli* meningitis. Antigen is usually absent from the fluid within 24 to 48 hours after treatment is begun, and its further presence is ominous.[329]

Organisms involved in the acute purulent meningitides include essentially the entire spectrum of known bacteria, but organisms tend to differ according to the patient's age and the clinical setting. In general, *Neisseria meningitidis, Hemophilus influenzae, Listeria monocytogenes, E. coli* and other Enterobacteriaceae, *Pseudomonas aeruginosa, Diplococcus pneumoniae, Staphylococcus* species, and *Streptococcus* species account for essentially all cases.[132,333,395] Acute syphilitic meningitis may rarely be seen, in which case a turbid fluid under increased pressure will be found, as will cell counts ranging from 100 to 500 (neutrophils or lymphocytes may predominate) and occasionally as high as 2000 white cells. Protein is increased and glucose is reduced. Gamma globulin is increased and the VDRL titer should be high (greater than 1:32).[99,269,292,294]

Increases in cerebrospinal fluid lactate seen in purulent meningitis remain unhelpful in differential diagnosis and of uncertain cause, although Fishman believes effects of both bacterial endotoxin and polymorphonuclear leukocytes on local central nervous system metabolism account for anaerobic glycolysis, with the increased lactate being a mirror of the hypoglycorrhachia.[143]

Chronic Infectious Meningoencephalitis

Central nervous system involvement with numerous disease processes may be manifested by the syndrome of chronic meningitis, with similar findings in the fluid.[128,174] The pressure may be, and the protein level is, elevated. The associated pleocytosis is predominantly lymphocytic, and hypoglycorrhachia may be present. Failure of clinical improvement or lack of amelioration in cerebrospinal fluid findings lasting longer than four weeks has been suggested as the basic characteristic of these entities.

Tuberculous Meningitis

The outstanding characteristics of the fluid are a predominantly lymphocytic pleocytosis (100 to 500 cells, up to 86 per cent lymphocytes), increased protein, and decreased glucose (less than 40 mg per 100 ml in two thirds of patients and less than 20 mg per 100 ml in one third; if untreated, 98 per cent of cases will develop a glucose value of less than 40 mg per 100 ml), and a low chloride value reflecting the low level of blood chlorides, an ominous sign. Early cases may present with polymorphonuclear predominance, but repeat taps will reveal the noted abnormalities, especially the hypoglycorrhachia. Diagnosis usually depends on demonstration of extraneural involvement. Cultures are positive in 38 to 88 per cent, and smears are positive in only 10 to 22 per cent of cases. Atypical mycobacteria have also been implicated.[223]

Cryptococcal Meningitis

In cryptococcal meningitis, caused by the yeastlike *Cryptococcus neoformans*, the cerebrospinal fluid findings resemble those of tuberculous meningitis. A large volume of fluid (around 20 ml) may be required to obtain enough sediment after centrifugation to yield a positive culture on Sabouraud's agar, but about half the time, encapsulated yeast can be seen in the India ink preparation. Identification of the yeasts is more frequently and convincingly done by utilizing the authors' method of Wright's staining of the centrifuged sediment in the presence of 20 per cent albumin. Additionally, if a patient is receiving amphotericin B, cultures may be negative at the same time that the organism can be recognized by the Wright's staining method.[404] Eighty-five per cent of patients have capsular anti gen demonstrable in the fluid, the antigen disappearing with cure of the infection.[128]

Coccidioidal Meningitis

Rarely, a smear of the fluid's sediment will reveal the spherules of *Coccidioides immitis;* the fungus may, however, be grown from it. This chronic infection will show a positive complement-fixation titer in 75 per cent of patients; a serum complement-fixation titer greater than 1:32 is diagnostic.[128]

Histoplasma Meningitis

Meningeal involvement occurs in about one fourth of cases of disseminated histoplasmosis. Cerebrospinal fluid fungal particles are sparse, however, and the diagnosis is difficult.[128]

Candida Meningitis

This infection is a late sequela of systemic candidemia. Pleocytosis, usually less than 500 leukocytes, elevated cerebrospinal fluid protein level, and hypoglycorrhachia are noted in about 50 per cent of patients. Since only half the cases will demonstrate a positive smear of the fluid sediment, it is diagnosed by culture.[128]

Blastomyces Meningitis

The cerebrospinal fluid usually demonstrates a lymphocytic pleocytosis and an elevated protein content. There may or may not be modest hypoglycorrhachia. Culture of the organism from the fluid is difficult.[128]

Paracoccidioides Meningitis

South American blastomycosis may present with findings in the fluid identical to those of tuberculous meningitis.[128]

Cerebral Dematiomycosis (Chromomycosis)

Although this infection may present with a profile of chronic meningitis, diagnosis has been made only from specimens obtained at operation.[128]

Actinomycotic Meningitis

Culture and smear of the cerebrospinal fluid has a low yield, and diagnosis is usually made from extraneural samples.[128]

Nocardia Meningitis

Occasionally *Nocardia* may be isolated from the cerebrospinal fluid.[128]

Neurobrucellosis

A lymphocytosis may occur in the fluid; neutrophils may predominate, however. Usually diagnosis depends on a history of exposure and serological identification, although 50 per cent of samples of fluid may grow the organism after three weeks of incubation.[128]

Toxoplasma Meningoencephalitis

This infection may present as a chronic meningitis, but more often it presents as a fulminant acute meningoencephalitis. Serological tests are suggestive, but brain biopsy remains diagnostic.[352]

Leptospiral Meningitis

Although in most cases the meningeal involvement in the syndrome of leptospirosis usually occurs as an aseptic meningitis, the course may be protracted (up to four months) with documented persistence of organisms in the fluid.[128]

Angiostrongylus Meningitis

Eosinophilic meningitis due to *Angiostrongylus cantonensis* occurs in the South Pacific and Southeast Asia. Although it usually is acute and self-limiting, protracted courses do occur. Eosinophilic meningitis is also seen with *Gnathostoma spinigerum* infection as well as with lymphoma. Eosinophilic pleocytosis has been seen in cysticercosis, paragonimiasis, schistosomiasis, and toxocariasis.[128]

Cysticercosis and Echinococcosis

Cerebrospinal fluid pleocytosis in cysticercosis may be lymphocytic, granulocytic, or eosinophilic; and glucose may be decreased.[242] Repeated leakage of an echinococcal cyst has been reported as a cause of recurrent aseptic meningitis.[128]

Multiceps multiceps Meningitis

Chronic lymphocytic meningitis may be seen with cerebral coenurosis (the larval form of the dog tapeworm *Multiceps multiceps*).[128]

Chronic Aseptic Meningoencephalitis

Noninfectious, nonparasitic causes of chronic lymphocytic response in the fluid are numerous.[128,174] In neoplastic involvement of the central nervous system, a cerebellar hemangioma has been associated with a lymphocytic, hypoglycorrhachic fluid without neoplastic cells.[128]

Superficial central nervous system hemosiderosis is a poorly understood entity that is associated with tumors. It involves pathological iron pigment deposition in glial and mesodermal cells in the meninges and ventricles and around cerebral blood vessels. Clinically it may resemble the chronic meningitides.[128]

Malignant hematological diseases may result in a profile of the fluid that resembles that of a chronic meningitis.[128] Diffuse lymphomatous or leukemic meningeal infiltration or diffuse histiocytic lymphoma is more frequently a cause of this finding than is undifferentiated lymphoma or Hodgkin's disease. Both Hodgkin's and non-Hodgkin's lymphoma may cause an eosinophilic meningitis. Meningeal leukemia has decreased with prophylactic treatment of the craniospinal axis with intrathecal methotrexate and irradiation of the central nervous system.

Meningeal carcinomatosis from metastatic spread may present a similar picture of chronic meningitis with findings in the fluid that include a minimal lymphocytic pleocytosis and hypoglycorrhachia. Numerous spinal taps may be necessary to obtain positive cytological confirmation. It is possible for the fluid to have a normal leukocyte count and still have malignant cells in it.[128]

In addition to the more classically recognized mass lesions, sarcoidosis may take the form of a chronic meningitis, in which case abnormalities of the fluid include a mild increase in protein, slight lymphocytic pleocytosis, and occasionally hypoglycorrhachia.[99,128]

Lymphocytic pleocytosis with increased protein may be seen as a prodrome of the Vogt-Koyanagi-Harada syndrome in 50 to 90 per cent of cases. The diagnosis is aided by the presence of severe granulomatous uveitis.[128]

In 20 per cent of patients with Behçet's disease the findings in the fluid include pleocytosis (lymphocytic or neutrophilic) and the clinical picture is consistent with chronic meningitis.[63,128]

Although dermoid or epidermoid cysts of childhood generally present as acute purulent meningitis, chronic leakage of irritative material may lead to a chronic progressive syndrome in adults.[99,128]

Granulomatous angiitis in the older age group has shown abnormalities of the fluid that include increased protein and a lymphocytic predominance, but the diagnosis is extremely difficult even with brain biopsy material available.[128]

Mollaret's meningitis (benign recurrent aseptic meningitis) demonstrates a mixed pleocytosis including large endothelial cells in the fluid during acute attacks.[128,174]

Chronic benign lymphocytic meningitis resembles the classically defined aseptic meningitis that is discussed later. It runs a course from nine months to three years.[128,174]

Some patients with pseudotumor cerebri will have a chronic low-grade lymphocytosis.[99,174]

A large group of entities may mimic chronic meningitis but have different diagnostic and therapeutic implications. These entities include aseptic meningitis, viral encephalitis, nonviral encephalitis-encephalopathy, partially treated bacterial meningitis, brain abscess, parameningeal focus of infection, subdural hematoma, subarachnoid hemorrhage, brain tumor, multiple sclerosis, malignant hypertension, thrombotic thrombocytopenic purpura, systemic lupus erythematosus, and temporal arteritis.[128,134,174]

In chronic meningitis, the cerebrospinal fluid profile is never diagnostic.[128] Hypoglycorrhachia is helpful, however, in limiting the differential diagnostic possibilities to tuberculosis, fungal infections, or bacterial infections (in which the hypoglycorrhachia frequently is marked, i.e., less than 25 mg per 100 ml), subarachnoid hemorrhage (with low glucose levels in about 10 per cent of cases), sarcoidosis, or viral meningoencephalitides. In herpes simplex meningoencephalitis, Mollaret's meningitis, chronic benign lymphocytic meningitis, and epidermoid cyst, hypoglycorrhachia may occur, but generally in only about 10 per cent of patients. A pleocytosis of less than 50 cells is characteristic of carcinomatous meningitis, sarcoid, and chronic benign lymphocytic meningitis, while more than 200 cells suggests an infectious cause.[128,174]

Serial spinal taps are extremely important. Wright's stain examination of the sediment should always be performed; and repeated large-volume taps to obtain a large amount of sediment for repeated cultures of cerebrospinal fluid must be done. A positive culture is the sine qua non.

Recent reports of persistent pleocytosis in the fluid of pediatric patients with bacterial meningitis who have been adequately treated and have shown good clinical response have appeared. There has also been a similar report of a lymphocytic pleocytosis lasting at least 102 days in the presence of complete clinical recovery in a pediatric patient after mumps meningoencephalitis. The significance of these findings remains unclear.[13,65]

Neurosyphilis

In the primary stage, the fluid may or may not be abnormal. In untreated secondary syphilis it is abnormal in 35 per cent of cases, the most frequent changes being pleocytosis (usually 500 but rarely up to 3000) and increased total protein; an increased percentage of IgG and oligoclonal IgG bands are also found in 53 to 70 per cent of patients with symptomatic neurosyphilis. The fluid always is abnormal in active progressive cases of meningovascular neurosyphilis, tabes dorsalis, and general paresis. The characteristic that distinguishes it from other meningeal infections is the positive serological tests. Gummas of the central nervous system may or may not produce a meningeal reaction, but the serological tests are positive. Except with a deep-seated gumma, a normal cell count is a good indication of arrested neurosyphilis (as is also true for congenital neurosyphilis). It takes the total protein longer to become normal in arrested neurosyphilis. With regard to the syphilitic serological tests, the longer they are positive before treatment, the longer they will remain positive after treatment, and quantitative examinations are important (see the section on serology). As implied earlier, pleocytosis in the fluid is useful in following the course of neurosyphilis. The course of cellular response of luetic meningitis resembles that of pyogenic meningitides, i.e., from exudative (acute) to proliferative and repair phases. While the cell count may exceed 3000, it usually is less than 500. In tabes and general paresis, fewer than 40 cells are usually found, or there may be no pleocytosis.[21,107,270,435]

Viral Meningoencephalitis

Viral infection of the central nervous system may cause several well-recognized syndromes, which comprise acute encephalitis, "aseptic" meningitis, postinfectious encephalopathies, and the "slow" viral illnesses.[163,196] Acute encephalitis may occur in epidemics or sporadically. The epidemic encephalitides are caused by the more than 350 identified arboviruses (*ar*thropod *bo*rne). Sporadic encephalitis may result from infection by enterovirus, mumps virus, adenovirus, or herpesvirus. Herpes simplex accounts for most cases of sporadic viral encephalitis. Measles, varicella, rubella, and mumps all cause a subclinical encephalitis in a significant proportion of patients with the usual clinical course, and a smaller number of patients develop a clinically apparent encephalitis. Infection with these same viruses may also result in a postinfectious demyelinating encephalopathy, as may vaccination. Reye's syndrome may also occur in these circumstances.

Aseptic Meningitis

The term "aseptic meningitis" is used to refer to a benign illness that is associated with fever, headache, meningismus, photophobia, and degrees of mental dysfunction, and usually runs its course in about two weeks.[455] The fluid is characterized by a pleocytosis that is polymorphonuclear within the first day but monocytic from that point onward. There is a small and variable increase in the fluid's protein. No organisms are demonstrable by smear or bacterial culture. The spinal fluid glucose is normal except in cases of mumps or viral lymphocytic choriomeningitis, in which cases hypoglycorrhachia may be found.[459] In general, the fluid returns to normal within 14 days. Three fourths of these cases are of viral etiology, and of these, 95 per cent are due to the following viruses in order of decreasing frequency: enteroviruses (echovirus, coxsackievirus, and nonparalytic poliovirus), which account for 75 per cent of all cases; mumps, herpes simplex type 2; adenovirus, lymphocytic choriomeningitis virus; California virus (an arbovirus); Leptospira (actually spirochetal organisms); and the encephalomyocarditis viruses.[382,455]

Less commonly, a meningitic syndrome with similar findings may be seen in the icteric stage of infectious mononucleosis (Epstein-Barr virus) and in cases of *Mycoplasma pneumoniae* infection.[455]

Epidemic Encephalitis

In epidemic (arbovirus) encephalitis, pleocytosis is also common, but cell counts in the cerebrospinal fluid reach higher levels, up to about 1000 leukocytes per cubic millimeter. Mononuclear cells usually predominate, although polymorphonuclear cells may predominate early in fulminant encephalitis. Glucose and chloride levels are normal. The protein content is usually increased. Serological tests have been helpful only retrospectively, but the specific diagnosis can usually be made in the context of the epidemic occurrence.

Sporadic Encephalitis (Herpes)

The availability and efficacy of adenine arabinoside for the treatment of herpes encephalitis has led to renewed efforts to elaborate a diagnostic test short of brain biopsy.[456a] Herpesvirus is almost never recovered from the cerebrospinal fluid. Most serological tests have remained unhelpful, although alteration of the ratio between anti–herpes IgM in the cerebrospinal fluid and in the serum, if an intact blood-brain barrier can be demonstrated, may prove to be helpful. The cerebrospinal fluid in herpes encephalitis is usually under increased pressure (up to 600 mm of water), has pleocytosis (average of 50 to 100 cells, up to 3000 cells) that is usually lymphocytic, contains red blood cells in about half the cases and is xanthochromic in somewhat fewer, and is characterized by increased protein levels (50 to 150 mg per 100 ml) in most cases.

Acute Anterior Poliomyelitis

In this viral illness the cerebrospinal fluid is abnormal in the early stages, with pleocytosis ranging from 10 to over 1000 predominantly polymorphonuclear cells. As the disease progresses and the convalescent phase ensues, the cells decrease in number and lymphocytes predominate. Concurrently the protein increases and values of 150 mg per 100 ml have been seen. This type of reaction may persist for several weeks.[99]

Herpes Zoster (Shingles)

Mild changes in the spinal fluid may precede or occur at the time of the cutaneous eruptions.[99]

Rabies

In rabies infection of the central nervous system, the cerebrospinal fluid is normal; its collection may be useful, however, since the virus may be isolated from the fluid.

Subacute Sclerosing Panencephalitis

Subacute sclerosing panencephalitis is a slow virus disease due to rubeola or, rarely, rubella and possibly other viruses.[22a] The serum and cerebrospinal fluid antibody titers may be normal early in the disease, but eventually they will become extremely high in the blood and proportionately higher in the fluid. The level of IgG is disproportionately high in relation to that of albumin, which is usually normal. The elevation has been shown to be due to in situ central nervous system synthesis of IgG, with the majority of the IgG being specific measles virus. Pleocytosis is unusual.[77,83,408,427]

Progressive Multifocal Leucoencephalopathy

In this opportunistic viral (papovavirus) encephalomyelopathy in which inflammatory changes are lacking, the cerebrospinal fluid is normal.[278a]

Creutzfeld-Jacob Disease and Kuru

In these slow virus diseases, characterized by spongioencephalopathy (clearing of neuronal cytoplasm and the formation of vacuoles in nerve terminals without an inflammatory response), the relationship between the transmissible agents is unknown. The fluid is rarely abnormal. There is no evidence that the central nervous system is synthesizing immunoglobulins.[22a]

Osteomyelitis of the Spine and Spinal Epidural Abscess

Both conditions may be associated with aseptic meningeal reaction, septic meningeal reaction, or a complete or incomplete subarachnoid block. If a subarachnoid block is present, the pressure may be normal, the Queckenstedt test may be abnormal, and the yellowish fluid may clot. There may or may not be pleocytosis, but with infected meninges, the cell count will be very high, with polymorphonuclear leukocytes predominating, and isolation of the microbe frequently is not successful.[99]

Meningism

Occurring most frequently in children, meningism is associated with acute febrile illnesses. It is manifested clinically by meningeal irritation with a slight elevation of pressure, but all constituents of the fluid are normal. This condition may be due to an increased rate of cerebrospinal fluid formation. The authors speculate that the arachnoid villi are functioning ineffectively.[99]

Acute Transverse Myelitis

This is a syndrome with many causes, for example, infections, demyelination, and trauma. The reaction of the fluid may be a manifestation of the cause. In idiopathic acute transverse myelitis (probably due to a virus), however, about half the cases have increases in pressure and in leukocyte count. If the edema is severe, subarachnoid block may result.[99]

Vascular Lesions

No significant abnormalities of the fluid are produced by vascular disease of the nervous system unless there has been a large infarction near the subarachnoid or ventricular spaces or both, a hemorrhage into the fluid, cerebral edema, or intracranial fluid collections producing increased intracranial pressure, or blockage of flow of the fluid.[99]

In cerebral arteriosclerosis and cerebrovascular insufficiency without cardiorenal vascular complications or cerebrovascular accident the spinal fluid is normal. Any significant abnormality should be investigated to rule out other diseases of the nervous system.[99]

Cerebral thrombosis and embolism are accompanied by a normal spinal fluid in the majority of cases. In recent infarction, pressure elevation over 300 mm of water is rare, and only occasionally is the protein increased to 75 mg per 100 ml. If a slight xanthochromia or a few erythrocytes or increased protein is found in the fluid, an infarct near the cerebrospinal fluid spaces should be suspected.[99]

In acute intracerebral hemorrhage the fluid is usually abnormal. A sustained increase of pressure on repeat taps is a grave prognostic sign. In over 85 per cent of cases the fluid is hemorrhagic with accompanying xanthochromia and a meningitic reaction (pleocytosis, increased total protein, and moderately low glucose level) that is roughly proportional to the degree of subarachnoid hemorrhage.[390,447] The authors' data suggest that the resolution of a subarachnoid hemorrhage associated with brain damage takes longer than resolution of a subarachnoid hemorrhage uncomplicated by brain damage.[425]

Spontaneous subarachnoid hemorrhage usually is due to rupture of an aneurysm or arteriovenous malformation.[362] Hemorrhagic fluid resulting from spontaneous subarachnoid hemorrhage must be distinguished from that caused by faulty lumbar puncture technique. Generally, for one or two hours after the ictus, the fluid is clear and the only abnormality is an increase in pressure.[447] Approximately two hours after the ictus, the fluid is persistently hemorrhagic and does not clot. Cell counts of the fluid may show several thousand to millions of erythrocytes. Xanthochromia may be obvious even at this early stage, especially if the red cell count is high. The xanthochromia is almost entirely due to oxyhemoglobin. The total protein concentration and leukocyte count are roughly proportional to the erythrocyte count at this early stage. The spontaneous subarachnoid hemorrhage clears at a varying rate probably dependent on the continuation of leakage from the site of the bleeding. The erythrocyte count may return to normal in 6 to 21 days. The xanthochromia increases for a few days, but its character changes. On the first day the oxyhemoglobin, which appears pink, increases precipitously, and as it decreases on the second and third days, the methemoglobin, which appears brownish, increases, as does the bilirubin (yellow). These components fall to normal within the first week except in patients with persistent hemorrhage. The total protein level and the pleocytosis follow the waxing and waning of the xanthochromia. In the first few days there is a polymorphonuclear leukocytosis followed by a mononuclear response. The leukocyte count is the last constituent to return to normal. It may remain abnormal for up to four weeks. This phase of resolution of a subarachnoid hemorrhage has been referred to as hematogenous meningitis, and its cerebrospinal fluid profile can be confused with one that is due to bacterial meningitis.[403,425,447]

With epidural and subdural hematomas, a lumbar puncture to determine pressure and obtain cerebrospinal fluid for analysis is contraindicated. If a puncture is performed, however, the fluid pressure is very high unless the patient is extremely dehydrated or in severe shock. Leukocyte and erythrocyte counts can also be increased. There may be xanthochromia due to methemoglobin, as has been mentioned earlier.[233]

Neoplastic Disease

Intracranial Tumors

When the patient has significant neurological signs, the pressure usually is elevated. When present, xanthochromia is related to high protein content or recent hemorrhage. If pleocytosis and an elevated protein level are found, this generally means the tumor is near the cerebrospinal fluid spaces, especially the ventricles. Acoustic neuromas invariably are accompanied by an elevated total protein level.[99]

Tumor cells may be detected in the cerebrospinal fluid. Frequently meningeal carcinomatosis is accompanied by a modest increase in protein and cells and a low glucose content, in which case the fluid's profile must be differentiated from that seen in tuberculous meningitis and other chronic meningitides.[25,39]

Spinal Cord Neoplasms

It is possible for a patient to have normal fluid in conjunction with spinal cord signs due to neoplasm. The fluid below a tumor that produces a complete block, however, may show a normal or low pressure, but removal of a few milliliters of the fluid will result in a precipitious drop in pressure. If the Queckenstedt test is normal at a time when the patient has significant focal spinal cord neurological signs, a diagnosis of spinal cord tumor is unlikely. The fluid may appear xanthochromic because of the high protein content. If the yellowish fluid clots, then the protein level is generally very high (Froin syndrome). Glucose content is usually normal.[99]

Neoplasms of the cauda equina may not be reflected in cerebrospinal fluid abnormalities, especially if the lumbar puncture is not accomplished below the tumor. Fluid from immediately above the tumor has, however, been reported to be yellow in color owing to increased protein.[99,174]

Leukemia

With subarachnoid hemorrhage secondary to defects in the clotting mechanism and with infiltration of the meninges with leukemic cells, there may be changes in the cerebrospinal fluid. The subarachnoid hemorrhage and its resolution are similar to those that occur in nonleukemic patients. Infiltration of the meninges with leukemic cells is associated with elevation of pressure, increase in the concentration of protein, and pleocytosis that is usually due to normal leukocytes (polymorphonuclear cells and lymphocytes). Leukemic cells may be found, however. Reduction in glucose may be seen. If the spinal cord is affected, a subarachnoid block may result.[99,143,174]

Trauma

In general, the amount of blood in the spinal fluid is roughly proportional to the severity of the cerebral or spinal cord trauma. Infections usually are complications of basilar skull fractures.[99,174]

Spinal Fracture

If the fluid is hemorrhagic, probably the spinal cord was injured by the trauma of the spine. If there is dislocation or fracture of a vertebra, a partial or complete subarachnoid block may be discovered. The Queckenstedt test may be abnormal, and a Froin syndrome may be present.[99]

Herniated Intervertebral Disc

In 50 per cent of cases there is a moderate increase of total protein (100 mg per 100 ml). A thoracic or cervical herniated disc may be associated with an abnormal Queckenstedt test.[99]

Developmental Defects

Congenital Hydrocephalus

In communicating hydrocephalus, the fluid is under increased pressure and all constituents may be decreased in concentration. In the noncommunicating type it may be impossible to get fluid via the lumbar route.

Basilar Impression

Signs of partial or complete subarachnoid block are occasionally present on lumbar puncture.[99]

Syringomyelia

At the time the clinical picture becomes classic, half the patients will have normal fluid. The other half may show an elevated total protein content with or without partial or complete spinal cord block and a modest pleocytosis.[99]

Inherited Diseases

Tay-Sachs Disease

The fluid is normal except for significant changes in the lipid profile and the appearance of foam cells similar in appearance to lipophages.[418,422,430] Since clinical signs of the disease are obvious when the changes occur, tests have limited diagnostic value.

Niemann-Pick Disease

Some studies on lipid profiles in this disease have shown an abnormality of the sphingomyelin fraction, with other constituents of the fluid being normal.[418]

Metachromatic Leukodystrophy (Sulfatide Sphingolipidosis)

Invariably, the total protein level is elevated in this condition. The lipid profiles have no obvious abnormality when the data are calculated on a per milligram of protein basis.[8]

Hereditary Ataxias

These include Friedreich's ataxia, Lévy-Roussy syndrome, Sanger-Brown and Marie syndromes, olivopontocerebellar atrophy, parenchymatous cerebellar degeneration, and familial spastic paraplegia. Occasionally there is a slight increase in the protein content of the cerebrospinal fluid, and rarely a slight pleocytosis.[99]

Metabolic Systemic Diseases

Cushing's Syndrome

The cerebrospinal fluid pressure may be greater than 200 mm of water, and more often the protein may be increased to over 100 mg per 100 ml.[99]

Thyroid Disease

Although normal cerebrospinal fluid has been reported, a slight increase in pressure and a total protein level elevated to more than 80 mg per 100 ml are common in hypothyroidism. This protein increase can only partly be accounted for by increased gamma globulin. The protein concentration returns to normal with thyroid therapy, although in some cases its return is greatly delayed.[314] Lipids in the fluid are increased in proportion to the total protein concentration.[367]

Parathyroid Disease

The pressure has been reported to be elevated above 400 mm of water, and the protein level may be elevated in some cases. The total calcium concentration may be depressed to a lesser degree than the serum level. In most cases, however, the diffusible calcium ion concentration is unchanged.[99,143]

Diabetes Mellitus

The spinal fluid is normal except that the glucose content is proportional to that in the blood. In diabetic coma the pressure may be low because of dehydration. Acetone bodies have been detected. In insulin shock the pressure may be low because of the fall in venous pressure secondary to vascular collapse.[99,143]

Pernicious Anemia

In most cases the cerebrospinal fluid is normal. It may, however, have a total protein content of less than 75 mg per 100 ml and pleocytosis of less than 10 leukocytes per cubic millimeter. The vitamin B_{12} level may be low.[99,143]

Osteitis Deformans (Paget's Disease)

The spinal fluid is normal unless the cerebral cortex, cranial nerves, or spinal cord are encroached upon by the bony changes. Under these circumstances, the total protein level may be elevated; and if a spinal subarachnoid block is present, the Froin syndrome may be found.[99]

Acute Porphyria

Except for an occasional moderate increase of protein, the cerebrospinal fluid is normal.[22]

Hepatic Diseases

The cerebrospinal fluid may show xanthochromia if the blood plasma bilirubin exceeds 10 to 16 mg per 100 ml.[28] In hepatic coma the ammonia level is about proportional to the serum value, while the high elevation of the fluid's glutamine level may be diagnostic.[199]

Cardiovascular Diseases

In congestive heart failure the pressure is increased in proportion to the increase in the venous pressure. In uncomplicated hypertension, the cerebrospinal fluid is normal. In hypertension encephalopathy the pressure can be high, the protein level may be elevated, and erythrocytes may be found in the fluid.[99]

Renal Disease

With generalized edema the pressure may be increased. In nephrosis associated with hyperlipemia the cerebrospinal fluid lipid profile is normal.[431a] In uremia the pressure is usually increased, and chlorides and nonprotein nitrogen concentration reflect the abnormalities of the serum.[156] In addition, abnormalities secondary to nephrogenic congestive heart failure and hypertensive encephalopathy may occur.

Immunological (Connective Tissue) Disease

Systemic Lupus Erythematosus

The major disease entity of concern in this group is systemic lupus erythematosus, in which neurological involvement is common and signs and symptoms are protean.[24,134,210,383] Examination of the cerebrospinal fluid alone is not useful in the diagnosis of involvement of the nervous system; examination of the fluid may, however, be helpful when combined with several other examinations. About half the patients with subacute systemic lupus erythematosus and neurological involvement have abnormal fluids, the most common findings being increased proteins (50 to 100 mg per 100 ml), pleocytosis (5 to 50 leukocytes, predominantly lymphocytes), and elevated pressures. Similar spinal fluid abnormalities also may be seen in patients with lupus erythematosus who do not have symptoms. The fourth component of complement (C4) may be reduced in the fluid during active involvement of the nervous system with the disease.[335] Also, the IgG-albumin quotient is elevated in about 70 per cent, and increased levels of deoxyribonucleic acid–binding antibodies are measured in the fluid of about two thirds of patients. The most striking abnormalities of the fluid are seen in patients with myelopathy or polyradiculopathy. Further abnormalities may be found if cerebral embolization secondary to verrucous endocarditis complicates the illness.[134]

Polyarteritis Nodosa

In polyarteritis nodosa, nervous system involvement tends to be restricted to the peripheral nerves. Of these patients, however, 20 per cent may have central nervous system involvement, with cerebrospinal fluid findings similar to those seen with lupus erythematosus. Radiculopathy will effect the most obvious abnormalities in the fluid.[24,134,335,383]

Demyelinating Diseases

Multiple Sclerosis

The cerebrospinal fluid profile of clinical definite multiple sclerosis is well known.* The de novo central nervous system IgG synthesis rate is elevated in 90 per cent of cases. The average patient with multiple sclerosis synthesizes 29 mg of IgG per day.[417] This is in contrast to the cerebrospinal fluid total protein or albumin, which is abnormal in about 20 per cent of cases.[406]

---

* See references 83a, 180, 215, 267, 324, 373, 401, 406, 409, 417, 463, 476.

If the total protein value is greater than 100 mg per 100 ml, doubt should be cast on the diagnosis of multiple sclerosis or it should suggest a complication.[406,409] Another sign of de novo central nervous system IgG synthesis is cerebrospinal fluid oligoclonal IgG. In 90 per cent of patients, two to four bands can be seen after electrophoresis.[417] This profile may be mimicked in part by neurosyphilis, subacute sclerosing panencephalitis, and certain othjer diseases, especially infections.* It is most helpful when they can be ruled out on the basis of their pathognomonic symptoms or signs, their pathognomonic laboratory tests, or both.

The cerebrospinal fluid leukocyte count is greater than 5 cells per cubic millimeter in about 30 per cent of cases, whether the patient is in relapse or remission. A count that exceeds 50 should cast doubt on the diagnosis of multiple sclerosis or suggest a complication. The differential cell count of the fluid is normal, and if polymorphonuclear cells are present, one should be wary of the diagnosis of multiple sclerosis or should suspect a complication.[406,409]

Measles antibodies are increased more in the fluid than in the blood, but many other common viral antibodies also are increased.[148,417] A myelinotoxic antibody has been detected in the fluid as well as in the blood.†

The cerebrospinal fluid lipid profiles (total phospholipids, cephalins, lecithins, sphingomyelin, cerebroside, total cholesterol, free cholesterol, neutral lipids, and total lipids) of 40 normal individuals were compared with those found in 156 multiple sclerosis patients and certain subgroups of patients.[409a] The cerebroside (a myelin lipid) was significantly increased in all categories of multiple sclerosis, and the percentage was much more elevated than those of all the other lipids. It was increased in every subgroup except the patients who had received ACTH and can thus be considered to be the lipid most characteristically elevated in the fluid in multiple sclerosis.

Radioimmunoassay shows myelin basic protein in the fluid of 60 per cent of patients with multiple sclerosis but of only 20 per cent of normal persons. More recent application of this method has increased its usefulness as a measure of active demyelination.[70,71]

* See references 26, 29, 185, 239, 240, 406, 427.
† See references 401, 405–409, 412–417, 419–421.

Retrobulbar Neuritis

Many reports have dealt with the cerebrospinal fluid changes in retrobulbar neuritis without any other present or past symptoms and signs suggestive of multiple sclerosis. In 1969 in the authors' report on lipids in the cerebrospinal fluid, they studied 14 patients with retrobulbar neuritis only. Significant abnormalities were noted in the cephalins and cerebrosides, a result similar to that found for multiple sclerosis.[409a] Additionally, in 1978, they found that 50 per cent of the patients had an increased rate of de novo central nervous sytem IgG synthesis.[417] These results may be of special interest because it is presumed that only a few milligrams of inflamed tissue near the subarachnoid space is capable of producing changes in the cerebrospinal fluid profile.

Schilder's Disease, Neuromyelitis Optica (Devic's Disease), Acute Disseminated Encephalomyelitis

In these diseases the changes in the cerebrospinal fluid are similar to those in multiple sclerosis. Higher cell counts (more than 50) and total protein concentrations (more than 100 mg per 100 ml) are common, however. Also, there may be spinal subarachnoid block in neuromyelitis optica secondary to edema of the spinal cord.[99]

Degenerative Diseases

Amyotrophic Lateral Sclerosis

A slight increase of total protein (less than 95 mg per 100 ml) is seen in the cerebrospinal fluid of one third of patients.[99]

Sydenham's Chorea

Usually the cerebrospinal fluid is normal, but a mild pleocytosis occurs in a small percentage of cases.[99]

Parkinsonism

Occasionally a mild increase in total cerebrospinal fluid protein (less than 75 mg per 100 ml) is found.[99]

Polyneuropathy

Polyneuropathy may have many different causes. It may occur with no indication of central nervous system involvement.[99,138,143,174] Anatomical considerations and the specific pathological process affecting the peripheral nerves will determine whether the cerebrospinal fluid reflects the presence of disease. For example, segmental demyelination of the nerve root occurs in Guillain-Barré syndrome, and the anatomical proximity of the spinal nerve roots and their proximal subarachnoid space extensions thus result in changes in the fluid. As mentioned elsewhere, all nerve roots possess this subarachnoid extension, at least as far out from the cord as to the dorsal ganglia, and for spinal nerves in the cauda equina, these extensions may reach centimeters.[143]

Chronic Alcoholism, Avitaminoses, Pregnancy, Heavy Metal Poisoning, Diabetes Mellitus, Diphtheria, Botulism

These diverse conditions may produce moderately elevated total protein values (less than 200 mg per 100 ml). Lead, arsenic, and other heavy metals have also been detected in the cerebrospinal fluid.[99,350]

Guillain-Barré Syndrome

The cerebrospinal fluid pressure may be elevated in the presence of respiratory dysfunction or in association with marked increase of the protein without a clot (fibrinogen). The total protein level may not reach its zenith until two or three weeks after the onset of the illness. Values as high as 1000 mg per 100 ml may be seen. A relative increase in gamma globulin has been noted, but all the fractions are increased.[244] In general, the leukocyte count is normal. Fifteen per cent of patients, however, may demonstrate a pleocytosis of the cerebrospinal fluid. Although the albuminocytological dissociation usually noted in the Guillain-Barré syndrome has been stressed as a diagnostic point, it remains a nonspecific laboratory finding, as discussed earlier. It is, however, supportive of the diagnosis when ascending paralysis is the prominent clinical presentation.[99]

Paroxysmal Disorders

During an attack or in the interval between attacks of headaches (migraine and other types), idiopathic convulsive disorders, carotid sinus syncope, Meniere's syndrome, and narcolepsy, the cerebrospinal fluid shows no constant deviation from normal.[99]

In convulsive seizures that are symptomatic of some structural cerebral disease, there may be abnormalities characteristic of the underlying condition. Pressure greater than 200 mm of water in the interval between attacks is suggestive of an expanding lesion.[99]

Hypoliquorrhea (Aliquorrhea)

In this condition the fluid is under low pressure, and occasionally no fluid may be obtained even with aspiration. The fluid may be xanthochromic and contain increased protein.[99]

Normal-Pressure Hydrocephalus

Many etiological factors can underlie normal-pressure (communicating) hydrocephalus, although most cases remain idiopathic.[3,80,141,261] The cerebrospinal fluid in idiopathic normal-pressure hydrocephalus is characterized by dynamic abnormalities that may be demonstrated by isotope cisternography, metrizamide computed tomographic cisternography, and cerebrospinal fluid infusion tests. Abnormalities of the cerebrospinal fluid chemical or cellular elements should raise the suspicion of a concurrent active disease process.

Benign Intracranial Hypertension

This syndrome, which is also referred to as tumor cerebri and otitic hydrocephalus, is manifested by increased intracranial pressure without evidence of an intracranial mass lesion or obstruction of the ventricular passages. The pressure may be as high as 600 mm of water.[209] The Queckenstedt response may be abnormal if thrombosis of the jugular vein or lateral sinus is present.

Rarely the leukocyte count is elevated. Most often the total protein content is normal or below normal.[99]

Cerebrospinal Fluid Response to Prior Lumbar Puncture

When a second diagnostic lumbar puncture is performed 48 hours after the first in an individual whose fluid was normal on the initial tap, the pressure is normal unless the patient has developed a post–lumbar puncture headache, in which case it is low.[424] There is no change in the cell count or other chemical constituents. Furthermore, if the initial puncture was traumatic, the second sampling will show normal fluid except for a minimal pleocytosis. If the hemorrhage induced by the needle continues, xanthochromia and a cellular reaction may be seen.[403]

The authors have studied patients undergoing twice-weekly lumbar punctures as a means of evaluating methods of treating multiple sclerosis. The various parameters studied (leukocyte total and differential counts, albumin, IgG, daily de novo central nervous system IgG synthesis rate, and cerebrospinal fluid IgG oligoclonal bands) showed no significant change that was solely the result of lumbar puncture, prior to initiation of treatment.[409,417]

Post–Lumbar Puncture Syndrome

If a repeat tap is done the day after lumbar puncture or at the height of the symptoms, the fluid pressure generally is low to unobtainable, but no other abnormalities are found.[247,251,252,424,432]

Pneumoencephalography

A progressive increase of mononuclear cells to over 100 per cubic millimeter occurs after exchange of 50 to 100 ml of fluid with air. Therefore it is recommended that cell counts be done on the first withdrawal if a baseline value is desired. The pleocytosis encountered during the course of a pneumoencephalogram may be a sterile inflammatory reaction. Another explanation is that leukocytes are present along the walls of the cerebrospinal fluid spaces and become exfoliated by the churning fluid during the procedure. The pleocytosis lasts for about one week.[99,397] During the course of a pneumoencephalogram, in which air is exchanged for cerebrospinal fluid, the fluid protein content normally decreases in each serial sample drawn. Variations from this pattern could be of diagnostic significance.[119]

Other Post–Injection Cerebrospinal Fluid Findings

If a sterile anesthetic agent is injected into the subarachnoid space, an inflammatory reaction results, but the patient rarely is aware of it.[99] The reaction may persist for a week. Apparently corticosteroids produce no reaction in the subarachnoid space and may suppress an existing one.[99] On the other hand, with iophendylate (Pantopaque), lipophages emerge and may be found as long as six weeks later.[136,403] Inflammatory-type changes in the fluid may also result from adhesive arachnoiditis.[381]

RHINORRHEA AND OTORRHEA

Occasionally there is a problem in distinguishing nasal secretions from cerebrospinal fluid escaping through a fractured cribriform plate. A glucose concentration of at least 40 mg per 100 ml, i.e., similar to that in the cerebrospinal fluid, is a strong indication that the fluid is escaping from the cerebrospinal fluid space. No modern study has been reported that deals with the problem, but it would appear that a high concentration of IgA would favor the fluid's being nasal secretions.

REFERENCES

1. Achar, V. S., Welch, K. M. A., Chabi, E., Bartosh, D., and Meyer, J. S.: Cerebrospinal fluid gamma-aminobutyric acid in neurologic disease. Neurology (Minneap.), *26*:777–780, 1976.
2. Ackermann, H., Rieder, H., and Wuthrich, R.: Absolute or relative values in CSF electrophoresis? An evaluation of the gammaglobulins in multiple sclerosis and other neurological diseases. Eur. Neurol., *13*:131–1943, 1975.
3. Adams, R. D., Fisher, C. M., Hakim, S., et al.: Symptomatic occult hydrocephalus with "normal" cerebrospinal fluid pressure. New Eng. J. Med., *273*:117, 1965.
4. Agarwal, G. C., Berman, B. M., and Stark, L.:

A lumped parameter model of the cerebrospinal fluid system. IEEE Trans. Biomed. Engin., *16*:45–53, 1969.

5. Allen, J. C., Sheremata, W., Cosgrove, J. B. R., Osterland, K., and Shea, M.: Cerebrospinal fluid T and B lymphocyte kinetics related to exacerbations of multiple sclerosis. Neurology (Minneap.), *26*:579, 1976.
6. Allen, R. J., McCusker, J. J., and Tourtellotte, W. W.: Metachromatic leukodystrophy: Clinical, histochemical, and cerebrospinal fluid abnormalities. Pediatrics, *30*:629–638, 1962.
7. Arieff, A. I., Llach, F., and Massry, S. G.: Neurological manifestations and morbidity of hyponatremia: Correlation with brain water and electrolytes. Medicine (Balt.), *55*:121–129, 1976.
8. Aristegui, J., Juan, S., Saitua, G., and Hernandez, M.: Limulus test in diagnosis of acute meningitis. An. Esp. Pediat., *10*:835, 1977.
9. Ashby, P., Verrier, M., Warsh, J. J., and Price, K. S.: Spinal reflexes and the concentrations of 5-HIAA, MHPG, and HVA in lumbar cerebrospinal fluid after spinal lesions in man. J. Neurol. Neurosurg. Psychiat., *39*:1191–1200, 1976.
10. Astaldi, A., Passino, M., Rosanda, C., and Massimo, L.: T and B cells in cerebrospinal fluid in acute lymphocytic leukemias. New Eng. J. Med., *294*:550, 1976.
11. Ayala, G.: Ueber den diagnostischen Wert des Liquordruckes and einer Apparat zu seiner Messung. Z. Ges. Neurol. Psychiat., *84*:42, 1923.
12. Ayer, J. B.: Puncture of the cisterna magna. Arch. Neurol. Psychiat., *4*:529, 1920.
13. Azimi, P. H., Shaban, S., Hilty, M. D., and Haynes, R. E.: Mumps meningoencephalitis. Prolonged abnormality of cerebrospinal fluid. J.A.M.A., *234*:1161–1162, 1975.
14. Bakay, L.: *In* Richter, D., ed.: Metabolism of the Nervous System. New York, Pergamon Press, 1957, p. 136.
15. Banik, N. L., Mauldin, L. B., and Hogan, E. L.: Activity of 2′,3′-cyclic nucleotide 3′-phosphohydrolase in human cerebrospinal fluid. Ann. Neurol., *5*:539–541, 1979.
16. Baringer, J. R.: Herpes simplex virus infection of nervous tissue in animals and man. Progr. Med. Virol., *20*:1–26, 1975.
17. Barnes, B. D., and Hoff, J. T.: Radionuclide cisternography after head injury. Arch. Neurol. (Chicago), *33*:21–25, 1976.
18. Barrows, L. J., Hunter, F. T., and Banker, B. Q.: The nature and clinical significance of pigments in the cerebrospinal fluid. Brain, *78*:59–80, 1955.
19. Batnitzky, S., Keucher, T. R., Mealey, J., and Campbell, R. L.: Iatrogenic intraspinal epidermoid tumors. J.A.M.A., *237*:148–150, 1977.
20. Bauer, H.: Die Cerebrospinalflussigkeit: Neuere Methoden und Forschungsergebnisse als Grundlage der Deutung von Liquorbefunden. Internist, *2*:85–94, 1961.
21. Beck, B.: Syphilis: Neurosyphilis, diagnosis and followup by lumbar puncture; interpretation of serology and treatment. Unpublished data.
22. Becker, D. M., and Kramer, S.: The neurological manifestations of porphyria: A review. Medicine (Balt.), *56*:411–423, 1977.

22a. Behan, P. O., and Currie, S.: Clinical Neuroimmunology. London, W. B. Saunders Co., Ltd., 1978.

23. Bell, W. E., Joynt, R. J., and Sahs, A. L.: Low spinal fluid pressure syndromes. Neurology (Minneap.), *10*:512, 1960.
24. Bennahum, D. A., and Messner, R. P.: Recent observations on central nervous system lupus erythematosus. Seminars Arthritis Rheum., *4*:253–266, 1975.
25. Berg, L.: Hypoglycorrhachia of non-infectious origin. Diffuse meningeal neoplasia. Neurology (Minneap.), *3*:811–824, 1953.
26. Bergmann, L., Gilland, O., Olanders, S., and Svennerhold, L.: Clinical profile and paper electrophoresis in multiple sclerosis. Acta Neurol. Scand., *40*:suppl. 10:33–48, 1964.
27. Bering, E. A., Jr.: Circulation of the cerebrospinal fluid. J. Neurosurg., *19*:405–413, 1962.
28. Berman, L. B., Lapham, L. W., and Pastore, E.: Jaundice and xanthochromia of the spinal fluid. J. Lab. Clin. Med., *44*:273–279, 1954.
29. Berner, J. J., Ciemins, V. A., and Schroeder, E. F., Jr.: Radial immunodiffusion of spinal fluid: Diagnostic value in multiple sclerosis. Amer. J. Clin. Path., *48*:145–152, 1972.
30. Biegeleisen, J. Z., Jr., Mitchell, M. S., Marcus, B. B., et al.: Immunofluorescence techniques for demonstrating bacterial pathogens associated with cerebrospinal meningitis. I. Clinical evaulation of conjugates on smears prepared directly from cerebrospinal fluid sediments. J. Lab. Clin. Med., *65*:976–989, 1965.
31. Bird, M., Ratcheson, R., Seigel, B., and Fishman, M.: The evaluation of arrested communicating hydrocephalus utilizing cerebrospinal fluid dynamics: A preliminary report. Develop. Med. Child. Neurol., *15*:474, 1973.
32. Bledsoe, S. W., and Mines, A. H.: Effect of plasma [K^+] on the DC potential and on ion distributions between CSF and blood. J. Appl. Physiol., *39*:1012–1016, 1975.
33. Bosch, I., and Oehmichen, M.: Eosinophilic granulocytes in cerebrospinal fluid: Analysis of 94 cerebrospinal fluid specimens and review of the literature. J. Neurol., *219*:93, 1978.
34. Bowers, M. B., Jr.: Central dopamine turnover in schizophrenic syndromes. J.A.M.A., *229*:480, 1974.
35. Bowsher, D.: Cerebrospinal Fluid Dynamics in Health and Disease. Springfield, Ill., Charles C Thomas, 1960.
36. Bradbury, M.: Electrolyte disorders and the brain. *In* Maxwell, M., and Kleeman, C., eds.: Clinical Disorders of Fluid and Electrolyte Metabolism. 2nd Ed. New York, McGraw-Hill Book Co., 1972.
37. Bradbury, M. W. B., Kleeman, C. R., Bagdoyan, H., and Berberian, A.: The calcium and magnesium content of skeletal muscle, brain and cerebrospinal fluid as determined by atomic absorption flame photometry. J. Lab. Clin. Med., *71*:884–892, 1968.
38. Bradley, K. C.: Cerebrospinal fluid pressure. J. Neurol. Neurosurg. Psychiat., *33*:387, 1970.
39. Bramlet, D., Gilberti, J., and Bender, J.: Meningeal carcinomatosis, case report and review of the literature. Neurology (Minneap.), *26*:287, 1976.

40. Breebaart, K., Becker, H., and Jongebloed, F.: Investigation of reference values of components of the cerebrospinal fluid. J. Clin. Chem. Clin. Biochem., *16*:561, 1978.
41. Brightman, M. W.: The distribution within the brain of ferritin injected into cerebrospinal fluid compartments. Part 2 (Parenchymal distribution). Amer. J. Anat., *117*:193–220, 1965.
42. Brightman, M., and Broadwell, R.: The morphological approach to the study of normal and abnormal brain permeability. *In* Levi, G., et al., eds.: Transport Phenomena in the Nervous System. New York, Plenum Publishing Corp., 1976, pp. 41–54.
43. Brightman, M., and Reese, T.: Membrane specializations of ependymal cells and astrocytes. *In* Tower, D., ed.: The Nervous System. Vol. 1, The Basic Neurosciences. New York, Raven Press, 1975, pp. 267–277.
44. Brightman, M., Prescott, L., and Reese, T.: Intercellular junctions of special ependyma. pp. 146–165 *In* Brain-Endocrine Interaction II. The Ventricular System. Second International Symposium, Tokyo, 1974. Basel, S. Karger, 1975.
45. Brightman, M., Shivers, R., and Prescott, L.: Morphology of the walls around fluid compartments in nervous tissue. *In* Cserr, H. F., et al., eds.: Fluid Environment of the Brain. New York, Academic Press, Inc., 1975, pp. 3–29.
46. Brightman, M. W., Klatzo, I., Olsson, Y., and Reese, T. S.: The blood-brain barrier to proteins under normal and pathological conditions. J. Neurol. Sci., *10*:215, 1970.
47. Bronnestam, R., Dencker, S., and Bengt, S.: Fibrinogen in cerebrospinal fluid. Arch. Neurol. (Chicago), *4*:288, 1961.
48. Brooks, C. M., Kao, F. F., and Lloyd, B. B., eds.: Cerebrospinal Fluid and the Regulation of Ventilation. Oxford, Blackwell Scientific Publications, Ltd., 1965.
49. Brownell, B., and Hughes, J. T.: Distribution of plaques in the cerebrum in multiple sclerosis. J. Neurol. Neurosurg. Psychiat., *25*:315–320, 1962.
50. Bruyn, H. B.: Purulent meningitis. *In* Brennemann's Practice of Pediatrics. Hagerstown, Md., Harper & Row, 1968, pp.1–39.
51. Bulat, M., Lacković, Z., Jakupčevič, M., et al.: 5-Hydroxyindoleacetic acid in the lumbar fluid: A specific indicator of spinal cord injury. Science, *185*:527–528, 1974.
52. Burch, E., and Sullivan, F., eds.: Trace Elements. Med. Clin. N. Amer., Vol. 60. Philadelphia, W. B. Saunders Co., 1976.
53. Burtin, P.: Les protéines du liquide céphalorachidien. *In* Grabar, P., and Burtin, P., eds.: Analyse Immuno-electrophoretique: Applications aux Liquides Biologiques Humains. Paris, Masson, 1960, p. 245.
54. Burtin, P.: The proteins of the cerebrospinal fluid. *In* Grabar, P., and Burtin, P., eds.: Immunoelectrophoretic Analysis. Amsterdam, Elsevier Publishing Co., 1964, pp. 244–251.
55. Cameron, A. T., and Moorhouse, V. H. K.: The relation between plasma and cerebrospinal fluid calcium. J. Physiol. (London), *91*:90–100, 1937.
56. Cameron, I. R.: Acid-base changes in cerebrospinal fluid. Brit. J. Anaesth., *41*:213–221, 1969.
57. Cappel, R., Thiry, L., and Clinet, G.: Viral antibodies in the CSF after acute CNS infections. Arch. Neurol. (Chicago), *32*:629–631, 1975.
58. Carey, M., and Vela, R.: Effect of systemic arterial hypotension on the rate of cerebrospinal fluid formation in dogs. J. Neurosurg., *41*:350, 1974.
59. Carlsson, C., and Dencker, S. J.: Cerebrospinal uric acid in alcoholics. Acta Neurol. Scand., *49*:39–46, 1973.
60. Carpenter, R. R., and Petersdorf, R. G.: The clinical spectrum of bacterial meningitis. Amer. J. Med., *33*:262, 1962.
61. Caspary, E. A.: Comparison of immunological specificity of gamma globulin in the cerebrospinal fluid in normal and multiple sclerosis subjects. J. Neurol. Neurosurg. Psychiat., *28*:61–64, 1965.
62. Cawley, L. P., Minard, B. J., Tourtellotte, W. W., Ma, B. I., and Chelle, C.: Immunofixation electrophoretic techniques applied to identification of proteins in serum and cerebrospinal fluid. Clin. Chem., *22*:1262–1268, 1976.
63. Chajek, T., and Fainaru, M.: Behçet's disease. Report of 41 cases and a review of the literature. Medicine (Balt.), *54*:179–196, 1975.
64. Chakrabarti, A.: Significance of raised protein content in cerebrospinal fluid (a review). Neurol. India, *23*:23, 1975.
65. Chartrand, S. A., and Cho, C. T.: Persistent pleocytosis in bacterial meningitis. J. Pediat., *88*:424–426, 1976.
66. Clarke, E., and O'Malley, C. D.: The Human Brain and Spinal Cord. Berkeley, University of California Press, 1968.
67. Clausen, J., Matzke, J., and Gerhardt, W.: Agar-gel micro-electrophoresis of proteins in the cerebrospinal fluid: Normal and pathological findings. Acta Neurol. Scand., *40*:suppl. 10:49–56, 1964.
68. Cohen, H.: The magnesium content of the cerebrospinal and other body fluids. Quart. J. Med., pp. 173–186, Jan. 1927.
69. Cohen, S., and Bannister, R.: Immunoglobulin synthesis within the central nervous system in disseminated sclerosis. Lancet, *1*:366–367, 1967.
70. Cohen, S. R., Herndon, R. M., and McKhann, G. M.: Radioimmunoassay of myelin basic protein in spinal fluid. An index of active demyelination. New Eng. J. Med., *295*:1455, 1976.
71. Cohen, S., Herndon, R., and McKhann, G.: Myelin basic protein in cerebrospinal fluid as an indicator of active demyelination. Trans. Amer. Neurol. Ass., *101*:45, 1976.
72. Corning, J. L.: Spinal anesthesia and local medication of the cord. New York Med. J., *42*:483, 1885.
73. Cosgrove, J. B. R., and Agius, P.: Studies in multiple sclerosis. Part 2 (Comparison of the β-γ globulin ratio, γ-globulin elevation and first-zone colloidal gold curve in the cerebrospinal fluid). Neurology (Minneap.), *16*:197–204, 1966.
74. Coxon, R. V.: Cerebrospinal fluid transport. Brain Res., *29*:135–146, 1968.

75. Curzon, G., Gumpert, J., and Sharpe, D.: Amine metabolites in the cerebrospinal fluid in Huntington's chorea. J. Neurol. Neurosurg. Psychiat., *35*:514–519, 1972.
76. Cushing, H.: Studies on the cerebro-spinal fluid I. Introduction. J. Med. Res., *31*:1, 1914.
77. Cutler, R., and Tourtellotte, W.: Synthesis of gamma globulin inside the blood-brain barrier in subacute sclerosing panencephalitis. Riv. Pat. Nerv. Ment., *92*:163–170, 1971.
78. Cutler, R. W. P., Keuel, R. K., and Barlow, C. F.: Albumin exchange between plasma and cerebrospinal fluid. Arch. Neurol. (Chicago), *17*:261–270, 1967.
79. Cutler, R., Murray, J., and Cornick, L.: Variations in protein permeability in different regions of the cerebrospinal fluid. Exp. Neurol., *28*:257, 1970.
80. Cutler, R., Murray, J., and Moody, R.: Overproduction of cerebrospinal fluid in communicating hydrocephalus—a case report. Neurology (Minneap.), *23*:1, 1973.
81. Cutler, R. W. P., Watters, G. V., and Hammerstad, J. P.: The origin and turnover rates of cerebrospinal fluid albumin and γ-globulin in man. J. Neurol. Sci., *10*:259–268, 1970.
82. Cutler, R. W. P., Page, L., Galicich, J., and Watters, G. V.: Formation and absorption of cerebrospinal fluid in man. Brain, *91*:707–720, 1968.
83. Cutler, R. W. P., Watters, G. V., Hammerstad, J. P., and Merlen, E.: Origin of cerebrospinal fluid γ-globulin in subacute sclerosing leukoencephalitis. Arch. Neurol. (Chicago), *17*:620–628, 1976.
83a. Cuzner, M. L., and Davison, A. N.: The scientific basis of multiple sclerosis. Molec. Aspects Med., *2*:147–248, 1979.
84. Dandy, W. E.: Experimental hydrocephalus. Ann. Surg., *70*:129, 1919.
85. Dandy, W. E.: Roentgenography of the brain after the injection of air into the spinal canal. Ann. Surg., *70*:397, 1919.
86. Daughaday, W. H., Lowry, O. H., Rosebrough, N. J., and Fields, W. S.: Determination of cerebrospinal fluid protein with the folin phenol reagent. J. Lab. Clin. Med., *39*:663–665, 1952.
87. Davidson, D., Pullar, I. A., Mawdsley, C., Kinloch, N., and Yates, C. M.: Monoamine metabolites in cerebrospinal fluid in multiple sclerosis. J. Neurol. Neurosurg. Psychiat., *40*:741–745, 1977.
88. Davison, A. N., and Cuzner, M. L.: Immunochemistry and biochemistry of myelin. Brit. Med. Bull., *33*:60–66, 1977.
89. Davson, H.: Physiology of the Ocular and Cerebrospinal Fluids. London, J. & A. Churchill, Ltd., 1956.
90. Davson, H.: *In* Field, J., Magoun, H. W., and Hall, V. E., eds.: Handbook of Physiology. Washington, D.C., American Physiological Society, 1960. Vol. 3. p. 1961.
91. Davson, H.: Physiology of the Cerebrospinal Fluid. London, J. & A. Churchill, Ltd., 1967.
92. Davson, H.: Dynamic aspects of cerebrospinal fluid. Develop. Med. Child Neurol., *14*:suppl. 27:1–16, 1972.
93. Davson, H., and Segal, M. G.: Effect of cerebrospinal fluid on volume of distribution of extracellular markers. Brain, *92*:131–136, 1969.
94. Davson, H., Domer, F., and Hollingsworth, J.: The mechanism of drainage of the cerebrospinal fluid. Brain, *96*:329, 1973.
95. Davson, H., Hollingsworth, G., and Segal, M. B.: The mechanism of drainage of the cerebrospinal fluid. Brain, *93*:665–678, 1970.
96. Davson, H., Kleeman, C. R., and Levin, E.: Quantitative studies of the passage of differential substances out of the cerebrospinal fluid. J. Physiol. (London), *161*:126, 1962.
97. Dayan, A. D.: Viral antigen in cells of lumbar cerebrospinal fluid. Lancet, *1*:437–438, 1973.
98. Dayan, A. D., and Stokes, M. I.: Rapid diagnosis of encephalitis by immunofluorescent examination of cerebrospinal fluid cells. Lancet, *1*:177, 1973.
99. DeJong, R. N., ed.: Cerebrospinal fluid syndromes. *In* The Neurologic Examination. 4th Ed. New York, Hoeber, Harper & Row, 1979.
100. Delmotte, P.: Analysis of complex protein mixtures by capillary isotachophoresis. Some qualitative and quantitative aspects. Science Tools, *24*: No. 3, 1977.
101. Delmotte, P.: Comparative results of agar electrophoresis and isoelectric focusing examination of the gammaglobulins of the cerebrospinal fluid. Acta Neurol. Belg., *72*:226, 1972.
102. Dencker, S. J.: Variation of total cerebrospinal fluid proteins and cells with sex and age. World Neurol., *3*:778–781, 1962.
103. Dencker, S. J.: Quantification of individual CSF proteins by immune precipitation in agar gel. J. Neurochem., *16*:465–466, 1969.
104. Dencker, S. J., and Swahn, B.: Clinical Value of Protein Analysis in Cerebrospinal Fluid, a Micro-Immunoelectrophoretic Study. Lund, AB C.W.K. Gleerup Bokförlag, 1961.
105. Dencker, S. J., Brönnestam, R. and Swahn, B.: Demonstration of large blood proteins in cerebrospinal fluid. Neurology (Minneap.), *11*:441–444, 1961.
106. Denis, W., and Ayer, J. B.: A method for the quantitative determination of protein in cerebrospinal fluid. Arch. Intern. Med. (Chicago), *26*:436, 1920.
107. Dewhurst, K.: Composition of cerebrospinal fluid in neurosyphilitic psychoses. Acta Neurol. Scand., *45*:119, 1969.
108. DiChiro, G.: Observations on the circulation of the cerebrospinal fluid. Acta Radiol. [Diagn.] (Stockholm), *5*:988–1002, 1966.
109. DiChiro, G., Hammock, M., and Bleyer, W.: Spinal descent of cerebrospinal fluid in man. Neurology (Minneap.), *26*:1, 1976.
110. DiGiovanni, A. J., and Dunbar, B. S.: Epidural injections of autologous blood for postlumbar-puncture headache. Anesth. Analg. (Cleveland), *49*:268–271, 1971.
111. DiMattio, J., Hochwald, G., Malhan, C., and Wald, A.: Effects of changes in serum osmolarity on bulk flow of fluid into cerebral ventricles and on brain water content. Pfluger. Arch., *359*:253, 1975.
112. Dohrmann, G. J.: The choroid plexus: Historical review. Brain Res., *18*:197, 1970.
113. Dommasch, D.: Monocytes and histiocytes in

cell cultures of cerebrospinal fluid. J. Neurol., *209*:103, 1975.

113a. Domschke, W., Dickschas, A., and Mitzness, P.: C.S.F. beta-endorphin in schizophrenia. Lancet, *2*:425, 1979.

114. Drayer, B. P., and Rosenbaum, A. E.: Pediatric metrizamide CT cisternography: Cerebrospinal fluid circulation and hydrocephalus. Neurology (Minneap.), *28*:71–77, 1978.

115. Drewinko, B., Sullivan, M. P., and Martin, T.: Use of the cytocentrifuge in the diagnosis of meningeal leukemia. Cancer, *31*:1331, 1973.

116. Duffy, P. E., Simon, J., Defendini, R., and Karalian, S.: The study of cells in cerebrospinal fluid by electron microscopy. A new method. Arch. Neurol. (Chicago), *21*:358–362, 1969.

117. Duma, R. J., Helwig, W. B., and Martinez, A. J.: Meningoencephalitis and brain abscess due to a free-living amoeba. Ann. Intern. Med., *88*:468–473, 1978.

118. DuPont, A., Villeneuve, A., Bouchard, J. P., et al.: Rapid inactivation of enkephalin-like material by C.S.F. in chronic schizophrenia. Lancet, *2*:1107, 1978.

119. Dykes, J. R. W., and Stevens, D. L.: Alterations in lumbar cerebrospinal fluid protein during air encephalography. Brit. Med. J., *1*:79–81, 1970.

120. Editors: Lymphatic drainage of the brain. Experientia, *24*:1283, 1968.

121. Editors: The outflow pathways of aqueous and cerebrospinal fluid. Lancet, *2*:31, 1973.

122. Editors: Cerebrospinal fluid: The lymph of the brain? Lancet, *2*:444, 1975.

123. Editors: Benign intracranial hypertension. Lancet, *2*:1007, 1976.

124. Editors: Intracranial pressure in childhood convulsions. Lancet, *1*:139, 1979.

125. Egg, D., Herold, M., and Rumpl, E.: Prostaglandin F_2 alpha in cerebrospinal fluid after stroke. Lancet, *1*:990, 1978.

126. Eisenberg, H., McComb, G., and Lorenzo, A.: Cerebrospinal fluid overproduction and hydrocephalus associated with choroid plexus papilloma. J. Neurosurg., *40*:381, 1974.

127. Ekstedt, J.: CSF hydrodynamic studies in man: 1. Method of constant pressure CSF infusion. J. Neurol. Neurosurg. Psychiat., *40*:105–119, 1977.

128. Ellner, J. J., and Bennett, J. E.: Chronic meningitis. Medicine (Balt.), *55*:341–369, 1976.

129. Engelhardt, P., and Avenarius, H. J.: Der diagnostische Wert von Enzymbestimmungen im Liquor cerebrospinalis. Med. Klin., *71*:699–702, 1976.

130. Esiri, M.: Immunoglobulin containing cells in multiple sclerosis plaques. Lancet, *2*:478–480, 1977.

131. Eveland, W. C.: Fluorescent antibody tests in medical diagnosis. Public Health Lab., *24*:41, 1966.

132. Fallon, R. J.: Diagnosis and prognosis in pyogenic meningitis. Lancet, *1*:1411, 1976.

133. Feinbloom, R. I., and Alpert, J. J.: The value of routine glucose determination in spinal fluid without pleocytosis. J. Pediat., *75*:121–123, 1969.

134. Feinglass, E. J., Amett, F. C., Dorsch, C. A., Zizic, T. M., and Stevens, M. B.: Neuropsychiatric manifestations of SLE. Medicine (Balt.), *55*:323–339, 1976.

135. Feldman, W. E.: Effect of prior antibiotic therapy on concentrations of bacteria in cerebrospinal fluid. J.A.M.A., *240*:399, 1978. (abstract)

136. Ferry, D. J., Gooding, R., Standefer, J. C., and Wiese, G. M.: Effect of Pantopaque myelography on cerebrospinal fluid fractions. J. Neurosurg., *38*:167–171, 1973.

137. Field, E.: The production of γ-globulin in the central nervous system. J. Neurol. Neurosurg. Psychiat., *17*:228–232, 1954.

138. Fisher, R.: The cerebrospinal fluid. Mayo Clin. Proc., *50*:482–486, 1975.

139. Fishman, R. A.: Exchange of albumin between plasma and cerebrospinal fluid. Amer. J. Physiol., *175*:96–98, 1953.

140. Fishman, R. A.: Carrier transport of glucose between blood and cerebrospinal fluid. Amer. J. Physiol., *206*:836, 1964.

141. Fishman, R. A.: Occult hydrocephalus. New Eng. J. Med., *274*:466, 1966.

142. Fishman, R. A.: Cerebrospinal fluid: A review of recent clinical advances. *In* Tower, D., ed.: The Nervous System. Vol. 2, The Clinical Neurosciences. New York, Raven Press, 1975, pp. 55–60.

143. Fishman, R. A.: Cerebrospinal Fluid in Diseases of the Nervous System. Philadelphia, W. B. Saunders Co., 1980.

144. Flexner, L. B.: The chemistry and nature of the cerebrospinal fluid. Physiol. Rev., *14*:161, 1934.

145. Foldi, M.: Lymphatic drainage of the brain. Lancet, *2*:930, 1975.

146. Forbes, I. J., and Henderson, D. W.: Globulin synthesis by human peripheral lymphocytes. In vitro measurements using lymphocytes from normals and patients with disease. Ann. Intern. Med., *65*:69–79, 1966.

147. Ford, D.: Blood-brain barrier: A regulatory mechanism. *In* Ehrenpreis, S., and Kopin, J. J., eds.: Reviews of Neuroscience. Vol. 2. New York, Raven Press, 1976.

148. Fraser, K. B.: Multiple sclerosis: A virus disease? Brit. Med. Bull., *33*:34–39, 1977.

149. Frick, E.: Lipid- und Kohlenhydratelektrophorese des Liquor cerebrospinalis. *In* Schmidt, R., ed.: Der Liquor Cerebrospinalis. Berlin, VEB Verlag, 1968.

150. Frick, E.: Immunologische Untersuchungen zur Identifizierung einzelner Liquoreiweisskörper. Klin. Wschr., *38*:1135–1139, 1960.

151. Frick, E., and Scheid-Seydel, L.: Untersuchungen mit J^{131}-markiertem Albumin über Austauschvorgänge zwischen Plasma und Liquor cerebrospinalis. Klin. Wschr., *36*:66–69, 1958.

152. Frick, E., and Scheid-Seydel, L.: Untersuchungen mit J^{131}-markiertem Globulin zur Frage der Abstammung der Liquoreiweisskörper. Klin. Wschr., *36*:857–863, 1958.

153. Frick, E., and Scheid-Seydel L.: Untersuchungen mit J^{131}-markiertem Globulin zur Frage der Abstammung der Liquoreiweisskörper. Klin. Wschr., *38*:1240–1243, 1960.

154. Froin, G.: Inflammations meningées avec reactions chromatique, fibrineuse, et cytologique

du liquide cephalorachidien. Gaz. Hôp., *76*:1005, 1903.

155. Fryden, A., Link, H., and Moller, E.: Demonstration of cerebrospinal fluid lymphocytes sensitized against virus antigens in mumps meningitis. Acta Neurol. Scand., *57*:396, 1978.

155a. Fumagalli, R., and Paoletti, P.: Sterol test for human brain tumors: Relationship with different oncotypes. Neurology (Minneap.), *21*: 1149–1156, 1971.

156. Funder, J., and Wieth, J. O.: Changes in cerebrospinal fluid composition following hemodialysis. Scand. J. Clin. Lab. Invest., *19*:301–312, 1967.

157. Gangji, D., Collard-Ronge, E., Balleriaux-Waha, D., et al.: T lymphocytes in cerebrospinal fluid. New Eng. J. Med., *294*:902, 1976.

158. Gilland, O.: Normal cerebrospinal fluid pressure. New Eng. J. Med., *280*:904, 1969.

159. Gilland, O., and Nelson, J. R.: Lumbar cerebrospinal fluid electromanometrics with a minitransducer. Neurology (Minneap.), *20*:103, 1970.

160. Gilland, O., Tourtellotte, W. W., O'Tauma, L., and Henderson, W. G.: Normal cerebrospinal fluid pressure. J. Neurosurg., *40*:587–593, 1974.

161. Glaeser, B. S., and Hare, T. A.: Measurement of GABA in human cerebrospinal fluid. Biochem. Med., *12*:274–282, 1975.

162. Glasner, H.: Barrier impairment and immune reaction in the cerebrospinal fluid. Europ. Neurol., *13*:304, 1975.

163. Glass, B., Collipp, P. J., and Waldman, M. A.: Viral and bacterial meningitis. New York J. Med., *71*:2182, 1971.

164. Goldstein, G. W., Chaplin, E. R., and Maitland, J.: Transient hydrocephalus in premature infants: Treatment by lumbar punctures. Lancet, *1*:512–514, 1976.

165. Goldstein, N. P., McKenzie, B. F., and McGuckin, W. F.: Changes in cerebrospinal fluid of patients with multiple sclerosis after treatment with intrathecal methylprednisolone acetate: A preliminary report. Proc. Staff Meet. Mayo Clin., *37*:657, 1962.

166. Goldstein, N., McKenzie, B., McGuckin, W., and Mattox, V.: Experimental, intrathecal administration of methylprednisolone acetate in multiple sclerosis. Trans. Amer. Neurol. Ass., *95*:243, 1970.

167. Gomez, D., Potts, D., and Deonarine, V.: Arachnoid granulations of the sheep, stuctural and ultrastructural changes with varying pressure differences. Arch. Neurol. (Chicago), *30*:169, 1974.

168. Gomez, D., Chamber, A., Di Benedetto, A., and Potts, D.: The spinal cerebrospinal fluid absorptive pathways. Neuroradiology, *8*:61, 1974.

169. Gondos, B.: Cytology of cerebrospinal fluid: Technical and diagnosis considerations. Ann. Clin. Lab. Sci., *6*:152, 1976.

170. Gondos, B., and King, E.: Cerebrospinal fluid cytology: Diagnostic accuracy and comparison of different techniques. Acta Cytol. (Balt.), *20*:542, 1976.

171. Gordon, E., and Rossanda, M.: The importance of the cerebrospinal fluid acid-base status in the treatment of unconscious patients with brain lesions. Acta Anaesth. Scand., *12*:51–73, 1968.

172. Grainger, R. G.: Lumbar myelography with metrizamide—a new nonionic contrast medium. Brit. J. Radiol., *49*:996–1003, 1976.

173. Greitz, T., and Hindmarsh, T.: Computer assisted tomography of intracranial CSF circulation using a water-soluble contrast medium. Acta Radiol. [Diagn.] (Stockholm), *15*:497, 1974.

174. Grinker, R. R., Bucy, P. C., and Sahs, A. L.: Neurology. Springfield, Ill., Charles C Thomas, 1960.

175. Hadler, N. M., Gerwin, R. D., Frank, M. M., et al.: The fourth component of complement in the cerebrospinal fluid in systemic lupus erythematosus. Arthritis Rheum., *16*:507–518, 1973.

175a. Haerer, A. F.: Pyruvate, citrate, alphaketoglutarate and glucose in the CSF and blood of neurologic patients. Acta Neurol. Scand., *48*:306–312, 1972.

176. Haerer, A. F., and Tourtellotte, W. W.: Postlumbar puncture headaches. New Eng. J. Med., *290*:1262, 1974.

177. Haerer, A. F., Tourtellotte, W. W., Richard, K. A., et al.: A study of the blood–cerebrospinal fluid–brain barrier in multiple sclerosis. I. Blood–cerebrospinal fluid barrier to sodium bromide. Neurology (Minneap.), *14*:345–354, 1964.

178. Haire, M.: Significance of virus antibodies in multiple sclerosis. Brit. Med. Bull., *33*:40–44, 1977.

179. Haire, M., Millar, J., and Merrett, J.: Measles virus–specific IgG in cerebrospinal fluid in multiple sclerosis. Brit. Med. J., *4*:192, 1974.

180. Halliday, A. M., and McDonald, W. I.: Pathophysiology of demyelinating disease. Brit. Med. Bull., *33*:21–27, 1977.

181. Hammock, M., and Milhorat, T.: The cerebrospinal fluid: Current concepts of its formation. Ann. Clin. Lab. Sci., *6*:22–26, 1976.

182. Hansen, E. B., Fahrendrug, A., and Praesthold, J.: Late meningeal effects of myelographic contrast media with special reference to metrizamide. Brit. J. Radiol., *51*:321, 1978.

183. Harris, W. H., and Sonnenblick, E. D.: A study of calcium and magnesium in the cerebrospinal fluid. Biol. Med., *27*:297–303, 1955.

184. Harter, D. H., and Yahr, M. D.: Cerebrospinal fluid changes in meningitis. Int. J. Neurol., *4*:113, 1964.

185. Harter, D. H., Yahr, M. D., and Kabat, E. A.: Neurological disease with elevation of cerebrospinal fluid γ-globulin: A critical review. Trans. Amer. Neurol. Ass., *87*:210–212, 1962.

186. Hass, W. K., and Hochwald, G. M.: Studies of cerebrospinal fluid proteins precipitated by zinc sulfate solutions. Neurology (Minneap.), *11*:1071–1075, 1961.

187. Hedlund, L., Lischko, M., Rollag, M., and Niswender, G.: Melatonin: Daily cycle in plasma and cerebrospinal fluid in calves. Science, *195*:686–687, 1976.

188. Heiblim, D. I., Evans, H. E., Glass, L., and Agbayani, M. M.: Amino acid concentrations in cerebrospinal fluid. Arch. Neurol. (Chicago), *35*:765–768, 1978.

189. Held, D., Fence, V., and Pappenheimer, J. R.: Electrical potential of cerebrospinal fluid. J. Neurophysiol., *27*:942–959, 1964.

190. Herndon, R. M., and Kasckow, J.: Electron microscopic studies of cerebrospinal fluid sediment in demyelinating disease. Ann. Neurol., *4*:515–523, 1978.

191. Herndon, R. M., and Johnson, J.: A method for the electron microscopic study of cerebrospinal fluid sediment. J. Neuropath. Exp. Neurol., *29*:320–330, 1970.

192. Hindersin, P., and Heidrich, R.: Fibrinogen degradation product concentration (SFP) as a diagnostic parameter for the differentiation of artificial and essential blood in cerebrospinal fluid. Psychiat. Neurol. Med. Psychol. (Leipzig), *30*:36–39, 1978.

193. Hochwald, G. M.: Influx of serum proteins and their concentration in spinal fluid along the neuraxis. J. Neurol. Sci., *10*:269, 1970.

194. Hochwald, G. M., and Wallenstein, M.: Exchange of albumin between blood, cerebrospinal fluid and brain in the cat. Amer. J. Physiol., *212*:1199– 1204, 1967.

195. Hochwald, G. M., and Wallenstein, M.: Exchange of γ-globulin between blood, cerebrospinal fluid and brain in the cat. Exp. Neurol., *19*:115–126, 1967.

196. Hoeprich, P.: Acute bacterial meningitis. *In* Hoeprich, R., ed.: Infectious Diseases. 2nd Ed. New York, Harper & Row, 1977.

197. Hoffman, A. A., Harbeck, R. J., Hoffman, S. A., and Shucard, D. W.: Altered cerebrospinal fluid (CSF) composition in experimental immune complex disease. Seventh Annual Meeting of Neuroscience, Anaheim, November 6–10, 1977.

198. Hosfield, W. B.: Management and complications of acute bacterial meningitis. Postgrad. Med., *50*:100, 1971.

199. Hourani, B. T., Hamlin, E. M., and Reynolds, T. B.: Cerebrospinal fluid glutamine as a measure of hepatic encephalopathy. Arch. Intern. Med. (Chicago), *127*:1033–1036, 1971.

200. Hughes, J., and Kosterlitz, H. W.: Opioid peptides. Brit. Med. Bull., *33*:157–161, 1977.

201. Huizinga, J. D., Teelken, A. W., Muskiet, F. A. J., Muellen, J. V. D., and Wolthers, B. G.: Identification of GABA in human CSF by gas liquid chromatography and mass spectrometry. New Eng. J. Med., *296*:692, 1977.

202. Hussey, F., Schanzer, B., and Katzman, R.: A simple constant-infusion manometric test for measurement of CSF absorption. II. Clinical Studies. Neurology (Minneap.), *20*:665–680, 1970.

203. Hyyppä, M. T., Långvik, V. A., Nieminen, V., and Vapalahta, M.: Tryptophan and monoamine metabolites in ventricular cerebrospinal fluid after severe cerebral trauma. Lancet, *1*:1367–1368, 1977.

204. Jaffe, H. W.: Laboratory diagnosis of syphilis. Ann. Intern. Med., *83*:846–850, 1975.

205. James, A., McComb, J., Christian, J., and Davson, H.: The effect of cerebrospinal fluid pressure on the size of drainage pathways. Neurology (Minneap.), *26*:659, 1976.

206. Janeway, C. A., Rosen, F. S., Merler, E., and Alper, C. A.: The Gamma Globulins. Boston, Little, Brown & Co., 1967.

207. Jeffcoate, W. J., Rees, L. H., McLoughlin, L., et al.: β-Endorphin in human cerebrospinal fluid. Lancet, *2*:119–121, 1978.

208. Jeffs, G., and Kaldor, J.: Cerebrospinal fluid fructose-biphosphate aldolase (aldolase) activity in infectious diseases of the central nervous system. Pathology, *8*:293, 1976.

209. Johnston, I.: Reduced CSF absorption syndrome, reappraisal of benign intracranial hypertension and related conditions. Lancet, *2*:418, 1973.

210. Johnson, R. T., and Richardson, E. P.: The neurological manifestations of systemic lupus erythematosus. Medicine (Balt.), *47*:337–369, 1968.

211. Johnson, R.: Cerebrospinal fluid. *In* Goldensohn, E. S., and Appel, S. H., eds.: Scientific Approaches to Clinical Neurology. Philadelphia, Lea & Febiger, 1977.

212. Jordan, R. M., Kendal, J. W., Seaich, J. L., et al.: Cerebrospinal fluid hormone concentration in the evaluation of pituitary tumors. Ann. Intern. Med., *85*:49–55, 1976.

213. Kabat, E. A., Glusman, M., and Knaub, V.: Quantitative estimation of the albumin and gamma-globulin in normal and pathologic cerebrospinal fluid by immunochemical methods. Amer. J. Med., *4*:653, 1948.

214. Kabat, E. A., Moore, D. H., and Landow, H.: An electrophoretic study of the protein components in cerebrospinal fluid and their relationship to the serum proteins. J. Clin. Invest., *21*:571–577, 1942.

215. Kabat, E. A., Freedman, D. A., Murray, J. P., and Knaub, V.: A study of the crystalline albumin, γ-globulin and total protein in the cerebrospinal fluid of 100 cases of multiple sclerosis and in other diseases. Amer. J. Med. Sci., *219*:55–64, 1950.

216. Katzenelbogen, S.: The Cerebrospinal Fluid and Its Relations to the Blood: A Physiological and Clinical Study. Baltimore, Md., The Johns Hopkins Press, 1935.

217. Katzman, R.: The distribution of inulin and sucrose in the brain, evidence against the sink action of the CSF. Trans. Amer. Neurol. Ass., *93*:128–132, 1968.

218. Katzman, R.: Blood-brain barriers. *In* Siegel, G. J., et al., eds.: Basic Neurochemistry. Boston, Little, Brown & Co., 1976.

219. Katzman, R., and Hussey, R.: A simple constant-infusion manometric test for measurement of CSF absorption: I Rationale and Method. Neurology (Minneap.), *20*:534–544, 1970.

220. Katzman, R., and Pappius, H. M.: Hydrocephalus. Chapter 17 *in* Brain Electrolytes and Fluid Metabolism. Baltimore, Md., Williams & Wilkins, 1973.

221. Katzman, R., and Pappius, H. M.: Formation, absorption, and circulation of the cerebrospinal fluid. Chapter 2 *in* Brain Electrolytes and Fluid Metabolism. Baltimore, Md., Williams & Wilkins, 1973.

222. Kaufman, R. E., Olansky, D. C., and Weisner, P. J.: FTA-ABS (IgM) test for neonatal congenital syphilis: A critical review. J. Amer. Vener. Dis. Ass., *1*:79–84, 1974.
223. Kennedy, D., and Fallon, R.: Tuberculous meningitis. J.A.M.A., *241*:264, 1979.
224. Kerenyi, L., Hegedus, K., and Palffy, G.: Characteristic gamma globulin subfractions of native CSF in multiple sclerosis. Brain Res., *87*:123, 1975.
225. Kjellin, K. G.: The CSF iron in patients with neurological diseases. Acta Neurol. Scand., *43*:299–313, 1967.
226. Kjellin, K. G., and Besterberg, O.: Isoelectric focusing of CSF proteins in neurologic diseases. J. Neurol. Sci., *23*:199, 1974.
227. Kjellin, K. G., and Stibler, H.: Isoelectric focusing and electrophoresis of cerebrospinal fluid proteins in muscular dystrophies and spinal muscular atrophies. J. Neurol. Sci., *27*:45, 1976.
228. Knight, S. C.: Cellular immunity in multiple sclerosis. Brit. Med. Bull., *33*:45–49, 1977.
229. Kolar, O., and Zeman, W.: Spinal fluid cytomorphology. Arch. Neurol. (Chicago), *18*:44, 1968.
230. Kolmel, H.: Atlas of Cerebrospinal Fluid Cells. Berlin, Springer Verlag, 1976.
231. Komorowski, R. A., Farmer, S. G., Hanson, G. A., and Hause, L. L.: Cerebrospinal fluid lactic acid in diagnosis of meningitis. J. Clin. Microbiol., *8*:89, 1978.
232. Krauss, A. N., Thibeault, D. W., and Auld, P. A. M.: Acid-base balance in cerebrospinal fluid of newborn infants. Biol. Neonat., *21*:25–34, 1972.
233. Kronholm, V.: Spectrophotometric investigation of spinal fluid. World Neurol., *2*:435–441, 1961.
233a. Kuberski, T.: Eosinophils in the cerebrospinal fluid. Ann. Intern. Med., *91*:70–75, 1979.
234. Kubinski, H., and Manucher, J.: Proteins from human cerebrospinal fluid: Binding with nucleic acids. Science, *182*:296, 1974.
235. Labadie, E. L., Hamilton, R. H., Lundell, D. C., and Bjelland, J. C.: Hypoliquorreic headache and pneumocephalus caused by thoraco-subarachnoid fistula. Neurology (Minneap.), *27*:993–995, 1977.
236. Laglia, A. G., Eisenberg, R. L., Weinstein, P. R., and Mani, R. L.: Spinal epidural hematoma after lumbar puncture in liver disease. Ann. Intern. Med., *88*:515–516, 1978.
237. Lakke, J. P. W. F.: Queckenstedt's Test. Amsterdam, Excerpta Medica Foundation, 1969.
238. Lakke, J. P. W. F., and Teelken, A. W.: Amino acid abnormalities in cerebrospinal fluid of patients with parkinsonism and extrapyramidal disorders. Neurology (Minneap.), *26*:489–493, 1976.
239. Lamoureux, G., Lolicoeur, R., Giard, N., St-Hilaire, M., and Duplantis, F.: Cerebrospinal fluid proteins in multiple sclerosis. Neurology (Minneap.), *25*:537, 1975.
240. Laterre, E. C.: Les Protéines du Liquide Céphalorachidien à l'Etat Normal et Pathologique. Bruxelles, Arscia, 1965.
241. Latner, A.: Some clinical biochemical aspects of isoelectric focusing. Ann. N.Y. Acad. Sci., *209*:281, 1973.
242. Latovitzki, N., Abrams, G., Clark, C., Mayeux, R., Ascherl, G., Jr., and Sciarra, D.: Cerebral cysticercosis. Neurology (Minneap.), *28*:838–842, 1978.
243. Lauwers, S.: Lactic-acid concentration in cerebrospinal fluid and differential diagnosis of meningitis. Lancet, *2*:163, 1978.
243a. Lee, T. J., and Sparling, P. F.: Syphilis: An algorithm. J.A.M.A., *242*:1187–1189, 1979.
244. Lemmen, L. J., Tourtellotte, W. W., Glimm, J. G., Higgins, J. E., and Parker, J. A.: Study of cerebrospinal fluid proteins with paper electrophoresis IV. Methods for concentrating dilute protein solutions. Univ. Mich. Med. Bull., *23*:135–138, 1957.
245. Lennette, D. A., Emmons, R. W., and Lennette, E. H.: Rapid diagnosis of mumps virus infections by immunofluorescence methods. J. Clin. Microbiol., *2*:81, 1976.
246. Lepkifker, E., and Lewin, L.: Elevated myo-inositol concentrations in cerebrospinal fluid of neonates and of patients with an impaired state of consciousness. Biomedicine [Express], *25*:368–371, 1976.
247. Levine, M. C., and White, D. W.: Chronic post-myelographic headache. A result of persistent epidural cerebrospinal fluid fistula. J.A.M.A., *229*:684–686, 1974.
248. Levinson, A. I., Lisak, R. P., and Zweiman, B.: Immunologic characterization of cerebrospinal fluid lymphocytes: Preliminary report. Neurology (Minneap.), *26*:693, 1976.
249. Levy, N. L., and Schoen, T. M.: Spinal fluid from patients with multiple sclerosis contains nucleotide-rich material associated with IgG. (Part 2) Neurology (Minneap.), *26*:62, 1976.
250. Lewis, A.: Mechanisms of Neurologic Disease. Boston, Little, Brown, & Co., 1976.
251. Lieberman, L. M., Tourtellotte, W. W., and Newkirk, T. A.: Prolonged post-lumbar puncture cerebrospinal fluid leakage from lumbar subarachnoid space demonstrated by radioisotope myelography. Neurology (Minneap.), *21*:925–929, 1971.
252. Liebeskind, A. L., Herz, D. A., Rosenthal, A. D., and Freeman, L. M.: Radionuclide demonstration of spinal dural leaks. J. Nucl. Med., *14*:356–358, 1973.
253. Link, H.: Immunoglobulin-G and low molecular weight proteins in human cerebrospinal fluid: Chemical and immunological characterization with special reference to multiple sclerosis. Acta Neurol. Scand., *43*:suppl. 28:1–136, 1967.
254. Link, H., and Tibbling, G.: Principles of albumin and IgG analyses in neurological disorders. III. Evaluation of IgG synthesis within the central nervous system in multiple sclerosis. Scand. J. Clin. Lab. Invest., *37*:397–401, 1977.
255. Link, H., Zettervall, O., and Blennow, G.: Individual cerebro-spinal fluid (CSF) proteins in the evaluation of increased CSF total protein. Z. Neurol., *203*:119, 1972.
256. Lippincott, S. W., Korman, S., Lax, L. C., and Corcoran, C.: Transfer rates of γ-globulin between cerebrospinal fluid and blood plasma (results obtained on a series of multiple sclerosis patients). J. Nucl. Med., *6*:632–644, 1965.
257. Lisak, R. P., and Zweiman, B.: In vitro cell-me-

diated immunity of cerebrospinal-fluid lymphocytes to myelin basic protein in primary demyelinating diseases. New Eng. J. Med., *297*:850, 1977.

258. Loewenich, V. V., and Konrath, B.: Neugeborenen-Meningitis: Prognose in Abhängigkeit von diagnostischem und therapeutischem Vorgehen. Mschr. Kinderheilk., *122*:405–406, 1974.
259. Logothetis, J.: Cerebrospinal fluid free amino acids in neurologic diseases. Neurology (Minneap.), *8*:374–376, 1958.
260. Lord, R. A., Goldblum, R. M., Forman, P. M., et al.: Cerebrospinal-fluid IgM in the absence of serum-IgM in combined immunodeficiency. Lancet, *2*:528–529, 1973.
261. Lorenzo, A., Bresna, M., and Barlow, C.: Cerebrospinal fluid absorption deficit in normal pressure hydrocephalus. Arch. Neurol. (Chicago), *30*:387, 1974.
262. Lowenthal, A.: Agar Gel Electrophoresis in Neurology. Amsterdam, Elsevier–North Holland Publishing Co., 1964.
263. Lowry, O. H., Rosebrough, N. H., Farr, A. L., and Randall, R. J.: Protein measurement with the Folin phenol reagent. J. Biol. Chem., *193*:265–275, 1951.
264. Lumsden, C. E.: *In* Wolstenholm, G. E. W., and O'Connor, C. M., eds.: The Cerebrospinal Fluid. Ciba Foundation Symposium. Boston, Little, Brown & Co., 1958, p. 97.
265. Lumsden, C. E.: Problems in the cytology of cerebrospinal fluid. Arch. De Vecchi Anat. Pat., *31*:319–338, 1960.
266. Lumsden, C. E.: The proteins of cerebrospinal fluid in multiple sclerosis. *In* McAlpine, D., Lumsden, C. E., and Acheson, E. D., eds.: Multiple Sclerosis: A Reappraisal. Baltimore, Md., Williams & Wilkins, 1965, pp. 252–299.
267. Lumsden, C. E.: The clinical immunology of multiple sclerosis. *In* McAlpine, D., Lumsden, C. E., and Acheson, E. D., eds.: Multiple Sclerosis: A Reappraisal. Baltimore, Md., Williams & Wilkins, 1965, pp. 345–380.
268. Lundberg, N.: Continuous recording and control of ventricular fluid pressure in neurosurgical practice. Acta Psychiat. Neurol. Scand., *36*:suppl. 149:1, 1960.
269. Lups, S., and Haan, A. M. F. H.: The Cerebrospinal Fluid., Amsterdam, Elsevier Publishing Co., 1956.
270. Luxon, L., Lees, A. J., and Greenwood, R. J.: Neurosyphilis today. Lancet, *1*:90–93, 1979.
271. Ma, B. I., and Tourtellotte, W. W.: A sensitive technic for identifying immunoglobulin-G oligoclones by immunofixation in cerebrospinal fluid (CSF). Amer. J. Clin. Path., *67*:210, 1977.
272. Maker, S. M., Clarke, D. D., and Lajtha, A. L.: Intermediary metabolism of carbohydrates and amino acids. *In* Siegel, G. J., et al., eds.: Basic Neurochemistry. 2nd Ed. Boston, Little, Brown & Co., 1976.
273. Manconi, P. E., Zaccheo, D., Bugiani, O., et al.: T and B lymphocytes in normal cerebrospinal fluid. New Eng. J. Med., *294*:49, 1976.
274. Manconi, P. E., Marrosu, M. G., Spissu, A., Todde, P. F., and Ferelli, A.: Plasma cell reaction in cerebrospinal fluid: An additional case report. Neurology (Minneap.), *28*:856, 1978.
275. Mann, J. D., Butler, A. B., Rosenthal, J. E., Maffeo, C. J., Johnson, R. N., and Bass, N. H.: Regulation of intracranial pressure in rat, dog, and man. Ann. Neurol., *3*:156, 1978.
276. Marks, V., and Marrack, D.: Tumor cells in the cerebrospinal fluid. J. Neurol. Neurosurg. Psychiat., *23*:194, 1960.
277. Marlin, A., Wald, A., Hochwald, G., and Malhan, C.: On the movement of fluid through the brain of hydrocephalic cats. Neurology (Minneap.), *26*:1159, 1976.
278. Marmarou, A., Shulman, K., and LaMorgese, J.: Compartmental analysis of compliance and outflow resistance of the cerebrospinal fluid system. J. Neurosurg., *43*:523, 1975.
278a. Marriott, P. J., O'Brien, M. D., Mackenzie, I. C. K., and Janota, I.: Progressive multifocal leucoencephalopathy: Remission with cytarabine. J. Neurol. Neurosurg. Psychiat., *38*:205–209, 1975.
279. Martin, G.: Lundberg's B-waves as a feature of normal intracranial pressure. Surg. Neurol., *9*:347–348, 1978.
280. Masserman, J. H.: Cerebrospinal hydrodynamics. IV. Clinical experimental studies. Arch. Neurol. Psychiat., *32*:523–553, 1934.
281. Masserman, J. H.: Correlations of the pressure of the cerebrospinal fluid with age, blood pressure, and the pressure index. Arch. Neurol. Psychiat., *34*:564–566, 1935.
282. Matakas, F., Waechter, R. V., Knupling, R., and Potolicchio, J.: Increase in cerebral perfusion pressure by arterial hypertension in brain swelling. J. Neurosurg., *42*:282, 1975.
283. Maurer, J., and Rieder, H. P.: Totalprotein und elektrophoretische Proteinfraktionen des Liquors im Kindesalter. Schweiz. Med. Wschr., *108*:1854–1860, 1978.
284. McCracken, G. H., and Sarff, L. D.: Endotoxin in cerebrospinal fluid. Detection in neonates with bacterial meningitis. J.A.M.A., *235*:617–620, 1976.
285. McDonald, J. V.: Persistent hydrocephalus following the removal of papillomas of the choroid plexus of the lateral ventricles. Report of two cases. J. Neurosurg., *30*:736–740, 1969.
286. McEntee, W. J., and Mair, R. G.: Memory impairment in Korsakoff's psychosis: A correlation with brain noradrenergic activity. Science, *202*:905–907, 1978.
287. McHugh, R., et al.: Dynamics of the Cerebrospinal Fluid in Health and Disease: Scientific Basics, Tests, and Models (Selected Reprints). VA Technical Book WT/AP VIII 77, Los Angeles, 1977.
288. McKenna, C., Schroeter, A., Kierland, R., Stilwell, G., and Pien, F.: The fluorescent treponemal antibody absorbed (FTA-ABS) test beading phenomenon in connective tissue diseases. Mayo Clin. Proc., *48*:545, 1973.
289. McKinley, M. J., Blaine, E. H., and Denton, D. A.: Brain osmoreceptors, cerebrospinal fluid electrolyte composition and thirst. Brain Res., *70*:532–537, 1974.
290. McMenemey, W. H.: Immunity mechanisms in neurological disease. Proc. Roy. Soc. Med., *54*:127–136, 1961.
291. McQueen, J. D., Northrup, B. E., and Leibrock, L. G.: Arachnoid clearance of red blood cells.

J. Neurol. Neurosurg. Psychiat., *37*:1316–1321, 1974.

292. Merritt, H. H.: A Textbook of Neurology. 6th Ed. Philadelphia, Lea & Febiger, 1979.
293. Merritt, H. H., and Fremont-Smith, F.: The Cerebrospinal Fluid. Philadelphia, W. B. Saunders Co., 1937.
294. Merritt, H. H., and Sciarra, D.: *In* Harvey, J. C., ed.: Tice's Practice of Medicine. Vol. 9. Hagerstown, Md., W. F. Prior Co., Inc., 1962, p. 271.
295. Mestrezat, W.: Le Liquide Cephalo-Rachidien Normal et Pathologique. Thèse de Montpelier, 1911.
296. Mestrezat, W.: Le Liquide Cephalorachidien Normal et Pathologique: Valeur Clinique de l'Examen Chimique; Syndromes Humoraux dans les Diverses Affections. Paris, A. Maloine, 1912.
297. Meyer, J. S., Stoica, E., Pascu, I., et al.: Catecholamine concentrations in CSF and plasma of patients with cerebral infarction and haemorrhage. Brain, *96*:277–288, 1973.
298. Milhorat, T.: The third circulation revisited. J. Neurosurg., *42*:628–645, 1975.
299. Millen, J. W., and Woollam, D. H. M.: The Anatomy of the Cerebrospinal Fluid. London, Oxford University Press, 1962.
300. Mingioli, E., Strober, W., Tourtellotte, W., Whitaker, J., and McFarlin, D.: Quantitation of IgG, IgA, and IgM in the CSF by radioimmunoassay. Neurology (Minneap.), *28*:991, 1978.
301. Misra, S. S., Singh, K. S., and Bhargawa, K. P.: Estimation of 5-hydroxy-tryptamine (5-HT) level in cerebrospinal fluid of patients with intracranial or spinal lesions. J. Neurol. Neurosurg. Psychiat., *30*:163–165, 1967.
302. Mitchell, M. S., Marcus, B. B., and Biegeleisen, J. Z.: Immunofluorescence techniques for demonstrating bacterial pathogens associated with cerebrospinal meningitis. II. Growth, viability, and immunofluorescent staining of *Hemophilus influenzae, Neisseria meningitidis* and *Diplococcus pneumoniae* in cerebrospinal fluid. J. Lab. Clin. Med., *65*:990–1003, 1965.
303. Moir, A. T. B., Ashcroft, G. W., Crawford, T. B., et al.: Cerebral metabolites in cerebrospinal fluid as a biochemical approach to the brain. Brain, *93*:357–368, 1970.
304. Morariu, M. A.: Transient spastic paraparesis following abdominal aortography: Management with cerebrospinal fluid lavage. Ann. Neurol. *3*:185, 1978.
305. Morton, C. A.: The pathology of tuberculous meningitis, with reference to its treatment by tapping the subarachnoid space of the spinal cord. Brit. Med. J., *2*:840, 1891.
306. Moser, R. P., Robinson, J. A., and Prostko, E. R.: Lymphocyte subpopulations in human cerebrospinal fluid. Neurology (Minneap.), *26*:726, 1976.
307. Mutani, R., Monaco, F., Durelli, L., and Delsedime, M.: Free amino acids in the cerebrospinal fluid of epileptic subjects. Epilepsia, *15*:593–597, 1974.
307a. Nagai, Y., Kanfer, J. N., and Tourtellotte, W. W.: Preliminary observations of gangliosides of normal and multiple sclerosis cerebrospinal fluid. Neurology (Minneap.), *23*: 945–948, 1973.
308. Naylor, B., and Path, M. C.: The cytologic diagnosis of cerebrospinal fluid. Acta Cytol. (Balt.), *8*:141–149, 1964.
309. Neame, K.: A comparison of the transport systems for amino acids in brain, intestine, kidney and tumour. Brain Res., *29*:185–199, 1968.
309a. Neethling, A. C., McCarthy, B., and Taljaard, J. J. F.: Gamma-aminobutyric acid in CSF. Lancet, *1*:211, 1980.
310. Nelson, J., and Goodman, S.: An evaluation of the cerebrospinal fluid infusion test for hydrocephalus. Neurology (Minneap.), *21*:1037–1053, 1971.
311. Nelson, P. V., Carey, W. F., and Pollard, A. C.: Diagnostic significance and source of lactate dehydrogenase and its isoenzymes in cerebrospinal fluid of children with a variety of neurological disorders. J. Clin. Path., *28*:828, 1975.
312. Netsky, M., and Shuangshoti, S.: The Choroid Plexus in Health and Disease. Charlottesville, Va., University Press of Virginia, 1975.
313. Newman, J., Josephson, A. S., Cacatian, A., et al.: Spinal-fluid lysozyme in diagnosis of central-nervous-system tumours. Lancet, *2*:756, 1974.
314. Nickel, S. N., Frame, B., Bebin, J., Tourtellotte, W. W., Parker, J. A., and Hughes, B. R.: Myxedema neuropathy and myopathy. A clinical and pathologic study. Neurology (Minneap.), *11*:125–137, 1961.
315. Nielsen, H. A., and Reyn, A.: A treponema pallidum immobilization test. Bull. W.H.O., *14*: 263–288, 1956.
316. Norrby, E., and Vandvik, B.: Relationship between measles virus–specific antibody activities and oligoclonal IgG in the central nervous system of patients with subacute sclerosing panencephalitis and multiple sclerosis. Med. Mecrobiol. Immun. (Berlin), *162*:63, 1975.
317. Oehmichen, M.: Characterization of mononuclear phagocytes in human CSF using membrane markers. Acta Cytol. (Balt.), *20*:548, 1976.
318. Oehmichen, M., and Gruninger, H.: Cytokinetic studies on the origin of cells of the cerebrospinal fluid with a contribution to the cytogenesis of the leptomeningeal mesenchyme. J. Neurol. Sci., *22*:165, 1974.
319. Oldendorf, W. H.: Why is cerebrospinal fluid? Bull. Los Angeles Neurol. Soc., *32*:169–179, 1967.
320. Oldendorf, W.: Cerebrospinal fluid formation and circulation. Progr. Nucl. Med., *1*:336, 1972.
321. Oldendorf, W.: Permeability of the blood brain barrier. *In* Tower, D., ed.: The Nervous System. Vol. 1: The Basic Neurosciences. New York, Raven Press, 1975, pp. 279–289.
322. Oldendorf, W.: Certain aspects of drug distribution to brain. *In* Levi, G., et al., eds.: Transport Phenomena in the Nervous System. New York, Plenum Press, 1976, pp. 103–109.
323. Oldendorf, W., and Davson, H.: Brain extracellular space and the sink action of cerebrospinal fluid. Trans. Amer. Neurol. Ass., *92*:122, 1967.
324. Olsson, J., and Link, H.: Immunoglobulin abnor-

malities in multiple sclerosis—relation to clinical parameters: Exacerbations and remissions. Arch. Neurol. (Chicago), *28*:392, 1973.

325. Olsson, J., Blomstrand, C., and Gaglid, K.: Cellular distribution of beta-trace protein in CNS and brain tumors. J. Neurol. Neurosurg. Psychiat., *37*:302, 1974.

326. Ouvrier, R. A.: Progressive dystonia with marked diurnal fluctuation. Ann. Neurol., *4*:412–417, 1978.

327. Papanicolaou, G. N.: Atlas of Exfoliative Cytology. Cambridge, Mass., Harvard University Press, 1954.

328. Papavasiliou, P. S., Cotzias, G. C., and Lawrence, W. H.: Levodopa and dopamine in cerebrospinal fluid. Neurology (Minneap.), *23*:756–759, 1973.

329. Pappagianis, D.: Serologic studies. Chapter 13 *in* Hoeprich, P., ed.: Infectious Diseases. 2nd Ed. New York, Harper & Row, 1977.

330. Pappenheimer, J., et al.: Perfusion of the cerebral ventricular system in unanesthetized goats. Amer. J. Physiol., *203*:763–774, 1962.

331. Pappius, H. M., Oh, J. H., and Dossetor, J. B.: The effects of rapid hemodialysis on brain tissue and cerebrospinal fluid of dogs. Canad. J. Physiol. Pharmacol., *45*:129, 1967.

332. Patel, Y. C., Rao, K., and Reichlin, S.: Somatostatin in cerebrospinal fluid. New Eng. J. Med., *296*:529–533, 1977.

333. Peterson, D. I., Voorhees, E. G., and Elder, H. A.: Bacteroides meningitis successfully treated with metronidazole. Ann. Neurol., *6*:364–365, 1979.

334. Petito, F., and Plum, F.: The lumbar puncture. New Eng. J. Med., *290*:225–226, 1974.

335. Petz, L. D., Sharp, G. C., Cooper, N. R., et al.: Serum and cerebral spinal fluid complement and serum autoantibodies in systemic lupus erythematosus. Medicine (Balt.), *50*:259–275, 1971.

335a. Pilz, H.: Die Lipide des Normalen und Pathologischen Liquor Cerebrospinalis. Berlin, Springer-Verlag, 1970.

336. Plum, C. M.: Biochemical studies of the composition of cerebrospinal fluid in multiple sclerosis. Int. J. Neurol., *2*:121–148, 1961.

337. Porter, J. M., Acinapura, A. J., Kapp, J. P., and Silver, D.: Fibrinolysis in the central nervous system. Neurology (Minneap.), *19*:47–52, 1969.

338. Posner, J. B., and Plum, F.: Spinal fluid pH and neurologic symptoms in systemic acidosis. New Eng. J. Med., *277*:605–613, 1967.

339. Posner, J. B., Swanson, A. G., and Plum, F.: Acid-base balance in cerebrospinal fluid. Arch. Neurol. (Chicago), *12*:479–496, 1965.

340. Prineas, J.: Multiple sclerosis: Presence of lymphatic capillaries and lymphoid tissue in the brain and spinal cord. Science, *203*:1123, 1979.

341. Prockop, L. D., and Fishman, R. A.: Experimental pneumococcal meningitis. Permeability changes influencing the concentration of sugars and macromolecules in cerebrospinal fluid. Arch. Neurol. (Chicago), *19*:449–463, 1968.

342. Queckenstedt, H.: Zur diagnose de Ruckenmarkskompression. Deutsch. Z. Nervenheilk., *55*:325, 1916.

343. Quincke, H.: Die Lumbalpunction des Hydrocephalus. Berlin. Klin. Wschr., *28*:929, 1891.

344. Quincke, H.: Ueber Lumbalpunction. Berlin. Klin. Wschr., *32*:889, 1895.

345. Rall, D.: Transport through the ependymal linings. Progr. Brain Res., *29*:159–172, 1968.

346. Rall, D. P., Oppelt, W. W., and Patak, C. S.: Extracellular space of brain as determined by diffusion of inulin from the ventricular system. Life Sci., *1*:43–48, 1962.

347. Rapoport, S.: Osmotic opening of the blood-brain barrier. Ciba Foundation Symposium 56. Amsterdam, Elsevier–North Holland Publishing Co., 1978, p. 237.

348. Rapoport, S. I.: Blood-Brain Barrier in Physiology and Medicine. New York, Raven Press, 1976.

349. Rathke, E., and Jones, M.: Serum cerebrosides in multiple sclerosis. J. Neurochem., *22*:311–313, 1974.

350. Reiner, E. R.: The cerebrospinal fluid in methylalcohol poisoning. Arch. Neurol. (Chicago), *64*:528–535, 1950.

351. Resurreccion, E. C., and Rosenblum, J. A.: Common causes of spurious xanthochromia in cerebrospinal fluid. Angiology, *23*:105–110, 1972.

352. Rhodes, R. H., Davis, R. L., Berne, T. V., and Tatter, D.: Disseminated toxoplasmosis with brain involvement in a renal allograft recipient. Bull. Los Angeles Neurol. Soc., *42*:16–22, 1977.

353. Riekkinen, P., and Rinne, U.: Proteinases in human cerebrospinal fluid. J. Neurol. Sci., *7*:97, 1968.

354. Roberts-Thomson, P., Esiri, M., Young, A., and Maclennan, I.: Cerebrospinal fluid immunoglobulin quotients, kappa/lambda ratios, and viral antibody titres in neurological disease. J. Clin. Path., *29*:1105, 1976.

355. Roboz, E., Hess, W. C., and Forster, F. M.: Quantitative determination of gamma globulin in cerebrospinal fluid. Its application in multiple sclerosis. Neurology (Minneap.), *3*:410–416, 1953.

356. Roost, K. T., Pimstone, N. R., Diamond, I., and Schmid, R.: The formation of cerebrospinal fluid xanthochromia after subarachnoid hemorrhage. Neurology (Minneap.), *22*:973–977, 1972.

357. Ronquist, G., Ericsson, P., Frithz, G., et al.: Malignant brain tumors associated with adenylate kinase in cerebrospinal fluid. Lancet, *1*:1284–1286, 1977.

358. Ross, S., Rodriguez, W., Controni, G., Korengold, G., and Watson, S.: Limulus lysate test for gram-negative bacterial meningitis. Bedside application. J.A.M.A., *233*:1366, 1975.

359. Rottenberg, D., Howieson, J., and Deck, M.: The rate of CSF formation in man: Preliminary observations on metrizamide washout as a measure of CSF bulk flow. Ann. Neurol., *2*:503, 1977.

359a. Rudolph, A. H.: Syphilis. *In* Hoeprich, P., ed.: Infectious Diseases. 2nd ed. New York, Harper & Row, 1979.

360. Rudman, D., Fleischer, A., and Kutner, M. H.: Concentration of 3′, 5′ cyclic adenosine monophosphate in ventricular cerebrospinal fluid of

patients with prolonged coma after head trauma or intracranial hemorrhage. New Eng. J. Med., *295*:635–638, 1976.

361. Rutter, N., and Smales, O. R. C.: Lumbar puncture in children with convulsions. Lancet, *2*:190–191, 1977.
362. Sahs, A. L.: Cooperative study of intracranial aneurysms and subarachnoid hemorrhage. Report on a randomized treatment study. I. Introduction. Stroke, *5*:550–551, 1974.
363. Sambrook, M. A.: The relationship between cerebrospinal fluid and plasma electrolytes in patients with meningitis. J. Neurol. Sci., *23*:265–273, 1974.
364. Sambrook, M. A., Hutchinson, E. C., and Aber, G. M.: Serial changes in cerebrospinal fluid and plasma urea electrolytes and osmolality. Brain, *96*:191–202, 1973.
365. Sambrook, M. A., Hutchinson, E. C., and Aber, G. M.: Metabolic studies in subarachnoid hemorrhage and strokes. I. Serial changes in acid-base values in blood and cerebrospinal fluid. Brain, *96*:171–190, 1973.
366. Sandberg-Wollheim, M., Zettervall, O., and Müller, R.: In vitro synthesis of IgG by cells from the cerebrospinal fluid in a patient with multiple sclerosis. Clin. Exp. Immun., *4*:401–405, 1969.
367. Schact, R. A., Tourtellotte, W. W., Frame, B., and Nickel, S. N.: Distribution of protein, lipid, and administered bromide between serum and CSF in myxedema. Metabolism, *17*:786–793, 1968.
368. Schinko, H., and Tschabitscher, H.: Der IgG-Quotient als differential-diagnostisches Kriterium zwischen Multipler Sklerose und degenerativen Erkrankungen des Nervensystems unter besonder Berücksichtigung der Krankheitsdauer. Wien. Klin. Wschr., *7*:417–422, 1959.
369. Schmidt, R.: Bestimmung organischer Sauren im Liquor cerebrospinalis. *In* Schmidt, R., ed.: Der Liquor Cerebrospinalis. Berlin, VEB Verlag, 1968.
370. Schmidt, R.: Liquorzuckerbestimmung. *In* Schmidt, R., ed.: Der Liquor Cerebrospinalis. Berlin, VEB Verlag, 1968.
371. Schoenen, J., Einaudi, N., and Delwaide, P. J.: L'Analyse cytologique qualitative du liquide céphalo-rachidien. Rev. Med. Liege, *31*:471, 1976.
372. Schossberger, P. F., and Touya, J. J.: Dynamic cisternography in normal dogs and in human beings. Neurology (Minneap.), *26*:254–260, 1976.
373. Schuller, E., Castaigne, P., and Lhermitte, F.: Les reactions immunitaires humorales au cours de la sclerose en plaques. INSERM, Colloque de synthèse 1974. Serie Action thematique Rapport No. 4: Immunopathologie du systeme nerveux. Annees 1971–1973.
374. Sellers, M. I., and Lavender, J.: Studies on the interrelationship between the blood brain barrier and entry of viruses into the central nervous system. I. The effect of carbon dioxide on type II poliovirus infection in mice. J. Exp. Med., *115*:107–137, 1962.
375. Selverstone, B.: *In* Wolstenholme, G. E. W., and O'Connor, C. M., eds.: The Cerebrospinal Fluid. Ciba Foundation Symposium. Boston, Little, Brown & Co., 1958 p. 147.
376. Shuttleworth, E. C., Parker, J. M., Wise, G. R., and Stevens, M. E.: Differentiation of early subarachnoid hemorrhage from traumatic lumbar puncture. Stroke, *8*:613–617, 1977.
377. Sicard, J. A., and Forestier, J.: Méthode générale d'exloration radiologique par l'huile iodée lipiodol. Bull. Soc. Méd. Hôp. Paris, *46*:463, 1922.
378. Siegel, G., et al., eds.: Basic Neurochemistry. 2nd Ed. Boston, Little, Brown & Co., 1976.
379. Siesjo, B. K.: The regulation of cerebrospinal fluid pH. Kidney Int., *1*:360–374, 1972.
380. Simpson, J. F., Tourtellotte, W. W., Kokmen, E., Parker, J. A., and Itabashi, H. H.: Fluorescent protein tracing in multiple sclerosis brain tissue. Arch. Neurol. (Chicago), *20*:373–377, 1969.
381. Skalpe, I.: Adhesive arachnoiditis following lumbar myelography, Spine, *3*:61, 1978.
382. Skoldenberg, B., Jeansson, S., and Wolontis, S.: Herpes simplex virus type 2 and acute aseptic meningitis. Clinical features of cases with isolation of herpes simplex virus from cerebrospinal fluid. Scand. J. Infect. Dis., *7*:227–232, 1975.
383. Small, P., Mass, M. F., Kohler, P. F., et al.: Central nervous system involvement in SLE. Arthritis Rheum. *20*:869–878, 1977.
384. Smith, J. A., Mee, T. J. X., Barnes, N. D., Thorburn, R. J., and Barnes, J. L. C.: Melatonin in serum and cerebrospinal fluid. Lancet, *2*:425, 1976.
385. Snead, O. C., III, Yu, R. K., and Huttenlocher, P. R.: Gamma hydroxybutrate. Correlation of serum and cerebrospinal fluid levels with electroencephalographic and behavioral effects. Neurology (Minneap.), *26*:51–56, 1976.
386. Sobotka, H., Baker, H., and Frank, O.: Vitamin levels in normal cerebrospinal fluid. Proc. Soc. Exp. Biol. Med., *103*:801, 1960.
387. Söderström, C. E., Kjellin, K. G., and Cronqvist, S.: Computer tomography compared with spectrophotometry of cerebrospinal fluid in cerebrovascular diseases. Acta Radiol. [suppl.] (Stockh.) *346*:130–142, 1975.
388. Sokolowski, S.: A new quantitative technique for the assessment of cerebrospinal fluid absorption in man. J. Neurol. Sci., *23*:37, 1974.
389. Sophian, L. H., and Connolly, V. J.: Ultraviolet absorption spectra of normal cerebrospinal fluid. J. Phys. Colloid Chem., *55*:712–716, 1951.
390. Sornas, R., et al.: Cerebrospinal fluid cytology after stroke. Arch. Neurol. (Chicago), *26*:489, 1972.
391. Sourkes, T. L.: Parkinson's disease and other disorders of the basal ganglia. *In* Siegel, G. J., et al., eds.: Basic Neurochemistry. 2nd Ed. Boston, Little, Brown & Co., 1976.
392. Spriggs, A. I., and Boddington, M. M.: The Cytology of Effusions in the Pleural, Pericardial, and Peritoneal Cavities and of the Cerebrospinal Fluid. 2nd Ed. London, William Heinemann, Ltd., 1968.
393. Stalder, H., Oxman, M. N., Dawson, D. M., and Levin, M. J.: Herpes simplex meningitis: Isolation of herpes simplex virus type 2 from cere-

brospinal fluid. New Eng. J. Med., *298*:1296–1298, 1973.

394. Stokes, H. B., O'Hara, C. M., Buchanan, R. D., and Olson, W. H.: An improved method for examination of cerebrospinal fluid cells. Neurology (Minneap.), *25*:901, 1975.
395. Swartz, M. N., and Dodge, P. R.: Bacterial meningitis—a review of selected aspects. I. General clinical features, special problems, and unusual meningeal reactions mimicking bacterial meningitis. New Eng. J. Med., *272*:725, 1965.
396. Sweet, W. H., Brownell, G. L., Scholl, J. A., Bowsher, D. R., Benda, P., and Stickley, E. E.: The formation, flow and absorption of cerebrospinal fluid; newer concepts based on studies with isotopes. Res. Publ. Ass. Res. Nerv. Ment. Dis., *34*:101, 1954.
397. Taveras, J. M., and Wood, E. H.: Diagnostic Neuroradiology. Baltimore, Md., Williams & Wilkins Co., 1964.
398. Thompson, E., et al.: The analysis of the cerebrospinal fluid. Brit. J. Hosp. Med., December 1975, pp. 645–652.
399. Tiselius, A.: Electrophorese. Med. Prisma 5. Ingelheim, C. H. Boehnunger, 1962.
400. Toomey, J. A.: Stiff neck and meningeal irritation. J.A.M.A., *127*:436, 1945.
401. Tourtellotte, W. W.: Multiple sclerosis and cerebrospinal fluid. Med. Clin. N. Amer., *47*:1619–1628, 1963.
402. Tourtellotte, W. W.: Cerebrospinal fluid and its reactions in diseases. *In* Minckler, J., ed.: Pathology of the Nervous System. McGraw-Hill Book Co., Inc., 1968, pp. 434–456.
403. Tourtellotte, W. W.: A selected review of reactions of the cerebrospinal fluid to disease. *In* Fields, W. S., ed.: Neurological Diagnostic Techniques. Springfield, Ill., Charles C Thomas, 1966, pp. 25–50.
404. Tourtellotte, W. W.: Cerebrospinal fluid examination in meningoencephalitis. Mod. Treatm., *4*:879, 1967.
405. Tourtellotte, W. W.: Multiple sclerosis—the hunt for etiology. Hosp. Practice, *4*:29–33, 1969.
406. Tourtellotte, W. W.: Multiple sclerosis cerebrospinal fluid. *In* Vinken, P. J., and Bruyn, G. W., eds.: Handbook of Clinical Neurology. Vol. 9. Amsterdam, Elsevier–North Holland Publishing Co., 1970, pp. 324–382.
407. Tourtellotte, W.: On cerebrospinal fluid immunoglobulin-G (IgG) quotients in multiple sclerosis and other diseases, a review and a new formula to estimate the amount of IgG synthesized per day by the central nervous system. J. Neurol. Sci., *10*:279, 1970.
408. Tourtellotte, W.: Cerebrospinal fluid immunoglobulins and the central nervous system as an immunological organ particularly in multiple sclerosis and subacute sclerosing panencephalitis. *In* Rowland, L. P., ed.: Immunological Disorders of the Nervous System. ARNMD Research Publication 49. New York, Raven Press, 1971, pp. 112–155.
409. Tourtellotte, W. W.: What is multiple sclerosis? Laboratory criteria for diagnosis. *In* Davison, A. N., et al., eds.: Multiple Sclerosis Research. Amsterdam, Elsevier–North Holland Publishing Co., 1975, pp. 9–26.

409a. Tourtellotte, W. W., and Haerer, A. F.: Lipids in cerebrospinal fluid. XII. In multiple sclerosis and retrobulbar neuritis. Arch. Neurol. (Chicago), *20*:605–615, 1969.

410. Tourtellotte, W. W., and Haerer, A.: Clinical Aspects of the Cerebrospinal Fluid and Relevant Basic Science Information (A Collection of Reprints and References). Los Angeles, VA Wadsworth Hospital Center Press, 1973.
411. Tourtellotte, W. W., and Parker, J. A.: Distribution and subfractionation of immunoglobulins in patients with multiple sclerosis. Trans. Amer. Neurol. Ass., *90*:107–112, 1965.
412. Tourtellotte, W. W., and Parker, J. A.: Multiple sclerosis: Correlation between immunoglobulin-G in cerebrospinal fluid and brain. Science, *154*:1044–1046, 1966.
413. Tourtellotte, W. W., and Parker, J. A.: Immunoglobulins in multiple sclerosis white matter. J. Neuropath. Exp. Neurol., *25*:167–169, 1966.
414. Tourtellotte, W. W., and Parker, J. A.: Multiple sclerosis: Brain immunoglobulin-G and albumin. Nature, *214*:683–686, 1967.
415. Tourtellotte, W. W., and Parker, J. A.: Some spaces and barriers in postmortem multiple sclerosis. Progr. Brain Res., *29*:493–522, 1967.
416. Tourtellotte, W. W., and Parker, J. A.: Postmortem evaluation of the blood brain barrier in multiple sclerosis. J. Neuropath. Exp. Neurol., *27*:159–163, 1968.
417. Tourtellotte, W. W., and Ma, B. I.: Multiple sclerosis: The blood-brain-barrier and the measurement of de novo central nervous system IgG synthesis. Neurology (Minneap.), *28*:76–83, 1978.
418. Tourtellotte, W. W., Allen, R. J., and DeJong, R. N.: A study of lipids in cerebrospinal fluid (and serum). VII. In several sphingolipidoses (Tay-Sachs' disease, metachromatic leucodystrophy, and Niemann-Pick disease). *In* Aronson, S. M., and Volk, B. W., eds.: Cerebral Sphingolipidoses: A Symposium on Tay Sachs' Disease and Allied Disorders. New York, Academic Press, Inc., 1962, pp. 317–326.
419. Tourtellotte, W. W., Itabashi, H. H., and Parker, J. A.: Multifocal areas of synthesis of immunoglobulin-G in multiple sclerosis brain tissue and the sink action of the cerebrospinal fluid. Trans. Amer. Neurol. Ass., *92*:288–290, 1967.
420. Tourtellotte, W. W., Parker, J. A., and Haerer, A. F.: Subfractionation of multiple sclerosis gamma globulin. Immunitäts forsch., *126*:85–103, 1964.
421. Tourtellotte, W. W., Parker, J. A., and Itabashi, H. H.: Source of elevation of γ-globulin in brain tissue from patients with multiple sclerosis. Trans. Amer. Neurol. Ass., *91*:351–352, 1966.
422. Tourtellotte, W. W., Allen, R. J., Haerer, A. F., and Bryan, E. R.: Study of lipids in cerebrospinal fluid and serum. X. In Tay-Sachs' disease. Arch. Neurol. (Chicago), *12*:300–310, 1965.
423. Tourtellotte, W. W., DeJong, R. N., Janich, S., and Gustafson, K.: A study of lipids in the cerebrospinal fluid (and serum). VIII. Further comments on the normal lipid profile. Univ. Mich. Med. Bull., *28*:114–126, 1962.
424. Tourtellotte, W. W., Haerer, A. F., Heller, G.

L., and Somers, J. E.: Post–Lumbar Puncture Headaches. Springfield, Ill., Charles C Thomas, 1964.

425. Tourtellotte, W. W., Metz, L. N., Bryan, E. R., and DeJong, R. N.: Spontaneous subarachnoid hemorrhage. Neurology (Minneap.), *14*:301–306, 1964.

426. Tourtellotte, W. W., Parker, J. A., Alving, R. E., and DeJong, R. N.: Determination of total protein in cerebrospinal fluid by an ultramicro-Kjeldahl nitrogen procedure. Anal. Chem., *30*:1563–1566, 1958.

427. Tourtellotte, W. W., Parker, J. A., Herndon, R. B., and Cuadros, C. V.: Subacute sclerosing panencephalitis: Brain immunoglobulin-G, measles antibody and albumin. Neurology (Minneap.), *18*:117–121, 1968.

428. Tourtellotte, W. W., Quan, K. C., Haerer, A. F., and Bryan, E. R.: Neoplastic cells in the cerebrospinal fluid. Neurology (Minneap.), *13*:866, 1963.

429. Tourtellotte, W. W., Tavaloto, B., Parker, J. A., and Comiso, P.: Cerebrospinal fluid electroimmunodiffusion. An easy, rapid, sensitive, reliable, and valid method for the simultaneous determination of immunoglobulin-G and albumin. Arch. Neurol. (Chicago), *25*:345–350, 1971.

430. Tourtellotte, W. W., Allen, R. J., Haerer, A. F., Kelly, S. A., et al.: A study of lipids in the cerebrospinal fluid. IX. Two new laboratory observations on the cerebrospinal fluid in Tay-Sachs disease. Trans. Amer. Neurol. Ass., *88*:104–107, 1963.

431. Tourtellotte, W. W., Somers, J. F., Parker, J. A., Itabashi, H. H., and DeJong, R. N.: A study on traumatic lumbar punctures. Neurology (Minneap.), *8*:129–134, 1958.

431a. Tourtellotte, W. W., Haerer, A. F., DeJong, R. N., Janich, S., and Gustafson, K.: Cerebrospinal fluid lipid profiles in various diseases. *In* Jacob, H., ed.: IV. Internationaler Kongress fur Neuropathologie, 4–8 September, 1961, Munchen. Proceedings Vol. I. Stuttgart, Georg Thieme Verlag, 1962, pp. 46–58.

432. Tourtellotte, W. W., Henderson, W. G., Tucker, R. P., Gilland, O., Walker, J. E., and Kokman, E.: A randomized, double-blind clinical trial comparing the 22 versus 26 gauge needle in the production of the post–lumbar puncture syndrome in normal individuals. Headache, *12*: 73–78, 1972.

433. Tower, D. B.: Neurochemistry—one hundred years, 1875–1975. Ann. Neurol., *1*:2–36, 1977.

434. Trabucchi, M., Cerri, C., Spano, P. F., et al.: Guanosine 3′-5′-monophosphate in the CSF of neurological patients. Arch. Neurol. (Chicago), *34*:12–13, 1977.

435. Traviesa, D. C., Prystowsky, S. D., Nelson, B. J., and Johnson, K. P.: Cerebrospinal fluid findings in asymptomatic patients with reactive serum fluorescent treponemal antibody absorption tests. Ann. Neurol., *4*:524–530, 1978.

436. Tripathi, B. J., and Tripathi, R. C.: Vacuolar transcellular channels as a drainage pathway for cerebrospinal fluid. J. Physiol. (Lond.), *239*:195–206, 1974.

437. Tripathi, R.: Ultrastructure of the arachnoid matter in relation to outflow of cerebrospinal fluid—a new concept. Lancet, *2*:8, 1973.

438. Tripathi, R.: Tracing the bulk outflow route of cerebrospinal fluid by transmission and scanning electron microscopy. Brain Res., *80*:503, 1974.

439. Truner, D. A., Brown, F., Ganz, E., and Huttenlocher, P. R.: Treatment of elevated intracranial pressure in Reye syndrome. Ann. Neurol., *4*:275, 1978.

440. Tsang, D., Lal, S., Sourkes, T. L., Ford, R. M., and Aronoff, A.: Studies on cyclic AMP in different compartments of cerebrospinal fluid. J. Neurol. Neurosurg. Psychiat., *39*:1186–1190, 1976.

441. Tschirgi, R. D.: Chemical environment of the central nervous system. *In* Field, J., Magoun, H. W., and Hall, V. E., eds.: Handbook of Physiology. Vol. 3. Washington, D.C., American Physiological Society, 1960, p. 1865.

442. Tuna, N., Logothetis, J., and Kammererck, R.: The fatty acids of the human cerebrospinal fluid: Their relation to the serum fatty acids. A study using gas-liquid chromatography. Neurology (Minneap.), *13*:331, 1963.

443. van Harrereld, A.: The extracellular space in the vertebrate central nervous system. *In* Borne, G. H., ed.: The Structure and Function of Nervous Tissue. Vol. 4. New York, Academic Press, Inc., pp. 447–511.

444. Vannucci, R. C., Dubynsky, O. D., Hellmann, J., and Maisels, M. J.: Cerebral oxidative metabolism in perinatal posthemorrhagic encephalopathy. Ann. Neurol. *4*:188, 1978.

445. Vapaatalo, H., Myllyla, V., Heikkinen, E., and Hokkanen, E.: Cyclic AMP in CSF of patients with neurologic disease. New Eng. J. Med., *296*:691, 1977.

446. Waddell, W. J.: A simple ultraviolet spectrophotometric method for the determination of protein. J. Lab. Clin. Med., *48*:311–314, 1956.

447. Walton, J. N.: Subarachnoid Haemorrhage. Edinburgh and London, E. & S. Livingstone Ltd., 1956.

448. Wassermann, A., et al.: Eine serodiagnostische Reaktion bei Syphilis. Deutsch. Med. Wschr., *32*:745, 1906.

449. Weed, L. H.: Certain anatomical and physiological aspects of the meninges and cerebrospinal fluid. Brain, *58*:383–397, 1935.

449a. Weil, M. L., Itabashi, H. H., Cremer, N. E., Oshiro, L. S., Lennette, E. H., and Carnay, L.: Chronic progressive panencephalitis due to rubella virus simulating subacute sclerosing panencephalitis. New Eng. J. Med., *292*: 994–998, 1975.

450. Weil-Malherbe, H., and Liddell, D. W.: Adrenaline and noradrenaline in cerebrospinal fluid. J. Neurol., *17*:247–249, 1954.

451. Weiner, W. J., and Klawans, H. L.: Failure of cerebrospinal fluid homovanillic acid to predict levodopa response in Parkinson's disease. J. Neurol. Neurosurg. Psychiat., *36*:747–752, 1973.

452. Weisner, B., and Bernhardt, W.: Protein fractions of lumbar, cisternal, and ventricular cerebrospinal fluid. Separate areas of reference. J. Neurol. Sci., *37*:205, 1978.

453. Weisz, R., and Mars, H.: Deoxyribonucleic acid

determination in human cerebrospinal fluid. Ann. Neurol. *2*:357, 1977.

454. Weller, R.: Mechanisms of cerebrospinal fluid absorption. Develop. Med. Child Neurol., *16*:85, 1974.

455. Wenner, H.: Viral meningitis. *In* Hoeprich, P., ed.: Infectious Diseases. 2nd Ed. New York, Harper & Row, 1977.

456. Westergaard, E., and Brightman, M.: Transport of proteins across normal cerebral arterioles. J. Comp. Neurol., *152*:17, 1973.

456a. Whitley, R. J., Seng-Jaw, S., Dolin, R., Galasso, G. J., Ch'ien, L. T., and Alford, C. A., and the Collaborative Study Group: Adenine arabinoside therapy of biopsy-proved herpes simplex encephalitis. New Eng. J. Med., *297*:289–294, 1977.

456b. Whitaker, J. N., Lisak, R. P., Bashir, R. M., Fitch, O. H., Seyer, J. M., Krance, R., Lawrence, J. A., Ch'ien, L. T., and O'Sullivan, P.: Immunoreactive myelin basic protein in the cerebrospinal fluid in neurological disorders. Ann. Neurol., *7*:58–64, 1980.

457. Widal, F., Sicard, J., and Ravaut, P.: Cytologie du liquide céphalorachidien. Au cours de quelques processus meninges chroniques (paralysie générale et tabes). Bull. Soc. Méd. Hôp. Paris (S. 3), *18*:31, 1901.

458. Wieme, R. J.: Agar Gel Electrophoresis. Amsterdam, Elsevier–North Holland Publishing Co., 1965.

459. Wilfert, C. M.: Mumps meningoencephalitis with low cerebrospinal fluid glucose, prolonged pleocytosis and elevation of protein. New Eng. J. Med., *280*:855–858, 1969.

460. Wilkinson, A. E.: Fluorescent treponemal antibody tests on cerebrospinal fluid. Brit. J. Vener. Dis., *49*:346–349, 1973.

461. Williams, A., Mingioli, H., McFarland, H., Tourtellotte, W., and McFarlin, D.: Increased CSF IgM in multiple sclerosis. Neurology (Minneap.), *28*:996, 1978.

462. Williams, B.: Cerebrospinal fluid pressure changes in response to coughing. Brain, *99*:331, 1976.

463. Willoughby, E.: Measurement of cerebrospinal fluid IgG in the diagnosis of multiple sclerosis. Proc. Aust. Ass. Neurol., *13*:127, 1976.

464. Winship, M. J., and Goldstein, E.: Diagnosis of CNS infections: Source of CSF. New Engl. J. Med., *288*:1080, 1973.

465. Wolf, S. M.: Decreased cerebrospinal fluid glucose level in herpes zoster meningitis. Arch. Neurol. (Chicago), *30*:109, 1974.

466. Wolfe, L. S.: Prostaglandins synaptic transmission. *In* Siegel, G. J., et al., eds.: Basic Neurochemistry. 2nd Ed. Boston, Little, Brown & Co., 1976.

467. Wolfson, L. I., Katzman, R., and Escriva, A.: Clearance of amine metabolites from the cerebrospinal fluid: The brain as a "sink." Neurology (Minneap.), *24*:772–779, 1974.

468. Wolinsky, J. S., et al: Diagnostic tests in normal pressure hydrocephalus. Neurology (Minneap.), *23*:706, 1973.

469. Wolstenholme, G. E. W., and O'Connor, C. M., eds.: The Cerebrospinal Fluid. Ciba Foundation Symposium. Boston, Little, Brown & Co., 1958.

470. Wood, J. H., Lake, C. R., Ziegler, M. G., Sode, J., Brooks, B. R., and Van Buren, J. M.: Cerebrospinal fluid norepinephrine alterations during electrical stimulation of cerebellar, cerebral surfaces in epileptic patients. Neurology (Minneap.), *27*:716–724, 1977.

471. Woodbury, J., Lyons, K., Carretta, R., Hahn, A., and Sullivan, J. F.: Cerebrospinal fluid and serum levels of magnesium, zinc, and calcium in man. Neurology (Minneap.), *18*:700–705, 1968.

472. Woodruff, K. H.: Cerebrospinal fluid cytomorphology using cytocentrifugation. Amer. J. Clin. Path., *60*:621, 1973.

473. Woof, J. H., Ziegler, M. G., Lake, C. R., et al.: Cerebrospinal fluid norepinephrine reductions in man after degeneration and electrical stimulation of the caudate nucleus. Ann. Neurol., *1*:94–99, 1977.

474. Woolam, D. H. M.: The historical significance of the cerebrospinal fluid. Med. Hist., *1*:91, 1957.

475. Wynter, W. E.: Four cases of tubercular meningitis in which paracentesis of the theca vertebralis was performed. Lancet, *1*:981–982, 1891.

476. Yahr, M. D., Goldensohn, S. S., and Kabat, E. A.: Further studies on the gamma globulin content of cerebrospinal fluid in multiple sclerosis and other neurological diseases. Ann. N.Y. Acad. Sci., *58*:613–624, 1954.

477. Yam, P., Petz, L. D., Ma, B., and Tourtellotte, W.: Synthesis of C3 within the central nervous system in multiple sclerosis (abstract). Clin. Res., *27*:40A, 1979.

478. Younes, F., Just, R., Ranganath, K. A., and Tourtellotte, W. W.: Lipid cerebrospinal fluid in a patient with cerebral hemorrhage. Neurology (Minneap.), *27*:701–703, 1974.

479. Young, S. N., Lal, S., Feldmuller, F., Sourkes, T. L., et al.: Parallel variation of ventricular CSF tryptophan and free serum tryptophan in man. J. Neurol. Neurosurg. Psychiat., *39*: 61–65, 1976.

480. Zivin, J.: Lateral cervical puncture: An alternative to lumbar puncture. Neurology (Minneap.), *28*:616–618, 1978.

481. Zwibel, H. L., and Schwartzman, R. J.: Evaluation of the nitroblue tetrazolium test as applied to polymorphonuclear leucocytes in the cerebrospinal fluid. Neurology (Minneap.), *24*: 995–998, 1974.

14

RADIOLOGY OF THE SPINE

A large body of knowledge concerning the radiology of the spine and its contents has accumulated over the years. For a more comprehensive review than is given in this chapter, the reader is referred to the standard texts on the subject.[13,21,30,33,42,45]

The examination of the spine should include views taken to outline the odontoid peg, the bodies of the vertebrae, the pedicles and laminae, the spinous processes, the articular facets, the spinal canal dimensions, the intervertebral spaces, the intervertebral foramina, and the lateral masses (Figs. 14–1, 14–2, and 14–3). These requirements should be met by the open-mouth view for the odontoid peg and oblique views for the intervertebral foramina, obtained by drawing the shoulders downward to visualize the lower cervical spine, and by angulation of the tube for a view of the lateral masses (see Fig. 14–16). For accurate assessment of the extent of the disc space, the x-ray beam must be directed through each intervertebral space individually. An extended Water's skull projection often will allow an unobstructed view of the odontoid process through the foramen magnum. Extension and flexion films may be indicated on occasion. This is particularly true in the cervical and lumbar region. Laminagraphy and cinematography will enhance the anatomical details and are helpful in diagnosis in some patients (see Figs. 14–13 and 14–18). Recently developed techniques of transverse axial tomography and computed tomographic scanning provide a new dimension in the study of the spine (see Fig. 14–31*C*).[16,22] The latter, when utilized with metrizamide (a water-soluble contrast agent) to enhance the spinal subarachnoid space, is a promising tool in the study of the spinal cord as well.

A valuable indication of the dimensions of the spinal canal may be obtained by using the following measurement. In the anteroposterior projection the interpedicular distances may be measured and compared with the charts compiled by Elsberg and Dyke and Schwarz.[12,43] Reference may also be made to Hinck and co-workers for spinal canal measurements in children.[26] In the measurement of the interpedicular distances, it should be noted that the shape of the pedicles normally changes from an indistinct round shadow in the cervical region to a kidney-shaped structure in the thoracic region and to a round structure in the lumbar region. The inner margin is always convex inward.

In the lateral projection, the sagittal diameter of the canal is measured by a line drawn from the middle of the posterior surface of the vertebral body to the closest point on the cortical line marking the fusion of the corresponding laminae and spinous process (Fig. 14–4).[13] This is easily accomplished on the lateral plain film of the cervical spine, but in the lumbar and thoracic regions laminagraphy may be needed to locate the posterior limits of the spinal canal precisely.

The intervertebral foramen at C2–C3 is usually larger than the other cervical foramina. This is important when evaluating the possible presence of a dumbbell tumor.

Smith has summarized the various figures presented in the literature concerning the dimensions of the cord and spine at various levels. As a general rule the interpedicular distance increases and becomes progressively wider from C2 to C6. From C6 to T4 there is progressive diminution, and from T4 downward another progressive increase. In the anteroposterior diameter

---

M. M. SCHECHTER AND E. SAJOR, II

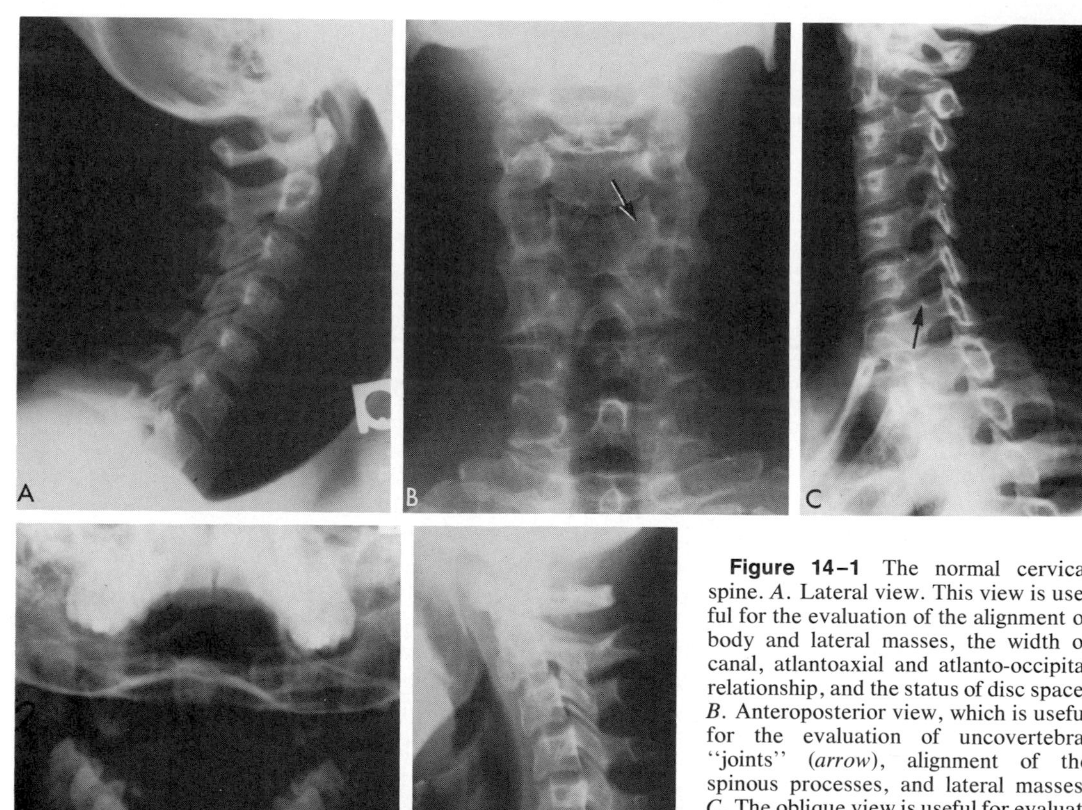

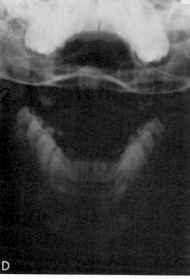

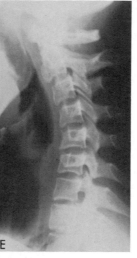

Figure 14–1 The normal cervical spine. *A*. Lateral view. This view is useful for the evaluation of the alignment of body and lateral masses, the width of canal, atlantoaxial and atlanto-occipital relationship, and the status of disc space. *B*. Anteroposterior view, which is useful for the evaluation of uncovertebral "joints" (*arrow*), alignment of the spinous processes, and lateral masses. *C*. The oblique view is useful for evaluating the intervertebral foramina, the uncovertebral "joints" (*arrow*), the lateral masses, and the pedicles. *D*. Open-mouth view. This view is useful for an evaluation of the odontoid peg and the atlantoaxial joints. *E*. Normal flexion film.

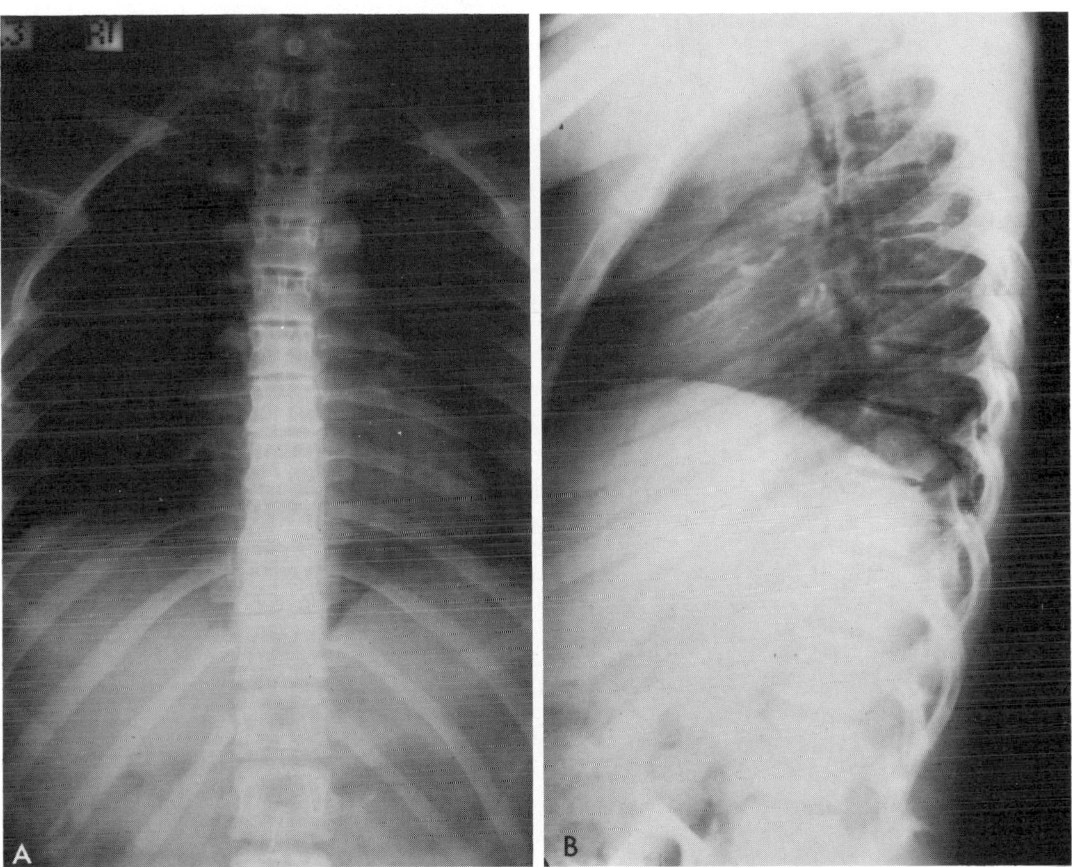

Figure 14–2 The normal thoracic spine. *A*. Anteroposterior projection. This view is useful for evaluation of the pedicles, interpedicular distances, alignment of spinous processes, paraspinal masses. *B*. Lateral projection. This view is useful for an evaluation of disc spaces and pedicles.

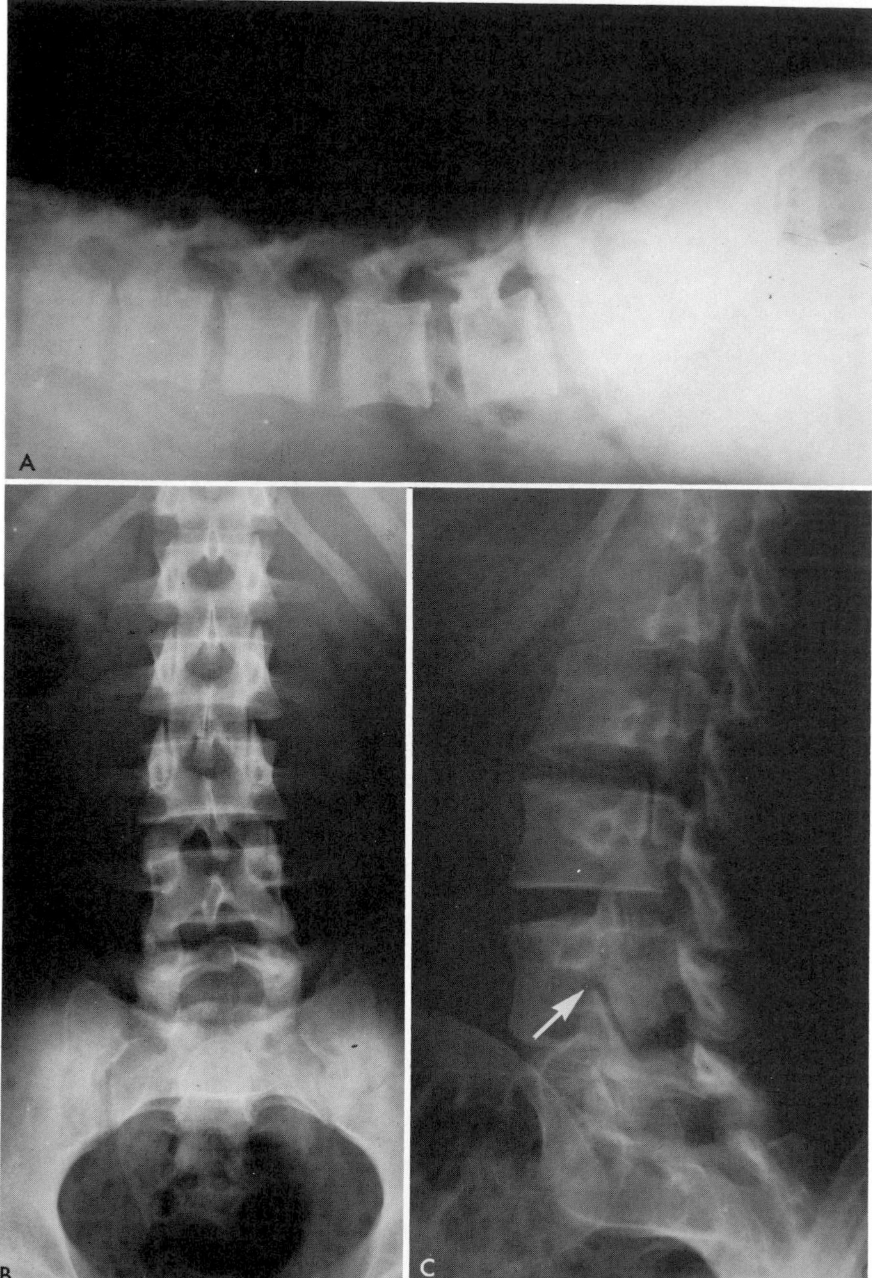

Figure 14–3 The normal lumbar spine. *A*. Lateral projection for evaluation of disc spaces, bodies, alignment. *B*. Anteroposterior projection for evaluating disc space, shape and integrity of pedicles and spinous processes, integrity of sacrum, and sacroiliac joints. *C*. Oblique view for pedicles, articular facets, pars interarticularis (*arrow*).

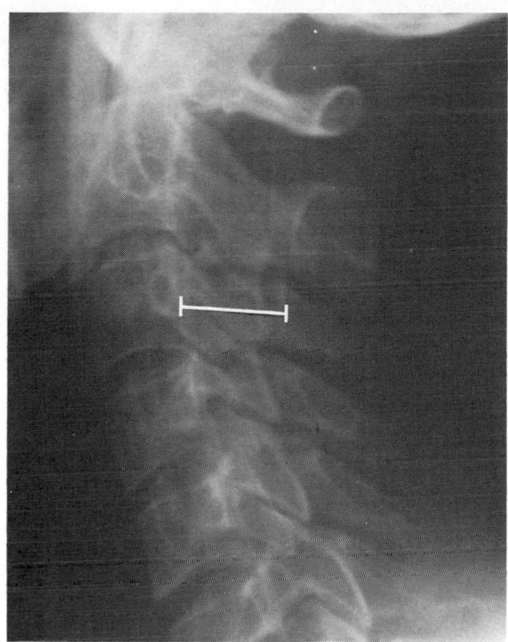

Figure 14–4 Lateral view of a normal cervical spine. Horizontal line marks the sagittal diameter of the cervical canal at C3.

the canal progressively narrows. Wolf and associates state that a sagittal diameter of 10 mm or less of the cervical spinal canal is likely to be associated with cord compression.[57] In the cervical region, however, a sagittal diameter of 12 mm or less becomes significant if coupled with relevant neurological findings. In the lumbar region, where correct measurement of the sagittal diameter may be prevented by the difficulty in adequately defining the posterior midline of the canal in the plain films, it may be helpful to look for changes such as vertical elongation of the neural foramina, vertical or convergent alignment of the laminae, and heavy thick pedicles when a narrow canal is suspected (cf. Fig. 14–25).[14]

ABNORMALITIES OF THE SPINE

Congenital Anomalies

In an evaluation of the cervical spine the following anomalies may be encountered. In basilar invagination there is indentation of the upper cervical vertebra into the base of the skull. Various lines and measurements are available in the literature to determine its presence. McGregor's line extends from the posterior margin of the hard palate to the inferior margin of the occipital squamae. The tip of the odontoid should not extend more than 5 mm above this line. Other measurements for evaluating basilar invagination have been described by Bull, by Chamberlain, and by others.[27,37] This condition may be congenital or acquired. It may be secondary to trauma or to various diseases that cause bone softening such as Paget's disease, osteomalacia, osteogenesis imperfecta, and fibrous dysplasia (Fig. 14–5).

In occipitalization of the atlas, the capacity of the foramen magnum is diminished as shown in Figure 14–5. The posterior arch of C1 is not visible but is assimilated into the occiput. The effective sagittal diameter of the foramen magnum is measured by a line from the posterior aspect of the tip of the dens to the posterior margin of the foramen magnum. McRae states that a sagittal measurement of 19 mm or less may predispose to neurological symptoms.[37] Partial absence of the arch of C1 should be considered in the evaluation of fractures in this region (Fig. 14–6).

Many anomalies of the odontoid may be encountered. The odontoid ossifies from five primary and two secondary centers. The ossification is not complete until the second year of life and occasionally remains incomplete. Ossification may be a prolonged process, and because of the many centers involved, anomalies do occur. These should not be interpreted as fractures or fracture-dislocations (Fig. 14–7). The dens may be congenitally absent or bifid, and the apex may be unossified or unfused to the rest of the odontoid. The odontoid may remain unfused to the body of C2.

Failures of normal segmentation will result in many anomalies, including the Klippel-Feil syndrome, Sprengel's deformity, hemivertebrae, and blocked vertebrae, all of which have classic appearances (Fig. 14–8). The blocked vertebrae should be distinguished from destruction of the disc space by infection and trauma. In acquired blocked vertebrae, other evidence of trauma or infection is present. In addition, the total height of the two fused vertebrae is less than that of the congenital blocked ver-

Text continued on page 496

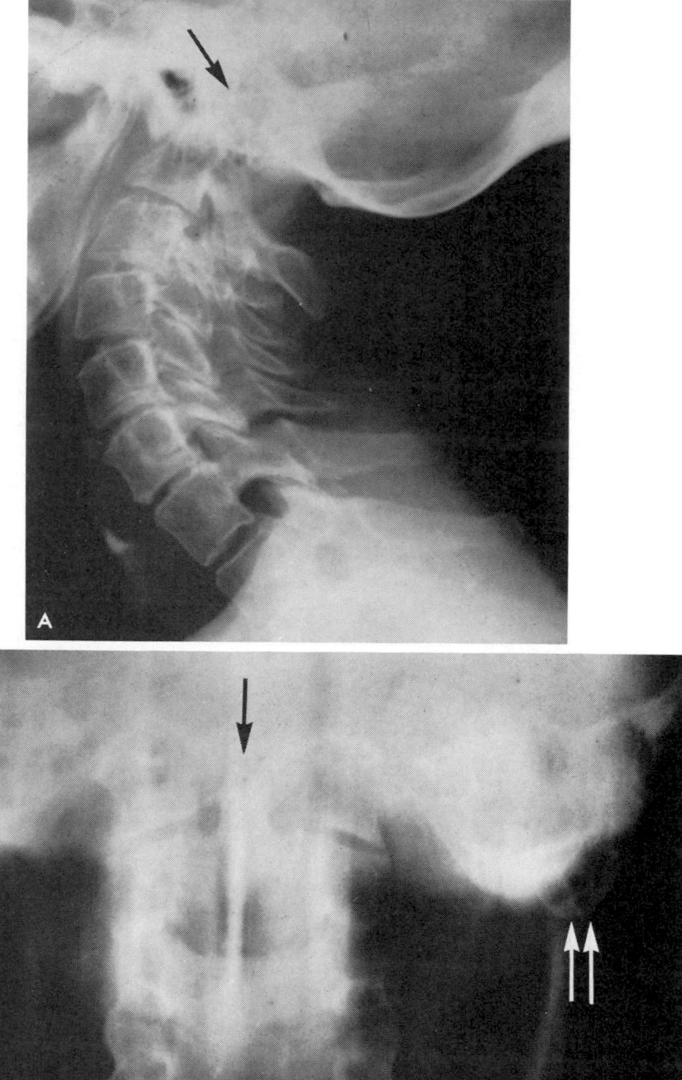

Figure 14–5 Basilar invagination (Paget's disease). *A*. Note that the odontoid peg (*arrow*) extends above the foramen magnum. There is occipitalization of the posterior arch of C1. *B*. Anteroposterior projection showing the odontoid peg (*black arrow*) high above the mastoid processes (*white arrows*).

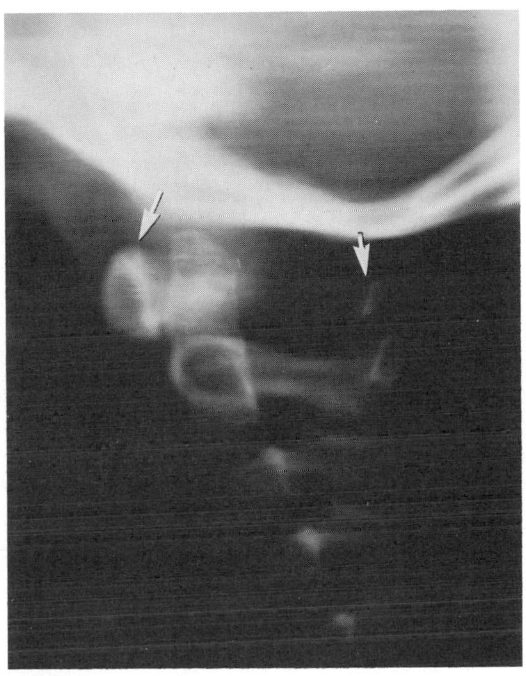

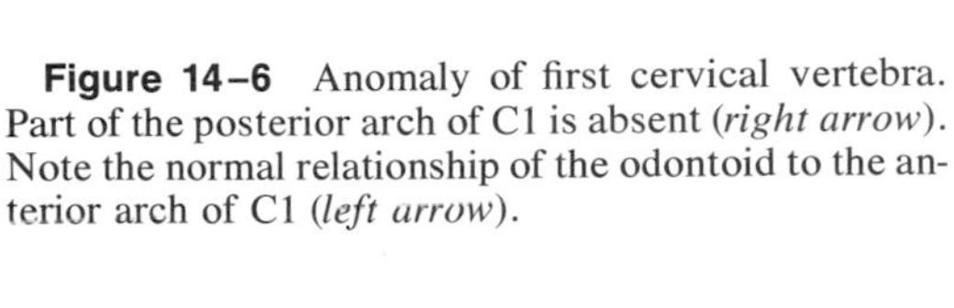

Figure 14–6 Anomaly of first cervical vertebra. Part of the posterior arch of C1 is absent (*right arrow*). Note the normal relationship of the odontoid to the anterior arch of C1 (*left arrow*).

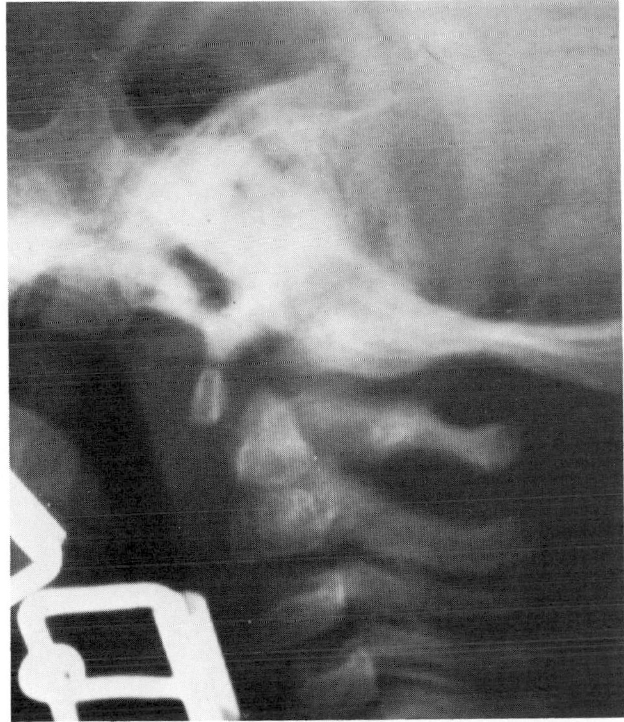

Figure 14–7 Infant cervical spine. Note the normally large distance between the incompletely ossified odontoid peg and the anterior arch of the atlas. The odontoid is not fused to the body of C2.

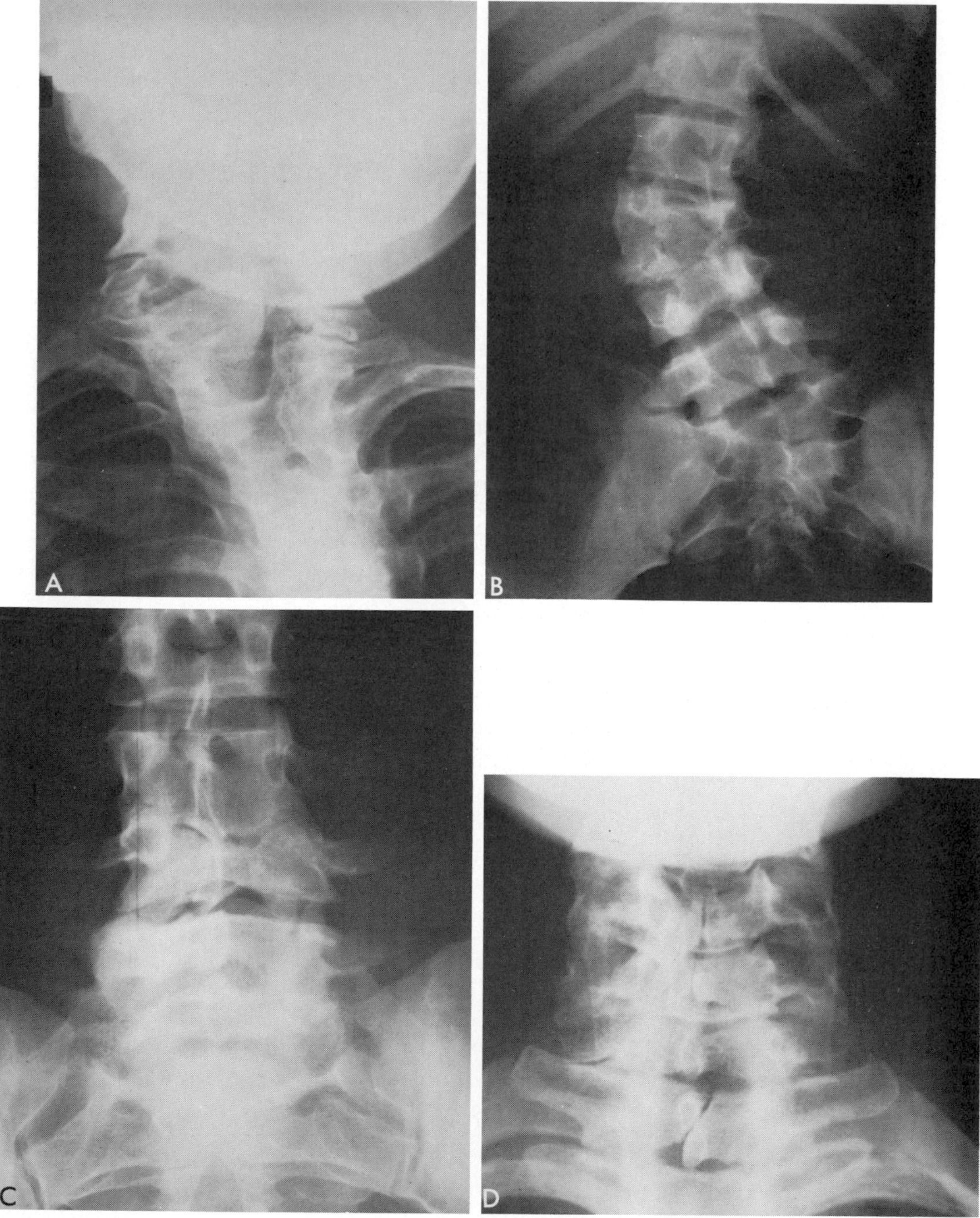

Figure 14–8 *A*. Klippel-Feil syndrome. *B*. Lumbar hemivertebra. *C*. Lumbar block vertebrae. *D*. Spina bifida occulta.

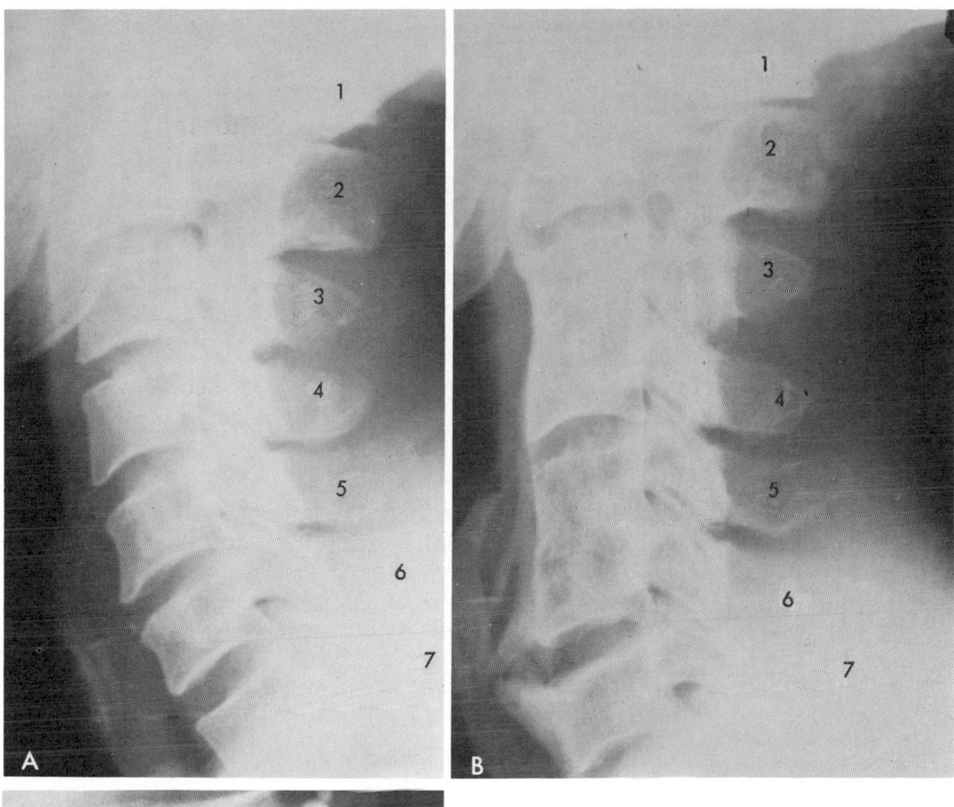

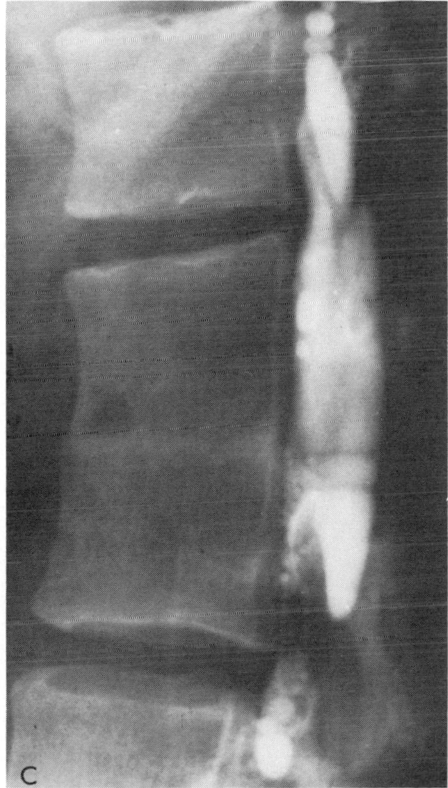

Figure 14–9 Acquired block vertebrae. *A* and *B*. Preoperative and postoperative views of cervical spine showing two pairs of block vertebrae from surgical fusion. *C*. Block vertebrae secondary to infection.

tebrae because of destruction of the disc space (Fig. 14–9).

Diastematomyelia is an unusual anomaly occurring mostly in the lower thoracic and lumbar regions and characterized by a midline cleft in the spinal cord or cauda equina. The midline cleavage may be marked by a bony spur visible in the plain x-ray and laminagrams, or by a fibrocartilagenous septum demonstrated only by myelography (Fig. 14–10). There is separation of the interpedicular spaces. Hemivertebrae, scoliosis, kyphosis, neural arch anomalies, and tethering of the cord are commonly present, and these may be primarily responsible for the patient's complaints.

Spina bifida may occur as an isolated defect in bony fusion, but it may also be associated with a congenital anomaly that may include a meningomyelocele, a lipoma, a dermoid, or any other defect associated with spinal dysplasia (Fig. 14–11). Segmentation anomalies of the lumbar sacral region may present as a sacralized L5 or a lumbarized S1. The only way to determine the exact structure is to count down from C1. The presence of a large sacral canal may suggest an occult sacral meningocele (Fig. 14–12).

Trauma

Fractures of the spinal column are usually associated with certain types of injuries. The cervical spine is most commonly involved in trauma. Certain types of trauma affect parts of the arch, making them vulnerable to further injury. The trauma may involve the odontoid peg, as shown in Figures 14–13 and 14–14, the body of the vertebrae, the intervertebral disc, the neural arch, or the transverse and spinous processes.

Fractures and subluxations of the lower cervical and upper thoracic vertebral bodies can be missed. In the anterior-posterior projection, subluxation is suspected when the vertical distance between the spinous processes of the involved vertebrae measures less than half the interspinous distances of the adjacent normal vertebrae.[39] Unless an effort is made to pull the shoulders down, these vertebrae will

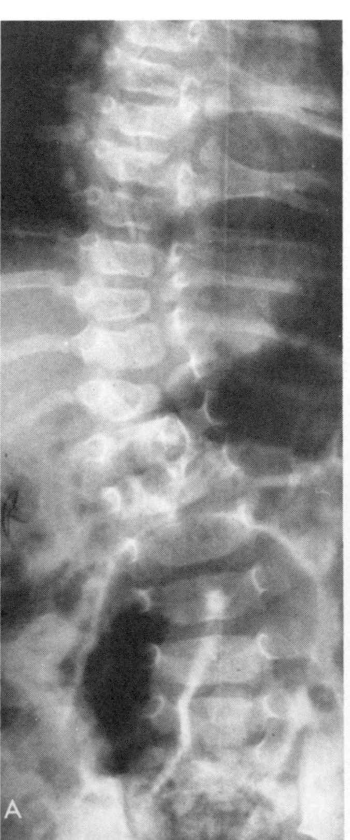

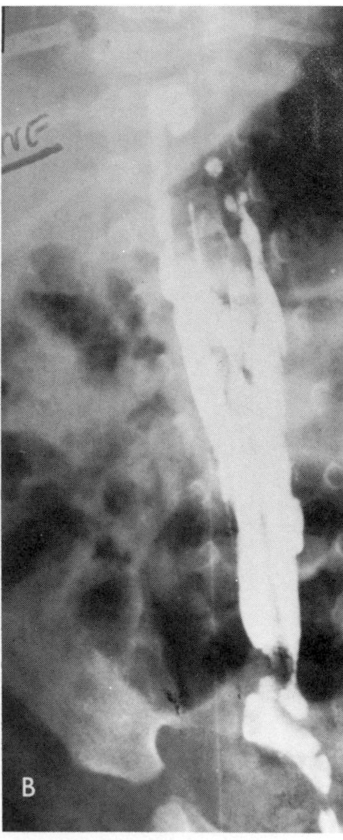

Figure 14–10 Diastematomyelia. *A*. Bony spur near midline at L1, multiple vertebral anomalies in the lower thoracic region, and fusion of left ribs. *B*. Bony spur separates the lower spinal cord, and filum terminale is enlarged.

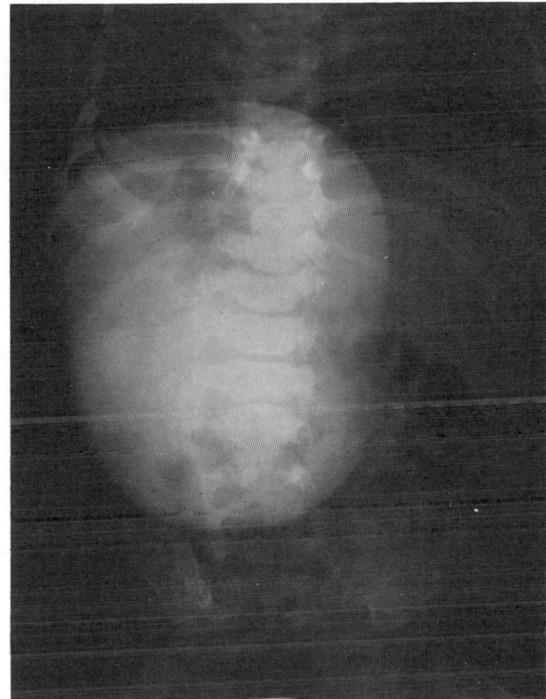

Figure 14–11 Meningomyelocele. The large soft-tissue density is obvious. Note multiple anomalies of the thoracolumbar spine.

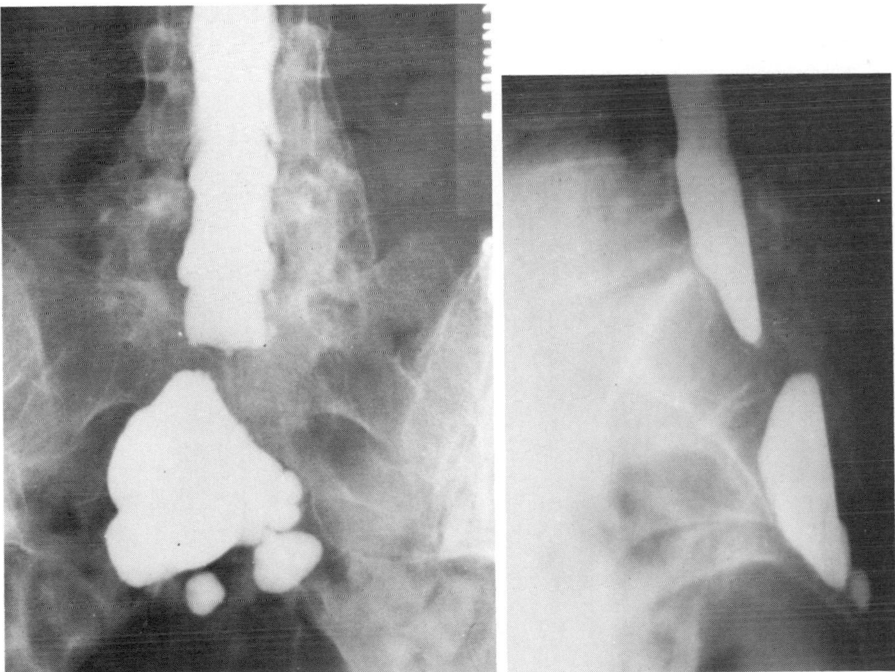

Figure 14–12 Occult sacral meningocele.

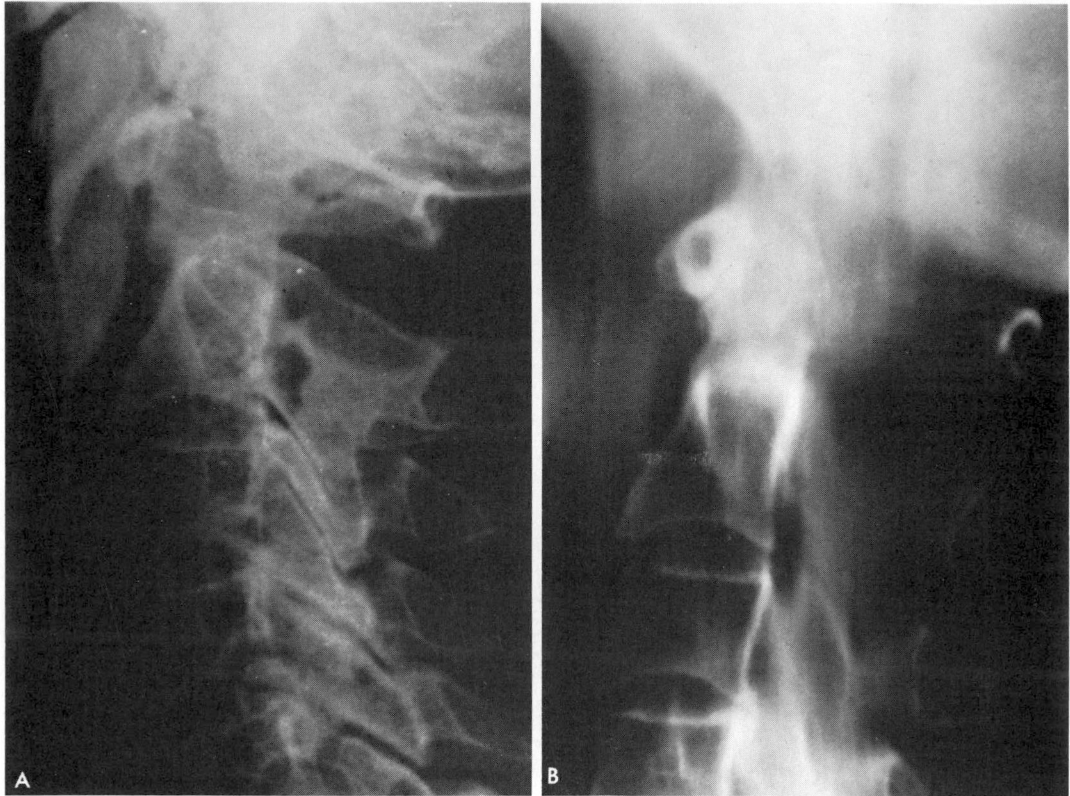

Figure 14–13 *A*. Fracture through the base of odontoid peg suspected on plain film. *B*. Confirmed on laminagraphy.

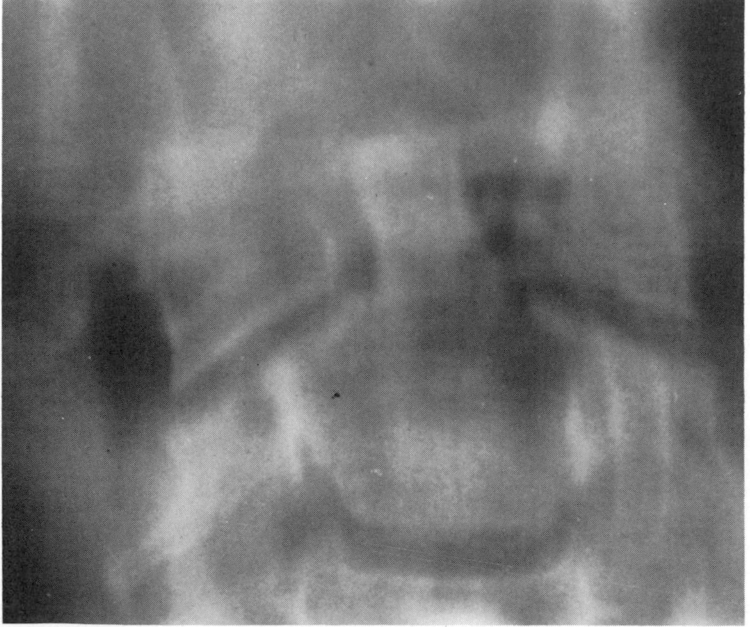

Figure 14–14 Fracture through base of odontoid peg seen on anteroposterior view. Note the atlantoaxial dislocation.

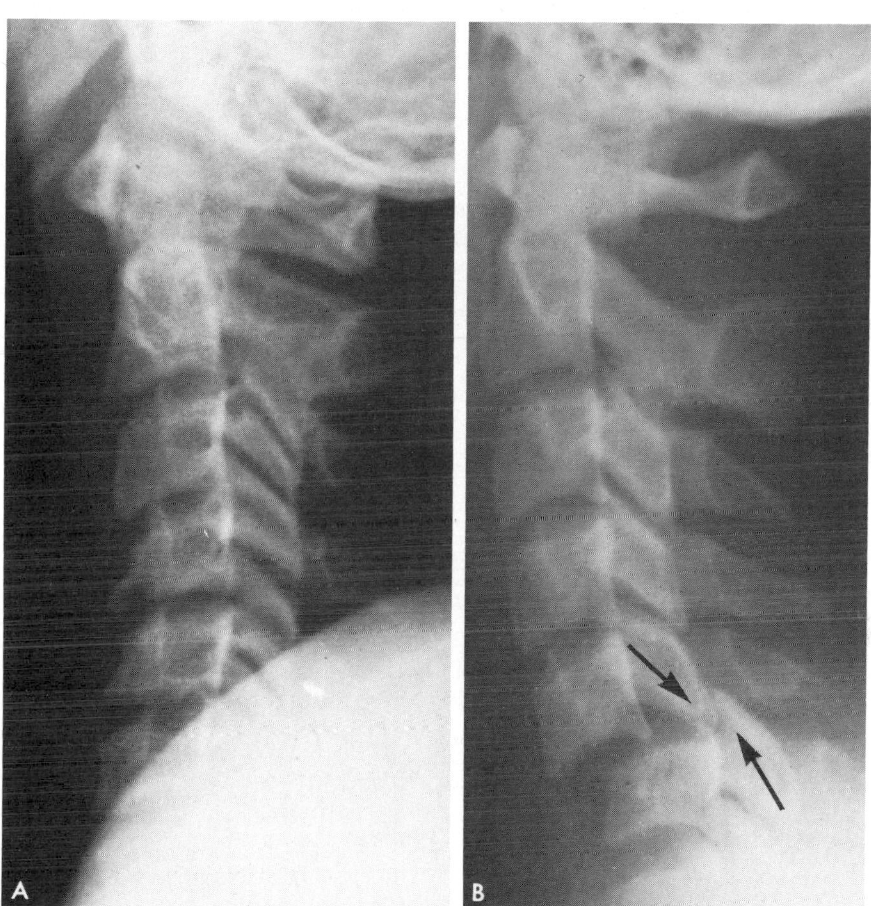

Figure 14–15 *A*. Compression fracture of C4 and C5. *B*. Fracture-dislocation of C5 and C6 with locking of articular facets (*arrows*).

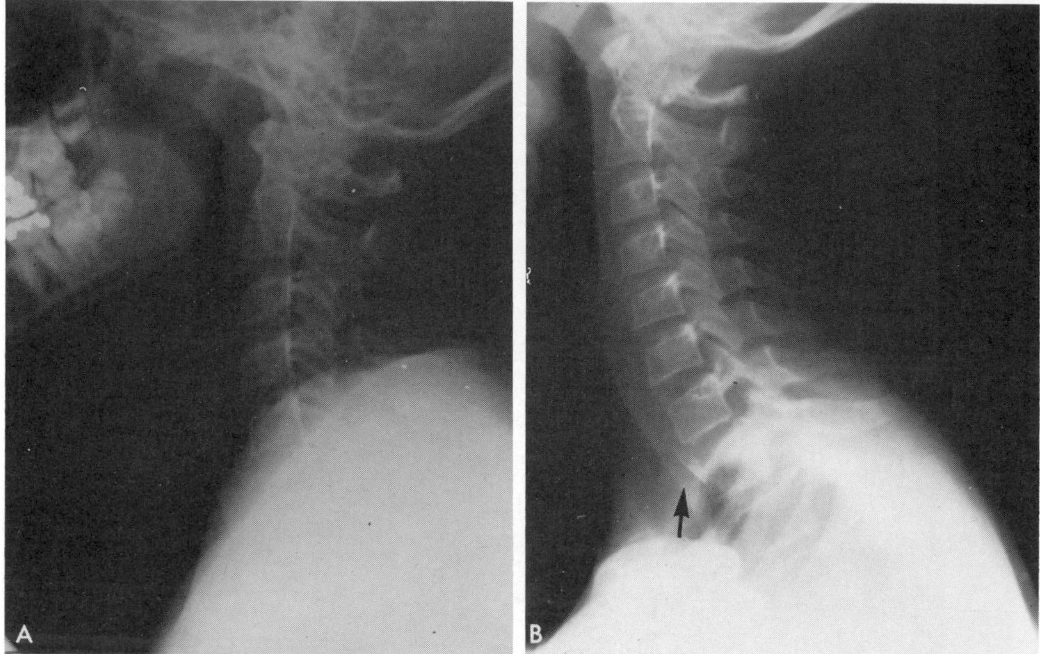

Figure 14–16 *A*. Compression fracture of T1 was missed on initial examination because shoulders were not pulled down. *B*. The fracture is obvious in the examination with the shoulders pulled down.

not be visualized in a large number of patients (Fig. 14–16). In the obese patient with a short neck, pulling the shoulders down is inadequate and spinal alignments are difficult to evaluate in the swimmer's projection. A special double-exposure technique is necessary to visualize the cervical thoracic junction.[15] It is imperative to make an all-out effort to visualize the lower cervical region, especially in the unresponsive patient. Occasionally an intoxicated patient admitted for trauma will be rendered quadriparetic as a result of manipulation that was considered safe because of a "negative" cervical spine examination that did not include the cervical-thoracic junction (Fig. 14–17). Blurring of the cervical prevertebral fat stripe may help in the detection of a fracture.[56] Oblique anteroposterior projections may demonstrate unsuspected fractures of the lateral masses. Laminagraphy may help to visualize fractures not apparent on plain x-ray (Fig. 14–18). Occasionally cervical spine trauma results from trauma to the skull. Thus, every patient with head trauma should have a careful examination of the cervical spine.

The following fractures occur in the cervical spine: (1) Jefferson's fracture of the atlas; (2) fractures of the axis at the base of the odontoid; fractures through laminae and pedicles; and (3) fractures through C3–C7, which may include a fracture-dislocation without vertebral body compression as well as fracture with body compression.

Fractures of the spinous processes and transverse processes may result from sudden traction of ligaments and muscles. These may be recognized in the routine projections, but special projections may be necessary.

The majority of thoracic-lumbar fractures involve T12, L1, and L2. These are increasing in frequency in automobile accidents involving cars in which abdominal seat belts are used (Figs. 14–19 and 14–20). Thoracic-lumbar fractures may result in wedging of the vertebral bodies, disruption of the posterior elements, and fractures of the transverse processes. Compression fractures may result in the extrusion of disc material through the disrupted posterior ligaments and annulus.

Dislocation occurs when the inferior articular facet of an upper cervical segment slides forward on the upper articulating facet of an adjacent lower cervical segment. These may be locked in this abnormal position (see Fig. 14–15*B*).

Atlantoaxial dislocation is commonly

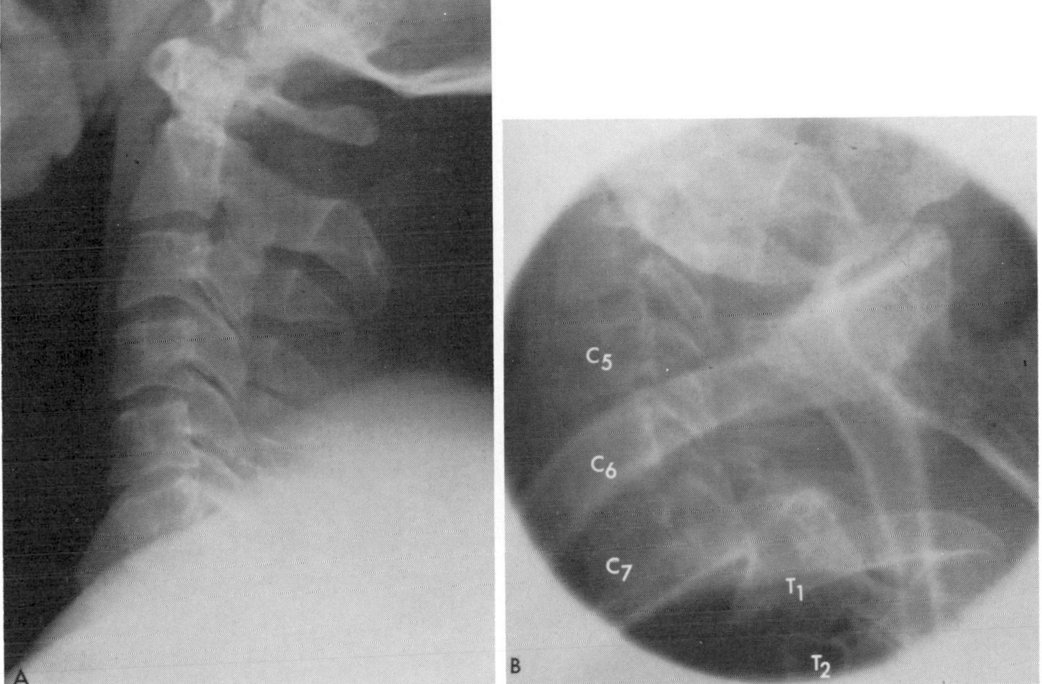

Figure 14–17 *A*. Severe fracture-dislocation of C7, T1 was missed. Since the fracture was not suspected after the initial roentgenogram, manipulations of the neck resulted in pressure on the cord and paraplegia. *B*. Double-exposure technique shows the severe fracture-dislocation.

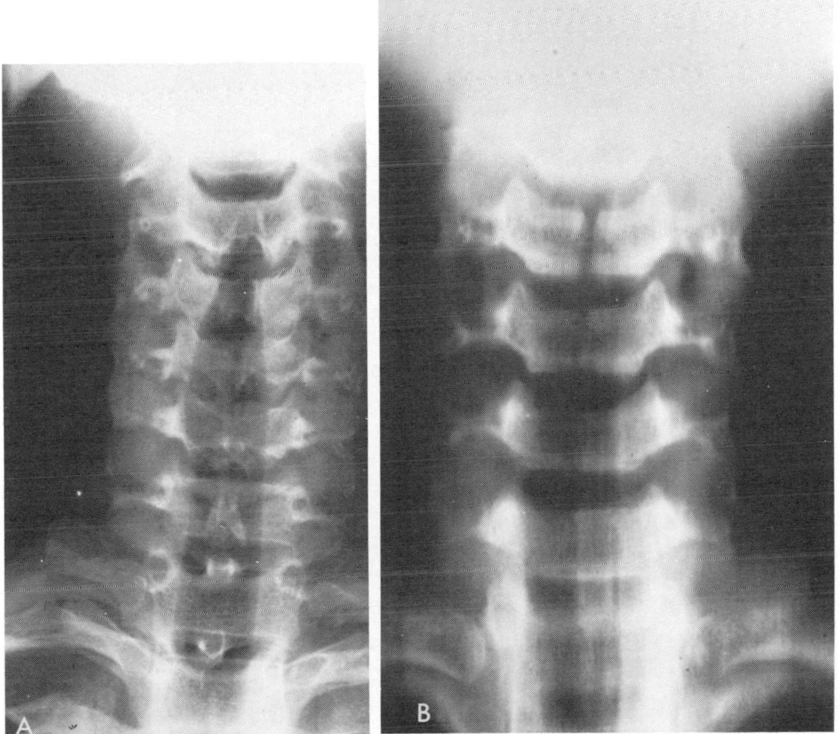

Figure 14–18 Rare vertical fracture through vertebral bodies of C4 and C5, not apparent on anteroposterior projection, *A*, and well shown on the frontal tomogram, *B*.

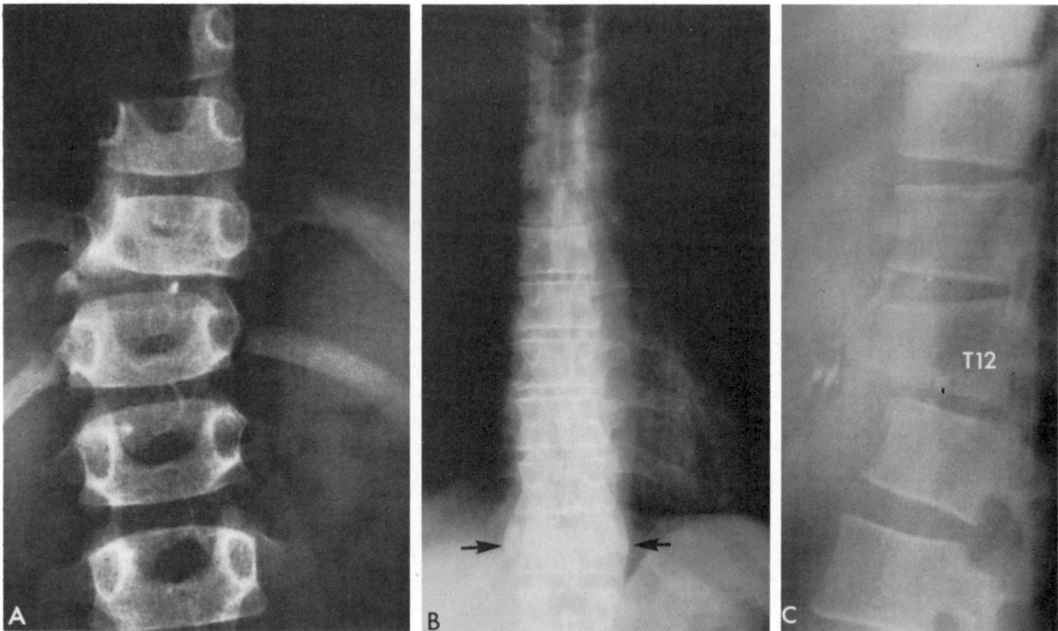

Figure 14–19 *A*. Fracture-dislocation T11, T12. *B*. T12 fracture recognized in chest film by paraspinal hematoma (*arrows*). *C*. Seat belt fracture of T12. Compression injury. Radiograph was taken with patient lying on her back and with a horizontal beam. The important trauma to the posterior elements was not detected. This illustrates the need to raise the patient off the table top to include these structures in the roentgenogram.

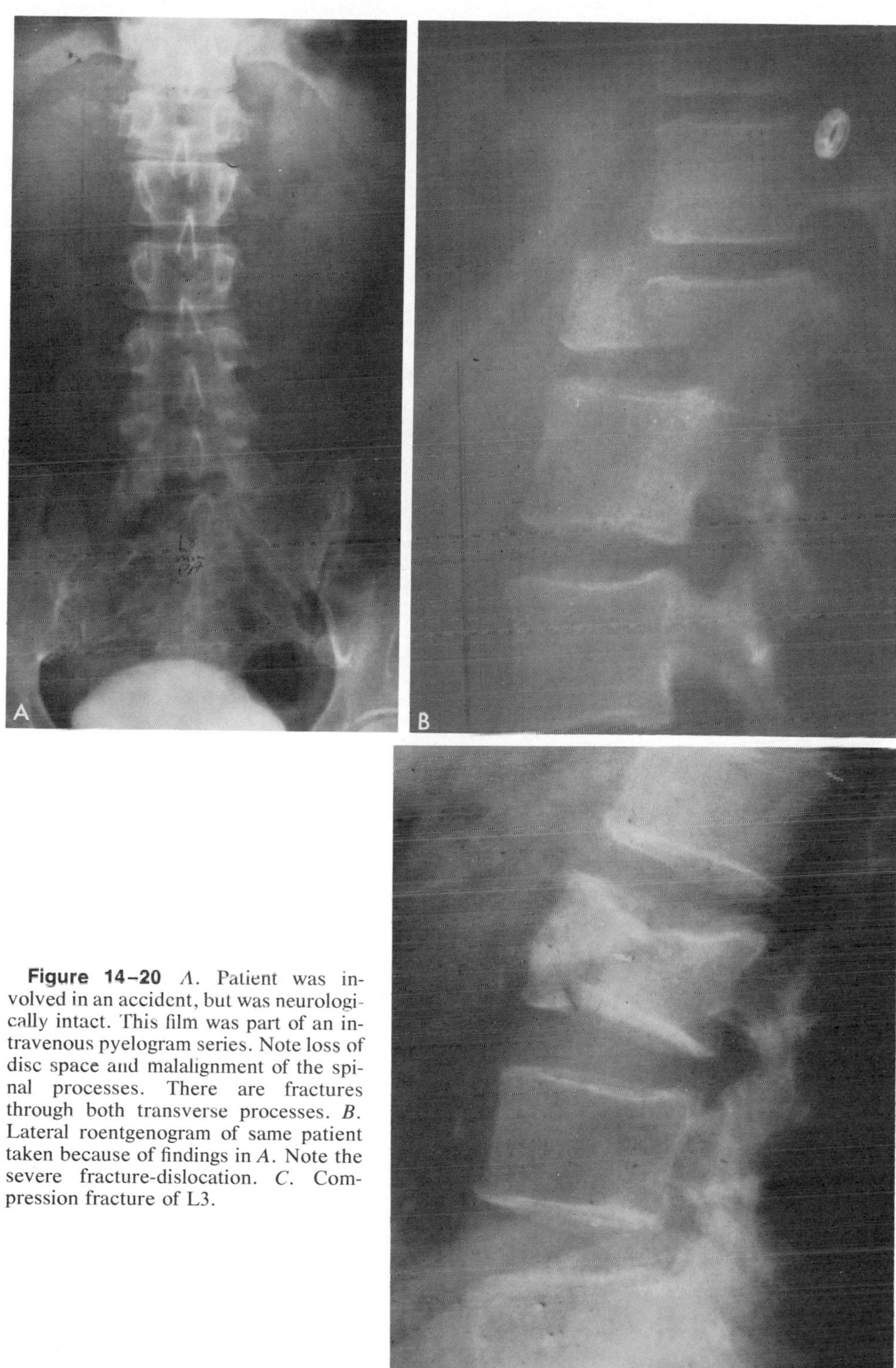

Figure 14–20 *A*. Patient was involved in an accident, but was neurologically intact. This film was part of an intravenous pyelogram series. Note loss of disc space and malalignment of the spinal processes. There are fractures through both transverse processes. *B*. Lateral roentgenogram of same patient taken because of findings in *A*. Note the severe fracture-dislocation. *C*. Compression fracture of L3.

caused by conditions that predispose to pathological laxity of the transverse ligament such as infection and rheumatoid arthritis (see Fig. 14–27).[19] It rarely results from trauma because of the tendency of the dens to fracture before the ligament ruptures.[45] The diagnosis is made by the increased distance between the anterior arch of the atlas and the dens, which normally should not exceed 2.0 mm in adults and 3.0 mm in children. Associated rotary dislocation at C1–C2 may also occur. To make a diagnosis of rotary dislocation, Shapiro emphasized, a pair of true right-angle films of the atlas is needed because the crucial finding is the distance of the dens from the anterior arch of the atlas on the lateral film.[46] To determine this distance, it is necessary to analyze the position of the articular facets of C1 and C2 and of the dens relative to the lateral masses of C1 on the anteroposterior film and to examine the relative position of

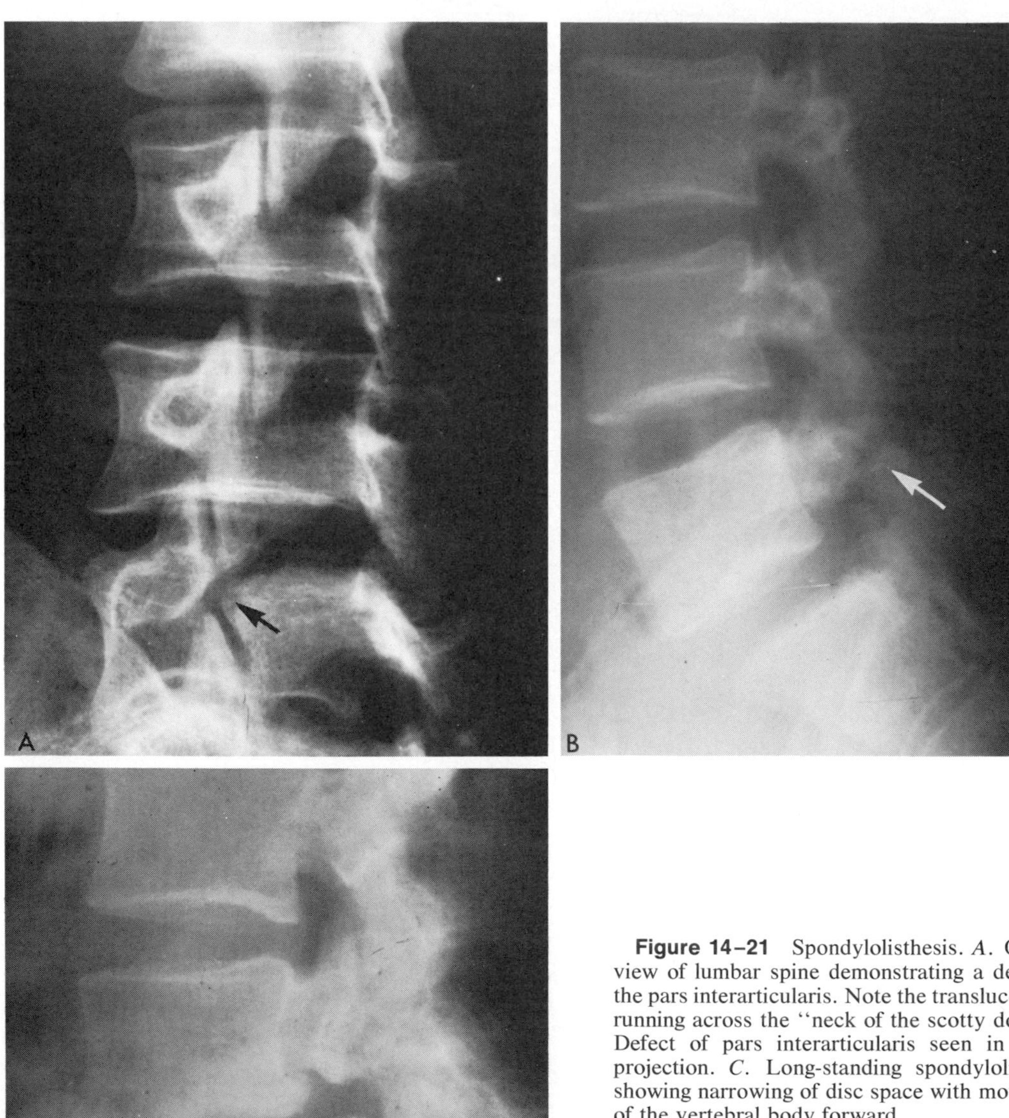

Figure 14–21 Spondylolisthesis. *A*. Oblique view of lumbar spine demonstrating a defect in the pars interarticularis. Note the translucent line running across the "neck of the scotty dog." *B*. Defect of pars interarticularis seen in lateral projection. *C*. Long-standing spondylolisthesis showing narrowing of disc space with movement of the vertebral body forward.

the head, neck, and trunk of the patient. Rotary fixation of C1–C2 is an unusual deformity thought to be due to a tear and invagination of the capsular ligament.[58] In this condition, the asymmetrical position of the dens relative to the lateral masses of C1 is fixed and cannot be corrected by counter rotation, as shown by the anteroposterior films taken with 15 degrees of rotation to each side.

Spondylolisthesis is considered to be a result of trauma (Fig. 14–21). The vertebral body moves forward, leaving the posterior elements behind. In the minor degrees no defect is present in the pars interarticularis and degeneration of the disc may be sufficient to allow the minor movements. When the dislocation is great, however, a defect may be recognized in the pars interarticularis. Oblique views should be taken routinely when this situation is suspected, and the defect should be searched for (Fig. 14–21*A*).

In lateral roentgenograms of the cervical spine with the neck flexed there is frequently a slight displacement anteriorly with respect to the subjacent vertebrae. In infants and children this displacement may be exaggerated (Fig. 14–22). This displacement should not be mistaken for a dislocation; flexion and extension of the neck will show that the movements are normal.[52]

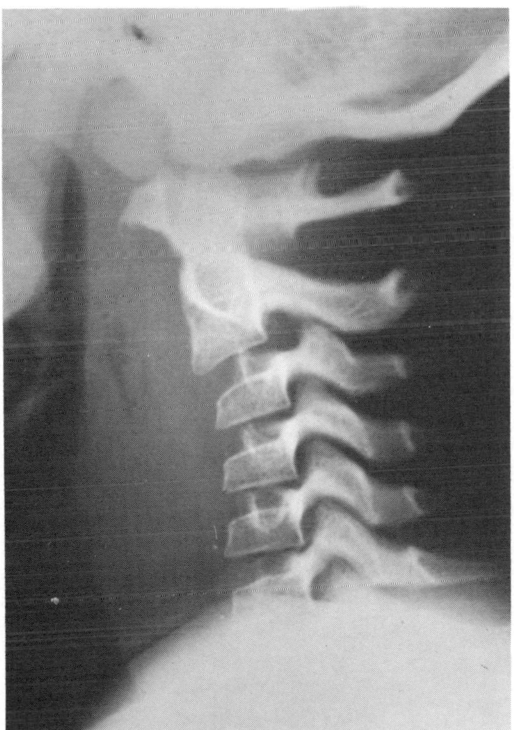

Figure 14–22 Retropharyngeal abscess and pseudo-subluxation at C2 and C3 in a child.

Various types of traumatic subarachnoid disruption may occur (see Fig. 14–52). Avulsion of the brachial nerve roots may occur as a result of severe trauma to the shoulder. The arachnoid and dura forming the nerve root sleeve are torn, leaving a pocket in which the contrast medium may collect. Various traumatic communications between the subarachnoid space and the thoracic and abdominal cavities may occur. Subarachnoid mediastinal fistulae are extremely rare.[59] Traumatic extradural cysts of the spine may result from tears of the dura during operations on lumbar discs.[44]

Infections

There is a tendency not to consider seriously the possibility of infectious diseases of the spine. This attitude has been propagated by the antibiotic era. Awareness of the possibility of an infectious process may, however, alert the physician to it in time to avoid the serious complications of spinal cord damage associated with it.

Of the organisms causing pyogenic infection of the vertebrae, *Staphylococcus aureus* is still the most common, though its incidence appears to be decreasing, and the gram-negative bacilli are second in frequency, but their incidence appears to be increasing. *Streptococcus* is still prevalent in children. The hematogenous route is the most frequent mode of spread, especially among drug addicts.[20] The radiological changes due to infection may manifest themselves weeks after the onset of symptoms. The infection usually begins in the vertebral body near the disc, which shows early involvement. The characteristic changes are loss of definition of the margins of the vertebral bodies with slight narrowing of the disc spaces (Fig. 14–23). Prolonged infection is marked by bony proliferation, which may end in fusion of the bodies. A paravertebral mass occasionally is seen and may be one of the early changes and the only clue to the bony disease. In the later stages the infected material may break down and calcify, leaving a signature of the

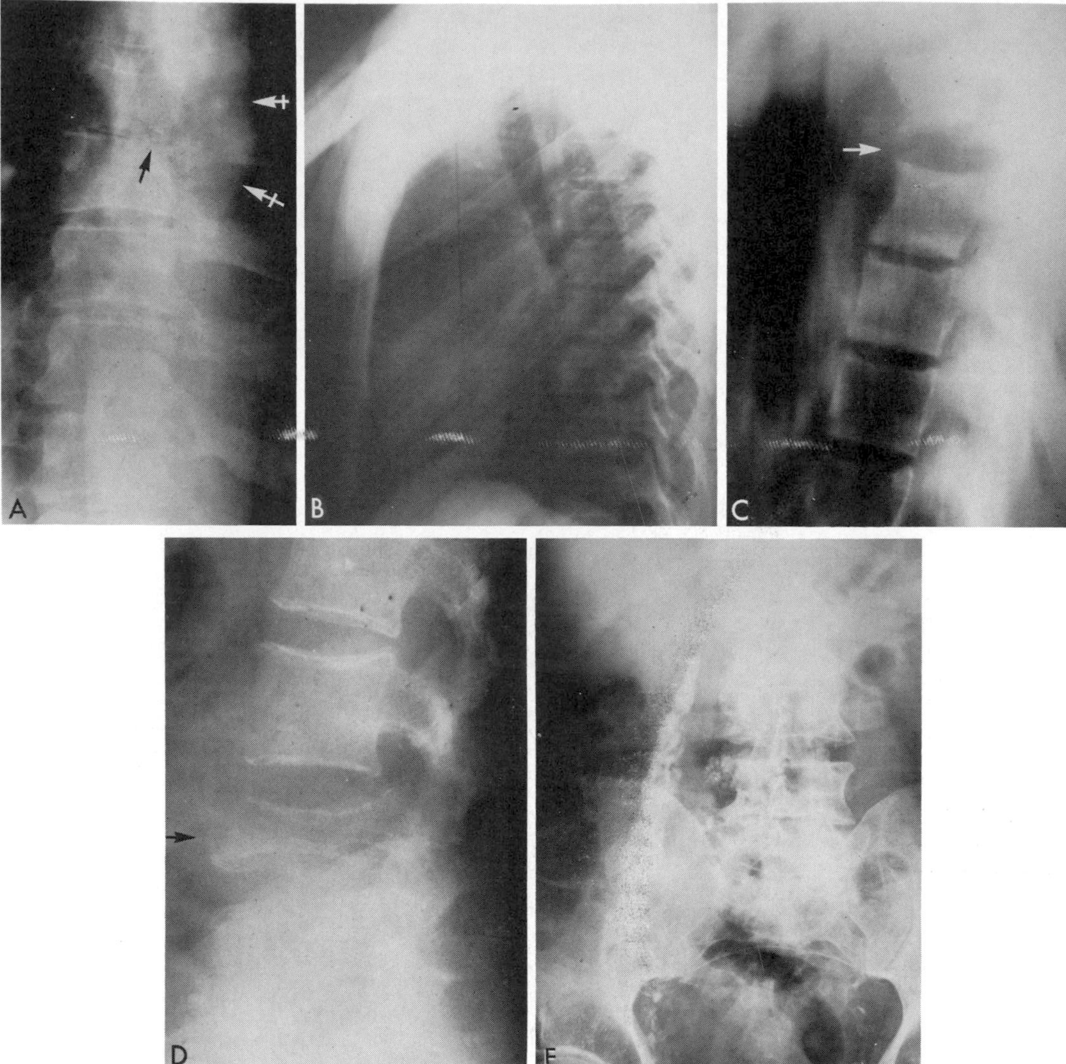

Figure 14–23 Infection. *A*. Pyogenic infection with loss of the disc space (*single arrow*) and a paraspinal mass (*arrows with crossed shaft*). *B*. Tuberculous destruction of a vertebral body was missed in the routine lateral chest film but recognized in the laminagram, *C*, in which the body is seen to have virtually disappeared, leaving what looks like a wide disc space (*arrow*). *D*. Pyogenic osteomyelitis simulating metastatic disease. Note collapse of the body (*arrow*) with intact disc spaces. *E*. Calcified psoas abscess, a late manifestation of tuberculosis osteomyelitis.

disease process. In tuberculous infection the process is much more prolonged, with caseation going on to granulomatous changes. Pus may rupture through the ligaments, tracking and forming a cold abscess. The abscess and tracks may later calcify. Severe spinal deformity may occur and may include scoliosis and a pronounced kyphoscoliosis. Other infectious processes such as syphilis, brucellosis, actinomycosis, toxoplasmosis, and typhoid may involve the spine without any specific characteristic changes. Charcot's spine, a neuropathic joint disease, is usually due to syphilis, diabetes, tumors, paraplegia, syringomyelia, or transverse myelitis. The neuropathic joint changes consist of marked articular cartilaginous destruction and haphazard proliferation of subchondral bone with osteophytes and complete disorganization of the joint.

Osteoarthritis

Osteoarthritis results from the aging process of the disc, which is the precipitating factor in the production of this condition.

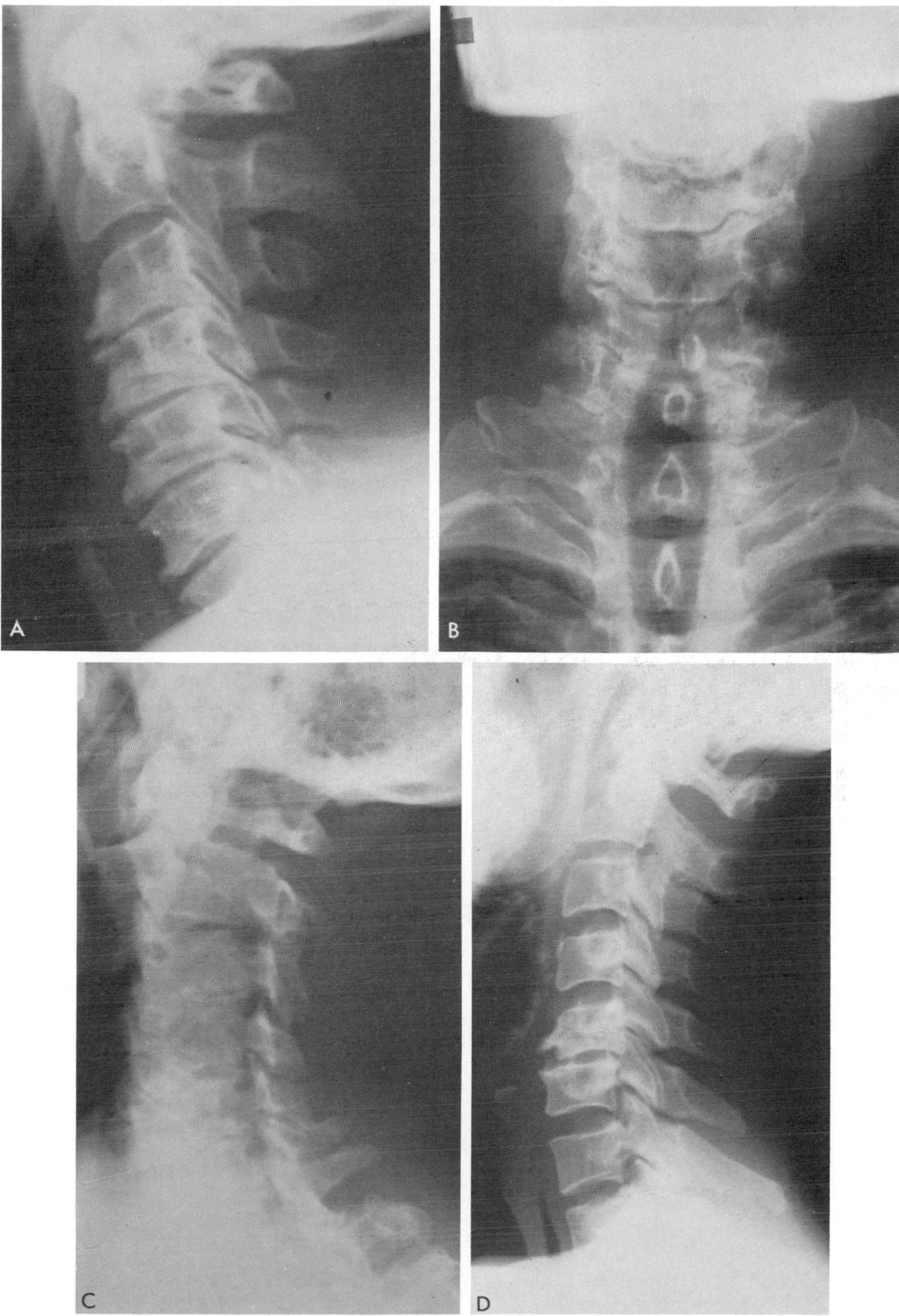

Figure 14–24 Osteoarthritis. *A, B,* and *C.* Note the diffuse narrowing of the disc spaces, spur formation, eburnation of bone, and encroachment on intervertebral foramina. *D.* Isolated involvement of C5 and C6.

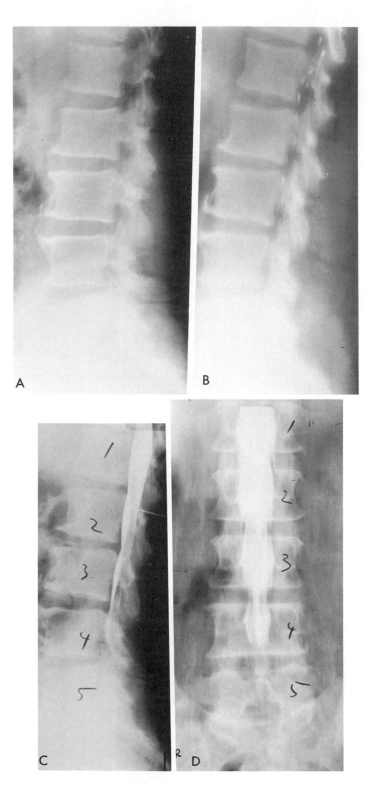

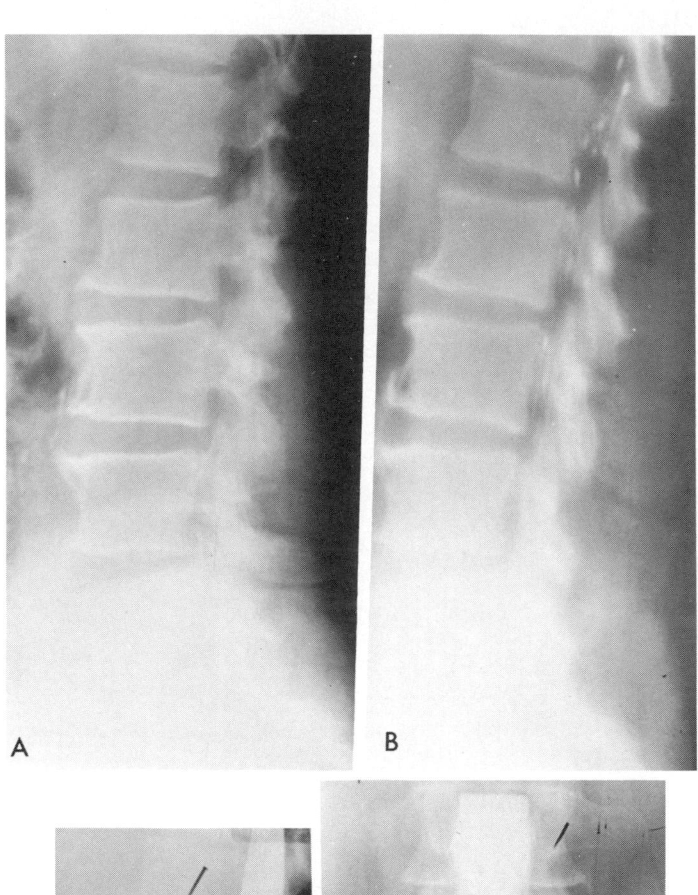

Figure 14–25 *A* and *B*. Narrow lumbar canal. Lateral tomogram, *B*, reveals narrowing of sagittal diameter in the lumbar region that is not so apparent on lateral plain x-ray, *A*. *C* and *D*. Complete extradural block at L4–L5.

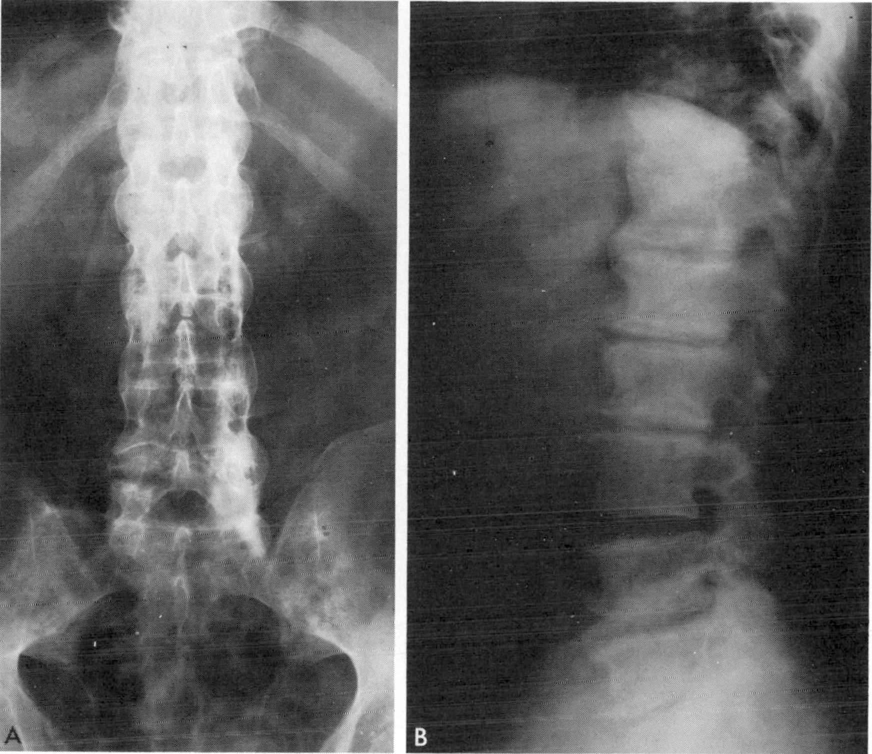

Figure 14–26 *A*. Ankylosing spondylitis–note changes in sacroiliac joints and the typical bamboo spine with ossification of the longitudinal ligaments. *B*. Advanced Paget's disease.

Dehydration, disintegration, and fragmentation of the disc cause it to bulge, increasing traction at the attachment of the longitudinal ligaments. As the disc continues to degenerate and narrow, abnormal movements and contact of exposed adjacent bony structures result in secondary formation of spurs and ridges. These ridges and spurs may encroach upon the spinal canal and the intervertebral foramina, causing cord compression or root compression respectively (Fig. 14–24). Individuals with congenitally narrow canals are predisposed to compression by ridges and spurs early in life, unlike those with capacious canals, who remain asymptomatic despite the presence of these bony processes (Fig. 14–25). Vertical elongation of the neural foramina, vertical or convergent alignment of the laminae, and heavy thick pedicles are changes suggestive of congenitally narrow canal. Rarely, the vertebral artery may be compromised by ridges encroaching upon its lumen, particularly when the head and neck are rotated. The most common sites of cervical disc degeneration are at C5–C6 and C6–C7. These bony ridges may be recognized in the plain radiographs. Oblique projections must be taken to outline the intervertebral foramina.

Ankylosing spondylitis is also known as Marie-Strumpell disease. The pathological process of this disease involves the sacroiliac and other spinous joints with eventual ligamentous ossifications (Fig. 14–26).

The most important aspect of rheumatoid arthritis of the spine is its effect on the synovial joint between the dens and the anterior arch of the atlas. The resulting ligamentous involvement, which at times is accompanied by odontoid peg destruction, may cause atlantoaxial dislocation. This condition should not be mistaken for trauma to this region (Fig. 14–27).

Paget's Disease

Paget's disease is often unsuspected and occurs mainly in the spinous body. Its cause is unknown. Pathological changes in

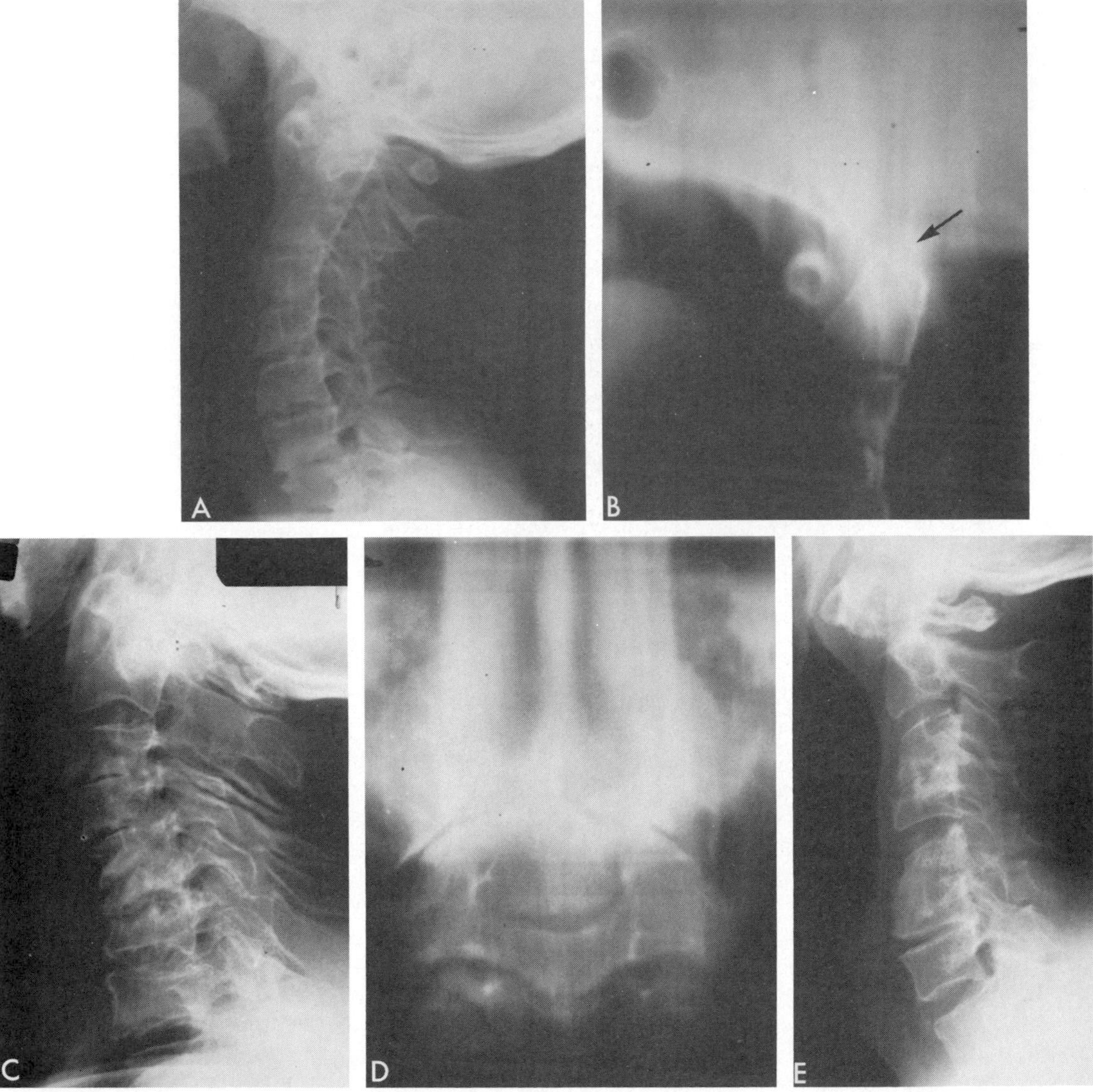

Figure 14–27 Rheumatoid arthritis. *A*. Rheumatoid arthritis with destruction odontoid process. *B*. Tomography shows the area of destruction to better advantage (*arrow*). *C*. Another case of rheumatoid arthritis showing less destruction of the odontoid peg but more changes in movement in the cervical spine. *D*. Tomography in the anteroposterior projection showing the odontoid changes. *E*. A third example showing C3-C4 and C5-C6 fusion secondary to rheumatoid arthritis.

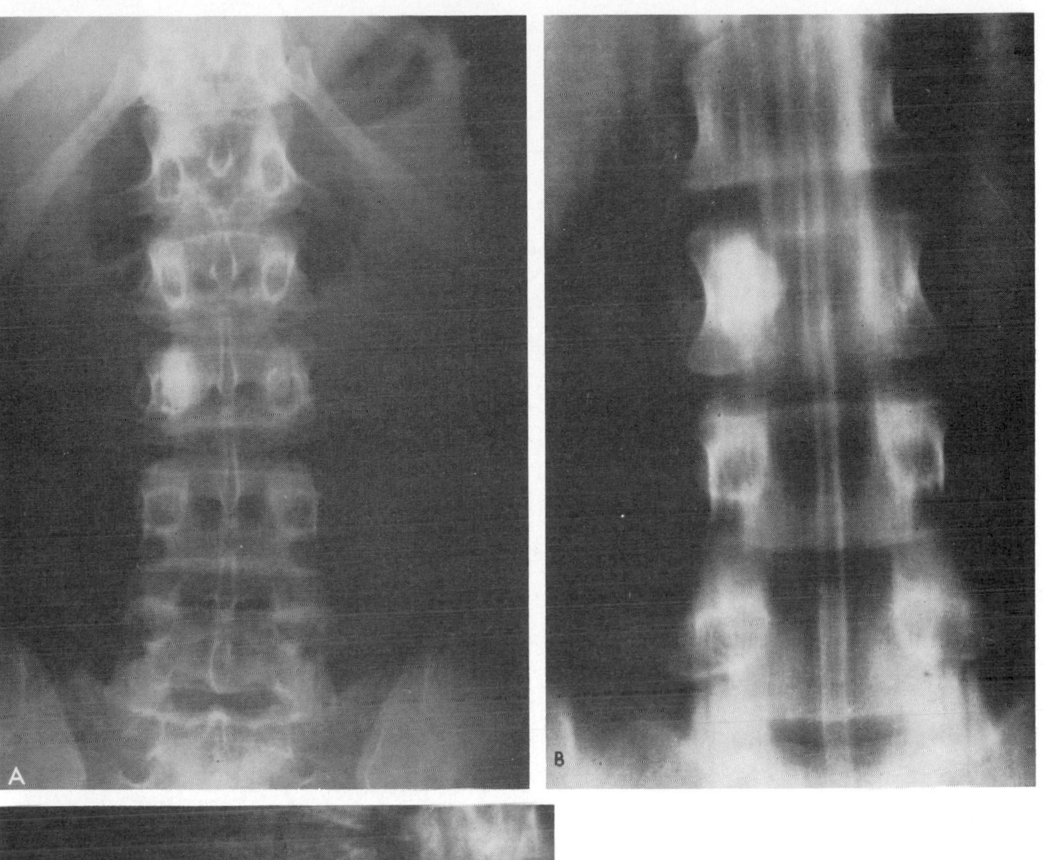

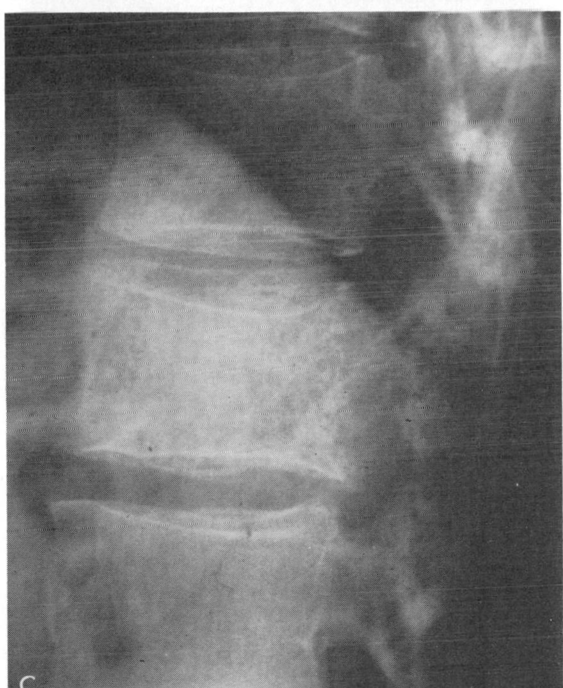

Figure 14–28 Metastatic disease. *A*. Blastic metastasis involving pedicle only. *B*. Tomogram showing the osteoblastic metastatic deposit to better advantage. *C*. Osteoblastic vertebral body metastasis from prostate.

the spine include bone softening, resorption, and disorganized bony reformation. The result is a widened, dense vertebral body that may fracture and may cause cord compression (see Fig. 14–26*B*). Malignant degeneration may occur but is rare. It must be differentiated from osteoblastic metastasis to the spine from carcinoma of the prostate or breast, or occasionally, malignant lymphoma (Fig. 14–28*C*).

Tumors

Although spinal cord tumors are only one sixth as common as brain tumors, over 50 per cent of them are benign, and great effort should be made to recognize them. The usual classification of spinal tumors is: extradural, intradural extramedullary, and intradural intramedullary. The myelographic criteria for deciding in which group a specific tumor belongs are discussed later. The grouping is not of academic interest alone, since the determination of the compartment involved usually gives a clue to the type of tumor. Over 90 per cent of extradural tumors are malignant, 75 per cent of extradural lesions are metastatic, and over 50 per cent of intradural lesions are benign.

Neurofibromas and meningiomas constitute more than 90 per cent of intradural lesions. Eighty per cent of spinal meningiomas occur in women of an average age of 50 years and favor the thoracic area. Calcification that can be detected in plain films is infrequent in meningiomas. Rarely meningiomas are extradural and occasionally they are multiple. When spinal meningiomas are multiple, it is nearly impossible to differentiate them from multiple neurofibroma prior to operation.[5]

Schwannomas are slightly more common than meningiomas. There is no sexual or site predilection. Occasionally they are multiple. Seventy per cent of schwannomas are intradural, 15 per cent are dumbbell (intradural and extradural), and 15 per cent are extradural. Bone changes are more frequent than in meningiomas and usually occur with the dumbbell tumors. The bony changes include erosion of the pedicles, widening of the interpedicular distance, and scalloping of the posterior surface of the vertebral body. These bony changes may be caused directly by adjacent schwannomas, but they may also be present without the tumor as part of the mesenchymal defect (dural ectasia) in this condition.

Over 95 per cent of intramedullary lesions are gliomas. These may cause a widening of the spinal canal involving more than one segment. Other causes of intramedullary mass are nonneoplastic conditions such as spinal cord contusion, hematomyelia, syringomyelia, and hydromyelia. Intramedullary metastatic lesions are rare, but 160 cases have been reported in the literature.[40] Half of these were from primary lung carcinoma (see Fig. 14–48).

Metastatic disease is the most common cause of tumor of the spine. As metastatic hematogenous spread affects the spongiosa first, and since the radiological density of the body resides in the cortical bone, a large part of the body may be involved without showing any radiological change. Only when the cortex is involved will radiological changes be appreciated.

The most common tumors to metastasize to the spine are those of the breast, prostate, thyroid, kidney, and lung. The bone reaction depends on the nature of the primary neoplasm. Breast and prostate tumors are usually osteoblastic (see Fig. 14–28). Those of the thyroid and kidney are usually osteolytic, and any combination may be present (Fig. 14–29). Pedicular involvement is important to recognize, since it may be associated with cord compression and is usually due to metastatic disease. Multiple myeloma may resemble metastatic disease closely, and sometimes it is not possible to distinguish between them.

Certain solitary tumors have characteristic changes, such as sarcomas, aneurysmal bone cyst, hemangiomas, osteoid osteomas and histiocytosis (Figs. 14–30 and 14–31). The diffuse disseminated diseases at times may have characteristic changes but often cannot be distinguished from one another or from metastatic diseases (Fig. 14–32).

A condition simulating an intraspinal neoplasm is the dural ectasia that may occur as an isolated manifestation of neurofibromatosis (Fig. 14–33). This ectasia with associated bone changes may involve one or several vertebral segments. The backs of the vertebral bodies assume a scalloped appearance, and there may also be thinning of the pedicles. Other manifestations of neurofibromatosis are severe kyphoscoliosis, spondylolisthesis, and intrathoracic meningoceles.

MYELOGRAPHY

Myelography may be performed with positive or negative contrast medium. Pantopaque (iodophenylundecylic acid) is

Text continued on page 517

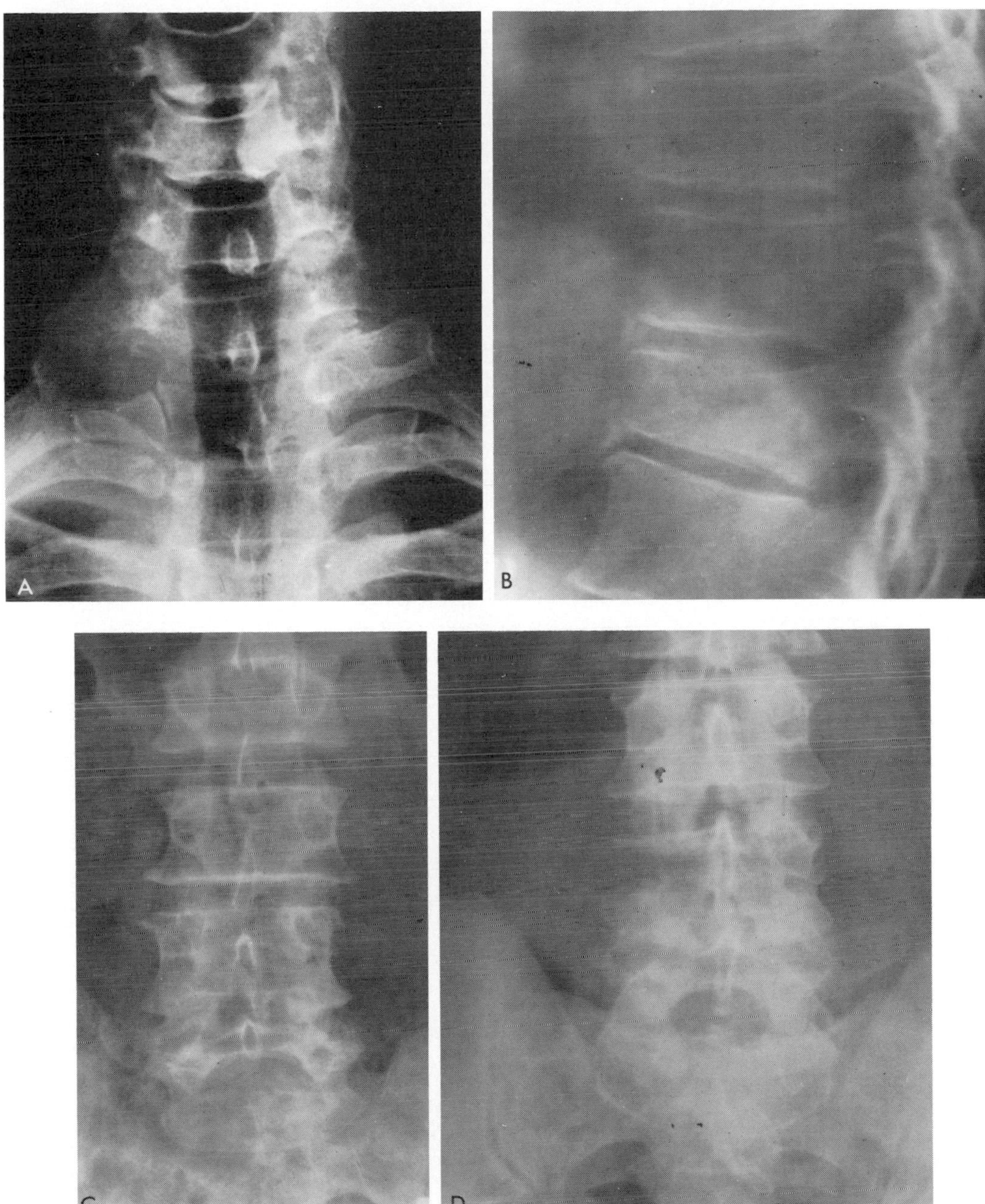

Figure 14–29 *A*. Osteolytic metastatic disease destroying the lateral transverse process of T1. *B*. Partial collapse of a vertebral body involved in metastatic disease. *C*. Unsuspected sacral and iliac destruction in patient with clinical diagnosis of herniated disc. *D*. Lytic vertebral body destruction secondary to adjacent soft-tissue sarcoma.

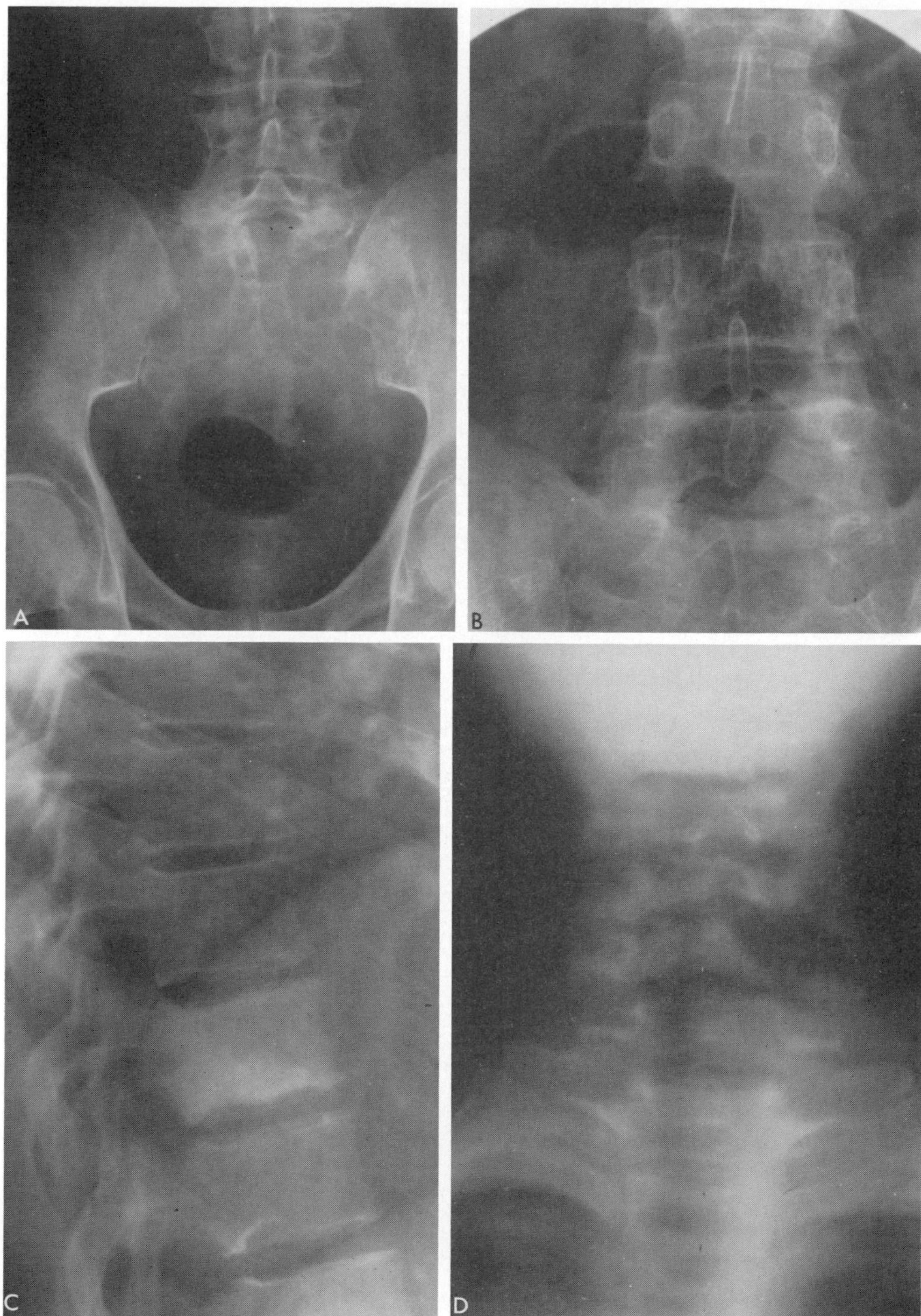

Figure 14–30 Solitary tumors of bone. *A*. Chordoma of the sacrum. *B*. Hemangioma of L4. *C*. Hodgkin's disease involving only T11 vertebral body. *D*. Reticulum cell sarcoma involving left side of vertebral body and pedicle of C6.

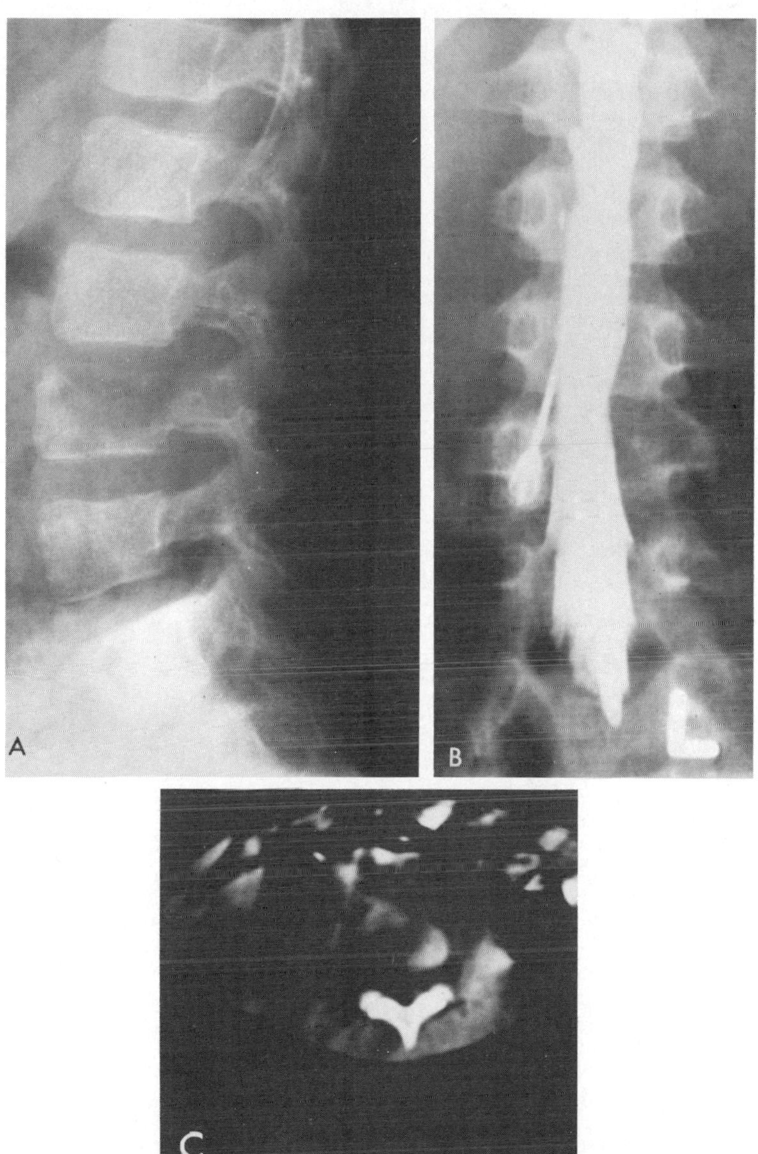

Figure 14–31 Eosinophilic granuloma. *A*. Lytic lesion of left pedicle and left side of vertebral body at L4. *B*. Lateral extradural defect on the left at L4. *C*. Coned down CT scan at L4 showing destruction of the left half of vertebral body.

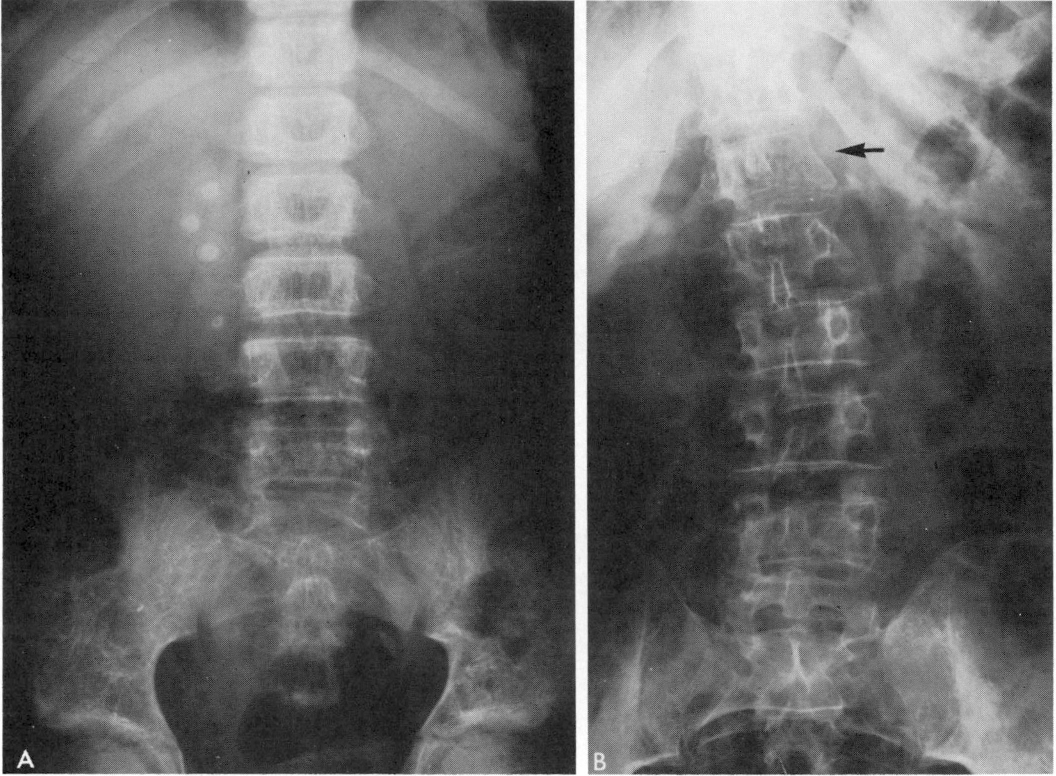

Figure 14–32 *A*. Sickle cell disease. *B*. Multiple myeloma. Note severe osteoporosis and absence of T12 pedicle.

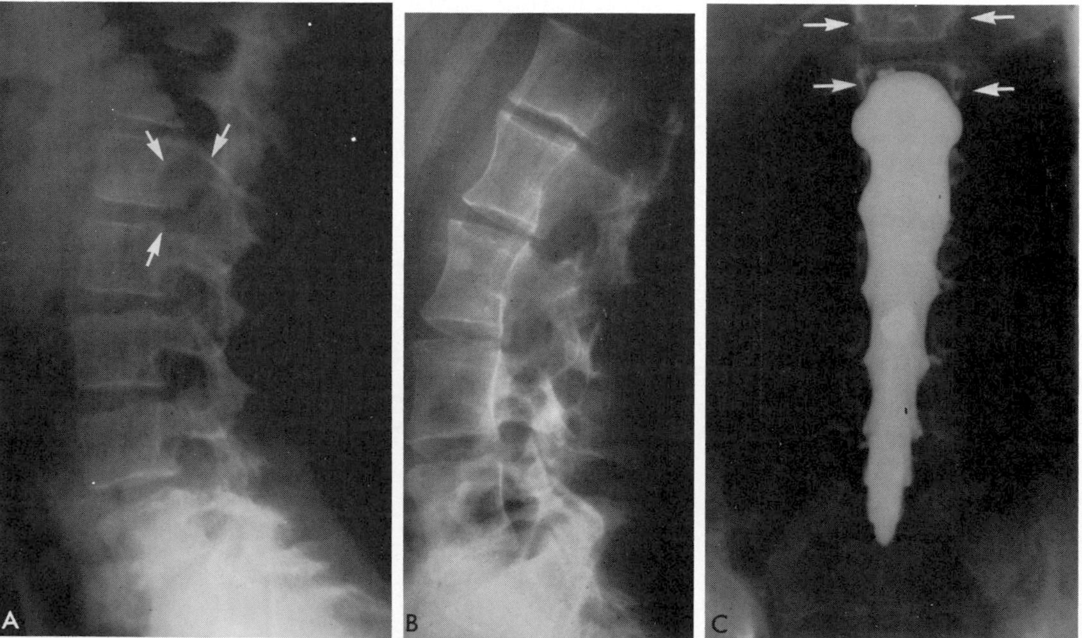

Figure 14–33 Neurofibromatosis. *A*. Enlarged intervertebral foramen (*arrows*) as a result of a dumbbell neurofibroma, *B*. Neurofibromatosis showing dysplasia of bone. The spinal canal is widened; there is pedicular erosion and scalloping of the posterior margins of the vertebral bodies simulating a spinal tumor. An intraspinal may resemble this. *C*. Dural ectasia showing thinning of pedicles (*arrows*) and outpouchings of contrast medium.

usually the contrast medium of choice although metrizamide myelography has increased in popularity. Pantopaque is not the ideal contrast medium, but it is the least irritating and the safest of the positive-contrast agents that are available at the present time. Systemic reactions and local reactions have been reported. Because of the irritating effects of the Pantopaque, it is important to remove it at the end of the procedure.

Since Pantopaque is hyperbaric, it must be manipulated into position. No other positive-contrast medium in use today may be passed from the sacral sac to the basilar subarachnoid system. Emulsified Pantopaque has not gained popularity because of the incidence of increased meningeal reactions.[36] One of the disadvantages of regular Pantopaque, which contains 30 per cent iodine by weight, is its potential for masking intraspinal masses because of its density. This prompted several investigators to use less dense Pantopaque.[25,32] The disadvantages of the less dense Pantopaque are its poor radiographic density and its reduced rate of flow, which make the examination tedious. A water-soluble contrast medium has been used extensively in Europe. Its major disadvantage is its irritant effect, necessitating spinal anesthesia. Another disadvantage is that it can only be used in the lumbar region.

Before the introduction of safer water-soluble contrast agents like metrizamide, gas myelography was used extensively in Scandinavia. The technique is much more exacting than Pantopaque myelography and requires more sophisticated equipment and meticulous care in performance and interpretation.[30,55] The gas produces little irritation, is completely absorbed in a short time, and may be used for any region of the spine. The examination can be repeated as often as desired, and there is no residual contrast agent present to obscure the picture. The discomfort some patients have may be a disadvantage of this technique. In experienced hands, gas myelography has shown its greatest versatility in demonstrating lesions that may not be recognized with other contrast media. This medium is of special value in the detection of cystic spinal cord lesions that communicate with the subarachnoid space and for detecting cord atrophy (see Fig. 14–55).[6]

Technique

Undoubtedly the most important aspect of myelography is the introduction of the entire amount of desired contrast agent into the subarachnoid space. This requires a meticulous technique. The patient may be placed in the lateral decubitus position with the knees drawn toward the forehead. In this position, the spinal spaces are opened to allow easiest introduction of the needle. The myelographer may prefer to place the patient prone on the table with a pillow under the abdomen or to have him sitting with the back flexed. The smallest possible gauge needle should be used, but the viscosity of the medium precludes using anything smaller than 20-gauge. A short-bevel needle is preferred because the contrast medium can be introduced into a single compartment. Furthermore, it facilitates the Pantopaque removal. The disadvantages of a short-bevel needle are that it is harder to introduce and may tear the arachnoid. Introducing the needle under fluoroscopic guidance assures a midline puncture, which facilitates removal of the Pantopaque. There are also various specialized myelographic needles that have inner cannulae with multiple holes designed for easier and complete removal of Pantopaque.

The site of puncture is usually at L2–L3, since this is below the level of the cord and above the majority of herniated discs. Occasionally the puncture site has to be lower when an upper lumbar lesion is suspected. In cases of total block or when the upper extent of a lesion is to be outlined, a cisternal puncture or a lateral cervical puncture may be used.[41] Fluoroscopic control of the entire procedure is absolutely essential. This monitors the position of the needle for the correct midline introduction and the desired level of puncture.

A small amount of Pantopaque should be introduced and its movement observed under screen control. If the Pantopaque remains around the needle tip when the patient is tilted, it is imperative to stop. The position of the test injection may then be ascertained by fluoroscopic visualization or by a cross-table roentgenogram. When the examiner is satisfied that the contrast is in the proper compartment and moving satisfactorily, the remainder of it can be introduced. It should be remembered that the flow may be slow in a spondylotic canal. By taking other views and ascertaining that the contrast is in the appropriate compartment, needless cancellation of the examination may be avoided.

It should be noted that a normal rate of flow of the Pantopaque can occur in the subdural space. A film to ascertain the position of the test dose will insure the correct placement of the contrast medium. When Pantopaque is outside the subarachnoid space, the needle should be withdrawn and a new puncture two spaces removed should be undertaken (Fig. 14–34). A myelogram should not be performed, if delay is at all possible, within seven days of a previous lumbar puncture because of collapse of the subarachnoid space.

The amount of Pantopaque to be used depends upon the personal preference of the examiner, the area of examination, and the width of the spinal canal. Usually 6 to 9 ml is used for the lumbar region, 12 to 15 ml for the cervical region, and 15 to 20 ml for the thoracic region. Other myelographers prefer a much larger volume that will fill up the region of interest completely, especially if a midline puncture assures them of its complete removal.

The routine examination of the lumbar region includes anteroposterior, oblique, and lateral projection films. Occasionally films are taken with the patient standing to demonstrate extension and flexion of the spine. The count of vertebral level should be included in each study (Fig. 14–35). In the thoracic region, fluoroscopy is more essential because the contrast medium usually passes fairly rapidly over the thoracic kyphosis. The best way to examine the thoracic cord is to place the patient in the supine position after removing the needle. Again anteroposterior and lateral projections should be taken. Lateral decubitus films may be useful to show filling of the nerve root pouches (Fig. 14–36).

In the cervical area, anteroposterior, lateral, and oblique views should be taken. Films may also be taken in extension and flexion of the neck. To fill the cervical subarachnoid canal the head must be well extended during the passage of the contrast medium from the lumbar region. The table is tilted head down, and the neck is extended maximally. After the contrast has pooled in the cervical region, the table may be placed horizontally and the neck placed in a neutral position between flexion and extension (see Fig. 14–34). Cervical myelography is incomplete if C7 is not outlined in the lateral projection. In order to see the C7 level, the shoulders may be pulled down or the swimmer's projection may be used. The double-exposure technique may be helpful in the lateral projection (Figs. 14–37 and 14–53).

When a vascular lesion of the cord is suspected, the patient must be examined in the supine position, since these lesions are predominantly on the back of the cord.[9] For lesions around the foramen magnum the patient must be examined in both the prone and the supine positions. An alternative method is to leave the lumbar puncture needle in place and to take right and left decubitus views of the craniocervical junction with the Pantopaque filling up the front and back of the foramen magnum.

Whenever possible an attempt should be made to remove the contrast medium. Removal is best achieved under fluoroscopic control, particularly when only a milliliter or two remains and may be pooled under the tip of the needle. The siphonage technique facilitates removal.[14] When a complete block is present, it is the usual practice not to attempt to remove the contrast medium. In the thoracic region a reference point on the skin is helpful to the surgeon to show the level of the block.

Metrizamide Myelography

Metrizamide, is a water-soluble triiodinated contrast agent that has proved to be quite useful in myelography.[1,18,23,28,38,47,48] It is a substituted amide and is not a salt, unlike previous water-soluble contrast agents such as meglumine iocarmate (Dimer-X) and meglumine iothalamate (Conray meglumin). Because of its chemical make-up, it is nonionic and does not dissociate (nonionizing) in solution. Consequently, its solution has a much lower osmolality than previous ionizing water-soluble media that are salts. With water-soluble contrast agents, lower osmolality is desirable, as many of their toxic effects

Text continued on page 525

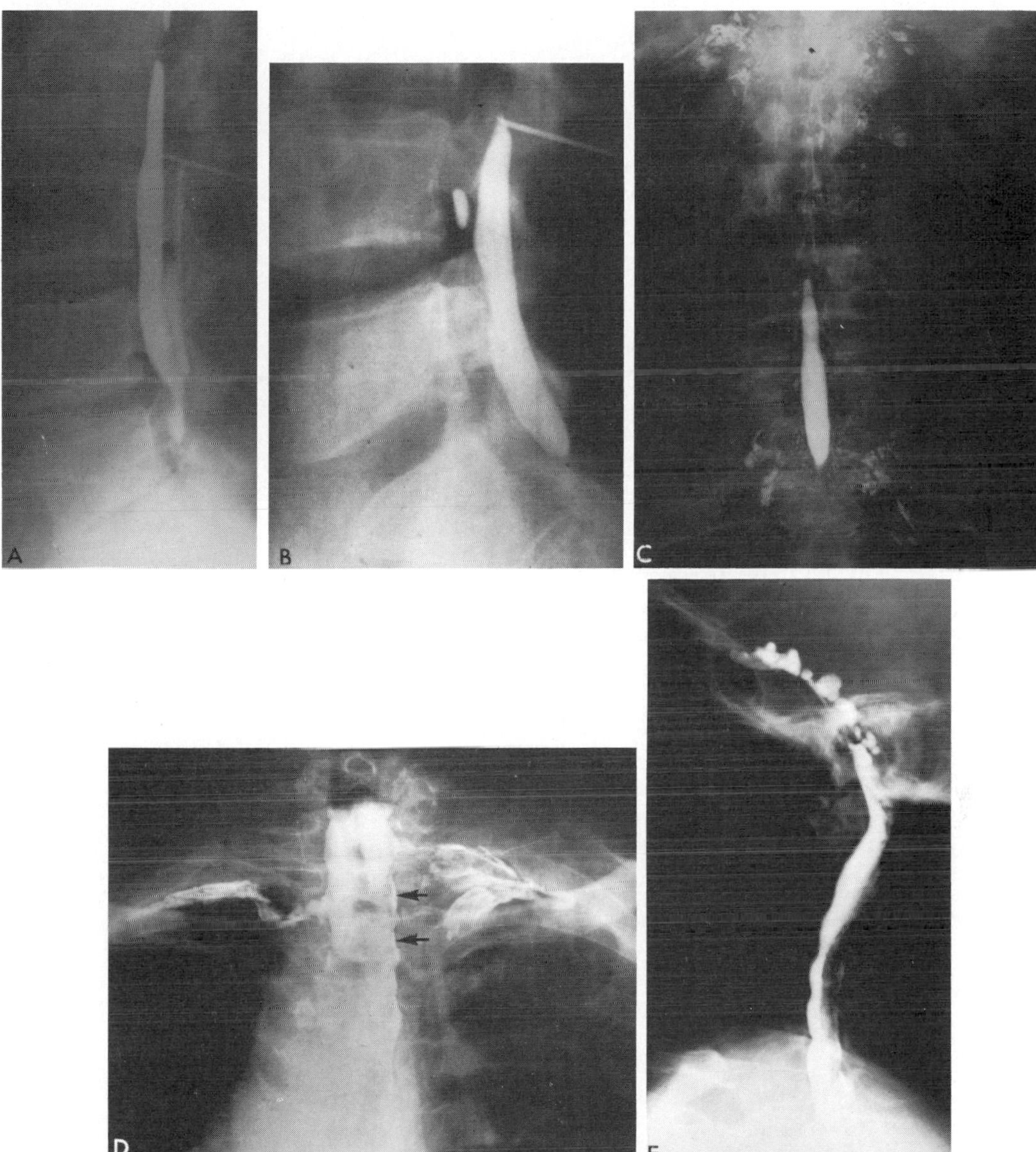

Figure 14–34 *A*. The patient is lying prone. The bulk of the contrast medium is in the subarachnoid space. A second collection is in the subdural space. *B*. The patient is lying prone, but the contrast medium is not against the back of the spinal bodies. This is the typical appearance of subdural contrast. A repeat myelogram with contrast medium in the subarachnoid space revealed the presence of a diseased lumbar disc missed on the first study. *C*. Epidural contrast medium showing the classic appearance of tracking along nerve roots. This may occur during the study or after the removal of the needle. *D*. Pantopaque in the three compartments–subarachnoid, subdural, and epidural. The arrows point to the subdural collection–the thin dense line. *E*. Cervical myelogram. Improper position of head has resulted in spillage of contrast into the middle fossa.

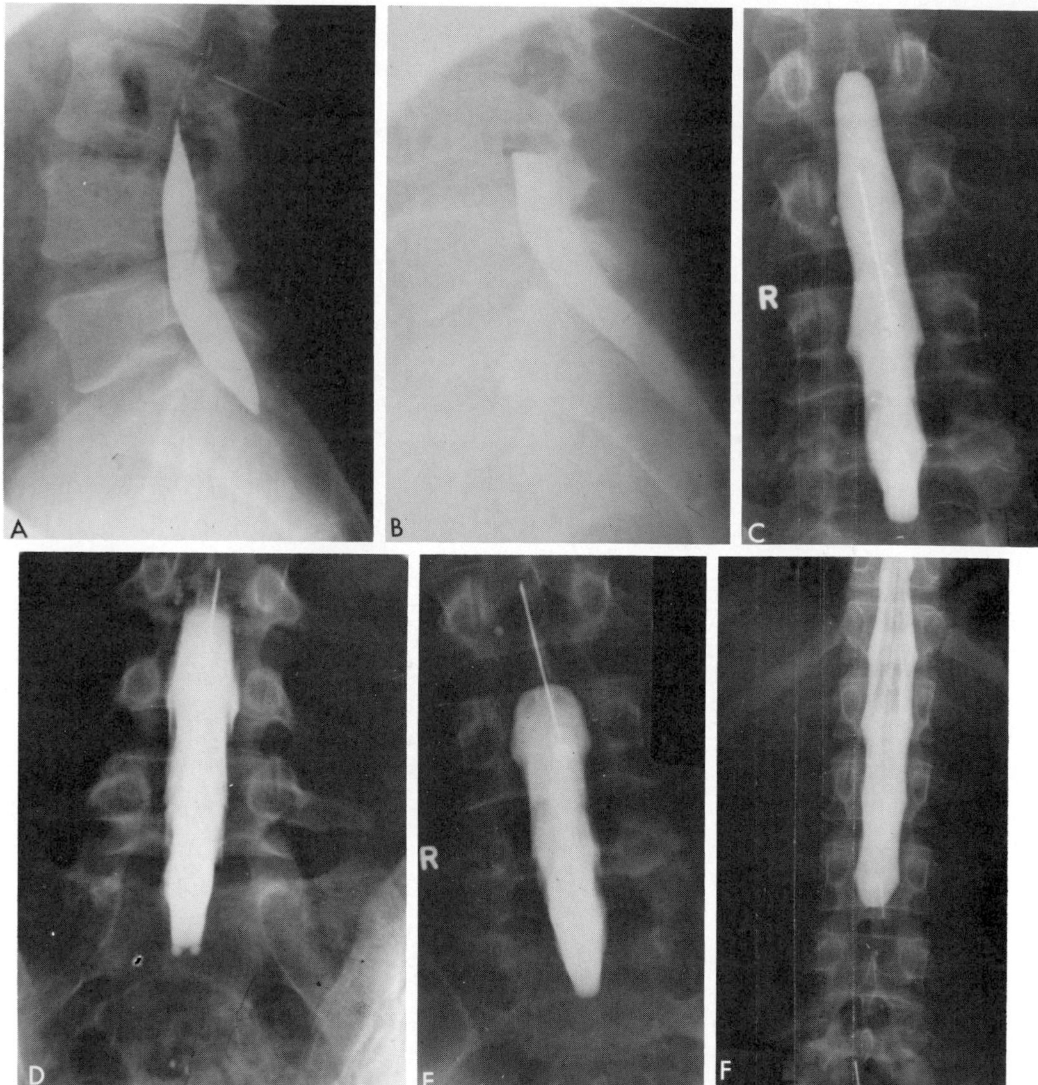

Figure 14–35 Lumbar myelogram. *A*. Lateral view. *B*. Lateral view with patient standing in hyperextension. This is done to accentuate bulge of anulus. *C*. Posteroanterior view. *D*. Posteroanterior view with tube angled toward feet. This is done for better visualization of sac. *E*. Posteroanterior view with patient erect. *F*. View of conus.

Illustration continued on opposite page

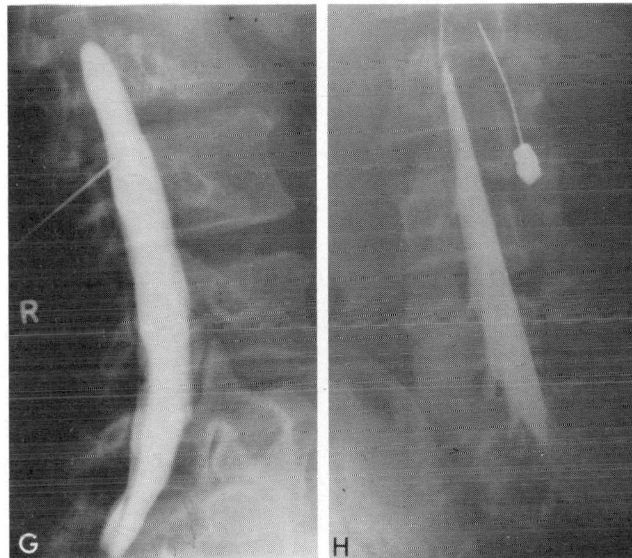

Figure 14–35 (*continued*) *G*. Oblique view. *H*. Lateral decubitus view.

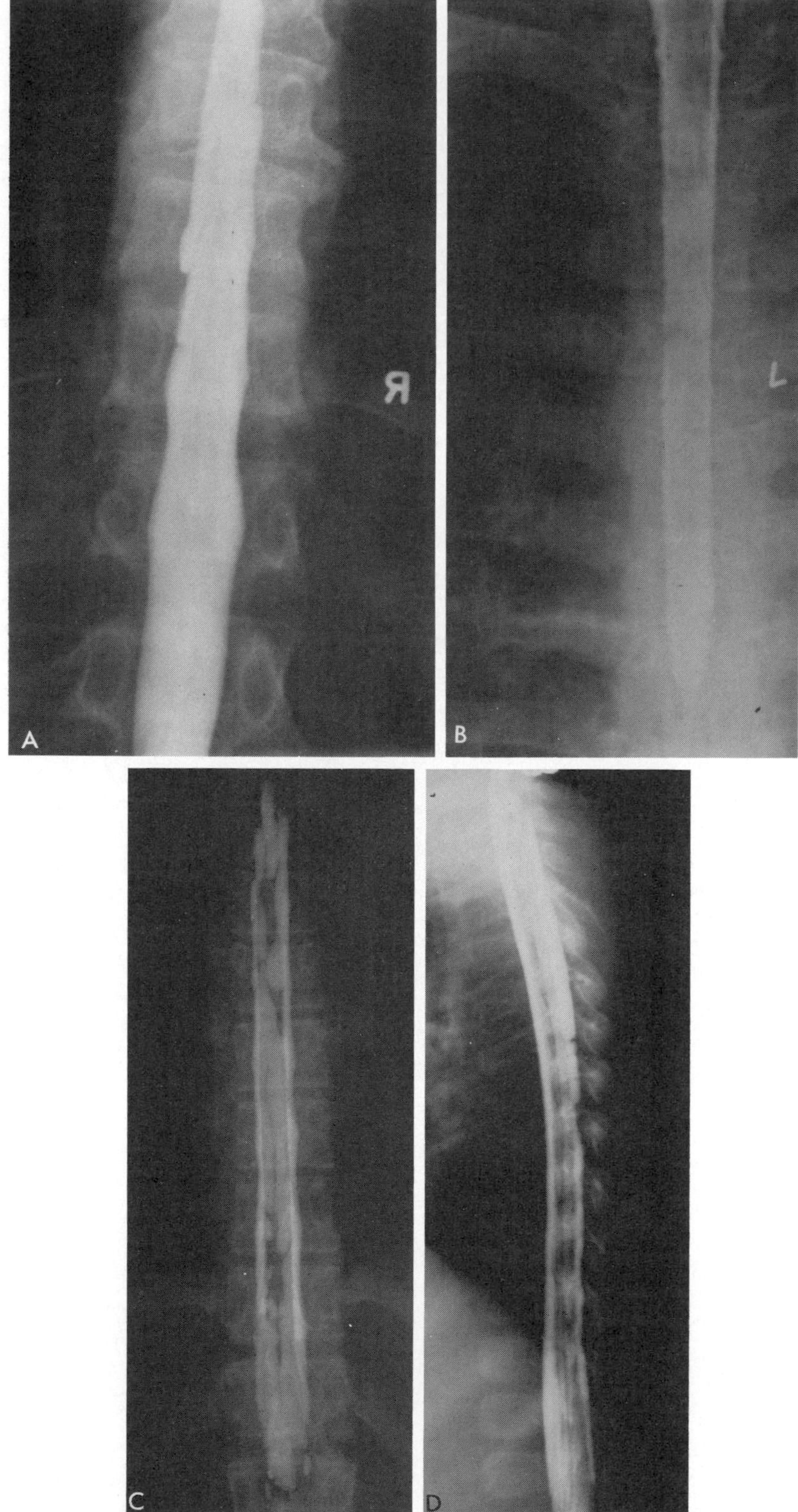

Figure 14–36 Thoracic myelogram. *A*. Prone position showing lower thoracic region. *B*. Prone position showing upper thoracic region. *C*. Anteroposterior projection with needle removed and patient supine. This is the best view for visualizing the thoracic cord and demonstrating abnormal vascularity. *D*. In decubitus film with vertical beam and with enough Pantopaque, the entire cord may be outlined. Overpenetration film may be taken to reveal anatomy obscured by dense Pantopaque.

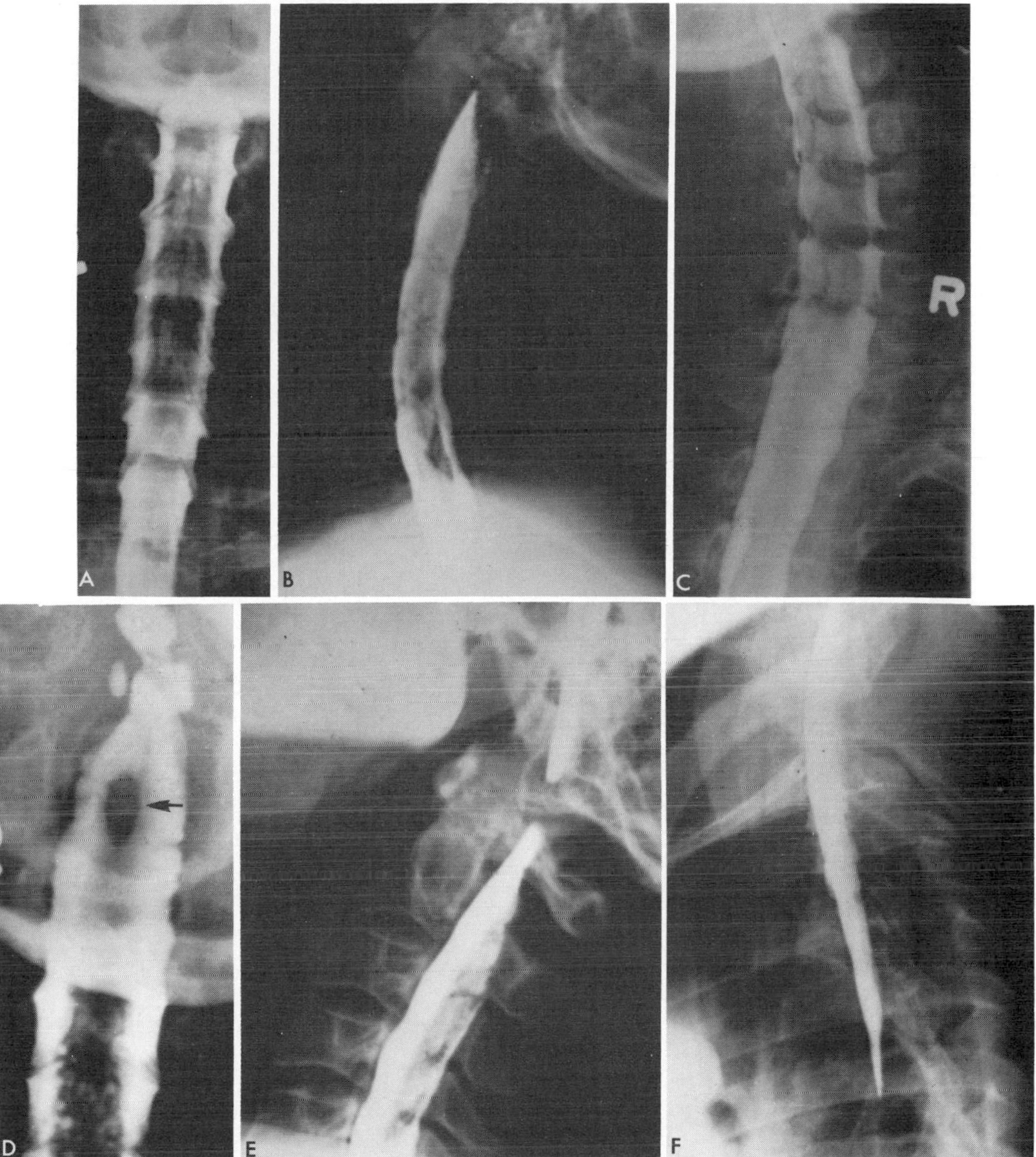

Figure 14–37 Cervical myelogram. *A*. Normal posteroanterior projection of cervical myelogram. *B*. Lateral cervical myelogram, *C*. Oblique projection. *D*. Upper cervical area. Note defect of odontoid peg (*arrow*). *E*. Lateral view showing the normal "skip area" around the odontoid peg and ligaments with some contrast medium on the clivus. *F*. Swimmer's position. A useful view for the cervicothoracic junction when obesity or the shoulder shadows might obscure the anatomy of this region.

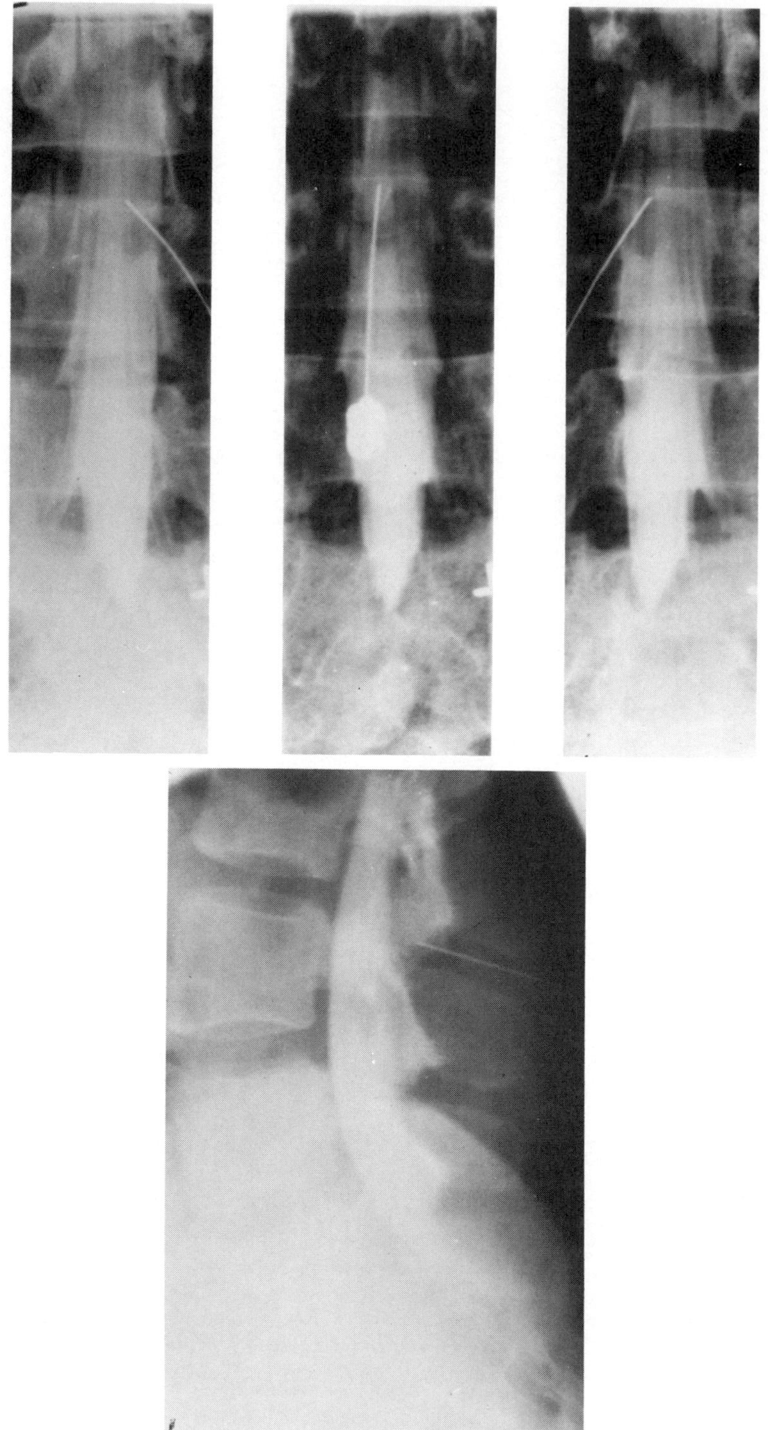

Figure 14–38 Normal metrizamide lumbar myelogram. The cauda equina and nerve roots are distinctly outlined.

are a result of their hypertonicity.[2] A metrizamide solution isotonic with cerebrospinal fluid contains 166 mg iodine per milliliter.

The concentration of the solution used depends upon the extent of myelography and ranges between 170 to 300 mg iodine per milliliter. Metrizamide is introduced by a lumbar puncture with a small-gauge needle and with the patient in the lateral decubitus or prone position with the head slightly elevated. A C1–C2 lateral puncture is preferred if only the cervical region is to be studied. The C1–C2 route permits use of a lower concentration than does the lumbar route, where a higher concentration is needed to compensate for dilution by cerebrospinal fluid before contrast reaches the cervical region. Usually, no more than mild sedation with diazepam is required for premedication. Better filling of nerve roots is accomplished if the area of interest is placed in the most dependent position with the aid of fluoroscopy and varying table tilt before metrizamide thoroughly mixes with the cerebrospinal fluid. Radiographic factors not exceeding 75 to 80 kv utilizing high milliamperage and short exposure times are essential in order to produce optimum details of the nerve roots and the spinal cord (Fig. 14–38).[18]

In the diagnosis of herniated discs, metrizamide has greater than 90 per cent reliability, which is comparable with previous water-soluble contrast agents.[23] Its diagnostic accuracy in herniated disc, however, is superior to Pantopaque and is undoubtedly related to its full miscibility with cerebrospinal fluid, allowing better filling in of the more distal portions of the nerve roots (Fig. 14–39). With other lesions in the three compartments elsewhere in the spinal canal, metrizamide and Pantopaque are equally reliable (Fig. 14–40). As contrast media in myelography, both metrizamide and Pantopaque have definitely produced clearer anatomical details than has air, even when excellent tomography was employed.

The principal advantage of metrizamide

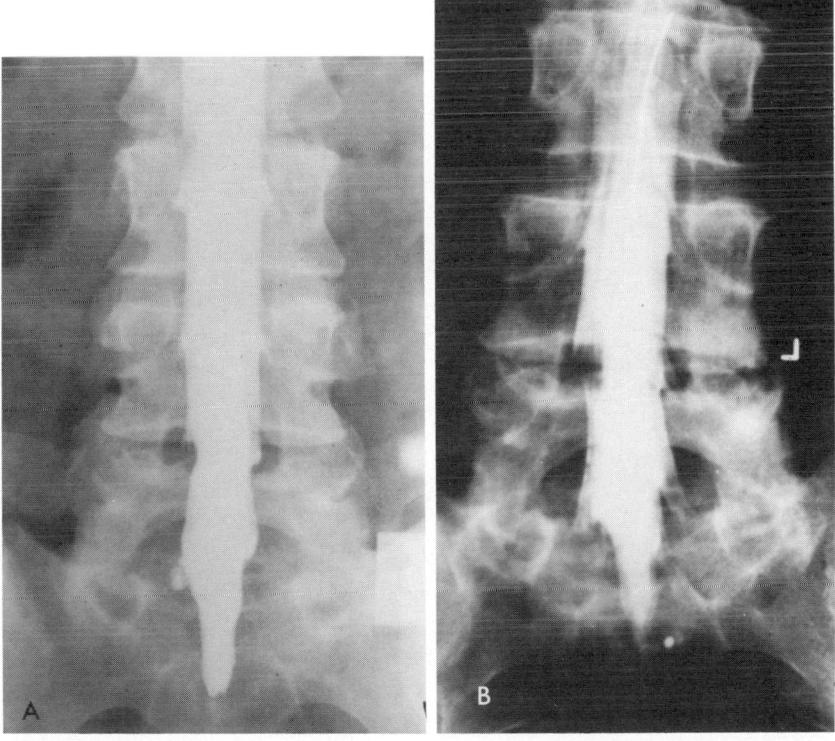

Figure 14–39 Lateral herniated disc at L4–L5 on the right side. Pantopaque, *A*, and metrizamide, *B*, myelograms of the same patient.

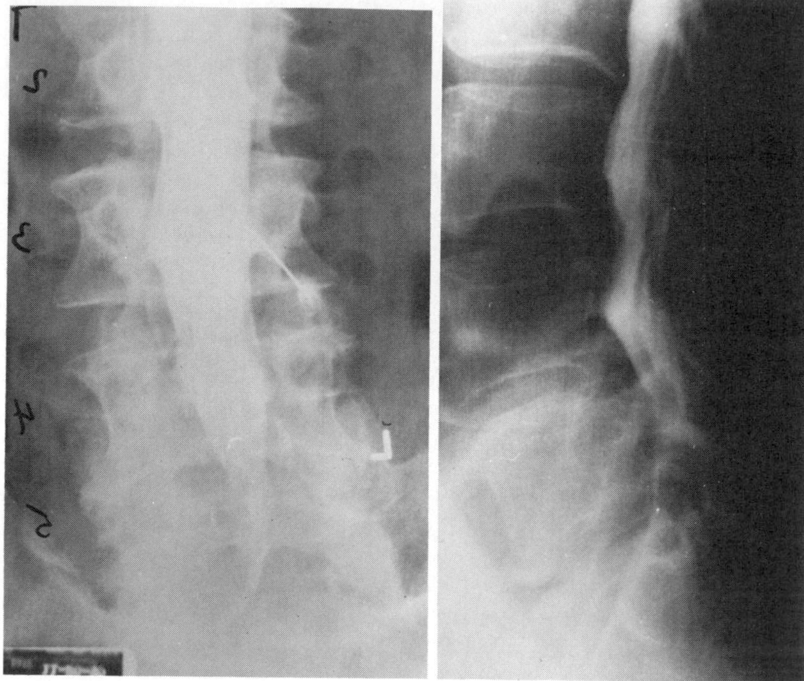

Figure 14–40 Metrizamide lumbar myelogram. Extradural lymphoma of L5.

over other water-soluble contrast media is its relative absence of serious side effects. Severe muscle spasms do not occur, and spinal anesthesia is not needed.[23,47] Very little epileptogenic activity is produced in experimental animals by intrathecal introduction of metrizamide in comparison with other water-soluble agents.[49,51] The isolated reports of seizure activity have been attributed to its interaction with neuroleptic drugs such as the phenothiazines, in both humans and experimental animals.[29,51]

Among the minor side effects, headache occurs in 29 to 51 per cent, nausea in 10 to 27 per cent, vomiting in 3 to 12 per cent, and dizziness in 4 to 14 per cent.[47,48] Headache appears to increase with the dose and when the horizontal position is assumed immediately after myelography.[18,23,28] It is often mild and, like other side effects, seldom lasts for more than 24 hours. Other recorded adverse effects are transient increase in back or leg pain, paresthesia, neck stiffness, tinnitus, and urinary retention. Slight to moderate pleocytosis can be seen if cerebrospinal fluid examination is repeated within 48 hours following myelography. Transient electroencephalographic abnormality occurs in 16 per cent.[31]

In more than 80 repeat metrizamide myelograms at intervals of 2 to 18 months, no arachnoidal changes could definitely be attributed to metrizamide.[1] There is however, recent experimental evidence using the primate model that metrizamide at 300 mg iodine per milliliter, like meglumine iocarmate (Dimer-X), can cause mild to severe arachnoid fibrosis.[24] The risk of arachnoiditis is probably minimized by the use of reduced volume and concentration.

Intrathecal metrizamide is probably absorbed mostly by arachnoid granulations over the cerebral convexities.[28] The rest probably diffuses through brain parenchyma (which may be responsible for the minor side effects and electroencephalographic changes) and spinal subarachnoid space.[31] Its intrathecal circulation has been the basis for its added use as a contrast enhancing agent for visualizing the spinal cord and canal, the subarachnoid cisterns, and the ventricles in the diagnosis of tumor or altered cerebrospinal fluid dynamics by means of the CT scan.[10,11,22] After 24 hours, more than 90 per cent of its iodine has been excreted in the urine.[3]

Cisternography

The value of positive-contrast cisternography resides in its applicability to the investigation of angle tumors. Tiny acoustic neuromas may defy recognition in air studies, even with careful laminagraphy.

Two milliliters of Pantopaque is introduced into the subarachnoid space and is manipulated into the internal auditory meatus, preferably under fluoroscopic control (Figs. 14–41 and 14–42).[4,53] Fluoroscopic guidance allows concurrent examination of the foramen magnum and clivus, where oc-

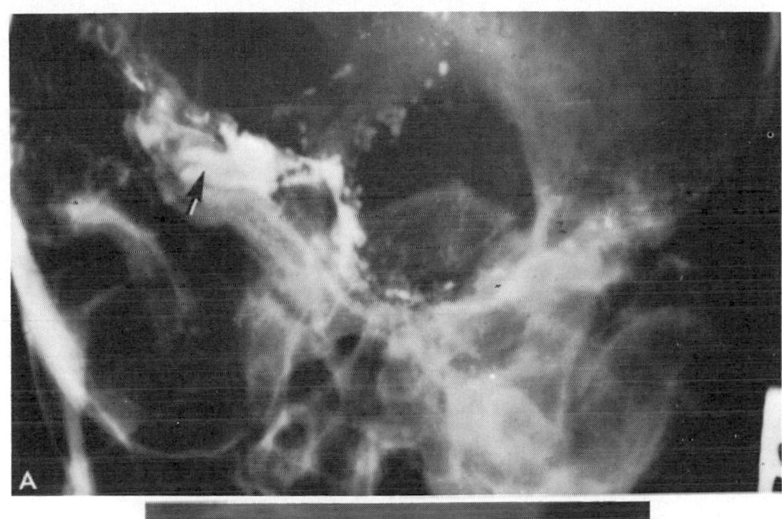

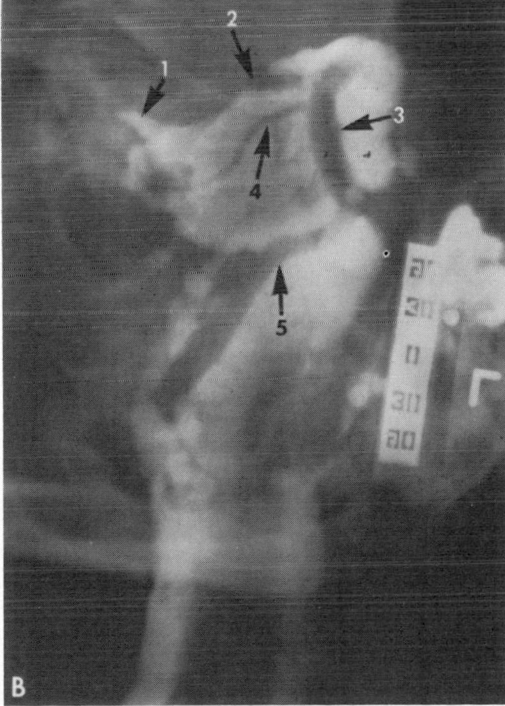

Figure 14–41 Normal cisternal myelography. *A*. Study with 2 ml of Pantopaque demonstrating contrast in internal auditory meatus. Note defect formed by crista (*arrow*). *B*. Large-volume cisternogram. Note the structures visualized: 1, internal auditory canal; 2, fifth cranial nerve; 3, basilar artery; 4, anterior inferior cerebellar artery; 5, vertebral artery.

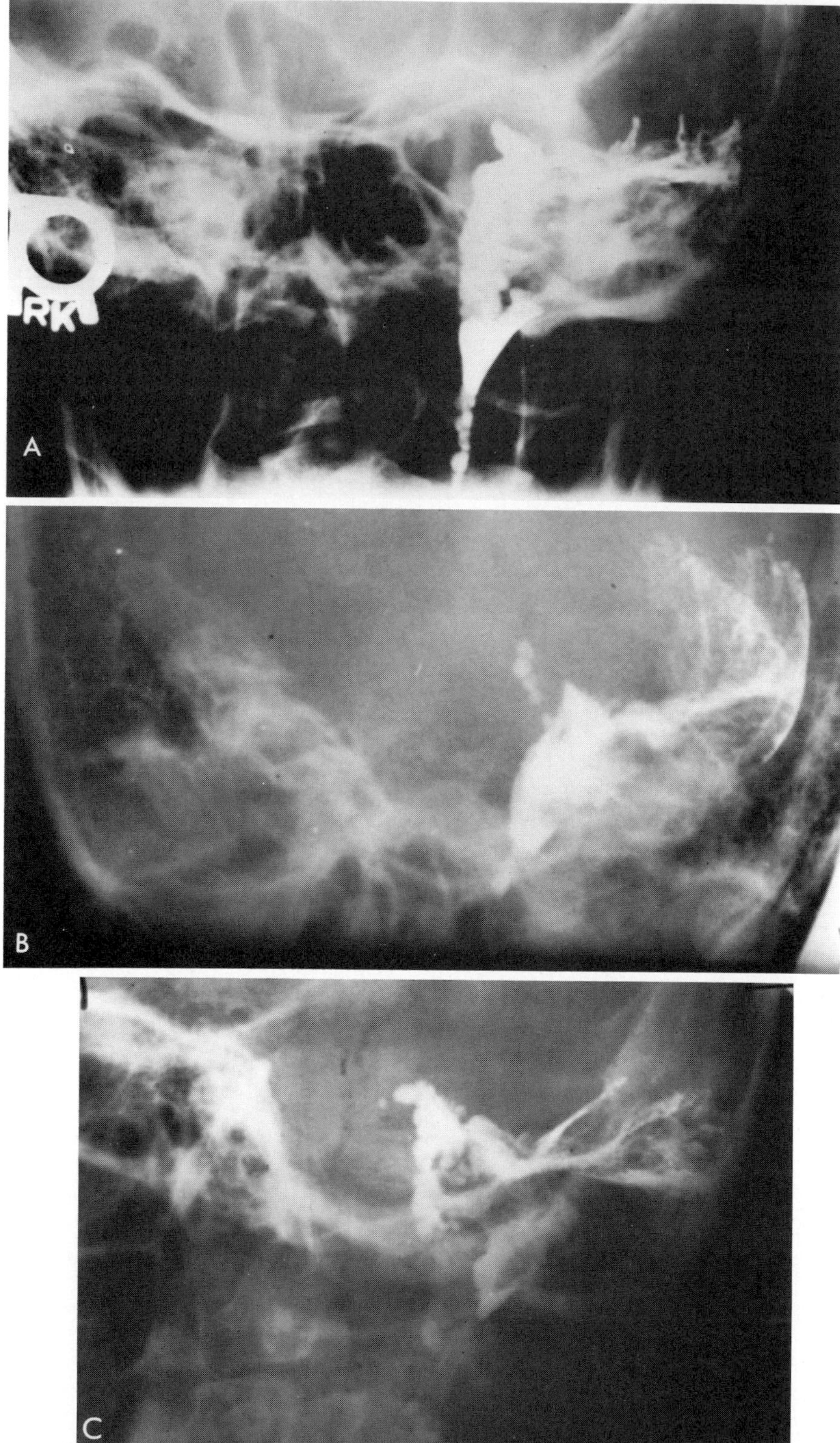

Figure 14–42 Cerebellopontine angle arachnoid cyst. Left decubitus films, in *A*, the anteroposterior, *B*, Towne's, and, *C*, Stenvers projections show a round filling defect at the left porus.

casionally a large cerebellopontine angle mass may extend or may cause tonsillar herniation. Conversely, masses from the clivus or foramen magnum can invade the cerebellopontine angle and present themselves clinically as a cerebellopontine angle syndrome. Both canals should be examined. Occasionally, the spinal canal may not fill because of its normally small size (less than 2.5 mm in diameter), large nerves, or a subarachnoid space that may not extend into the canal. The use of tomography during Pantopaque cisternography may sometimes clarify the problem of partial or asymmetrical filling of the canals.[53] Large angle masses may, rarely, be missed with 2-ml Pantopaque cisternography.[35] It is no longer necessary, however, to use the larger volume advocated by Gold and Kieffer.[17] When a large cerebellopontine angle tumor is suspected clinically and on the plain x-ray and tomography, the radiological investigation can proceed immediately with computed tomography and vertebral angiography if indicated.[7]

Air Myelography

Air myelography entails replacing the spinal subarachnoid fluid with air. The technique as first described by Lindgren involves puncturing the cisterna magna with the patient in the lateral decubitus position and the table tilted head down 30 to 40 degrees.[34] The cerebrospinal fluid is replaced by air, and the space is distended by the introduction of air to a pressure of 200 mm of water. Tomographic cuts are then undertaken to include the whole length of the cord. Other modifications for the cervical region include using a lumbar puncture rather than a cervical puncture and trapping air in the cervical subarachnoid space.[30] Air myelography is useful in differentiating a cavitary intramedullary lesion from a solid intramedullary mass (the "collapsing cord" sign of syringomyelia or hydromyelia) (Figs. 14–43 and 14–55). In high cervical, craniocervical, and posterior fossa lesions it may be combined with pneumoencephalography. It is also used in studying cord atrophy and, occasionally, in defining cystic lesions communicating with the spinal canal.

Myelographic Appearance of Specific Lesions

The width of the shadow of the cord is an important indicator of spinal cord disease.[8]

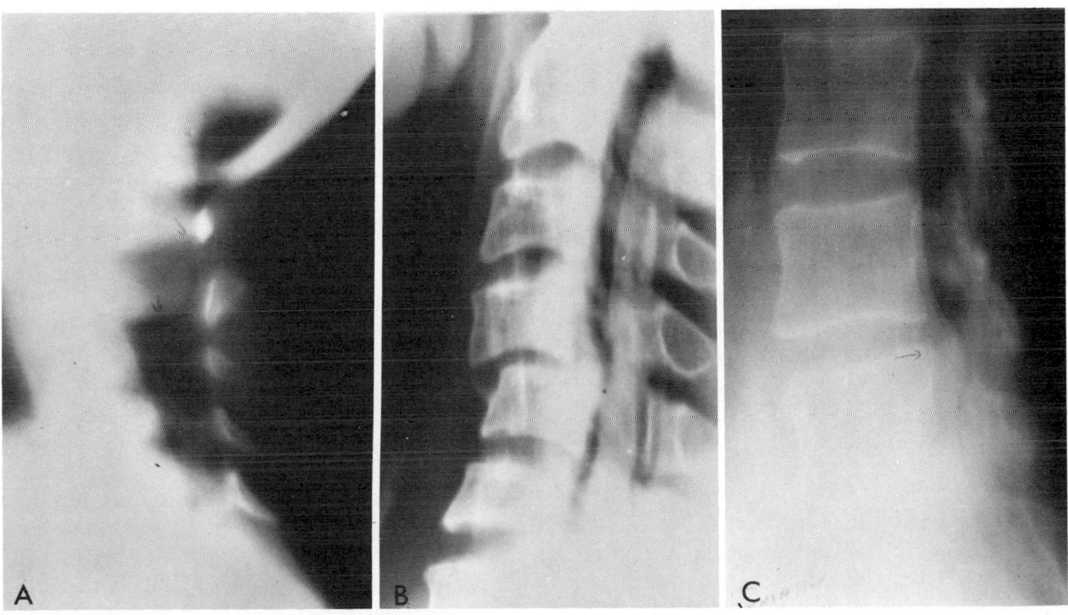

Figure 14–43 Gas myelography. *A*. Foramen magnum meningioma. *B*. Dislocation and disc herniation at C4–C5. *C*. Herniated disc at L4–L5.

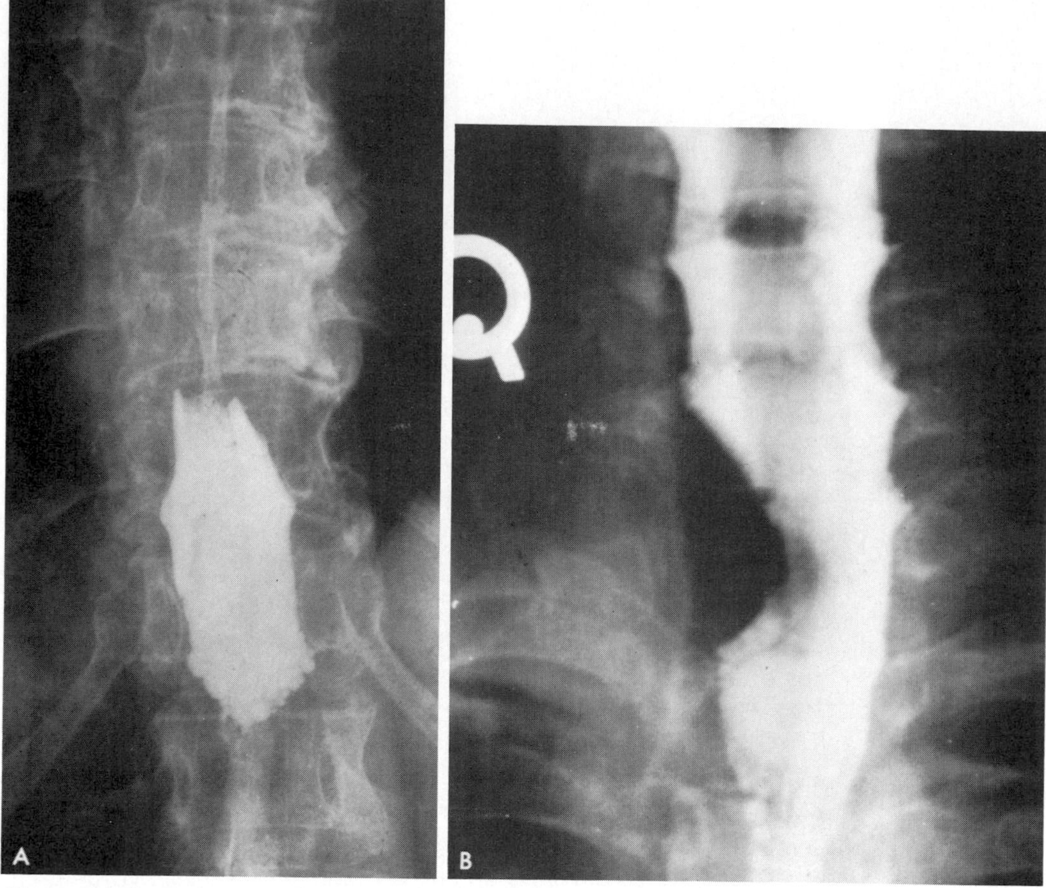

Figure 14–44 Tumors. *A*. Epidural metastases showing the column of contrast displaced medially with tapering of the column of contrast showing the "bundle of faggots" appearance and displacement of the cord. *B*. Metastatic deposit. An epidural lesion showing medial displacement of the Pantopaque column.

Because of magnification factors, the proportionate size relative to the width of the subarachnoid space is a much better indicator of cord abnormalities than the absolute measurements. Space-taking lesions may be epidural, subdural, subarachnoid, or intramedullary. Each has a characteristic appearance in the myelogram (Figs. 14–44 and 14–62). Occasionally the lesion may be in more than one compartment (Fig. 14–45).

Spondylosis usually occurs in the cervical and lumbar regions.[50] The familiar myelographic appearance is the "stepladder" appearance caused by multiple bulgings of the disc space (Figs. 14–54 and 14–57). The lateral projection will show this to best advantage. Occasionally spondylosis may occur at one level with a single defect.

Recognition of herniated disc material depends upon certain changes in the Pantopaque column. These appearances vary with the level of the pathological changes. Thus in the low lumbar region there may be amputation of nerve roots. At higher levels there may be amputation of a nerve root with encroachment on the major column of contrast suggesting root involvement and cord involvement (Fig. 14–61). In the cervical region compression of the column of contrast in the anteroposterior diameter may widen the cord shadow and suggest an intramedullary lesion. The lateral projection will reveal the extradural nature of the compressive lesion. It should be mentioned that a large disc fragment may be extruded without deforming the myelographic picture and also that deformities may be present in the Pantopaque column in the absence of symptoms.

References on page 549

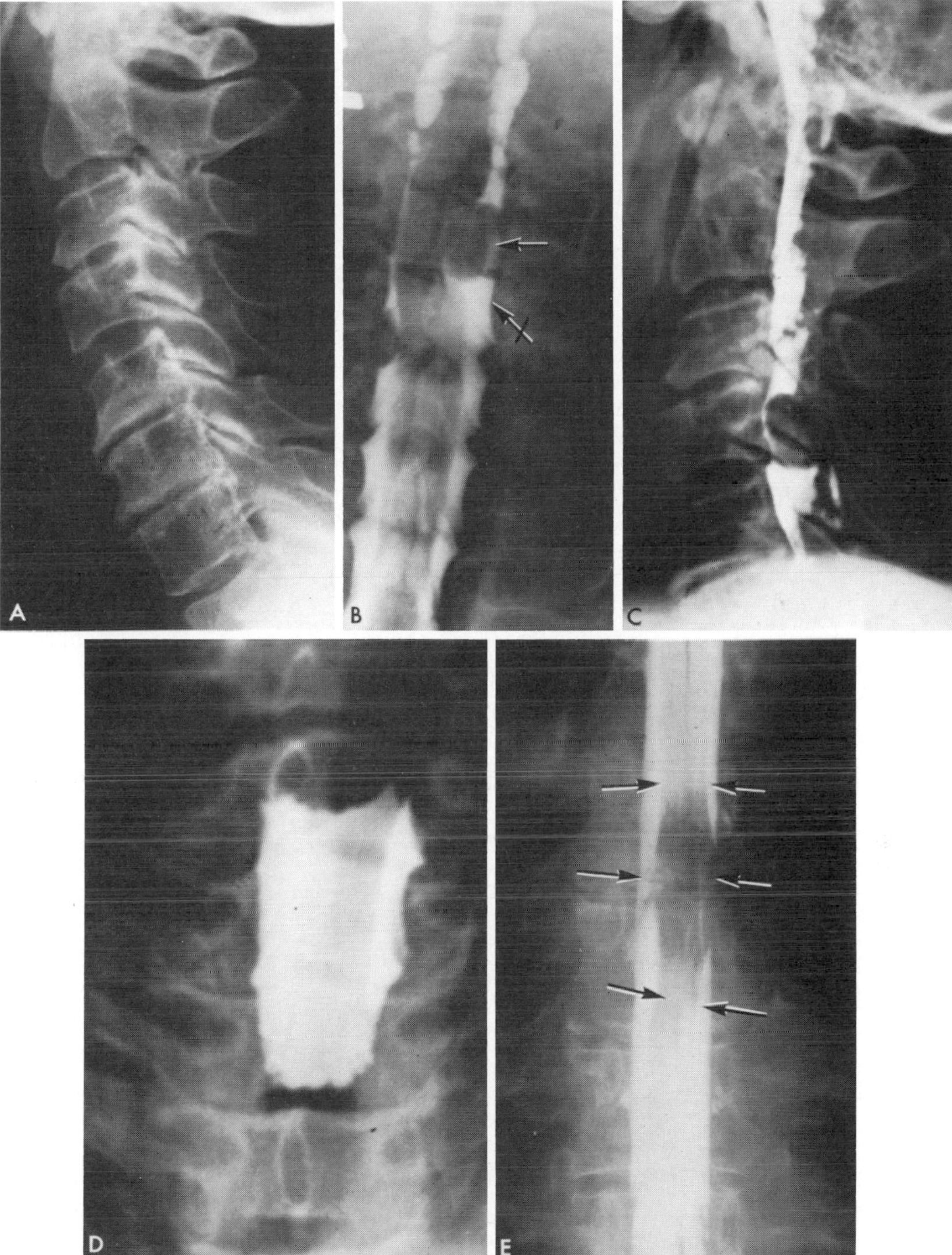

Figure 14–45 Intradural tumor. *A*. The plain x-rays of this patient and the clinical picture suggested the diagnosis of osteoarthritis. *B*. The myelogram reveals the classic appearance of an intradural extramedullary lesion with displacement of the cord and widening of the subarachnoid space (*arrow with crossed shaft*) at the level of the lesion (*arrow*), which is capped by contrast medium. There was a partial block permitting contrast medium to pass beyond this point, and an effort was made to cap the upper extent of the tumor. *C*. Lateral projection demonstrating the capped lesion. *D*. Unusual case of an intradural metastatic deposit with capping, displaced cord, and widened subarachnoid space. Metastatic disease may simulate a benign lesion myelographically when it is located in the intradural compartment. *E*. Thoracic disc in which widening of the cord shadow in the anteroposterior projection simulates an intramedullary lesion.

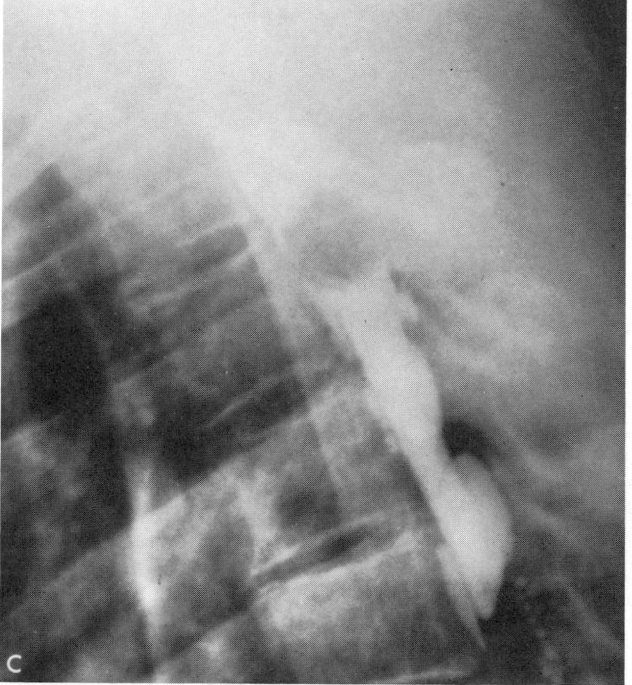

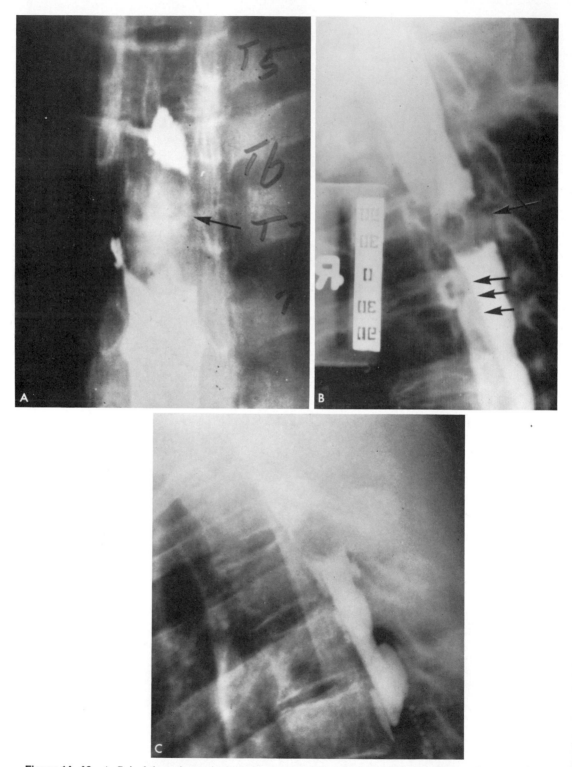

Figure 14–46 *A*. Spinal thoracic meningioma in a woman. Film shows calcification of tumor (*arrow*) and capping with Pantopaque. *B* and *C*. Thoracic meningioma in a woman showing characteristic displacement of the cord (*arrows*) with widening of the subarachnoid space and capping of the lesion (*arrow with crossed shaft*).

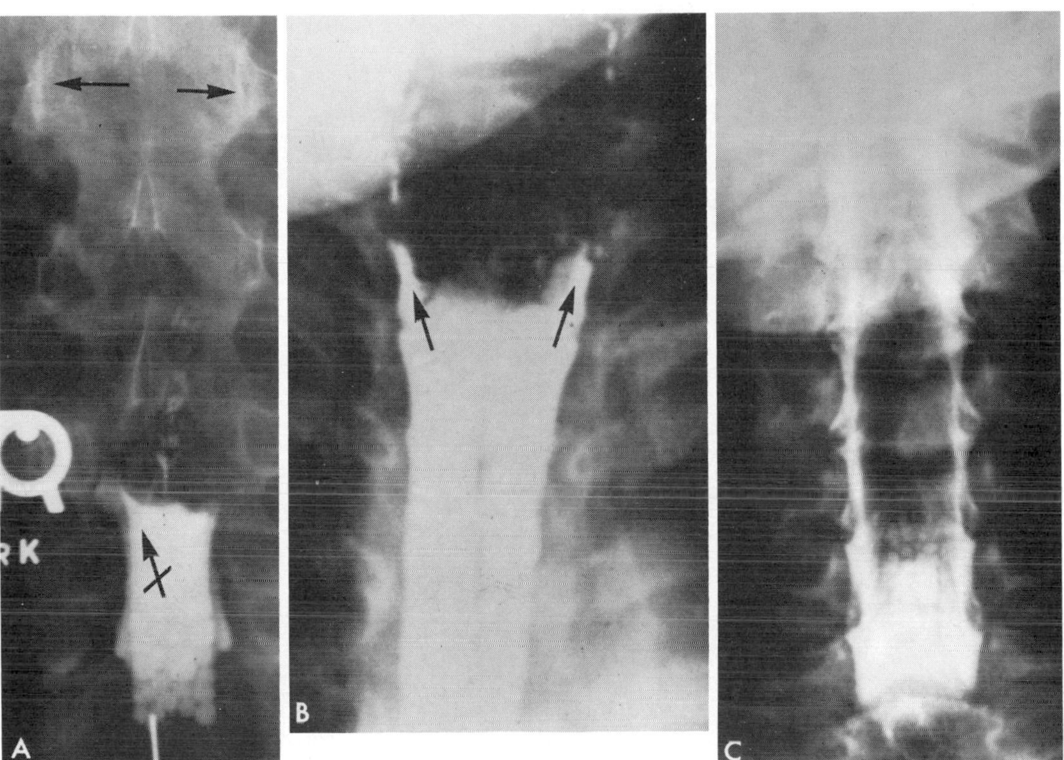

Figure 14–47 Intramedullary lesions. *A*. Ependymoma of the conus with a total block. There is marked thinning of the pedicles (*arrows*) above the level of the Pantopaque block, evidence of the extent of the tumor. Margins of the contrast medium are displaced outward (*arrow with crossed shaft*). *B*. Glioma of cervical cord with almost total block but showing the extreme narrowing of the Pantopaque column with its margins displaced laterally (*arrows*). *C*. Spinal cord hematoma from a diving accident. Note wide shadow of cord.

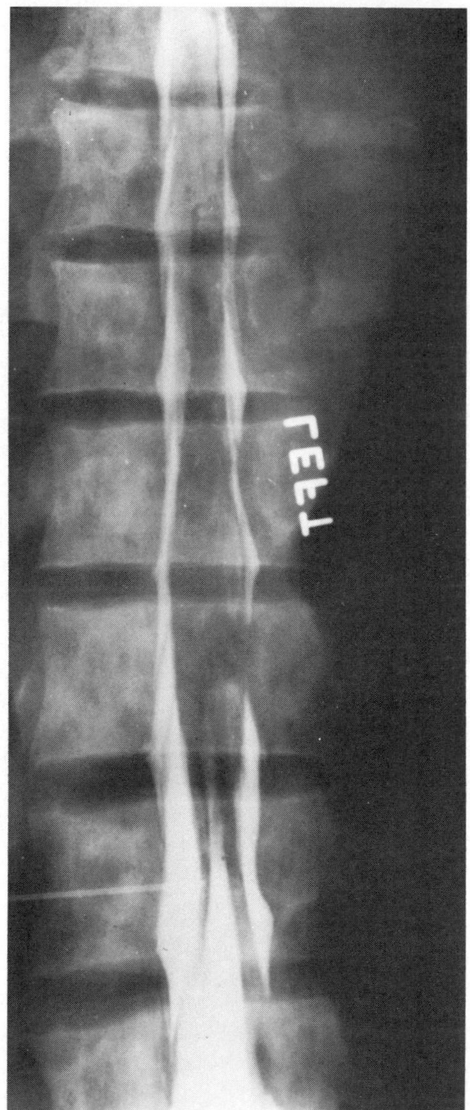

Figure 14–48 Intramedullary metastatic bronchogenic carcinoma of the conus.

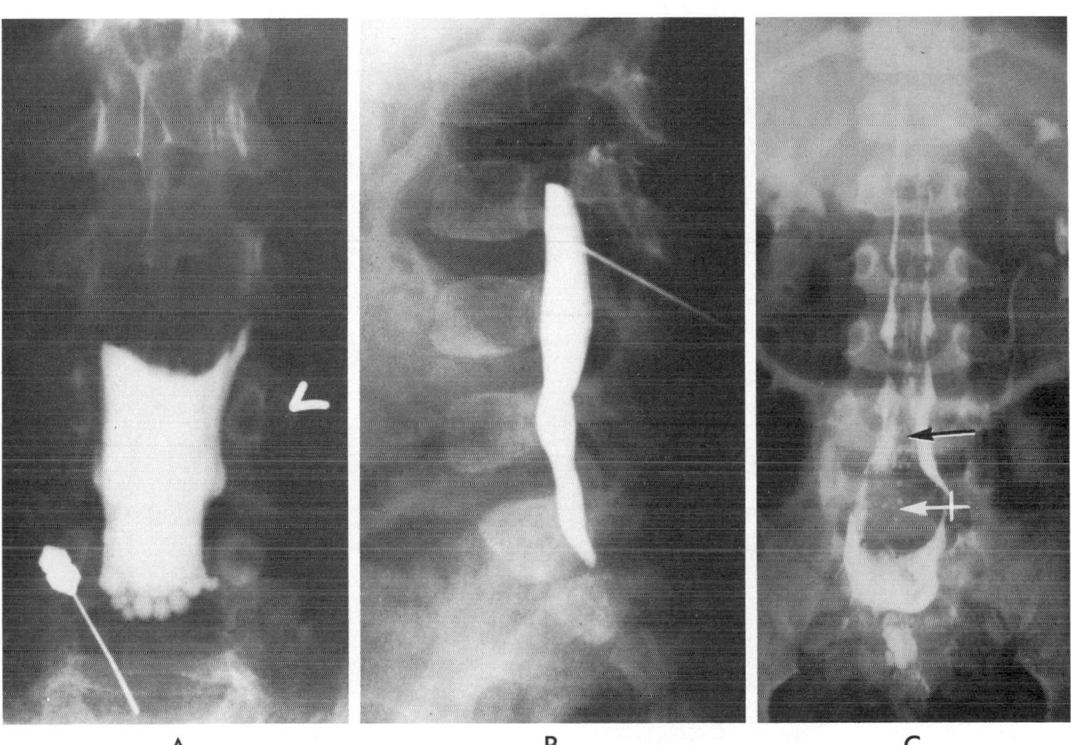

Figure 14–49 *A*. Epidermoid. Multiple lumbar punctures were performed in the past. The Pantopaque reveals a large round tumor lying within the dura. *B*. Spinal lipoma with tethering of cord. Patient was erect, and the lesion was not demonstrated. *C*. Same case as *B* with patient supine following removal of needle. The lipoma (*arrow with crossed shaft*) was now visualized. Note the low tethered cord.

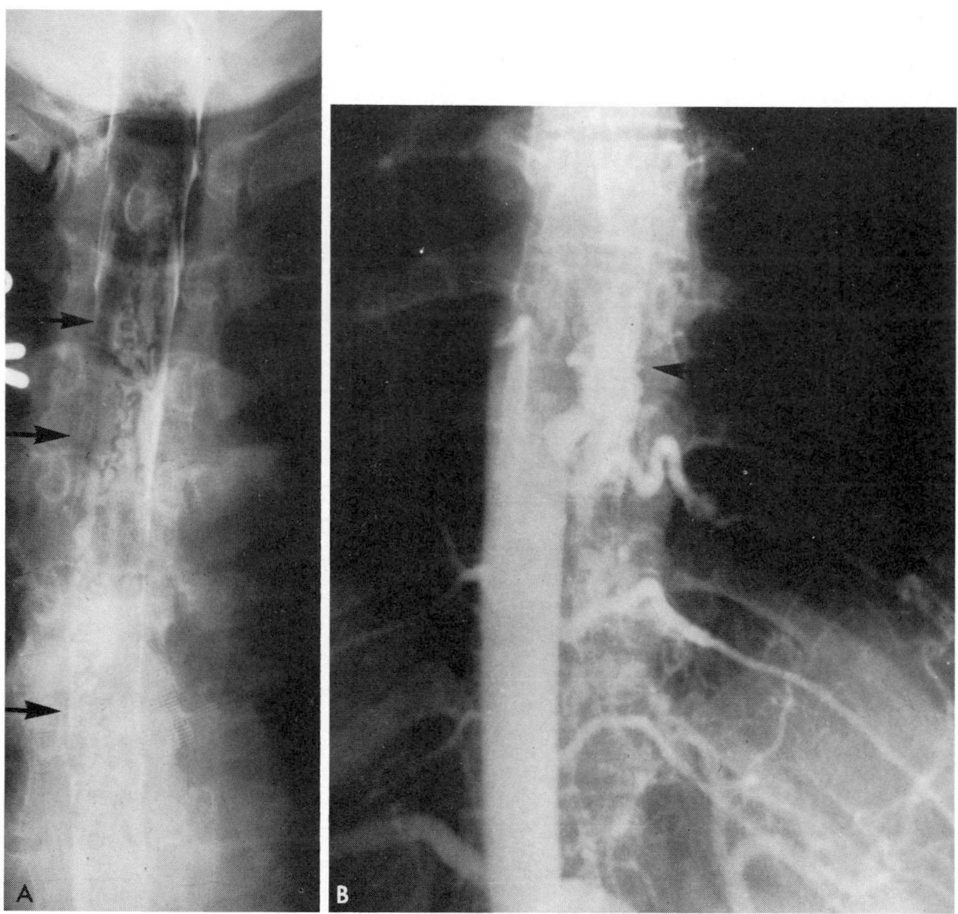

Figure 14–50 Spinal angioma. *A*. Supine myelogram demonstrating a widened cord and serpiginous shadows representing tortuous large spinal vessels (*arrows*). *B*. An aortogram showing the large spinal angioma (*arrow*).

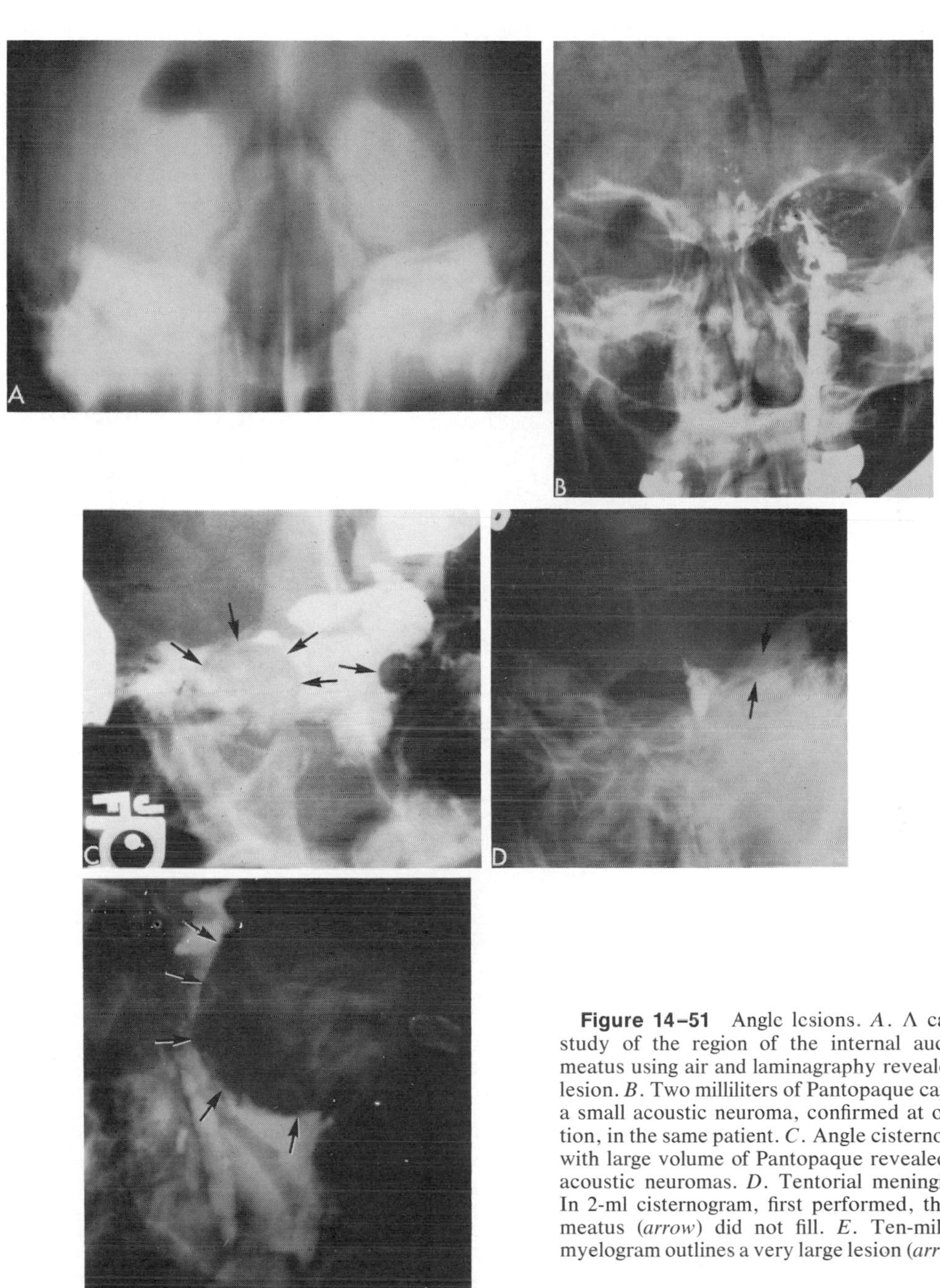

Figure 14–51 Angle lesions. *A*. A careful study of the region of the internal auditory meatus using air and laminagraphy revealed no lesion. *B*. Two milliliters of Pantopaque capping a small acoustic neuroma, confirmed at operation, in the same patient. *C*. Angle cisternogram with large volume of Pantopaque revealed two acoustic neuromas. *D*. Tentorial meningioma. In 2-ml cisternogram, first performed, the left meatus (*arrow*) did not fill. *E*. Ten-milliliter myelogram outlines a very large lesion (*arrows*).

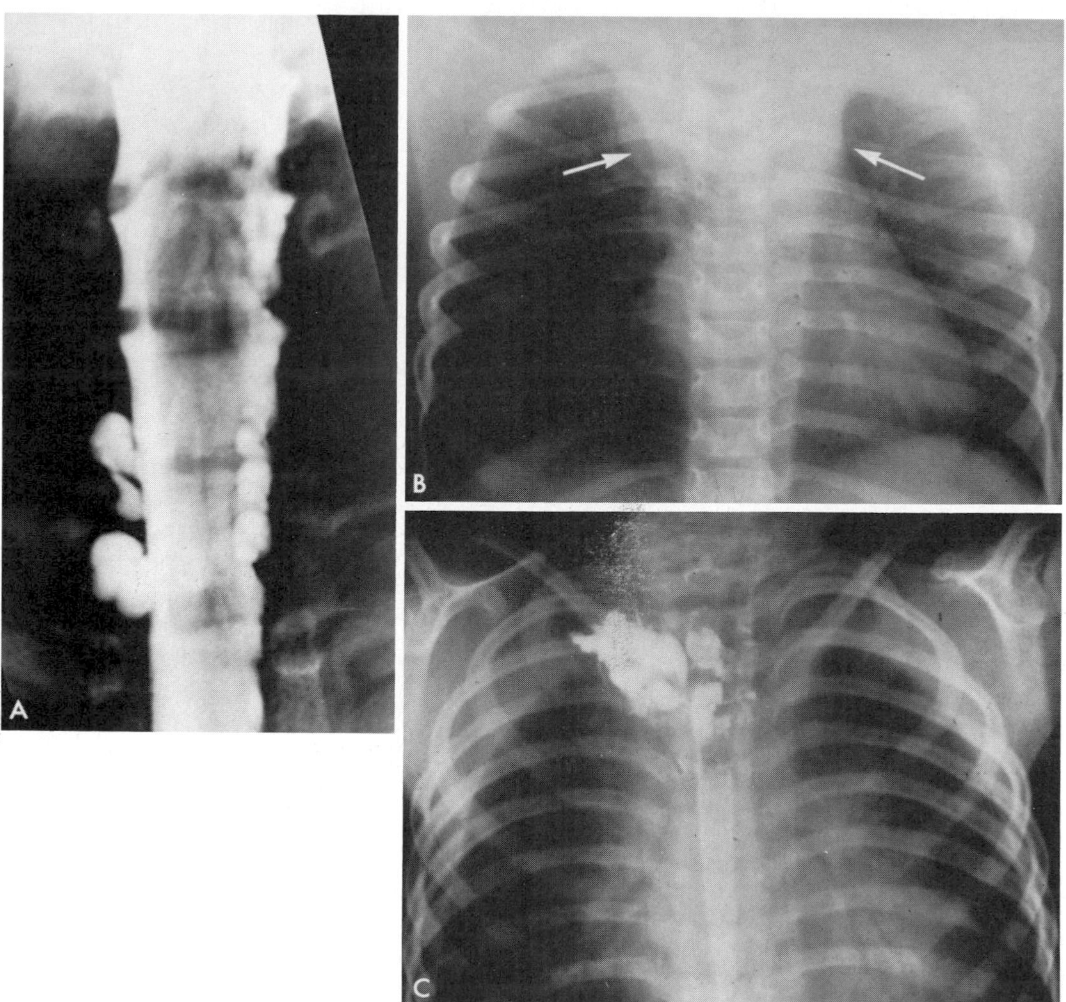

Figure 14–52 *A*. Brachial plexus avulsion with subarachnoid diverticula. *B* and *C*. Chest x-ray showing an abnormal density (*arrows*) in the upper mediastinum in a child who suffered severe trauma. The myelogram shows Pantopaque outside the subarachnoid space and loculated within the mediastinum.

Illustration continued on opposite page

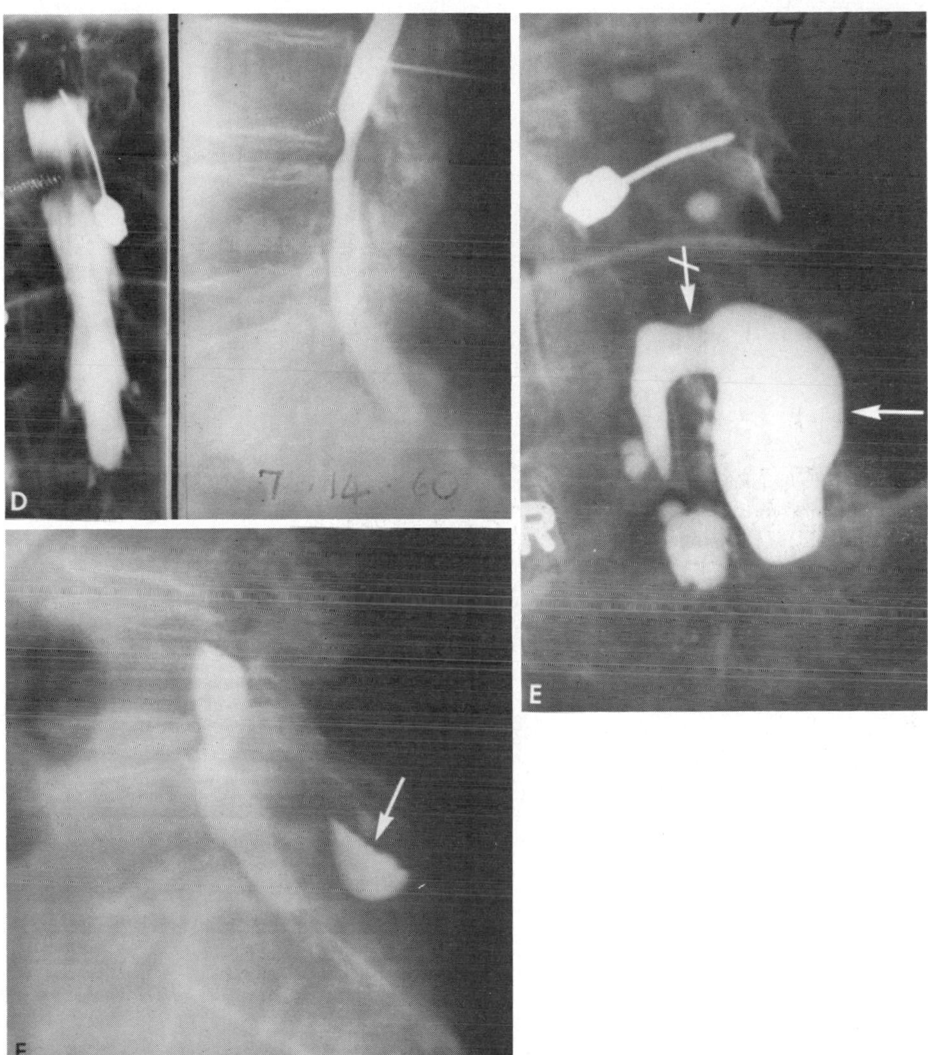

Figure 14–52 (*continued*) *D*. Myelogram showing disc protrusion. A laminectomy showed a large protruded disc, which was removed. *E* and *F*. Myelogram made three years later showing large extradural cyst (*arrow*) communicating with the lumbar subarachnoid space (*crossed-shaft arrow*). Confirmed at operation.

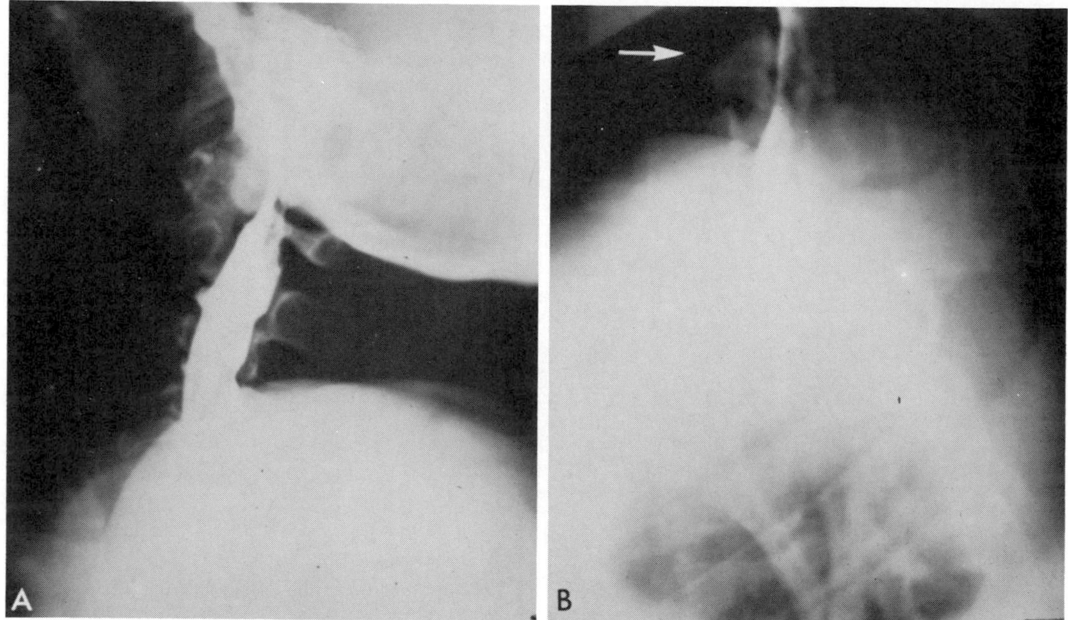

Figure 14–53 *A*. Spinal trauma with cord compression was missed on first myelogram because no attempt was made to visualize the lower cervical region. *B*. A repeat myelogram with the double-exposure technique revealed a compression fracture of a lower cervical body compressing the cord.

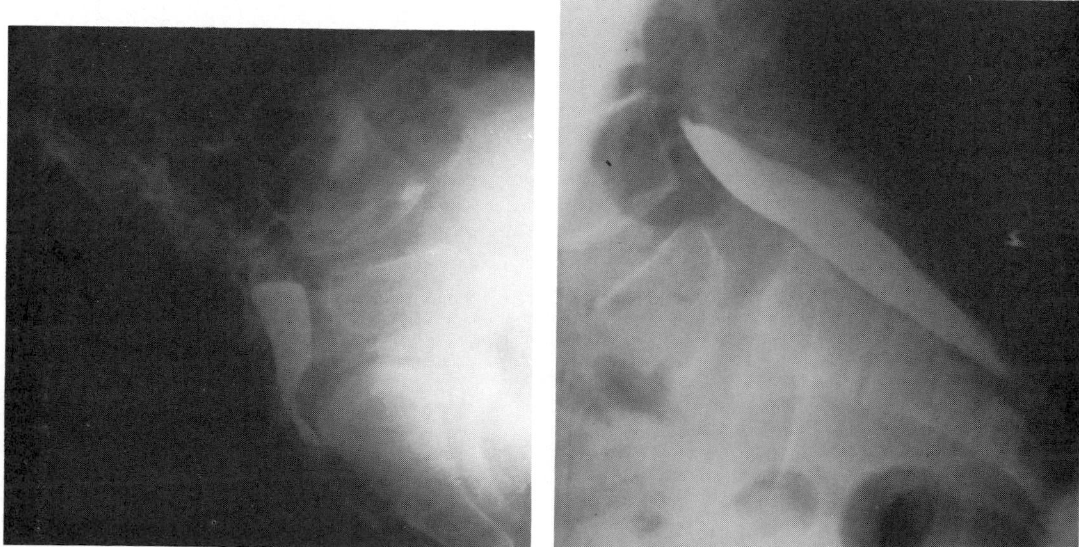

Figure 14–54 Myelographic appearance of spondylolisthesis at L5–S1.

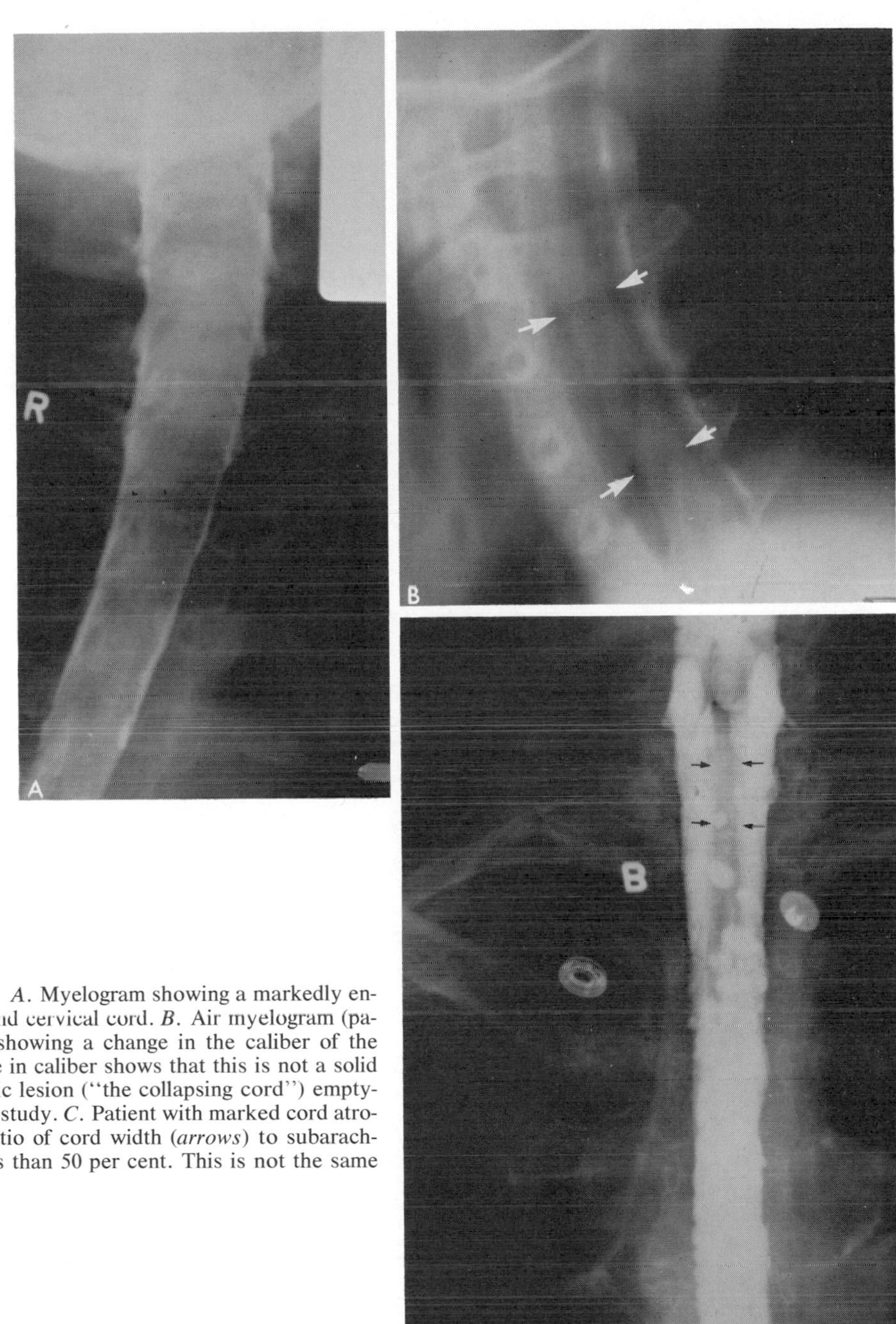

Figure 14–55 *A*. Myelogram showing a markedly enlarged thoracic and cervical cord. *B*. Air myelogram (patient semierect) showing a change in the caliber of the cord. The change in caliber shows that this is not a solid tumor but a cystic lesion ("the collapsing cord") emptying during the air study. *C*. Patient with marked cord atrophy. Note the ratio of cord width (*arrows*) to subarachnoid width is less than 50 per cent. This is not the same case as *A* and *B*.

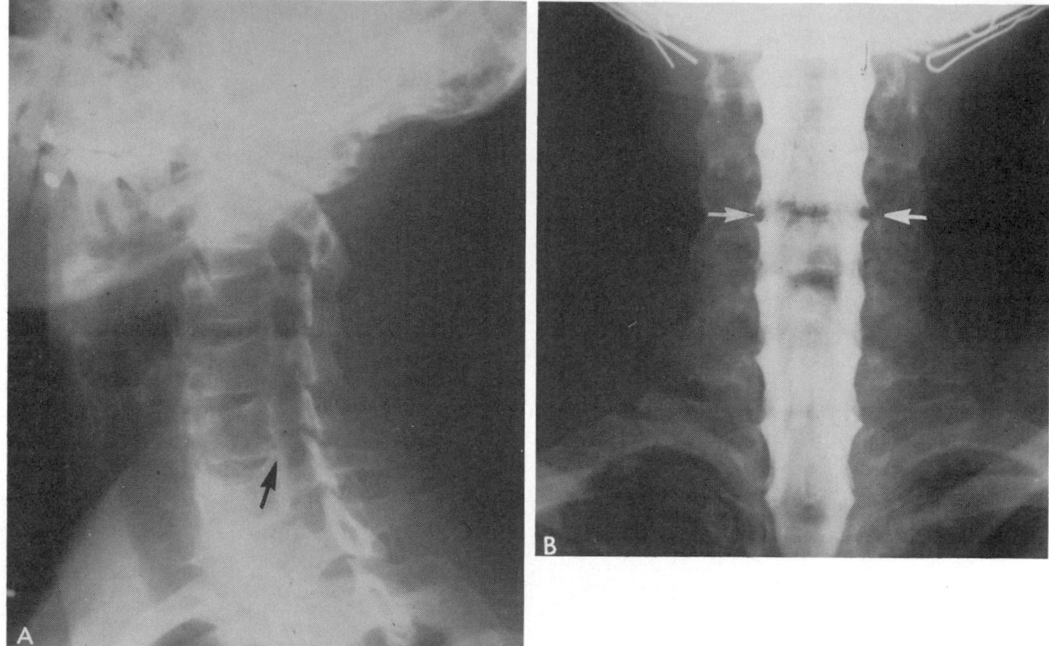

Figure 14–56 *A*. Forty-year-old woman referred with a diagnosis of amyotrophic lateral sclerosis. Note uncovertebral osteophytes in this oblique projection at the C5–C6 level. *B*. Myelogram. Note the presence of a bar defect and nerve root amputations at the same level. Patient markedly improved following operation.

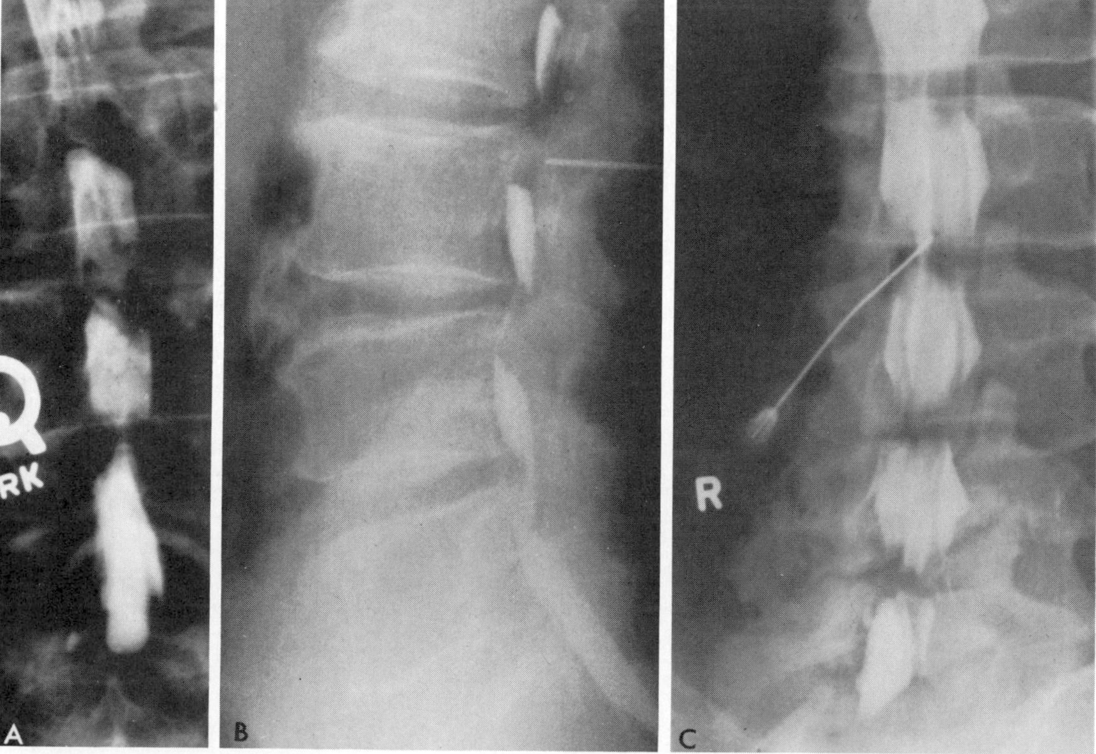

Figure 14–57 Lumbar spondylosis. Washboard appearance in the lumbar region is due to lumbar spondylosis. Although this is considered a classic picture, multiple discs may resemble this closely. The flow may be slow during myelography, since the Pantopaque has to negotiate each hump opposite the disc spaces.

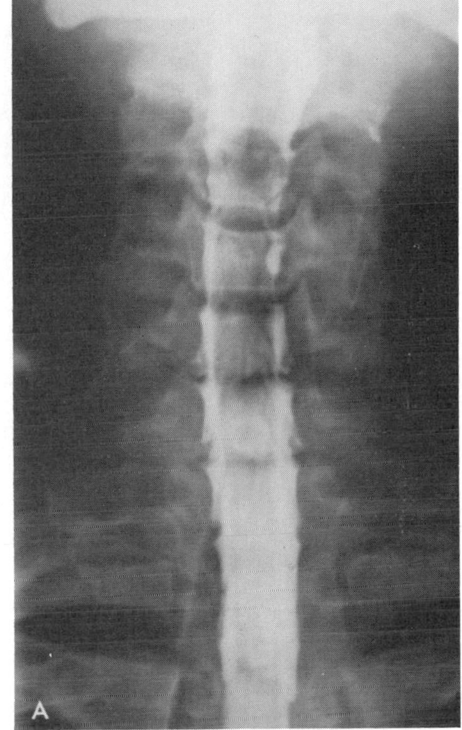

Figure 14–58 Cervical spondylosis. *A*. Cervical spondylosis with multiple bar defects and encroachment on nerve root sleeves. *B* and *C*. Severe spondylosis with cord compression.

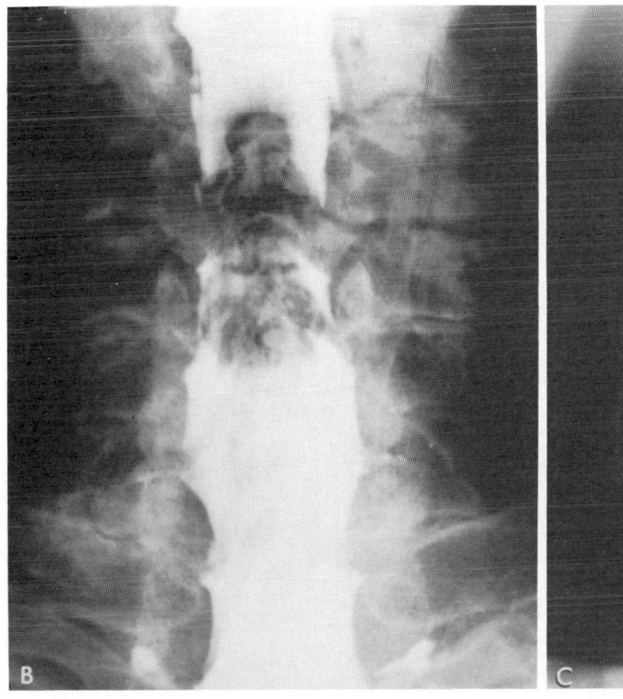

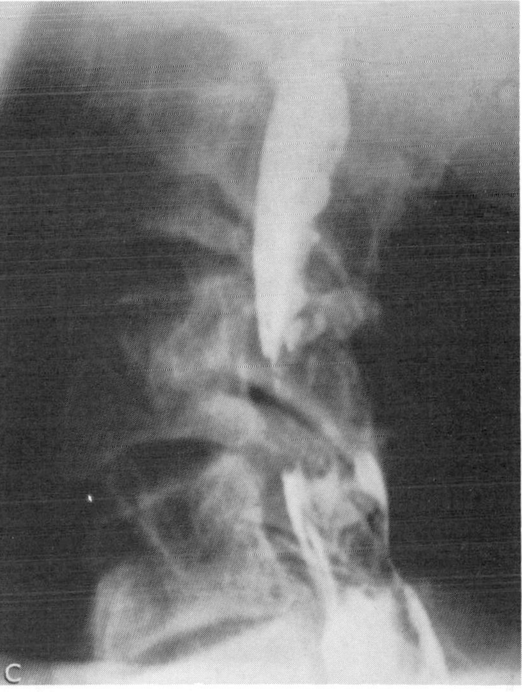

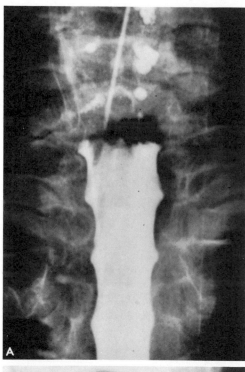

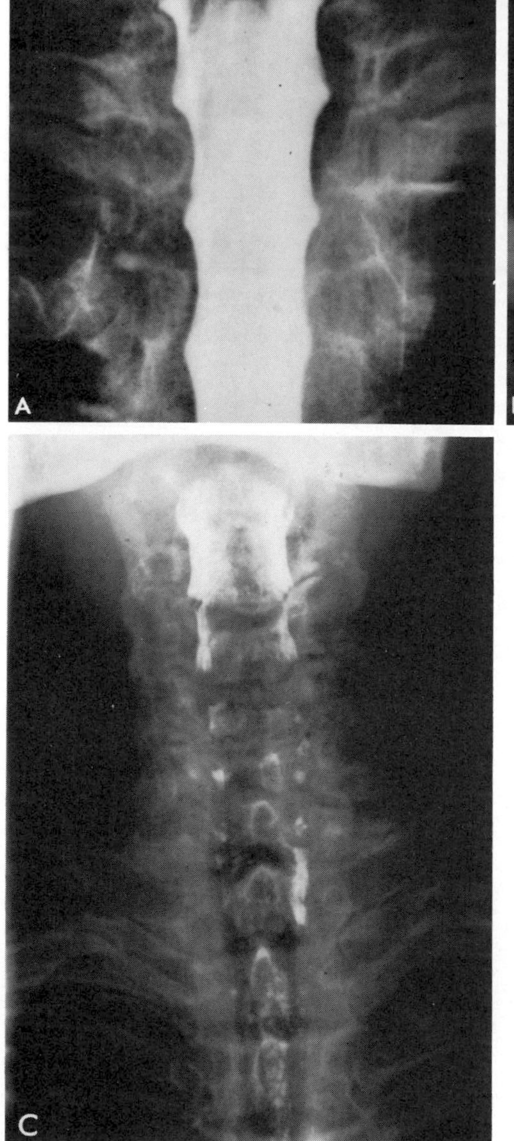

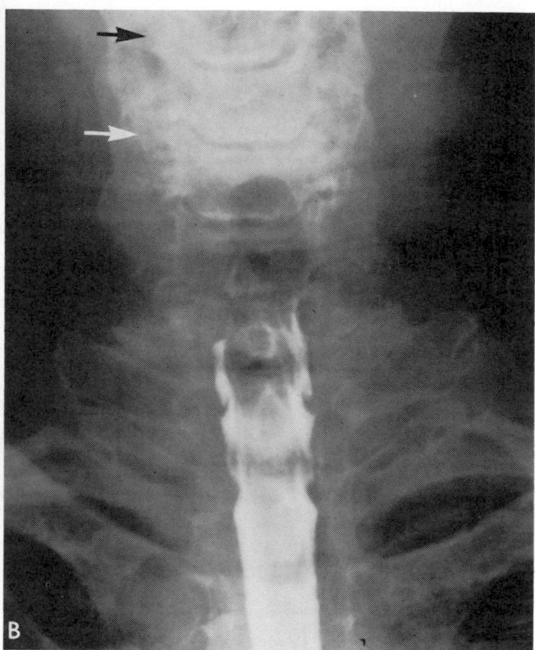

Figure 14–59 *A*. Myelogram from below showing complete block at C7–T1 due to severe spondylosis with disc herniation. An exploratory operation at this level produced no improvement. A re-exploration revealed a disc herniation two spaces higher. *B* and *C*. A patient with extensive cervical spondylosis showed a block at C6–C7 when Pantopaque was introduced from the lumbar region, *B*. Only after introduction of Pantopaque from above was another block outlined at C3–C4. Note the uncovertebral "joints" (*arrows*), associated with the degeneration of the disc and collapse of the disc space.

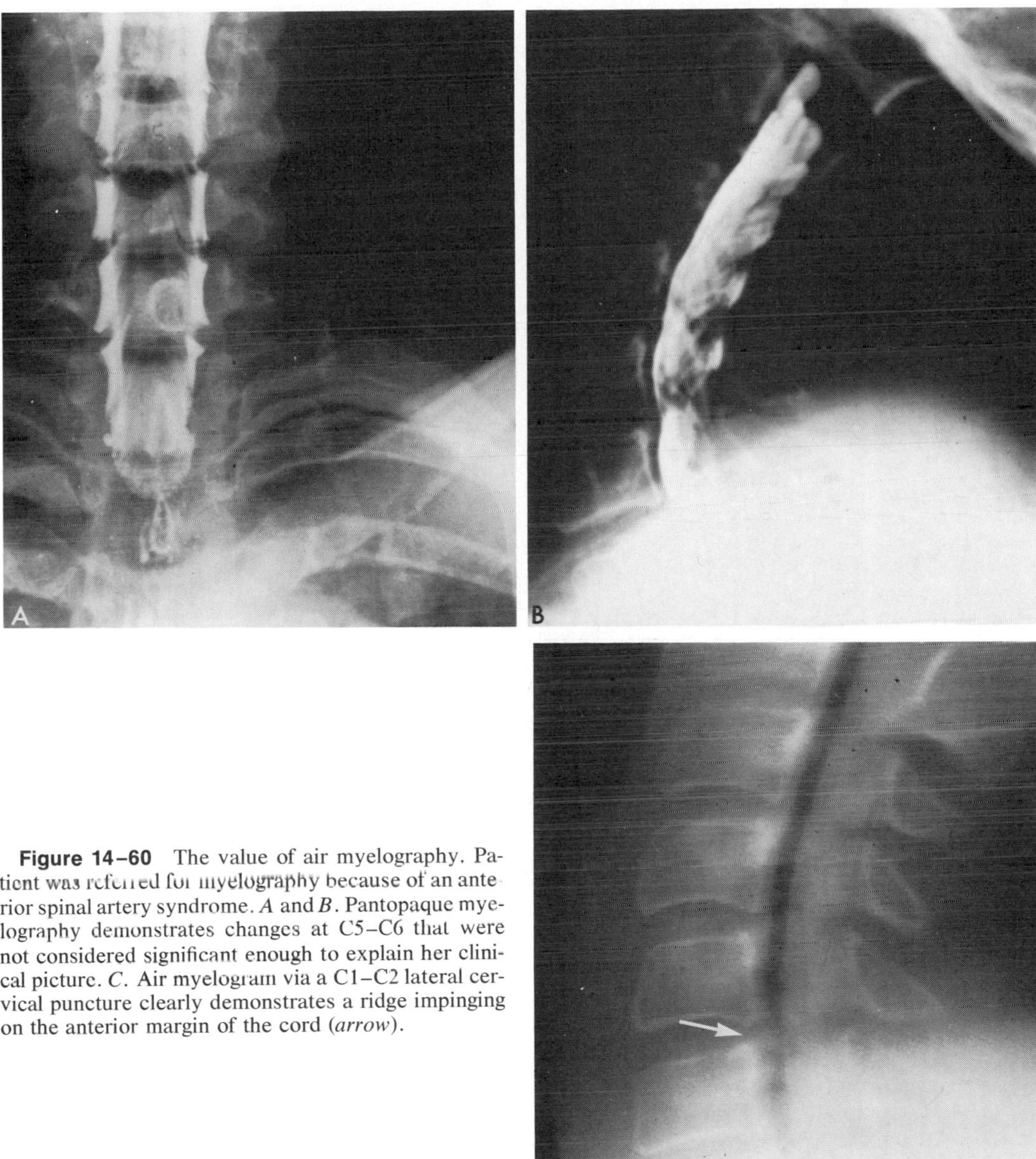

Figure 14–60 The value of air myelography. Patient was referred for myelography because of an anterior spinal artery syndrome. *A* and *B*. Pantopaque myelography demonstrates changes at C5–C6 that were not considered significant enough to explain her clinical picture. *C*. Air myelogram via a C1–C2 lateral cervical puncture clearly demonstrates a ridge impinging on the anterior margin of the cord (*arrow*).

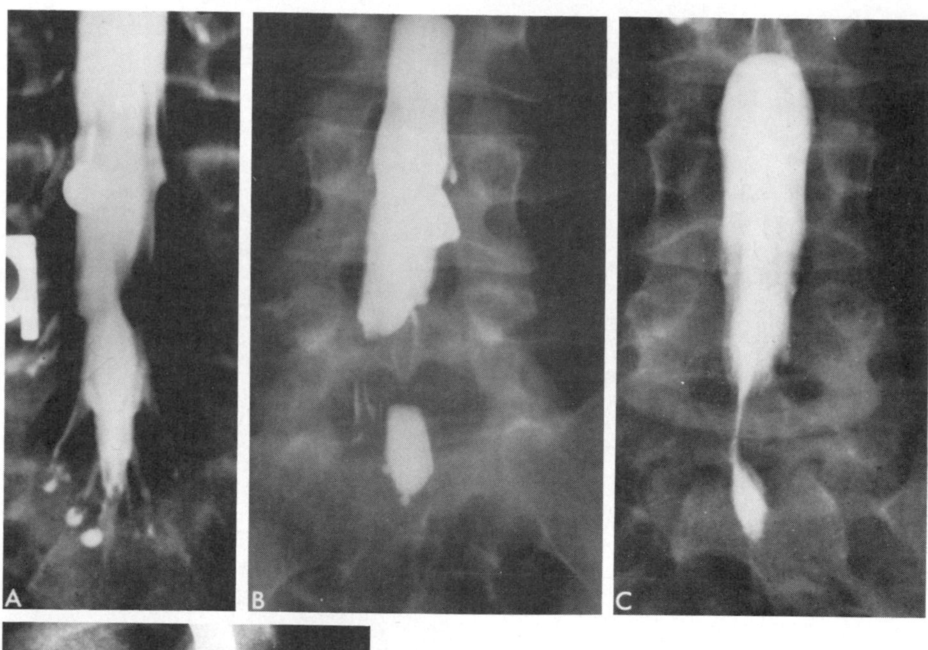

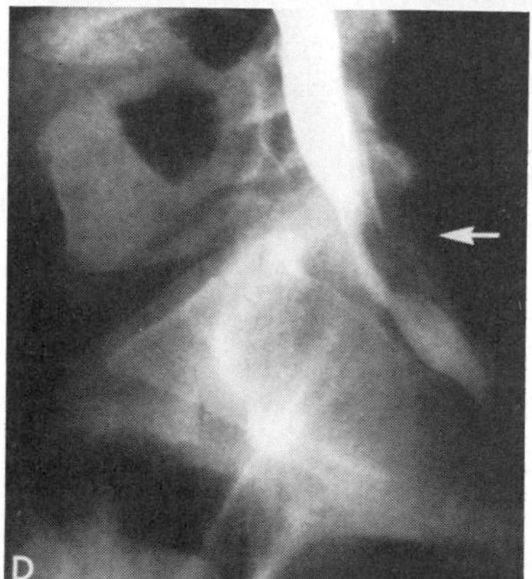

Figure 14–61 *A*. Lumbar myelogram showing amputation of a nerve root sleeve and a lateral defect in the column of contrast. A few sacral diverticula are seen. *B*. Lumbar myelogram showing L5–S1 disc with almost total block. *C* and *D*. Disc extrusion at L5–S1 with posterior migration and presenting with a posterior defect (*arrow*).

Illustration continued on opposite page

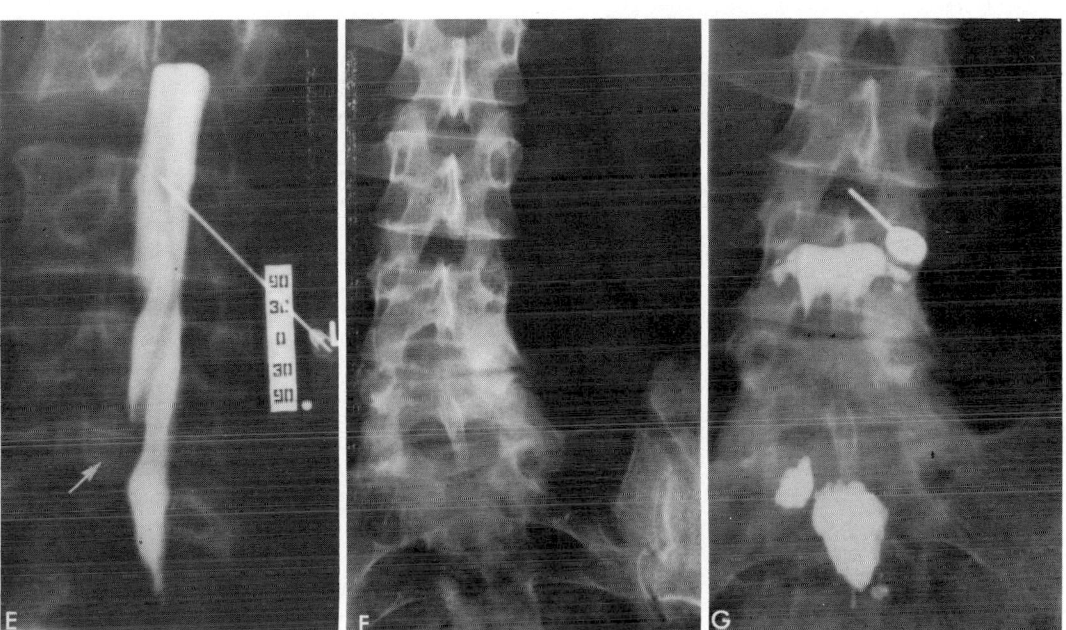

Figure 14–61 (*continued*) *E*. Oblique view demonstrating L4–L5 disc (*arrow*). *F* and *G*. Patient with marked L4–L5 disc space narrowing and vertebral body sclerosis. Myelography demonstrates almost complete block secondary to large herniated disc.

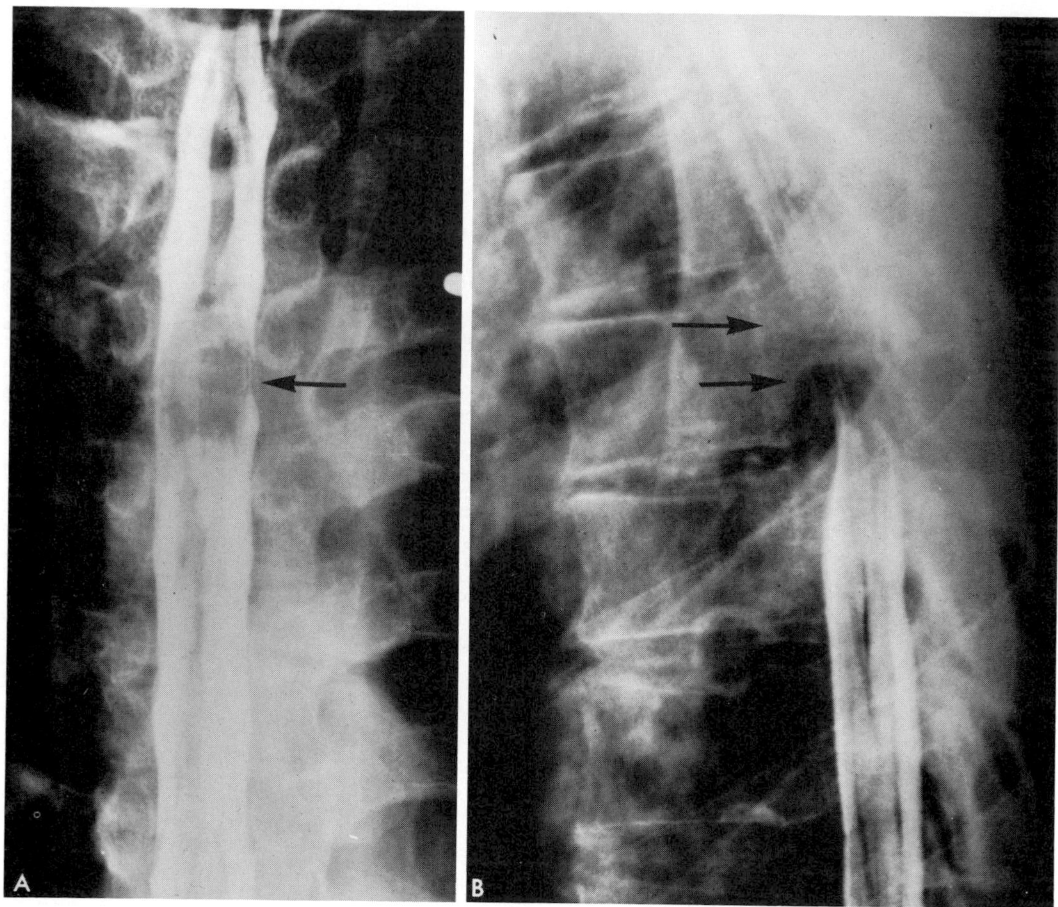

Figure 14–62 *A*. Thoracic disc widening the cord (*arrow*), simulating an intramedullary lesion in the anterior projection. *B*. The lateral projection shows posterior displacement of the cord and Pantopaque opposite a disc space.

REFERENCES

1. Ahlgren, P.: Amipaque myelography. Neuroradiology, *9*:197–202, 1975.
2. Almen, T., and Wiedeman, M. P.: Application of contrast media to the external surface of the vasculature. Invest. Radiol., *3*:151, 1968.
3. Amundsen, P., Foss, O. P., Godal, H. C., and Nitter-Hauge, S.: Intravenous injections of metrizamide into human volunteers. Acta Radiol. (Diagn.) Suppl. 335:339–345, 1973.
4. Britton, B. H., Hitselberger, W. E., and Hurley, B. J.: Iophendylate examination of posterior fossa in diagnosis of cerebellopontine angle tumors. Arch. Otolaryng. (Chicago), *88*:608–617, 1968.
5. Bull, J. W. D.: Spinal meningiomas and neurofibromas. Acta Radiol., *40*:283, 1953.
6. Conway, L. W.: Hydrodynamic studies in syringomyelia. J. Neurosurg., *27*:501–514, 1967.
7. Davis, K. R., Parker, S. W., New, P. F. J., et al.: Computed tomography of acoustic neuroma. Radiology, *124*:81–86, 1977.
8. DiChiro, G., and Fisher, R. L.: Contrast radiography of the spinal cord. Arch. Neurol. (Chicago), *11*:125–143, 1964.
9. Djindjian, R.: Angiography of the Spinal Cord. Baltimore, Md., University Park Press, 1970.
10. Drayer, B. P., Rosenbaum, A. E., and Higman, H. B.: Cerebrospinal fluid imaging using serial metrizamide CT cisternography. Neuroradiology, *13*:7–17, 1977.
11. Drayer, B. P., Rosenbaum, A. E., Kennerdell, J. S., Robinson, A. G., Bank, W. O., and Deeb, Z. L.: Computed tomographic diagnosis of suprasellar masses by intrathecal enhancement. Radiology, *123*:339–344, 1977.
12. Elsberg, C. A., and Dyke, C. G.: The diagnosis and localization of tumors of the spinal cord by means of measurements made on the x-ray films of the vertebra and the correlation of clinical and x-ray findings. Bull. Neurol. Inst. N. Y., *3*:359, 1934.
13. Epstein, B. S.: The Spine. 4th Ed. Philadelphia, Lea & Febiger, 1969.
14. Epstein, B. S., Epstein, J. A., and Lavine, L.: The effect of anatomic variations in the lumbar vertebrae and spinal canal on cauda equina and nerve root syndromes. Amer. J. Roentgen., *91*:1055, 1964.
15. Febbroriello, M.: Double exposure of the lateral cervical spine. Presented at the Connecticut Society of X-ray Technologists, 1963.
16. Gargano, F. P., Meyer, J., Houdek, P. V., and Charyuhe, K. K. N.: Transverse axial tomography of the cervical spine. Radiology, *113*:363, 1974.
17. Gold, L. A., and Kieffer, S. A.: Positive contrast evaluation of the posterior cranial fossa. Radiology, *102*:63–70, 1972.
18. Grainger, R. D., Kendall, B. E., and Wylie, J. G.: Lumbar myelography with metrizamide—a new non-ionic contrast medium. Brit. J. Radiol., *49*:996–1003, 1976.
19. Greenberg, A. D.: Atlanto-axial dislocation. Brain, *91*:655, 1968.
20. Griffiths, H. E. D., and Jones, D. M.: Pyogenic infection of the spine. J. Bone Joint Surg., *53B*:383, 1971.
21. Hadley, L. A.: Anatomico-Roentgenographic Studies of the Spine. Springfield, Ill., Charles C Thomas, 1964.
22. Hammerschlag, S. B., Wolpert, S. M., and Carter, B. L.: Computed tomography of the spinal canal. Radiology, *121*:361–367, 1976.
23. Hanson, E. B., Praestholm, J., Fahrenkrug, A., and Berrum, J.: A clinical trial of Amipaque in lumbar myelography. Brit. J. Radiol., *49*:34–38, 1976.
24. Haughton, V. M., Ho, K. C., Larson, S., Unger, G. F., and Correa Pas, F.: Experimental production of arachnoiditis with water-soluble myelographic media. Radiology, *123*:681–685, 1977.
25. Heinz, E. R., Brinker, R. A., and Taveras, J. M.: Advantages of a less dense Pantopaque contrast for myelography. Acta Radiol. (Diagn.), *5*:1024–1031, 1966.
26. Hinck, V. C., Clark, W. M., and Hopkins, C. E.: Normal interpediculate distances (minimum and maximum) in children and adults. Amer. J. Roentgen., *97*:141–153, 1966.
27. Hinck, V. C., Hopkins, C. E., and Savara, B. S.: Diagnostic criteria of basilar impression. Radiology, *76*:572, 1961.
28. Hindmarsh, T.: Myelography with the non-ionic soluble contrast medium metrizamide. Acta Radiol. (Diagn.), *16*:417–435, 1975.
29. Hindmarsh, T., Grepe, A., and Widen, L.: Metrizamide-phenothiazine interaction. Report of a case with seizures following myelography. Acta Radiol. (Diagn.), *16*:129–131, 1975.
30. Jirout, J.: Pneumomyelography. Springfield, Ill., Charles C Thomas, 1969.
31. Kaada, B.: Transient EEG abnormalities following lumbar myelography with metrizamide. Acta Radiol. (Diagn.) Suppl. *335*:380–386, 1973.
32. Kieffer, S. A., Peterson, H. O., Gold, L. H. A., and Binet, E. F.: Evaluation of dilute Pantopaque for large volume myelography. Radiology, *96*:69 74, 1970.
33. Koehler, A.: Borderlands of the Normal and Early Pathologic in Skeletal Roentgenology. 10th Ed., New York, Grune &Stratton, 1956.
34. Lindgren, E.: Radiologic examination of brain and spinal cord. Acta Radiol. Suppl. 151, 1957.
35. Long, J. M., Kier, E. L., and Hilding, D. A.: Pitfalls of posterior fossa cisternography using 2 ml. of iophendylate (Pantopaque). Radiology, *102*:71–75, 1972.
36. Maupin, R. A., Baker, H. L., and Kerr, F. W. L.: Emulsified Pantopaque: Its possible application for myelography. Radiology, *86*:509–514, 1966.
37. McRae, D. L.: The significance of abnormalities of the cervical spine. Caldwell Lecture, 1959. Amer. J. Roentgen., *34*:3–25; 1960.
38. Metrizamide. A non-ionic water-soluble contrast medium. Experimental and preliminary clinical investigation. Acta Radiol. Suppl. 335, 1973.
39. Naidich, J. M., Naidich, T. P., Garfan, C., Liebeskind, A. L., and Hyman, R. A.: The widened interspinous distance. A useful sign of anterior cervical dislocation in the supine frontal projection. Radiology, *123*:113–116, 1977.
40. Puljic, S., Batnitzky, S., Yang, W. C., and Schechter, M. M.: Metastases to the medulla of the spinal cord. Myelographic features. Radiology, *117*:89–91, 1975.

41. Rosomoff, H. L., Carroll, F., Brown, J., and Sheptak, P.: Percutaneous radiofrequency cervical cordotomy: Technique. J. Neurosurg., *23*:639–644, 1965.
42. Schmorl, G., and Junghanns, H.: The Human Spine in Health and Disease. New York, Grune & Stratton, 1959.
43. Schwarz, G. S.: The width of the spinal canal in the growing verebra with special reference to the sacrum. Maximal interpedicular distances in adults and children. Amer. J. Roentgen., *76*:476, 1956.
44. Shahinfar, A. H., and Schechter, M. M.: Traumatic extradural cysts of the spine. Amer. J. Roentgen, *98*:713–719, 1966.
45. Shapiro, R.: Myelography. 3rd Ed. Chicago, Year Book Medical Publishers, 1975.
46. Shapiro, R., Youngberg, A. S., and Rothman, S. L. G.: The differential diagnosis of traumatic lesions of the occipito-atlanto-axial segment. Radiol. Clin. N. Amer., *11*:505–526, 1973.
47. Skalpe, I. O., and Amundsen, P.: Lumbar radiculography with metrizamide. Radiology, *115*:91–95, 1975.
48. Skalpe, I. O., and Amundsen, P.: Thoracic and cervical myelography with metrizamide. Radiology, *116*:101–106, 1975.
49. Skalpe, I. O., and Torvik, A.: Toxicity of metrizamide and meglumine iocarmate in the spinal subarachnoid space. Invest. Radiol., *10*:154–159, 1975.
50. Smith, B. H.: Cervical spondylosis and its neurological complications. Springfield, Ill., Charles C Thomas, 1968.
51. Sowhnoy, B. B., and Oftedal, S. I.: Reaction to suboccipital injection of water-soluble contrast media in rabbits. Acta Radiol. (Diagn.), Suppl. *335*:67–83, 1973.
52. Swischuk, L. E.: Radiology of the Newborn and Young Infant. Baltimore, Md., Williams & Wilkins Co., 1973.
53. Valvassori, G. E.: Myelography of the internal auditory canal. Amer. J. Roentgen., *115*:575–586, 1972.
54. Vines, F. S.: The significance of "occult" fractures of the cervical spine. Amer. J. Roentgen., *107*:493–504, 1969.
55. Westberg. G.: Gas myelography and percutaneous puncture in the diagnosis of spinal cord cysts. Acta Radiol. (Diagn.), Suppl. *252*:1–67, 1966.
56. Whalen, J. P., and Woodruff, C. L.: The cervical prevertebral fat stripe. Amer. J. Roentgen., *109*:445–451, 1970.
57. Wolf, B. S., Khilnani, M., and Malis, L.: The sagittal diameter of the bony cervical spinal canal and its significance in cervical spondylosis. J. Mount Sinai Hosp., N.Y., *23*:283–298, 1956.
58. Wortzman, G., and Dewar, F. P.: Rotary fixation of the atlantoaxial joint: Rotational atlantoaxial subluxation. Radiology, *90*:479–487, 1968.
59. Zilkha, A., Reiss, J., Shulman, K., and Schechter, M. M.: Traumatic subarachnoid mediastinal fistula. J. Neurosurg., *32*:473, 1970.

15

ANGIOGRAPHY OF THE SPINAL CORD

The radiographic evaluation of the spinal cord vasculature is a difficult procedure at best. In the past, paraplegia has been produced by opacifying the spinal cord arteries that are the principal interest of the angiographic study. In addition, the multiplicity of arteries supplying the cord and the obscuration of the angiographically opacified vessels by the enclosing vertebral column have impeded the development of useful and successful cord angiography.

Since 1966, more than 3000 arteriographic examinations of the spinal cord have been performed at the Lariboisière Hospital in Paris. Profiting from an improved knowledge of spinal cord vascular anatomy, technical advances (such as high-milliamperage generators, smaller catheter materials, improved contrast agents, and image subtraction techniques), and improved anesthetic agents, spinal cord angiography has advanced to include the study of all ischemic, vascular, and neoplastic processes. In some patients, treatment of lesions by transcatheter embolization and angioplastic techniques is now possible.

ANATOMICAL REVIEW OF CORD VASCULATURE

The spinal cord is supplied in front by the anterior spinal artery lodged in the anterior median fissure, and in back by two posterolateral arteries located in the dorsolateral sulci on either side of the spinal cord.

Arterial Network Within the Cord

The anterior four fifths of the cord, of major functional importance, is supplied by sulcocommissural arteries arising from the anterior spinal artery, whereas the two posterolateral arteries supply only a small part of the posterior funiculi and the posterior horns, which have less functional importance (Fig. 15–1). Thus, the anterior spinal artery serves as the principal blood supply of the cord.[7]

Arterial Network Outside the Cord

The thoracolumbar and thoracic portions of the anterior spinal artery are formed by

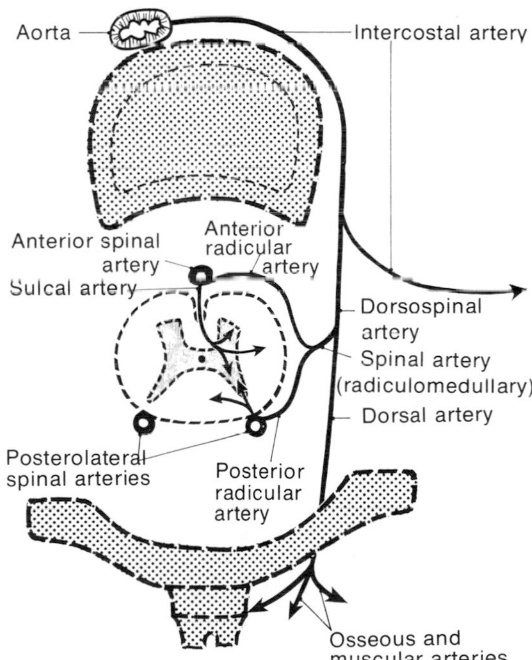

Figure 15–1 A cross-sectional display of the spinal cord arterial anatomy. (From Djindjian, R., Hurth, M., and Houdart, R.: Angiography of the Spinal Cord. Paris, Masson & Cie; Baltimore, Md., University Park Press, 1970. Reprinted by permission.)

R. DJINDJIAN, A. DUBLIN, AND M. DJINDJIAN

anastomoses between the two branches of the ascending and descending divisions of certain arteries (called anterior radiculospinal arteries) arising from intercostal arteries. The cervical portion of the anterior spinal artery is formed from branches of the subclavian and vertebral arteries. These anterior radicular arteries are quite few in number; two or three for the cervical region, one for the superior thoracic region, and one large one called the artery of Adamkiewicz for the thoracolumbar cord (Fig. 15–2). The description of this artery by Adamkiewicz in 1882 modified the initial concept of a segmental spinal vasculature in favor of a concept of regional vascular territories.[1]

These functional vascular territories

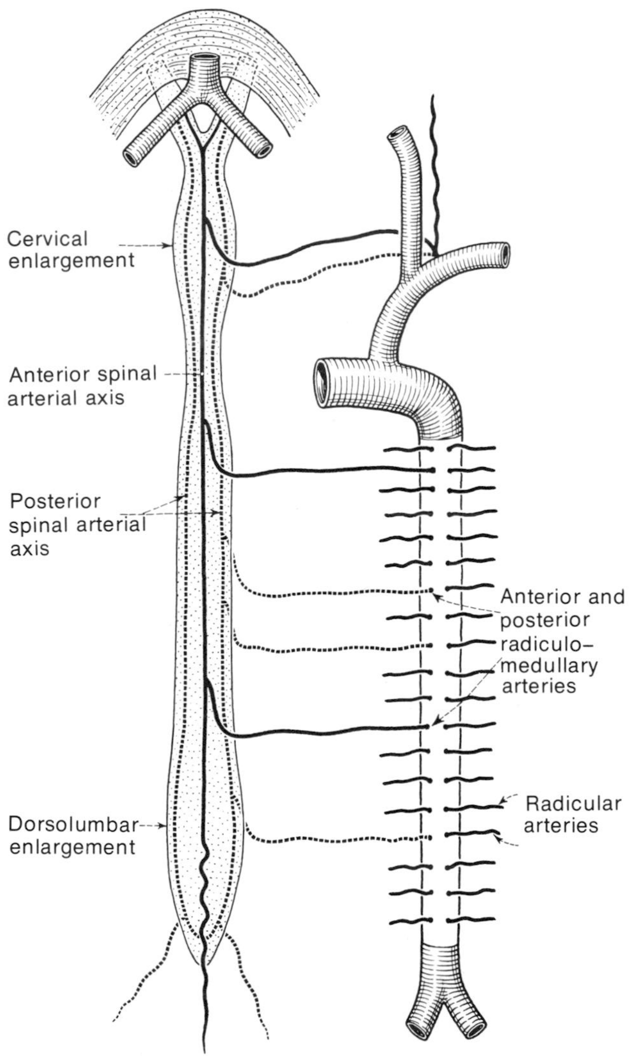

Figure 15–2 Anterior and posterior radiculomedullary arteries. *A.* Frontal view.

Illustration continued on opposite page

were demonstrated by Lazorthes and coworkers.[17] Each of these three arteries, the cervical artery, the superior thoracic artery, and the artery of Adamkiewicz, supplies by itself the territory that is attributed to it, with poor cephalad-caudal anastomoses with the territory of another (Fig. 15–3). Thus, the artery of Adamkiewicz has as its principal territory a very important segment extending from T5 to the conus medullaris. A lesion in this artery will cause massive ischemia of this region, since the collateral circulation is poorly formed.

DiChiro and associates suggest, however, that there is probably sufficient vertical collateral flow to explain the smaller incidence of paraplegia and paralysis as side effects with selective arterial segmental injection

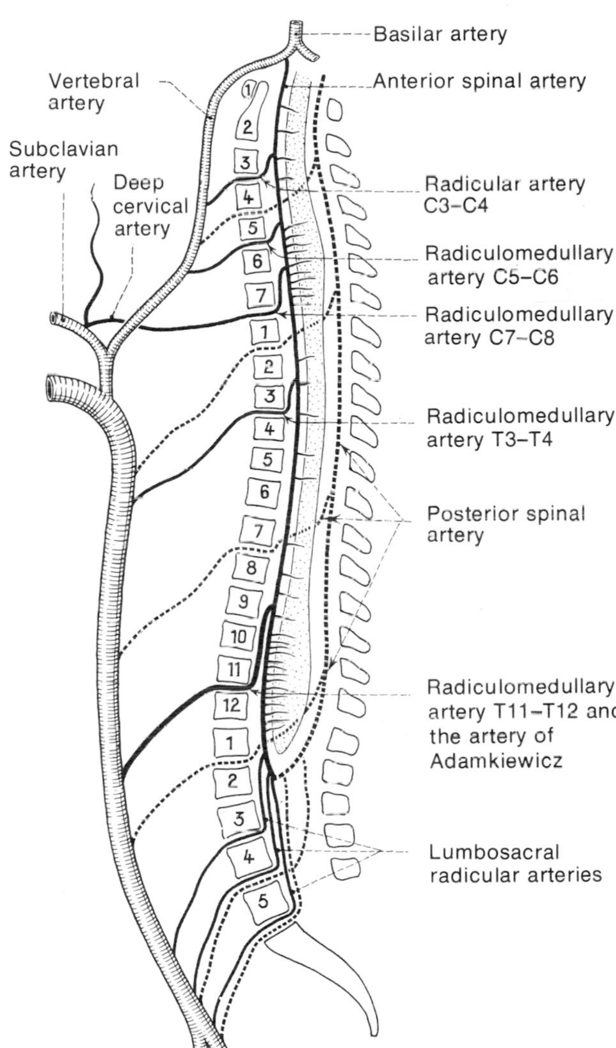

Figure 15–2 (*continued*) *B*. Lateral view (From Djindjian, R., Hurth, M., and Houdart, R.: Angiography of the Spinal Cord. Paris, Masson & Cie; Baltimore, Md., University Park Press, 1970. Reprinted by permission.)

than there is with an aortic flush. In the latter situation, all the vascular channels are flooded with contrast material. With selective arterial injection, the cephalad-caudal collateral flow in the cord will be sufficient to allow adequate wash-out by more oxygenated blood. The amount of contrast medium injected should be kept to a minimum; it is especially important to use small amounts of contrast, as selective bronchial artery injections in the midthoracic region have been shown to cause paraplegia.[4] The vulnerability of the T4 to T7 region is related to the fact that it has the smallest vessels and is the least richly supplied area of the spinal cord.[16]

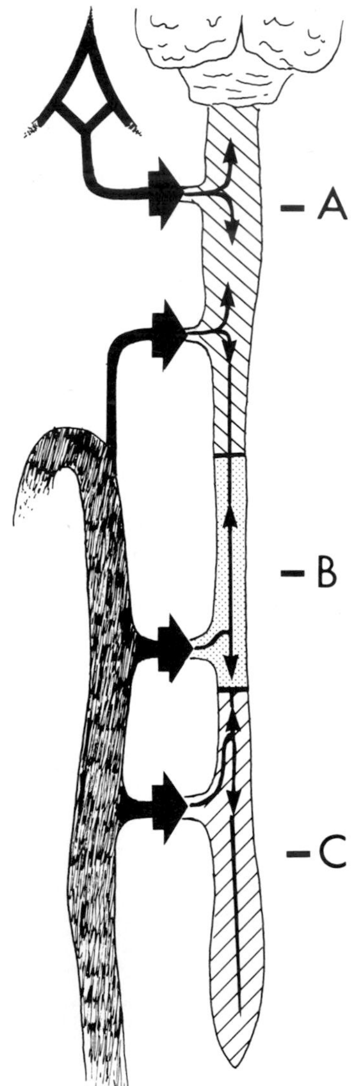

Figure 15–3 Schematic representation of the three major regional arterial supplies to the spinal cord. The flow patterns to, A, the cervical and upper thoracic; B, the midthoracic; and, C, the lower thoracic and lumbar regions are represented by arrows.

If paraplegia does occur, rapid removal of aliquots of cerebrospinal fluid by spinal puncture may help to reverse or improve paralytic complications, probably by decreasing abnormally high iodine levels in the cerebrospinal fluid bathing the spinal cord.[18]

The posterior spinal arteries are fed largely by the numerous posterior radiculospinal vessels arising from intercostal arteries and, furthermore, are widely anastomosed between themselves. Their functional territory is much smaller than that of the anterior spinal artery, and injury to one of them will not necessarily cause cord ischemia.

The Anterior Spinal Artery

This artery frequently is not continuous in the midcervical and upper thoracic regions. It is fed by several anterior radicular arteries, which from cephalad to caudad are: (1) a branch arising from the terminal portion of the vertebral artery and rejoining its fellow from the other side at C2 to form a single trunk, from which springs the origin of the anterior spinal artery; (2) at the level of C3–C4, one or two radicular arteries arising from the cervical vertebral artery; and (3) at the lower cervical (usually C6) portion, a large artery arising most frequently from the deep cervical artery (Fig. 15–4). Often this last is called the artery of the cervical enlargement (or cervical artery of Lazorthes). Many variations in the number of arteries (ipsilateral or contralateral), their origin (vertebral right or left, deep cervical right or left, the scapular thyrocervical trunk), and their route of penetration (C5, C6, C7) are observed. In the thoracic region the anterior spinal artery is reinforced by a small radicular artery arising from the third or fourth intercostal artery, most often on the left. In the thoracolumbar region, the anterior spinal artery consists of the artery of Adamkiewicz, diagrammed in Figure 15–5, the largest of the anterior radicular arteries, whose site of origin is variable (75 per cent from the left), as is the level of origin (75 per cent from the eighth to the twelfth intercostals, 25 per

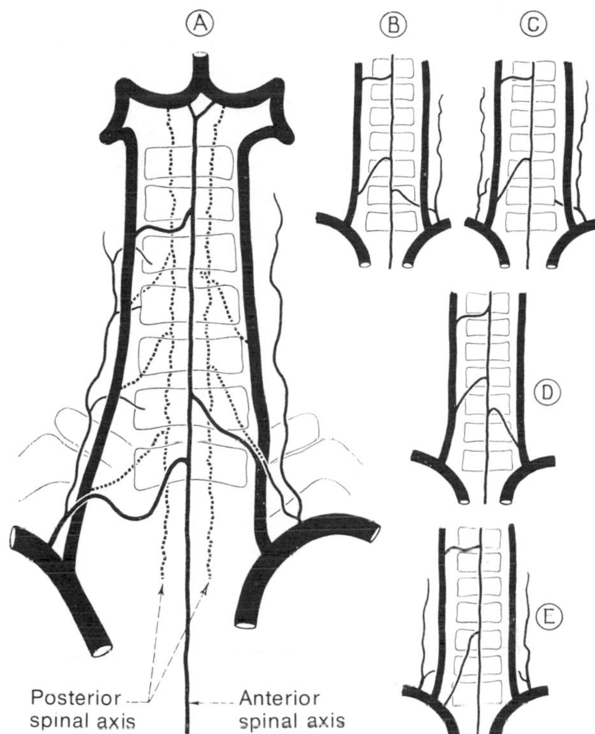

Figure 15–4 Anterior and posterior cervical radiculomedullary arteries and their variations. *A*. C3 radiculomedullary artery arising from the vertebral; C5–C6, from the left deep cervical; C6–C7, from the first right intercostal, supplying the anterior axis. *B*. Cervical enlargement supplied by the right vertebral and the left deep cervical. *C*. Cervical enlargement supplied by the right vertebral. *D*. Cervical enlargement supplied by both vertebrals. *E*. Cervical enlargement supplied by branch from the subclavian. (From Djindjian, R., Hurth, M., and Houdart, R.: Angiography of the Spinal Cord. Paris, Masson & Cie; Baltimore, Md., University Park Press, 1970. Reprinted by permission.)

cent from the fifth to the seventh intercostals and from the first to the third lumbar arteries.)[8]

Lazorthes and co-workers maintain that the artery of Adamkiewicz gives rise to both a large anterior and a large posterior root artery. Thus, they suggest, the term "artery of the lumbar enlargement" might be more appropriate.[17] Jellinger believes that these two arterial feeders are most often separate trunks, while Corbin suggests that there is no proof of the existence of a particularly consistent or large feeder to the dorsal aspect of the cord from the artery of Adamkiewicz.[2,13] For the purposes of this presentation, the term "artery of Adamkiewicz" is used to imply the arterial blood supply to the thoracolumbar cord.

Alternative vessels to the anterior spinal artery are important. They do not exist at the level of the upper thoracic region, which probably explains the frequency of ischemic accidents in the region T4. At the level of the cervical cord, the alternative supply (in case of subclavian or vertebral obstruction) may, in the superior third, be by way of the anastomotic meshwork behind the atlas and axis formed from muscular branches of the vertebral artery, the deep and ascending cervical arteries, and the occipital artery. In the lower two thirds of the cervical cord, the alternative supplies are derived from the two vertebral arteries by way of the superior and inferior thyroid arteries and the internal mammary arteries, as well as from branches of the deep and ascending cervical arteries. In the thoracolumbar region, the territory of the artery of Adamkiewicz may be supplied by the development of radicular lumbosacral arteries that empty into the anastomotic loop of the conus medullaris formed by the union of the two posterior spinal arteries and the terminal portion of the artery of Adamkiewicz.

TECHNIQUE OF SPINAL CORD ANGIOGRAPHY

Pre-Study Evaluation of the Patient

A careful work-up including electrocardiography (when indicated by advanced age or cardiovascular history), chest x-ray, and urinalysis should be performed before arteriography. Two important contraindications to arteriography are a recent anticoagulant treatment and the presence of renal damage that will preclude the use of a large load of contrast material. Advanced age is not an obstacle except when atherosclerotic stenosis of both iliac arteries makes the study impossible by the femoral route.

Anesthesia

At the Lariboisière Hospital, spinal angiography is done under general anesthesia with tracheal intubation, assisted respiration, and careful monitoring. The "dissociated" anesthetics used are chloroprocaine, pethidine (meperidine), and sodium 4-dihydroxybutylnitrate carried in liquid containing low molecular weight dextran. The controlled breathing is stopped at the time each series of pictures is taken to block movement and to aid in the use of subtraction methods. DiChiro and Wener prefer the use of local anesthesia to allow continuous observation of a patient's neurological status and the detection of early spinal cord ischemia, the latter of which

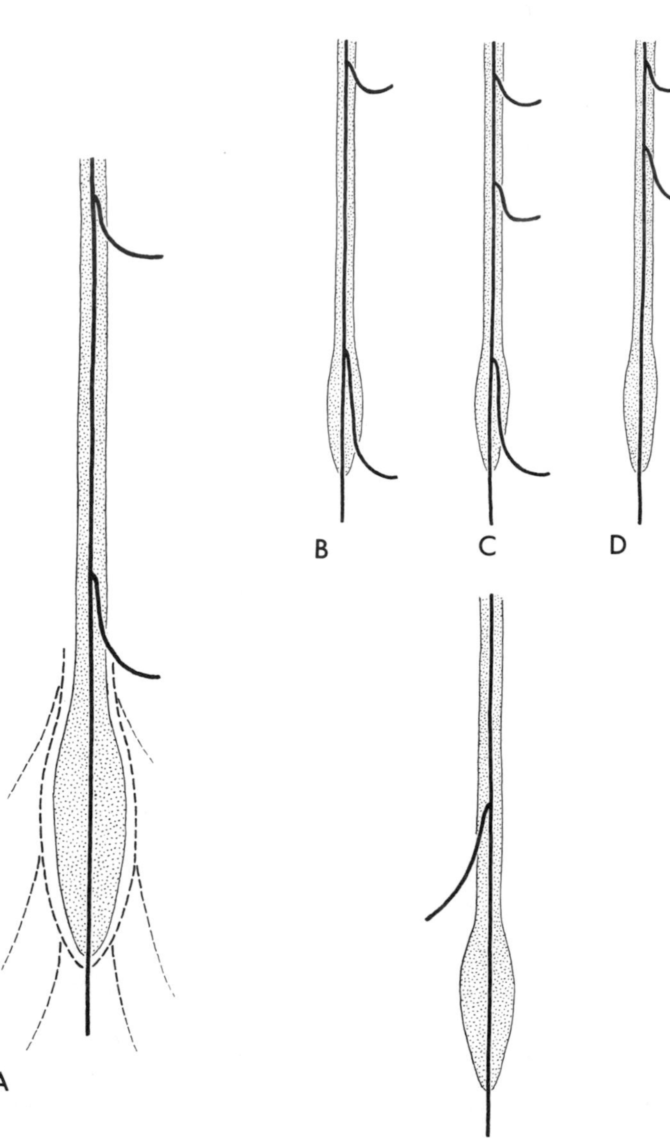

Figure 15–5 Variations in the origin of the artery of Adamkiewicz. *A*. From left side: *A*, T3–T4; *B*, L1–L2; *C* and *D*, T5–T6–T7–T8. *E*. From right side. (From Djindjian, R., Hurth, M., and Houdart, R.: Angiography of the Spinal Cord. Paris, Masson & Cie; Baltimore, Md., University Park Press, 1970. Reprinted by permission.)

would mean termination of the radiological examination.[4]

Radiographic Equipment

The radiological equipment is composed of a movable extension with coupled Potter grid that allows the exposure of three successive films, a television monitor, biplane film changers, and a videodisc for producing immediate subtraction on the television screen. The latter is especially useful for monitoring the effectiveness of embolization procedures.

Magnification techniques, especially using microfocal x-ray tubes (0.05 mm), promise to improve the visualization of normal and pathological vascular structures.[20]

Arterlography

A green Odman 160 catheter or similar catheter material, bent back at the tip to allow easy entrance into the lumina of the intercostal lumbar arteries, is introduced by Seldinger femoral puncture. Selective catheterization as close as possible to vessels feeding the cord produces a much better radiological image as well as reducing cord damage because of the small amount of material injected and the low pressure with which it is manually introduced. Methylglucamine iothalamate preparations are recommended. The greater safety of these materials has been suggested by several authors.[4,11,15] In uncomplicated cases, a maximum of 8 ml per injection has been suggested by DiChiro and associates.[4] However, 15 ml or more may be required to opacify highly vascular angiomas or tumors.[8]

The arteriographic technique differs according to the spinal segment to be examined. At the cervical level, it is possible to distinguish the vessels feeding the cord by selective catheterization of the vertebral arteries, branches of the thyrocervical, the scapular trunk, and the cervical intercostal trunk. The methods of mass exploration (humeral, subclavian, and aortic) are unsatisfactory and can only constitute an orienting examination. At the thoracolumbar level, orientation aortography has proved

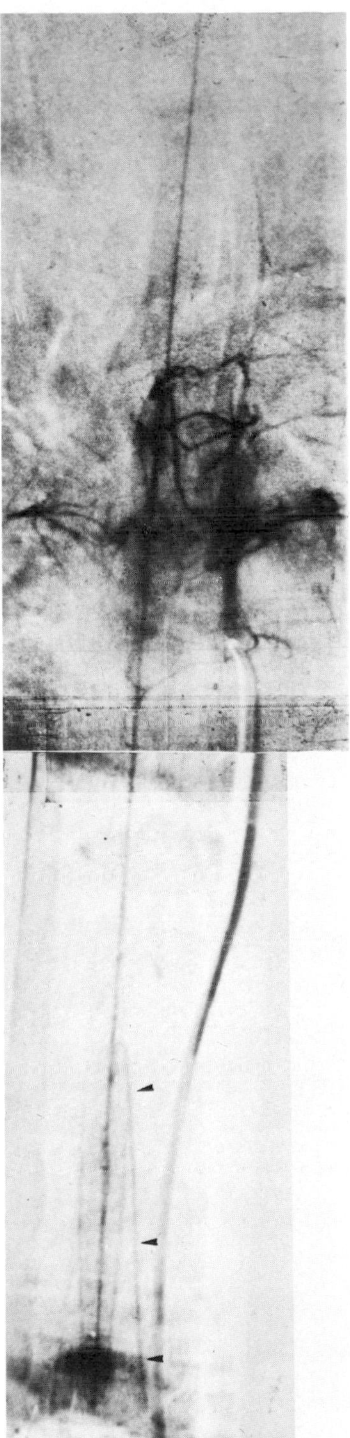

Figure 15–6 A bipolar injection catheter in the second left lumbar artery opacifying the artery of Adamkiewicz (*arrows*) and a second catheter in the left sixth intercostal artery produced complete opacification of the anterior spinal arterial axis by means of simultaneous injection in both catheters.

to be not only insufficient but also dangerous because of the risk of injection under great pressure to vessels that lead to the cord. Spinal cord angiography has been improved by bipolar arteriography, which consists of introducing a catheter via each femoral artery and simultaneously and selectively opacifying the artery of Adamkiewicz and the anterior superior thoracic artery on the one hand, and the artery of the cervical enlargement on the other (Fig. 15–6). Simultaneous injections of contrast material in these two arteries allow the opacification of the entire anterior spinal pathway. Although this seems in contradiction to the classic notion of interruption of this important arterial axis, clinically significant cord ischemia usually is not a serious contraindication to this technique.

Venography

In normal situations, angiographic confirmation of classic anatomical studies is not obtained because of the small caliber of the veins of the spinal cord and the degree to which the contrast is diluted in the veins during the late phase of spinal angiography. Also, it is not possible to inject into the veins of the cord in a retrograde fashion except for azygography or cavography. In angiomas, however, the presence of dilated veins draining the spinal cord does allow such a comparative study. These angiomatous veins confirm anatomical studies demonstrating a smaller number of radiculospinal veins (six to eight), as compared to the arterial supply to the cord. The drainage of these spinal veins is cephalad into the vein of Galen by way of the bulbopontomesencephalic veins, caudally into the inferior vena cava by way of the sacral veins, and laterally into the azygous system by way of the radiculospinal veins.

THE NORMAL ANGIOGRAM

The opacification of the network surrounding the cord varies as a function of the caliber of the vessel into which the contrast is injected and the level considered. Usually, this network of external cord vessels can be visualized with a high degree of frequency. On the other hand, the intramedullary arterial network cannot be angiographically demonstrated with the present state of radiographic technique. It is only when there is a pathological dilatation of

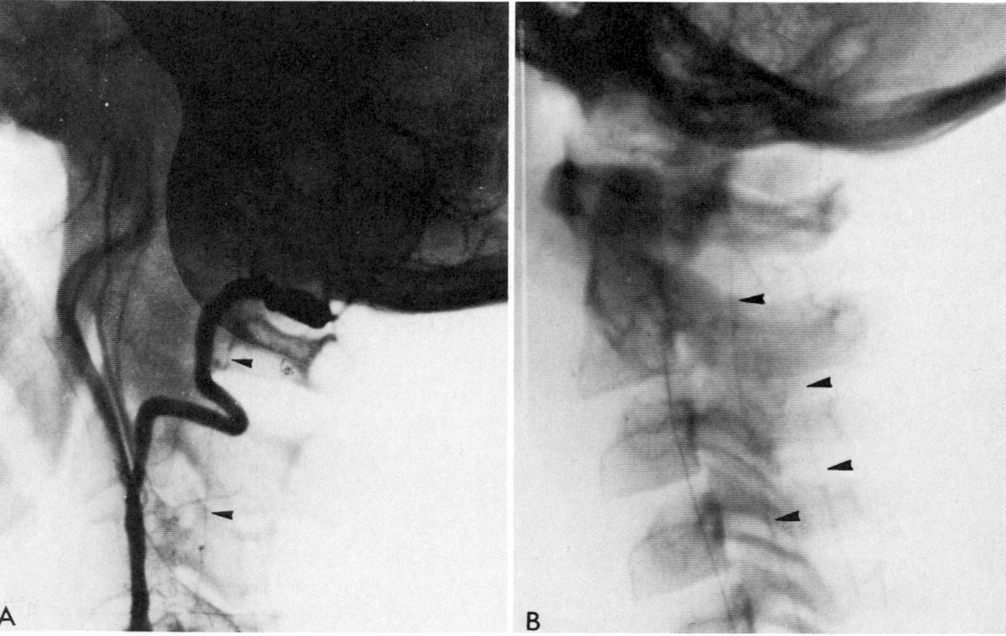

Figure 15–7 Lateral vertebral arterial injections. *A*. Anterior spinal artery originating from the vertebral artery (*arrows*). *B*. Anterior and posterior spinal arteries (*arrows*) outlining the upper part of the cervical cord. (From Djindjian, R., Hurth, M., and Houdart, R.: Angiography of the Spinal Cord. Paris, Masson & Cie; Baltimore, Md., University Park Press, 1970. Reprinted by permission.)

the central arteries (as in angiomas), that the structures can be identified by angiography.

Anterior Spinal Arteries

The anterior spinal artery arising from the intracranial vertebral artery is opacified in half of the cases of direct vertebral puncture angiography. The percentage is increased further if a catheter is placed higher in the vertebral artery via the femoral route. In the anteroposterior (AP) projection, the anterior spinal artery progresses caudally and may often be followed to C3 or C5. From the side, it descends in a straight line parallel to the posterior surface of the vertebral bodies, marking the anterior border of the spinal cord (Fig. 15–7). The anterior branch to the cord from the vertebral artery at the C3–C4 level is as a general rule not seen (Fig. 15–8). The artery of the cervical enlargement is variable in origin (most frequently the deep cervical artery or the first intercostal artery) in the normal state (Fig. 15–9).

The anterior branch to the first thoracic segments of the cord arises from the third or fourth intercostal artery and joins the anterior spinal axis after a short ascending course. It is frequently thin and, with its median descending branch, forms a tight hairpin loop. Its ascending branch is filiform and never rejoins the descending branch of the artery of the cervical enlargement.

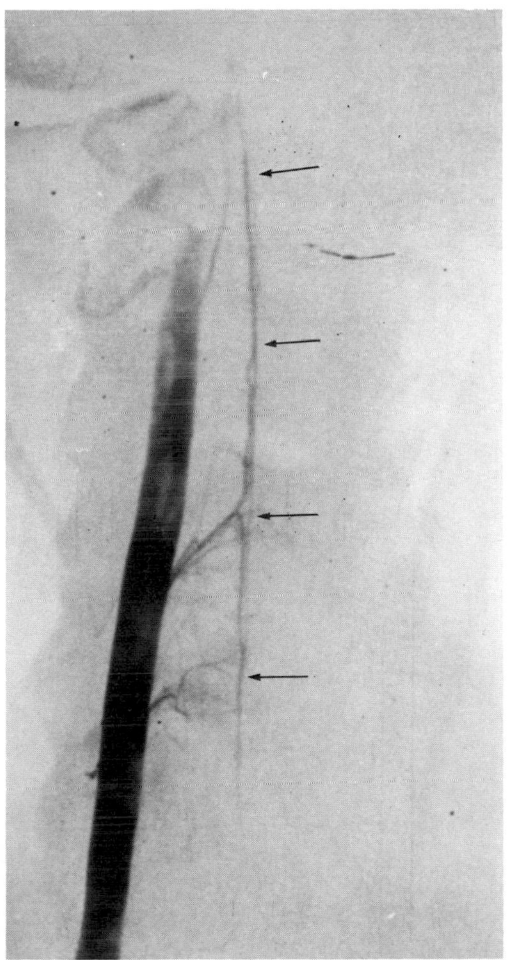

Figure 15–8 Artery of the cervical enlargement (*arrows*) originating from the right vertebral artery.

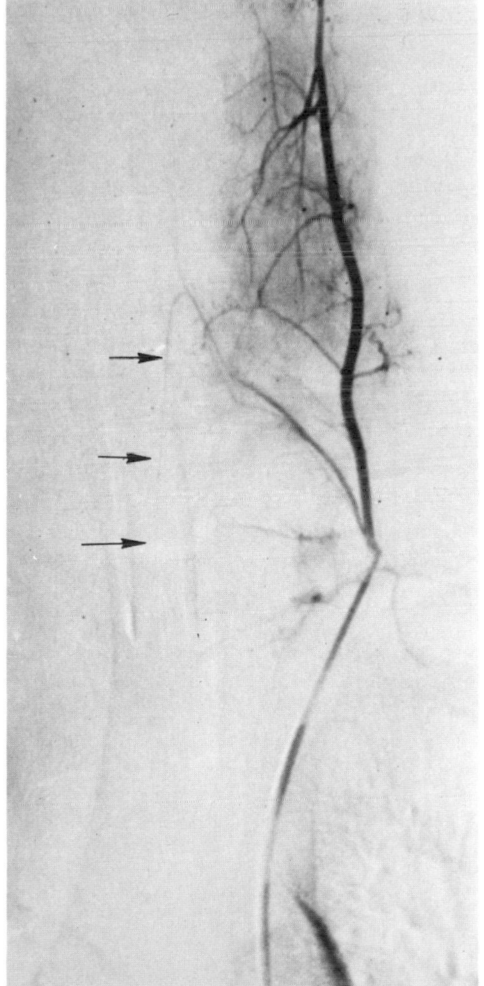

Figure 15–9 Artery of the cervical enlargement (*arrows*) originating from the left deep cervical artery.

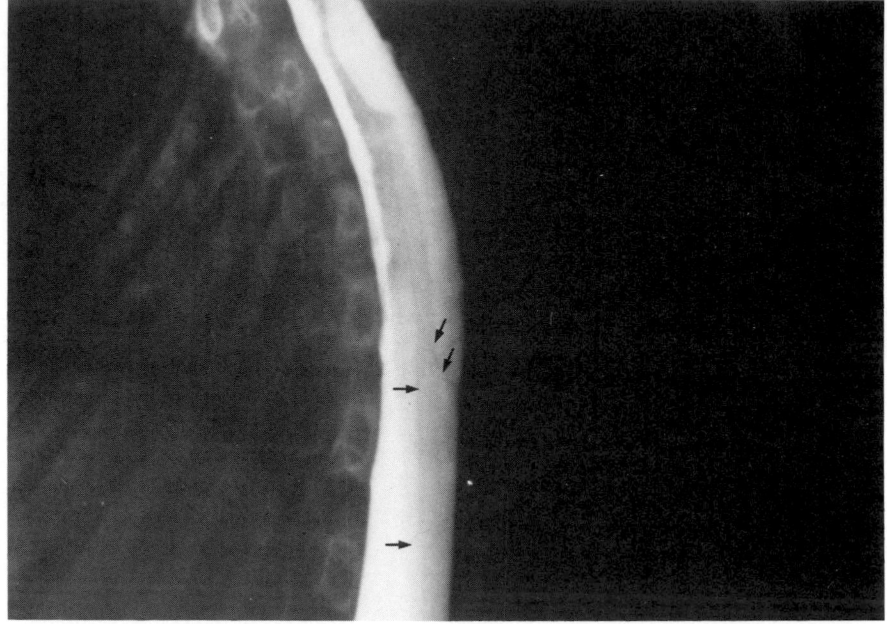

Figure 15–10 Pantopaque myelogram. Frontal projection demonstrating the artery of Adamkiewicz (*arrows*).

Figure 15–11 Artery of Adamkiewicz originating from the left twelfth intercostal artery. (From Djindjian, R., Hurth, M., and Houdart, R.: Angiography of the Spinal Cord, Paris, Masson & Cie; Baltimore, Md., University Park Press, 1970. Reprinted by permission.)

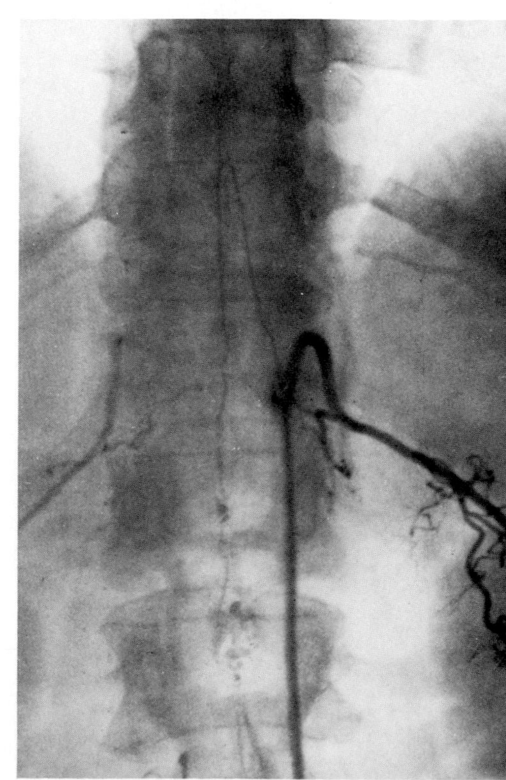

At the thoracolumbar level, the artery of Adamkiewicz has two branches with a strictly median division, a thin and straight ascending division, and a descending one that is larger and often tortuous (Figs. 15–10, 15–11, and 15–12). In the frontal projection, this vessel takes a characteristic hairpin curve. In the lateral view, the artery of Adamkiewicz runs in a straight line a short distance from the posterior vertebral border, which forms the anterior limit of the cord. Total opacification of the anterior spinal artery from the artery of Adamkiewicz or from the superior thoracic artery is not observed except in pathological cases. The end "basket" or anastomotic loop of the conus medullaris is not visualized in the normal subject.

Posterior Spinal Arteries

In the cervical region one cannot, except for very rare exceptions, opacify the normal posterior afferent vessels or the spinal axis. In the thoracic and thoracolumbar regions, on the other hand, it is not rare to visualize one or more posterior spinal arteries of which the two branches of the ascending and descending division constitute the posterolateral spinal axis (Fig. 15–13).

Other Arterial Branches

Arteriography may opacify muscular arteries at different levels, and these must be differentiated from the spinal arteries. Selective arteriography may visualize normal

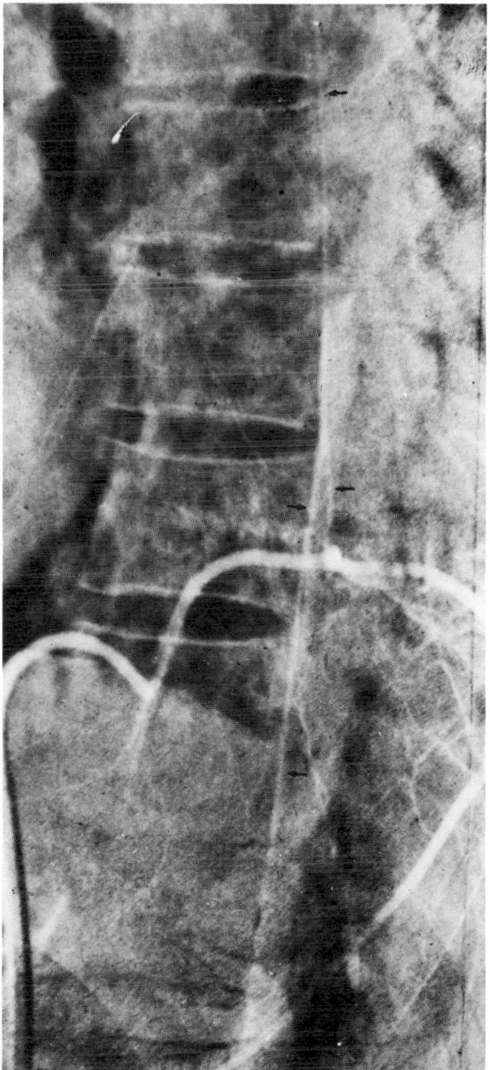

Figure 15–12 Artery of Adamkiewicz, lateral projection (*arrows*). (From Djindjian, R.: Angiography of the spinal cord. Surg. Neurol., *2*:179–185, 1974. Reprinted by permission.)

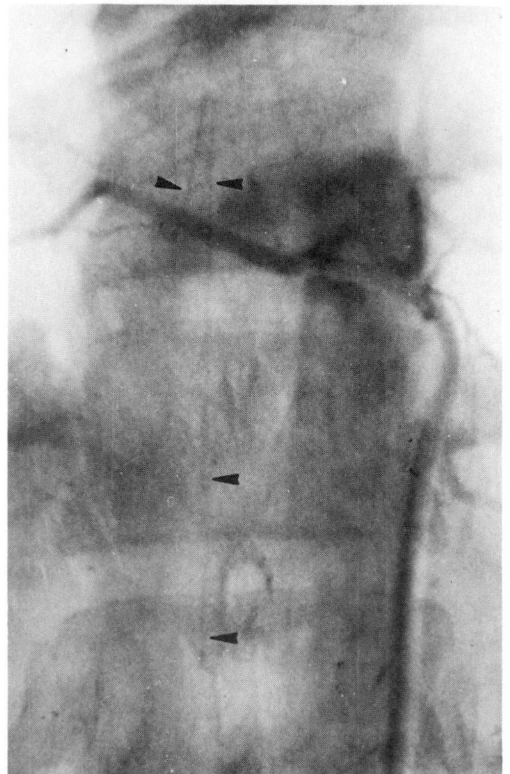

Figure 15–13 Posterior spinal artery originating from the right tenth intercostal artery (*arrows*). (Adapted from Djindjian, R., Hurth, M., and Houdart, R.: Angiography of the Spinal Cord. Paris, Masson & Cie; Baltimore, Md., University Park Press, 1970.)

vertebrae, producing a dense homogeneous opacification strictly limited to the corresponding hemivertebra of the site of injection (Fig. 15–14). Dural arteries are not observed except in pathological conditions such as spinal angiomas.

ANGIOGRAPHY IN SPINAL ANGIOMAS

Angiomas, or arteriovenous malformations, of the spinal cord are more commonly encountered than is usually believed. Selective spinal angiography has allowed very small malformations to be detected, which are not visualized by myelography or nonselective aortography. In addition, selective angiography has corrected erroneous diagnoses of multiple sclerosis or myelitis in several individuals. In a 10-year period, 175 cases of angiomas were seen in 3000 patients who had spinal cord angiography at the Lariboisière Hospital.

Clinical Classification

The spinal arteriovenous malformations called angiomas fall into two distinct groups: those within the cord with an exclusively or predominantly anterior supply, evolving clinically in a stepwise fashion, with onset in childhood or young adulthood; and those located behind the cord with a posterior blood supply, of later clinical onset, producing steadily progressive clinical signs and symptoms (Fig. 15–15). With both types, the risk of progressing to total paralysis is the same, and only an early diagnosis and appropriate treatment can avoid such a prognosis.

Arteriovenous malformations of the spinal cord, as well as intracerebral lesions, are more frequent in males (73 per cent); for both, the age of appearance favors childhood and young adulthood. A third of cases of each were diagnosed before 20 years, between 20 and 40 years, and between 40 and 60 years of age. A tenth were discovered in the group aged 60 to 74 years. The extreme ages in the authors' series were 1½ years and 74 years. The time from onset of symptoms to establishment of a diagnosis is

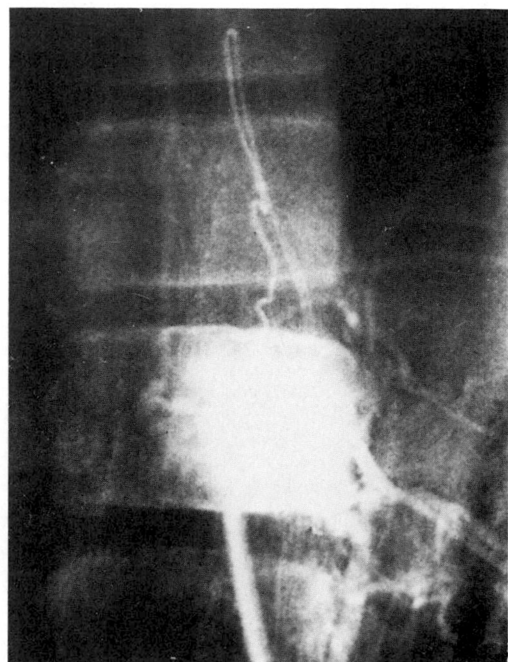

Figure 15–14 Normal opacification of a hemivertebra by injection of an intercostal artery. (Adapted from Djindjian, R., Hurth, M., and Houdart, R.: Angiography of the Spinal Cord. Paris, Masson & Cie; Baltimore, Md., University Park Press, 1970.)

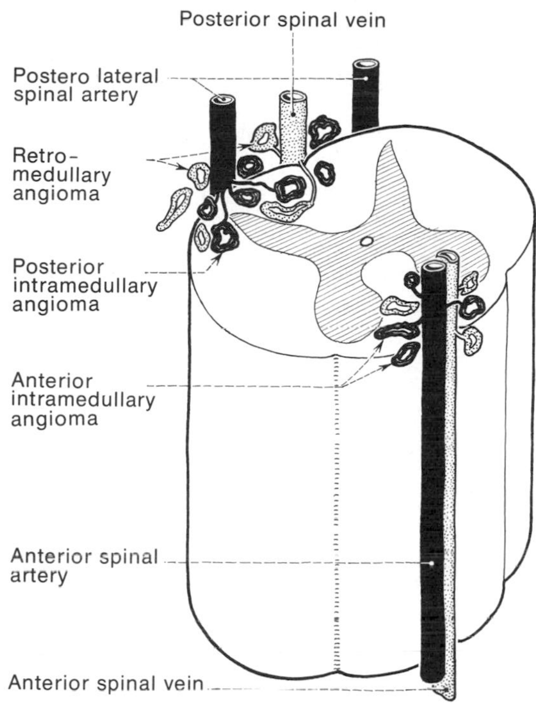

Figure 15–15 Schema of intramedullary angiomas fed by the anterior spinal arterial axis, and retromedullary angiomas fed by the posterolateral arterial axis. (Modified from Djindjian, R., Hurth, M., and Houdart, R.: Angiography of the Spinal Cord. Paris, Masson & Cie; Baltimore, Md., University Park Press, 1970.)

variable. The diagnosis is considered to be early if it is made at less than one year after the beginning of symptoms (26 per cent of the authors' cases). It is late if made more than 10 years after the beginning of symptoms (14 per cent of cases). The remaining 60 per cent of cases were discovered between 1 and 10 years after symptoms began.

Clinical Symptoms

These malformations may be localized within the spinal cord or on its surface. Owing to the diverse topography of these lesions, the clinical symptoms may take many forms. The symptoms are influenced by the spinal level where they occur, the age of the patient, and the mechanism of decompensation, whether due to rupture, compression, thrombosis, hematomyelia, softening, or hemodynamic imbalance. Among the clinical pictures of angiomatous malformation, however, two are characteristic: meningeal hemorrhage and the localized radiculospinal syndromes evolving in a stepwise fashion.[8]

Spinal Meningeal Hemorrhage

Rapid onset of spinal cord symptoms combined with pain should suggest the diagnosis of an angioma with hemorrhage. Bleeding, however, is less frequent as a presenting sign of spinal cord angioma than it is in the cerebral forms. It was seen in only three fourths of the authors' cases. DiChiro reports an even lower incidence of 10 per cent.[3]

These hemorrhages can be seen at all ages. In 33 cases in which symptoms started before 15 years, 16 hemorrhagic episodes were noted. Recurrent hemorrhages are the rule because of delay in diagnosis (on the average of 12 years). The recurring forms are not rare. Recurrence has been seen 13 times, and in five cases has occurred more than 3 times. Recurrence is often accompanied by associated root signs (six cases). Nevertheless, the recurrent hemorrhages do not cause a severe effect on the life course: Only one patient died (as a result of intracranial hypertension); two other patients received shunts for hydrocephalus that was presumably secondary to hemorrhage.

Hemorrhages usually occur in angiomas that are totally or predominantly within the cord (83 per cent). The rarity of hematomyelia should be emphasized. This latter diagnosis was suggested preoperatively in only five patients. While the diagnosis of spinal meningeal hemorrhage may be easy when well-developed spinal cord and nerve root changes are present, it is important to be able to recognize the subtler forms of this entity when only back or root pain is evident. In retrospect, in only 27 of 36 cases could appropriate symptoms be elicited by questioning the patient or established by objective signs on the examination.

Syndromes of Spinal Root Deficit

In contrast to intracranial angiomas, which usually present with signs of subarachnoid hemorrhage or epileptic seizures, spinal angiomas may progress from minimal paresis to total paraplegia.

Different syndromes may occur. The most striking is that of a local root syndrome that evolves in a stepwise fashion (69 per cent of cases). This stepwise evolution is variable and is often associated with precipitating factors such as strenuous physical exercise or pregnancy. Frequently, the first attack is associated with a meningeal hemorrhage, which may recur. Rarely, the first hemorrhagic episode occurs unexpectedly in one of the later episodes of the syndrome. The level of cord disease is always the same for each patient, a fundamental fact to note in ruling out multiple sclerosis as a basis for the symptoms. In the initial stages of this syndrome, partial or, much less likely, total regression of symptoms may occur. As a rule, however, each hemorrhage is usually followed by a less complete recovery than the previous bleeding episode.

The radiculomedullary syndromes with progressive evolution were noted in 30 per cent of the cases in the authors' series. Their onset is least suggestive of spinal angioma. The peak age of the first occurrence of symptoms is 38 years. These lesions occur most frequently at the thoracolumbar level (23 cases) and often are posterior in location (15 cases). Two cervical and three low thoracic angiomas (T5 to T7) were also observed.

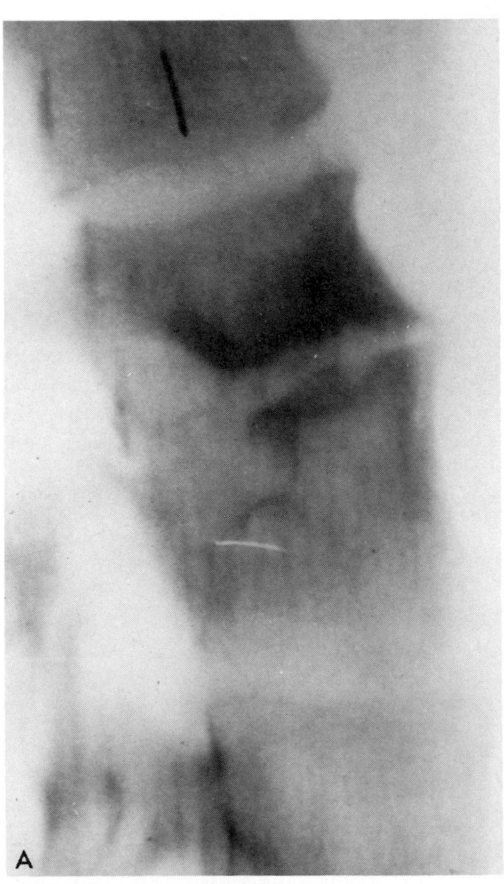

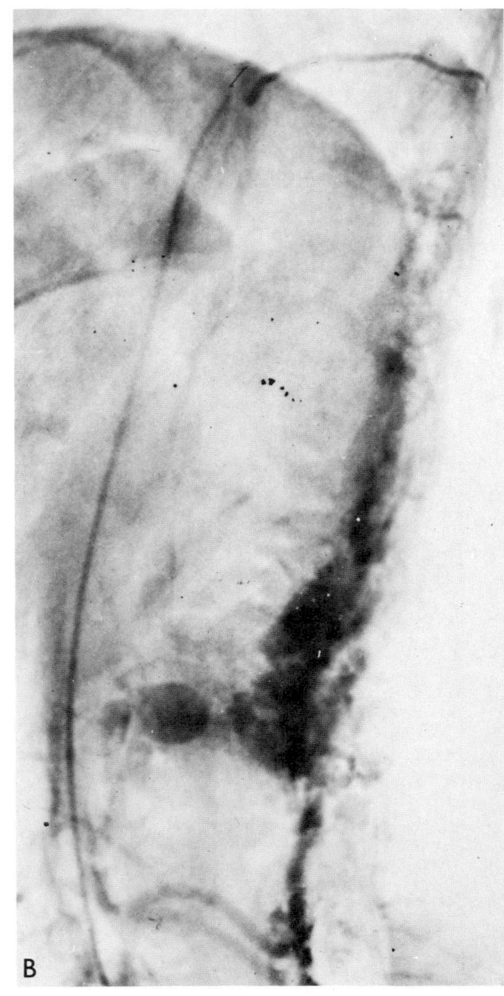

Figure 15–16 *A*. Cobb's syndrome: posterior vertebral destruction by an osseous and spinal angioma. *B*. In the same case, angiography demonstrates an angioma corresponding to the area of osseous destruction seen in *A*. (From Djindjian, R., Hurth, M., and Houdart, R.: Angiography of the Spinal Cord. Paris, Masson & Cie; Baltimore, Md., University Park Press, 1970. Reprinted by permission.)

In older patients, a combined effect of hemostatic steal by a malformation and atheromatous involvement of the intercostal nutrient vessels probably accounts for the symptoms observed.

Radiculomedullary syndromes of sudden onset were recognized in 7 per cent of cases and produced a picture of myelomalacia within several hours.

Associated Dysplasias

The diagnosis of medullary angiomas may be aided by the presence of associated dysplasias. Since arteriovenous malformations are developmental defects in spinal cord tissue, it is not unexpected that associated dysplasias (34 cases) may be present. Cutaneous angiomas (12 cases, in 5 of which the cutaneous angioma was not metameric and had no localizing value), vertebral angiomas (5 cases), and the triple cutaneous-vertebral-medullary association of Cobb's syndrome (2 cases) were noted (Fig. 15–16). Rendu-Osler angiomatosis was observed in eight cases (Figs. 15–17 and 15–18). A complex malformation of the lymphatic system was noted in one case of von Recklinghausen's disease (Fig. 15–19). Five cases of Klippel-Trenaunay syndrome and one of hepatic angiomatosis, were observed (Figs. 15–20 and 15–21).

Cerebrospinal Fluid Findings

Study of the cerebrospinal fluid may reveal three things: hemorrhage, albumocytological disturbances, or no abnormality at all. Hemorrhage into the cerebrospinal fluid may be indicative of a spinal cord angioma. A high protein level and normal or near normal cell count are not against this diag-

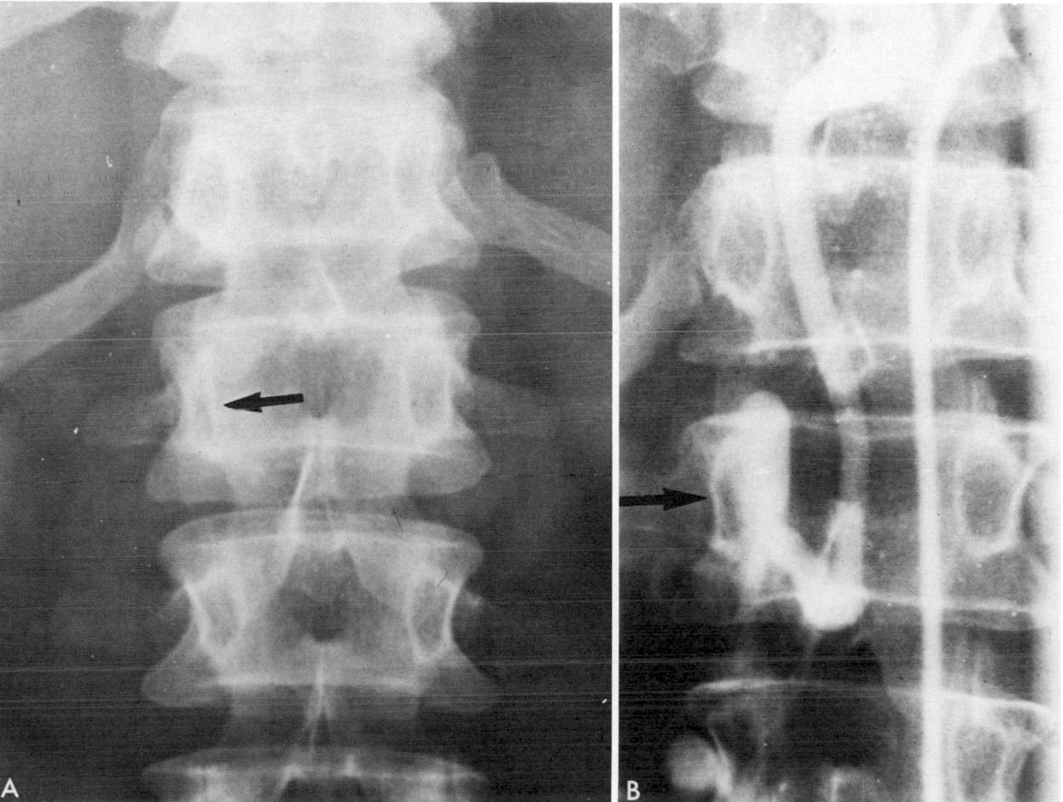

Figure 15–17 Rendu-Osler angiomatosis. *A*. Vertebral column shows erosion of the right T1 pedicle (*arrow*). *B*. In the same case, pedicular angioma is fed by the dilated artery of Adamkiewicz originating from the ninth right intercostal artery. The draining vein responsible for erosion of the T1 pedicle (*arrow*) is demonstrated.

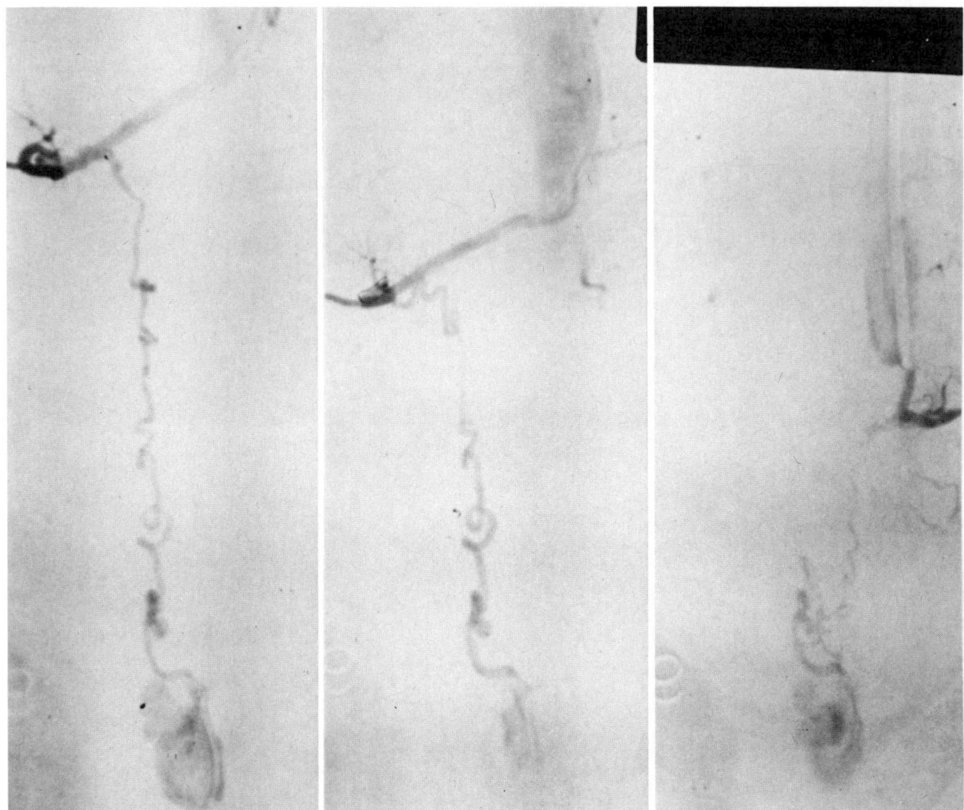

Figure 15–18 Rendu-Osler angiomatosis. Posterior spinal pedicles are seen (T10 right, T9 right, T7 left).

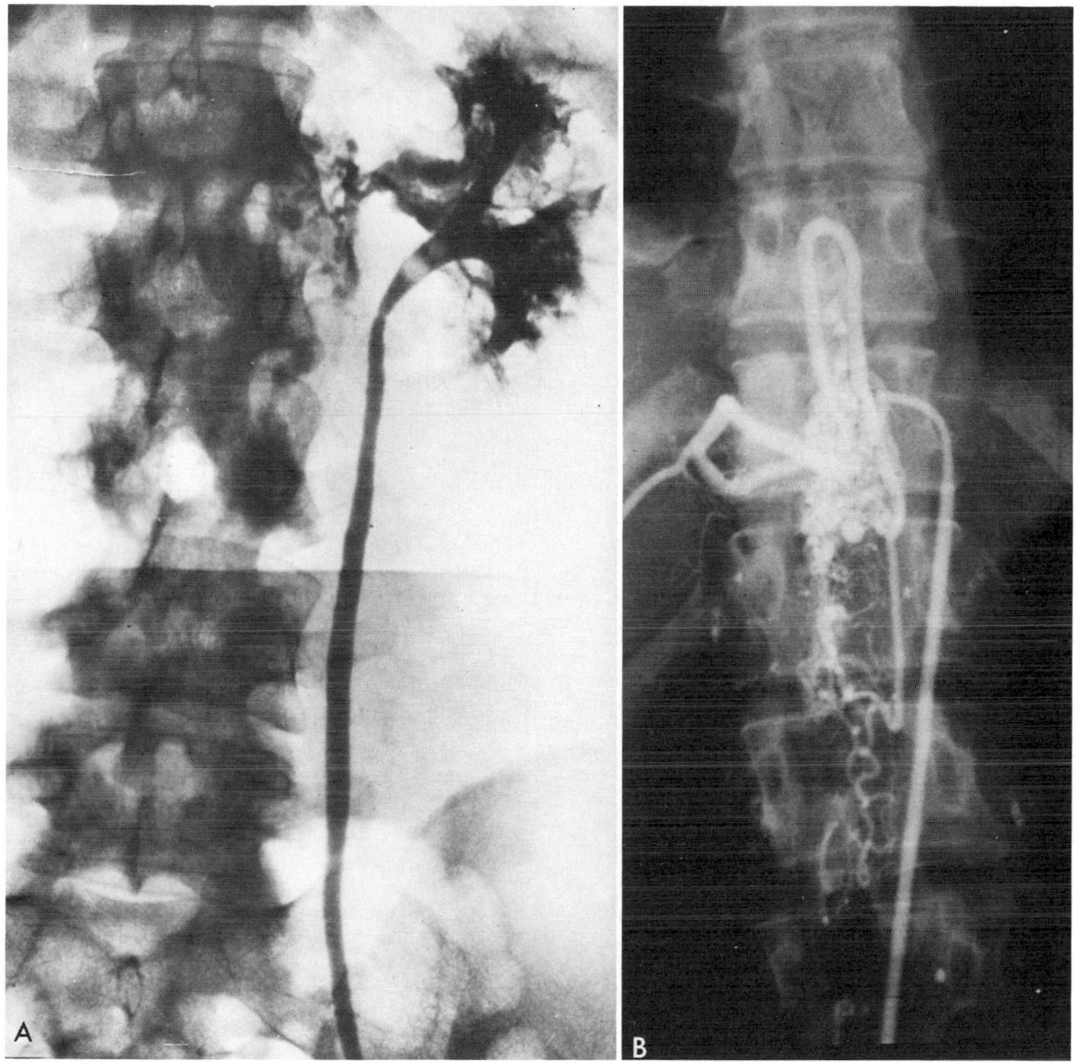

Figure 15–19 Von Recklinghausen's disease with a lymphatic system malformation. *A*. Abnormal communication between the renal pelvis and the vertebral lymphatics is seen. *B*. In the same case, an intramedullary angioma is fed by a voluminous artery of Adamkiewicz originating from the eleventh right intercostal artery. (From Djindjian, R., Hurth, M., and Houdart, R.: Angiography of the Spinal Cord. Paris, Masson & Cie; Baltimore, Md., University Park Press, 1970. Reprinted by permission.)

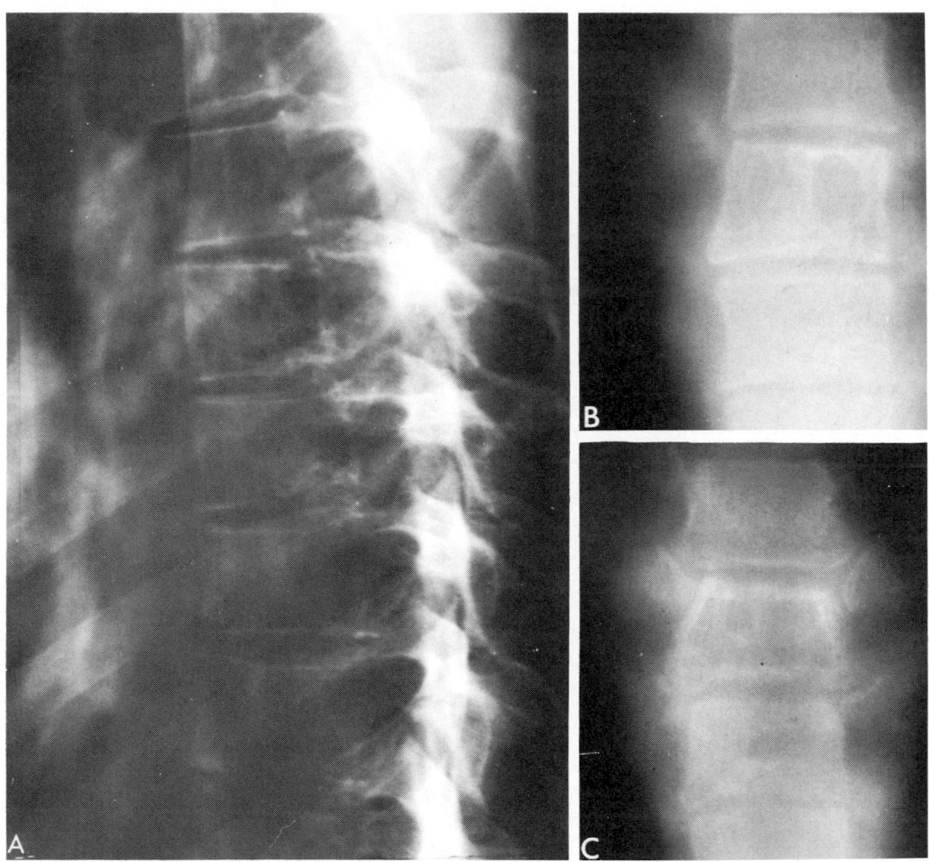

Figure 15–20 Klippel-Trenaunay syndrome. *A*. Lateral thoracic spine. *B* and *C*. Frontal tomograms demonstrate multiple large lytic lesions of the sixth and seventh thoracic vertebral bodies.

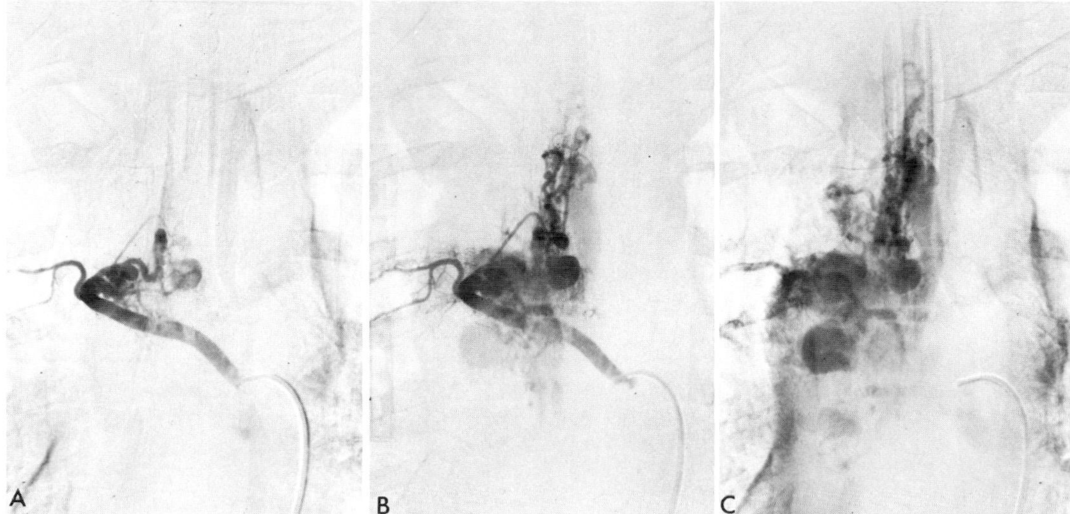

Figure 15–21 Klippel-Trenaunay syndrome. A vertebral epidural angioma fed by the dilated sixth intercostal artery on the right with drainage into the azygous system is seen. *A* and *B*. Early arterial and midarterial phases. *C*. Venous phase.

nosis, and in fact, about one third of the patients with angiomas have normal cerebrospinal fluid.

Radiological Evaluation

Plain and Tomographic X-Rays

Plain and tomographic x-rays may indicate an expanding intraspinal process. Widening of the spinal canal was the most frequently observed plain radiographic finding in the authors' series (15 cases). In 6 of these 15 cases the lesion was in the cervical region (Figs. 15–22 and 15–23). Erosion of the pedicle (11 cases) is often secondary to enlarged draining veins. Erosion of the posterior aspect of the vertebral body is more rarely seen (three cases) (Figs. 15–24 and 15–25). Scoliosis or kyphoscoliosis was seen in 15 patients (Fig. 15–26). Spina bifida in the region of an angioma was identified in five cases. Calcification within the angioma was observed in one case (Fig. 15–27). In summary, plain films may be helpful, and in a third of the cases these studies were extremely useful for proper orientation for further studies such as tomography, myelography, and especially angiography.

Positive Contrast Myelography

Pantopaque studies were abnormal in 93 per cent of angiomas that were investigated. In 62 per cent, the myelographic pattern was specific for an angiomatous malformation (Figs. 15–28 and 15–29). In 31 per cent, a partial or total block was observed, without characteristics pathognomonic for angioma (Fig. 15–30). The remaining 7 per cent of angiomas demonstrated no myelographic abnormality, in spite of detailed and careful examinations in both supine and prone positions. This latter group represents very small lesions, demonstrable only by selective angiography.

Nonionic myelography with metrizamide, a new water-soluble contrast material, provides a myelographic tool to visualize better the detailed structures of the spinal cord. Unlike that with Pantopaque, metrizamide myelography may be performed before angiography without compromising the angiographic subtraction images.

It has been suggested by DiChiro that not all angiomatous lesions should be myelographically evaluated. Some angiomas may be so large as to prevent successful subarachnoid puncture, and penetrating them during such a puncture may increase the risk of hemorrhage and cord damage. In the presence of appropriate signs and symptoms such as subarachnoid hemorrhage, paraplegia syndromes, and particularly, an audible bruit over the back, angiography alone may be warranted.[3] Confirmation of

Text continued on page 578

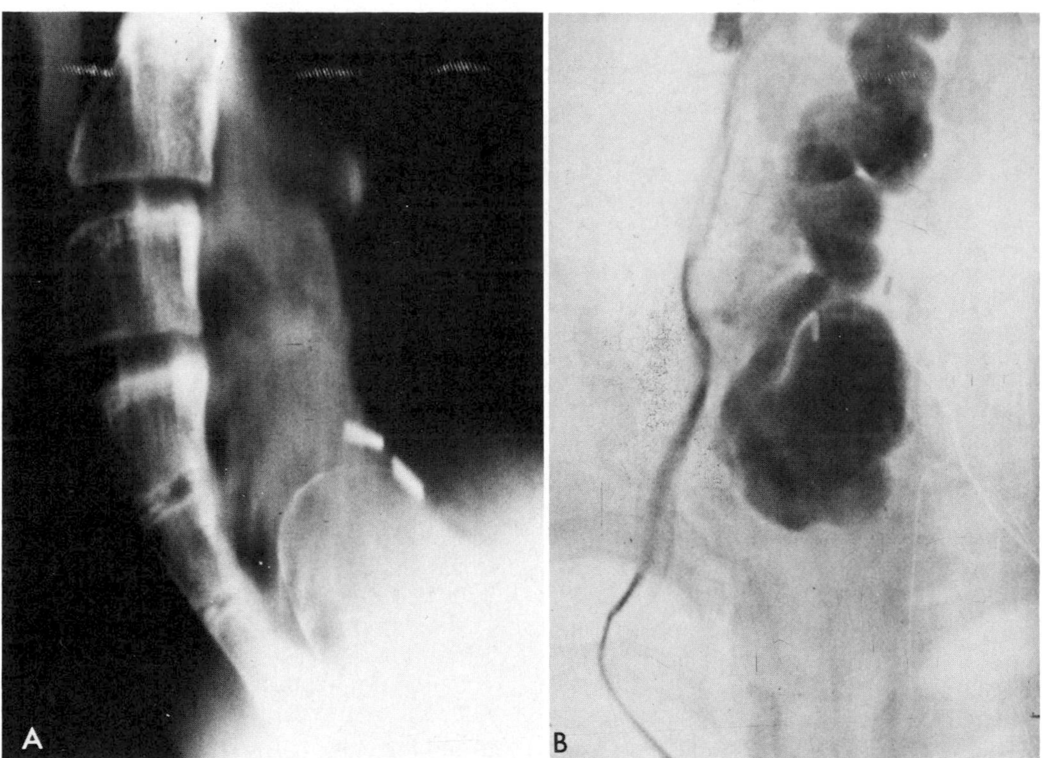

Figure 15–22 *A*. Destruction of the posterior edge of the fourth, fifth, and sixth cervical vertebrae, with a curvilinear calcification projecting into the dilated spinal canal. *B*. In the same case, angiography shows the cervical angioma, opacified via the right vertebral artery, that is producing the osseous changes of *A*. (From Djindjian, R., Hurth, M., and Houdart, R.: Angiography of the Spinal Cord. Paris, Masson & Cie; Baltimore, Md., University Park Press, 1970. Reprinted by permission.)

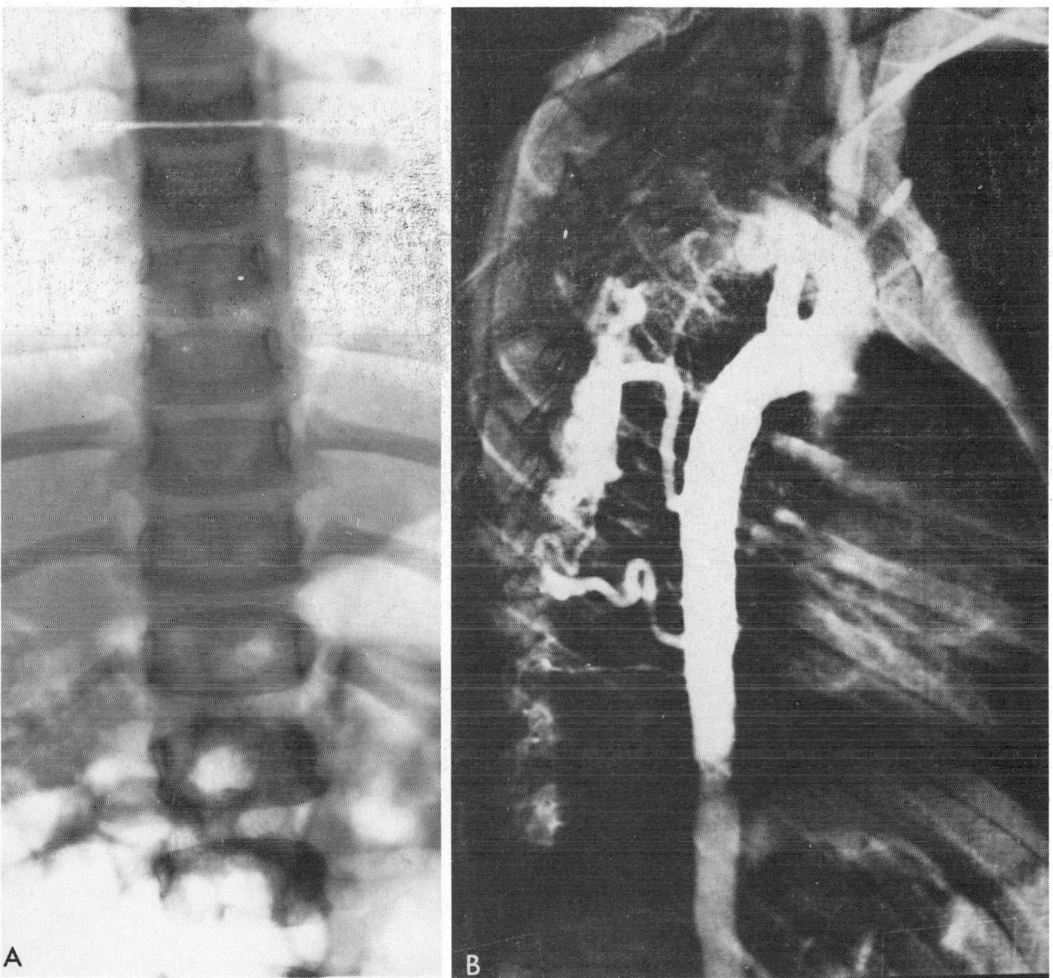

Figure 15–23 *A*. Widening of the spinal canal in a small child. *B*. In the same case, intramedullary angioma fed by two dorsal pedicles. (From Djindjian, R., Hurth, M., and Houdart, R.: Angiography of the Spinal Cord. Paris, Masson & Cie; Baltimore, Md., University Park Press, 1970. Reprinted by permission.)

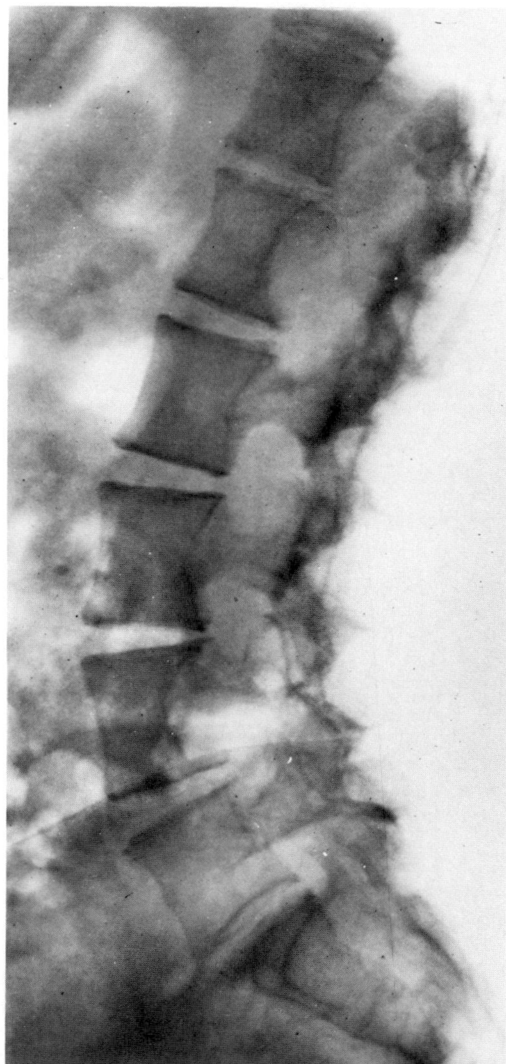

Figure 15–24 Significant erosion of the posterior aspect of the vertebral bodies of L1–L4.

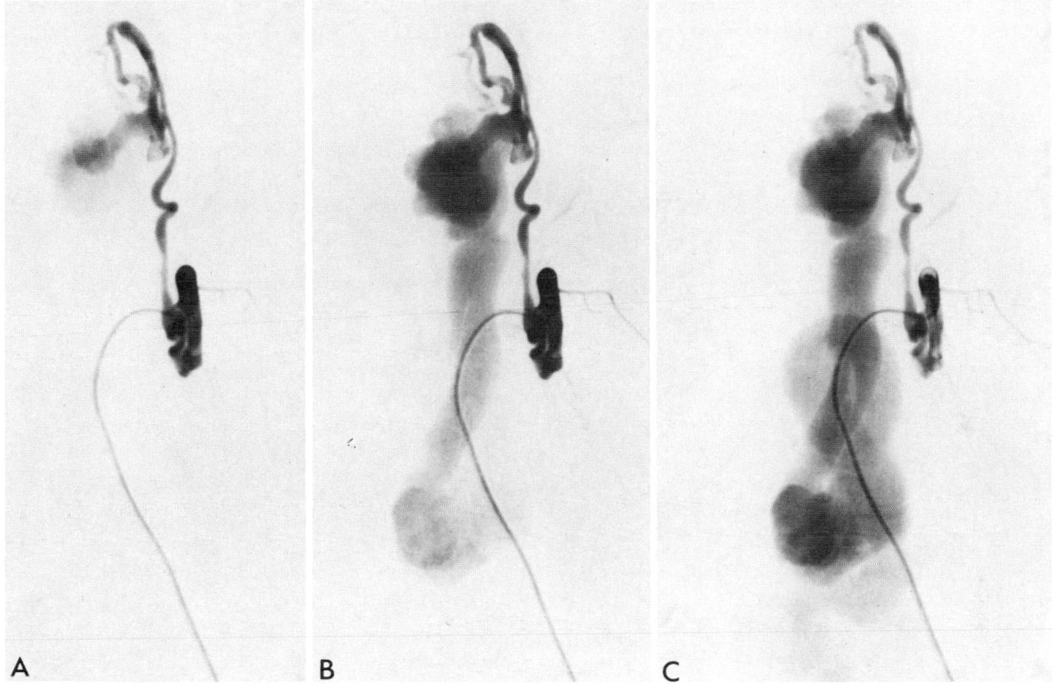

Figure 15–25 *A, B,* and *C*. Sequential filling of a grossly dilated angioma that produced the osseous changes seen in Figure 15–24.

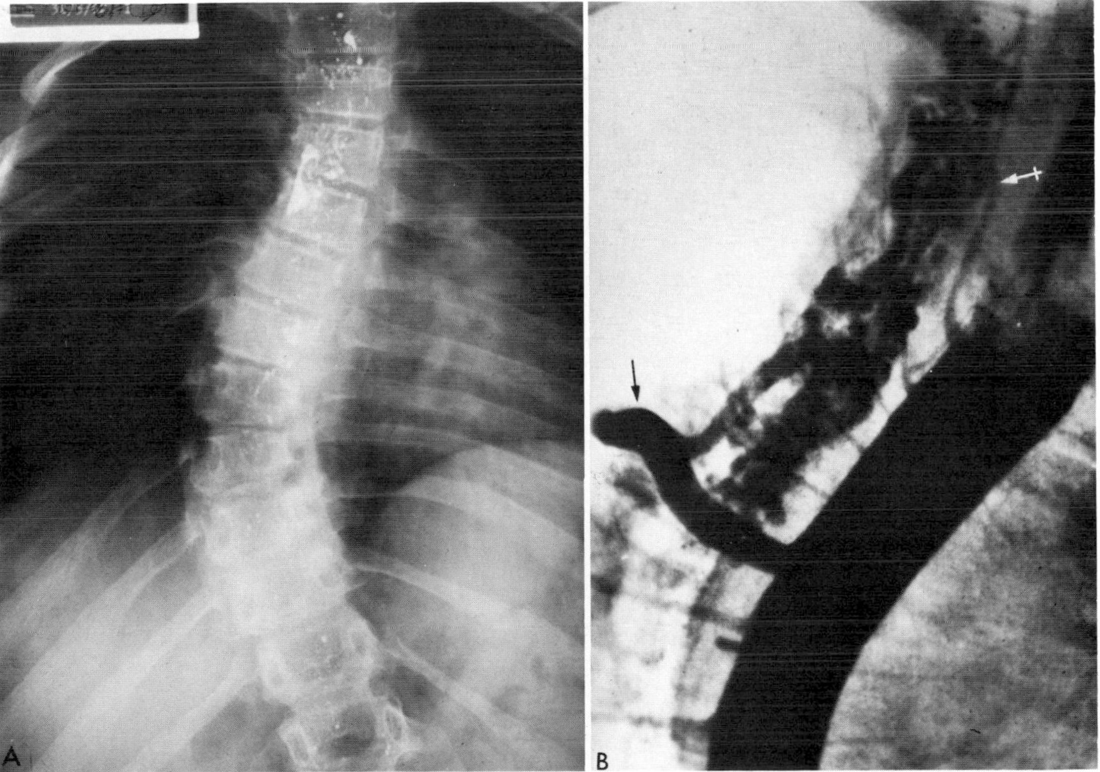

Figure 15–26 *A*. Significant scoliosis in a boy, age 14. *B*. In the same case, voluminous dorsal angioma supplied from the right sixth (*black arrow*) and third intercostal (*white arrow*) arteries is seen. (From Djindjian, R., Hurth, M., and Houdart, R.: Angiography of the Spinal Cord. Paris, Masson & Cie; Baltimore, Md., University Park Press, 1970. Reprinted by permission.)

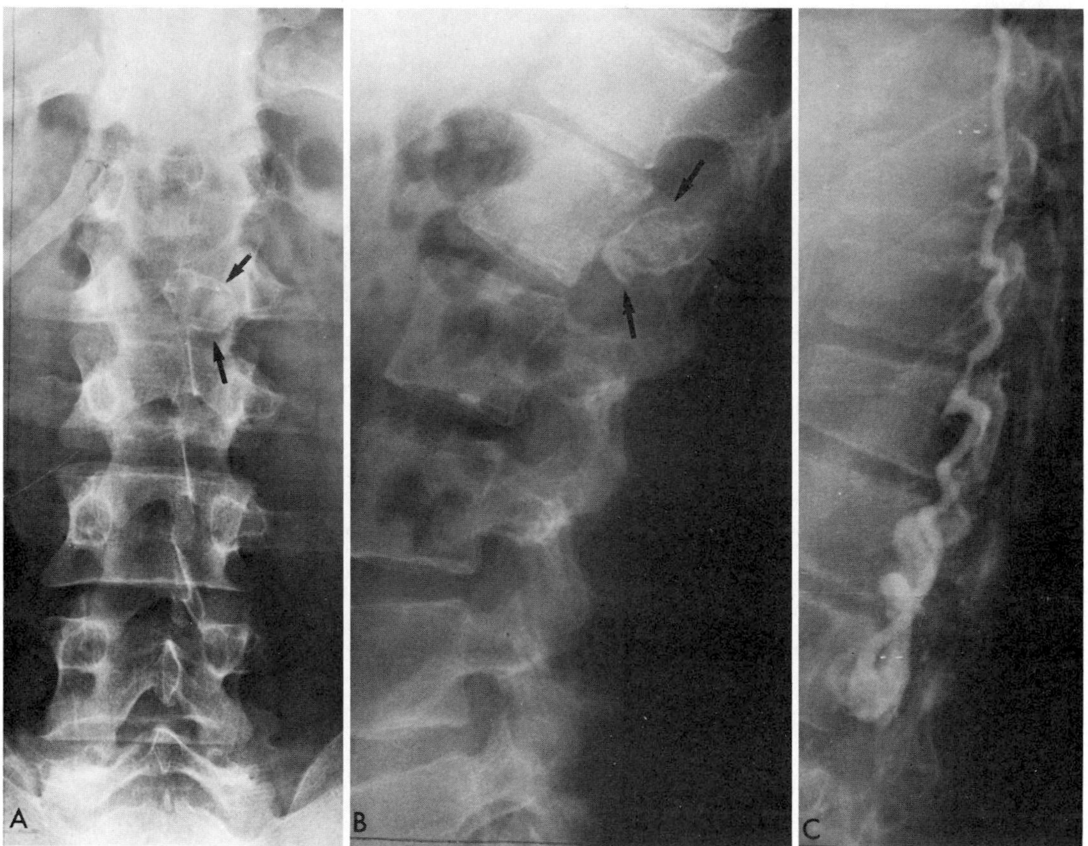

Figure 15–27 A round calcification (*arrows*) at the level of the L1 vertebral body. *A*. Frontal view. *B*. Lateral view. *C*. Lateral view angiogram, showing an angioma corresponding in part to the calcification seen in *A* and *B*.

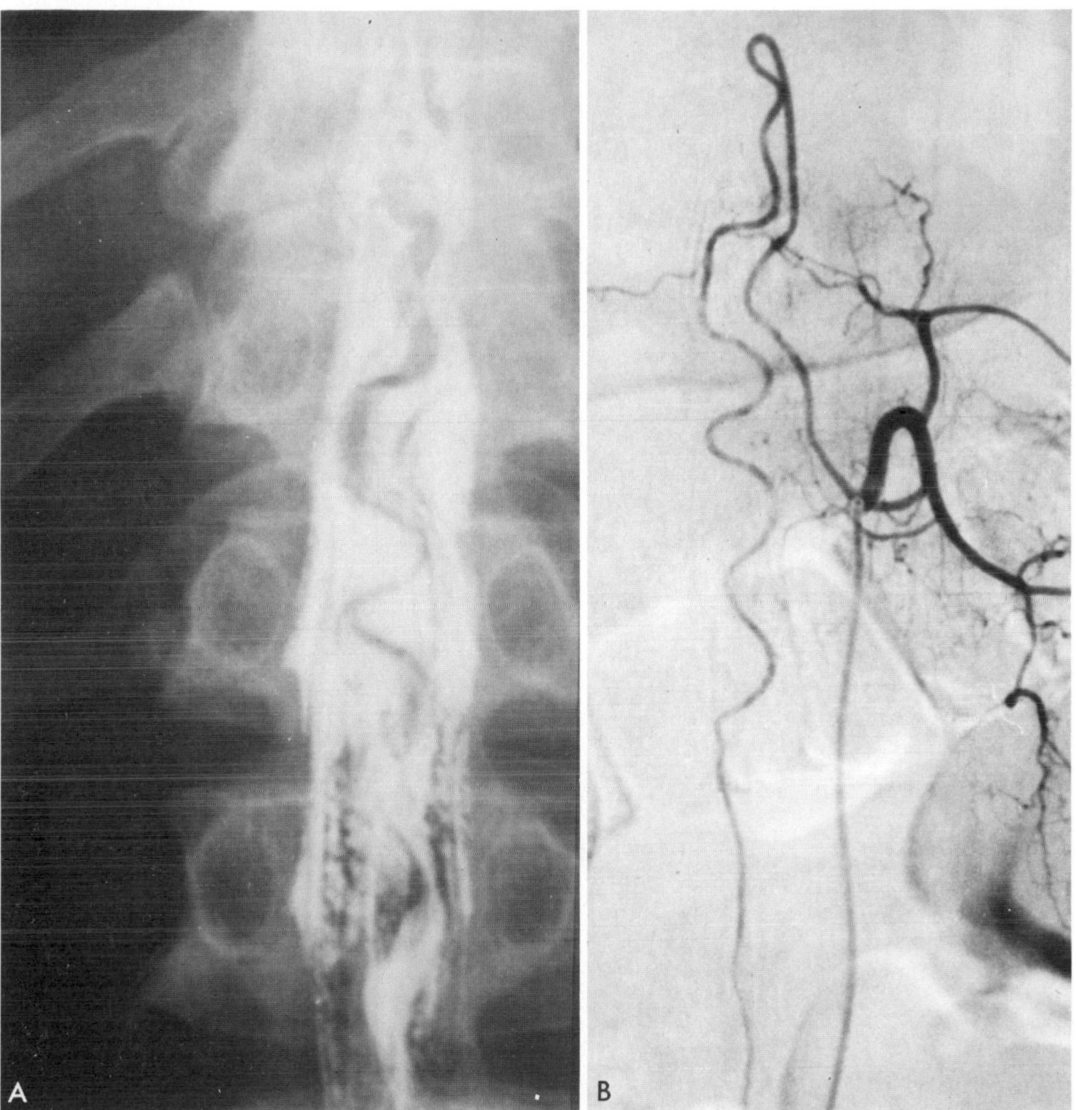

Figure 15–28 *A*. Pantopaque myelography demonstrating enlarged vascular structures. *B*. Angiography reveals an arteriovenous fistula supplied by the artery of Adamkiewicz corresponding to the vascular structures seen in *A*.

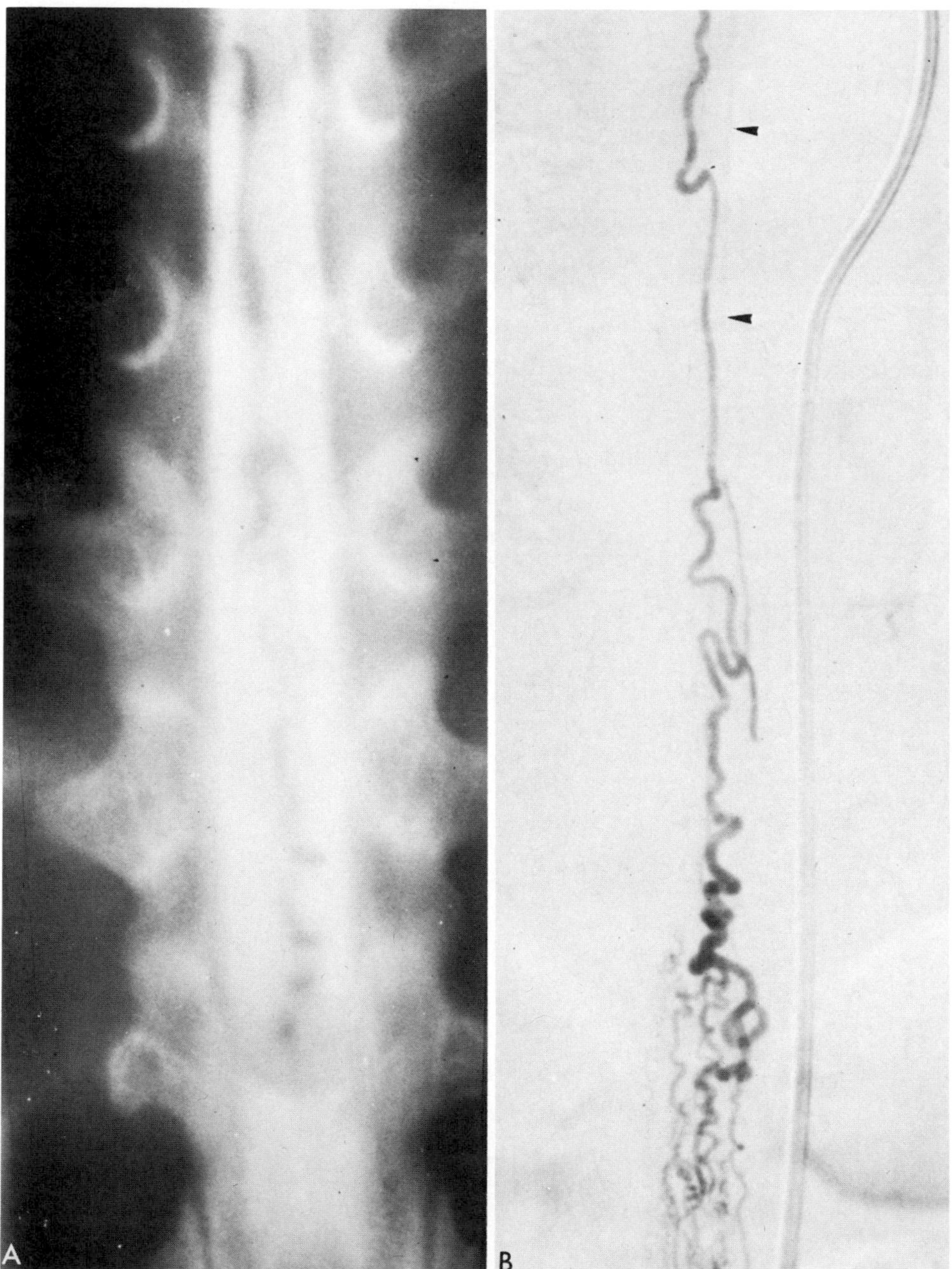

Figure 15–29 *A*. Metrizamide myelography with tomography. Serpiginous vascular structures are seen. *B*. Spinal angiography reveals an angioma fed by the anterior thoracic superior spinal artery arising from the sixth right intercostal artery. The artery of Adamkiewicz (*arrows*) and large draining veins are demonstrated, the latter representing the vascular structures seen in *A*. (*B* from Djindjian, R., et al.: Intradural extramedullary spinal arterio-venous malformations fed by the anterior spinal artery. Surg. Neurol., *8*:85–93, 1977. Reprinted by permission.)

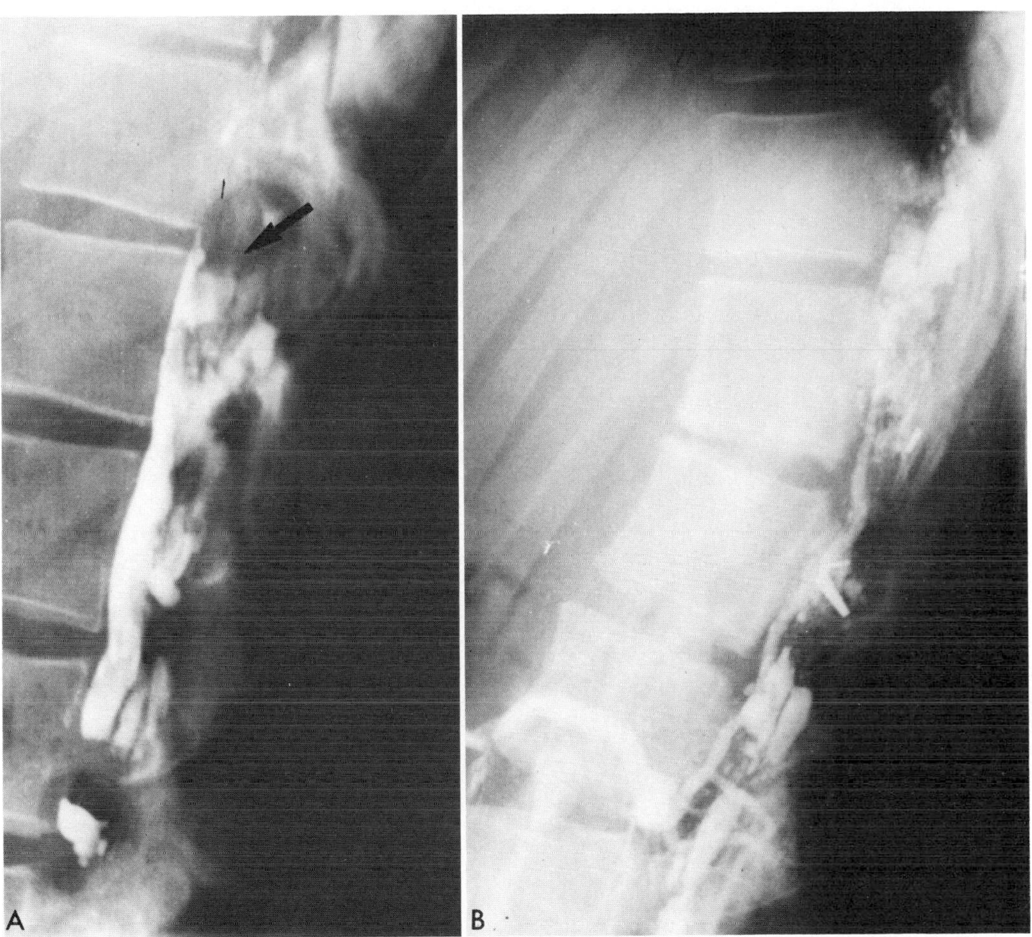

Figure 15–30 *A*. Pantopaque myelography, lateral view. Enlarged vascular structures with a high-grade block (*arrow*) to Pantopaque flow are demonstrated. *B*. Spinal angiography reveals a dorsolumbar angioma supplied by a dilated radicular artery originating from L2 with large vascular lakes, corresponding to the area of block in *A*. (From Djindjian, R., Hurth, M., and Houdart, R.: Angiography of the Spinal Cord. Paris, Masson & Cie; Baltimore, Md., University Park Press, 1970. Reprinted by permission.)

the preangiographic diagnosis may be aided in two thirds of cases by employing radioisotopic angiography, as described by Di-Chiro and co-workers.[6]

In rare cases, serpiginous dilated vessels mimicking an arteriovenous malformation may be appreciated cephalad to areas of severe spinal stenosis. These vessels may change with the Valsalva maneuver and probably represent dilated and partially occluded venous structures.[19]

Gas Myelography

The gas myelogram, illustrated in Figure 15–31, is contraindicated whenever the diagnosis of an angioma is suspected, since the massive withdrawal of cerebrospinal fluid usually required in these studies may lead to deterioration of the patient's neurological status. This procedure drastically compromised the clinical condition of two of three patients in the authors' series.

In conclusion, plain radiographic and myelographic studies may be very helpful in the initial evaluation of an angioma, particularly in ascertaining the degree of cerebrospinal fluid block and for localizing the level of a lesion. Radioisotopic angiography and metrizamide myelography may be especially useful in evaluating these an-

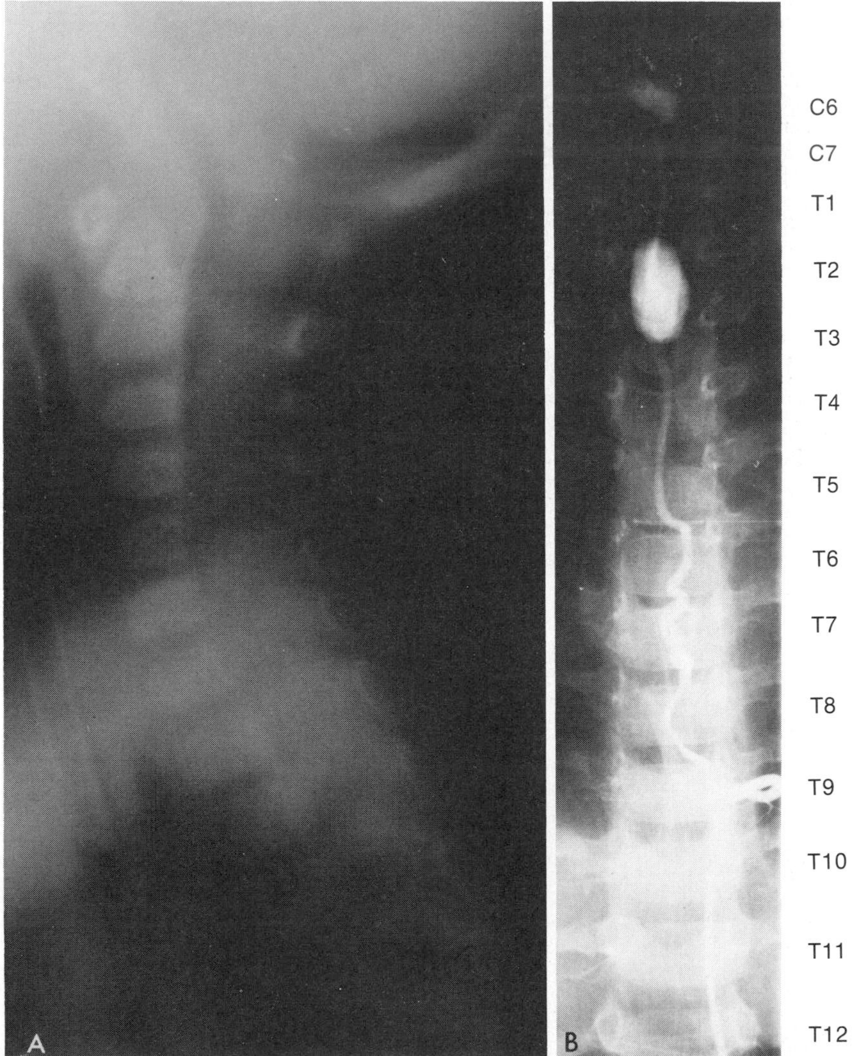

Figure 15–31 *A*. Gas myelography. Enlargement of the lower part of the cervical canal with an enlarged spinal cord and associated mass lesion is seen. *B*. An intramedullary angioma fed by the ninth left intercostal artery with two dilated vascular pouches in the vicinity of the ascending draining vein explains the blockage of gas seen in the cervical canal in *A*.

giomas. Angiographic evaluation is mandatory, however, for the true appreciation of the anatomical extent and possible therapy of these vascular lesions.

Angiography

Angiographic evaluation of an angiomatous malformation is essential. A schematic drawing representing a compilation of the various angiographic sequences is helpful and should comprise the afferent arterial supply, the various levels of its penetration into the spinal cord, and the appropriate anterior and posterior terminations; the origin, penetration, and appearance of the radiculospinal arteries in the vicinity of the angioma; the malformation itself; and the extent of the main venous and associated efferent channels (Fig. 15–32).

General Characteristics of Angiomas

NUTRIENT VESSELS

Number. There was only one nutrient artery in 30 per cent of cases, multiple arteries being demonstrated in the remaining 70 per cent. In unusual cases, up to 10 nutrient arteries have been observed. In the midthoracic region, nutrient vessels ascending from the first lumbar artery or descending from the vertebral artery have been observed.

Diameter of vessels. In general, the cervical, intercostal, or lumbar arteries supplying the anterior or posterior nutrient radiculomedullary pedicle are dilated, becoming at times dolichomegalic arteries (Fig. 15–33).

The ascending or descending branches of the nutrient pedicles are often very tortuous and are superimposed upon dilated anterior or posterior spinal veins. This explains the images that are sometimes observed on myelographic examination.

Occasionally, the pedicle and the medullary artery are of normal caliber, usually in angiomas of *moderate size*. Identification of a bifid intercostal artery with a common trunk should raise the suspicion of an angiomatous malformation. Very rarely, the nutrient pedicle is narrowed (Fig. 15–34). In these cases it is necessary to perform an-

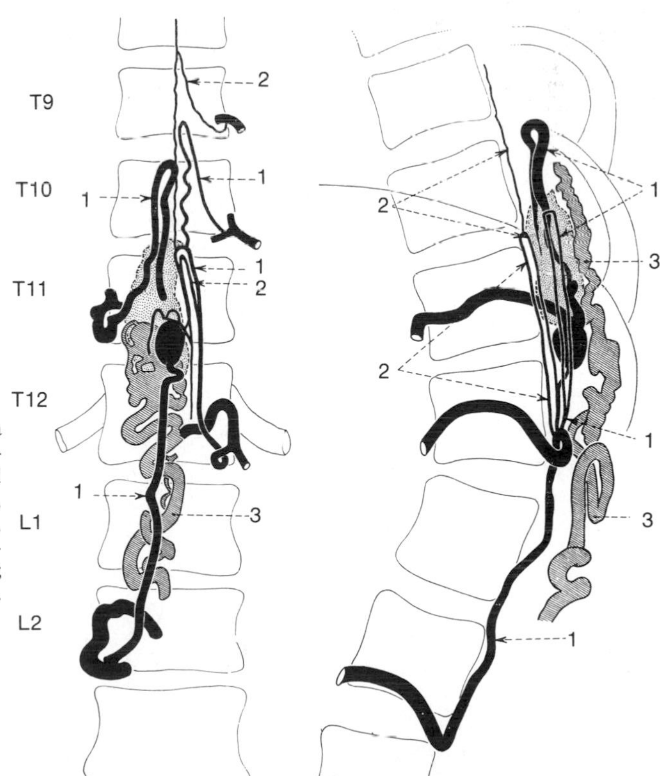

Figure 15–32 Composite drawing of a typical angioma with (1) posterolateral spinal arteries, (2) anterior spinal arteries, and (3) draining veins. *A.* Frontal projection, and *B.* Lateral projection. (From Djindjian, R., Hurth, M., and Houdart, R.: Angiography of the Spinal Cord. Paris, Masson & Cie; Baltimore, Md., University Park Press, 1970. Reprinted by permission.)

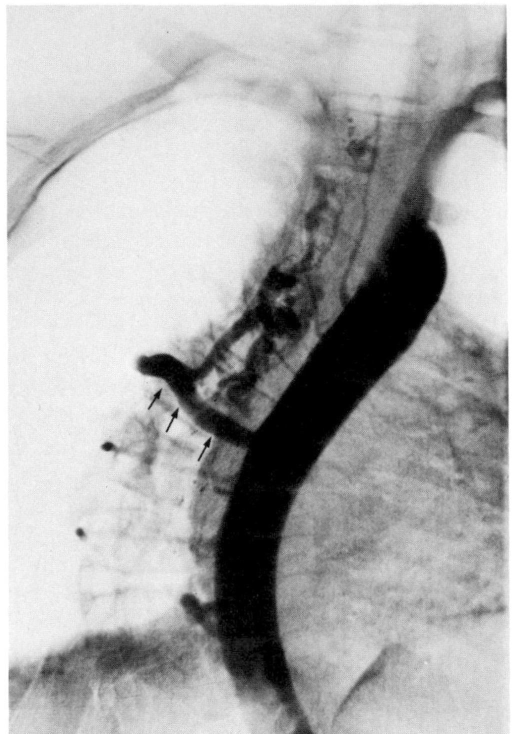

Figure 15–33 Mixed thoracic superior angioma nourished by several pedicles, one of which is the posterior spinal artery originating from a dilated intercostal artery on the right (*arrows*). (From Djindjian, R., Hurth, M., and Houdart, R.: Angiography of the Spinal Cord. Paris, Masson & Cie; Baltimore, Md., University Park Press, 1970. Reprinted by permission.)

giography with delayed sequential filming in order to appreciate the late-appearing draining veins.

Origin. Anterior spinal arteries supply intramedullary angiomas. The increase in caliber of these arteries permits the opacification of the dilated sulcocommissural arteries. Lateral projections permit one to see these latter vessels, in general numbering three to six, penetrating the anterior surface of the spinal cord, ultimately opacifying the intramedullary angioma (Fig. 15–35).

Visualization of the sulcocommissural arteries is more than academic. In the future, advances in micro-operative techniques may permit ligation of these vessels by myelocommissurotomy without damage to the anterior spinal pathway or the spinal cord.

In the cervical region the anterior nutrient arteries are the anterior spinal artery arising from the terminal portion of the vertebral arteries and the artery of the cervical enlargement, which may arise from either the vertebral or the deep cervical arteries (Fig. 15–36). In addition, it is not unusual to find, in the inferior two thirds of the cord, some anterior afferents arising from the first intercostal arteries and ending at the inferior pole of the malformation. As a general rule, cervical angiomas are multipedicled, and frequently new pedicles develop after ligation or embolization when the angiomatous mass has not been completely excised or obliterated.

In the thoracic region, the main nutrient artery is the superior thoracic anterior radiculospinal artery, which can arise on the

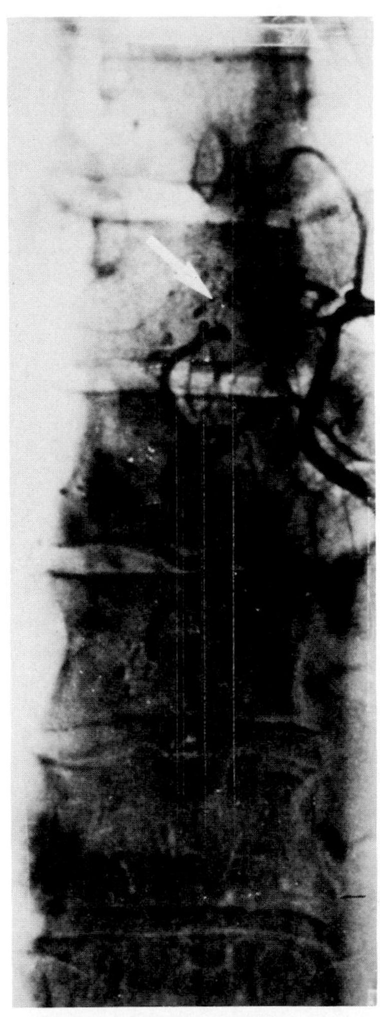

Figure 15–34 A stenotic pedicle of a thoracic angioma is seen (*arrow*). (From Djindjian, R., Hurth, M., and Houdart, R.: Angiography of the Spinal Cord. Paris, Masson & Cie; Baltimore, Md., University Park Press, 1970. Reprinted by permission.)

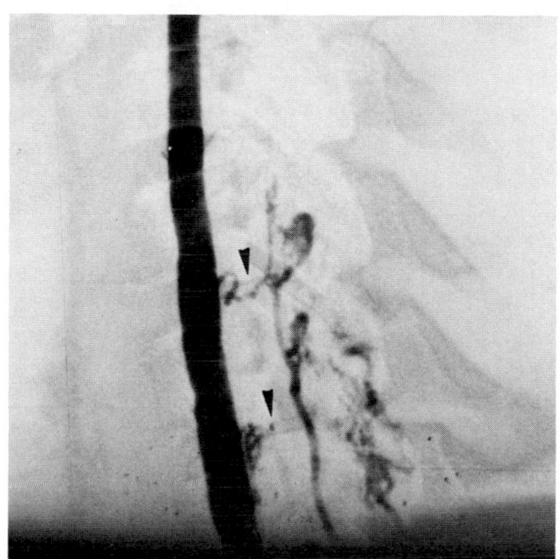

Figure 15–35 A cervical angioma nourished by a sulcocommissural artery that arises from the artery of the cervical enlargement. Dilatation of radicular artery (*arrows*) arising from the vertebral artery reinforces the arterial supply from the cervical enlargement.

right or on the left from the third, fourth, or fifth intercostal arteries. Very often, these arteries arise from a common ascending trunk from the fourth or fifth intercostal artery, and from this trunk arise the fourth, third, and second intercostal arteries.

The radiculospinal artery is often dilated, and its ascending branch can opacify an angioma located as far cephalad as C6 to C7; its descending branch can opacify an intramedullary angioma sometimes as far caudally as T6 or T7. This emphasizes the need to visualize this artery for the complete evaluation of thoracic angiomas. Opacification of the artery of the cervical enlargement and of the artery of Adamkiewicz will not demonstrate a superior thoracic angioma.

In the thoracolumbar region, the nutrient artery is the artery of Adamkiewicz (Fig. 15–37). Sometimes a true dolichomegalic artery, this vessel can opacify an intramedullary angioma from T5 to the conus medullaris. Existence of a supplemental artery in the region of T7 or T9, when the artery of Adamkiewicz is in a low position, is often difficult to demonstrate because of the vascular neck created by the angioma. In the low thoracolumbar region, angiomas may be supplied both by the artery of Adamkiewicz arising from an intercostal or lumbar artery and by a lumbosacral radicular artery arising from the iliac artery.

Posterior spinal arteries supply the retromedullary angiomas. The arterial pedicle may be dilated and tortuous or, in small angiomas, may have an almost normal caliber.

In the cervical region the nutrient pedicles are multiple, usually occurring bilaterally from the vertebral arteries and from the deep cervical arteries. The nutrient vessel in the superior third of the cervical cord is most often the posterior spinal artery, which in turn arises from the vertebral artery. In the lower two thirds of the cervical cord, the most important tributaries are the ascending branches of the posterior spinal arteries from the first intercostal arteries.

In the thoracic region it is not unusual to note several posterior spinal pedicles, as shown in Figure 15–38, but in occasional cases, a single posterior spinal nutrient pedicle opacifying an angioma can be demonstrated. This underlines the importance of injecting contrast medium into the intercostal arteries bilaterally from T2 to T7.

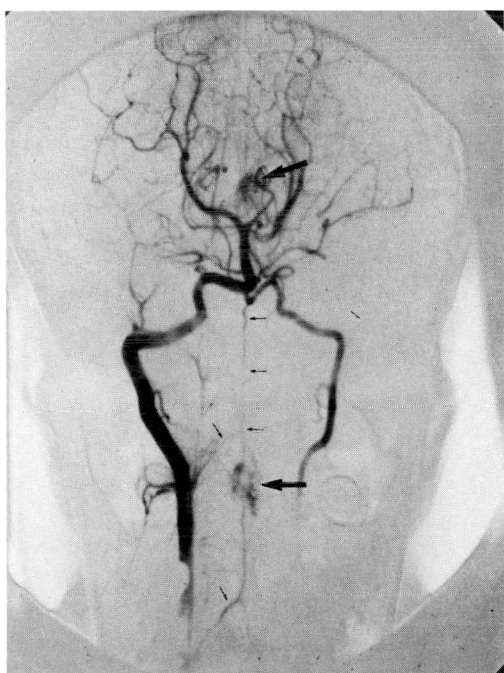

Figure 15–36 Cervical and intracerebral angiomas (*large arrows*). The cervical angioma is fed by the anterior spinal axis formed by the anterior spinal artery (*small arrows*), a radicular artery that arises from the vertebral artery (*superior slanted arrow*), and the artery of the cervical enlargement (*inferior slanted arrow*).

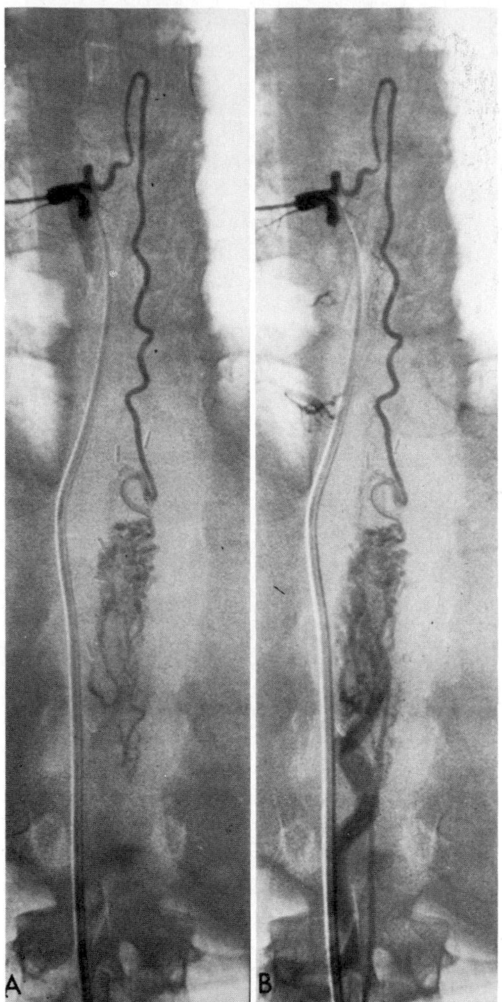

Figure 15–37 *A*. Intramedullary angioma supplied by dilated artery of Adamkiewicz arising from the sixth left intercostal artery. *B*. A voluminous inferior draining vein is demonstrated.

In the thoracolumbar region the small malformation may be supplied by an isolated posterior spinal artery (Figs. 15–39 and 15–40). More bulky malformations usually are supplied by multiple spinal arteries. Given the frequency of retrocorporeal anastomoses, connections between the posterior spinal arteries are not unusual in this region.

Mixed angiomas are lesions combining intra- and retromedullary features in the same voluminous angiomatous mass. In the lateral projection, this mass may be separated into two portions, the anterior part supplied by an anterior radiculospinal artery, and the posterior part supplied by a posterior spinal artery. The mixed angioma may be supplied by an artery from the lumbar or cervical enlargement, composed of an anterior spinal artery and a posterior spinal artery arising from the same trunk, or possibly supplied by one or multiple posterior spinal arteries and an artery of Adamkiewicz, the latter of which may arise at a level far removed from the angioma itself.

THE ANGIOMATOUS MASS. Usually, the angioma is of medium and discernible mass. When small, however, it may be difficult to recognize, especially if obscured by residual Pantopaque droplets from a pre-

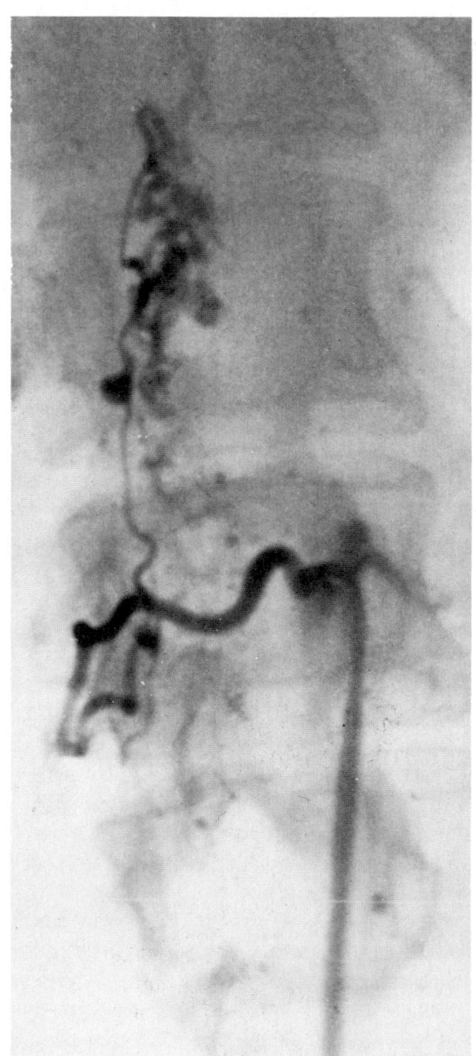

Figure 15–38 A dilated posterior spinal artery nourishing a retromedullary angioma. (From Djindjian, R., Hurth, M., and Houdart, R.: Angiography of the Spinal Cord. Paris, Masson & Cie; Baltimore, Md., University Park Press, 1970. Reprinted by permission.)

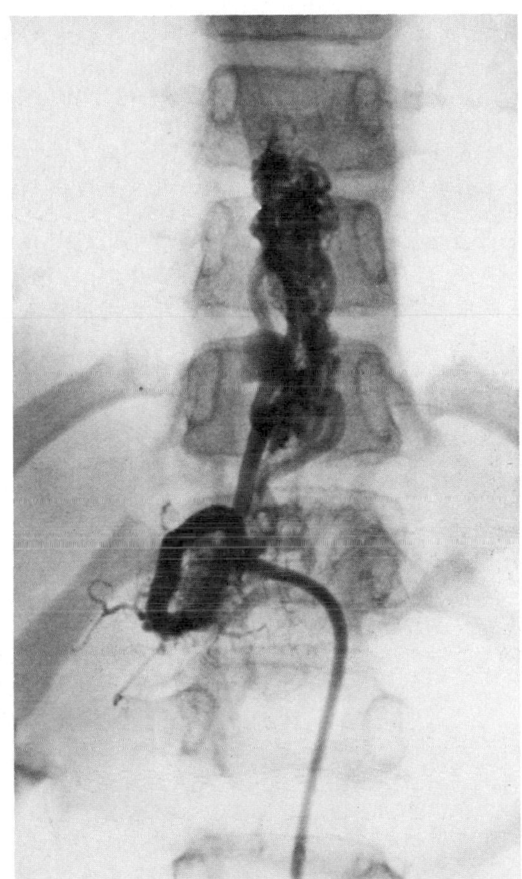

Figure 15–39 Retromedullary thoracolumbar angioma fed by a posterior spinal artery arising from the twelfth right intercostal artery. (From Djindjian, R., Hurth, M., and Houdart, R.: Angiography of the Spinal Cord. Paris, Masson & Cie; Baltimore, Md., University Park Press, 1970. Reprinted by permission.)

vious myelogram. Sometimes it is massive, covering several arterial and osseous segments. In these cases, the nutrient pedicles are multiple and may number up to 10 different tributaries.

In the Rendu-Osler syndrome (six cases), the angiomatous mass is often voluminous, with very dilated nutrient arteries and draining veins, covering the whole length of the spinal cord; in all of these cases, large venous lakes have been demonstrated, eroding the bony pedicles and occasionally even hollowing out the posterior surface of two or three vertebrae.

In the authors' series of 90 intramedullary arteriovenous malformations, 18 (20 per cent) pseudoaneurysmal lesions have been demonstrated. This pattern was present angiographically in 10 cases treated by palliative methods, and verified histologically in the other 8. In three of the latter cases, the arteriographic and operative appearance was that of an aneurysm connected to a contiguous arteriovenous malformation. In the other five cases, the aneurysm represented the heart of the arteriovenous malformation (Fig. 15–41). The authors have been able to observe angiographically a morphological modification of an intramedullary angioma. Initially, the location of the angiomatous mass on the anterior spinal axis precluded operative intervention or embolization. Two years later, the patient presented with complete flaccid paraplegia, and at arteriography, the angioma had an aneurysmal appearance (Fig. 15–42). In one of eight cases verified histologically, an association between a true arterial aneurysm and an arteriovenous malformation could be demonstrated (Fig. 15–43).

Draining Veins. The draining veins of angiomas covering the entirety of the spinal cord are always voluminous and extensive

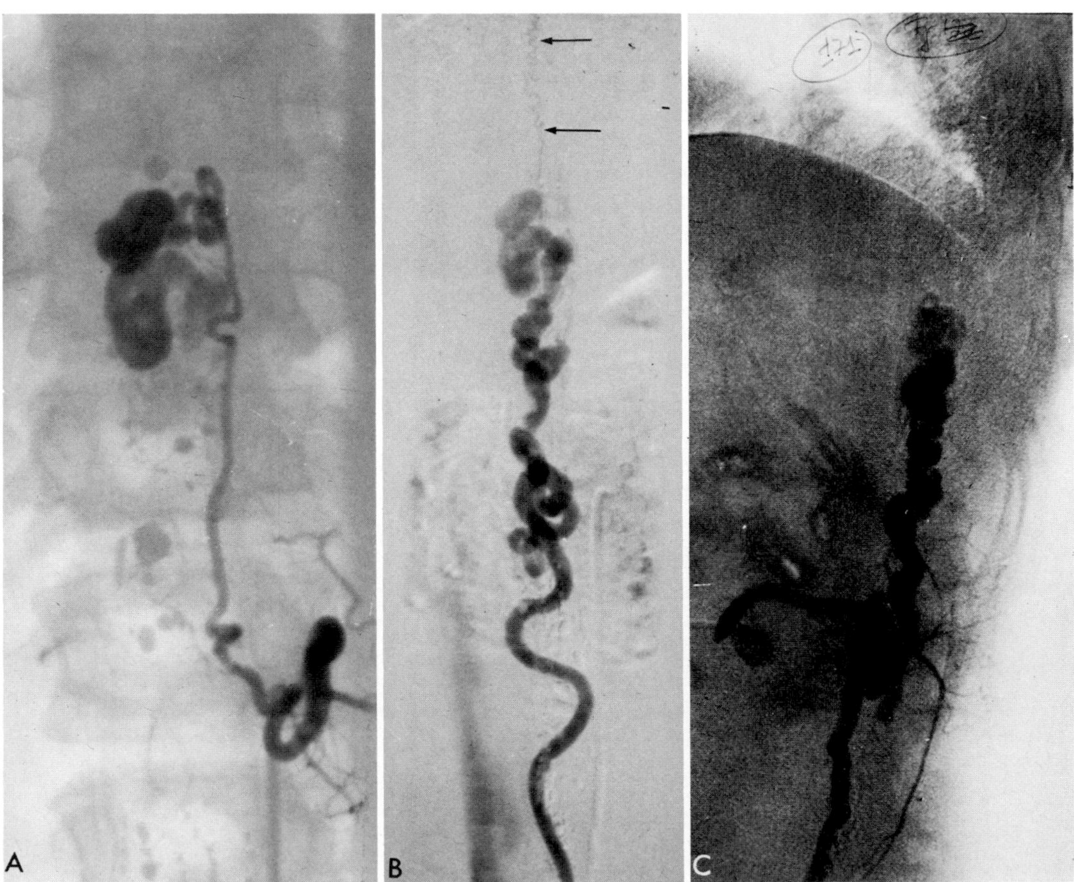

Figure 15–40 *A*. Retromedullary angioma fed by a voluminous dilated posterior spinal artery arising from the first left lumbar artery. *B*. Voluminous inferior draining veins. *C*. Lateral view of same case.

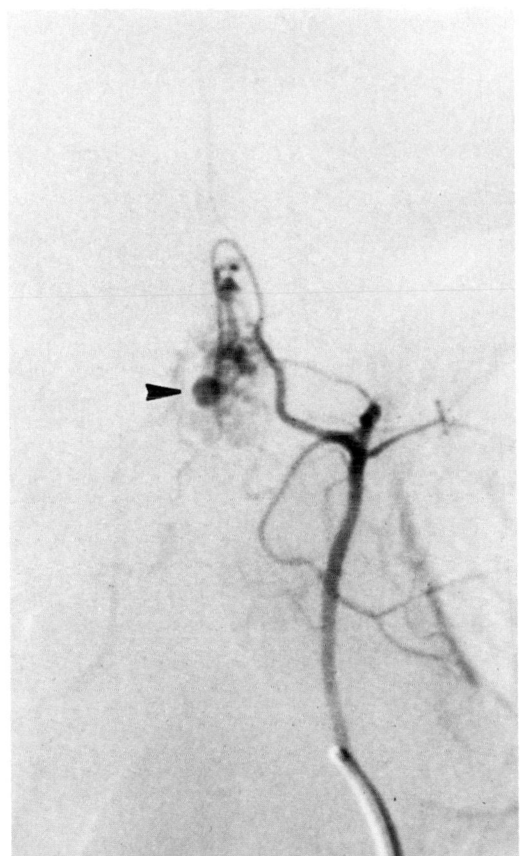

Figure 15–41 Pseudoaneurysmal form of a superior thoracic intramedullary angioma fed by a dilated superior thoracic anterior spinal artery.

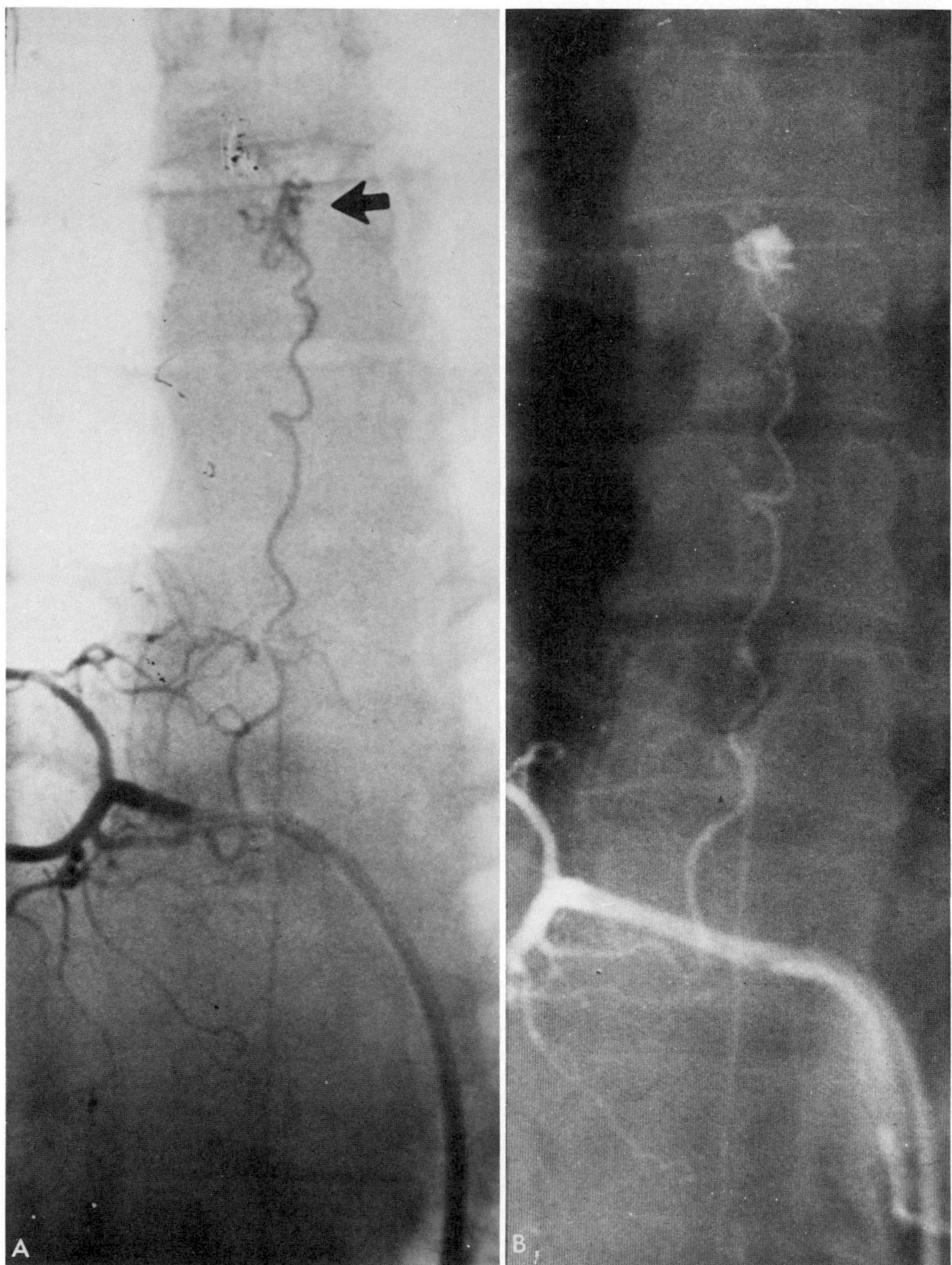

Figure 15–42 *A*. An intramedullary thoracic angioma (*arrow*) fed by a dilated ascending branch of the artery of Adamkiewicz arising from the ninth right intercostal artery. *B*. Arteriography two years later. The angioma has changed into a pseudoaneurysmal form. (From Djindjian, R., Hurth, M., and Houdart, R.: Angiography of the Spinal Cord. Paris, Masson & Cie; Baltimore Md., University Park Press, 1970. Reprinted by permission.)

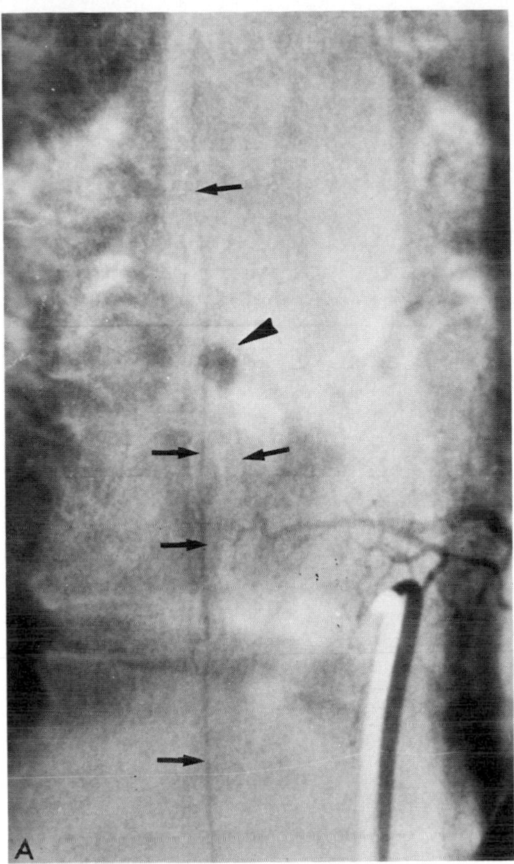

Figure 15–43 A true arterial aneurysm (*arrowhead*) is situated at the bifurcation of the ascending and descending branches of the artery of Adamkiewicz (*arrows*). There are no draining veins.

in a caudal-cephalic direction. These dilated veins may present as pseudoaneurysms, varying from the size of a pea to large vascular masses such as those seen in the Rendu-Osler syndrome (Fig. 15–44). The draining veins are the dilated normal veins of the spinal cord. They therefore may have the same topography: (1) The anterior spinal vein traverses the anterior surface of the cord behind the anterior spinal artery in the median groove. It drains the intramedullary angiomas. (2) The posterior spinal vein courses medially on the posterior surface of the cord without arterial equivalent. It drains the retromedullary angiomas. The spinal veins superimposed on anteroposterior views are readily visible on the lateral views (Fig. 15–45). In the thoracic region, they may be divided and are angiographically poorly separated from one another.

A communication between anterior and posterior spinal veins is not unusual. Thus, certain retromedullary and intramedullary angiomas are drained not only by posterior spinal veins but also by anterior ones. While these communications are most often located circumferentially around the cord, intramedullary venous channels traversing the cord may provide communication between the anterior and posterior spinal veins.[21]

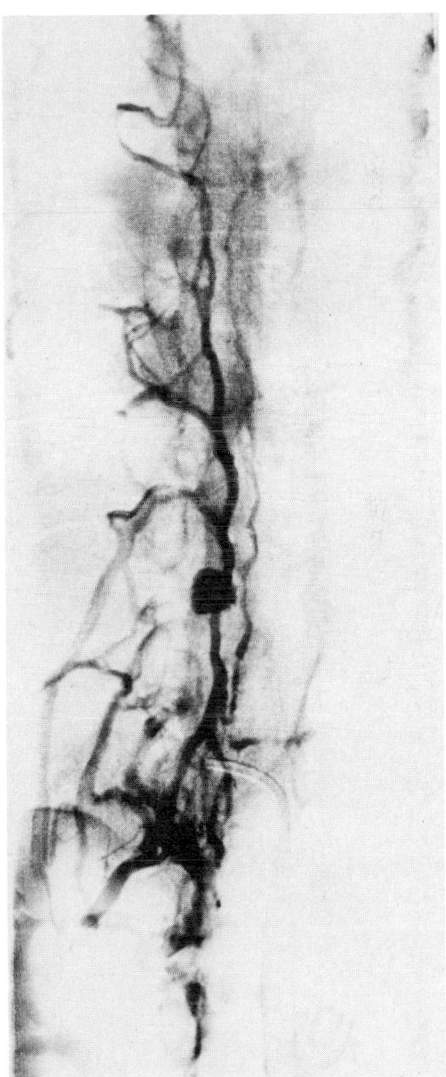

Figure 15–44 A venous vascular pouch simulates an aneurysmal pouch. (From Djindjian, R., Hurth, M., and Houdart, R.: Angiography of the Spinal Cord. Paris, Masson & Cie; Baltimore, Md., University Park Press, 1970. Reprinted by permission.)

Classification Based on Topography

A classification of spinal angiomas may be made on the basis of spinal topography: (1) caudal-cephalic extent—cervical, upper and midthoracic, and dorsolumbosacral types corresponding to the three vascular spinal cord territories; and (2) the degree of penetration into the spinal cord—intramedullary lesions with anterior vascularization, retromedullary lesions, and mixed types.

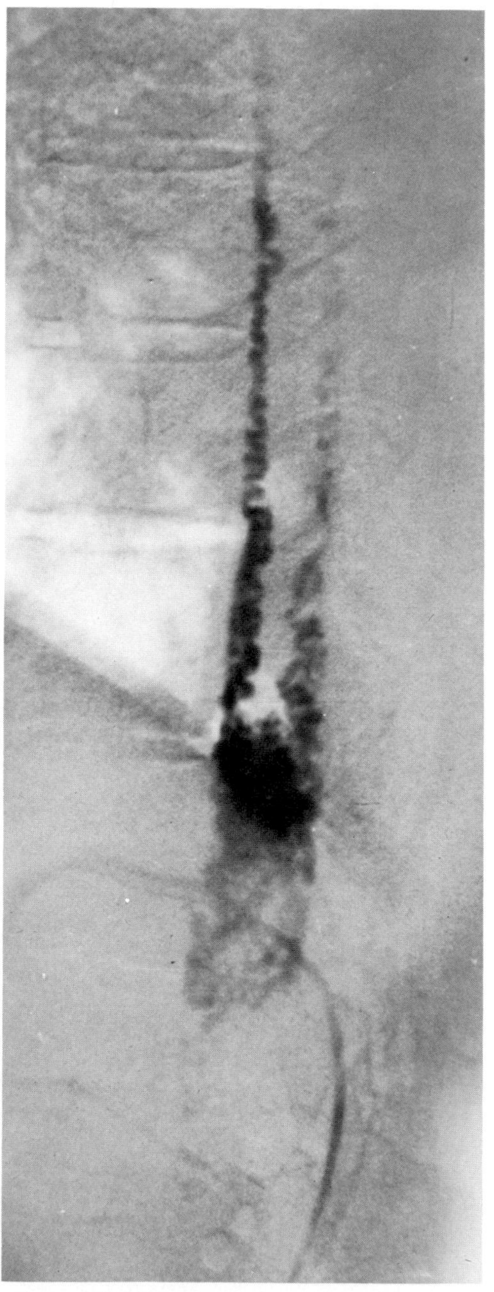

Figure 15–45 A thoracolumbar intramedullary angioma with pre- and postmedullary ascending draining veins. Lateral projection.

Distribution of Angiomas of the Spinal Cord

CERVICAL ANGIOMAS. In 21 cases (14 per cent) the lesion was localized at the level of the cervical enlargement and in all cases spared the upper segments. The nutrient arteries originated from the vertebral artery and from the cervicointercostal trunk of the subclavian artery. All but one case had anterior afferent arteries. The nutrient pedicles frequently numbered more than three. The efferent vessels were voluminous, a function of the size of the malformation, and drained into the venous system of the posterior fossa. Diagnosis of these lesions was most often made early because of the obvious neurological signs. On the other hand, six cases were not recognized as angiomas for more than 10 years. Spinal root signs and symptoms were unusual (three cases) and when present were always unilateral and often purely subjective. The cord signs and symptoms dominated the clinical picture, usually related to the degree of intramedullary involvement. The Brown-Séquard syndrome (five cases), syringomyelia syndrome (five cases), paraplegia (two cases), and tetraplegia (three cases) were seen. Associated meningeal hemorrhage was very frequent, present in eight cases.

THORACIC ANGIOMAS Thirty-three cases (22 per cent) were localized to the first six or seven thoracic segments, supplied by cervical branches of the subclavian arteries, thoracospinal branches of the first six or seven intercostal aortic arteries, and the terminal cord tributary of the artery of Adamkiewicz, the latter of which can originate as far cephalad as the fifth thoracic segment.

Twenty-one of thirty-three cases (two thirds) demonstrated intramedullary penetration. The volume of these malformations was intermediate between the cervical and thoracolumbar forms, owing to the smaller number of nutrient pedicles. The afferent vessels occasionally drained toward the cranio-occipital junction, or toward the vena cava–azygous system.

These thoracic forms often have an obvious symptom complex, explaining their early diagnosis. The frequency of meningeal hemorrhage is less important (four cases). Five cases manifested themselves by a cauda equina syndrome due to a diversion of blood flow at the expense of the lumbar enlargement.

DORSOLUMBOSACRAL ANGIOMAS. In 96 cases (64 per cent) these angiomas were located at the level of the last segments of the thoracic cord, the conus, and the roots of the cauda equina (two cases), depending on the vascular territory of the artery of Adamkiewicz.

The nutrient arteries arose from the last intercostal and the first lumbar vessels. The preponderantly posterior intramedullary location of these angiomas (67 cases) made this group eminently favorable for therapy. The malformation usually was of small size and unipedicular. The venous drainage was as a rule, but not constantly, into the vena cava–azygous system.

The clinical latency of this type of angioma is characteristic. The average age at time of discovery of these lesions is 51 years, as opposed to a mean age of 33 years for malformations that include a direct supply from the artery of Adamkiewicz. This is because, in the latter group, the arterial flow favors hemorrhage, and the arterial steal expresses itself readily. The clinical quiescence of the posterior forms becomes conspicuous when one studies the topography of the angiomas. In subjects 60 years or older (11 cases), however, the clinical picture of the more quiescent posterior intramedullary forms is similar to that of the rapidly evolving thoracolumbar types; this pattern of the former type is explained by the stasis of blood aggravated by atheromas. Almost all the posterior lesions have presented themselves in a stepwise clinical fashion, with the exclusion of two cases of mixed angiomas.

The first symptoms of thoracolumbosacral lesions are usually radicular manifestations associated with a more advanced stage of medullary syndrome. This group as a whole is amenable to therapy, owing mainly to the frequency with which they are posterior lesions. This advantage is offset, however, by the gravity of the neurological picture at the time of diagnosis.

Classification of Intramedullary Angiomas by Lateral Angiography

Eighty-six cases were evaluated by lateral angiography, and three subtypes were derived. These are outlined in Table 15–1, with some mention of appropriate operative intervention. A diagrammatic representation of this classification is presented in Figure 15–46, and the angiographic appearance of the various types is illustrated in Figures 15–47 through 15–54.

TABLE 15–1 CLASSIFICATION OF INTRAMEDULLARY ANGIOMAS BY LATERAL ANGIOGRAPHY

Type 1a	An intramedullary angioma supplied by sulcocommissural arteries; operative intervention may result in a cure (Fig. 15–47)
Type 1b	A diffuse angioma developed around the anterior arterial spinal axis, without a plane of cleavage; operative intervention is contraindicated (Fig. 15–48)
Type 2a	A diffuse spinal cord arteriovenous malformation; operative intervention is contraindicated (Fig. 15–49)
Type 2b	An isolated "aneurysmal ball" may be demonstrated angiographically; total excision is recommended (Fig. 15–50)
Type 2c	An intramedullary arteriovenous malformation (pseudoaneurysmal form) associated with an angiomatous malformation ("ball" angioma); partial excision is indicated (Fig. 15–51)
Type 3	Mixed arteriovenous malformation; intramedullary angioma with large extramedullary vascular lakes
Type 3a	Arteriovenous malformation with median vascular lake ("like an iceberg") (Fig. 15–52)
Type 3b	Arteriovenous malformation with a vascular lake laterally placed (Fig. 15–53)
Type 3c	Extramedullary arteriovenous malformation (Fig. 15–54)

Embolization of Spinal Cord Angiomas

Spinal cord angiomas were embolized in 45 cases that were divided as follows: posterior or retromedullary angiomas (16 cases), intramedullary angiomas (14 cases), and mixed angiomas (15 cases). Gelfoam emboli of various sizes were used primarily in these procedures.[12] Liquid polymers such as cyanoacrylate are useful in embolizing the interior of angiomas while preserving the normal spinal cord arterial branches.[14]

General Indications

The indications for embolization rather than operative extirpation of spinal cord angiomas are: (1) multiplicity of nutrient pedicles, (2) a large angiomatous mass, (3) previous and repeated operative interventions

Text continued on page 596

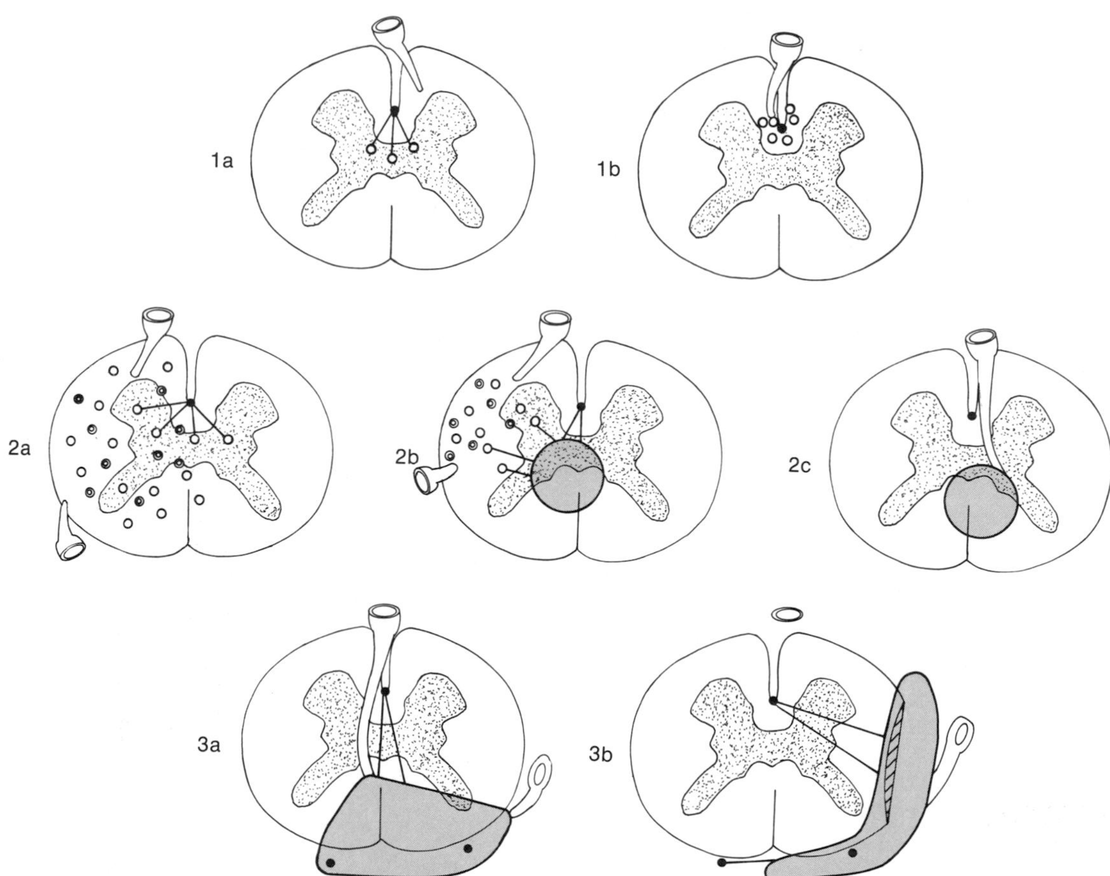

Figure 15–46 A schema for types of intramedullary angiomas as listed in Table 15–1. (Modified from Djindjian, R., et al.: Intradural extramedullary spinal arterio-venous malformations fed by the anterior spinal artery. Surg. Neurol., *8*:85–93, 1977.)

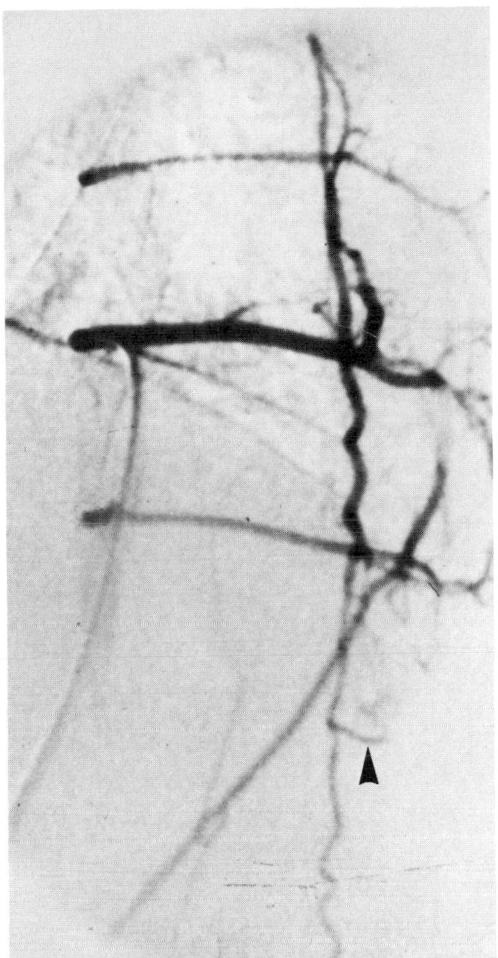

Figure 15–47 Angioma type 1a. Intramedullary angioma fed by a sulcocommissural artery (*arrow*) arising from the artery of Adamkiewicz.

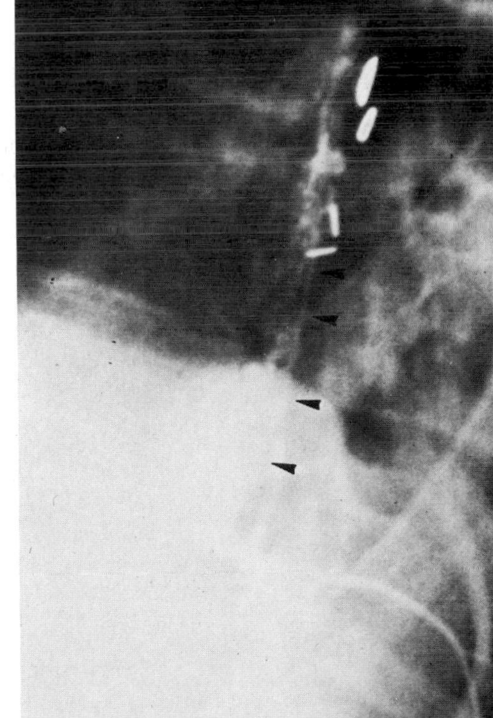

Figure 15–48 Angioma type 1b. Diffuse intramedullary angioma (*arrows*) has developed around the anterior spinal arterial axis (a portion of the retromedullary artery has been extirpated (*clips*).

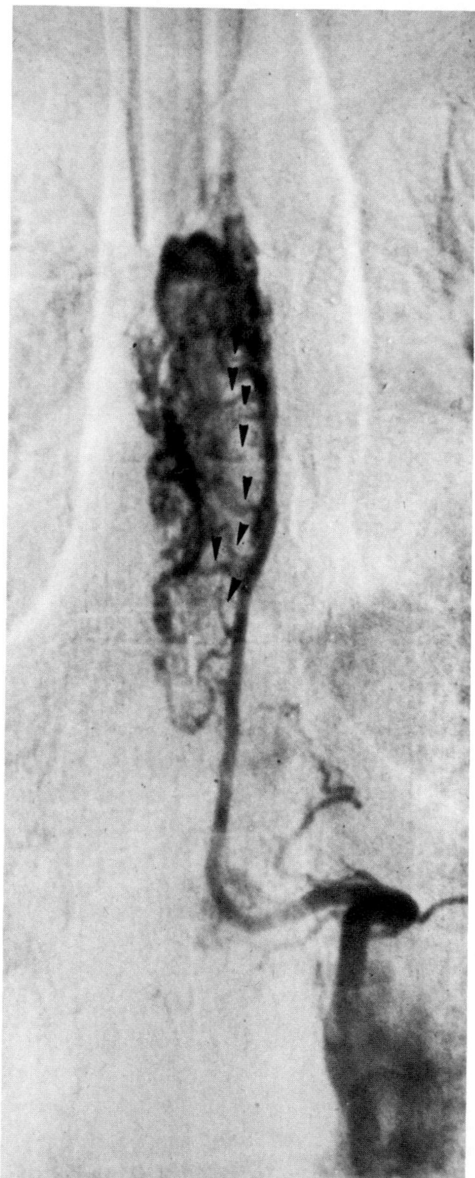

Figure 15–49 Angioma type 2a. A diffuse intramedullary angioma fed by numerous sulcocommissural arteries (*arrows*).

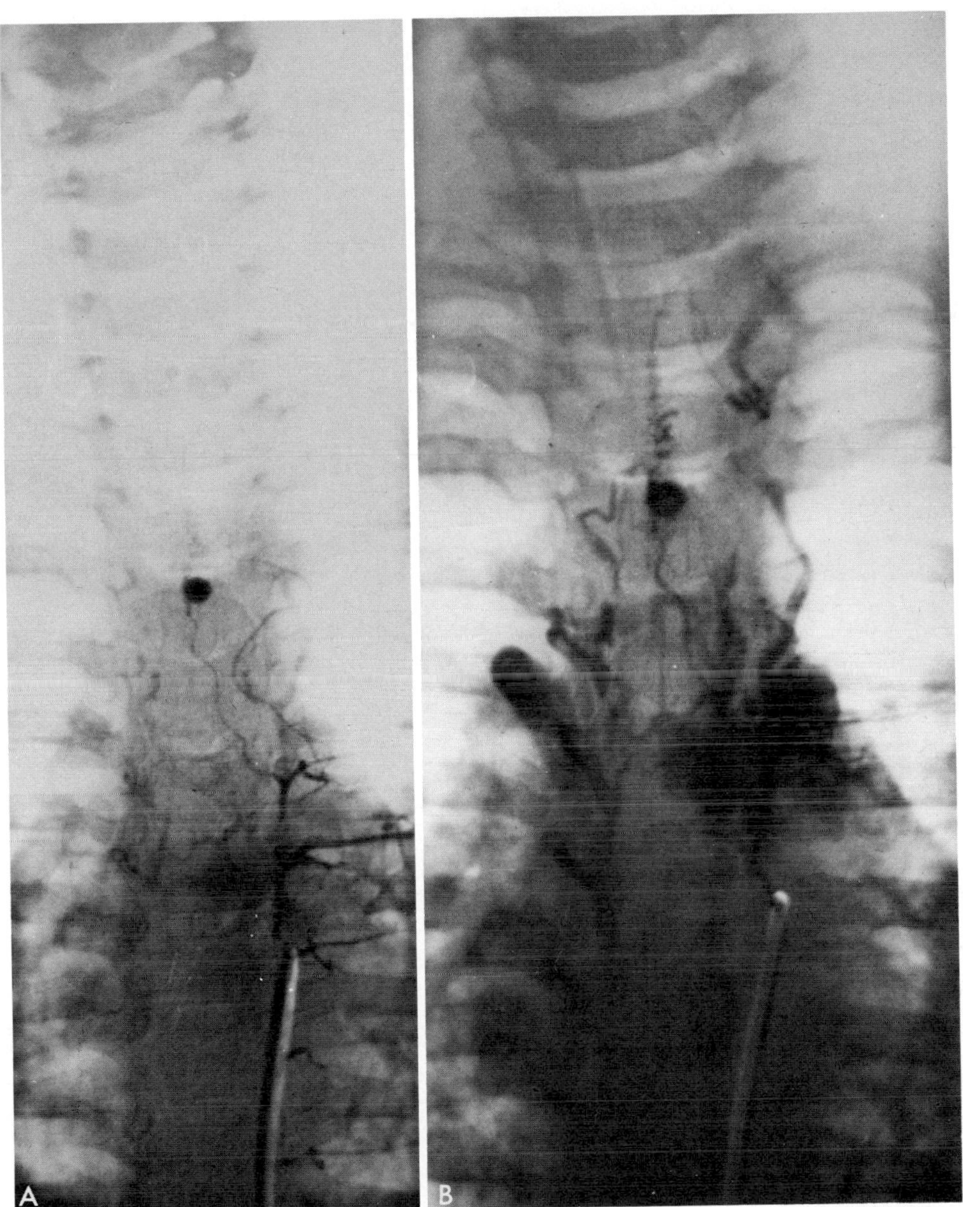

Figure 15–50 Angioma type 2b. The isolated angioma of the pseudoaneurysmal form. *A*. Early arterial phase. *B*. Late arterial phase.

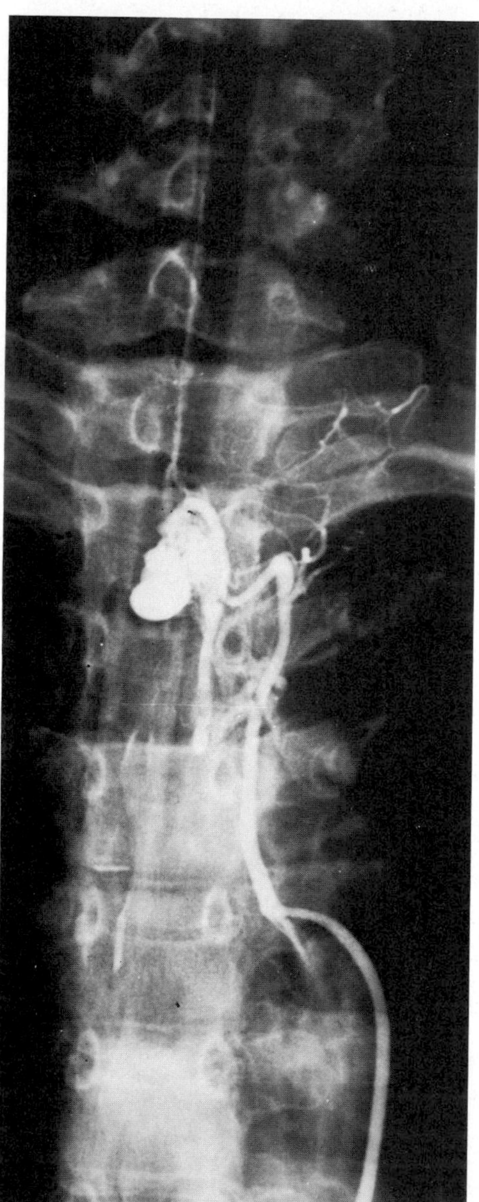

Figure 15–51 Angioma type 2c. A pseudoaneurysmal form of angioma associated with an angiomatous malformation (ball and angioma).

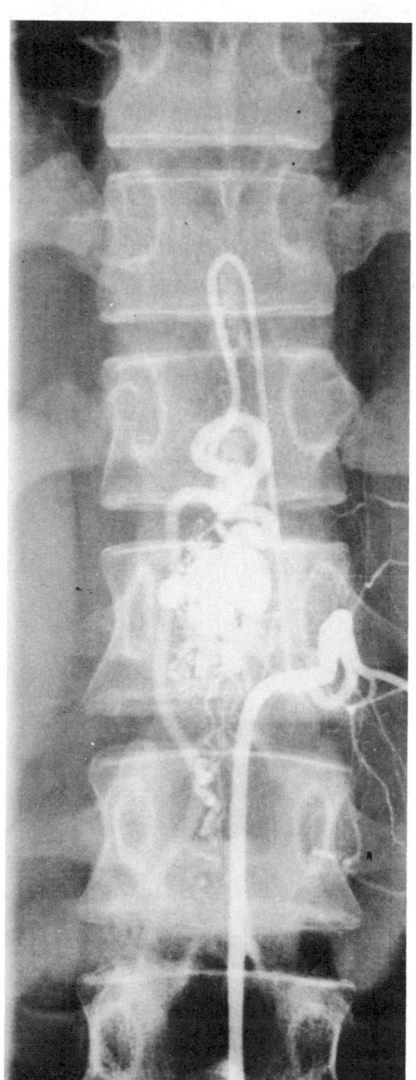

Figure 15–52 Angioma type 3a. An intramedullary angioma with large median vascular lakes.

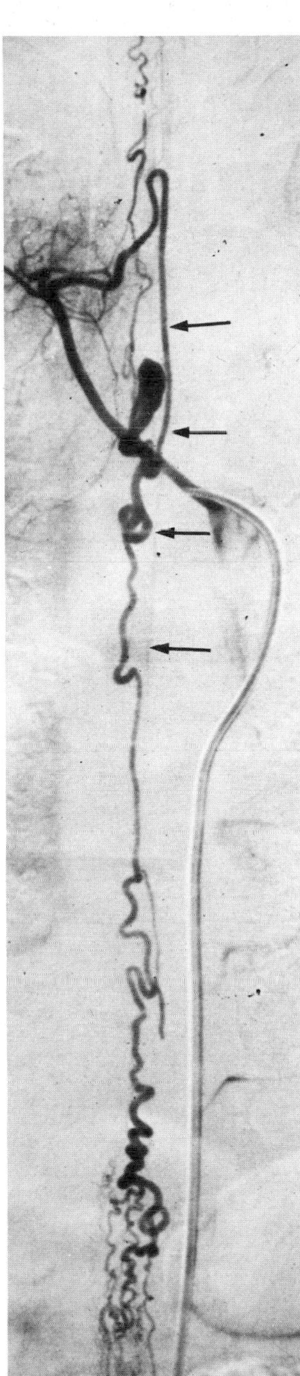

Figure 15–53 Angioma type 3b. The artery of Adamkiewicz (*arrows*) is thin following opacification of the laterally placed vascular lake.

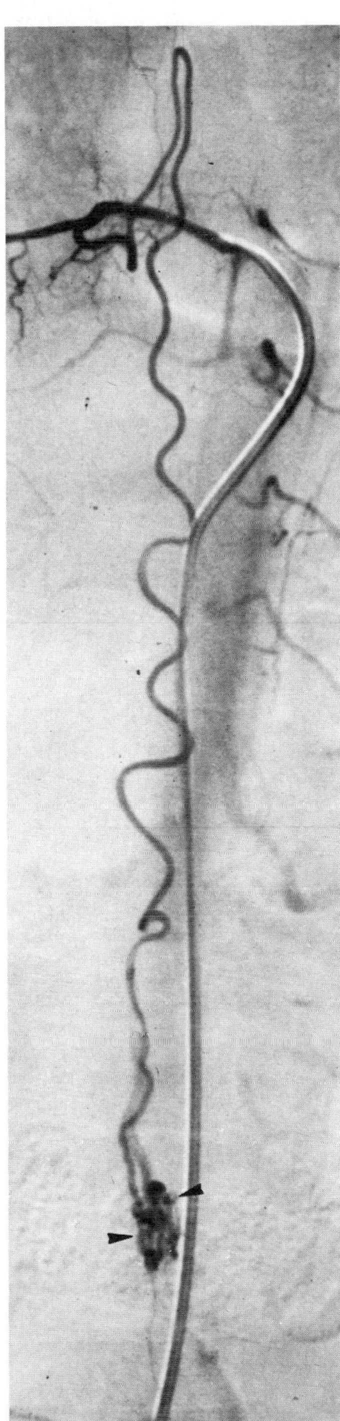

Figure 15–54 Angioma type 3c. An extramedullary angioma fed by the artery of Adamkiewicz projects at the level of L3 (*arrows*). (From Djindjian, R., et al.: Intradural extramedullary spinal arteriovenous malformations fed by the anterior spinal artery. Surg. Neurol., *8*:85–93, 1977. Reprinted by permission.)

with subtotal removal of angioma, and (4) the clinical state of the patient (in particular, the presence of cutaneous sores, phlebitis, or somatic damage.)

Paraspinal muscle infarction with transient (three to five days' duration) and intermittently severe back pain, among other complications, has been reported.[10]

Retromedullary Angiomas

Embolization in these cases carries little risk of spinal cord ischemia (Fig. 15–55). Ideally, one would like to embolize the posterior spinal artery as close to the angiomatous mass as possible. Therefore, it is important to distinguish enlarged posterior arterial components from the anterior spinal artery, which is sometimes very thin, embedded in the voluminous draining veins of the angioma, and thus poorly visualized. In cases of doubt, a lateral arteriogram is necessary to sort out the appropriate anatomical arterial relationships.

It is also necessary to identify the muscular anastomoses between the supra- and subjacent intercostal arteries and the retrocorporeal anastomosis by the intercostal or lumbar artery of the opposite side. In case of effective anastomosis, embolization is imperative.

Failure occurs when only the intercostal

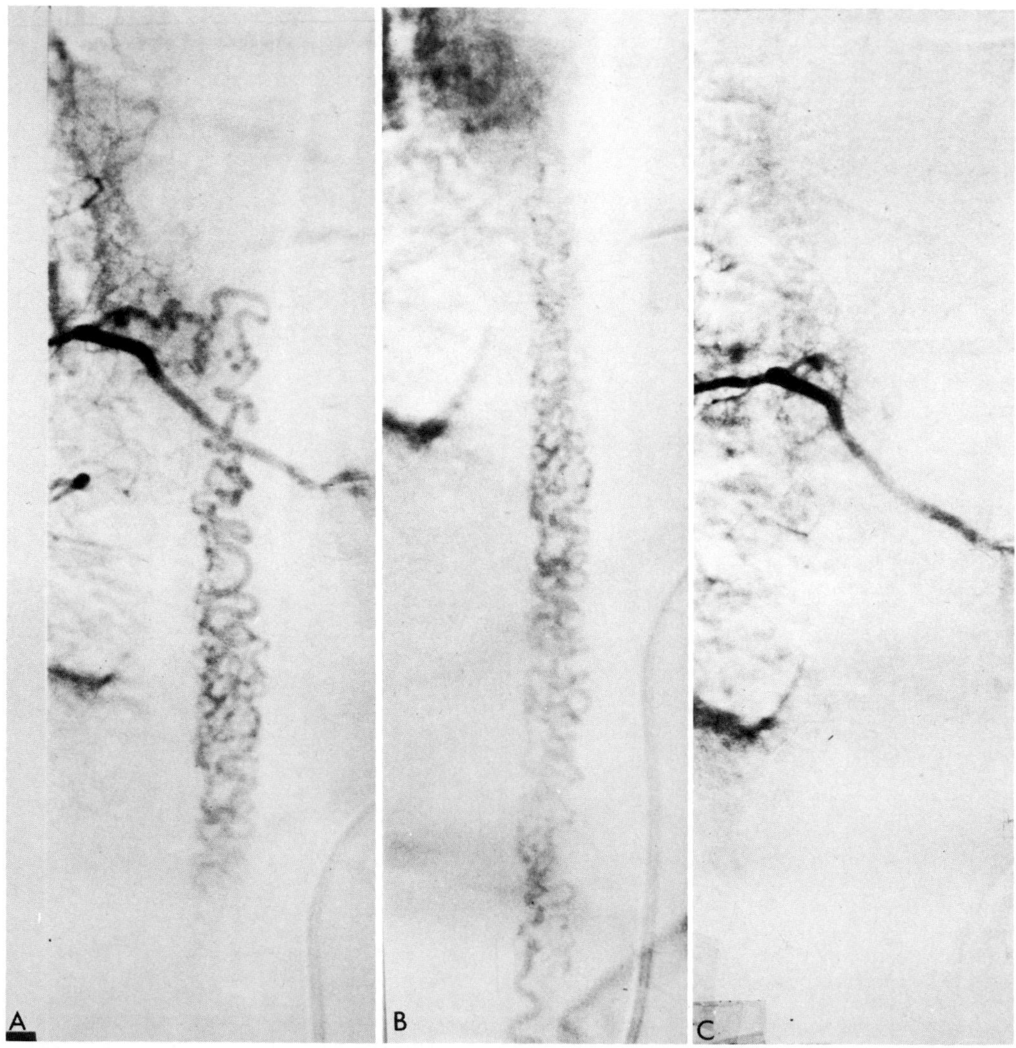

Figure 15–55 A retromedullary angioma fed by a posterior spinal artery arising from a right superior intercostal artery. *A* and *B*. Early and late angiographic phases. *C*. Following embolization. (*A* and *C* from Djindjian, R., et al.: Treatment of angiomas of the spinal cord. Surg. Neurol., *2*:186–194, 1974. Reprinted by permission.)

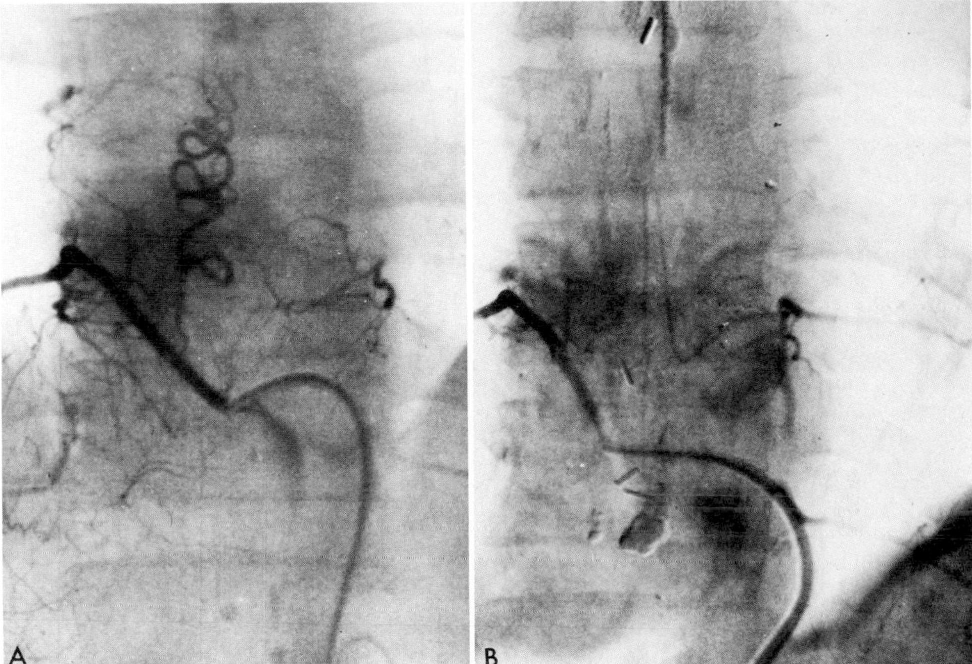

Figure 15–56 Operative treatment of a retromedullary angioma fed by a posterior spinal artery arising from the right tenth intercostal artery. *A*. Early arterial phase. *B*. Postoperative view after total removal of the angioma and opacification of the artery of Adamkiewicz by the opposite intercostal vessel. (From Djindjian, R., Hurth, M., and Houdart, R.: Angiography of the Spinal Cord. Paris, Masson & Cie; Baltimore, Md., University Park Press, 1970. Reprinted by permission.)

artery has been embolized, and not the main nutrient pedicle. Ipsilateral and contralateral muscular anastomoses may then develop. In such cases, a repeat embolization should be undertaken unless the ipsilateral or contralateral intercostal arteries supply the artery of Adamkiewicz.

If clinical improvement is rapid, then the embolization procedure generally can be called successful. If, at the time of follow-up arteriography, pedicles are again seen opacifying the malformation, a repeat procedure is desirable if the subject is young and in generally good condition (Fig. 15–56). On the other hand, in aged subjects or subjects presenting with poor clinical states (malnutrition, cutaneous sores, phlebitis), multiple embolization procedures may be contraindicated.

Intramedullary Angiomas

The excision of angiomas supplied by the anterior spinal pathway carries great risk because of the primordial functional role of the associated sulcocommissural arteries. Sooner or later, however, progressive neurological deterioration is bound to occur. Paraplegia secondary to intramedullary hemorrhage (pseudoaneurysmal appearance on the angiogram), death from meningeal hemorrhage, and death from intracranial hypertension (occlusion of the basal cisterns by recurrent hemorrhages—seven meningeal hemorrhages in one example) may be encountered. Therefore, some form of therapy, in this case intra-arterial embolization, offers a valuable tool that may be utilized in the presence of a rapidly progressive angioma. It is possible, by adjusting the size of the emboli, to obstruct nutrient vessels quite near to the arteriovenous shunt, which reduces the risk of iatrogenic neurological damage.

The primary indication for embolization is the neurological state of the patient. It is useful to divide patients into two groups, paraplegic and nonparaplegic patients (the latter who have had one or two episodes of regressive paraplegia).

Paraplegic Patients

If a severe deficit has occurred recently, it is wise to wait 8 to 15 days in hopes of a progressive spontaneous recovery from this deficit—and entrance into the category of nonparaplegia. Quite a different problem is presented by the patient who has an old well-defined paraplegia with sphincter problems, bedsores, wasting of muscles, and especially spinal automatism with hyperspasticity that makes mobilization impossible and prevents the patient from sleeping (Fig. 15–57). This automatism should be distinguished from pseudotetanoid contractures related to obstruction of the artery of Adamkiewicz. It is possible for one phenomenon to be superimposed on the other.

Embolization may suppress the sometimes intolerable root pain and enable the patient to discontinue opiates; it prevents repeated and sometimes fatal meningeal hemorrhage; and finally it diminishes the phenomena of spinal automatism, sup-

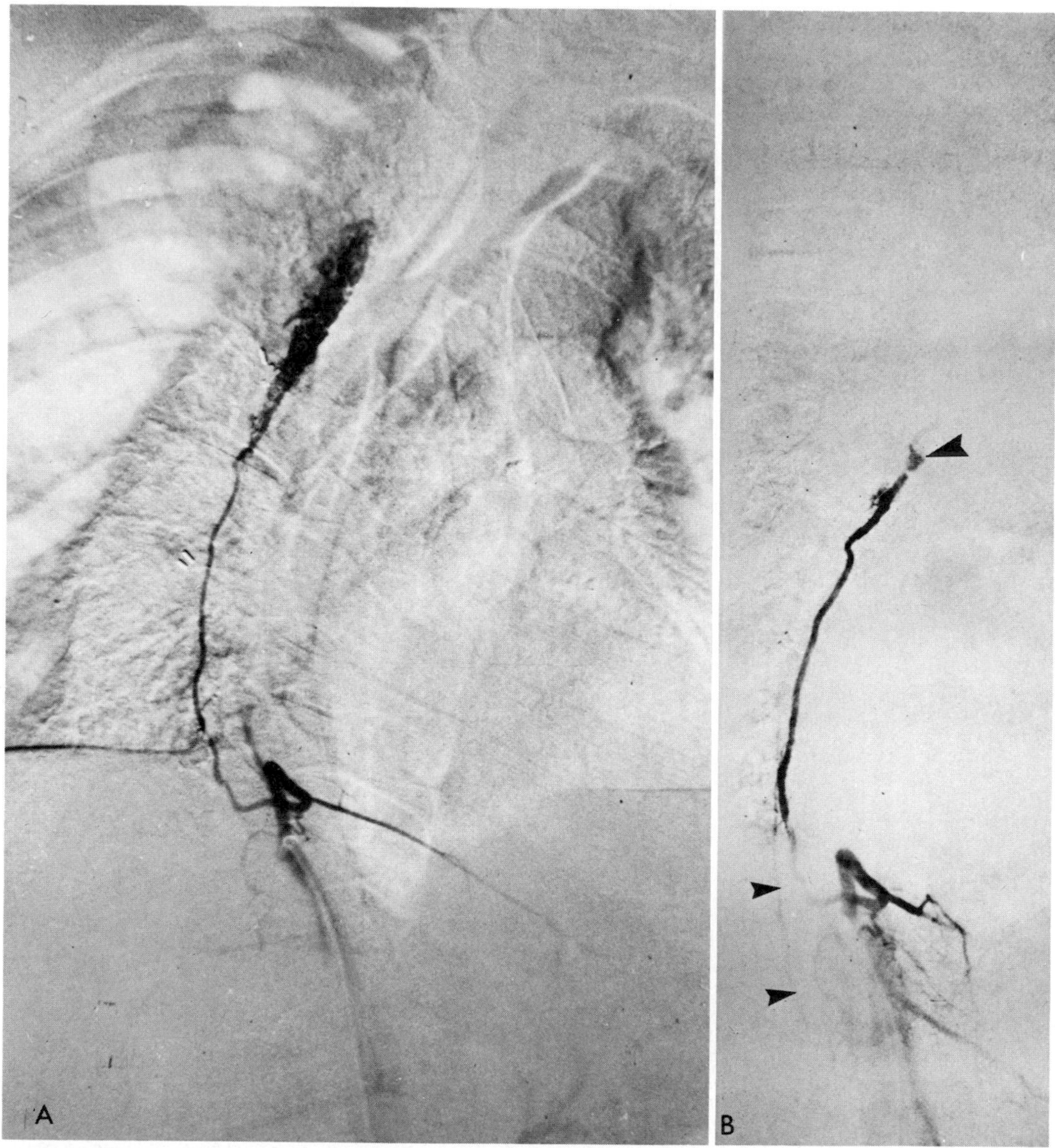

Figure 15–57 *A*. An intramedullary angioma fed by an ascending dilated branch of the artery of Adamkiewicz is seen to arise from the left ninth intercostal artery. *B*. Following embolization, there is no opacification of the angioma (*large arrowhead*), and opacification of the descending branch of the artery of Adamkiewicz (which was not visible before embolization) is now seen (*small arrowheads*). (*A* and *C* from Djindjian, R., et al.: Superselective arteriographic embolization by the femoral route in neuroradiology. Neuroradiology, *6*:132–142, 1973. Reprinted by permission.)

presses muscle spasm, permits mobilization, and makes sleep possible.

Nonparaplegic Patients

Two factors should be considered: the level of embolization contemplated (cervical, thoracic, or thoracolumbar), and the caliber of the radiculomedullary afferent vessels.

AT THE CERVICAL LEVEL. In the authors' experience the cervical malformations always include an intramedullary component exclusively or predominantly. The anterior spinal pathway is supplied by several anterior radiculomedullary arteries, of which the largest is the artery of the cervical enlargement. These arteries arise from the two vertebral arteries and the two deep cervical arteries. The function of the artery of the cervical enlargement can be partially replaced by other radiculomedullary arteries. To prevent interruption of the anterior spinal arterial pathway, the embolus should be lodged as close as possible to the angioma (Figs. 15–58 and 15–59).

AT THE THORACIC AND THORACOLUMBAR LEVELS. At these levels, embolization of the artery of Adamkiewicz is feasible because of the caliber of the enlarged, dilated artery. Thus the embolus may be lodged close to or within the angioma without interrupting the main Adamkiewicz arterial supply. It is necessary to monitor the progressive diminution of the opacity of the angioma angiographically during embolization (Fig. 15–60). Sometimes the artery of Adamkiewicz is in spasm, and the emboli may lodge in the proximal portion of this artery, which can lead to paraplegic complications. Reversal of paraplegias produced by embolization of the artery of Adamkiewicz is less likely than in other areas, because of suboptimal collateral flow to this vessel. Intramedullary angiomas of small size supplied by an artery of Adamkiewicz of normal caliber constitute a major contraindication to embolization, for the em-

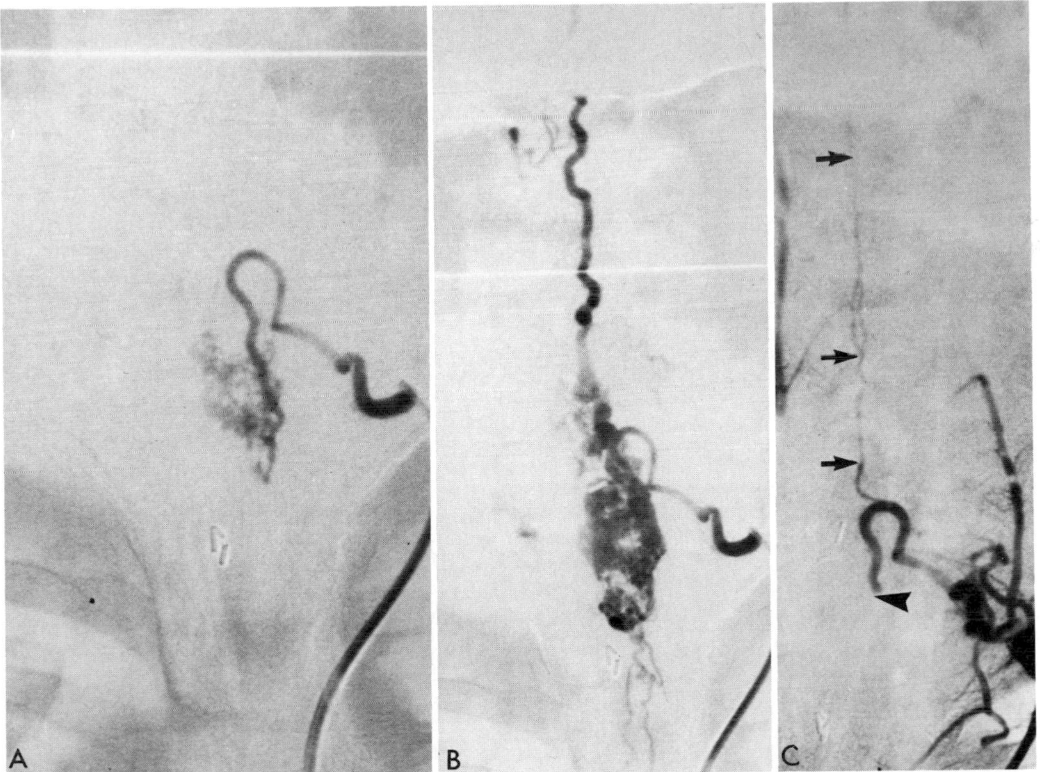

Figure 15–58 Cervical angioma fed by the artery of the cervical enlargement. *A*. No opacification of the ascending branch of the artery of the cervical enlargement is seen. *B*. An angioma and ascending draining vein are demonstrated. *C*. Following embolization of the angioma (*arrowhead*) and disappearance of the "steal" syndrome, opacification of the anterior spinal axis (*arrows*) is appreciated. (From Djindjian, R., et al.: Superselective arteriographic embolization by the femoral route in neuroradiology. Neuroradiology, *6*:132–142, 1973. Reprinted by permission.)

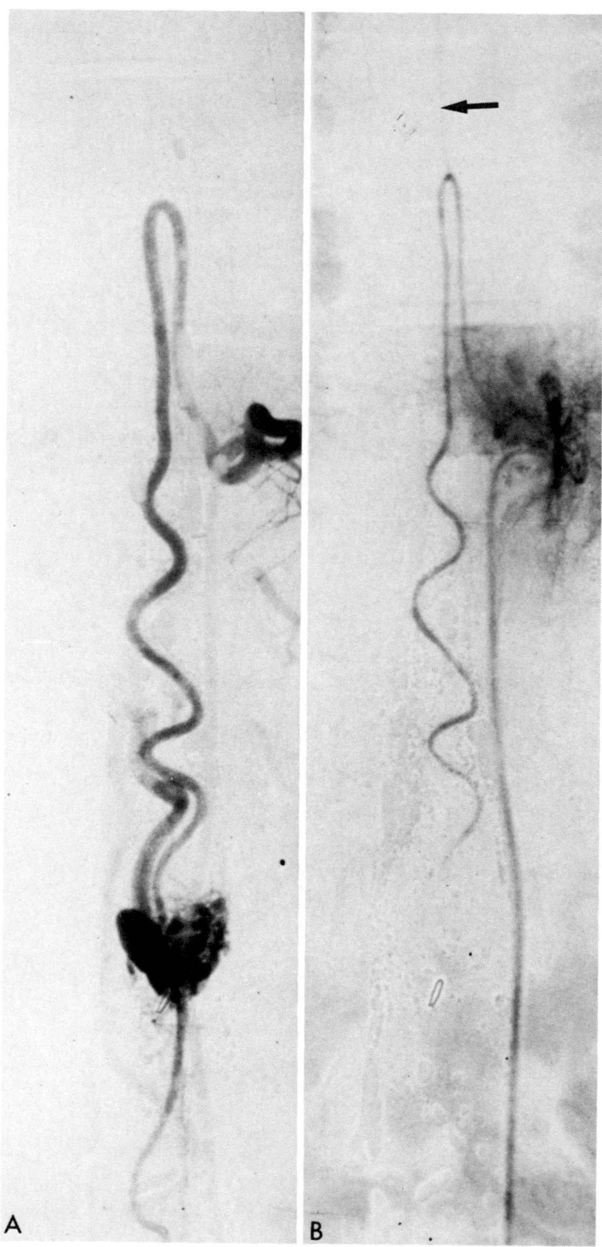

Figure 15–59 *A*. A cervical angioma fed by the artery of the cervical enlargement. The anterior spinal artery axis is visualized. A radicular artery opacifies the right vertebral artery and draining veins. *B*. Following embolization, neither the angioma nor the anterior spinal axis (*arrow*) is opacified. (From Djindjian, R., et al.: Superselective arteriographic embolization by the femoral route in neuroradiology. Neuroradiology, *6*:132–142, 1973. Reprinted by permission.)

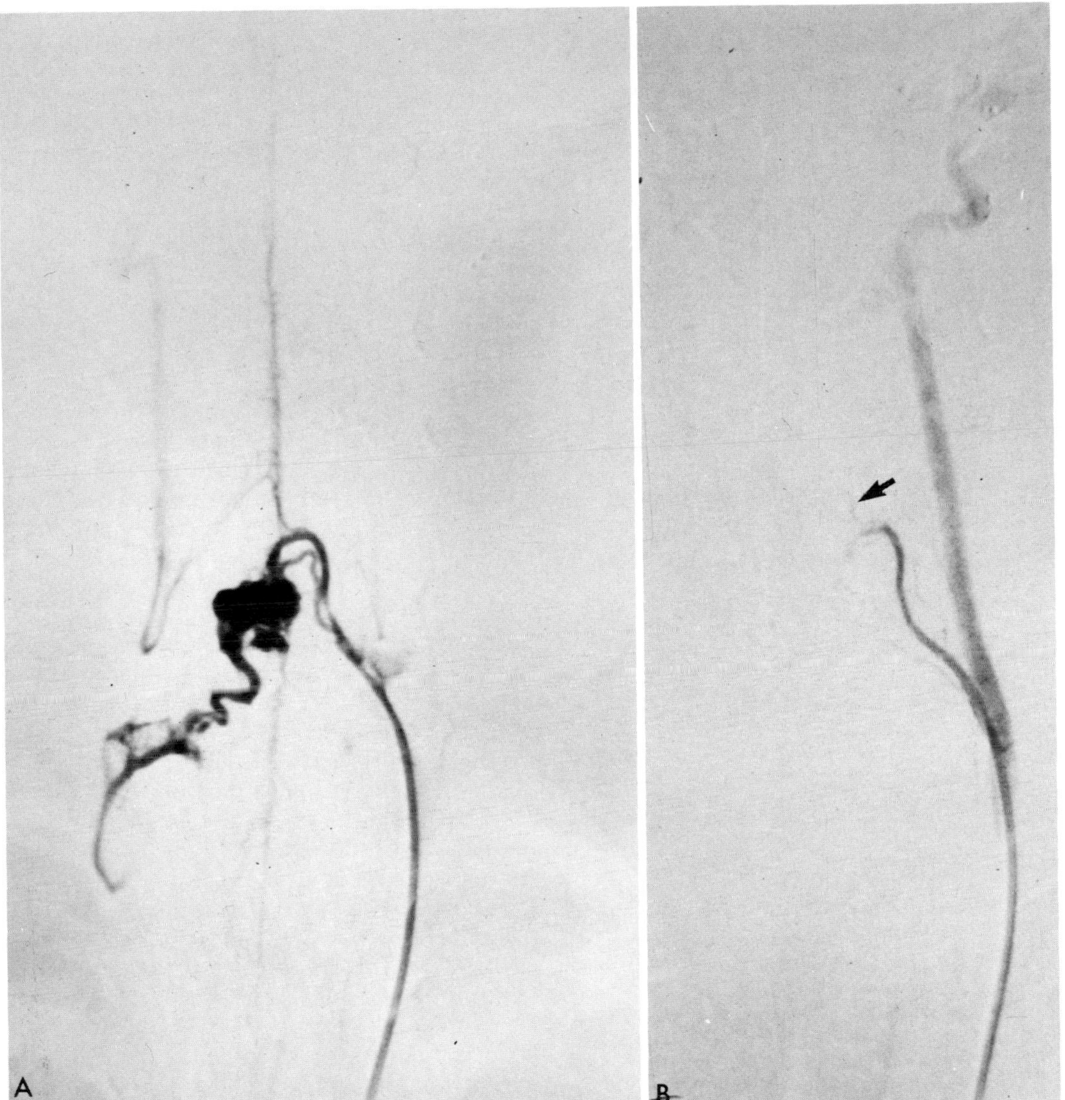

Figure 15–60 *A*. A thoracolumbar angioma is fed by the artery of Adamkiewicz. *B*. Following embolization, there is no opacification of the angioma (*arrow*), and a normal caliber of the artery of Adamkiewicz and opacification of the ascènding branch and the artery of Adamkiewicz because of disappearance of the "steal" syndrome are demonstrated. (From Djindjian, R., et al.: Superselective arteriographic embolization by the femoral route in neuroradiology. Neuroradiology, *6*:132–142, 1973. Reprinted by permission.)

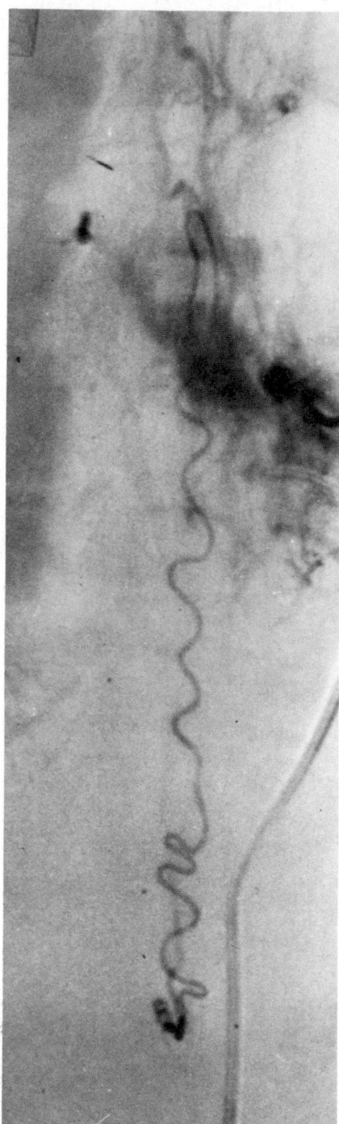

Figure 15–61 A medullary angioma fed by the slightly dilated and very sinuous artery of Adamkiewicz. In this case, embolization is contraindicated. (From Houdart, R., Djindjian, R., Hurth, M., et al.: Treatment of angiomas of the spinal cord. Surg. Neurol., *2*:186–194, 1974. Reprinted by permission.)

bolus will lodge in the proximal segment of this vessel (Fig. 15–61).

Mixed Treatment: Embolization Plus Operation

Operative excision is necessary to relieve compression produced by intramedullary angiomas that have large vascular draining lakes. Preliminary embolization facilitates the operation by thrombosing the angiomatous mass. Since 1973, new advances have been made with respect to intramedullary angiomas. These advances have to do with angiographic diagnosis and operative treatment. Precise angiographic analysis of intramedullary angiomas has permitted operation by posterior commissural myelotomy without posterior complications (Fig. 15–62). At the Lariboisière Hospital, posterior commissural myelotomy is now preferred to embolization of the malformation. Arteriographic control is necessary in order to verify the total removal of the malformation. Embolization can then be attempted in cases of incomplete excision.

Results of Treatment

Therapeutic results in 150 consecutive cases of spinal angiomas have been analyzed. Treatment of this group consisted of embolization only, of embolization combined with operative extirpation, and of operative extirpation alone. In a few cases, no embolic or operative therapy was undertaken. Because of the differences in the treatment of angiomas before and after 1968, discussion of these results is divided into two parts. In the first series of 50 cases (before 1968), complete avoidance of the anterior afferent vessels dominated the conduct of treatment. No therapy was undertaken in 21 cases, the results being inexorable evolution toward paraplegia and, in 1 case, death from massive hemorrhage. In the 29 cases treated, 19 angiomas were completely excised, and 10 were incompletely removed or treated (ligation of the posterior pedicles, excision of the posterior portion, or both). Six cases were totally cured. Great improvement in clinical condition was noted in 11 cases, 3 were moderately improved, and in the remaining 9 no or very minimal improvement was noted. In summary, only 34 per cent of the patients treated (before 1968) benefited by operative therapy or embolization therapy or both.

In the second series of 100 cases (after 1968), active treatment of anterior angiomas was undertaken, adopted on the basis of the neurological picture of the patient at the time of angiography. Eighty-six cases were treated by excision or total embolization, and 10 cases were incompletely treated. Only four cases were not treated. Sixty-six cures, 20 ameliorations, and 10 failures or semifailures with one death from cardiac arrest at the emergence from anesthesia were noted. In summary, 86 per cent of the treatments were effective for the 92 per cent of cases treated.

If the progress seems moderate with respect to the number of subjects cured, it should be emphasized that the number of patients older than 60 years of age increased from 1 to 10 between the two series. Of these, two were cured, whereas the eight others were failures, or only very slightly improved.

Conclusion

Early diagnosis before irreversible spinal cord lesions have occurred produces a favorable prognosis. Neither age nor a variable neurological picture can exclude the possibility of an angioma. Angiography is necessary both for specific diagnosis and as

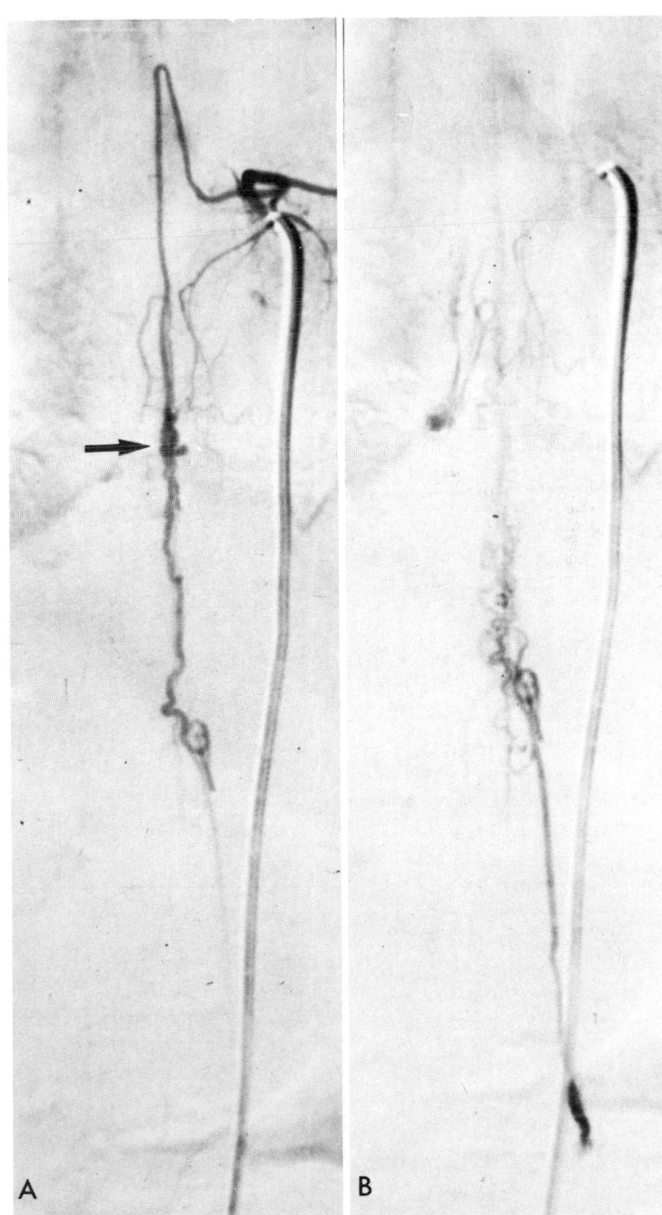

Figure 15–62 Operative treatment of an intramedullary angioma by means of a posterior commissural myelotomy. *A*. An angioma (*arrow*) fed by an artery of Adamkiewicz, is appreciated. *B*. Inferior draining veins are demonstrated. (From Djindjian, R., et al.: Les angiomes antérieurs de la moelle et leur traitement. Rev. Neurol., *133*:13–21, 1977. Reprinted by permission.)

a prelude to operative extirpation or embolic therapy.

ANGIOGRAPHY IN VERTEBROMEDULLARY TUMORS

Since 1964, 105 tumors have been angiographically evaluated at the Lariboisière Hospital and are the basis for this discussion. While myelography may suggest the presence of a neoplasm, angiography may allow an etiological diagnosis and permit precise identification of tumor vascularity.

Intraspinal Hemangioblastoma (13 Cases)

A highly vascular tumor, the hemangioblastoma is ideally suited for angiographic evaluation. Several features of these neoplasms should be emphasized: (1) The angiographic appearance of spinal hemangioblastoma is identical to that of cerebellar hemangioblastoma. (2) The arteriographic image of spinal hemangioblastoma is different from that of angiomas of the spinal cord. (3) These lesions very often are multiple, and sometimes very small, and therefore may be clinically silent (Fig. 15–63). (4) Angiography of the cerebellum, cerebrum, and retina permits one to localize multiple, often clinically silent, lesions associated with von Hippel–Lindau disease (Fig. 15–64). Circular calcifications of the ocular globe have been previously described in association with well-developed retinal lesions, but none were identified within the retina or spinal cord in the authors' series. (5) Angiographic evaluation of abdominal viscera (kidneys, pancreas, and adrenals) may demonstrate lesions morphologically identical with central nervous system hemangioblastomas and the possible coexistence of other entities (von Recklinghausen disease, Sturge-Wever syndrome).

Standard and Tomographic Study of the Spine

Like any expanding process, an intraspinal hemangioblastoma can initially present as a nonspecific osseous or myelographic abnormality. The plain and tomographic characteristics of hemangioblastoma were as follows: (1) Abnormalities of the spine were found in 40 per cent of these cases. Deformities such as a scoliosis (usually in younger individuals) were seen in 38 per cent of the abnormal subjects. (2) A diffuse or rather symmetrically enlarged

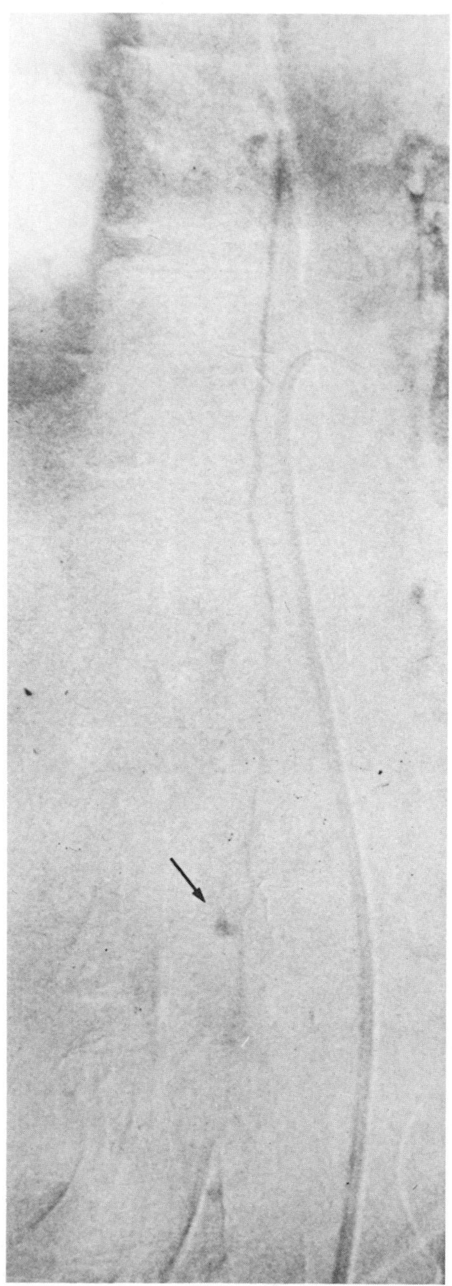

Figure 15–63 A small asymptomatic hemangioblastoma (*arrow*) is fed by the anterior spinal artery (T10).

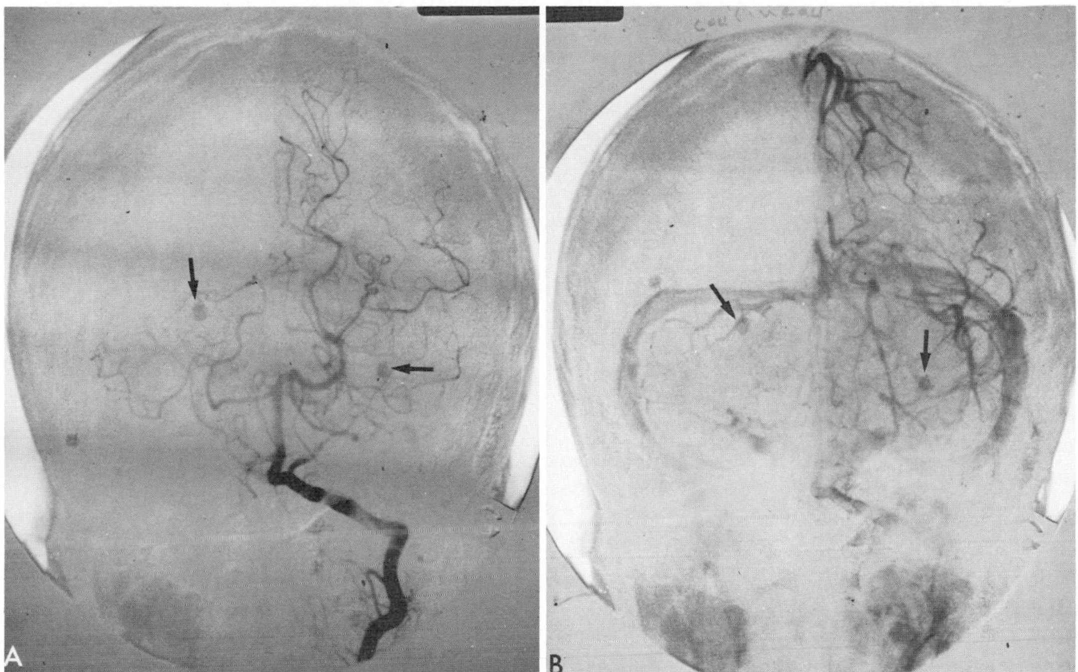

Figure 15–64 An asymptomatic subtentorial collection of hemangioblastomas (*arrows*). *A*. Arterial phase. *B*. Venous phase.

spinal canal, as evidenced by an increase in the interpedicular distance or by the sagittal diameter, was noted in 30 per cent of pathological spines. (3) A localized erosion of a pedicle, of a vertebral body, or of a lamina accounted for 25 per cent of the anomalies. This was usually seen in extradural hemangioblastomas. In one case an enlarged intervertebral neural foramen due to an hourglass-shaped hemangioblastoma was noted. Spina bifida and cervical ribs may be seen, but are probably incidental findings. (4) One case of an angiographically suggested hemangioblastoma was associated with a metameric "lattice work" vertebra not previously described in the literature.

Spinal Angiography

Spinal angiography is the only examination that permits a preoperative diagnosis of hemangioblastoma. Angiography allows the study of the form and structure and size of the tumor, the existence of single or multiple tumors, the nutrient arterial pedicles, the draining veins, and the extent of associated intracranial and abdominal lesions.

Technique of Spinal Angiography

Study of the entire spinal cord is indicated if a lesion is detected, because of the frequency of multiple hemangioblastomas (25 per cent). The value of delayed angiographic sequence filming (up to 30 to 35 seconds), in order to visualize draining veins optimally, should be emphasized. One film per second during the first 10 seconds, followed by one film per 2 or 3 seconds for 20 to 25 seconds is recommended.

Image subtraction by photographic or electronic processes (single or double mask) is indispensable, especially when Pantopaque oil droplet residues are present. Again, water-soluble myelographic agents are recommended to prevent suboptimal subtraction results.

Angiographic Appearance of the Hemangioblastomic Tumor

Regardless of its location along the neural axis, the hemangioblastoma has a pathognomonic angiographic appearance that is a direct reflection of its histological structure. This structure consists of intermingled vascular lakes in the form of multiple bunches of dilated capillaries, which are responsible for the early and dense angiographic opacification. Intravascular tumorous islets produce a picture of coherent regularly circumscribed lesions that compress neighboring normal vascular structures. Thus, early opacification (from the third second) progresses to a steadily increasing dense homogeneous blush that persists for a long time (mean 16.9 seconds) and has distinct boundaries (Fig. 15–65). This appearance is in contrast with the rapid arteriovenous shunting of the medullary angioma. Anatomically, hemangioblastomas present as well-circumscribed tumors, rounded or oval and rarely multilobuled, well encapsulated, and easily separable from the normal cord parenchyma.

The presence of cystic or pseudosyringomyelic cavities appears angiographically as an irregular area of tumor opacification with more or less marked notches connected to the cyst. A small hemangioblastoma demonstrated angiographically may be associated with a paradoxical complete block of myelographic material due to a large associated cyst. A cystic hemangioblastoma may rarely manifest itself angiographically by simple arterial displacement without tumor "blush." It is possible that the presence of a cyst may hinder the arteriographic opacification of spinal cord hemangioblastomas in the same way that intracranial hypertension can thwart the identification of cerebral hemangioblastomas.

SIZE OF THE TUMOR. The size of these tumors is variable, but usually they are me-

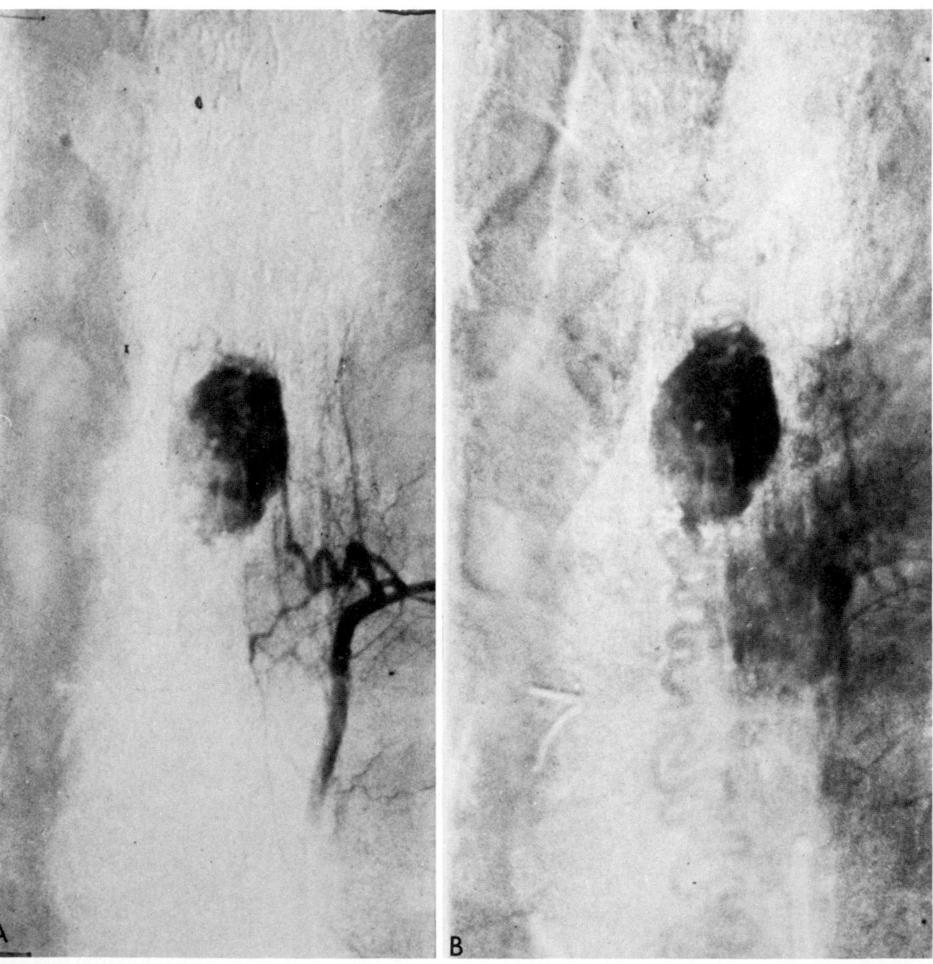

Figure 15–65 Intramedullary hemangioblastoma at T5–T6. *A*. Early arterial phase. *B*. Later angiographic phase. (From Djindjian, R., et al.: Superselective arteriographic embolization by the femoral route in neuroradiology. Neuroradiology, *6*:132–142, 1973. Reprinted by permission.)

dium-sized (less than 8 cm) or small lesions. The large tumors (sometimes 8 to 10 cm) involve several vertebral segments; in the cervical region it is not unusual to see two vertebral, deep cervical, and some superior intercostal arteries supplying these larger lesions.

Even small tumors may have recognizable draining veins, and it is this feature that permits them to be identified angiographically. Arteriography is capable of detecting with precision some tumors less than 3 mm in diameter. Only the microscopic hemangioblastomas (generally no larger than the head of a pin) do not show angiographically recognizable draining veins, but these are fortunately asymptomatic.

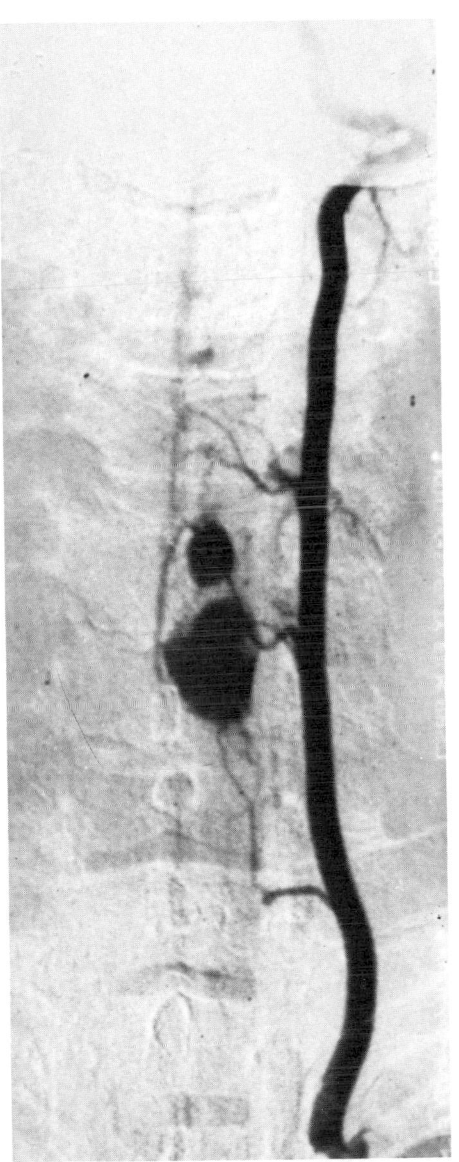

Figure 15–66 Vertebral angiogram. Multiple hemangioblastomas of the cervical region are appreciated.

NUMBER OF TUMORS. Multiplicity of lesions is not unusual (Fig. 15–66). It is not rare to find five or six hemangioblastic tumors in the same individual. In one of the authors' cases, 10 lesions were scattered from the cervical cord to the conus medullaris.

SITE OF THE TUMOR. The typical intramedullary hemangioblastoma (66 per cent, or 97 of 138 cases) is a fleshy mass located posterior to the central canal, flush with the cord surface, and covered by a thin leptomeningeal membrane. This is particularly true of small tumors. Its identification at operation is therefore easy. The large tumors, however, occupy the greater part of the spinal cord, leaving intact only a small peripheral portion of medullary tissue.

The intradural, extramedullary tumors (10 of 138 cases) are lesions independent of the spinal cord and its nerve roots. They are often in a more or less lateralized retromedullary site.

The radicular hemangioblastomas (28 tumors) develop among the root filaments at the level of the spinal cord, or at the level of the cauda equina, and can be quite large. These tumors almost always develop on the posterior roots. They may include an hourglass extension through the neural foramen. It is usually possible to identify a radicular hemangioblastoma angiographically, including its draining veins, especially the hourglass type.

It is difficult to differentiate the intradural extramedullary from the intramedullary hemangioblastomas, inasmuch as combined types are frequent. Tumoral opacification in the posterior half of the cord and abuttment on the surface of the cord by the tumor in the lateral projection should suggest an intramedullary tumor. Angiotomography and computed tomography (CT) can provide supplementary information.

The presence of extradural hemangioblastomas is less frequently seen (12 per cent), and its existence as a well-defined entity is debated by some.

CRANIOCAUDAL DISTRIBUTION. The tumors are located preferentially at places of normal cord enlargement (50 per cent). Tumors of the thoracic and thoracolumbar regions predominate over tumors of the cervical spinal cord. These findings are in accord with the maturation of the spinal vascular system.

THE NUTRIENT ARTERIES. These are enlarged but otherwise normal arteries of the anterior and posterior lateral spinal arterial axes. These vessels never attain the size of the dolichomegalic arteries of angiomas of the spinal cord.

As a general rule, the small intramedullary hemangioblastomas are supplied by only one anterior spinal artery, while the medium-sized tumors may be supplied by either one anterior or one posterior spinal artery. Large tumors are supplied by both anterior and posterior arteries. In the latter case, these vessels are very well developed and are widely anastomotic with the contralateral and ipsilateral sub- and suprajacent posterior spinal arteries. The anterior portion of the intramedullary hemangioblastoma is supplied by dilated sulcocommissural arteries, which are quite visible in the lateral projections.

In the high cervical region it is necessary to study vertebral and deep cervical arteries bilaterally. Superficial or inferiorly situated cerebellar hemangioblastomas may be supplied by meningeal branches of the ascending pharyngeal, occipital, or middle meningeal arteries. Therefore, it is neces-

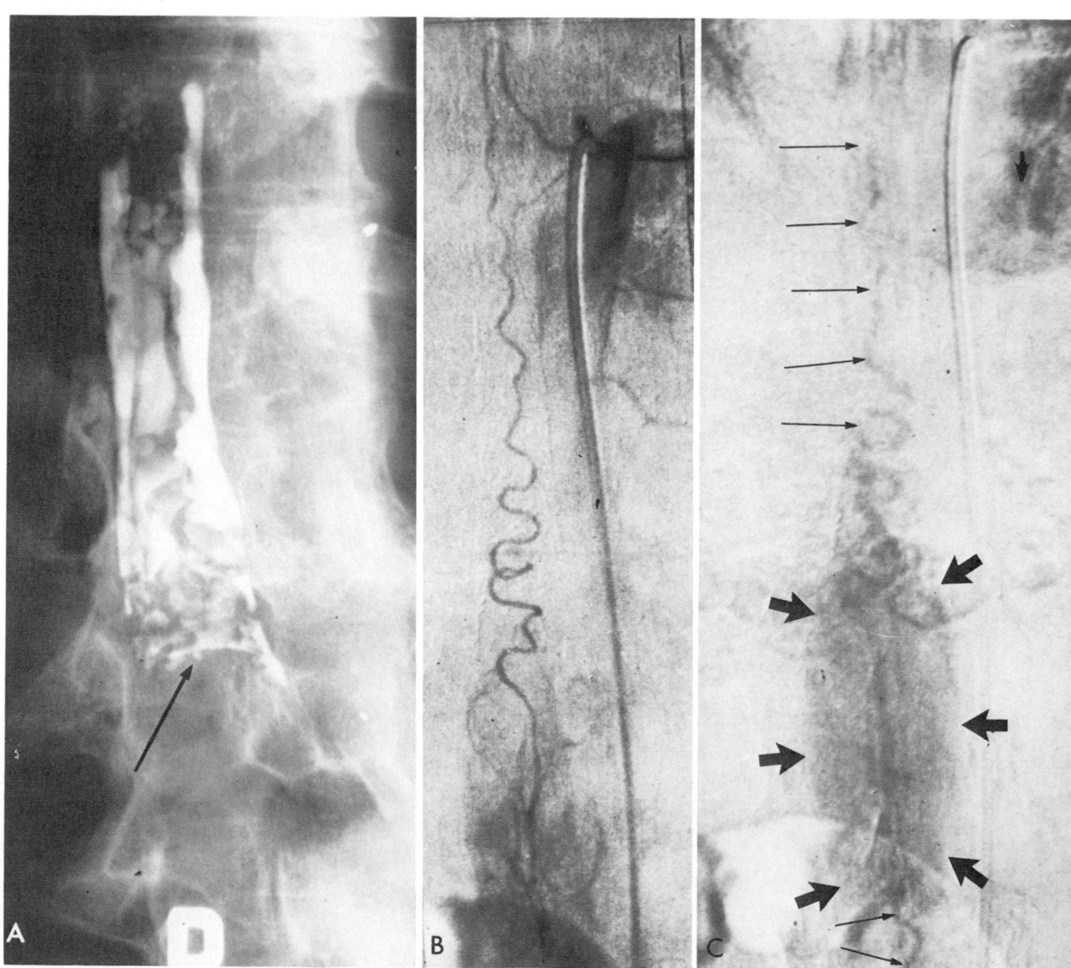

Figure 15–67 An ependymoma of the cauda equina. *A*. Pantopaque myelography demonstrates subjacent vascular imprints and a complete block (*arrow*). *B*. Arteriography shows a tumor blush supplied by the artery of Adamkiewicz. *C*. Later arterial phase: Tumor opacification is better appreciated (*large arrows*) with ascending and descending venous drainage (*small arrows*). (*B* and *C* from Djindjian, M., et al.: Subarachnoid hemorrhage due to intraspinal tumors. Surg. Neurol., *9*:223–229, 1978. Reprinted by permission.)

sary to study not only the cervical arteries but also the branches of the external carotid if high cervico-occipital lesions are suspected. The nutrient branches of radicular hemangioblastomas are often difficult to demonstrate.

THE DRAINING VEINS. These vessels are seen in 43 per cent of cases and are often large, sometimes even monstrous in size. In order to demonstrate them, it is necessary to perform serial angiography with long-sequence filming, for they may not be seen until after 25 to 35 seconds or even longer. The slow circulation contrasts with that in medullary angiomas, in which the draining veins may appear from six seconds onward and disappear rapidly. These neovessels form a network of greater density at the level of the tumor itself with some intramedullary extensions.

The draining veins of hemangioblastomas are primarily retromedullary in location and can extend along the entirety of the spinal cord from the cervical region to the conus medullaris. It is thus understandable that at operation without angiography one can confuse them with the draining veins of a medullary angioma if the laminectomy window demonstrates only the veins and not the tumor mass.

The radiculomedullary veins drain laterally toward the intercostal veins and the azygous system, inferiorly toward the spinal venous plexus, and from these into the vena cava. Superiorly they drain by the pontomesencephalic veins into the jugular system.

Spinal Cord Tumors of Glial Origin

Ependymomas may produce a faint tumor blush. In one case, posterolateral spinal arteries were displaced, suggesting a widened cord (Fig. 15–67). Dilated intramedullary veins have also been observed.[8] DiChiro and co-workers have also described nonpathognomonic changes in ependymomas, including displaced and somewhat pathological vessels, with large draining veins.[5,10]

Except for the ependymomas, the authors have never obtained definite tumoral opacification of a glial cell tumor, but arteriography may nevertheless be advantageous in two ways: first, to rule out an angioma, and second, to confirm the existence of a tumor and its intramedullary localization by the type or manner of displacement of spinal cord vessels.

Both the anterior spinal arteries (artery of the cervical enlargement, superior dorsal artery, and artery of the lumbar enlargement) and the posterior spinal arteries are larger and therefore more easily opacified than in normal subjects. On the anteroposterior projection, the anterior and posterior spinal arteries may be compressed laterally, which indicates the existence of an expanding lesion without localizing it. On the lateral views, an increase in spinal cord diameter will be demonstrated by compression of the anterior spinal artery against the posterior vertebral border and posterior displacement of the posterior spinal arteries.

Neuromas

While some of these tumors are not opacified by angiography (two cauda equina neuromas and one located in the thoracolumbar region close to the artery of Adamkiewicz), the majority of these tumors do demonstrate a tumor blush that is discrete, homogeneous, dense, and ovoid during the capillary phase (Fig. 15–68). This appearance is similar to that of neuromas of the cerebellopontine angle. During the capillary phase fine trabeculations with a bordering edge are present. There are no early arteriovenous fistulae, which suggests the benign histological nature of these tumors. The extraspinal extension of the neoplasms is accompanied by a deformation of the vertebral artery in the cervical region, of the intercostal and lumbar arteries in the lower regions. In the lateral projection, the tumor mass appears superimposed on the intervertebral foramina.

Thoracolumbar neuromas may displace the kidneys and ureters by extraspinal tumor spread. Thus, lateral films of the abdomen to visualize such displacements are useful. Invasion of the inferior vena cava may be present, and cavography is also recommended.

Meningiomas

These neoplasms usually demonstrate a moderate homogeneous blush with poorly

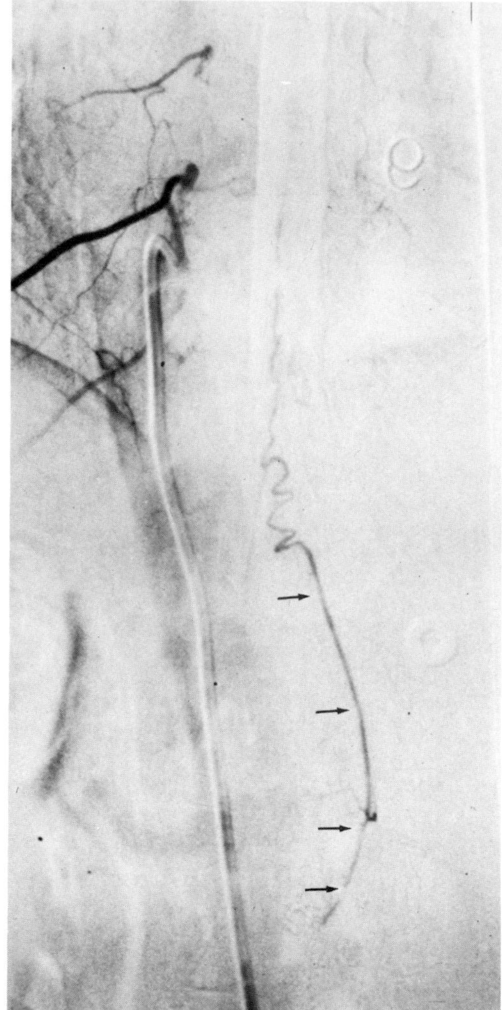

Figure 15–68 A giant neuroma of the cauda equina. Dilatation of the anterior spinal axis is appreciated (*arrows*). (From Djindjian, M., et al.: Subarachnoid hemorrhage due to spinal tumors. Surg. Neurol., 9:223–229, 1978. Reprinted by permission.)

defined limits, supplied by multiple dilated branches of duromeningeal, radicular, muscular, or osseous arteries.

Vertebroepidural Tumors

Vertebral hemangiomas demonstrate classic *plain radiographic* findings with a latticed appearance of the vertebral body that is often accompanied by characteristic hypertrophy of the posterior arch (Fig. 15–69*A*).

The *angiographic* findings demonstrated by angiomatous vertebrae are also characteristic, consisting of confluent vascular lacunae of variable size occupying the *whole* of the vertebra and extending to the vertebral lamina (Fig. 15–69*B*). In the late capillary phase the tumor blush loses its lacunar character, becoming diffuse, dense, and homogeneous. This pattern of opacification allows one to differentiate angiomatous vertebrae from normal osseous structures. In the latter, the opacification is homogeneous and always limited to *one half* of the vertebral body, corresponding to the side of injection. Pathological vertebrae often demonstrate one or two sinuous dilated arterials supplying these structures during the arterial phase. They arise from the intercostal or lumbar arteries a little way beyond the origin of the muscular branches and before the medullary arteries, where they penetrate at the same level. Such arteries are never encountered in the normal individual.

Lateral angiography demonstrates the extraosseous extension of an angiomatous tumor, notably posteriorly toward the spinal canal. This associated epidural extension will be confirmed by myelography.

Finally, the level of penetration of the spinal arterial supply in relationship to the pathological vertebra can be precisely demonstrated. This is valuable information, not only if operative intervention is considered but also for any decision involving radiation therapy. The proximity of the spinal artery to an involved vertebra is important when the risk of postradiation vascular necrosis and spinal cord ischemia is being considered. Examples of such complications are not lacking in the literature and are explained by the continuity existing between the irradiated vertebrae and the arterial afferent to the cord.

Aneurysmal Bone Cysts

Arteriography shows a more or less sharply delineated area of opacification ranging from a faint density in some cases to veritable vascular lakes. In one study by Voigt and co-workers, two lesions were demonstrated in the cervical area, two in the lumbar region, and five in the thoracic spine. Of these, two cases were angiographically normal, one demonstrated mild displacement of arterial structures, four demonstrated a benign diffuse and homogeneous pattern, and in two the lesions could not be distinguished from malignant bone tumors.[22]

Malignant Tumors

Vertebral medullary and epidural metastases usually are evident and well opacified. Early arteriovenous fistulae, poor edge definition, blood pools, and pathological vessels, may suggest their malignant nature.[22] The extraspinal extension of the tumor, which is sometimes considerable, can easily be defined. The identification of feeding vessels may be helpful in palliative embolization procedures, alone or as an adjunct to operative intervention.

Miscellaneous Osseous Lesions

In *chronic inflammatory disease* (80 per cent of the cases of tuberculosis), a persistent late arterial capillary phase stain was

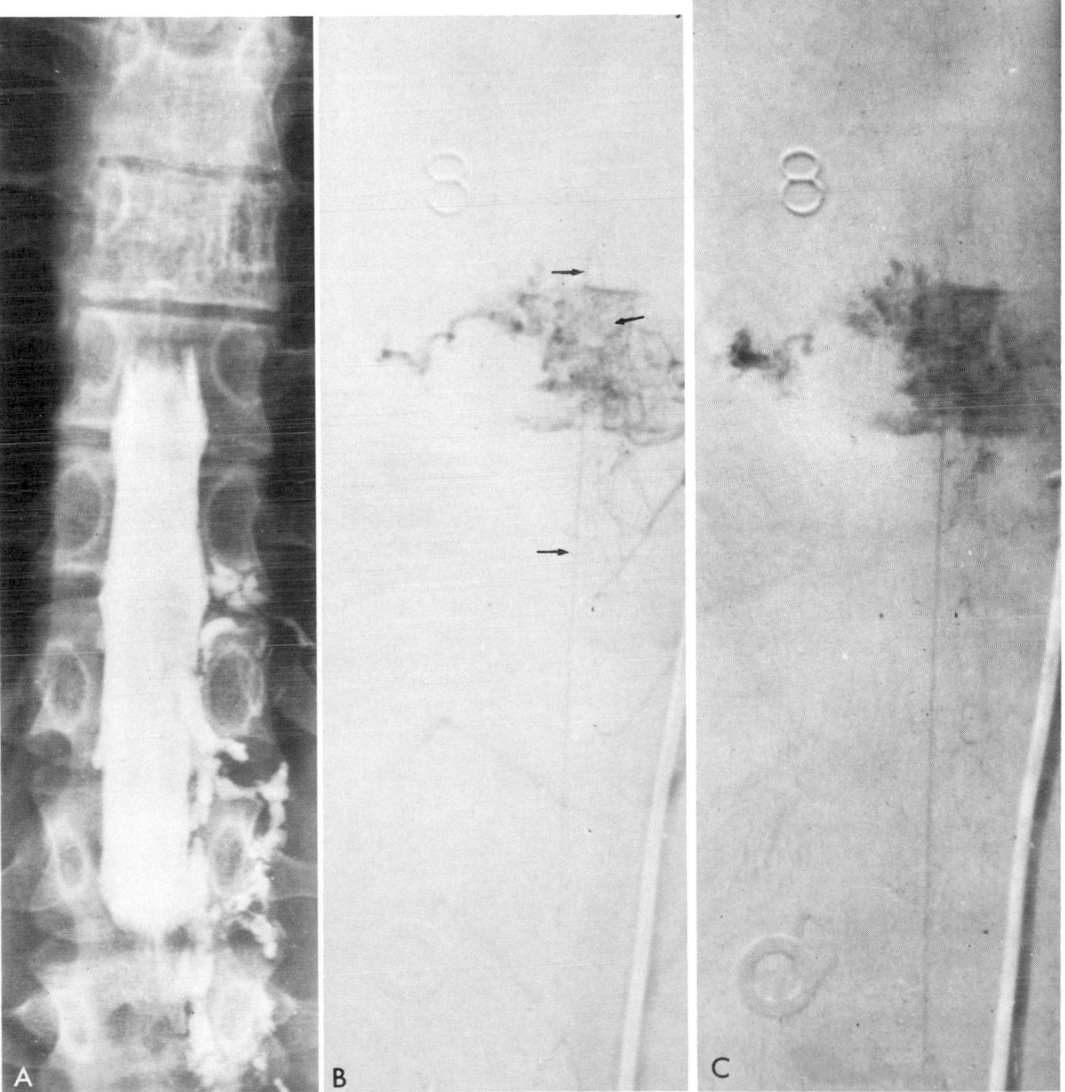

Figure 15–69 Vertebral hemangioma with paraplegia. *A*. Pantopaque myelography shows a block caudal to the vertebral hemangioma. *B* and *C*. Subtraction angiography. Injection of the left T9 intercostal vessel opacifies the vertebral hemangioma and also demonstrates the anterior spinal axis (*arrows*). In this case, embolization is contraindicated.

present, occasionally extending into the paravertebral region.[22]

Two cases of *chondroma* demonstrated nonspecific avascular displacement of the artery of Adamkiewicz, while two showed no angiographic abnormality whatsoever. Two of three cases of *giant cell tumors* were normal angiographically, with one demonstrating changes that could not be distinguished from frankly malignant lesions.[22]

ANGIOGRAPHY IN SPINAL CORD ISCHEMIA FROM ATHEROMATOUS OR DISC LESIONS

Because of the suboptimal collateral flow between the three major anterior spinal arterial territories, the zones between these areas are especially prone to ischemic insults and are often the first regions of the cord to demonstrate such changes clinically.

Total or partial intrinsic or extrinsic obstruction of the arterial supply to an area of spinal cord, regardless of localization, may manifest itself by two angiographic signs: a direct sign represented by deviation or narrowing of the vessel by vertebral disc protrusion or stenosis secondary to atheromatous thrombosis; and an indirect sign, which is the demonstration of collateral circulation in an area of ischemia that tends to compensate for the absence of normal vascular supply.

Cervical Spinal Cord

The opacification of the complete anterior spinal arterial network is very unusual in the normal subject, since the anterior spinal artery (a branch of the vertebral artery) is visible in only 50 per cent of cases. This network appears on the arteriogram when there is a compromise of the normal vasculature and thus, paradoxically, is the pathological pattern.

Thoracolumbar Spinal Cord

Lazorthes, Gouaze, and co-workers showed that the inferior lumbosacral arteries "constitute a potential arterial supply on which the lumbar enlargement can call in case of deficiency of the artery of the lumbar enlargement" (Adamkiewicz).[17] Selective arteriography of the arterial afferents of the dorsolumbosacral spinal cord has permitted confirmation of these anatomical studies in vivo by opacifying the lumbosacral radicular arteries when an ischemic process is present that involves the artery of Adamkiewicz. Thus, the territory usually supplied by the artery of Adamkiewicz can be covered by the substitute radicular lumbosacral network in the anastomotic loop of the conus.

Thoracolumbar Disc Herniations

Compression by a herniated disc without arteriographic displacement of the artery of Adamkiewicz may occur close to the latter's origin from the intercostal artery at the level of the intervertebral foramen. Thus, a contralateral and very lateralized operative approach in such cases would be indicated. Compression of the descending branch of the artery of Adamkiewicz by median dorsal disc protrusion will, by contrast, show arterial deformations. On the anteroposterior projections, one will observe a discrete displacement of the artery of Adamkiewicz or perhaps a major compression of that artery at the level of the pathological interspace. In the lateral projection, the descending branch of the artery of Adamkiewicz will be displaced posteriorly according to the size of the disc protrusion (Fig. 15–70). Knowledge of the exact position of the artery of Adamkiewicz will prevent its injury at the time of operative intervention.

Aortic Atheromatous Lesions

These lesions are limited in size, and are proximal in location, involving the first 2 cm of the intercostal artery or, occasionally, only the first few millimeters around the ostium (Fig. 15–71). Rarely the lesion may extend over 3 to 4 cm. The degree of obstruction is variable, ranging from simple stenosis to total arterial obstruction. Atheromatous lesions of the artery of Adamkiewicz are exceptional. Selective arteriography of this vessel may demonstrate the presence of a proximal stenosis of the inter-

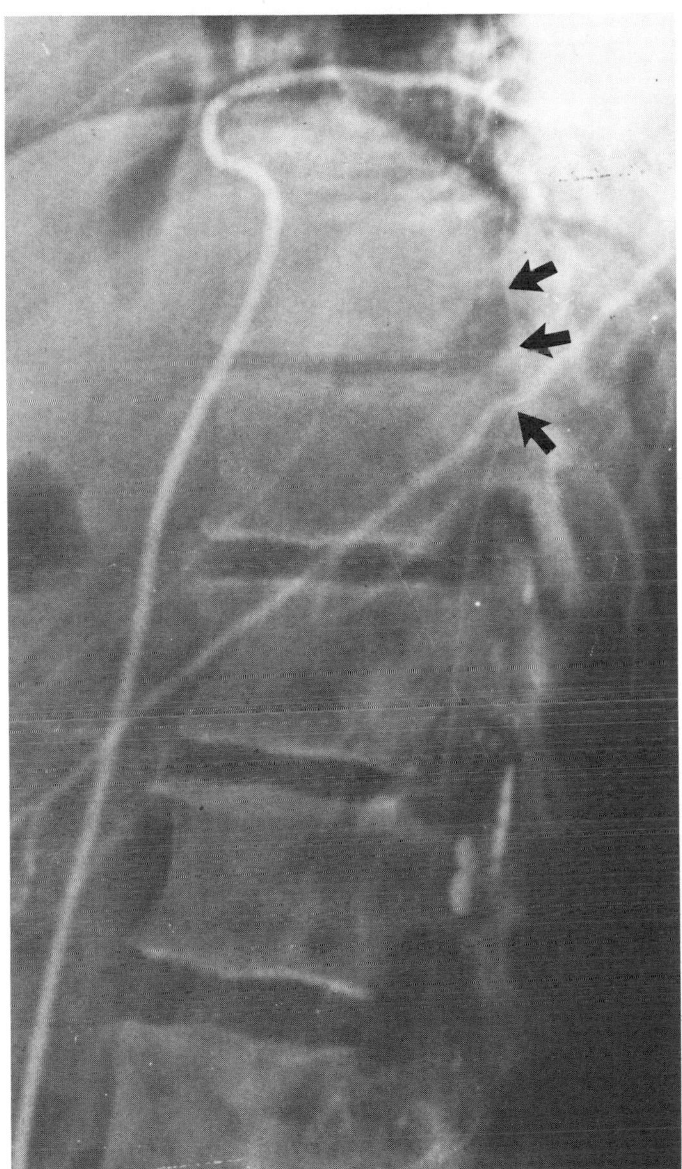

Figure 15–70 Angiography, lateral view, of a dorsal disc herniation. The artery of Adamkiewicz is reduplicated or bent at the level of discopathy (*arrows*). (From Djindjian, R., Hurth, M., and Houdart, R.: Angiography of the Spinal Cord. Paris, Masson & Cie; Baltimore, Md., University Park Press, 1970. Reprinted by permission.)

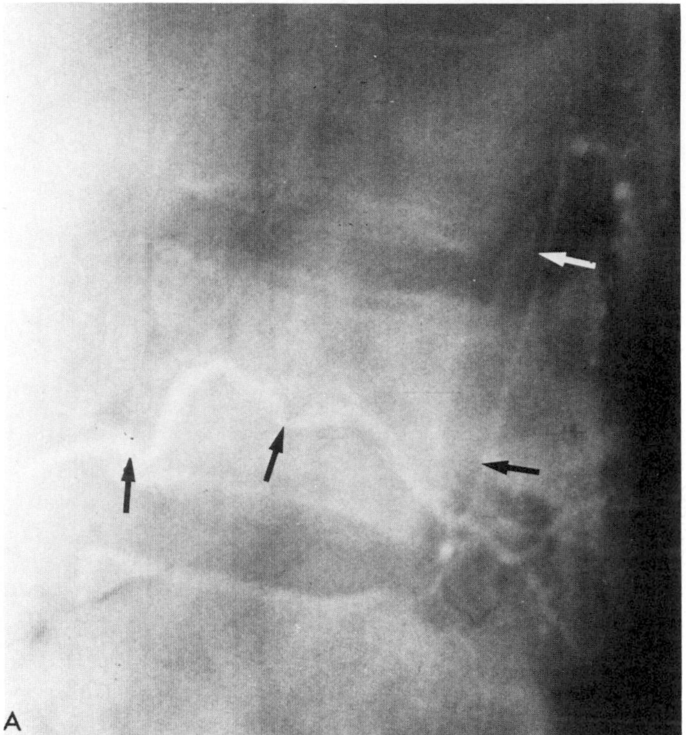

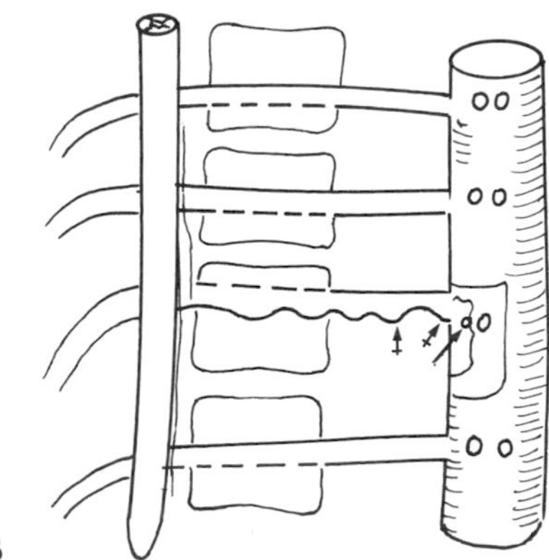

Figure 15–71 Lateral angiography, left T12. *A*. Stenosis of the intercostal artery and a sinuous trajectory and atheromas of this artery are appreciated (*black arrows*). The anterior spinal artery is faintly visualized (*white arrow*). *B*. Diagrammatic representation of the arteriostenosis (*barred arrows*). (*A* from Djindjian, R., Hurth, M., and Houdart, R.: Angiography of the Spinal Cord. Paris, Masson & Cie; Baltimore, Md., University Park Press, 1970. Reprinted by permission. *B* modified from Djindjian, R., et al.: Angiography of the spinal cord. Yield and orientation of the research after 10 years' experience. Acta Radiol. [Diagn.] (Stockholm), *13*:771–791, 1972.)

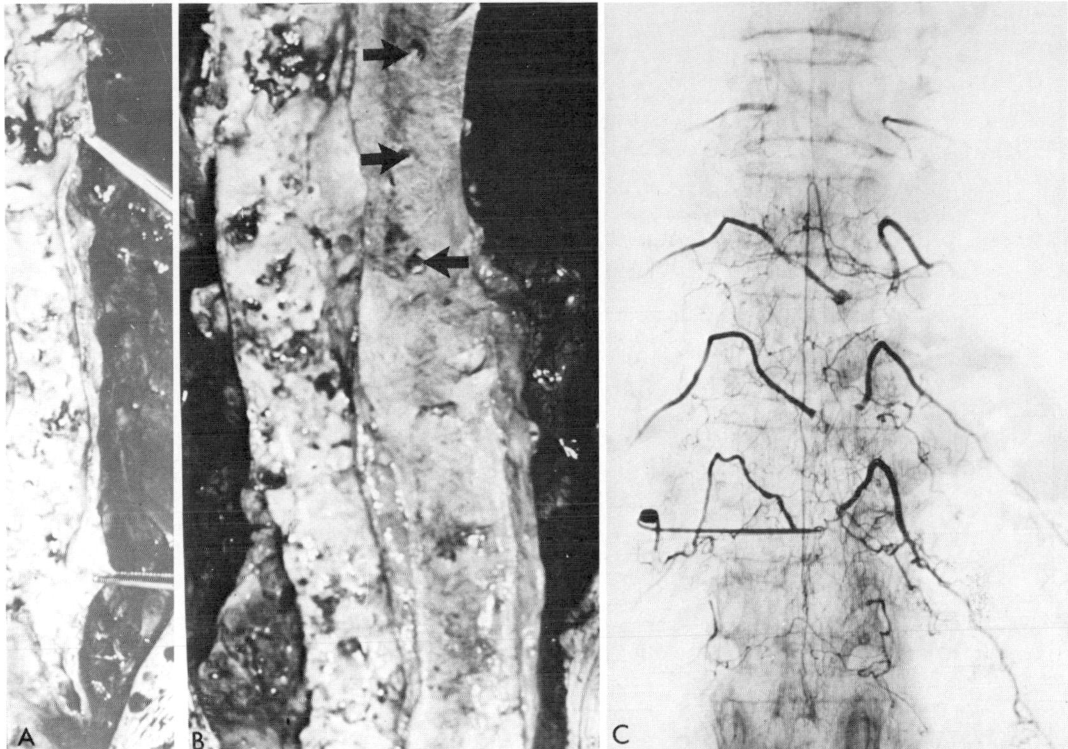

Figure 15–72 *A*. Dissection of the thoracolumbar aorta in an elderly patient who had succumbed following flaccid paraplegia of sudden onset. The significance of the atheromatous obstruction of the intercostal ostia and the lumbar arteries is not appreciated on this preparation. *B*. After endarterectomy, the wall of the aorta and the various ostia (*arrows*) are appreciated. *C*. Selective postmortem angiography demonstrates the origin of the artery of Adamkiewicz arising from the eleventh left intercostal artery, where the ostium had been obstructed prior to endarterectomy. (From Djindjian, R., Hurth, M., and Houdart, R.: Angiography of the Spinal Cord. Paris Masson & Cie; Baltimore, Md., University Park Press, 1970. Reprinted by permission.)

costal or lumbar carrier artery (Fig. 15–72). This narrowing can lie in the ostium itself, flush with the aorta, or a little downstream from the orifice.

These lesions may be the etiological agents in a number of "myelopathies of undetermined origin." Transcatheter angioplasties of the atheromatous aortic plaque at the level of the stenotic ostium, have been accomplished in four cases to date.

REFERENCES

1. Adamkiewicz, A.: Die Blutgefässe des menschlichen Rückenmarkesoberflache Sitzung. Akad. Wissensch. Wien. Math. Natur. Klasse, 1882–1885.
2. Corbin, J. L.: Anatomie et Pathologie Arterilles de la Moelle. Paris, Masson & Cie, 1961.
3. DiChiro, G.: Recent successes and failures in radiographic and radioisotopic angiography of the spinal cord. Brit. J. Radiol., *45*:533–560, 1972.
4. DiChiro, G., and Wener, L.: Angiography of the spinal cord. A review of contemporary techniques and applications. J. Neurosurg., *39*:1–29, 1973.
5. DiChiro, G., and Wener, L.: Angiography of ependymomas of the spinal cord and filum terminale. Amer. J. Roentgen., *122*:628–633, 1974.
6. DiChiro, G., Jones, A. E., Johnston, G. S., et al.: Value and limits of radionuclide angiography of the spinal cord. Radiology, *109*:125–130, 1973.
7. Djindjian, R.: Angiography of the spinal cord. Surg. Neurol., *2*:179–185, 1974.
8. Djindjian, R., Hurth, M., and Houdart, R.: Angiography of the Spinal Cord. Baltimore, University Park Press, 1970.
9. Doppman, J. L., and DiChiro, G.: Paraspinal muscle infarction. A painful complication of lumbar artery embolization associated with pathognomonic radiographic and laboratory findings. Radiology, *119*:609–613, 1976.
10. Doppman, J. L., DiChiro, G., and Ommaya, A. K.: Selective Arteriography of the Spinal Cord. St. Louis, Warren H. Green Inc., 1969.
11. Fauré, C., Djindjian, R., and Lefebvre, J.: A propos du risque médullaire de l'aortographie abdominale. Ann. Radiol. (Paris), *9*:523–530, 1966.
12. Houdart, R., Djindjian, R., Hurth, M., et al.:

Treatment of angiomas of the spinal cord. Surg. Neurol., *2*:186–194, 1974.
13. Jellinger, K.: Zür Orthologie und Pathologie der Ruckenmarksdurch blutung. Vienna, Springer-Verlag, 1966.
14. Kerber, C. W., Cromwell, L. D., and Sheptak, P. E.: Intra-arterial cyanoacrylate: An adjunct in the treatment of spinal/paraspinal arteriovenous malformations. Amer. J. Roentgen., *103*:99–103, 1978.
15. Killen, D. A., and Foster, J. H.: Spinal cord injury as a complication of contrast angiography. Surgery, *59*:969–981, 1966.
16. Lazorthes, G.: Pathology, classification and clinical aspects of vascular diseases of the spinal cord. *In* Vinken, P. J., and Bruyn, G. W., eds.: Handbook of Clinical Neurology. Vol. 12, Part II. New York, American Elsevier Publishing Co., 1972, p. 492.
17. Lazorthes, G., Gouaze, A., Bastide, G., et al.: La vascularization artérielle du renflement lombaire. Etude des variations et des suppleances. Rev. Neurol. (Paris), *114*:109–122, 1966.
18. Mishkin, M. M., Baum, S., Ng, L., et al.: Cerebrospinal fluid iodine levels in uncomplicated and complicated angiography. Invest. Radiol., *7*:439, 1972 (abstract).
19. Newton, T. H.: Personal communication, 1979.
20. Shiozawa, Z., Tankaka, Y., Makino, N., et al.: Spinal cord angiography using four times magnification. Radiology, *127*:181–184, 1978.
21. Suh, T. H., and Alexander, L.: Vascular system of the human spinal cord. Arch. Neurol. Psychiat., *41*:659–677, 1939.
22. Voigt, K., Hooglard, P. H., Stoeter, P., et al.: Diagnostic value and limitations of selective spinal angiography in different lesions of the vertebral bones. Radiol. Clin. (Basel), *47*:73–90, 1978.

16

NEUROMUSCULAR ELECTRODIAGNOSIS

While techniques for the recording of electrical activity from nerves and muscles have been available for many years, they were used mainly in research until relatively modern times. The large number of peripheral nerve injuries seen in World War II stimulated interest in electrodiagnostic techniques, and the field of modern electrodiagnosis was born.

Currently there are three types of electrodiagnostic tests that are routinely available. These are electromyography (EMG), nerve conduction velocity (NCV) studies of both motor and sensory nerve fibers, and repetitive nerve stimulation studies that assess the function of the neuromuscular junction. With the development of reliable techniques for electromyography and nerve conduction velocity testing, the earlier techniques such as the determination of chronaxie, rheobase, and strength-duration curves are rarely performed.

INDICATIONS FOR ELECTRODIAGNOSTIC TESTING

As a general rule, electrodiagnostic testing is of little or no value in the evaluation of disorders of the central nervous system above the foramen magnum and of only limited value in the evaluation of upper motor neuron spinal cord disorders. The few exceptions are discussed later.

Electrodiagnostic testing is useful in the evaluation of disorders involving the motor unit, i.e., the anterior horn cell, its axon, the neuromuscular junction, and all the muscle fibers supplied by the anterior horn cell. Thus, on the motor side, disorders of the lower motor neuron, neuromuscular junction, and muscle itself are easily investigated. The addition of sensory nerve conduction velocity testing to the available test panel makes it possible to evaluate peripheral sensory mechanisms as well.

Taking into account the anatomical limitations of electrodiagnosis, it is apparent that its greatest value lies in the evaluation of weakness, fatigue, decreased muscle tone, and muscular atrophy. Furthermore, the sensitivity of procedures allows the detection of minimal dysfunction of the motor unit in the absence of clinical signs or in the presence of equivocal clinical findings. Also, functional weakness, e.g., hysteria or malingering, usually can be differentiated from organic dysfunction, and lower motor neuron disease can be detected even in the presence of concurrent upper motor neuron dysfunction. The value of electrodiagnostic techniques in the evaluation of sensory disturbances is much more limited at present and is mainly concerned with disturbed sensation in a peripheral nerve distribution, or in some cases, in a root distribution.

One important point must be kept in mind. Electrodiagnostic tests are capable of evaluating only the functional status of structures to which they are applicable. They do not provide an etiological diagnosis and they must be correlated with other information such as history, physical examination, and other laboratory data.

A list of the most common problems seen by a neurosurgeon for which electrodiagnostic tests are needed would be headed by root syndromes, usually associated with a herniated nucleus pulposus. In addition,

J. S. LIEBERMAN

the entrapment neuropathies and neural trauma are common problems that are easily investigated.

ELECTRICAL CHANGES AFTER ACUTE NERVE INJURY

After an acute nerve injury in which there is minimal damage to the neural tissue, very little is noted in the electromyogram. There may be a drop out of the number of motor units firing, but even this change may be difficult to detect. With more severe damage or complete injury, very few or no motor units can be found. At the same time, for the first several days, the muscle can and does respond normally to stimulation of its nerve supply distal to the injury site. Stimulation proximal to the injury site gives variable results depending on lesion type and severity. After three to four days, those axons that will not survive the injury begin to degenerate.

Eight to twenty-one days following the injury, electromyographic examination reveals abnormal irritability in those muscles whose nerve supply is affected. This abnormal activity is described in more detail later.

Abnormal rest activity, also described later, appears 14 to 35 days following injury to muscles of the extremities. With injuries to short nerves, such as those to the paraspinous muscles, these changes may occur as early as 8 to 10 days later. Basically, the appearance of abnormal rest activity is dependent on the axonal length between the injury site and the muscle that is studied: The closer a tested muscle is to the site of the lesion, the earlier the electromyographic changes will be seen.

Electrodiagnostic studies should be ordered no earlier than the mean time for appearance of electromyographic changes, which in most cases is 21 days after the injury. The same holds true for studies involving nerve conduction velocity changes. The *exceptions* include acute peripheral nerve trauma. The value and limitations of immediate studies in this type of injury are discussed in the section on clinical applications.

Like abnormal insertional and rest activity, abnormal motor unit potentials have a certain time course for their development. Several months must elapse before absolutely typical changes are seen with great frequency. When regeneration has occurred or is occurring, the electromyogram can detect its appearance before it is revealed by the clinical examination.

THE ELECTRODIAGNOSTIC STUDY

Requesting the Study

Care in ordering an electrodiagnostic study will help to insure that maximum information is obtained. As mentioned earlier, the timing of the study is important. In most conditions of importance to the neurosurgeon, an average of 21 days should elapse between insult and investigation in order to maximize the chance of finding abnormal electrical signs. Studies that are ordered too early often will provide false negative results, and retesting will be required at a later date. Studies ordered late in the course of a problem may likewise fail to yield all of the desired information that could be obtained from a study at the proper time. With an acute problem, electrodiagnosis is of limited value. The major exception in acute problems is the ability to show whether a peripheral nerve is functionally or anatomically intact after trauma to an extremity. This is discussed in greater detail in the section on nerve injuries.

The physician requesting the study should provide as much clinical information as possible to the electromyographer. At the very least, the diagnostic problem that the clinician suspects should be stated. Most electromyographers take a brief history and do a brief examination in order to plan the study properly. Their history taking and examination, however, are no substitute for adequate clinical information. It should be realized that unlike an electrocardiogram or electroencephalogram, the electromyogram follows no set procedure and each examination is an individual one, tailored to the patient's problems. Further, it is a dynamic study that is modified as the examination proceeds and the results become available.

To illustrate the foregoing discussion, it is not unusual for the clinician to suspect a carpal tunnel syndrome and to ask for appropriate motor and sensory nerve conduction studies. Should these be negative, but the patient have appropriate signs, the experienced electrodiagnostician will also do an electromyogram to find the possible C6 root lesion. Conversely, it is not unusual to see a request for an electromyogram and nerve conduction velocity study in all four extremities to confirm the suspicion of a right L5 root lesion. If the electromyogram shows that there is indeed only the suspected root lesion, the patient should not be subjected to a long, expensive, uncomfortable, and fruitless study.

The patient must be prepared for the test. All the tests are time consuming and usually require a minimum of 30 minutes for a simple problem and longer than one hour for more complex ones. Both needle electromyographic studies and electrical stimulation studies are uncomfortable and sometimes are painful. The patient should understand that the tests will cause pain and that no sedation or anesthetic will be given because his cooperation is needed during the tests. When the tests are to be done on a child, the parents must be told about patient discomfort even though the child is not told until their arrival at the laboratory.

Most electromyographic studies are done with monopolar needles, although bipolar or coaxial needles are still in use. The monopolar needles are thinner and cause less discomfort. They may make the test more bearable for a patient with little pain tolerance. There is, however, no choice of technique with respect to nerve stimulation studies.

Electromyography

The essential apparatus for both electromyography and nerve conduction studies includes electrodes, a preamplifier, a loud speaker and audio amplifier, and an oscilloscope. A physiological stimulator is required for nerve conduction and repetitive nerve stimulation studies. Permanent records of the tests usually are not made, but tape recorders, cameras, and photographic recorders are available for this purpose.

On the assumption that the proper equipment is available, the electromyogram is planned so that the information derived will give a diagnostic impression of the type of abnormality and its anatomical distribution.

Each study will be slightly different, but the basic concept is to study an appropriate number of muscles so that any possible combination of peripheral nerve, root, or part of plexus can be covered. Whenever possible, at least two muscles are studied for each peripheral nerve, and each root level studied is derived from at least two peripheral nerves. Furthermore, when root or cord lesions are suspected, erector spinae muscles are included to localize the site of disease accurately. Tables 16–1 and 16–2 show typical upper and lower extremity nerve and root patterns and give examples of a typical screening electromyogram for both arm and leg. As more information is derived from the study, more muscles can be added to, for example, pinpoint a lesion along a particular peripheral nerve.

For each muscle that is studied, the report should give information in four spheres: (1) insertional activity, i.e., that electrical activity caused by insertion of the electrode or needle movement; (2) spontaneous activity, the presence or absence of electrical activity with the muscle at rest without needle movement or contraction, (3) motor unit action potential description during minimal contraction of the muscle being studied; and (4) motor unit action potential description during maximum contraction, the so-called interference pattern. This material may be presented either in tabular or narrative form, depending on the reporting style of the individual laboratory. A discussion of each phase of the report follows. In any case, all muscles studied should be listed and the technique should be described.

Insertional Activity

When a muscle is penetrated by a needle electrode, a brief burst of electrical activity occurs that lasts 10–300 msec. This activity probably is caused by mechanical stimulation or transient fiber injury. This activity *should* be present. It should have a crisp sound on the speaker, a sharp onset with needle insertion or movement, and an equally sharp cessation when needle movement stops. Insertional activity that normally is present is reported simply as such

TABLE 16–1 UPPER EXTREMITY MUSCLES NERVE AND ROOT SUPPLY

MUSCLE	MYO-TOME	PERIPHERAL NERVE
Sternocleidomastoid	C2, C3	Accessory
Trapezius	C2, C3, C4	Accessory
Rhomboid	C4, C5	Dorsal scapular
Supraspinatus	C5	Suprascapular
Infraspinatus	C5, C6	Suprascapular
Serratus anterior	C5, C6, C7	Long thoracic
Deltoid*	C5, C6	Axillary
Biceps*	C5, C6	Musculocutaneous
Brachioradialis	C5, C6	Radial
Supinator	C5, C6	Radial
Triceps*	C6, C7, C8	Radial
Extensor carpi radialis*	C6, C7, C8	Radial
Pronator teres	C6, C7	Median
Flexor carpi radialis*	C6, C7, C8	Median
Extensor digitorum communis	C7, C8	Radial
Flexor digitorum sublimis	C7, C8, T1	Median
Flexor digitorum profundus	C7, C8, T1	Median-ulnar
Flexor carpi ulnaris*	C8, T1	Ulnar
Thenar muscles*	C8, T1	Median
Dorsal interossei*	C8, T1	Ulnar
Hypothenar muscles*	C8, T1	Ulnar

* Minimum screening electromyogram for upper extremity.

without further detailed description. Absence of electrical activity on insertion indicates the absence of functioning muscle fibers or that the electrode is not in muscle tissue. It is also possible to have decreased insertional activity when a muscle is atrophied. This finding is reported as decreased insertional activity and is nonspecific, since either neuropathic or myopathic disease can cause it. Conversely, insertional activity can be increased, which means that it persists too long after movement of the needle. It, likewise, is a nonspecific finding in many cases. It is seen in inflammatory myopathies such as polymyositis and also early in neuropathic disorders. It may be reported simply as *increased irritability* or *increased insertional activity*. When it is in the distribution of only one root or peripheral nerve it may be considered the minimal or earliest abnormality present. The reliability of increased irritability as the sole diagnostic finding is directly proportional to the experience and judgment of the electromyographer. The extreme example of increased insertional activity is found in myotonia, e.g., in myotonic dystrophy, in which in many cases it is almost continuous after insertion of the needle. It is also, on occasion, difficult to separate increased insertional activity from certain types of bizarre spontaneous activity that are described later.

TABLE 16–2 LOWER EXTREMITY MUSCLES NERVE AND ROOT SUPPLY

MUSCLE	MYO-TOME	PERIPHERAL NERVE
Iliopsoas	L2, L3, L4	Femoral
Quadriceps femoris*	L2, L3, L4	Femoral
Sartorius	L2, L3	Femoral
Gluteus medius*	L4, L5, S1	Superior gluteal
Gluteus maximus	L5, S1, S2	Inferior gluteal
Tensor fasciae latae	L4, L5, S1	Superior gluteal
Hamstrings	L5, S1, S2	Sciatic
Adductor	L2, L3, L4	Obturator
Tibialis anterior*	L4, L5, S1	Peroneal
Peroneus longus*	L5, S1	Peroneal
Medial gastrocnemius*	S1, S2	Tibial
Lateral gastrocnemius	L5, S1, S2	Tibial
Tibialis posterior	L5, S1	Tibial

* Minimum screening electromyogram for lower extremity.

Resting or Spontaneous Activity

If the patient is properly relaxed, the normal muscle usually is silent at rest. This is a feature of the electronic engineering of the electromyograph. The amplifier measures only changes in voltage, and because at rest there is no electrical potential change, silence is present. The electromyograph, therefore, does not show the membrane potential.

The two exceptions to the rule of silence at rest concern activity in proximity to the neuromuscular junction. This activity is called either end-plate noise or nerve potentials, depending on the type of activity. The presence of either of these two types is not reported by the electromyographer, as they are normal findings. Their only significance is that nerve potentials may be confused with an abnormality, the fibrillation potential, although their wave forms are different.

Excluding poor patient relaxation and end-plate activity, spontaneous electrical activity at rest is usually but not always abnormal. It is of four types: fibrillations, positive sharp-wave potentials, fasciculations, and bizarre high-frequency potentials. Drawings of fibrillations, nerve potentials, and positive sharp-wave potentials are shown in Figure 16–1.

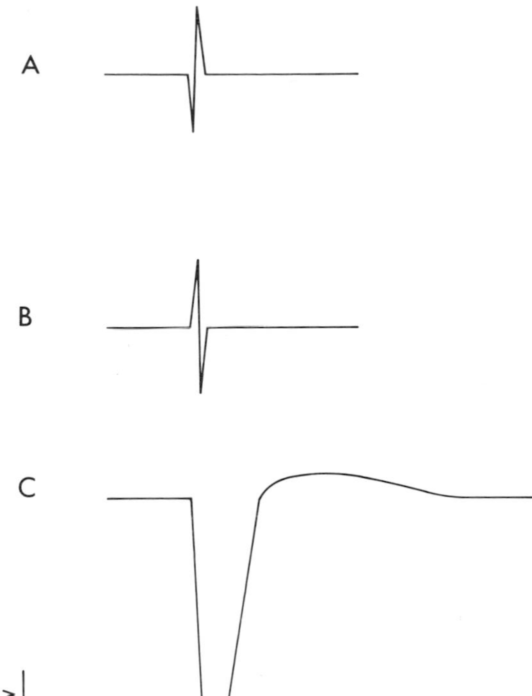

Figure 16–1 *A*. Drawing of "idealized" fibrillation potential. *B*. "Idealized" nerve potential showing similarity to fibrillation potential but with opposite initial polarity. *C*. "Idealized" positive sharp-wave potential.

Fibrillation Potentials

Under normal circumstances muscle fibers are under neural control and do not depolarize without an appropriate neural impulse. With the loss of proper circuitry, as in lower motor neuron dysfunction, neural control of the muscle fiber is lost. The muscle fiber is capable of independent physiological activity and it assumes its own inherent bioelectric rhythmicity. This inherent rhythmicity results in spontaneous depolarization of a single muscle fiber. The resulting electrical activity is a fibrillation potential. These potentials are diphasic or triphasic with an initial positive deflection. They are 1 to 5 msec in duration and vary in amplitude from 20 to 300 μv. Their frequency usually is less than two per second.

In order to be considered significant, they should be found at more than one site in a muscle and away from the end-plate area. These requirements aid in eliminating local muscle trauma as a cause of the potentials and help to eliminate the presence of nerve potentials as a possible source of confusion.

It has long been thought that fibrillation potentials were pathognomonic of denervation. Often they have been called "denervation potentials." It is now clear that they can be seen in myopathies such as polymyositis, in which their presence is believed to be due to involvement of intramuscular nerve twigs.[4] They have also been reported in upper motor neuron lesions, but the reason for their occurence is not clear.[15]

Although fibrillation potentials are most often associated with lower motor neuron disorders, it is necessary to correlate them with abnormalities of motor unit action potentials or with a specific neural anatomical distribution to be sure that they represent denervation.

Fibrillation potentials are graded subjectively as 1+ to 4+ depending upon their numbers. One scheme uses 1 or 2 per minute as 1+, 2 to 10 per minute as 2+, 10 to 30 per minute as 3+, and more than 30 per minute as 4+.[2] The system of grading is more useful for following the course of a lesion than for deciding whether an abnormality is present. The use of fibrillation potentials versus positive sharp-wave potentials to date a lesion is discussed next.

Positive Sharp-Wave Potentials

These potentials are diphasic with a sharp initial positive deflection followed by a long-lasting negative phase. They are 50 to 1000 μv in amplitude and usually more than 10 msec in duration. Their frequency varies from 2 to 100 per second, and they are graded as for fibrillation potentials, i.e., 1+ to 4+.

Since these potentials may be seen as a normal phenomenon with needle insertion, they are considered abnormal only if they persist after electrode movement stops. When they occur in a muscle at rest, they are analogous to fibrillation potentials and are seen in the same disorders.

While a combination of fibrillation potentials and positive sharp-wave potentials usually is seen, there are numerous cases in which a preponderance of one or the other is present. Many electromyographers believe that a preponderance of positive sharp waves suggests a more recent lesion, e.g., less than 6 to 12 months old, while a preponderance of fibrillations suggests an older lesion.[2,6,10] While this difference is not diagnostic, it is very useful in evaluating patients with recurrent problems such as exacerbations of disc disease that have occurred over a sufficient time to allow this type of differentiation. It is especially useful when serial electromyograms are available.

Fasciculations

Fasciculations represent the spontaneous involuntary depolarization and twitch of an entire motor unit, that is, a twitch of multiple muscle fibers. In contrast to fibrillations, fasciculations may be seen through the skin. As viewed on the oscilloscope, the fasciculation potential is diphasic, triphasic, or often polyphasic. Its amplitude, duration, and wave form are identical to a motor unit action potential (MUP). The rhythm, however, is irregular, and the rate varies. Fasciculations are graded similarly to fibrillations and positive sharp waves.

Care must be used in interpreting the significance of fasciculations. They may be completely normal or may represent serious disease states such as amyotrophic lateral sclerosis. They must be correlated with the remainder of the electromyographic findings and, of course, with the clinical situation. When they represent a disease state, it is neuropathic in origin.

The presence of fasciculations either clinically or electrically does not necessarily mean anterior horn cell disease, although they are seen frequently in these disorders. They are, however, seen in root disease and less often in peripheral nerve disorders.

Bizarre High-Frequency Potentials

There are a number of types of repetitive electrical discharges that are spontaneous, are not related to needle movement, and occur without muscle contraction. They are not made up of fibrillations, positive sharp waves, or fasciculations.

True myotonia is both a form of increased insertional activity and a spontaneous bizarre high-frequency potential. It consists of high-frequency discharges of trains of potentials of different amplitude, duration, and configuration (wave form). These discharges wax and wane and make a characteristic sound like a "dive bomber," which is a slang term for them.

True myotonia is thought to occur because of an unstable muscle fiber membrane that is able to depolarize muscle fibers in a repetitive manner. It occurs in myotonic dystrophy, congenital myotonia, paramyotonia, hyperkalemic periodic paralysis, and in patients receiving certain anticholesterol agents.

Neuromyotonia consists of intense, highly repetitive discharges similar to true myotonia except for being present for prolonged periods without waxing and waning. They are seen in odd disease states such as Schwartz-Jampel syndrome.

The third type of bizarre high-frequency potential has no special name. The discharges are brief, at a constant frequency, and have been described in patients with acute rapidly progressive disorders involving the anterior horn cells or peripheral nerves or roots. They also are seen in acute metabolic myopathies such as hypothyroidism. When this type is in a specific anatomical distribution, e.g., one root, it may be highly significant and represent the sole early abnormality.

The fourth type, again with no special name, has all the characteristics of motor unit potentials. These are seen in tetanus, stiff man syndrome, tetany, and cramps.

Except for the true myotonic discharge, the remaining types of bizarre high-frequency discharges are again relatively nonspecific and must be correlated with other electrical findings.

Minimal Contraction Pattern

After examining the insertional and spontaneous activity in a muscle, attention is turned to the electrical activity generated during contraction. Initially a weak contraction is observed to check the following parameters of individual motor units.

For each muscle studied, the amplitude, duration, configuration (shape, wave form), and recruitment of individual motor unit potentials should be reported. There are a number of variables that affect these parameters regardless of whether a disease state is present. They include: (1) type and size of recording electrode, (2) distance of the electrode from the motor unit potential being studied, (3) number of muscle fibers near the needle tip, (4) geometry of the motor unit, (5) size of muscle, (6) muscle fiber type, (7) patient age, (8) body temperature, (9) patient cooperation or fatigue or both, and (10) strength of contraction.

Normal motor unit potentials usually are diphasic or triphasic and do not have more than four phases. They usually are 5 to 15 msec in duration and 300 to 5000 μv in amplitude. They have a relatively specific recruitment pattern of from 6 to 12 impulses per second during weak contraction to 20 to 50 impulses per second during maximal contraction.

Maximum Contraction

The final step in examining a muscle is to request a maximum effort by the patient. As the strength of contraction is increased to maximum, the individual motor unit potentials run together on the oscilloscope screen, producing an electrical picture called the interference pattern. With lower motor neuron disorders causing weakness of the muscle, a full interference cannot be seen. Maximum contraction patterns with a waxing and waning picture and those in which firing rates are less than 20 per second are nonorganic.

Abnormal Motor Unit Potentials

Earlier, it was stated that electromyography is of little benefit in assessing upper motor neuron disease. With upper motor neuron weakness, however, decreased numbers of motor unit potentials will be seen, but those that are seen will be normal. There will be no abnormal insertional or spontaneous activity in most cases. Exceptions to this are reported, however.[15]

With total denervation of a muscle, no motor unit potentials will be seen. The presence of abnormalities during insertion or rest depend on the time that has elapsed since the injury. Far more common are situations with partial denervation and reinnervation. After a proper lapse of time, appropriate insertional activity and spontaneous activity will be noted. For a period the potentials will be reduced in numbers, but other parameters will be normal. As the process progresses or reinnervation occurs, remaining nerve fibers from still-functioning anterior horn cells undergo branching and add muscle fibers from other motor units that have lost their own nerve supply. This branching of fibers leads to more fibers per given motor unit in those that remain viable, and they may be spread over a greater territory spatially.

By oversimplifying events, it may be said that the amplitude of a given motor unit potential is dependent on the number of fibers contained within the unit, and the duration is dependent upon the spatial arrangement around the needle electrode. The configuration (wave form) of the potential is dependent upon the geometry to the degree that a smooth summated action potential is the result of orderly depolarization about the electrode.

In the case of partial denervation, the motor units have reached a point at which they have excess fibers per unit in a larger territory. This change leads to a wide-amplitude, prolonged-duration motor unit potential, frequently polyphasic because its summation is not smooth. Numbers are reduced because too few potentials are present. This combination of changes is the typical picture in lower motor neuron disease and has been referred to as the "neuropathic motor unit potential.'' It must be realized, however, that these potentials take time to develop, and even though reduced numbers are seen early, the large, broad polyphasic potentials do not appear until about six months following insult. It should be noted that such potentials may occur in normal patients. They cannot be considered to be abnormal unless they constitute more than 15 per cent of the muscle's motor unit potentials or occur in a specific anatomical distribution.

In cases of partial denervation with reinnervation or after operative repair of nerve, the electromyogram will show motor unit potentials associated with regeneration before clinical evidence of recovery is present. These so-called regeneration potentials are of low amplitude, frequently prolonged, polyphasic, and present where a different pattern existed previously. Their appearance will follow the proper time sequence for reinnervation from a pathological standpoint. This ability to show reinnervation is extremely useful in following the course of nerve injuries.

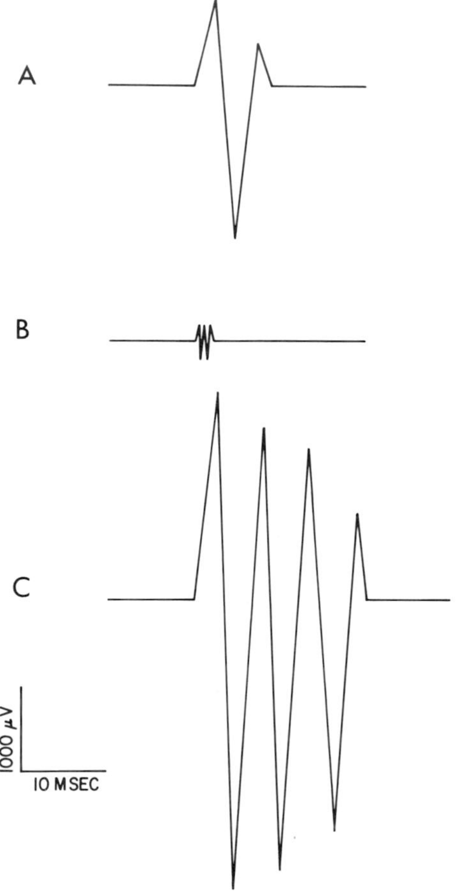

Figure 16–2 *A*. Drawing of normal motor unit potential *B*. Typical low-amplitude, brief-duration polyphasic motor unit potential seen in myopathic disorders. *C*. Typical large-amplitude, prolonged-duration polyphasic motor unit potential seen in neuropathic disorders.

In myopathies a different pattern emerges. There is loss of individual muscle fibers. Thus, there are fewer fibers per motor unit, resulting in a potential of decreased amplitude (usually less than 1000 μv). Duration is also reduced, perhaps because the unit territory has shrunk. The potential may be polyphasic as well. Since neural control is still intact, more than the usual number of motor unit potentials are recruited to perform a muscular contraction. This recruitment results in an excess of potentials in relation to the strength of the contraction. These potentials have been called ''myopathic.'' Current usage has advanced the acronym ''BSAP potentials'' (brief, small, abundant, polyphasic potentials).

In summary, then, the motor unit potential changes in neuropathic disorders could be classed as too big, too broad (long), and too few. In contrast, in the myopathies they would be too small, too narrow (short), and too many. Drawings of normal, ''myopathic,'' and ''neuropathic'' potentials are shown in Figure 16–2.

Conduction Velocity Studies

Motor Nerve Conduction

Motor nerve conduction velocities may be obtained easily only from those nerves that are readily accessible to stimulation through the skin in at least two locations along their course. In the extremities these nerves are the median, ulnar, radial, posterior tibial, and peroneal. Femoral nerve studies are performed but present many technical and anatomical problems. In the cranial nerve distribution, facial nerve studies are available even though only one stimulus point is used. Special studies to be mentioned later include those developed for phrenic, accessory, laryngeal, and sciatic nerves.

In all motor nerve conduction studies in the extremities a similar procedure is fol-

TABLE 16–3 NORMAL ADULT MOTOR NERVE CONDUCTION VALUES

NERVE	RECORDED FROM	MEAN VELOCITY (m/sec ± 2 S.D.)	LOWER LIMIT OF NORMAL	MEAN DISTAL LATENCY (msec ± 2 S.D.)	UPPER LIMIT OF NORMAL
Ulnar	Abductor digiti minimi	56 ± 10	45	2.9 ± 0.8	4
Median	Opponens pollicis	57 ± 8	47	3.8 ± 1.0	5
Radial	Extensor indicis	58 ± 14	45	2.4 ± 1.0	4
Peroneal	Extensor digitorum	50 ± 10	40	5.0 ± 2.0	7
Posterior tibial	Abductor hallucis	50 ± 14	37	5.0 ± 2.0	7
Facial	Orbicularis oris	—	—	3.4 ± 1.6	5

lowed. A surface recording electrode is placed over the belly of a muscle innervated by the nerve in question. This electrode is the active one, while an indifferent or reference electrode is placed 2 to 4 cm from the muscle belly. A ground electrode is appropriately placed.

With the cathode of the stimulating electrode placed distally, the nerve is stimulated at two points along its course. Two points are used to obtain the conduction velocity along the nerve itself, since the system has a neuromuscular junction and muscle fibers supervening. Using two points eliminates conduction delay of an undetermined amount through these structures.

For each stimulation point a time value is derived for conduction between that point and the muscle electrode. By convention, this value is from the stimulus to the initial negative deflection of the evoked muscle action potential and is referred to as the *conduction* or *latency* time for that segment. The distance between the two stimulus points is then measured and the time for the impulse to travel that distance is derived by utilizing the difference between latency times.

The *conduction velocity* is expressed in meters per second. It is the distance in millimeters between the two stimulation points divided by the time difference in milliseconds. Normal values for the commonly studied peripheral nerves in adults are shown in Table 16–3 and in children in Table 16–4.

Other useful values in clinical electrodiagnosis include the distal motor latencies and the evoked potential amplitude. The report of these studies should include the proximal latency, distal latency, interelectrode distance, and evoked potential amplitude.

Sensory Nerve Conduction

The development of sensory nerve conduction testing as a routine procedure has greatly advanced the field of electrodiagnosis. A number of clinical conditions, both medical and surgical, show abnormalities only in this sphere. Those sensory nerves that can be studied, however, are far fewer than are motor nerves for study.

Two basic techniques are in common use today: orthodromic and antidromic recording. Each technique has its advocates.

Orthodromic conduction studies utilize impulse propagation in the normal physiological direction in the axon or nerve fiber. The sensory fibers are stimulated in the periphery and recorded proximally over a larger segment of mixed nerve. For example, the median nerve would be stimulated at the index finger and recorded at the wrist. These potentials are small in amplitude, but usually are recordable from the wrist. Frequently special electronic averag-

TABLE 16–4 NORMAL PEDIATRIC MOTOR NERVE CONDUCTION VALUES

	MEAN VELOCITY (m/sec ± 1 S.D.)					
NERVE	*Birth to 1 Week*	*1 Week to 4 Months*	*4 Months to +1 Year*	*1 to 3 Years*	*3 to 8 Years*	*8 to 16 Years*
Ulnar	32 ± 4	42 ± 8	50 ± 7	60 ± 8	65 ± 8	67 ± 6
Median	29 ± 4	34 ± 9	40 ± 5	49 ± 6	58 ± 5	64 ± 6
Peroneal	29 ± 4	37 ± 7	48 ± 8	54 ± 8	57 ± 7	57 ± 7

TABLE 16–5 NORMAL ADULT SENSORY NERVE CONDUCTION VALUES

NERVE	TEST TYPE	MEAN VELOCITY (m/sec ± 2 S.D.)	LOWER LIMIT OF NORMAL	MEAN DISTAL LATENCY (msec ± 2 S.D.)	UPPER LIMIT OF NORMAL
Ulnar	Orthodromic	57 ± 8	45	3 ± 0.4	4
	Antidromic	55 ± 8	45	3 ± 0.6	4
Median	Orthodromic	58 ± 10	47	3 ± 0.4	4
	Antidromic	57 ± 8	47	3 ± 0.4	4
Sural	—	46	40	—	—

ing equipment is needed. More proximal impulses are harder to record by this method, but they are more likely to be from purely sensory fibers.

The antidromic method utilizes the physiological principle that impulses can travel in either direction in an axon regardless of the normal direction of travel during normal function. Thus, while normal sensory pathways are afferent from distal to proximal, impulses may be propagated in sensory fibers from proximal to distal points. In the antidromic method, the mixed nerve is stimulated proximally, say at the wrist in the median nerve example just cited, but only sensory potentials are recorded distally, say at the finger. A larger amplitude response usually is obtained with this method and usually is easier to obtain without averaging equipment. The major disadvantage, however, lies in the fact that a conducted motor response may be seen at the pick-up and mistaken for a sensory response. It is for this reason that some authorities favor only the orthodromic method. With an examiner experienced in the technique, however, antidromic results are as reliable as orthodromic results.

The usual principles apply with respect to calculating sensory conduction velocity (NCV = distance/time). While two stimulus points usually are used when a motor conduction velocity is reported, a *distal sensory latency* usually is reported with only one stimulation site, and it is worthwhile to realize that with sensory conduction studies only one stimulus point is needed because impulses are recorded over nerve from nerve stimulation without a synapse or muscle fiber conduction time to confuse the issue. In this case, all that is needed is the distance from stimulus point to pick-up divided by the latency.

In most laboratories, median and ulnar nerve sensory conduction is routinely studied. Radial nerve studies can be done but require special equipment. In the lower limb, sural nerve conduction studies usually are available in most laboratories. Sensory conduction studies for other lower limb nerves are being developed. Because of technical problems, sensory conduction studies are more difficult in the lower limbs than in the upper limbs. Examples of normal values for sensory conduction are given in Table 16–5.

Abnormalities of Conduction

Current routine techniques utilize the fastest-conducting fibers as the index of measurement of conduction time. Conduction along peripheral nerves depends upon the integrity of the myelin sheath. When this structure is injured, conduction is appreciably impaired.

With a partial nerve injury, the insult may affect motor or sensory fibers. Until significant denervation has occurred, motor conduction velocities or latencies may remain normal. The amplitude of the evoked response, however, is usually decreased and prolonged in duration early in a peripheral denervating process. Thus, change in evoked potential amplitude and duration is the earliest sign of motor impairment. Sensory conduction usually is impaired or abolished quite early. The motor conduction velocity will become slow later in the course when sufficient involvement has occurred.

With a complete nerve injury, such as the traumatic severing of a nerve, normal responses and conduction may be obtained from the distal segment for up to seven days following injury. Care must be taken to be sure that the stimulation is above the site of injury. In contrast to most electrodiagnostic situations, immediate studies of these lesions are of value, since there will be normal distal conduction below a site of injury but none above, in combination with no motor unit potentials on attempted contraction.

Besides showing general slowing within

one or more nerves, nerve conduction studies are used to show sharply focal areas of involvement, as in the entrapment neuropathies. This is discussed later.

Some disorders of peripheral nerves involve axons instead of myelin. These disorders, such as toxic neuropathies from thallium or acrylamide, do not show slowing of conduction until late in their course. Evoked potential amplitude changes will be seen. Also, it should be noted that some more proximal disorders such as anterior horn cell disease may cause mild slowing of motor conduction in peripheral nerves. The entire panel of electromyographic and nerve conduction findings must be considered in correctly evaluating this type of problem to avoid the erroneous conclusion that a peripheral neuropathy exists.

Repetitive Nerve Stimulation Studies

These studies utilize the same techniques as those used for motor nerve conduction studies. Their objective is to test the integrity and proper function of the neuromuscular junction. Normally they are used in the diagnostic evaluation of patients who are suspected of having myasthenia gravis or the myasthenic syndrome.

Routine studies usually utilize the upper extremity and the median nerve–thenar muscle complex, or the ulnar nerve–hypothenar muscle complex. The nerve is stimulated distally, and the evoked potential amplitude is recorded and measured during each of several serial stimuli. Stimulus rates are usually 2 and 20 impulses per second.

The rationale is that a patient with myasthenia gravis will show an abnormal decrement in the evoked potential amplitude with repeated stimuli. This decrement can be reversed by edrophonium given intravenously. Conversely, the patient with the myasthenic syndrome may show a mild decrement at low-frequency stimulation and an abnormal increment at high rates of stimulation, beginning with subnormal amplitude of the first evoked potential.

Numerous variants of these techniques are now in use and are described in standard textbooks of electrodiagnosis.[2,6,10,14] All physicians treating patients with myasthenia gravis should, however, know that anticholinesterase drugs interfere with an accurate assessment of repetitive nerve stimulation studies. All medications for myasthenia gravis must be withdrawn for several days prior to the testing. Therefore, the need for testing must be weighed carefully against the risk to the patient.

Special Procedures

As with any diagnostic service, certain procedures are routine, certain are rarely done, and certain are experimental but possibly of use in a particular situation. A few of these are described as follows.

Muscle Studies

Most muscle studies by needle electrode are routine. Some laboratories, however, may be able to study muscles that are not commonly studied. Examples include intercostal and abdominal musculature and deep and barely accessible muscles. Only in rare cases is this type of skill needed. Two special electromyographic procedures are deserving of specific mention, however.

Anal Sphincter

Information about the S2, S3, and S4 spinal segments can be obtained with anal sphincter needle studies. This study is easy to perform but very difficult to evaluate. First, this sphincter is normally in a tonic state, and abnormal rest activity is almost impossible to see and assess in patients who do not have severe loss of function. Second, assessment of voluntary activity requires patient cooperation, which is difficult at best under the circumstances. This technique should be requested only after discussion with the electromyographer. Its yield is low, and few electromyographers are skilled in performing it.

Extraocular Muscles

These studies are available in some medical centers. They require the cooperation and joint efforts of both the electromyographer and an ophthalmologist who will place the electrodes.

The procedure has important clinical applications. For example, it can without difficulty be used for kineseology studies.

Studying the extraocular muscles is much harder than the other body muscles. The motor unit potentials are different, and the identification of abnormal potentials and rest activity is difficult even with experience in the field. Experts claim the ability, however, to detect the difference between neuropathic and myopathic processes in the extraocular muscles.[6]

The most useful role of extraocular muscle electromyography lies in the diagnosis of ocular myasthenia. In this condition, routine repetitive nerve stimulation studies of the extremities frequently are normal. In addition, the clinical edrophonium test often is normal.

An extraocular electromyogram before and after administration of edrophonium is quite reliable in diagnosing ocular myasthenia, however. The special feature of this study is that an enhancement of activity may be seen even without clinical evidence of eye movement.

Nerve Conduction Studies

Besides those studies already described as routine, nerve conduction techniques can be applied to studies of accessory, phrenic, intercostal, laryngeal, and sciatic nerves. Many of these are not "routine" because their usefulness is limited and because needle electrodes are needed for stimulation or recording, thus increasing the patient's discomfort and risk.

These studies are of value in those cases in which damage to a specific peripheral nerve is suspected. Phrenic nerve studies have a special value in evaluating quadriplegics, and this is discussed later in the clinical section.

Reflex Studies

THE H REFLEX. The H reflex, or the electrically induced analog of the monosynaptic stretch reflex, usually is obtainable from the posterior tibial nerve–medial gastrocnemius complex. Less frequently it is available from other nerve-muscle combinations.

The technique allows the selective excitation of muscle spindle afferent fibers prior to excitation of large alpha motor fibers by using appropriate stimuli. When properly done, an evoked potential is noted at a latency of about 30 to 35 msec poststimulus. Other measurable parameters include the amplitude and relation to the evoked direct muscle response. This technique has been used to study various central neural functions such as reflex excitability. In clinical electromyography, however, its main use is in evaluating proximal sensory conduction, especially in the S1 root distribution, where it is an adjunct in the diagnosis of S1 root disease.

Some investigators believe that a side-to-side H reflex latency measurement of more than 2.5 msec is significant.[11] Others believe that only the absence of the H reflex on the affected side is significant.[17] This latter is a more conservative viewpoint and possibly a wiser one.

THE F WAVE. When supramaximal stimuli are applied, another late wave form, the F wave, can be seen at approximately the same latency as the H reflex seen with submaximal stimuli. The F wave is not a true reflex, but probably represents antidromic activation of alpha motor neurons that has a long latency because of distance travelled from stimulus site to cord to recording site. This study usually is not done, although the F wave can be seen in any routine motor conduction study. Recent pilot studies suggest that a side-to-side latency difference of more than 2 msec may be very helpful in assessing root syndromes or entrapment neuropathies.[3,12] This study may soon become a routine one.

CLINICAL APPLICATIONS

The majority of cases referred to an electrodiagnostic laboratory by the neurosurgeon or orthopedic surgeon are for either disc disease, entrapment neuropathies, or traumatic neuropathies. The electrodiagnostic results that are achieved in these situations are covered in some detail, while other conditions amenable to electrodiagnostic evaluation are briefly reviewed.

Disc Disease

Electromyographic studies are especially valuable in assessing patients with root syndromes, provided that the study is requested at a time when abnormalities can be seen. The studies should be ordered approximately 21 days after an acute insult, even though abnormalities in posterior primary ramus–innervated muscles (erector spinae group) may be seen earlier.

The electromyographic changes seen are those noted in any neuropathic disorder. In a root compression syndrome, the compression of the motor root leads to irritation followed by destructive changes within the root.

Frequently, the earliest change seen is increased irritability or insertional activity localized to the structures innervated by one particular root. Following this phase, or concurrently with it, one may see sharply focal bizarre high-frequency potentials or fasciculations in a root distribution.

When actual axonal damage has occurred the electromyographer begins to detect the presence of positive sharp waves and fibrillations. These appear at 14 to 30 days in extremity muscles and at about 8 to 10 days in the paraspinal muscles. Late in the course of the disease, abnormal motor unit potentials appear.

The paraspinal muscle electromyogram is of vital importance in the evaluation of any root syndrome. When a patient has not had a prior operation, the test is not complete unless these structures have been studied. The electrical changes usually appear first in the erector spinae group, and in many cases are limited to these structures at any stage in the disease. The limiting factor in paraspinal electromyography is a previous laminectomy. In these cases paraspinal muscles will show abnormalities for many years, and the diagnostic value of the study is lost. Because of the importance placed on paraspinal electromyographic studies, it is preferable to study patients with lumbosacral disc disease prior to myelography. This precaution eliminates one possible source of a false positive test, i.e., minimal electrical changes from a paramedian myelogram needle placement. If difficulty is encountered during the myelogram and several insertions of the needle are made, electrical changes may persist for a few days.

The key to accurate electrodiagnosis in disc disease is showing a root distribution for the changes seen, rather than a peripheral nerve distribution. An example illustrates the deductive reasoning process and can be viewed as representative of all electromyographic localization studies:

The following muscles have the L5 root as a common denominator: peroneus longus, tensor fasciae latae, tibialis posterior, gluteus medius, biceps femoris, and tibialis anterior. These muscles have different peripheral nerve supplies, however: peroneus longus and tibialis anterior from the peroneal nerve, gluteus medius and tensor fasciae latae from gluteal nerves, tibialis posterior from the tibial nerve, and biceps femoris from the sciatic nerve–peroneal portion. If an electrical abnormality is seen in two of the muscles that are supplied by the L5 root but have different nerve supplies, a root lesion is suggested. The exception, of course, would be if a sciatic nerve lesion were responsible, e.g., changes were recorded in tibialis posterior and tibialis anterior. At that point the gluteus medius might be used, since it has proximal innervation and is not innervated by the sciatic nerve. Finally, the paraspinal muscles should be studied. If they are abnormal, the lesion must be proximal to the division of anterior and posterior primary rami, i.e., proximal to the intervertebral foramen. Should the paraspinal findings be normal, however, the answer can usually be deduced from the extremity electromyogram. In interpreting an electromyogram, it is essential to know the root overlap to assess localization. For example, changes in quadriceps and anterior tibial muscles suggest L4, anterior tibial and peroneus longus L5, and peroneus longus and medial gastrocnemius S1.

Even with disease states, the electromyogram of the extremities and back muscles may be normal. If the clinical story is sufficient to warrant a strong suspicion of a root lesion, another test, the H reflex, is available. This test is able to measure the proximal sensory arc, at least for the S1 root, and its absence on the proper side may be considered reasonable evidence for an S1 root lesion. Since the H reflex is good for S1 only and only the dorsal root is involved, there will be some valid cases of root compression in which the studies are normal. The exact percentage is unknown.

The accuracy of electromyography has been compared with that of myelography in order to determine the diagnostic reliability of each test.[8] It would appear that the electromyogram frequently is more accurate than the myelogram at the L5–S1 interspace with S1 involvement. When root disease is suspected at this level, both studies should be done, since a normal myelogram does not rule out a significant disc protrusion. At the L4–L5 interspace with L5 involvement there is no advantage to electromyography, and the scales of accuracy tip somewhat to myelography. The consensus at the present time favors the idea that the electromyogram more accurately identifies the root that is involved, and the myelogram the interspace that is involved. The combination of both techniques is useful and helps to eliminate an operation for a myelographic defect of unknown or of doubtful clinical significance.

Recurrent disc disease poses a special problem in analyzing the electromyogram. As noted, the paraspinal study has lost its value because of prior laminectomy. Furthermore, many patients do not have an electromyogram until after a recurrence of the problem, and no earlier data are then available—in itself, a compelling argument for baseline electromyographic recordings in almost all disc cases.

The electromyogram can provide reasonable evidence that an electrical abnormality is new or old if sufficient time—approximately 12 months—has elapsed between the first disc problems and the recurrence. For this purpose, the ratio of fibrillations to positive waves, and changes in motor unit potentials are used. Since myelography may be confusing after laminectomy, electromyography is of great value at this time.

While most of the emphasis has been on lumbosacral disc disease, the electromyogram also is highly accurate in cervical disc disease. In view of the incidence of cervical degenerative disease leading to a positive myelogram, the ability of paraspinal studies to localize the problem accurately as proximal or distal to the intervertebral foramen is especially useful.

In thoracic disc disease, the electromyogram is more limited. A careful study of the thoracic paraspinal muscles and intercostal nerve conduction studies may be of value, however.

Peripheral Entrapment Neuropathies

By definition, an entrapment neuropathy is a localized area of nerve injury caused by impingement and continued irritation from a neighboring anatomical structure. These usually occur where a nerve passes through a fibro-osseous tunnel, acutely angulates over a structure such as a tendon insertion, or passes between two fibrous structures as the median nerve does between the heads of the pronator teres. Many of these entrapment neuropathies lend themselves to accurate diagnosis by electrodiagnostic means. The prototype, the carpal tunnel syndrome, is discussed in most detail. Others are considered briefly, however.

Median Nerve

The carpal tunnel syndrome, impingement on the median nerve as it traverses the carpal tunnel, can occur from many causes: trauma, occupational irritation, tenosynovitis, and as a complication of diabetes, pregnancy, hypothyroidism, and rheumatoid arthritis.

Not all needle electromyographic studies are rewarding in this condition. The electrical changes are those of any neuropathy and are localized to thenar muscles. At the time of early clinical suspicion of the syndrome, a normal electromyogram is much more common than an abnormal one; 10 years ago, the literature quoted a rate of 55 to 60 per cent.[7,9,12,16] Because of the higher index of suspicion of the problem at present, the studies are being done earlier, and the percentage of normal studies is even higher.

The earliest technique for studying median nerve conduction through the carpal tunnel used distal motor latencies. Abnormalities of conduction were found in as many as 67 per cent of patients with symptoms, but there still were a number of false negative studies. New techniques for sensory conduction studies through the carpal tunnel, however, have drastically improved the reliability of electrical testing. Since sensory fibers show an early abnormality in this syndrome, the accuracy of sensory conduction studies is close to 95 per cent. Interestingly, some cases are now being reported in which sensory conduction is normal but motor conduction abnormal. In addition, F wave studies are now being reported as valuable in the entrapment neuropathies. When a carpal tunnel syndrome is proved on one side, the other hand should be studied as well. The asymptomatic hand also may show electrical evidence of involvement. Upper limits of normal for distal motor and sensory latencies are shown in Tables 16–3 and 16–5.

After baseline studies are obtained, repeat studies after an operation provide a good follow-up for objective evidence of recovery.

It should be noted that the carpal tunnel syndrome may occur in conjunction with other lesions such as root disease or a thoracic outlet syndrome. Careful and complete electrodiagnosis will provide the clinician with information on this situation and allow for early planning of appropriate therapy.

The median nerve also is subject to entrapment at the pronator teres, the "pronator syndrome," and even more proximally at the ligament of Struthers. Both of these entrapments can be diagnosed and differentiated from the carpal tunnel syndrome by careful analysis of both conduction studies and electromyograms. In the pronator syndrome there may be a slight slowing of conduction in the forearm segment of the median nerve and the electromyogram will show changes in the flexor carpi radialis as well as the thenar muscles. The pronator teres will be spared. A ligament of Struthers entrapment will add electrical changes in the pronator teres.

Ulnar Nerve

The ulnar nerve is subject to entrapment at the elbow, wrist, and palm. Lesions at the elbow are the most common. The anatomy of the ulnar nerve allows determination of conduction velocities for a number of segments that include distal latency across the wrist, below the elbow to the wrist, across the elbow, above the elbow to the wrist, the axilla to the wrist, the axilla to above the elbow, Erb's point to the wrist, and Erb's point to the axilla. This variety of test points allows accurate localization in ulnar nerve problems.

Entrapment at the wrist occurs where the nerve traverses Guyon's canal. The electromyogram, if abnormal, will be so only in ulnar intrinsic muscles. Nerve conduction studies should show only prolonged distal sensory or motor latencies. With a palmar lesion, the changes may be localized to muscles supplied by one branch.

With an entrapment at the elbow, the conduction velocity should be slowed across the elbow segment. Because there is slight slowing across the elbow in many asymptomatic subjects, the two arms should be compared, especially if no electrical abnormality is seen. With lesions at the elbow, there will be electromyographic changes in the forearm and hand muscles that are innervated by the ulnar nerve. The interpretation of conduction changes at the elbow is made much easier if there are marked amplitude differences between the right and left sides or above and below the elbow on the symptomatic side.

Examination of ulnar nerve conduction from Erb's point to the axilla (thoracic outlet) is of great value in diagnosing the thoracic outlet syndrome. Technically, it is easy to study ulnar nerve conduction in this segment, but assessing the results is difficult. Originally, a value of less than 70 meters per second across the outlet was believed to represent significant slowing, but asymptomatic patients are seen with lower values across the outlet.[1] If the symptoms are unilateral, a definite difference in conduction velocity, probably greater than 15 meters per second, must be shown between the right and left sides. Usually neurological signs are present when slowing of conduction is seen. A normal study, however, does not rule out the presence of the syndrome, especially a primarily vascular one. Bilateral thoracic outlet syndromes are difficult to evaluate by current techniques.

Radial Nerve

In lesions of the radial nerve, electromyographic findings usually are more reliable than nerve conduction studies, since the anatomy of the radial nerve allows conduction to be readily studied only in the segment from the spiral groove to the elbow. If the appropriate time has elapsed, however, the electromyogram can reliably locate radial nerve damage.

Posterior Tibial Nerve

Entrapment neuropathies are much less common in the leg than in the arm. They do occur, however. The posterior tibial nerve can be entrapped in the popliteal fossa by an arterial aneurysm or compressed by a cast. Entrapment at the ankle in the tarsal tunnel is more usual. Diagnosis rests upon showing a prolonged distal motor latency in either the medial or lateral plantar nerves or in both, since each is liable to an independent entrapment neuropathy. Sensory conduction studies for both the medial and lateral plantar nerves are being developed.

Peroneal Nerve

The peroneal nerve is most subject to a compressive neuropathy at the head of the fibula where the common peroneal nerve is very superficial—the so-called "crossed leg palsy." Peroneal nerve conduction studies can be extended to include a more proximal segment from popliteal fossa to fibular head, thus allowing the electromyographer to show very focal slowing. Likewise, in branch damage, electrical changes will show a differentiation between common, deep, and superficial peroneal nerve lesions.

Sciatic Nerve

While the sciatic nerve is injured in trauma, it is also subject to entrapment where it crosses the sciatic notch. Sciatic nerve conduction studies normally are not feasible, as they require a needle stimulating electrode. A complete leg electromyogram will, however, show involvement of hamstring muscles and leg muscles in a sciatic rather than nerve root, peroneal nerve, or tibial nerve pattern.

In general, the differentiation of an entrapment neuropathy from a more diffuse process involving the same nerve requires the demonstration of normal function above and below the lesion.

Peripheral Nerve Trauma

The same principles that apply to the entrapment neuropathies apply to electrodiagnosis of acute nerve injuries. The combination of electromyography and nerve conduction velocity testing permits accurate assessment of degree and location of the injury if the appropriate time has elapsed. In this situation, immediate or early testing is valuable. Immediately, there may be little useful evidence, since abnormal activity such as fibrillation potentials or positive sharp-wave potentials will be missing. If the patient can develop motor unit potentials on voluntary attempts at muscle contraction, however, the lesion must, by definition, be incomplete. The potentials may be seen even in the absence of clinically detectable movement, so this can be helpful in some cases. If no potentials are seen immediately, no assessment can be made until the period of neurapraxia is over; thus, their absence does not mean a complete lesion.

The early use of nerve conduction studies may or may not be of value. If a stimulus applied proximal to the injury site can cause a muscle to contract, the lesion can be considered incomplete. As in electromyography, however, the failure of a proximal stimulus to cause contraction does not necessarily mean that complete neurapraxia is present. Thus, the value of electrodiagnosis in acute nerve trauma lies in its ability to predict the incompleteness rather than the completeness of the lesion.

Trauma to the median, anterior interosseous, ulnar, radial, femoral, tibial, peroneal, sciatic, facial, accessory, and phrenic nerves can be assessed reliably in the proper time sequence. Serial studies are an excellent way of following the course after operative or conservative treatment.

Brachial plexus lesions are readily amenable to electrodiagnostic testing. The key lies in showing a distribution of changes compatible with a plexus lesion. Confirming a lesion of the brachial plexus is easier than confirming one of the lumbosacral plexus because the muscles in the arm are more easily tested and have a more specific innervation. In studying brachial plexus lesions, electromyography is the basic tool. The electrodiagnostic literature does, however, show many "normal values" for nerve conduction latencies to various muscles from various plexus segments.[2] Unfortunately these latencies are usually normal even with severe plexus lesions and may be "normal" because of purely technical reasons. Even though conduction is rarely slowed in plexus trauma, however, it is often slowed in plexus tumor infiltration.

An example of localizing a lesion to the plexus would be as follows: In an upper trunk lesion, all C5–C6 innervated muscles in the arm would be involved regardless of nerve supply. The rhomboids, however, would be spared because their nerve supply is formed at root levels proximal to the formation of the upper trunk. The erector spinae group at the appropriate level would also be normal, since the lesion is distal to the division of anterior and posterior primary rami. Should the lesion be more proximal and involve the rhomboids as well but spare the erector spinae, it would be localized at a very proximal root level but outside the foramina at the very origin of the plexus. Such patterns exist for all portions of the plexus.

Phrenic Nerve Viability

Reasonably reliable conduction studies can be performed on the phrenic nerve. The presence or absence of conduction along the nerve can be tested with ease. Serial studies can be used to show changes for the better or worse with time. In those patients being considered for an implanted phrenic nerve stimulator, knowledge about the viability of the phrenic nerve in which it is to be implanted may prove vital to the success of the procedure.

Functional Weakness

In a patient with functional weakness, nerve conduction velocity studies of both motor and sensory types will be normal, as will repetitive nerve stimulation studies. During electromyography, insertional activity will be normal, and no abnormal spontaneous activity will be seen. During muscle contraction, the motor units will be of normal amplitude, duration, and configuration. The members of motor units seen will be proportional to the strength of the patient's contraction, but may be reduced in number on so-called "maximum effort" by the patient. The recruitment pattern will be submaximal, indicating subnormal voluntary effort, and bizarre waxing and waning firing patterns are seen.

Upper Motor Neuron Lesions

In typical upper motor neuron lesions such as cerebral vascular accident or spinal cord injury, nerve conduction studies will be normal unless a particular peripheral nerve has been subjected to compression, as in a bedridden patient. Repetitive nerve stimulation studies are normal.

The electromyogram shows insertional activity to be normal. Abnormal spontaneous activity usually is absent, although as noted earlier, fibrillations and spontaneous positive waves are noted at times. The motor units seen during contraction have normal parameters, but they will be reduced in numbers in weak muscles.

Anterior Horn Cell Disease

In conditions such as amyotrophic lateral sclerosis or progressive spinal muscular atrophy, nerve conduction studies usually are normal, although slightly slow motor conduction velocities may be seen. Also, repetitive nerve stimulation studies usually are normal.

Electromyography shows increased insertional activity soon after the injury; when severe atrophy has occurred, it will be reduced. Bizarre high-frequency potentials are noted at times. Fibrillations and positive sharp waves appear diffusely, and marked fasciculations often are seen. During muscle contraction, the motor units are of increased duration and amplitude, frequently being so-called "giant" potentials. There are many polyphasic potentials. The numbers of units are greatly reduced. At times the fasciculations may occur as trains of potentials firing as doublets or triplets. This is rare in other conditions.

Diffuse Polyneuropathies

In disorders such as those caused by diabetes, ethanolism, and the like, motor or sensory conduction will be slowed. In a particular neuropathy, either one or the other will be more involved, depending on the pathologic changes of the lesion. Slowing of conduction in the peroneal nerve occurs so regularly with diffuse mixed neuropathy that caution should be exercised in making the diagnosis if it is absent. Very early, some nerves may show only impairment of evoked potential amplitude. Repetitive nerve stimulation studies will be normal.

During electromyography, insertional activity may be slightly increased. At rest, fibrillations and positive sharp waves may be seen. A rare fasciculation may be noted. During contraction, motor units will be nor-

TABLE 16–6 ELECTRODIAGNOSTIC

	FUNCTIONAL DISORDERS	UPPER MOTOR NEURON LESION	ANTERIOR HORN CELL DISEASE	ROOT LESION
Electromyography				
Insertional activity	Normal	Normal	Increased early Decreased late	Increased
Rest (spontaneous) activity				
Fibrillations	None	Sometimes present	Present	Present
Positive sharp waves	None	Sometimes present	Present	Present
Fasciculations	None	None	Present	Occasionally present
High-frequency discharges	None	None	Often present	Often present
Voluntary contraction				
Motor unit potentials				
Amplitude	Normal	Normal	Increased	Normal or increased
Duration	Normal	Normal	Increased	Normal or increased
Configuration	Normal	Normal	Polyphasic	Polyphasic
Recruitment	Reduced firing or waxing and waning	Normal or decreased	Normal or decreased	Normal
Interference pattern	Normal	Reduced	Reduced	Reduced
Nerve conduction studies				
Motor nerve conduction velocity	Normal	Normal	Usually normal, rare slight slowing	Normal
Distal motor latency	Normal	Normal	Normal	Normal
Sensory latency	Normal	Normal	Normal	Normal
Repetitive nerve stimulation	Normal	Normal	Normal	Normal
Miscellaneous	Often bizarre firing	When present abnormal rest activity diffuse	Giant motor unit potentials Doublets, triplets	Findings in root pattern Paraspinal muscles abnormal early

mal in amplitude and duration early, but polyphasic potentials will be seen. The total number of motor unit potentials seen on maximum contraction will be reduced. Recruitment will be normal, but with time, some large, prolonged motor unit potentials may develop.

Disorders at the Neuromuscular Junction

While these disorders have been described to some degree in preceding sections, the electromyogram in myasthenia gravis has not been described.

A patient with myasthenia gravis will have normal insertional and rest activity. During muscle contraction, the motor units are of normal amplitude, duration, and configuration. Occasionally, however, a somewhat myopathic pattern of motor unit potentials is observed. The contraction pattern frequently declines with prolonged effort as the patient's contraction fatigues.

Repetitive nerve stimulation studies in myasthenia gravis show decrementation of the evoked response with repeated stimuli if the patient has not had recent anticholinesterase therapy. The myasthenic syndrome has been described previously.

Myopathies

In general, myopathies produce a similar pattern regardless of their type. Nerve conduction studies usually are normal unless pressure neuropathies are superimposed. Also, repetitive nerve stimulation studies usually are normal.

Electromyography demonstrates normal insertional activity in dystrophies unless marked atrophy is present, in which case the activity will be reduced. In an inflammatory myopathy such as polymyositis, a marked increase in insertional activity may be seen and bizarre high-frequency potentials are common. Abnormal spontaneous activity is unusual in the dystrophies, although fibrillations and positive sharp-wave potentials are noted in rare cases. These abnormal spontaneous potentials are common in polymyositis.

During contraction, the motor units seen in all types of myopathy are of decreased amplitude and shortened duration with a polyphasic configuration a common finding. The rate of firing is rapid, and an increased number of motor unit potentials is seen for a given strength of muscle contraction.

Table 16–6 summarizes electrodiagnostic findings for various types of disorders.

FINDINGS IN VARIOUS CONDITIONS

PLEXUS LESIONS	PERIPHERAL NEUROPATHY	ENTRAPMENT NEUROPATHY	MYASTHENIA GRAVIS	INFLAMMATORY MYOPATHY	NONINFLAMMATORY MYOPATHY
Increased	Increased	Increased	Normal	Increased	Normal or decreased
Present	Present	Present	None	Present	Rare
Present	Present	Present	None	Present	Rare
Rare	Very rare	Very rare	None	None	None
Occasional	Occasional	Occasional	None	Present	Myotonia if appropriate
Normal or increased	Normal or increased	Normal or increased	Normal	Decreased	Decreased
Normal or increased	Normal or increased	Normal or increased	Normal	Decreased	Decreased
Polyphasic	Polyphasic	Polyphasic	Normal	Polyphasic	Polyphasic
Normal	Reduced	Reduced	Fatiguing	Rapid	Rapid
Reduced	Normal	Normal	Declines	Excessive motor unit potentials for contraction	Excessive motor unit potentials for contraction
Normal	Prolonged	Normal	Normal	Normal	Normal
Normal	Often prolonged	Normal or prolonged	Normal	Normal	Normal
Prolonged or absent	Prolonged or absent	Prolonged or absent	Normal	Normal	Normal
Normal	Normal	Normal	Decrementation	Normal	Normal
Plexus pattern "Plexus" motor latencies usually normal	Sensory conduction usually affected first Evoked potential amplitude changes often first finding	Evoked potential amplitude changes often first finding See sharply focal slowing on nerve conduction velocity studies	Abnormal incrementation with myasthenic syndrome Medicated myasthenics may show normal repetition stimulation	If mild, changes may not be distinguishable from dystrophy, etc., by electrodiagnosis	Changes nonspecific except for myotonia; cannot make specific etiological diagnosis

REFERENCES

1. Caldwell, J. W., Crane, C. R., and Krusen, E. W.: Nerve conduction studies: An aid in the diagnosis of the thoracic outlet syndrome. Southern Med. J., *64*:210–212, 1971.
2. Cohen, H. L., and Brumlik, J.: Manual of electromyography. 2nd Ed. Hagerstown, Md., Harper & Row, 1976.
3. Egloff-Baer, S., Shahani, B. T., and Young, R. R.: Usefulness of late response studies in diagnosis of entrapment neuropathies. Presented at the 24th Annual Meeting of The American Association of Electromyography and Electrodiagnosis, Salt Lake City, October, 1977.
4. Gamstorp, I.: Normal conduction velocity of ulnar, median, and peroneal nerves in infancy, childhood and adolescence. Acta Pediat. Scand. Suppl., *146*:68–76, 1963.
5. Goodgold, J.: Anatomical Correlates of Clinical Electromyography. Baltimore, Williams & Wilkins Co., 1974.
6. Goodgold, J., and Eberstein, A.: Electrodiagnosis of Neuromuscular Diseases. Baltimore, Williams & Wilkins, 1972.
7. Jonsson, B.: Morphology, innervation, and electromyographic study of the erector spinae. Arch. Phys. Med., *50*:638–641, 1969.
8. Knuttson, B.: Comparative values of electromyographic, myelographic and clinical-neurological examinations in diagnosis of lumbar root compression syndrome. Acta Orthop. Scand. Suppl., *49*:1–135, 1961.
9. Kopell, H. P., and Goodgold, J.: Clinical and electrodiagnostic features of carpal tunnel syndrome. Arch. Phys. Med., *49*:371–375, 1968.
10. Licht, S., ed.: Electrodiagnosis and Electromyography. 3rd Ed. Baltimore, Waverly Press, 1971.
11. Shahani, B. T.: Personal communication.
12. Shivde, A. J., Teixeira, C., and Fisher, M. A.: The F response—a clinically useful physiological parameter for the evaluation of back pain. Presented at the 24th Annual Meeting of The American Association of Electromyography and Electrodiagnosis, Salt Lake City, October, 1977.
13. Smorto, M., and Basmajian, J. V.: Clinical Electroneurography. Baltimore, Williams & Wilkins, 1972.
14. Smorto, M., and Basmajian, J. V.: Electrodiagnosis: A Handbook for Neurologists. Hagerstown, Md., Harper & Row, 1977.
15. Taylor, R. G., Kewalramani, L. S., and Fowler, W. M., Jr.: Electromyographic findings in lower extremities of patients with high spinal cord injuries. Arch. Phys. Med., *55*:16–23, 1974.
16. Thomas, J. E., Lambert, E. H., and Cseuz, R. A.: Electrodiagnostic aspects of the carpal tunnel syndrome. Arch. Neurol., *16*:635–641, 1967.
17. Visser, S. L.: The significance of the Hoffman reflex in the EMG examination of patients with herniation of the nucleus pulposus. Psychiat. Neurol. Neurchir., *68*:300–305, 1965.

Index

In this index page numbers set in *italics* indicate illustrations. Page numbers followed by (t) refer to tabular material. Drugs are indexed under their generic names when dosage or action or special use is given. The abbreviation vs. is used to indicate differential diagnosis.

INDEX

INDEX

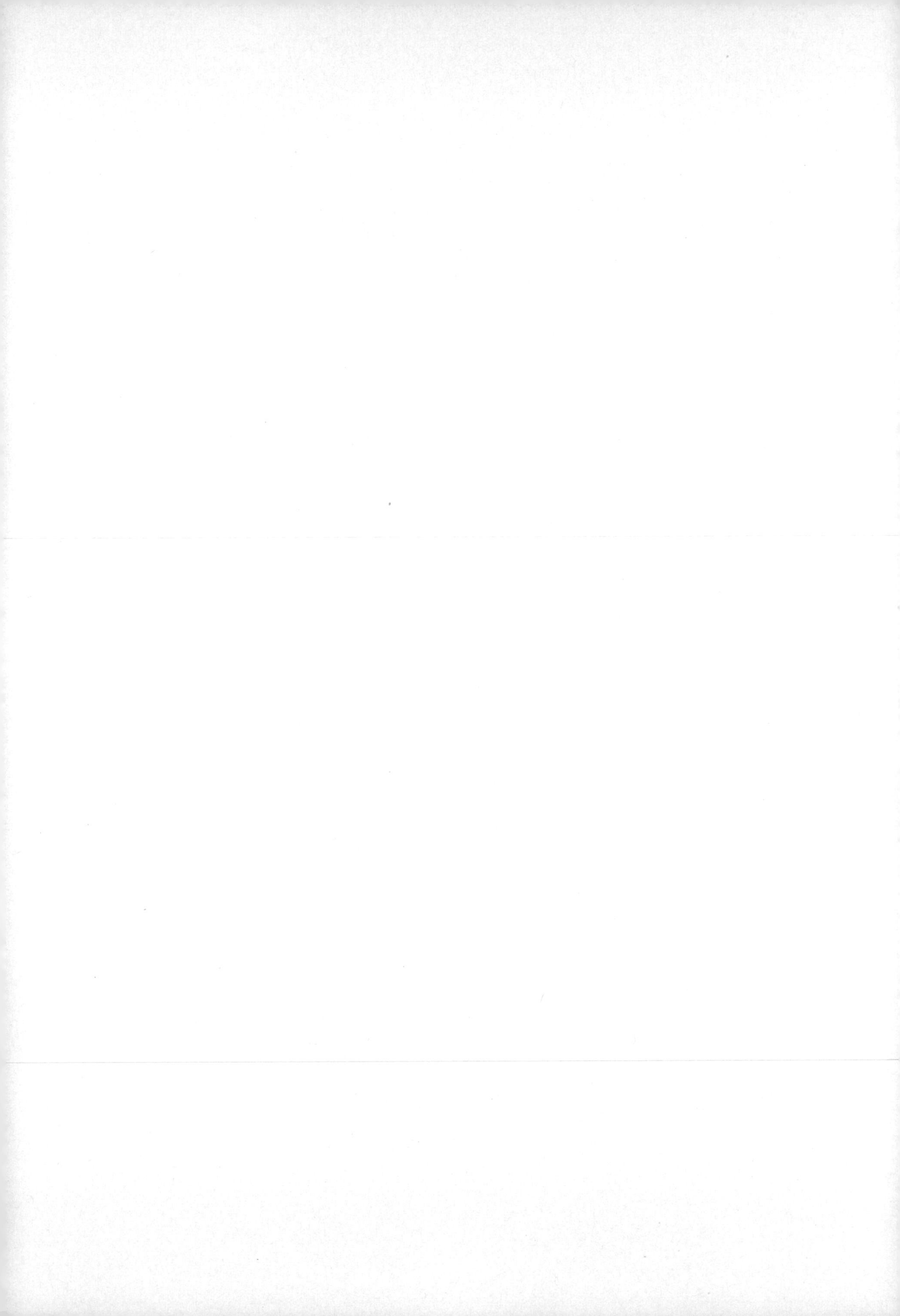